SI Units in Hematology

Parameter	Present Units	Conversion Factor	SI Unit
RBC	$6.0 \times 10^6/mm^3$	10^6	$6.0 \times 10^{12}/L$
Hematocrit	45%	0.01	0.45 L/L
Hemoglobin	15.0 g/dl (%)	10	150 g/L
MCV	$75 \mu^3$	1.0	75 fl
MCHC	33 g/dl (%)	10	330 g/L
MCH	$25 \mu\mu g$	1.0	25 pg
WBC	$15.0 \times 10^3/mm^3$	10^6	$15.0 \times 10^9/L$
Platelets	$250 \times 10^3/mm^3$	10^6	$250 \times 10^9/L$

RBC = red blood cell; MCV = mean corpuscular volume; MCHC = mean corpuscular hemoglobin concentration; MCH = mean corpuscular hemoglobin; WBC = white blood cell.

Key: $\mu\mu g$ = micromicrogram; mm^3 = cubic millimeter; fl = femtoliter; pg = picogram; U = unit; mEq = milliequivalent; μg = microgram; $\mu mol/L$ = micromole per liter; mmol/L = millimole per liter; nmol/L = nanomole per liter; mOsm = milliosmole.

Small Animal
MEDICINE

Small Animal MEDICINE

Editor
DANA G. ALLEN
DVM, MSc., DIPLOMATE ACVIM (INTERNAL MEDICINE)

Associate Professor; Associate Chair, Department of Clinical Studies;
Ontario Veterinary College; University of Guelph; Guelph, Ontario

Consulting Editors
Stephen A. Kruth
DVM, DIPLOMATE, ACVIM (INTERNAL MEDICINE)
Associate Professor; Ontario Veterinary College; Guelph, Ontario

Michael S. Garvey
DVM, DIPLOMATE, ACVIM (INTERNAL MEDICINE)
Chairman, Department of Medicine; The Animal Medical Center; New York, New York

With 31 Contributors

J.B. LIPPINCOTT COMPANY
Philadelphia
New York   St. Louis
London   Sydney   Tokyo

Acquisitions Editor: Nancy Mullins
Developmental Editor: Richard Winters
Project Editor: Melissa McElroy
Indexer: Barbara Littlewood
Designer: Doug Smock
Production Manager: Helen Ewan
Production Coordinator: Kathryn Rule
Compositor: Circle Graphics
Printer/Binder: Arcata Graphics/Halliday

6 5 4 3 2 1

Library of Congress Cataloguing-in-Publication Data

Small animal medicine / editor, Dana Allen;
   consulting editors, Michael Garvey, Stephen Kruth;
   with 31 contributors
       p.   cm.
   Includes bibliographical references and index.
   ISBN 0-397-51025-X
   1. Dogs–Diseases. 2. Cats–Diseases. 3. Pet medicine
I. Allen, Dana G. (Dana Gray) II. Garvey, Michael
(Michael S.)
III. Kruth, Stephen A.
SF991.S594   1991
636.089–dc20   90-6073
                                              CIP

The author and publisher have exerted every effort to
ensure that drug selection and dosage set forth in this text
are in accord with current recommendations and practice
at the time of publication. However, in view of ongoing
research, changes in government regulations, and the
constant flow of information relating to drug therapy and
drug reactions, the reader is urged to check the package
insert for each drug for any change in indications and
dosage and for added warnings and precautions. This is
particularly important when the recommended agent is a
new or infrequently employed drug.

To my parents, Frank and Barbara,
who gave me direction

To my wife, Lorraine,
who gave me love, understanding, and
reason

To my children, Erica and Kirsten,
who gave me purpose

CONTRIBUTORS

Dana G. Allen, DVM, MSc
Diplomate ACVIM (Internal Medicine)
Associate Professor
Associate Chair
Department of Clinical Studies
Ontario Veterinary College
University of Guelph
Guelph, Ontario

Clarke Atkins, DVM
Diplomate ACVIM (Internal Medicine)
Associate Professor of Medicine and Cardiology
College of Veterinary Medicine
Veterinary Teaching Hospital
North Carolina State University
Raleigh, North Carolina

Rebecca Baker, DVM, DVSc
Diplomate ACVP
Clinical Pathologist
Department of Pathology
Ontario Veterinary College
University of Guelph
Guelph, Ontario

Jeanne Barsanti, DVM, MS
Diplomate ACVIM (Internal Medicine)
Professor
Department of Small Animal Medicine
College of Veterinary Medicine
University of Georgia Veterinary Medical Teaching
Hospital
Athens, Georgia

Susan Cochrane, DVM, MSC, DVSc
Diplomate ACVIM (Neurology)
Staff Veterinarian, Neurology Department of
Clinical Studies
Ontario Veterinary College
University of Guelph
Guelph, Ontario

C. Guillermo Couto, DVM
Diplomate ACVIM (Internal Medicine and Oncology)
Associate Professor
Department of Veterinary Clinical Sciences
College of Veterinary Medicine
Chief, Oncology/Hematology Service
Veterinary Teaching Hospital
Ohio State University
Columbus, Ohio

Laine Cowan, DVM, MS
Diplomate ACVIM (Internal Medicine)
Assistant Professor
Department of Surgery and Medicine
College of Veterinary Medicine
Kansas State University
Manhattan, Kansas

Cynthia Culham, DVM
Research Associate
Department of Medical Sciences
School of Veterinary Medicine
University of Misconsin–Madison
Madison, Wisconsin

Duncan Ferguson, DVM, PhD
Diplomate ACVIM (Internal Medicine)
Associate Professor of Physiology and Pharmacology
Department of Small Animal Medicine
College of Veterinary Medicine
The University of Georgia
Athens, Georgia

Gregory Grauer, DVM, MS
Diplomate ACVIM (Internal Medicine)
Associate Professor
Department of Clinical Sciences
College of Veterinary Medicine and Biomedical
Sciences
Veterinary Teaching Hospital
Colorado State University
Ft. Collins, Colorado

Alan Hammer, DVM
Clinical Oncology Resident/Instructor
Department of Veterinary Clinical Sciences
College of Veterinary Medicine
Ohio State University
Columbus, Ohio

Margarethe Hoenig, DVM, PhD
Associate Professor
Department of Physiology and Pharmacology
Department of Small Animal Medicine
College of Veterinary Medicine
The University of Georgia
Athens, Georgia

David Holmberg, DVM, MVSc
Diplomate ACVS
Associate Professor
Department of Clinical Studies
Ontario Veterinary College
University of Guelph
Chief of Small Animal Surgery
Head of Small Animal Clinic
Veterinary Teaching Hospital
Guelph, Ontario

Doreen Houston, DVM, DVSc
Associate Professor
Department of Veterinary Internal Medicine
Western College of Veterinary Medicine
University of Saskatchewan
Saskatoon, Saskatchewan

Robert Jacobs, DVM, PhD
Diplomate ACVP
Associate Professor
Clinical Pathology Service Chief
Department of Pathology
Ontario Veterinary College
University of Guelph
Guelph, Ontario

Shirley Johnston, DVM, PhD
Diplomate ACT
Associate Professor
Department of Small Animal Clinical Sciences
College of Veterinary Medicine
University of Minnesota
St. Paul, Minnesota

Stephen Kruth, DVM
Diplomate ACVIM (Internal Medicine)
Associate Professor
Department of Clinical Studies
Ontario Veterinary College
University of Guelph
Guelph, Ontario

Ned Kuehn, DVM, MS
Diplomate ACVIM (Internal Medicine)
Chief of Staff
Specialists Center
Professional Veterinary Hospital
Allen Park, Michigan

Susan Longhofer, DVM, MS
Medicine Resident
Department of Medical Sciences
School of Veterinary Medicine
University of Wisconsin–Madison
Madison, Wisconsin

John Lumsden, DVM, MSc
Diplomate ACVP
Professor
Department of Pathology
Ontario Veterinary College
University of Guelph
Guelph, Ontario

Amy Marder, VMD
Clinical Assistant Professor
Tufts University School of Veterinary Medicine
Animal Behavior Consultant
Angell Memorial Animal Hospital
Cambridge, Massachusetts

Diane Mason, DVM, MS
Diplomate ACVA
Assistant Professor
Department of Surgical Sciences
School of Veterinary Medicine
University of Wisconsin–Madison
Madison, Wisconsin

Joane Parent, DVM, MVSc
Diplomate ACVIM (Neurology)
Associate Professor
Department of Clinical Studies
Ontario Veterinary College
University of Guelph
Guelph, Ontario

Peter Pascoe, DVM, DVA
Diplomate ACVA
Assistant Professor
Department of Surgery
School of Veterinary Medicine
University of California
Veterinary Medical Teaching Hospital
University of California
Davis, California

Stafano Romagnoli, DVM, MS
Department of Small Animal Clinical Sciences
College of Veterinary Medicine
University of Minnesota
St. Paul, Minnesota

Edmund Rosser, Jr., DVM
Diplomate ACVD
Assistant Professor of Dermatology
Department of Small Animal Clinical Sciences
Veterinary Clinical Center
Michigan State University
East Lansing, Michigan

Philip Roudebush, DVM
Diplomate ACVIM (Internal Medicine)
Mark Morris Associates
Topeka, Kansas

John Rush, DVM, MS
Diplomate ACVIM (Cardiology)
Assistant Professor
Staff Cardiologist
School of Veterinary Medicine
Tufts University
North Grafton, Massachusetts

Ann Washabaugh Sams, DVM
Resident/Instructor, Dermatology
Veterinary Clinical Center
Small Animal Clinical Sciences
Michigan State University
East Lansing, Michigan

Patti Snyder, DVM, MS
Diplomate ACVIM (Internal Medicine)
Assistant Professor
Cardiology/Internal Medicine
School of Veterinary Medicine
University of Wisconsin–Madison
Madison, Wisconsin

Michael Willard, DVM, MS
Diplomate ACVIM (Internal Medicine)
Professor of Small Animal Medicine and Surgery
Texas A & M University
Texas Veterinary Medical Center
College Station, Texas

PREFACE

Small Animal Medicine is designed to be a textbook and general reference for the veterinary student and the small animal general practitioner. It is intended to be a comprehensive guide to the diagnosis and management of the problems and diseases most often in small animal practice.

Small Animal Medicine is organized according to a consistent, problem-oriented approach so that it is practical and easy to use in the clinical setting. A key feature of this book is that its information can be located and understood quickly. Thus, the text of this book is richly complemented with flow diagrams, tables, and illustrations for maximum accessibility and visual enhancement of points of special importance.

The first section of the book, General Clinical Problems, discusses those clinical signs with which animals often are initially presented. The chapters in the following sections of the book deal with diseases or clinical signs of specific body systems. All of these chapters are structured according to a consistent, problem-oriented format that organizes the material according to the needs of the practitioner:

The *introduction* defines the problem or disease to be discussed and explains its clinical significance.

The *causes* then outlines the known and likely etiologies of the problem or disease. A table that lists the known causes is included for quick reference.

Pathophysiology is discussed with sufficient depth of coverage to ensure understanding of the problem and recommended management.

In the *clinical signs* section, the history and physical examination of the animal is discussed.

The *diagnostic approach* section summarizes the assessment of the problem, including the laboratory work-up and other appropriate diagnostic tests. It also addresses the findings of the history and physical examination.

Management of the problem is presented in depth, including both well established modes of therapy and possible new approaches.

The *patient monitoring* section discusses follow-up and prognosis. The prognosis is based on refereed material, or, if such information is lacking, on clinical experience.

All chapters conclude with a list of easily located reference material that can be used to obtain additional information.

The final section of the book, Special Techniques, lists the procedures most often used in private practice. The description of each technique includes diagrams and a table outlining the interpretation of data gained from the procedure.

The Appendices list the dosages, indications, and side effects of each drug mentioned in the book. A screened border on the Appendices' pages makes this often-used section easy to find.

Dana G. Allen, DVM, MSc,
Diplomate ACVIM (Internal Medicine)

ACKNOWLEDGMENTS

I wish to thank the consulting editors, Stephen A. Kruth and Michael S. Garvey, and the contributors to this book. All are leading veterinary practitioners, and their clinical expertise and experience have been invaluable in the successful completion of Small Animal Medicine. I would also like to thank the people at J.B. Lippincott Company—Nancy Mullins, Richard Winters, Susan Blaker, and Melissa McElroy—whose continued effort, guidance, and confidence helped me through the development and production of this book.

CONTENTS

THE PROBLEM-ORIENTED APPROACH

1

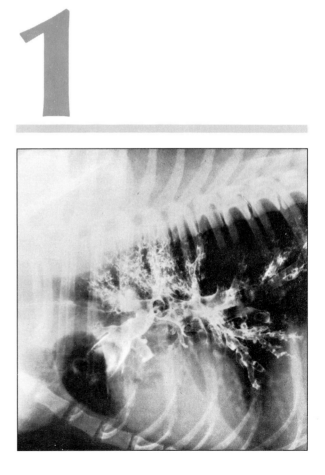

INTRODUCTION: THE PROBLEM-ORIENTED APPROACH

Stephen A. Kruth

The clinical veterinarian, regardless of the type of practice he or she works in, spends a lifetime solving problems for animals and their owners. A vomiting cat, a lame dog, an animal that is unable to conceive—these are all animals with medical problems, and the veterinarian is requested to set things right again. The thought processes of clinicians are usually centered around these types of problems. The first section of this book is organized according to problems, that is, why the animal is presented or abnormalities identified during the workup, rather than by diseases.

The years in veterinary school are spent acquiring the tools necessary to solve problems; however, one must also develop a method of applying that information in a logical and efficient manner. A structured approach to diagnosis and management has been developed that uses clinical "problems" (the presenting complaint, a physical finding, a laboratory abnormality, and so on) as the fulcrum for clinical decision making. This technique is called the problem-oriented approach, and is the basis of the problem-oriented veterinary medical record (POVMR).

FUNCTIONS OF THE MEDICAL RECORD

The medical record should accurately define the health of the patient. The approach to the medical record must be systematic, simple to use, and flexible enough to be modified to every practice. It is essential that receptionists, technical staff, and clinicians are consistent in their approach to the record. Clinicians often view the medical record as a time-consuming exercise in paper shuffling; reviewing the functions of the medical record may make the time spent writing records less objectionable to busy clinicians. The functions are as follows:

1. Record of client information
2. Record of the animal's medical history and a place to solve problems
3. Legal document, should a grievance or litigation occur
4. Source material for retrospective studies, especially in university hospitals

The general practitioner has a crucial role as clinical investigator. Those in private practice are in an excellent position to answer the common, and therefore the most important questions in veterinary medicine. What is the incidence of adverse reactions to a new vaccine one is using? How often does trimethoprim-sulfa cause keratoconjunctivitis sicca in dogs? The availability of computerized medical records should make clinical investigation much easier in general practice.

COMPONENTS OF THE PROBLEM-ORIENTED VETERINARY MEDICAL RECORD

The POVMR has been defined in several ways by various authors. The following is a description of how it is used at the Ontario Veterinary College. Our goal has been to develop a system that is easy to use and that can be utilized in private practice as well as in the teaching hospital. The POVMR consists of several components:

1. History and physical examination
2. Master problem list
3. Initial assessment and plan
4. Progress notes, composed of:
   a. Data
   b. Assessment
   c. Plan
      ▪ Diagnostic plans
      ▪ Therapeutic plans
      ▪ Client education
5. Laboratory, radiographic, biopsy reports
6. Case summary
7. Fee information

Collecting Information: The Data Base

The signalment, history, and physical examination will reveal a sign or group of signs. For instance, a 15-year-old intact male dog has a history of *anorexia* and *weight loss;* abnormal physical findings include a *mass in the abdomen.*

Based on the signs present, a variety of diagnostic aids (hematology, serum chemistry profiles, urinalysis, electrophysiology, diagnostic imaging, biopsy) may be used to arrive at a diagnosis and management plan. The signalment, history, physical examination, and diag-

nostic tests are collectively referred to as the data base. The data base is used to identify problems, which are then solved using a logical approach that relies on a sound understanding of pathophysiology and therapeutic principles, rather than memorized information about specific diseases.

The data base collected depends on the type of patient, the nature of the problem, and the environment in which one works. The signalment, history, and physical examination are always a part of the data base. A fecal floatation may be included with puppy and kitten examinations, a heartworm test with the routine yearly vaccination and checkup, a packed-cell volume and dipstick blood urea nitrogen as the preanesthetic data base for animals younger than 5 years of age undergoing elective surgery, and so on. More complex cases will require a more complex data base, such as a complete blood count, serum chemistry profile, urinalysis, thoracic radiographs, lymph node biopsy, and bone marrow aspirate for a dog with lymphoma. A predetermined data base for each type of patient or problem helps minimize diagnostic errors, saves time, and is usually more economical and better tolerated by clients.

Master Problem List

The problem-oriented approach begins with the acquisition of appropriate client information and the signalment (age, sex, breed) of the animal. This information is usually collected by lay personnel. The primary reason for the visit (sometimes called the chief complaint) is identified. The veterinarian then obtains a history and performs an examination (see Chapter 1).

At this point one or more "problems" have been identified, which are entered onto the master problem list. The master problem list is always the first page of the record, and problems are listed in numerical order and by the date first identified. The date of resolution of problems is also noted. More problems may be identified (and possibly resolved) throughout the workup. The master problem list is an index of the animal's medical history. The vaccination history is often indicated on the same page.

In the context of the POVMR, a problem is anything that may interfere with the patient's well-being and that will require further evaluation or management. Problems include:

1. Historical abnormalities (*e.g.*, vomiting)
2. Physical findings (*e.g.*, dehydration)
3. Laboratory abnormalities (*e.g.*, elevation of blood urea nitrogen level)
4. Syndromes (*e.g.*, uremic syndrome)
5. Specific diagnoses (*e.g.*, acute tubular necrosis due to ethylene glycol toxicosis)

Nonlocalizing problems (depression, anorexia, weight loss) can be "lumped" as one problem, as can obviously related problems (truncal alopecia and hyperpigmentation). The decision to combine problems is based on experience and personal approach; some clinicians are "lumpers," while others are "splitters." It is best to organize the master problem list however one finds it makes the most sense.

Problems may also be resolved into another problem. For instance, the separate problems of polyuria and alopecia may eventually resolve into the new problem hyperadrenocorticism as more information becomes available.

Two aspects of the master problem list should be emphasized: first, problems should be written at the current level of understanding (start initially with polyuria, then resolve it to hyperadrenocorticism later as more data becomes available). Second, the master problem list will always be evolving.

Initial Assessment

Some problems have now been identified. How should they be solved? We suggest starting with an initial assessment. This is the critical step in the problem-oriented approach, and relies on an understanding of pathophysiology and the use of logic and common sense. Attempt to generate the following, as the situation requires:

1. What organ system(s) is involved?
2. What pathophysiologic mechanism(s) explains the problem? (*e.g.*, What are the basic causes of alopecia, jaundice, or polyuria?) The strategy is to work from signs to a diagnosis and management plan; considering pathophysiologic mechanisms of disease may help to focus your effort.

3. What differential diagnoses ("rule-outs") can be considered for this patient? Using further investigation, one can rule out or rule in these possibilities. For example, the differential diagnoses of renal insufficiency, hyperadrenocorticism, and diabetes mellitus may be considered for a 12-year-old male poodle with polyuria. Knowing what to include in this list depends on how much information was generated by the history and physical examination and on the veterinarian's experience. Always start with the common conditions—the clinical adage "when you hear hoofbeats in your backyard, don't look for zebras" usually rings true. One may not be able to list differential diagnoses until much later in the workup; the important thing is to recognize the basic mechanisms of disease and to work from there.
4. How sick is the animal at this time, and what is the prognosis? (For a provocative appraisal of how veterinarians arrive at a prognosis see Crowe, Additional Reading.) A prognosis may not be possible this early in the clinical workup; however, the client will need to have a feeling from the onset whether it is worth pursuing the problems, both from a humane and an economic standpoint.

When the POVMR was initially developed, the idea was to write an assessment and plan for every problem on the master problem list. This approach can lead to a lot of paperwork. An alternative is to write one assessment and plan for the animal as a whole. The decision on which way to go depends on the case, and on what one defines as a problem. Some problems can probably be handled under one assessment (anorexia, nasal discharge, ocular discharge in a young unvaccinated cat); some problems require individual assessments and plans (pneumothorax and compound femoral fracture in a dog that was hit by a car). These formats may be combined, and may change from day to day as the case progresses. The important point is that the thought processes are sorted out and that the record retains efficiency.

Initial Plan

Once an assessment has been made, a plan of approach can be constructed. It is important to differentiate between diagnostic and therapeutic efforts, and to record one's discussions with the client. We set the plan up as follows:

Diagnostic plans (Dx): This is often called the workup. The diagnostic tests chosen are dictated by the assessment.

Therapeutic/management plans (Rx): Therapy can be symptomatic (gastrointestinal motility-modifying drugs), supportive (fluids), or specific (metronidazole for giardiasis). In many instances no therapy is appropriate until more information is available.

Client education (CE): This consists of what the client is told regarding fees, logistics, prognosis, and so on.

It is essential that one be as specific as possible when writing plans. If a urinalysis is needed, indicate if it is to be collected by catch or cystocentesis. Fluid orders must include the type, amount, rate of delivery, and route by which the fluid is to be given. Communication skills within the medical record, with clients, and with other veterinarians cannot be overemphasized. A veterinarian's ability to communicate clearly will largely dictate the success of his or her practice career.

Progress Notes

As information is generated about the case, the assessment and plan will need to be updated. This is done in the progress notes, which are a variation on the initial assessment format. Example progress notes for a 9-year-old male German shepherd are written as

Data (new information): Moderate regenerative anemia, splenic mass present on ultrasound, no abnormalities seen on thoracic radiographs, clotting profile normal

Assessment: The anemia is consistent with a bleeding splenic mass. In this patient hemangiosarcoma is likely. There does not appear to be gross pulmonary metastasis at this time.

Plan:

- Dx: Exploratory laparotomy
- Rx: Nothing now
- CE: Discuss risks of surgery, prognosis, and cost

We often refer to progress notes as the *DAP* (Data, Assessment, Plan).

How often should one write progress notes? Each problem should be assessed at least once daily while the animal is hospitalized. Some cases will require more frequent progress notes, such as an animal in intensive care whose physiologic parameters are changing quickly (*e.g.*, acute renal failure). Outpatient visits may (reassessment of a dog with diabetes mellitus) or may not (suture removal, vaccination, other routine consultations) require progress notes. Write progress notes whenever they will be helpful in organizing data or when a new assessment is needed. Flow charts are helpful when serial data are collected.

Case Summary

A case summary is written at the time the animal is discharged. This is a concise summary of the workup, diagnosis, and management of the animal during that hospitalization. Clinicians working in referral hospitals usually write a formal referral letter, which can also act as a case summary.

Written instructions should be given to the client. Be sure that they are written clearly at a level that is understood by a lay person. A copy of all correspondence should be kept in the record.

WHO NEEDS THE PROBLEM-ORIENTED VETERINARY MEDICAL RECORD?

Whenever there are multiple clinicians working on a case, or when a case is complex (as defined by the attending clinician), the POVMR is likely to be helpful. University teaching hospitals and large private hospitals usually require some variation of this system. The private practitioner is encouraged to keep a master problem list for each patient and to use the POVMR format for anything other than the most routine case.

ADDITIONAL READING

Crowe SE. Usefulness of prognosis: Qualitative terms vs. quantative designations. J Am Vet Med Assoc 1985; 187:700.

1

HISTORY AND PHYSICAL EXAMINATION OF THE DOG AND CAT

Stephen A. Kruth

In the problem-oriented approach to small animal medicine, emphasis is placed on the collection of data and the development of a minimum data base. The foundation of all data bases is the history and physical examination.

In our shiny world of automated serum chemistry profiles, ultrasound machines, endoscopes, and other technologies, it is easy to understand how the clinician can be seduced into relying on the "hard" data that these tests provide and placing less importance on the more mundane history and physical examination. We suggest that the clinical examination is far more important than it initially appears.

How powerful are the history and physical examination? Information on this area in veterinary medicine is scarce, if it exists at all. If we turn to the human literature, we may find a hint of the answer. In a study performed in a general hospital in the United States, 56% of cases had been assigned correct diagnoses by the end of a brief history, and this figure rose to 73% by the end of the physical examination (Sandler, Additional Reading). Several other studies have yielded similar results, and there is no reason to believe that the veterinary situation should be any different.

Further diagnostic and therapeutic plans, as well as prognostic information, rely on the initial clinical examination. In some instances, the usefulness of prognostic information acquired through the clinical examination may surpass that of complicated and invasive staging systems (Boyd, Additional Reading).

It is clear that the clinical examination has great potential power with regard to diagnosis, prognosis, and management decisions. It is also obvious that the examination must be accurate and reliable.

How accurate are our clinical observations? In the human literature we find that there is great variation between examiners (as well as between repeated examinations by the same examiner) in the accuracy of palpation, auscultation, the reading of radiographs and electrocardiograms, and other examinations. There is no reason to suspect that it is any different for veterinarians. We suggest that while the power of the clinical examination is great, the accuracy of examination can

7

Table 1–1 *Suggestions for the Improvement of the Clinical Examination*

THE EXAMINER

Record evidence, not inference ("the dog is pale," rather than "the dog is anemic")

Recognize how prior expectation influences the examination (you tend to find what you are looking for)

Recognize how fatigue and stress alter perception, cognition, and mood

THE EXAMINED

Recognize variations in the system examined, not only among breeds, but among individuals

Recognize the effect of medications and illnesses

Recognize the effect of rumination on the client—repeat the history at a later date

THE EXAMINATION

Make sure that the examination area is quiet and well lighted

Make sure that diagnostic tools function properly

Repeat key findings

(Modified from Sackett DL, Haynes RB, Tugwell P, eds. Clinical Epidemiology: A basic science for clinical medicine. Toronto: Little Brown & Co, 1985: 33.)

---

stand improvement. Table 1-1 lists some ways to improve the accuracy of the clinical examination.

THE HISTORY

The history begins with the description or signalment of the animal. Age, sex, and breed are always included (*e.g.*, "7-year-old spayed female Irish setter"). Many disorders have tendencies to occur at certain ages (congenital vs. degenerative and neoplastic disorders) or in certain breeds (aortic stenosis in Newfoundland dogs). Sex associations may be obvious (mammary cancer, prostatic disease); however, many disorders tend to occur more frequently in one sex than another (cardiomyopathy in male Doberman pincher dogs, pancreatitis in obese middle-aged female dogs). The sex of the animal may also be important when making therapeutic decisions (the administration of megestrol acetate for a skin disorder to an intact female may lead to the development of pyometra; the effective regulation of an intact female diabetic is more difficult).

The history is the information that is generated from the client interview, from reading the pre-

vious medical record, or from talking to other veterinarians. It begins with a problem as seen through the client's eyes (sometimes called the chief complaint), such as "My dog has diarrhea." The history is then developed by asking questions about the chief complaint; for example, "When did the diarrhea start?"; "How often does it occur?"; or "What does the stool look like?". The experienced clinician has predetermined history subroutines for common chief complaints (the cough history, the diarrhea history, the new puppy history, the well geriatric history, and so on).

The way questions are framed can bias the owner's response. To avoid this, ask neutral questions such as "Has there been a *change* in your dog's water consumption?" rather than leading questions such as "Is your dog drinking more?". Also, be sure that the client is not making a diagnosis for you—the animal that is "vomiting" may actually be regurgitating or even expectorating. Ask the client to *describe* what he or she sees (evidence is less misleading than inference!).

After the chief complaint has been developed, obtain a complete general history. Just because a client does not mention something does not mean that it is not occurring—the clinician must ask. The history should include questions regarding activity pattern, appetite, diet, the presence of vomiting, diarrhea, coughing, or sneezing, changes in water consumption, lameness, vaccine history, past medical problems, and treatment history. Other areas to investigate may include the presence and health of other animals, the environment in which the animal is kept, what the uses of the animal are, travel history, reproductive history, and so on as the situation dictates.

The question of whether animals have signs or symptoms sometimes arises. In humans, the term symptom refers to a subjective observation made by the patient, such as "It hurts here." A sign is an objective finding made by the examiner, such as "The dog tried to bite me when I palpated his distal femur; therefore, it must be painful." It would seem that animals are limited to having signs and not symptoms, thus testing the diagnostic skill of the veterinarian.

Good communication is essential to successful case (and client) management. Communicate at a level that your client understands (be careful with jargon such as "put to sleep"!). Listen actively, and interrupt when appropriate. It is helpful to summarize the history for the owner, to be sure that the history is complete and that there are no misunderstandings.

THE PHYSICAL EXAMINATION

In clinical practice there is no such thing as a "complete" physical examination. As with history taking, the examiner has a repertoire of subroutines to draw from as the situation requires. Thus, the examination of the neonate may include looking for a cleft palate and umbilical hernia, the examination of the vomiting juvenile dog may focus on abdominal palpation for a foreign body or intussusception, and the examination of the geriatric cat includes palpation of the neck for a thyroid nodule. Although animals may present with what appears to be a localizing sign (cough, diarrhea), we emphasize that a general examination should be performed on all ill animals.

This chapter will present a version (there are as many versions are there are clinicians) of a general examination and will identify other subroutines that may be indicated by the chief complaint. Subroutines are usually system-oriented (rather than animal-oriented) and are presented in other sections of this book. This general examination is designed for adult animals of either sex; the examination of the neonate, juvenile, and geriatric is modified to identify age-related abnormalities (Table 1-2).

Each practitioner must develop his or her own approach to the general physical examination. It is important that a routine be established and adhered to. The examination should be performed actively, not passively (Is there a cardiac murmur? Can I palpate a mass in the area of the thyroid? Are the kidneys small?). The techniques of inspection, palpation, and auscultation are learned through practice and experience, and the clinician should continually try to improve his or her examination skills.

Vital signs are generally obtained at the beginning of the examination, and include body weight, degree of hydration, temperature, respi-

Table 1–2 *Evaluation for Abnormalities in Different Age Groups to be Included in the General Examination*

NEONATE TO TWO MONTHS
Cleft palate
Umbilical hernia
Dewclaws
Unusual size and body weight relative to siblings

TWO TO SIX MONTHS
Cardiac murmurs
Crytorchidism
Improper position of permanent teeth

GERIATRIC (AGE DEPENDS ON BREED)
Obesity
Mass lesions, especially skin, mammary glands, mouth
Cataracts
Dental abnormalities
Thyroid nodule (cat)
Cardiac murmurs
Prostate

ratory rate, and heart rate. Systemic arterial blood pressure is a routine measurement in humans, and alterations in blood pressure abnormalities are becoming more frequently recognized in veterinary medicine. At this time, the determination of arterial blood pressure in animals is a subroutine.

Inspection of the animal from a distance is important, and can usually be done while obtaining the history. Observations regarding the animal's temperament, level of mentation, conformation, and ambulation are made as the animal moves around the examination room. The animal can then be examined more closely.

I start by reassuring the animal, and then examine the head, unless the dog looks like he wants to bite; then I start at the tail! The teeth, tongue, and pharynx are inspected, and the color of the oral mucous membranes is evaluated (see Chapter 2). Nasal discharge and abnormalities of the rhinarium are identified at this time (see Chapter 27). The ocular adnexa are inspected, and the anterior chamber is evaluated using a pen light (subroutines: examination of cornea, fundus, tear production, ocular pressure). The external ear canals are inspected (subroutine: otoscopic examination of tympanic membranes and proximal canals).

The submandibular and prescapular lymph nodes are palpated, as well as the ventral cervical region. Special attention is paid to the region of the thyroid in cats older than 7 years. I usually palpate the thoracic limbs and inspect the feet, pads, and nails.

I palpate the thorax next, and then begin examining the abdomen (I will auscultate the chest later). A two-handed technique is encouraged while palpating. Gentle, continuous digital pressure will usually cause the muscles of the abdomen to relax. Structures that are normally identifiable include the urinary bladder, loops of small intestine, the colon, and (in the cat) the kidneys. The liver, pancreas, spleen, and reproductive tract are not usually palpable. Learning palpation is sometimes simplified if the examiner visualizes an abdominal radiograph for use as a road map. Visualizing the various structures improves the likelihood of finding them.

Next, the pelvic limbs are examined in a similar manner to the thoracic limbs. The popliteal lymph nodes are palpated at this time.

I then examine the anus, perineum, and external reproductive organs. The prostate should be examined by digital rectal examination in any male dog older than 5 years of age (see Chapter 57).

The skin is examined along with each body section. In female dogs, the mammary chain is palpated for tumors.

I usually examine the thorax last. Auscultation is, in the minds of many clinicians, not a highly diagnostic technique in small animals. Difficulties arise from a long history of confusing terminology, the small body size and rapid respiratory rates of many patients, and reliance on radiographs. However, we feel that auscultation can be a valuable diagnostic technique, and challenge the clinician to develop his or her auscultatory skills.

Auscultation must be carried out in a quiet environment. It is a waste of time to try to evaluate the lung and heart sounds of an animal in a noisy ward or treatment room (an expensive "cardiology" stethoscope will not save your examination). The animal should be standing quietly, with its mouth held closed. Purring can sometimes be controlled by turning on a water tap in the room (first tell the owner what you are going to do!). The clinician will learn to recognize auscultatory artifacts, including the noise of hair moving across the diaphragm of the stethoscope, muscular contractions, the sniffing that animals do in a new environment, and purring. The following descriptions of sounds are based on an animal that is taking deep breaths; few sounds are generated if the animal is breathing shallowly. The external nares can be held shut for several seconds and then released to induce the animal to inspire deeply.

Respiratory sounds are classified as normal breath sounds and adventitious (added or abnormal) sounds. The lack of lung sounds, "silent lung," may also be a significant finding. Normal breath sounds are those sounds that are auscultated in the normal animal. Normal sounds may be the only auscultatory finding of the animal with respiratory disease. These sounds are generated by the vibration of solid respiratory tissues and the fluctuations in gas pressure in airways. Normal breath sounds are divided into tracheal (or bronchial), vesicular, and bronchovesicular sounds. Tracheal sounds are those sounds heard when the stethoscope is placed over the cervical trachea. Relatively loud inspiratory and expiratory sounds of equal duration are heard. Vesicular sounds are heard when the stethoscope is placed on the thoracic wall over normal lung tissue. These sounds consist of a quiet inspiratory sound followed by a quiet, shorter expiratory sound; it is not known how these sounds are produced. The alveoli and terminal airways are silent in normal animals.

Bronchovesicular sounds are intermediate in quality between tracheal and vesicular sounds. Normal breath sounds may be more intense than expected in young or underweight animals. The change in airflow velocity associated with exercise, anxiety, pain, hyperthermia, acidemia, or lung disease may also change the intensity of normal breath sounds ("rough" or "harsh" lung sounds).

Adventitious lung sounds are sounds that are suggestive of pulmonary pathology. Three types of sounds are defined: crackles, wheezes, and pleural friction rubs. These sounds are best heard when the animal is induced to breathe deeply. Crackles are intermittent, discrete sounds that have no musical tone. They are generated by two mechanisms, the first being the explosive, sudden opening of airways. This occurs in a variety of lung diseases in which the lung does not inflate evenly. Thus, high-pitched crackling (similar to a velcro zipper being slowly pulled open) may be a sign of pulmonary fibrosis, interstitial pneumonia, or interstitial edema. The second mechanism causing crackles is the bursting of bubbles in airway secretions. In this instance, low-pitched crackles are associated with severe pulmonary edema and bronchopneumonia. A "wet" sound or a "dry" sound has little if any meaning regarding the actual pathologic process in the lung.

The wheeze is the second adventitious sound. Wheezes are caused by the vibration of airway walls as air passes through a narrowed airway. A continuous whistling sound is thus a sign of obstructive lung disease. The pitch of the wheeze is largely independent of the size of the affected airway.

The third adventitious sound is not produced in the lung, but by inflamed parietal and visceral pleura rubbing against each other. A sound suggestive of creaking leather is generated by the fibrin-covered surfaces. Pleural friction rubs can be associated with septic pleural effusions, but are uncommonly heard in small animals.

A lack of audible lung sounds is common in small animals that are breathing shallowly, especially cats. Some conditions, however, dampen lung sounds, causing the finding of silent lung. This can be associated with obesity, pleural effusion, pneumothorax, diaphragmatic hernia, thoracic masses, severe emphysema, and diffuse terminal airway disease.

To complete the general examination, I auscultate the heart. The chest is palpated for the strongest precordial impulse ("heart beat"); this is the "point of maximum intensity," which is usually associated with the region of the mitral valve. The various valvular areas (or each hemithorax in cats or small dogs) are listened to. The heart sounds are evaluated, and murmurs identified (see Chapter 17). The femoral pulses are evaluated while listening to the heart; heart sounds occurring without a femoral pulse are called pulse deficits, and identify the presence of an arrhythmia (see Chapter 18).

This completes the basic examination; other subroutines (*e.g.,* lameness examination [Chapter 63], neurologic examination [Chapters 53–55], and dermatologic examination [Chapters 49–52]) can be performed as indicated by the chief complaint.

SUMMARY

We hope that this chapter has caused the clinician to reassess not only his or her clinical examination ability, but also the value of the examination itself. Physical diagnosis is a learned skill that improves with practice. One's ability improves when the examination is performed in the correct environment, with the correct instruments, and when the examiner is in the correct frame of mind. As clinicians in a referral veterinary hospital, we are constantly asked for assistance on "hard" cases. Many of the answers are found not after performing sophisticated and exotic diagnostic tests, but after interviewing the owner and performing a careful examination. The most important diagnostic tool we have is the clinical examination.

ADDITIONAL READING

Bistner S, Shaw D. Examination of the eye. Vet Clin North Am 1981; 11:595.

Boyd NF, Feinstein AR. Symptoms as an index of growth rates and prognosis in Hodgkin's disease. Clin Invest Med 1978; 2:25.

Kruth SA. Systemic hypertension. In: Allen DG, Kruth SA (eds). Small animal cardiopulmonary medicine. Toronto: BC Decker, 1988: 119.

Roudebush P. Lung sounds. J Am Vet Med Assoc 1982; 181:122.

Sackett DL, Haynes RB, Tugwell P, eds. Clinical epidemiology: A basic science for clinical medicine. Toronto: Little, Brown & Co, 1985: Chapter 2.

Sandler G. The importance of the history in the medical clinic and the cost of unnecessary tests. Am Heart J 1980; 100:931.

GENERAL
CLINICAL
PROBLEMS

2

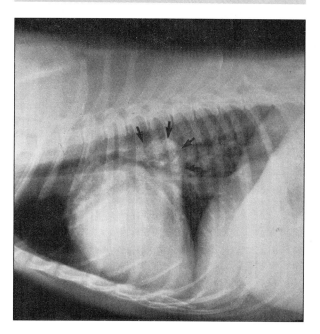

2

CYANOSIS, PALLOR, AND ERYTHEMA
Dana G. Allen

Examination of the color of the skin and mucous membranes provides insight into the general health of the patient. Normal mucous membranes are pink and moist. Abnormalities in skin and mucous membrane color include blue–gray (cyanotic), white (pale), red (erythemic), or yellow (icteric). Thin-skinned areas, unpigmented skin or mucous membranes, and areas with sparse hair cover are best for evaluation of color. Cyanosis, pallor, and erythema are discussed here. Jaundice is discussed in the following chapter.

Examination of mucous membrane color is best done under natural light. Fluorescent or incandescent light tends to obscure subtle changes in color.

CAUSES

Cyanosis

Diseases causing cyanosis are a common cause of color change of the mucous membranes. Cyanosis is categorized into central and peripheral causes. Central cyanosis results in the delivery of unoxygenated blood to the peripheral tissues. Cardiovascular disease, including tetralogy of Fallot and Eisenmenger's syndrome (pulmonary hypertension, ventricular septal defect, atrial septal defect,

or patent ductus arteriosus (PDA) and right-to-left shunting of unoxygenated blood), respiratory disease causing hypoxemia, and conditions leading to methemoglobinemia are associated with central cyanosis (Fig. 2-1).

In peripheral cyanosis fully oxygenated blood leaves the heart, but delivery to the peripheral tissues is hampered by poor blood flow secondary to a fall in cardiac output and vascular stasis, arterial or venous thrombosis, or local vasoconstriction. Peripheral cyanosis secondary to a fall in cardiac output alone is rare. Pallor is more common.

Differential cyanosis occurs in animals with PDA complicated by pulmonary hypertension. Unoxygenated blood flows from the pulmonary artery through the ductus arteriosus and enters the descending aorta caudal to the brachiocephalic trunk and left subclavian artery. These animals have normal coloration of the head and neck, but are cyanotic from the neck caudad.

Pallor

Animals presenting with pale mucous membranes have poor peripheral perfusion or anemia (including acute blood loss). In the cat feline leukemia virus (FeLV), hemobartonellosis, and

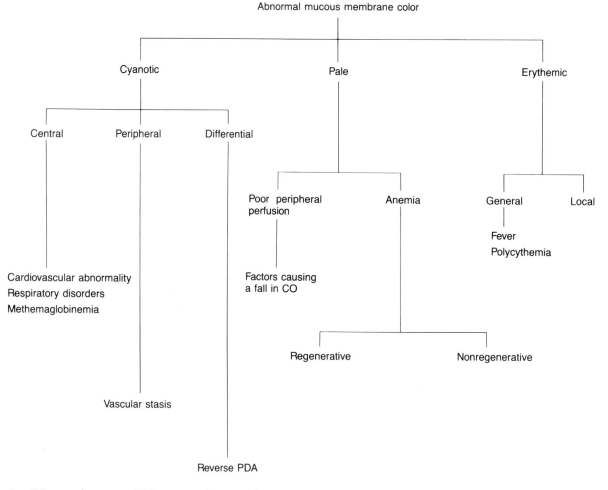

Key: CO = cardiac output; PDA = patent ductus arteriosus

Figure 2–1. *Approach to abnormalities of mucous membrane color. (Modified from Allen DG. Cyanosis, pallor and erythema. In: Allen DG, Kruth SA, eds. Small animal cardiopulmonary medicine. Philadelphia: BC Decker, 1988: 35.)*

Heinz-body anemias are common causes of anemia. Poor peripheral perfusion may be associated with any disease process that leads to a fall in cardiac output. Hypoadrenocorticism may also be associated with pale mucous membranes.

Erythema

Bright red skin or mucous membranes may be limited to an area of the body associated with localized hyperemia and vasodilation or may be generalized and associated with fever and gen- eral vasodilation or an increase in red cell mass (polycythemia) (see Fig. 2-1).

PATHOPHYSIOLOGY

Cyanosis

Central cyanosis is caused by cardiovascular or respiratory disease or methemoglobinemia. Cardiovascular disease causing cyanosis may be associated with an intracardiac defect and arterio- venous admixture of blood (tetralogy of Fallot or

Eisenmenger's syndrome). Cyanosis becomes clinically apparent when there is in excess of 5 g/dl (50 g/L) of reduced or unoxygenated hemoglobin present in the blood. Because of the lower hemoglobin content, severely anemic animals do not readily show physical evidence of cyanosis. Conversely, animals with polycythemia are more apt to show physical evidence of cyanosis.

Oxygen is carried primarily (97%) by hemoglobin. Only 3% is dissolved in plasma. With normal pulmonary blood flow and inspired oxygen content, hemoglobin is fully saturated with oxygen by the time it has passed only one third of the way through the pulmonary capillaries. Normal arterial oxygen tension (PaO_2) at sea level ranges from 85 to 100 mmHg in an animal breathing room air. Arterial oxygen saturation must fall lower than a PaO_2 of 50 mmHg (correlating to an arterial oxygen saturation of 80%) before cyanosis becomes clinically apparent. Hypoxemia may be associated with reduced inspired oxygen (anesthetic accident, laryngeal or tracheobronchial obstruction), hypoventilation (drug- or central nervous system-induced respiratory depression, thoracic disease limiting chest expansion), arteriovenous shunt, factors affecting alveolar membrane permeability, or ventilation perfusion mismatch with insufficient pulmonary blood flow or oxygen delivery to the lungs (pneumonia, atelectasis, pulmonary edema, aspiration pneumonia, pulmonary contusion). Cyanosis associated with hypoxemia is a late finding in the course of respiratory disease.

Functional hemoglobin is composed of a globin molecule and heme units containing iron. Iron must be in the ferrous (Fe^{+2}) form to bind and transport oxygen. In the ferric state (Fe^{+3}; methemoglobin) it cannot bind with or transport oxygen. The severity of cyanosis is proportional to the percent methemoglobin present within the circulation. Methemoglobinemia may be caused by exposure to oxidizing agents (nitrites, nitrates, phenacetin, sulfonamides, benzocaine, aniline dyes as used in laundry markers and crayons, and dapsone), a deficiency of reduced nicotinamide–adenine dinucleotide methemoglobin reductase (NADH-MR), or the presence of an abnormal hemoglobin structure (hemoglobin M). Congenital NADH-MR deficiency is rare in dogs, and abnormal hemoglobin structures have not been documented in small animals. Cats are especially sensitive to oxidant chemicals. Benzocaine-containing sprays (*e.g.,* Cetacaine) used to induce topical laryngeal anesthesia have been associated with methemoglobinemia in the cat. Similarly, dogs and cats with active skin lesions have developed methemoglobinemia following topical application of 5% benzocaine. Cats are deficient in glucuronyl transferase, which effectively delays the rate of glucuronide conjugation of drugs. Cats also have a limited ability to conjugate phenolic compounds with sulfate. Only half a tablet (163 mg) of acetaminophen may cause methemoglobinemia and cyanosis. Dogs may tolerate up to 200 mg/kg of acetaminophen before signs of toxicity become apparent.

Carbon monoxide competes with oxygen for binding sites on the hemoglobin molecule. The affinity of hemoglobin for carbon monoxide is 250 times greater than that for oxygen. As a result, animals exposed to carbon monoxide are incapable of transporting oxygen, and tissue anoxia follows. The mucous membranes in animals with acute toxicity, however, appear pink, and the blood from affected animals appears cherry red.

Peripheral cyanosis is due to the decreased delivery of blood to tissues or to the delayed transit of blood through capillary beds, allowing for the excessive extraction of oxygen. Shock, arterial or venous thrombosis, local arteriovenous shunts, vasoconstriction, and exposure to cold may cause peripheral cyanosis.

Pallor

Anemia or poor peripheral perfusion are associated with pale mucous membranes. Conditions that decrease peripheral perfusion are those associated with a fall in cardiac output. Cardiac output is a function of stroke volume and heart rate and rhythm. Stroke volume is decreased by decreases in preload (pericardial effusion, peripheral vasodilation, and shock), increases in afterload (arterial vasoconstriction), or decreases in myocardial contractility (cardiomyopathy). Alterations in heart rate and rhythm may also decrease cardiac output to a level contributory to pallor. It is clinically rare in conditions solely affecting stroke volume or heart rate or rhythm.

Erythema

Bright red mucous membrane color may be a localized phenomenon associated with inflammation, vasodilation, and an increase in local red cell mass. It may also reflect a systemic problem such as fever or polycythemia. Polycythemia is classified as relative (dehydration) or absolute (primary and secondary) (see Chapter 74). Primary polycythemia is a myeloproliferative disorder. Secondary polycythemia is related to oxygen deficiency (appropriate), erythropoietin-producing tumors, or increased blood levels of adrenal corticosteroids. Polycythemia may also be associated with cyanosis. In this case the markedly increased red cell mass and hemoglobin content predispose to cyanosis. Hyperthermia, including fever with peripheral vasodilation and flushing of the skin, may cause erythema. It is often accompanied by panting and shivering. Causes of fever include infectious disease, autoimmune disease and neoplasia (see Chapter 6).

CLINICAL SIGNS

Cyanosis

Clinical signs of central cyanosis are often related to the cause of the problem. Cardiovascular cases may present with histories that include coughing, poor exercise tolerance, and fainting. On physical examination a murmur, adventitial lung sounds, ascites, abnormalities in heart rate and rhythm, and poor pulse amplitude may be noted. Cases with respiratory disease often present with similar histories (other than fainting). Dyspnea, fever, adventitial lung sounds, and a productive cough may be additional findings.

The severity of clinical signs associated with methemoglobinemia correlates more with the chronicity of the disease rather than the degree of methemoglobinemia. Acute toxic methemoglobinemia is associated with a more severe clinical picture. In cases with markedly elevated methemoglobin levels (more than 50%), lethargy, ataxia, poor exercise tolerance, exertional dyspnea, and coughing have been recorded. Death occurs at methemoglobin levels exceeding 80%. Methemoglobinemia is most often associated with exposure to oxidant chemicals. Cats with acetaminophen toxicosis may be presented with cyanosis, tachycardia, tachypnea, vomiting, and depression. Edema of the face and extremities, icterus, and hemoglobinuria or hematuria may also be present. Congenital NADH-MR deficiency is rarely associated with clinical signs other than cyanosis. Anesthesia and surgery have been performed in NADH-MR cases without complication.

Peripheral cyanosis is clinically uncommon. It is most often associated with peripheral vascular stasis. Cats with iliac thromboembolic disease are presented lame with cold, firm, and painful hindlimb(s). No pulse is palpable in the affected limb(s) and the nailbed fails to bleed if it is purposely cut short. Cardiac murmurs and abnormalities in rate and rhythm secondary to the primary cause of cardiomyopathy may be evident. Pulmonary edema or pleural effusion may also be present. Other conditions predisposing to thromboembolic events (hyperadrenocorticism, glomerulonephropathies, bacterial endocarditis) and peripheral cyanosis are discussed in detail in their respective chapters.

Animals with reverse PDA (differential cyanosis) are typically normal for the first to fifth year of life, when weakness and collapse of the hind legs may become apparent. Other clinical signs may include decreased exercise tolerance, stunted growth, and dyspnea. A murmur is not audible because the volume of shunted blood is too small to generate sufficient turbulent flow. Accentuation and splitting of the second heart sound is, however, common. The disease has been recognized as a congenital problem in a number of breeds of dog, including the collie, poodle, Pomeranian, Shetland sheepdog, cocker spaniel, miniature schnauzer, and golden retriever. It is inherited as a polygenic trait in the poodle. A case has also been reported in the cat.

Carbon monoxide poisoning occurs most commonly in animals transported in the trunk of cars with faulty exhaust systems or housed in poorly ventilated areas with faulty fuel-generated heating equipment. Nausea, vomiting, lethargy, disturbances in gait, progressive depression, collapse, or acute coma and death occur.

Pallor

The severity of clinical signs related to anemia is more a reflection of the acuteness of onset of the problem rather than its magnitude. Animals with a hematocrit of 10% (0.10 L/L) may be clinically well if not subjected to stress. Animals suffering an acute fall in packed cell volume (acute blood loss) are apt to show signs of shock with or without hemoglobinemia and hemaglobinuria, depending on the cause. The classic signs of shock are tachypnea, tachycardia, decreased pulse amplitude, prolonged capillary refill time, pallor, weakness, and depression. Acute blood loss may be associated with vascular trauma, an acute decrease in platelet numbers or function, or a loss of factor function or concentration. Signs of external hemorrhage may not be evident in cases of acute anticoagulant toxicity (coumarins, indanediones). In these cases bleeding often occurs into the abdomen or chest. Other signs that may accompany anemia include lethargy, fainting with exercise, and anorexia.

Animals with cardiovascular causes of pallor have physical and historical signs compatible with the nature of the inciting disease. Rapid heart rates and weak, thready pulses characterize poor peripheral perfusion. Animals with hypoadrenocorticism, however, have slow heart rates and a poor pulse amplitude. They may also present with vomiting, weakness, depression, polyuria, polydipsia, and weight loss. Patients with anemia commonly have increased peripheral pulse amplitudes in the absence of historic or physical evidence of cardiovascular disease.

Erythema

Localized causes of erythema include conditions causing inflammation. Characteristic skin lesions, pruritis, swelling, local heat, or pain may accompany hyperemia and aid in differentiating its cause.

More generalized causes of erythema include fever and polycythemia. Clinical signs associated with fever include panting, shivering, and, depending on the etiology of the hyperemia, arrhythmias (bacterial endocarditis) and lameness (autoimmune disease, bacterial endocarditis). Neoplastic disease is associated with disorder of the organ system involved.

Animals with polycythemia have clinical signs related to elevations in red cell mass and an increase in blood viscosity (see Chapter 74). Bleeding diathesis with epistaxis, melena or hematuria, central nervous system signs (including ataxia, lethargy, weakness, seizure, or blindness), and polyuria and polydipsia may be noted.

Animals with pheochromocytoma, a rare catecholamine-secreting neoplasm of the adrenal medulla, may present with intermittent episodes of flushing, blanching, or cyanosis of the skin accompanied by tachypnea, weakness, muscle tremor, polyuria, polydipsia, and epistaxis. In most cases mucous membrane color is normal.

DIAGNOSTIC APPROACH

The diagnostic approach and a list of suggested laboratory tests to aid in the differentiation of causes associated with changes in color of the skin and mucous membranes appears in Table 2-1.

Cyanosis

Cardiovascular disease, respiratory disorders, and methemoglobinemia are the most common causes of central cyanosis. A thorough history and physical examination should help separate these three areas. Determination of the etiology of cardiovascular disease is made with electrocardiography (ECG), chest radiography, echocardiography, arterial blood gas analysis, and angiocardiography. Nonselective angiocardiography may be used to confirm the presence of a right-to-left intracardiac shunt in cats and small dogs (see Nonselective Angiocardiography in Chapter 80). Contrast material is injected into the cephalic or jugular vein. Simultaneous opacification of the right and left sides of the heart (right

Table 2–1 *Differential Diagnosis for Abnormalities in Mucous Membrane and Skin Color, and Suggested Laboratory Procedures*

Color Abnormality	Differential Diagnosis	Laboratory Tests
CYANOSIS		
Central	Cardiovascular problem (tetralogy of Fallot, Eisenmenger's syndrome)	ECG, chest radiographs, echocardiogram, arterial blood gas, angiocardiogram
	Pulmonary problem (causes leading to hypoxemia)	Chest radiographs, arterial blood gas, tracheobronchoscopy
	Methemaglobinemia	Blood test: does it remain brown when dropped onto filter paper or exposed to air?
	Carbon monoxide toxicity	Carboxyhemoglobin levels (Note that PaO_2 levels may be normal)
Peripheral	Thromboembolic disease, cardiomyopathy	ECG, chest radiographs, echocardiogram
	Nephrotic syndrome, bacterial endocarditis	Serum chemistry, U/A, urine protein to creatinine ratio, ECG, echocardiogram, blood culture
	Amyloidosis	Protein electrophoresis, serum chemistry, U/A, urine protein to creatinine ratio, biopsy
	Hyperadrenocorticism	CBC, serum chemistry, ACTH stimulation, dexamethasone suppression
	Tumor	Angiogram
Differential	Reverse patent ductus arteriosus	ECG, chest radiographs, echocardiogram, angiocardiogram
Pallor	Anemia	CBC; reticulocyte count; Coomb's test; search for Heinz bodies and *Leptospira, Babesia, Haemobartonella,* and Cytauxzoon organisms; U/A; serum chemistry; +/− marrow aspirate; feline leukemia virus test; feline immunodeficiency virus test; coagulation screen
	Poor peripheral perfusion	ECG, chest radiographs, echocardiogram, arterial blood pressure, serum electrolytes
ERYTHEMA		
General	Polycythemia	CBC, serum chemistry, U/A, ECG, chest radiographs, arterial blood gas, marrow aspirate
	Fever, infection	CBC, serum chemistry, culture and sensitivity test
	Autoimmune disease	CBC, Coomb's test, ANA, LE prep
	Neoplasia	CBC, chest radiographs, tumor biopsy
Peripheral	Inflammation	Skin scraping, skin biopsy, allergy testing

ECG = electrocardiogram; U/A = urinalysis; CBC = complete blood count; ANA = antinuclear antibody; LE = lupus erythematosus preparation
(Modified from Allen DG. Cyanosis, pallor and erythema. In: Allen DG, Kruth SA, eds. Small animal cardiopulmonary medicine. Philadelphia: BC Decker, 1988: 39.)

ventricle, left ventricle, aorta, and pulmonary arteries) may be seen with right-to-left intracardiac shunts. Most animals with right-to-left intracardiac shunts have a significant elevation in packed cell volume in response to tissue hypoxemia.

Respiratory diseases causing cyanosis are often accompanied by dyspnea. Inspiratory dyspnea is suggestive of upper airway pathology, and expiratory dyspnea of chest pathology. Examination of the upper airway is completed by auscultation, radiography, and endoscopy (see Thoracic Radiography and Tracheobronchoscopy in Chapter 80). Chest radiographs help evaluate the lung field and establish the nature and extent of pathology present. Blood gas analysis is used to evaluate the functional capacity of the lungs. Blood oxygen levels are a measure of the interaction of alveolar oxygen and pulmonary blood flow. Arterial blood samples must be taken to evaluate blood oxygen levels. Carbon dioxide levels are primarily determined by alveolar ventilation. Arterial or venous samples can be used to evaluate carbon dioxide levels in blood. Hypercapnea is observed with severe lung disease or hypoventilation. Chest radiography and blood gas analysis are not sensitive tests. Significant disease may be present and not be detected by analysis of these tests.

A presumptive test for methemoglobinemia is the spot filter test. A drop of blood with significant methemoglobin levels turns the filter paper brown. When blood from patients with cardiopulmonary causes of cyanosis is shaken with air it turns red because the hemoglobin molecule is functionally normal. Conversely, if blood taken from patients with methemoglobinemia is shaken with air it remains brown. Methemoglobin levels can be measured and reported as a percentage of total hemoglobin concentration. Normal dogs may have up to 2.5% methemoglobin concentration, and cats approximately 1%. Cyanosis may become clinically apparent when methemoglobin levels exceed 2.5%. However, in a report by Krake (Additional Reading) cyanosis was not clinically obvious in cats with methemoglobin levels as high as 6%. Dogs with NADH-MR deficiency have methemoglobin values of 30% to 40% without significant clinical effects. Levels exceeding 50% are associated with ataxia, lethargy, and semistupor. The laboratory diagnosis of NADH-MR deficiency is based on an assay of NADH-MR activity and the demonstration of methemoglobinemia.

Peripheral cyanosis is a rare clinical entity by itself. The most common clinical manifestation is thromboembolic disease in the cat secondary to cardiomyopathy. Vascular stasis, endothelial damage, and hypercoagulability predispose the cat to thrombosis. Cats are commonly presented with hindlimb paresis. The limb is cold, pulseless, firm, and painful. Bleeding does not readily occur if a nailbed is purposely cut short. Angiography can by used to localize the vascular occlusion, but this procedure can be justified only in cases that warrant surgery (see Chapter 24). Other diseases that decrease cardiac output and predispose to peripheral cyanosis lead to prolongation of capillary refill time.

Differential cyanosis (reverse PDA) is marked by severe right ventricular hypertrophy on chest radiographs and ECG. The hematocrit is elevated (60% to 65% and higher). Angiocardiography reveals simultaneous opacification of the pulmonary arteries, ductus arteriosus, and descending aorta.

Patients with carbon monoxide poisoning classically have cherry red blood. This finding, however, is inconsistent. The clinician should rely more on a history of likely exposure. Carboxyhemoglobin levels can be measured.

Pallor

Animals with pale mucous membranes are anemic or in a state of cardiovascular compromise. A thorough history, physical examination, and hematocrit level will readily differentiate these two causes. Animals with only anemia do not have histories consistent with cardiovascular disease (murmur, cough, syncope). Murmurs may be auscultated, however, if the hematocrit falls lower than 18% (0.18 L/L). A hematocrit less than 37% (0.37 L/L) in the dog and less than 24% (0.24 L/L) in the cat is considered clinically significant. Once a diagnosis of anemia has been made, the anemia is further classified into regenerative and nonregenerative forms based primarily on the presence (regenerative) or absence (nonregenerative) of reticulocytes, polychromasia, and an increase in mean cell volume (see Chapter 73). Causes of anemia are pursued with a Coomb's test, screening for Heinz bodies or *Hemobartonella* organisms (regenerative anemias), or a bone marrow biopsy (nonregenerative causes, *e.g.*, feline leukemia virus; see Table 2-1). Patients may present with cardiovascular disease and anemia. In these a history consistent with cardiovascular disease will also be present. Decreased exercise tolerance may be present with anemia or cardiovascular disease. An ECG, chest radiograph, and echocardiogram will help define the cardiovascular disease responsible for the pallor.

Hypoadrenocorticism is established on the basis of a complete blood count, urinalysis, serum electrolyte levels, and ACTH stimulation test (see Chapter 60).

Erythema

Generalized erythema is associated with fever or polycythemia. Core body temperature and hematocrit levels separate these causes. The approach to fever is discussed in detail in Chapter 6. The differential diagnosis includes infectious, autoimmmune, or neoplastic causes. Polycythemia is discussed in Chapter 74.

MANAGEMENT

Cyanosis

Animals with central cyanosis of cardiovascular origin (tetralogy of Fallot) are best handled by total surgical correction. This, however, is an impractical solution for the general practitioner. Medical management usually provides only temporary relief. Propanolol has been proven to be of some benefit to humans with tetralogy of Fallot. It reduces outflow tract obstruction, increases peripheral vascular resistance, increases the availability of oxygen to tissues, and improves myocardial oxygen consumption. Its value in the management of these cases in the dog is unknown. Phlebotomy should be used only to alleviate signs related to polycythemia. Oxygen therapy is of little help because much of the blood from the heart bypasses the lungs. The prognosis in most dogs with tetralogy of Fallot is poor. Right ventricular outflow obstruction tends to worsen with time. Death from thromboembolic disease, hypoxemia, and complications of polycythemia is common.

Management of patients with cyanosis of respiratory origin is directed to alleviation of the primary cause (edema, pneumonia, contusion, airway obstruction, and supplementation with oxygen).

Vomiting should be induced in animals presented with toxic methemoglobinemia if ingestion of the offending chemical occurred within the previous 4 hours. Emesis can be induced with apomorphine 0.04 mg/kg IV, 0.08 mg/kg IM, or subcutaneously (where available); syrup of ipecac 1 to 2 ml/kg orally; hydrogen peroxide 5 to 10 ml orally every 15 minutes until emesis occurs;

or xylazine in cats 0.44 mg/kg IM. Gastric lavage may be used to eliminate the absorption of any further drug. Gastric emptying is followed by the oral administration of activated charcoal (2 g/kg) to bind any drug remaining in the gastrointestinal tract. Supportive therapy includes intravenous fluid administration and oxygen. In some cases whole blood transfusion is required.

Methemoglobinemia due to acetaminophen toxicity is managed with acetylcysteine (140 mg/kg orally or IV of a 5% solution followed by 70 mg/kg every 4 hours for 3 to 5 treatments). Cats are deficient in glucuronyl transferase. As a result the rate of glucuronide conjugation and elimination of drugs is slow. Cats also have a limited ability to conjugate and eliminate phenolic compounds with sulfate. A large part of acetaminophen is metabolized to a glutathione conjugate. After hepatic stores of glutathione are exhausted the reactive metabolite is free to bind to cellular proteins. Methemoglobinemia and hepatic cell necrosis follows. Acetylcysteine increases the synthesis of glutathione in the liver and can also be oxidized in the liver to inorganic sulfate. Even though facial edema may occur, antihistamines should be avoided because they increase acetaminophen toxicity. If acetylcysteine is not available, sodium sulfate is an excellent alternative. It has been shown to be equally as effective as acetylcysteine. It is administered at a rate of 50 mg/kg (1.6% solution) every 4 hours for a total of 6 treatments.

Cimetidine (10 mg/kg orally initially, followed by 5 mg/kg every 6 hours for 48 hours) has also been proposed as an adjunct to acetylcysteine therapy. It promotes the generation and elimination of nontoxic metabolites. Methylene blue has also been used in the dog and cat for the treatment of toxic methemoglobinemia and NADH-MR deficiency syndromes (1 to 2 mg/kg of a 1% solution IV over a 5-minute period, repeated as indicated or given orally at 100 to 300 mg daily). Methylene blue reduces iron in the ferric form to the ferrous form capable of transporting oxygen. It is not effective for the treatment of abnormal hemoglobin structures (hemoglobin M) or sulfhemoglobinemia. Because it may induce Heinz-body anemia, animals should be screened for the presence of the condition prior to its use, and the blood should be monitored while the agent is in use. Ascorbic acid (30 mg/kg orally every 6 hours for a total of 7 treatments) is also of value in the reduction of methemoglobin. The reaction, however, is too slow to be of use in acute toxic methemoglobinemia and does not appear to be effective in the dog. It was believed to have been effective in a cat with benzocaine-induced methemoglobinemia (Wilkie, Additional Reading).

Animals with differential cyanosis (reverse PDA) rarely develop congestive heart failure. Medical therapy is therefore not warranted. Surgery is contraindicated because the ductus acts as an overflow valve permitting blood to flow from the pulmonary artery to the aorta. Ligation of the ductus would lead to massive overperfusion of the lungs and death. Those animals suffering from polycythemia and cyanosis may find some relief with periodic phlebotomy and concurrent fluid therapy in an effort to decrease the hematocrit and improve circulatory flow.

Animals with carbon monoxide poisoning are removed from the inciting cause and given oxygen therapy (preferably with 5% carbon dioxide).

Peripheral cyanosis is most commonly a reflection of thromboembolic disease. These cases are best managed by defining the primary cause of the thromboembolic event (cardiomyopathy, hyperadrenocorticism, bacterial endocarditis, glomerulonephropathy) and treating it appropriately. The thrombus is managed with rest and a platelet inhibitor (aspirin; see Chapter 24). Surgery is warranted only in cases of major organ impairment.

Pallor

The management of anemia is directed at its cause (see Chapter 73). Responsive and non-responsive cases of anemia often benefit from immunosuppressive doses of corticosteroids. In some cases whole blood transfusion is indicated (see Chapter 16).

Animals with cardiovascular disease causing pallor are managed with inotropic support and fluid volume replacement (Chapter 4).

Hypoadrenocorticism is managed with mineralocorticoid and sometimes glucocorticoid therapy (see Chapter 60).

Erythema

Management of cases of erythema is directed to the primary cause. Infectious causes of fever will benefit from antibiotic support. Immune-mediated causes may improve with the use of immunosuppressive agents, and those suffering from neoplasia improve with treatment of the cancer. Primary cases of polycythemia are treated with phlebotomy and concurrent fluid therapy (to decrease the hematocrit) and hydroxyurea (a myelosuppressive agent; see Chapter 74). Secondary cases of polycythemia are treated according to their etiology (hypoxemia or corticosteroid excess). Treatment of localized cases of erythema is based on analysis of skin scrapings and biopsy of the lesion.

PATIENT MONITORING

Specific guidelines are addressed in the respective chapters.

ADDITIONAL READING

Allen DG. Cyanosis, pallor and erythema In: Allen DG, Kruth SA, eds. Small animal cardiopulmonary medicine. Philadelphia: BC Decker, 1988: 35.

Atkins CE, Kaneko JJ, Congdon LL. Methemoglobin reductase deficiency and methemoglobinemia in a dog. Journal of the American Animal Hospital Association 1981; 17:829.

Harvey JW, Sameck JH, Burgard FJ. Benzocaine induced methemoglobinemia in dogs. J Am Vet Med Assoc 1979; 175:1171.

Hjelle JJ, Grauer GF. Acetaminophen induced toxicosis in dogs and cats. J Am Vet Med Assoc 1986; 188:742.

Krake AC, Arendt TD, Teachout DJ et al. Cetacaine induced methemoglobinemia in domestic cats. Journal of the American Animal Hospital Association 1985; 21:527.

Krotje LJ. Cyanosis: Physiology and pathogenesis. Compendium of Continuing Education 1987; 9:271.

Peterson ME, Randolph JF. Diagnosis of canine primary polycythemia and management with hydroxyurea. J Am Vet Med Assoc 1982; 180:415.

St. Omer VV, McKnight ED. Acetylcysteine for treatment of acetominophen toxicosis in the cat. J Am Vet Med Assoc. 1980; 176:911.

Wilkie DA, Kelly R. Methemoglobinemia associated with dermal application of benzocaine cream in a cat. J Am Vet Med Assoc 1988; 192:85.

3

JAUNDICE
Dana G. Allen

The accumulation of excessive levels of bilirubin in tissues or the bloodstream is termed *jaundice* or *icterus*. The degree of tissue staining is affected by the duration of the causative illness, the degree of bilirubinemia, and the type of bilirubin present. Conjugated bilirubin is water soluble and stains tissues more readily than unconjugated bilirubin, especially tissues high in elastic fiber content (skin and sclera). Jaundice becomes clinically obvious when serum bilirubin levels exceed 2 to 3 mg/dl (35–50 μmol/L). Bilirubinuria may precede hyperbilirubinemia in the dog. Significant bilirubinemia and yellow discoloration of plasma occurs before the staining of tissues becomes obvious. The best areas to visualize jaundice are the sclerae, pinnae, soft palate, mucous membranes, unpigmented skin, and areas of skin sparsely covered by hair.

CAUSES

Most cases of jaundice are hepatocellular in origin. In the cat the most common causes of jaundice are cholangitis or cholangiohepatitis, neoplasia, hepatic lipidosis, and feline infectious peritonitis. In the dog acute and chronic cholangiohepatitis, cirrhosis, chronic active hepatitis of Doberman pinschers, idiopathic chronic active hepatitis, and copper-associated hepatitis of Bedlington terriers represent the most common causes of intrahepatic cholestasis. Hyperadrenocorticism, diabetes mellitus, and starvation are less frequent causes. Hyperbilirubinemia and jaundice in the absence of hemolytic disease and histologic evidence of liver pathology has been documented in cats with hyperthyroidism (Meyer, Additional Reading). Fasting hyperbilirubinemia has not been documented in the cat. Neoplasia and pancreatitis causing compression of the bile duct or the porta hepatis are the most common causes of extrahepatic jaundice in the dog. Chronic pancreatitis and secondary bile duct obstruction is another important consideration in the dog. Causes of jaundice in dogs and cats are listed in Tables 3-1 and 3-2, respectively.

PATHOPHYSIOLOGY

The production, transport, and metabolism of bilirubin has been well described (Cornelius; Rogers and Cornelius; Pulley, Additional Reading). It is summarized here.

The production of bilirubin is primarily derived from the metabolism of hemoglobin from senescent red blood cells in the reticuloendothelial system (Fig. 3-1). Only 10% to 20%

Table 3–1 *Causes of Jaundice in Dogs*

Source	Causes
Prehepatic jaundice	Autoimmune hemolytic anemia
	Heinz-body anemia (onion ingestion)
	Hemolytic bacteremia
	Septicemia
	Transfusion reaction
	Heartworm
	Postcaval syndrome
Hepatic jaundice	Idiopathic hepatic necrosis
	Hepatic neoplasia
	Primary or metastatic cholangitis or cholangiohepatitis
	Chronic active hepatitis
	Hepatic fibrosis or cirrhosis
	Drugs or toxins (thiacetarsamide sodium, mebendazole, alflatoxins [moldy grain])
	Bacteremia
	Septicemia (usually gram-negative)
	Leptospirosis
	Hepatic copper accumulation (Bedlington terrier)
	Infectious canine hepatitis
Posthepatic jaundice	
Intrahepatic	Cholangitis or cholangiohepatitis
	Neoplasia
	Hepatic fibrosis or cirrhosis
Extrahepatic	Acute or chronic pancreatitis causing compression of bile duct
	Neoplasm compressing bile duct
	Traumatic rupture of bile duct or gallbladder
	Cholelithiasis

(Cornelius LM. Pathophysiological mechanisms of problems in internal medicine: Icterus. Proceedings of the American Animal Hospital Association 1982.)

Table 3–2 *Causes of Jaundice in Cats*

Source	Causes
Prehepatic jaundice	Infection with *Hemobartonella* organisms
	Babesiosis (rare)
	Cytauxzoonosis
	Heinz-body anemia
	Drugs (acetominophen, methylene blue)
	Bacteremia or septicemia
	Transfusion reaction
	Neonatal erythrocytolysis
Hepatic jaundice	Feline leukemia virus-associated diseases (lymphosarcoma, myeloproliferative disorders [including reticuloendotheliosis], immunosuppression and subsequent bacterial infection)
	Cholangitis or cholangiohepatitis
	Idiopathic hepatic lipidosis and lipidosis secondary to diabetes mellitus
	Feline infectious peritonitis
	Bacteremia or septicemia (usually gram-negative)
	Toxoplasmosis
	Histoplasmosis
	Drugs or toxins (acetominophen, methimazole)
	Neoplasia
Posthepatic jaundice	
Intrahepatic	Cholangitis or cholangiohepatitis
	Primary or metastatic neoplasia
Extrahepatic	Acute necrotizing pancreatitis
	Neoplasm compressing bile duct
	Traumatic rupture of bile duct or gallbladder
	Cholelithiasis (usually secondary to chronic colestasis and inspissation of bile associated with cholangiohepatitis)

(Modified from Cornelius LM. Pathophysiological mechanisms of problems in internal medicine: Icterus. Proceedings of the American Animal Hospital Association 1982.)

comes from the degradation of maturing red blood cells, myoglobin, and the hepatic hemoproteins cytochrome P-450, catalase, and peroxidase.

The hemoglobin molecule is split into globin and heme. The heme portion is further metabolized to free iron that can be stored in the reticuloendothelial system as ferritin or hemosiderin, or reused for the formation of hemoglobin. The remainder of the heme molecule is converted to biliverdin and then reduced to bilirubin. From the reticuloendothelial system bilirubin is transported to the liver, tightly bound to albumin. The large albumin–bilirubin complex prevents diffusion from the vascular space across cell membranes. The affinity of albumin for bilirubin is decreased by low serum albumin levels, competition for binding sites on the albumin molecule by drugs (*e.g.,* salicylates, thyroxine, heparin, digoxin, diazepam, hydrocortisone, sulfonamides) and by acidosis. In this form bilirubin is referred

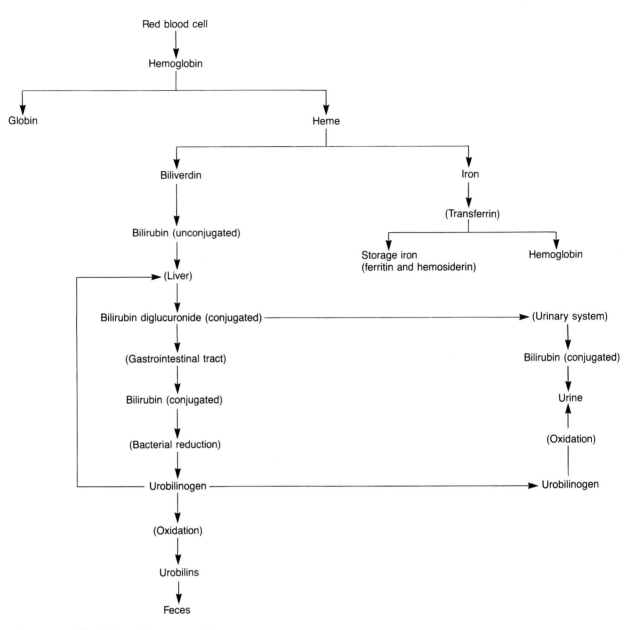

Figure 3–1. *Bilirubin formation and excretion.*

to as unconjugated, free, or indirect bilirubin. It is formed in the reticuloendothelial system, is water insoluble and fat soluble, is not filtered by renal glomeruli, and does not appear in the urine. Unconjugated bilirubin constitutes the principal form of bilirubin present in normal serum.

Prior to entry into the liver cell, albumin is separated from bilirubin. In the liver cell bil-

irubin combines with a Y or Z protein that traps it there. The bilirubin molecule is soon freed of this protein and becomes conjugated by glucuronyl transferase to form bilirubin diglucuronide. Conjugated bilirubin is water soluble, fat insoluble, filtered by renal glomeruli, and detected in the urine. In this form it can be excreted into the bile. In the dog, glucuronyl transferase is also found in the kidney and intestine. Conjugation of bilirubin occurs here to a lesser extent. Conjugated bilirubin is excreted in the bile complexed with phospholipids, cholesterol, and bile salts. The excretion of conjugated bilirubin into bile is the rate-limiting step in the course of its metabolism. Hepatic uptake and conjugation of bilirubin is less susceptible to dysfunction with hepatocellular injury than the excretory portion of metabolism. With hepatocellular injury regurgitation of conjugated bilirubin into plasma is common.

Bacterial enzymes in the ileum and large intestine reduce about half of the conjugated bilirubin to urobilinogen, most of which is excreted in the stool. Some of the urobilinogen is reabsorbed in the colon and transported back to the liver. Most of this is reexcreted into the bile (enterohepatic circulation). About 5% appears in the urine. Urobilinogens that remain in the intestine are oxidized to urobilins, which give the stool its characteristic color. The amount of urobilinogen that appears in the urine depends on the amount excreted into the intestine, the activity of the intestinal flora, and the intestinal transit time. An increase in urinary urobilinogen occurs with hemolysis, gastrointestinal hemorrhage, and constipation, which allows for increased urobilinogen formation and absorption. It may also increase with hepatocellular disease. In this case hepatic uptake and reexcretion into the bile is impaired. The absence of urobilinogen in urine may be associated with total biliary obstruction, dilution from polydipsia and polyuria, antibiotic inhibition of intestinal bacteria, diarrhea, or aciduria.

Increases in serum bilirubin may be associated with increased production of bilirubin, decreased hepatic uptake and conjugation, or decreased excretion into bile due to intrahepatic or extrahepatic cholestasis. Increases in unconjugated serum bilirubin are most often due to increased production subsequent to the increased destruction of red blood cells and the release of hemoglobin. If red blood cell destruction proceeds slowly, hepatic conjugation and excretion of bilirubin continues without significant elevations in serum bilirubin. Less frequent causes of jaundice appear in Tables 3-1 and 3-2. Increases in conjugated serum bilirubin most often reflect hepatic or biliary

tract disease. Various classification schemes in the approach to jaundice have been described (Pulley, Additional Reading). In this book, jaundice is classified as prehepatic, hepatic, and posthepatic.

CLINICAL SIGNS

Clinical signs associated with jaundice depend on the cause, duration of the illness, and etiology. It is difficult to differentiate intrahepatic from extrahepatic jaundice on the basis of clinical signs alone.

Prehepatic Jaundice

Prehepatic jaundice is most often associated with hemolytic anemia. The anemia must be acute and severe in onset to overwhelm the remarkable uptake and conjugating capacity of the liver. Animals may present with weakness, increased heart and respiratory rates, cardiac murmurs due to anemia, and dark brown stools. Urine with excessive amounts of hemoglobin appears red or port wine in color.

Hepatic Jaundice

Animals with hepatocellular jaundice may have general signs of liver disease, including ascites, diarrhea, vomiting, weight loss, change in liver size or conformation, bleeding tendencies, weakness, polydipsia, polyuria, or signs of hepatic encephalopathy (depression, stupor, seizure, blindness, coma).

Hepatomegaly is common in many of the disorders causing jaundice in the cat and dog. Microhepatia is uncommon in the cat. Melena, and hematochezia secondary to gastrointestinal ulceration and a tendency for bleeding may be noted. Urine with excessive amounts of bilirubin appears dark brown or orange. Ophthalmologic examination in cats may reveal changes consistent with lymphosarcoma, feline infectious peritonitis, or toxoplasmosis.

Posthepatic Jaundice

Cases of posthepatic jaundice are often caused by neoplasia or chronic pancreatitis causing compression of the bile duct. Dogs with pancreatic adenocarcinoma may not present with signs of severe pancreatic disease. More often they exhibit jaundice. Dogs with chronic pancreatitis have histories of intermittent vomiting and diarrhea. With complete biliary obstruction, steatorrhea and acholic or gray stools may be noted. Partial obstruction does not cause a change in stool color. Complete biliary obstruction also results in the decreased absorption of vitamin K. Clotting factors II, VII, IX, and X require vitamin K for their formation. A lack of vitamin K may be associated with bleeding tendencies. Parenteral administration of vitamin K_1 bypasses the biliary system and normalizes coagulation factor function within 24 to 48 hours. Other clinical signs are rare.

DIAGNOSTIC APPROACH

In this section the approach to jaundice is discussed on the basis of prehepatic, hepatic, and posthepatic causes. A minimum laboratory data base, including a complete blood count, packed-cell volume, serum biochemistry profile, serum T4 (older cats), urinalysis including urobilinogen levels, and visual inspection of stool color, should be completed on animals presenting with jaundice. The history, physical examination, and minimum laboratory data base should help delineate the three major areas of jaundice. Once the specific causative area is determined, an extended data base is completed (Table 3-3).

Prehepatic Jaundice

The most common cause of prehepatic jaundice is acute, severe hemolytic anemia. In dogs the anemia is often due to idiopathic autoimmune hemolytic anemia, and in cats to infection with *Hemobartonella* organisms. The anemia is further classified into regenerative anemia (significant increase in reticulocyte numbers, polychromasia,

Table 3–3 Diagnostic Approach to Animals with Jaundice

MINIMUM DATA BASE	Complete blood count
	Serum biochemistry profile
	Serum T4 (older cats)
	Urinalysis (including urobilinogen)
	Stool color
EXTENDED DATA BASE	
Prehepatic jaundice	Rapid slide agglutination or Coomb's test
	Check for red cell parasitism (cat)
	Check for Heinz bodies
	Blood culture
	Heartworm test (dog)
Hepatic jaundice	Plasma ammonia +/− ammonia tolerance test
	Serum bile acids
	Abdominal radiographs
	Abdominal ultrasound
	Coagulation screen
	Liver biopsy
	Culture of bile
	Feline leukemia virus test (cat)
	Feline infectious peritonitis titer (cat)
Posthepatic jaundice	Serum amylase and lipase
	Abdominal radiographs
	Abdominal ultrasound
	Abdominal paracentesis and lavage
	Laparotomy and biopsy

increased mean corpuscular volume, anisocytosis) or nonregenerative anemia (lack of an adequate response to the anemia) (see Chapter 73). If the anemia is acute, there may not have been sufficient time for an adequate response. A minimum of 4 days is required for the bone marrow to mount an adequate response to anemia. A concurrent leukocytosis is common in the dog with responsive anemias. It is less dramatic in the cat. Unresponsive anemias should be evaluated with bone marrow biopsy (see Bone Marrow Aspiration and Biopsy in Chapter 80). Poikilocytosis has been documented in dogs and cats with jaundice and portosystemic shunts. Microcytosis and a decreased mean corpuscular volume is documented in more than 65% of dogs with portosystemic shunts. An increase in white cell numbers may also accompany bacteremia or septicemia. In these cases blood cultures are indicated.

The serum biochemisty profile is generally unremarkable. Mild to moderate increases in alanine aminotransferase and aspartate aminotransferase may be seen secondary to tissue hypoxia associated with anemia and bilirubin overload. Van den Bergh's test measures serum levels of total and direct-acting (conjugated) bilirubin. Unconjugated bilirubin levels are calculated by subtracting the conjugated levels from the total levels. Unconjugated bilirubin levels increase with prehepatic jaundice and subsequent defective hepatic conjugation of bilirubin. Initially in hemolytic disease, hyperbilirubinemia is almost purely unconjugated bilirubin. After a day or two, levels of conjugated bilirubin also increase due to liver cell damage secondary to tissue hypoxia and overloading of the excretory capacity of the liver. At this point the levels of unconjugated and conjugated bilirubin are approximately equal. An increase in unconjugated bilirubin with a concurrent increase in excretion of urobilinogen (and conjugated bilirubin in the dog) is consistent with a hemolytic disorder. Van den Bergh's test actually has limited value in the diagnosis of jaundice (Zawie and Garvey, Additional Reading) for the following reasons: it is not required to make a diagnosis of hemolytic anemia; at low serum bilirubin concentrations the test is inaccurate; most liver diseases are a combination of intraheptic and extraheptic cholestasis; and as the disease progresses the quantity of conjugated and unconjugated bilirubin tends to equilibrate.

Hemoglobinuria is most often associated with intravascular hemolysis, although it can accompany extravascular hemolysis as well. Hemolysis does not initally result in bilirubinuria because unconjugated bilirubin is not filtered by renal glomeruli. With hemolysis the hemoglobin that is not bound to plasma haptoglobin is extracted by renal tubular epithelial cells, where it is converted to bilirubin, conjugated, and excreted in the urine. If the hemolytic event is acute and severe, the renal tubular cells may not be able to manage all the hemoglobin presented to them and hemoglobinuria will occur. Excessive amounts of hemoglobin impart a red or port wine color to urine. Stools may appear dark brown or orange. Stool color is affected by a number of factors and should not be considered a reliable test.

Hepatic Jaundice

Changes in the complete blood count are not specifically indicative of liver disease. In many cases the complete blood count is normal. In others a nonresponsive anemia of chronic or inflammatory disease may be present. Poikilocytosis has been documented in dogs and cats with jaundice and portosystemic shunts. The mean corpuscular volume is decreased in most dogs with with portosystemic shunts. Microcytosis may also be present in these patients. When present, leukocytosis may reflect inflammatory or infectious disease or stress.

The serum biochemistry profile is often helpful in the evaluation of jaundice. The enzymes of most use in small animal medicine are alanine aminotransferase (ALT), aspartate aminotransferase (AST), alkaline phosphatase (ALP), and τ-glutamyltransferase. Serum ALT is liver-specific in the dog and cat. It is confined to the cytoplasm of the hepatocyte. It readily leaks from the cytoplasm with minor cellular trauma. Serum ALT may remain elevated for up to 3 weeks following an acute bout of toxic hepatitis in the dog. It is thought that this continued elevation may represent a contribution of the enzyme to protein synthesis and the repair of liver damage. Serum ALT levels are highest in cats with cholangitis or cholangiohepatitis and lowest in those with feline infectious peritonitis.

Serum AST is also a leakage enzyme. It is found primarily in liver and muscle. In contrast to ALT, it is present in the cell cytoplasm and the mitochondria. Hepatocellular injury results in leakage of ALT and some AST. The magnitude of increase of serum ALT is generally greater than AST. Disruption of mitochondria results in further increases in AST. Consequently, significant increases in AST are suggestive of greater liver disease. The reported serum half life of ALT is 2 to 4 hours. The half life of AST is 5 hours in the dog and 77 minutes in the cat. Serum AST levels return to normal faster than ALT with repair of hepatic tissue.

Normal ALP activity is derived principally from the liver. Mild elevations in ALP activity from bone may be evident in puppies and kittens. Other sources, including the kidney, placenta, and intestine, are inconsequential. Increases in ALP follow intrahepatic and extrahepatic cholestasis. Cholestasis induces an increase in the production of the enzyme, and blocked bile canaliculi impair its excretion. Normal hepatic ALP concentration in the cat is one third that of dogs, and the serum half-life is 6 hours in the cat vs. 72 hours in the dog. Any increase in ALP activity is considered significant in the cat. Alkaline phosphatase levels are highest in cats with hepatic lipidosis and lowest in those with feline infectious peritonitis. Increases in serum τ-glutamyltransferase activity are also indicative of cholestatic disease in the dog and cat. Anticonvulsant drugs and corticosteroids increase serum ALT and ALP in dogs. A similar frequency of increase in ALP levels is not apparent in the cat.

Due to the large size and regenerative capabilites of the liver, more than half of the total functional mass must be impaired before changes in hepatic function tests become evident. Sulfobromophthalein sodium and indocyanine green excretion do not offer additional information in the jaundiced animal. Fasting blood ammonia levels can be measured in animals with suspect liver disease. If fasting ammonia levels are normal, an ammonium chloride tolerance test may yield more information. Conjugated serum bilirubin levels increase before unconjugated levels in hepatocellular and posthepatic biliary obstructive disease. In some cases of toxic or infectious hepatopathy, however, levels of unconjugated and conjugated bilirubin increase due to inadequate uptake, conjugation, and excretion of bilirubin.

Although both conjugated and unconjugated bilirubin levels are increased in hepatocellular disease, conjugated bilirubin predominates because hepatic excretion is affected to a greater degree than conjugating ability. However, in many animals, conjugated bilirubin spontaneously deconjugates in plasma over time, and equal levels of conjugated and unconjugated bilirubin are often found.

Serum bile acids are a useful assay in the assessment of liver pathology. Levels are highest in dogs with extrahepatic biliary obstruction, cirrhosis, and portosystemic vascular shunts.

Hypoalbuminemia is a late finding in chronic liver disease. Elevations in serum globulin concentration often accompany chronic liver disease.

Hyperglycemia may be found in animals with hepatic lipidosis secondary to diabetes mellitus. Hypoglycemia is rare.

The liver synthesizes most of the coagulation factors. Coagulation abnormalites may be present with liver disease; therefore, a coagulation screen should be completed prior to any invasive procedure, such as biopsy. Platelet function may also be adversely affected in jaundiced animals.

Conjugated bilirubin is filtered by renal glomeruli. Normal dogs have a low renal threshold for conjugated bilirubin. It may be present in normal urine in trace to 1+ amounts (specific gravity 1.040 or greater). A few bile crystals may also be present. Urine bilirubin levels of 2+ to 3+ suggests hyperbilirubinemia, and in the absence of red cell hemolysis, is indicative of hepatocellular or posthepatic jaundice. Bilirubin can also be formed in the renal tubules following reabsorption of filtered hemoglobin. Glucuronyl transferase present in renal tubules permits bilirubin conjugation. In contrast to the dog, cats do not normally excrete bilirubin in the urine; thus bilirubinuria is not a normal finding. Urinary bilirubin may be tested for with Ictotest reagent tablets (Ames). Normal urine forms a white foamy layer if shaken. Urine containing significant amounts of bilirubin turns the foamy layer yellow, yellow-green, or brown. False-positive color changes are noted in cases with excessive urobilinogen. Mild bilirubinuria may be associated with starvation or fever in dogs.

Posthepatic Jaundice

The complete blood count is most often normal in animals with posthepatic jaundice. Serum biochemistry is similar to that found in animals with hepatic jaundice and it cannot be relied on to differentiate the two. Dogs with chronic pancreatitis most often have significant elevations in

ALP, ALT, and total bilirubin. Serum amylase and lipase are often elevated, but may be normal.

Serum conjugated bilirubin is increased and excreted in the urine of patients with posthepatic obstruction. The presence of urobilinogen in the urine implies that the enterohepatic biliary system is patent. Hemolysis increases urobilinogen levels associated with the reexcretion of urobilinogen into the bile. Urobilinogen is absent with complete biliary obstruction. Even when present it may not be detected if there is a delay in the testing of the urine sample or if the sample is exposed to fluorescent lighting.

Vitamin K, a fat-soluble vitamin, is required for the activation of factors II, VII, IX, and X. Bleeding tendencies secondary to malabsorption of vitamin K may follow biliary obstruction. The coagulation screen will return to normal within 24 to 48 hours if these animals are treated with parenteral vitamin K_1.

Steatorrhea and acholic or gray stools may be present in animals with complete biliary obstruction. Stool color may be normal with partial biliary obstruction.

Other tests useful in the diagnosis of jaundice and liver disease include abdominal radiography (evaluation of liver size and conformation and the presence of abdominal fluid), abdominal ultrasonography (evaluation of the biliary system and liver parenchyma), hepatic biopsy (see Liver Biopsy in Chapter 80), and culture of bile. Transfusion of fresh whole blood or plasma is required prior to liver biopsy in those patients who do not respond to parenteral vitamin K_1. Additionally, feline leukemia virus testing and titers for feline infectious peritonitis and toxoplasmosis should be completed in the jaundiced cat. A retinal examination may reveal changes consistent with lymphosarcoma, feline infectious peritonitis, or toxoplasmosis.

MANAGEMENT

Once jaundice has been localized to a given area (prehepatic, hepatic, or posthepatic), efforts are made to determine the etiology. The primary goal of treatment is the elimination or management of that cause. Rest, the avoidance of stress, and adequate caloric and fluid supplementation constitute additional supportive measures. Patient care is often intense, time-comsuming, and costly.

Treatment of hemolytic anemia is discussed in detail in Chapter 73. Generally, immunosuppressive doses of corticosteroids (2–4 mg/kg/day of prednisone or prednisolone) with or without cyclophosphamide or azathioprine are required. To avoid sensitization of red blood cells and further hemolysis, whole blood transfusion is given only if clinical signs warrant it.

Intravenous fluid therapy is supplemented with glucose (10%) and potassium (20 mEq/L) where required. Supplemental potassium is not required if the animal is receiving its nutrition orally.

Initially, a diet high in fat should be Hill's Prescription Diet k/d. If fat restriction is required to maintain normal stools, Hill's Prescription Diet Canine i/d or Feline c/d may be used. Small amounts of the food are fed four to five times daily. For those patients with hepatic encephalopathy, diets should be high in carbohydrates and low in fat, with a restricted protein content of high biologic value. Cottage cheese is an excellent source of protein, and boiled white rice is high in carbohydrates. B complex and fat-soluble vitamins (A, D, E, and K) should be added to the diet. Lipotrophic agents containing choline or methionine have no place in the management of animals with liver disease. They have questionable efficacy and may potentiate hepatic encephalopathy (see Chapter 40).

Antibiotic therapy is indicated in animals with infectious causes of cholangitis, hepatitis, or cholangiohepatitis. Antibiotics that are concentrated in the bile include gentamicin, ampicillin, amoxicillin, and the cephalosporins. Antibiotics that should be avoided in hepatic patients include chlortetracycline, oxytetracycline, neomycin, streptomycin, and the sulfonamides. Chloramphenicol is a wide-spectrum anibiotic that is excreted in the bile. It may exacerbate anorexia. Metronidazole (Flagyl) is often used in combination with ampicillin or chloramphenicol (see Chapter 40).

Lactulose is indicated in animals with hepatic

encephalopathy. It is an osmotic cathartic agent. It also decreases the number of ammonia-producing bacteria.

Hydrochloretic agents such as dehydrocholic acid (Decholin) may improve biliary flow in animals with cholestasis. The recommended dose of this drug is 10 to 15 mg/kg orally three times daily for 7 to 10 days.

In addition, cimetidine, ranitidine hydrochloride, or sucralfate may be indicated in patients with gastrointestinal ulceration.

PATIENT MONITORING

Patient monitoring is tailored according to the specific cause. The prognosis depends on the cause of jaundice. Cats with cholangitis, hepatitis, or cholangiohepatitis have a fair to guarded prognosis for long-term survival. More than 77% of cats with hepatocellular jaundice in one retrospective study died or were euthanized (Cornelius, Additional Reading). In this study only those cats with cholangitis, hepatitis, or cholangiohepatitis had a potentially better prognosis (10 of 24 were discharged alive). Most icteric cats were young (mean age 3.8 years). Cats with cholangiohepatitis or hepatic lipidosis were older (5.1 years and 5.8 years, respectively). Almost half of all icteric cats were feline leukemia virus-positive. Those with hepatic lipidosis were not. In another study, 65% of cats with bilirubinuria died or were euthanized (Lees, Additional Reading). With the use of enteral tube feeding (see Nasoesophageal Intubation, Pharyngostomy Tube Placement, and Tube Gastrostomy Techniques in Chapter 80), the prognosis in cats with idiopathic hepatic lipidosis is good, and a greater than 50% survival rate can be expected.

ADDITIONAL READING

Center SA. Feline liver disorders and their management. Compendium of Continuing Education 1986; 8:889.

Center SA, Baldwin BH, Erb HN, Tennant BC. Bile acid concentrations in the diagnosis of hepatobiliary disease in the dog. J Am Vet Med Assoc 1985; 187:935.

Cornelius LM. Pathophysiological mechanisms of problems in internal medicine: Icterus. Proceedings of the American Animal Hospital Association 1982.

Cornelius LM, DeNovo RC. Icterus in cats. In: Kirk RW, ed. Current veterinary therapy VIII. Philadelphia: WB Saunders, 1983: 822.

Cribb AE, Burgener DC, Reimann KA. Bile duct obstruction secondary to chronic pancreatitis in seven dogs. Canadian Veterinary Journal 1988; 29:654.

Engelking LR. Disorders of bilirubin metabolism in small animal species. Compendium of Continuing Education 1988; 10:711.

Lees GE, Hardy RM, Stevens JB, Osborne CA. Clinical implications of feline bilirubinuria. Journal of the American Animal Hospital Association 1984; 20:765.

Meyer DJ, Center SA. Approach to the diagnosis of liver disorders in dogs and cats. Compendium of Continuing Education 1986; 8:880.

Osborne CA, Stevens JB, Lees GE, Barlough JE et al. Clinical significance of bilirubinuria. Compendium of Continuing Education 1980; 2:897.

Pulley LT. Jaundice. In: Ettinger SJ, ed. Textbook of veterinary medicine. Philadelphia: WB Saunders, 1983: 110.

Rogers KS, Cornelius LM. Feline icterus. Compendium of Continuing Education 1985; 7:391.

Zawie DA, Garvey MS. Feline hepatic disease. Vet Clin North Am 1984; 14:1201.

4

SHOCK
Dana G. Allen

Any condition that leads to a significant decrease in tissue perfusion, cellular hypoxia, metabolic acidosis, and cellular dysfunction may result in shock. Shock leads to multiple organ system failure and death if not recognized and treated early. Shock is classified as cardiogenic, hypovolemic, and vasculogenic (including septic and neurogenic) depending on the principal location of activity within the cardiovascular system. The pathophysiologic effect is the same in each.

CAUSES

Any condition that predisposes to a decrease in tissue perfusion may lead to cellular hypoxia and cell death (Table 4-1). Cardiogenic shock is characterized by a fall in cardiac output secondary to impaired systolic ejection of blood (arrhythmias, ruptured chordae tendinae cordis, aortic or pulmonic stenosis, primary cardiomyopathy, toxic cardiomyopathy, acute peripheral vasoconstriction) or secondary to impaired cardiac filling in diastole (cardiac tamponade, tension pneumothorax, positive pressure ventilation).

Hypovolemic shock is likely the most commonly encountered form of shock in veterinary medicine. It is caused by acute and severe losses of blood, plasma, or water and electrolytes, leading to a decrease in venous return, central venous pressure, and cardiac output. The normal blood volume in the dog is 90 ml/kg, and in the cat is 55 ml/kg. A loss of 30% in circulating blood volume will cause shock. Losses of 30% to 40% of circulating blood volume can be compensated for by peripheral vasoconstriction and fluid replacement with little or no mortality. Only half of the patients suffering losses of 40% or more survive without intense medical intervention. A loss of more than half of the circulating blood volume is almost always fatal.

Vasculogenic shock occurs with acute vasodilation and hypotension secondary to sepsis, central nervous system vasomotor paralysis, anaphylaxis, spinal shock, or high epidural local anesthesia. Circulating bacteria or endotoxins cause the hemodynamic changes seen in septic shock. Endotoxins are released principally from gram-negative bacterial cell walls upon the death of the organism or during the acute growth phase of replication. Gram-negative bacteria are the most common cause of endotoxic shock. Grampositve bacteria, yeast, fungi, and viruses are less common causes. Septic shock may also occur secondary to delayed or inadequate treatment of hypovolemic shock.

Table 4–1 *Causes of Shock*

CARDIOGENIC SHOCK

Systolic dysfunction (impaired left ventricular ejection)
  Cardiac rate or rhythm abnormalities
  Ruptured chorda tendineae cordis
  Primary cardiomyopathy
  Toxic cardiomyopathy (anesthetic overdose, endotoxemia)
  Cor pulmonale
  Aortic or pulmonic stenosis
  Acute vasoconstriction (methoxamine, epinephrine)
Diastolic dysfunction (impaired cardiac filling)
  Cardiac tamponade
  Tension pneumothorax
  Positive pressure ventilation
  Gastric dilation or volvulus (compressing caudal vena cava)

HYPOVOLEMIC SHOCK

Blood loss
  Hemorrhage from trauma
  Coagulopathies (platelet, factor, or vascular abnormalities)
  Coumarin, indanedione toxicity
Plasma loss
  Severe burns
  Effussive or exudative lesions (pyothorax, peritonitis)
Water and electrolyte loss
  Severe vomiting and diarrhea
  Intestinal obstruction
  Heat stroke
  Marked diuresis

VASCULOGENIC SHOCK

Endotoxic shock
  Infection with *Escherichia coli*
  Infection with *Klebsiella*
  Infection with *Proteus* organisms
  Infection with Pseudomonas
  Infection with *Enterbacter* organisms
  Infection with Bacteroides sp.
Neurogenic shock
  Spinal shock (acute cervical cord lesions)
  Sympathetic blockade (local anesthetic)
  Vasomotor paralysis (central nervous system trauma, deep
    anesthesia [halothane, methoxyflurane])
  Drug-induced vasodilation (phenothiazines, vasodilatory
    agents)
Other causes of shock
  Hypoadrenocorticism
  Massive histamine release (mast cell tumor)
  Anaphylaxis

PATHOPHYSIOLOGY

Although the precipitating causes of shock may vary, the pathophysiologic events that may terminate in the death of the animal are the same (Fig. 4-1). The precipitating cause leads to a fall in cardiac output and arterial blood pressure. The body responds through stimulation of the sympathoadrenal system. This results in an increase in heart rate and cardiac contractility, decreased peripheral resistance, splenic contraction, glycogenolysis, and the renal conservation of sodium and water, the purpose of which is to maintain blood pressure and blood flow to vital organs (heart, brain, lung). This is the hyperdynamic or hyperkinetic phase of shock. Cardiac output is normal or increased, and the animal is able to maintain normal blood pressure. Splenic contraction can replace up to 20% of a dog's circulating blood volume.

Hyperglycemia may be present initially. Glucose serves as a substrate for cellular metabolism, increases plasma osmolality, helps maintain blood pressure, prevents fluid extravasation, and helps increase extravascular fluid resorption. As shock progresses, glucose stores are depleted and hypoglycemia occurs. Hypoglycemia is a grave sign.

The kidney conserves salt and water through the actions of renin–angiotensin, aldosterone, and antidiuretic hormone. The result is a decrease in urinary output.

The hyperdynamic phase may resolve with treatment. If compensatory efforts do not improve peripheral perfusion, the animal may progress to the hypodynamic or hypokinetic phase and irreversible shock (see Fig. 4-1). This is characterized by a fall in cardiac output, hypotension, increased systemic arterial resistance, a decrease in central venous pressure, and hypothermia. It generally follows the hyperdynamic phase, but may occur independently.

Vasoconstriction at the level of the arteriole and precapillary sphincter in conjunction with arteriovenous shunting leads to tissue ischemia, anaerobic glycolysis, the accumulation of lactic acid and hydrogen ions, and the depletion of intracellular adenosine triphosphate. At the point that capillary pH becomes acidotic, shock is said to be irreversible. Cellular dysfunction and death result in the release of lysozymes, adenosine diphosphate, serotonin, prostaglandins, myocardial depressant factor, reticuloendothelial depressant factor, and tissue thromboplastin (see Fig. 4-1). This results in increased capillary permeability, cardiovascular depression, decreased

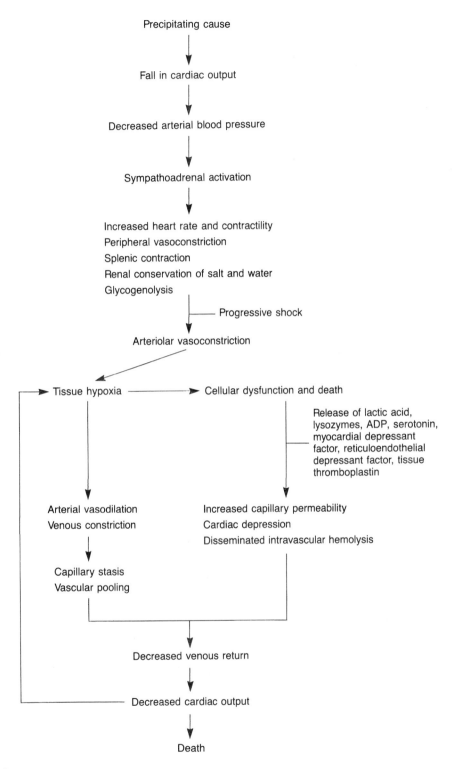

Figure 4–1. *Pathophysiology of shock.*

venous return, and a perpetuation of the shock state. Endotoxins activate the complement, kinin, and fibrinolytic systems, causing increased capillary permeability and a decrease in venous return. Tissue hypoxia leads to arterial vasodilation, venous constriction, capillary stasis, and decreased venous return and cardiac output. Cardiac function can be maintained only if venous return is adequate.

Vascular stasis, endothelial damage, severe acidosis, release of tissue thromboplastin, platelet injury, and the release of catecholamines predispose to an increased tendency for coagulation abnormalities and disseminated intravascular coagulation. Death in all shock states is due to cardiac failure from decreased coronary perfu-sion, myocardial hypoxia, acidosis, and the accumulation of myocardial depressant factor. Myocardial depressant factor has a potent negative inotropic effect; it intensifies vasoconstriction of splanchnic vessels and depresses phagocytosis by the reticuloendothelial system.

Prostaglandins (PG) play an important role in shock. Tissue hypoxia and cellular membrane injury lead to the activation of phospholipase A_2 and the release of arachidonic acid (Fig. 4-2). Arachidonic acid is metabolized by cyclooxygenase and lipoxygenase to the cyclic endoperoxides and the hydroperoxides, respectively. Hydroperoxides are converted to the leukotrienes and hydroperoxyarachidonic acid. Cyclic endoperoxides are converted to prostacyclin, thromboxane,

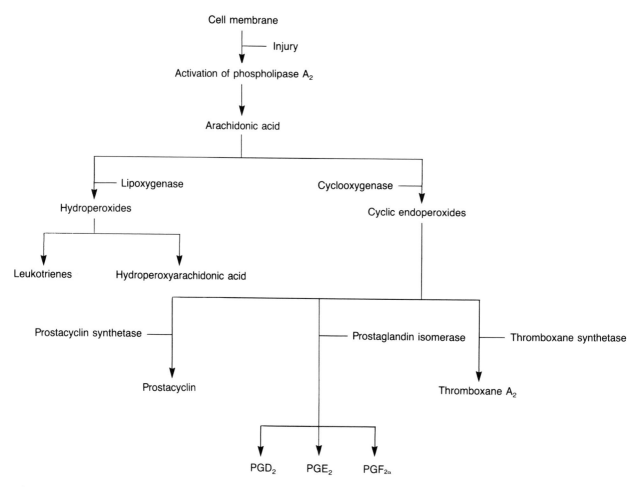

Figure 4–2. Arachidonic acid pathway.

PGE$_2$, PGD$_2$, and PGF$_2$. Prostacyclin induces smooth muscle relaxation and inhibits platelet aggregation. Thromboxane causes smooth muscle contraction and platelet aggregation. Normally, arachidonic acid metabolism favors the production of prostacyclin. In shock the pathway is shifted in favor of thromboxane production. Thromboxane levels are highest early in shock. Endotoxins directly injure vascular endothelium, expose collagen, and increase the production of thromboxane. Platelet adhesion, aggregation, and vasoconstriction lead to ischemia and disseminated intravascular coagulation. High levels of thromboxane and PGF$_2$ are associated with pulmonary hypertension, respiratory failure, a fall in cardiac output, and hypotension. High levels of prostacyclin and PGE$_2$ are associated with terminal hypotension.

Reticuloendothelial system function is impaired by histamine, serotonin, bradykinin, reticuloendothelial depressant factor, and hypoxia. Fibronectin, a plasma-opsonizing agent important for normal phagocytic function, is markedly depleted in shock.

CLINICAL SIGNS

It is important to recognize the clinical signs of shock so that immediate therapy can be instituted (Table 4-2). Although the causes of shock differ, the end result in all forms is a fall in the circulating blood volume. Tachycardia, decreased pulse amplitude, increased capillary refill time, pale mucous membranes, rapid respiratory rate, hypothermia, weakness, and depression are the hallmarks of shock. Decreased urinary output, pupillary dilation, and coma may also be noted. Vasculogenic (septic) shock initially differs from other forms of shock. In the early stages of septic shock, mucous membranes are hyperemic, cardiac output is normal or increased, capillary refill time is decreased, and the animal may be hyperthermic. It may resolve with treatment or progress to the hypodynamic phase.

Poor peripheral perfusion leads to multiple organ failure. Blood flow is maintained to the brain, heart, and kidney as long as arterial blood pressure remains above 50, 60, and 70 mmHg, respec-

Table 4–2 *Clinical Signs of Shock*

ALL FORMS OF SHOCK

Tachycardia
Poor peripheral pulse
Increased capillary refill time
Pale mucous membranes
Rapid respiratory rate
Hypothermia
Decreased urinary output
Weakness
Depression
Pupillary dilation
Coma

SEPTIC SHOCK

Hyperdynamic phase
  Tachycardia
  Brick red mucous membranes
  Rapid respiratory rate
  Decreased capillary refill time
  Fever
Hypodynamic phase
  Tachycardia or bradycardia
  Pale mucous membranes
  Rapid respiratory rate
  Increased capillary refill time
  Hypothermia

tively. Peripheral pulse is palpable at arterial pressures of 70 mmHg and above.

Hemorrhagic gastroenteritis is one of the earliest recognized clinical syndromes of irreversible shock in the dog. Vascular stasis, ischemia, platelet aggregation, the release of vasoactive agents, and endotoxic injury lead to villous hypoxia, necrosis, mucosal sloughing, and hemorrhage. Gastric hydrochloric acid and pancreatic proteases contribute to the disease process.

Acute renal failure is uncommon in dogs with shock. It is more common in older animals with preexisting renal disease, in animals with crush injuries and significant myoglobinuria and hemoglobinuria, or in animals with a combination of hypovolemic and septic shock. Persistent oliguria, glucosuria, and a decrease in urine specific gravity is indicative of tubular injury.

Respiratory distress syndrome, shock lung, or pulmonary insufficiency may occur 24 to 72 hours following the resuscitation of a shock patient. It is uncommon in the dog. Clinically, it is characterized by hyperventilation, adventitial lung sounds, and respiratory alkalosis that is unresponsive to oxygen therapy. An albumin-rich alveolar extravasate caused by microvascular injury secondary to complement activation and neutrophil migration, degranulation, and the release of lysozymes is evident histologically. Overhydration, embolization, sepsis, and oxygen therapy may contribute to the disease process. Animals that clear bacteria in the lungs are predisposed to respiratory distress syndrome. The dog clears bacteria primarily in the liver and spleen and is not very susceptible to the development of respiratory distress syndrome.

Liver dysfunction is common in dogs in septic shock from hypoxia owing to the inability to utilize gluconeogenetic substrates for glucose production and vascular pooling of blood in the mesenteric, gastrointestinal, splenic, and hepatic circulation. Cholestasis and jaundice may be seen with endotoxemia.

Endotoxemia, hypotension, increased levels of tissue thromboplastin, capillary stasis, platelet aggregation, and metabolic acidosis predispose to disseminated intravascular coagulation. Disseminated intravascular coagulation should be suspect in animals with severe, protracted bleeding (see Chapter 16).

DIAGNOSTIC APPROACH

The diagnosis is based on the history and clinical signs. The minimum data base in animals presented in shock includes a packed-cell volume; white cell count; total protein; serum urea, glucose, sodium, chloride, and potassium; and urine specific gravity (Table 4-3). Hemoconcentration is common. Splenic contraction and fluid extravasation from the vascular space leads to an increase in the packed-cell volume. Neutropenic leukopenia is common in early septic shock. Neutrophilic leukocytosis occurs subsequently and is common in all phases of hypovolemic shock.

Prerenal azotemia (increased serum urea in the face of adequate urine concentrating ability) is common. If peripheral perfusion is not restored within 12 to 24 hours, acute renal failure may occur. Hypoglycemia and hypokalemia may occur with shock. Hypoglycemia is a grave prognostic sign. Hypoalbuminemia may be noted in pa-

Table 4–3 *Diagnostic Approach to Animals in Shock*

Minimum data base	Packed cell volume
	White cell count
	Total plasma protein
	Serum urea, glucose, sodium,
	chloride, potassium
	Urine specific gravity
Extended data base	Complete blood count
	Serum biochemistry panel
	Complete urinalysis
	Central venous pressure
	Blood gas and acid-base analysis
	Chest radiographs
	Electrocardiogram
	Coagulation screen (prothrombin
	time, partial thromboplastin time,
	fibrin degradation product, clot
	retraction, platelet numbers)
Where indicated	Blood cultures
	Abdominal or cervical radiographs
	Echocardiogram

tients with severe burns, chronic hemorrhage, or effusive lesions.

Oliguria, isosthenuria, glucosuria, progressive increases in serum urea concentration, and the presence of renal tubular cells in the urine sediment are indicative of a deterioration in renal function. Normal urine output in a normally hydrated dog is 1 to 2 ml/kg/hour. Values less than 1 ml/kg/hour may be consistent with renal dysfunction.

The extended data base helps define the cause of shock and is useful for monitoring the progression of the disease and its treatment. It includes a complete blood count, full serum biochemistry panel, complete urinalysis, central venous pressure measurement, arterial blood gas and acid-base analysis, chest radiographs, an electrocardiogram, a coagulation screen, and, where indicated, blood cultures, abdominal or cervical radiographs, and an echocardiogram.

The liver enzymes alanine aminotransferase, aspartate aminotransferase, and alkaline phosphatase are usually increased. Central venous pressure is elevated in cardiogenic shock due to pericardial effusion, pneumothorax, and positive pressure ventilation (see Central Venous Pressure in Chapter 80). Central venous pressure is often decreased in severe hypovolemic or vasculogenic shock. Blood gas analysis frequently indicates metabolic acidosis. In the advanced stages of respiratory distress syndrome, hypoxemia and hypercapnea that is unresponsive to oxygen therapy is present. The measurement of blood gas better defines the patient's metabolic requirements. Chest radiographs may be indicative of pneumothorax, pericadial effusion, or primary cardiac disease. Arrhythmias may be diagnosed and monitored following therapy. Prolonged prothrombin time, partial thromboplastin time, clot retraction time, thrombocytopenia, and increased levels of fibrin degradation products are characteristic of disseminated intravascular coagulation.

Endotoxemia has been diagnosed in the dog from the measurement of circulating plasma endotoxin lipopolysaccharide concentration (Wessels, Additional Reading).

MANAGEMENT

Recognition of the clinical signs of shock, elimination of the cause, ventilatory support, and restoration of the circulating blood volume remain the cornerstones of shock therapy (Fig. 4-3). An indwelling intravenous catheter is placed in the jugular vein to the level of the right atrium for the administration of fluids and the monitoring of central venous pressure during fluid replacement. In the event that a venous access cannot be secured, fluids and drugs can be administered into the medullary cavity of the femur, tibia, or iliac crest (Otto, Additional Reading). A urinary catheter attached to a closed collection system is used to monitor urinary output.

Patients should be warmed slowly to prevent peripheral vasodilation and hypotension. Intravenous fluids are warmed (37°C) prior to infusion, and animals are covered with blankets. Oxygen therapy is indicated in patients with respiratory distress or hypoxemia. Oxygen therapy decreases anaerobic tissue metabolism, increases tissue viability, and increases the response to endogenous catecholamines.

Crystalloids, including lactated Ringer's injection, normal saline, Plasma-lyte 148, or Normosol R, are administered at a rate of 20 to 90 ml/kg

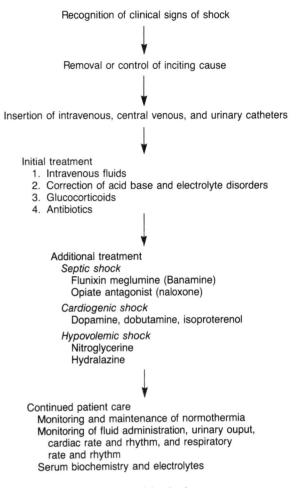

Figure 4-3. *Treatment protocol for shock.*

(dog) and 10 to 60 ml/kg (cat) over the first 15 to 30 minutes (Table 4-4). The requirements for each case vary. At higher flow rates, monitoring central venous pressure, body weight, total protein, packed-cell volume, and lung sounds becomes more critical if fluid overload is to be avoided. Central venous pressure measurements greater than 10 cm H_2O are associated with increased circulating blood volume or heart failure. The gain or loss of 1 kg of body weight is equivalent to the gain or loss of 1 L of fluid. Fluid overload can lead to pulmonary edema, hemodilution, and decreased tissue oxygen delivery. Intravenous fluid maintenance rates of 80 ml/kg/day are recommended. Flow rates may be decreased as homeostasis is approached (1–3 days). The success of

Table 4-4 *Drugs, Routes of Administration, and Dosage in the Management of Shock*

FLUID THERAPY

Ringer's injection, Normosol R, normal saline, Plasma-lyte 148 injection—dog (20 to 90 ml/kg over the first 15 to 30 minutes), cat (10 to 60 ml/kg over the first 15 to 30 minutes), recommended maintenance rates = 80 ml/kg/day (Normosol M, 2.5% dextrose in 0.45% saline, Plasma-lyte 56 with 5% dextrose)

Sodium bicarbonate (1 to 2 mEq/L slowly IV and add 1 to 4 mEq/L sodium bicarbonate/L of fluids)

Potassium (40 mEq/L) and glucose (50 ml of 50% dextrose/L of fluids)

GLUCOCORTICOIDS

Methylprednisolone sodium succinate [Solu-Medrol] (30 mg/kg IV)
Dexamethasone sodium phosphate [Decadron phosphate] (3 mg/kg IV)
Dexamethasone [Decadron] (5 mg/kg IV)
Hydrocortisone sodium succinate [Solu-Cortef] (8 to 20 mg/kg IV)
Prednisolone sodium succinate [Solu-Delta-Cortef] (10 to 30 mg/kg IV)

FLUNIXIN MEGLUMINE [BANAMINE]

1 to 2 mg/kg IV twice only at 3- or 12-hour intervals; none in the cat

ANTIBIOTICS

Gentamicin sulfate (2 mg/kg IM t.i.d.)
Trimethoprim-sulfadiazine (initially 120 mg/kg IV, then 60 mg/kg IV b.i.d.); none in the cat
Ampicillin (10 mg/kg IV, IM q.i.d.)

OTHER AGENTS

Dobutamine (5 to 20 μg/kg/min IV)
Dopamine hydrochloride (5 to 10 μg/kg/min IV)
Furosemide—dog (2 to 4 mg/kg IV, IM), cat (2 mg/kg IV, IM)
Heparin sodium (mini dose = 10 units/kg t.i.d.–q.i.d. subcutaneously; low dose = 150 to 250 units/kg t.i.d. subcutaneously)
Hydralazine hydrochloride (0.25 mg/kg IV; repeat every 4 to 6 hours as required)
Isoproterenol hydrochloride (0.1 to 0.2 mg/kg IM; q.i.d.)
Mannitol (20% solution: dilute with an equal volume of saline and give it IV at 1 to 2 g/kg q.i.d.)
Morphine sulfate—dog (1 mg/kg IM), cat (0.1 mg/kg IM)
Naloxone hydrochloride (2 to 2.5 mg/kg/hour IV)
Nitroglycerine ointment (4 to 8 mg; repeat every 4 hours as required)

---

fluid replacement can be judged by an increase in the amplitude of the peripheral pulse, decreased capillary refill time, pink and moist mucous membranes, warming of the skin and extremities, and an improvement in mental status. If diuresis in not initiated with fluid replacement, furosemide (2–4 mg/kg) is given intravenously and repeated in 15 to 30 minutes if diuresis does not occur. If furosemide fails, mannitol or liquid glucose may be effective. Mannitol increases renal blood flow, decreases renal cellular edema, and initiates diuresis. If these measures are unsuccessful, dopamine hydrochloride is administered (see Table 4-4).

Lactate in lactated Ringer's injection requires hepatic metabolism before effective buffering action occurs. Following rapid rehydration, sodium bicarbonate is administered slowly at a rate of 1 to 2 mEq/kg in a single intravenous injection. In addition, 1 to 4 mEq/kg sodium bicarbonate is added to each liter of fluids. Cats appear to be more sensitive to intravenous bicarbonate and should be monitored for central nervous system signs. During the maintenance phase of therapy, the addition of 50 ml/L of 50% dextrose and 40 mEq/L of potassium chloride is recommended to decrease peripheral resistance, improve myocardial oxygen availability and contractility, improve peripheral blood flow, and counteract hypoglycemia. Hypotonic solutions (5% dextrose in Water and 0.45% saline) should be avoided because less of these solutions remains within the vascular space and they do not expand the circulating blood volume as effectively.

It has been shown that a relatively small volume of extremely hypertonic saline solution (2400 mOsm/L or 7.2% sodium chloride at 4–5 ml/kg, administered slowly IV) may be sufficient to reverse the pathophysiologic effects of severe hemorrhagic shock in dogs (Fettman, Additional Reading). Compared with isotonic saline infusion, hypertonic saline solution reduced heart rate, decreased peripheral vascular resistance, and increased cardiac contractility, cardiac output, arterial blood pressure, and peripheral blood flow.

Colloids osmotically expand the circulating blood volume more effectively than crystalloid solutions. Dextran 40, dextran 70, plasma protein and gelatins are examples of colloids. However, these agents are expensive and have a tendency to induce an antigenic response that may result in anaphlyaxis.

Some patients require emergency surgery and general anesthesia. The precipitating cause should be controlled and the patient should be stabilized with the rapid infusion of intravenous fluids as previously described. The minimum data base as well as an electrocardiogram and arterial blood gas analysis should be obtained, and measures made to correct any abnormalities prior to anesthetic induction. The hematocrit should be 25% (0.25 L/L) or higher. Animals with an arterial Po_2 less than 65 mmHg or a Pco_2 greater than 50 mmHg are generally considered poor anesthetic risks. Preoxygenation with face mask oxygen is recommended in all animals with cardiopulmonary comprimise. Premedication with diazepam (0.2 mg/kg IV) or acepromazine (0.03 mg/kg IM) is indicated in animals with ventricular arrhythmias. Agents considered safe in animals with compromised cardiovascular function are listed in Table 4-5. These drugs must be used with caution. Although premedication with acepromazine is useful in animals with ventricular arrhythmias, it may potentiate hypotension and should be avoided in animals with overt heart failure (see Chapter 26). Other agents with potentially adverse cardiovascular effects that should be used with caution in shock patients include atropine (heart block, premature ventricular contractions), halothane (hypotension, arrhythmias—especially in conjunction with epinephrine and the thiobarbiturates), thiamylal sodium (premature ventricular contractions), and xylazine (bradycardia, heart block, decreases in myocardial contractility, sensitization of the heart to epinephrine in the face of halothane leading to arrhythmias).

If the packed-cell volume falls lower than 20% (0.20 L/L) in the dog or 12% to 15% (0.12–0.15 L/L) in the cat and shock is clinically apparent,

Table 4–5 *Anesthetic Agents of Choice in the Shock Patient*

Agent	Dosage and Route of Administration
Acepromazine	0.03 mg/kg IM or 0.01 to 0.03 mg/kg IV
Diazepam	0.2 mg/kg IV
Fentanyl droperidol (Innovar) without atropine	0.05 ml to 0.1 ml/kg IM (dog)
Isoflurane	1% to 1.5% in fresh gas flow of 50 to 130 ml/kg/min
Ketamine hydrochloride (with diazepam)	100 mg/ml ketamine and 5 mg/ml diazepam mixed 1 : 1 and given at 0.1 to 0.15 ml/kg IV
Morphine sulfate	0.5 mg/kg IM
Nitrous oxide	66% (oxygen flow 30 ml/kg/min) Do not use if pneumothorax or gastric dilation or volvulus is likely to be present
Oxymorphone	0.05 to 0.2 mg/kg IM or IV (dog—with diazepam if it is used for induction) Not to exceed 4.5 mg

(Allen DG. Anesthesia and the cardiopulmonary patient. In: Allen DG, Kruth SA, eds. Small animal cardiopulmonary medicine. Philadelphia: BC Decker, 1988: 135.)

infusion of whole blood is indicated. Whole blood is administered simultaneously with isotonic crystalloids to prevent microvascular sludging and to limit the negative inotropic effects that accompany transfusions (see Chapter 16). Solutions containing calcium, such as lactated Ringer's injection, should not be administered with a single intravenous tube with a "Y" connector because of the possibility of initiating clotting within the tube. The volume of blood required can be calculated from the formula:

$$\text{Volume of blood required (in anticoagulant)} = \\ \text{recipient weight (kg)} \times 90 \text{ (dog) or } 70 \text{ (cat)} \times \\ \frac{\text{desired PCV} - \text{recipient PCV}}{\text{PCV of donor}}$$

Plasma therapy is indicated in animals with significant hypoalbuminemia (less than 3.5 g/dl or 35 g/L). Hypoproteinemic animals may develop pulmonary edema during fluid therapy. In these cases plasma therapy may be combined with the administration of crystalloids. The plasma increases oncotic pressure and reduces the volume of crystalloid required. Plasma also serves as a source for amino acids and energy. The disadvantages of plasma therapy include induction of allergic reactions and interference with clotting. Plasma is administered at a dose of 10 to 20 ml/kg IV.

The use of glucocorticoids in shock is controversial. They appear to be beneficial in septic and cardiogenic shock if used within 1 to 2 hours following the onset of shock. Their use in hypovolemic shock is equivocal, and they do not appear to be of benefit in neurogenic shock. The beneficial effects of glucocorticoids include preservation of vascular and lysozymal membranes, decreased activation of the complement and clotting cascades, decreased platelet and neutrophil aggregation, binding of endotoxins, positive inotropic effect, dilation of precapillary sphincters, decreased release of arachidonic acid, prevention of gastrointestinal mucosal ischemia, increased gluconeogenesis, increased metabolism of lactic acid, decreased central nervous system edema, and a decrease in the release of antidiuretic hormone. Respiratory distress syndrome may be prevented if glucocorticoids are given before pulmonary damage occurs. Glucocorticoids are not useful once pulmonary edema has occurred. Their use has been associated with an increased incidence of gastrointestinal hemorrhage, ulceration, and impaired immune function. Glucocorticoids cause vasodilation and should be given only following adequate fluid replacement. Hydrocortisone sodium succinate (Solu-Cortef) and prednisolone sodium succinate have a rapid onset of action (4 minutes) and can be repeated every 3 to 4 hours until clinical signs of shock abate. Dexamethasone sodium phosphate (Decadron Phosphate) has a slower onset of action (up to 3 hours). Survival rates were dramatically improved with the use of prednisolone sodium succinate as opposed to dexamethasone sodium phosphate in dogs subjected to septic shock (White, Additional Reading).

Antibiotics are indicated in all forms of shock (see Table 4-4). Only bactericidal antibiotics have been shown to be useful in cases of septic shock. They should be given in conjunction with glucocorticoids because of the rapid bacterial death and massive release of endotoxin that accompany antibiotic use. The first drug of choice is gentamicin and the second drug of choice is trimethoprim sulfadiazine. Ampicillin is commonly added to this regimen to kill anaerobic bacteria. The combination of antibiotics and glucocorticoids increases survival times.

Several agents have been shown to increase survival rates in animals subjected to endotoxic shock. Flunixin meglumine (Banamine) blocks cyclooxygenase, the formation of thromboxane and prostacyclin, and the release of PGI_2 in endotoxic shock. It increases cardiac output and blood pressure, delays the onset of hypoglycemia, decreases hemoconcentration and metabolic acidosis, and improves tissue aerobic metabolism. Aspirin has also been shown to increase survival rates in endotoxic dogs and might be a suitable alternative to flunixin in the cat. Survival times have been shown to increase and mortality rates to decrease in animals with endotoxic shock when they are given the opiate antagonist naloxone. Naloxone increases cardiac output and arterial blood pressure, decreases hemoconcentration and metabolic acidosis, and helps prevent hypoglycemia. The drug is very expensive. A polyvalent equine antilipopolysaccharide hyperimmune serum, Atoxin (Atox Pharmaceutical Co.), is available for dogs with endotoxemia. It contains specific immunoglobulins that bind to circulating lipopolysaccharide, opsonize it, and destroy gram-negative bacteria. Wessels and associates (Additional Reading) claim the drug reduces endotoxemia and death associated with hemorrhagic enteritis.

Other forms of therapy recommended in the treatment of cardiogenic shock include morphine sulfate and catecholamine agents. Morphine sulfate decreases anxiety and respiratory rates and improves peripheral blood flow. Catecholamines, including dopamine hydrochloride, dobutamine, and isoproterenol hydrochloride, are indicated in patients who, in spite of adequate fluid replacement, show no improvement in cardiovascular function. Catecholamines improve cardiovascular function by increasing venous return through alpha-mediated vasoconstriction, decreasing peripheral resistance, and increasing peripheral blood flow by dopaminergic or beta-2 vasodilation. These drugs should be used only following adequate fluid replacement. Their use may be associated with cardiac arrhythmias.

Vasodilatory agents have been successfully used in the management of hemorrhagic shock to improve peripheral blood flow. Nitroglycerine ointment (4–8 mg applied topically and repeated every 4 hours as needed) and hydralazine hydrochloride (0.25 mg/kg IV every 4–6 hours as required) are the agents of choice. These drugs are used only after initial fluid therapy has been instituted.

Disseminated intravascular coagulation is treated with fresh whole blood, heparin (mini-dose regimen 10 units/kg three–four times daily subcutaneously, or low-dose regimen 150–250 units/kg three times daily subcutaneously), and fluid replacement (see Chapter 16).

PATIENT MONITORING

Animals in shock should not be moved or given sedative agents that may potentiate hypotension. Vital signs, including pulse rate and rhythm, respiratory rate and rhythm, and body temperature, should be monitored at least every 15 minutes. An electrocardiogram more accurately defines cardiac rate and rhythm. Changes in cardiac rate or rhythm should be treated as indicated in Chapter 18. Changes in respiratory rate or rhythm may be indicative of hypoxia, acid-base abnormalities, pulmonary edema, or respiratory distress syndrome. These cases should be pursued with arterial blood gas analysis and chest radiographs. Gradual rewarming of the patient and maintenance of normothermia is recommended. Body temperature correlates well with cardiac output and peripheral blood flow. Mucous membrane color is a poor indicator of peripheral perfusion and tissue oxygenation. Cyanosis associated with hypoxemia is a late finding in the course of pulmonary disease (see Chapter 2).

Animals must be closely observed for signs of fluid overload. Central venous pressure, body weight, urine ouput, packed-cell volume, total protein, and lung sounds are monitored. Adequate red cell mass and protein content are present if the packed-cell volume is greater than 25% (0.25 L/L) and the total protein is greater than 3.0 g/dl (30 g/L). Packed-cell volume and total protein levels are usually normal in the early stages of shock. The values decrease as the disease progresses, in association with fluid redistribution in response to the loss of blood volume and concurrent fluid replacement. If the packed-cell volume remains higher than 50% (0.50 L/L) and there is no indication of fluid overload, fluid replacement is inadequate. A fall in total protein concentration implies overhydration or continued protein loss. If total protein and packed-cell volume increase, this implies fluid loss. Urine output is quantified. Normal urinary output is 1 to 2 ml/kg/hour. Measures to increase urinary output were discussed previously.

Serum blood chemistry is monitored as indicated. Indices requiring special attention include serum urea, creatinine, glucose, and potassium, aspartate aminotransferase, alanine aminotransferase, and alkaline phosphatase.

Measures should be taken to lessen the opportunity for the development of septic shock in patients predisposed to it. Predisposing factors include old age, poor nutritional status, dehydration, the presence of indwelling catheters, immunosuppressive drug therapy, and immunosuppressive disease. General anesthetics, especially halothane and nitrous oxide, may impair the migration and phagocytic capabilites of leukocytes.

ADDITIONAL READING

Allen DG. Anesthesia and the cardiovascular patient. In: Allen DG, Kruth SA, eds. Small animal cardiopulmonary medicine. Philadelphia: BC Decker, 1988: 133.

Bottoms GD, Johnson MA, Roesel OF. Endotoxin induced hemodynamic changes in dogs: Role of thromboxane and prostaglandin I_1. Am J Vet Res 1983; 44:1497.

Bowen JM. Are corticosteroids useful in shock therapy? J Am Vet Med Assoc 1980; 177:453.

Dyson DH. Circulatory shock. In: Allen DG, Kruth SA, eds. Small animal cardiopulmonary medicine. Philadelphia: BC Decker, 1988: 41.

Fettman MJ. Hypertonic crystalloid solutions for treating hemorrhagic shock. Compendium of Continuing Education 1985; 7:915.

Guyton AC. Circulatory shock and physiology of treatment. In: Guyton AC, ed. Textbook of medical physiology. Philadelphia: WB Saunders, 1986: 326.

Hardie EM, Rawlings CA. Septic shock. Part I: Pathophysiology. Compendium of Continuing Education 1983; 5:369.

Hardie EM, Rawlings CA. Septic shock. Part II: Prevention, recognition, and treatment. Compendium of Continuing Education 1983; 5:483.

Hardie EM, Rawlings CA, Collins LG. Canine *Escherichia coli* peritonitis: Long term survival with fluid, gentamicin sulfate and flunixin meglumine treatment. Journal of the American Animal Hospital Association 1985; 21:691.

McAnulty JF. Septic shock in the dog: A review. Journal of the American Animal Hospital Association 1983; 19:827.

Morgan RV. Shock. Compendium of Continuing Education 1981; 3:533.

Otto CM, Kaufman GM, Crowe DT. Intraosseous infusion of fluids and therapeutics. Compendium of Continuing Education 1989; 11:421.

Stephens KA. Catecholamines and their use in shock. Compendium of Continuing Education 1983; 5:671.

Webb AI. Fluid therapy in hypotensive shock. Vet Clin North Am 1982; 12:515.

Wessels BC, Gaffin SL, Wells MT. Circulating plasma endotoxin (lipopolysaccharide) concentrations in healthy and hemorrhagic enteric dogs: Antiendotoxin immunotherapy in hemorrhagic enteric endotoxemia. Journal of the American Animal Hospital Association 1987; 23:291.

White GL, White GS, Kosanke SD et al. Therapeutic effects of prednisolone sodium succinate versus dexamethasone in dogs subjected to *E. coli* septic shock. Journal of the American Animal Hospital Association 1982; 18:639.

5

WEAKNESS, SYNCOPE, AND SUDDEN DEATH

Dana G. Allen

The clinical syndromes of generalized muscle weakness, syncope, and sudden death are often a diagnostic and therapeutic challenge. Syncope is more common in the dog than in the cat. In the dog it has been documented most frequently in the poodle, Chihuahua, Boston bull, boxer, pug, Pekingese, English bull, and Pomeranian.

CAUSES

Weakness includes the syndromes of generalized muscle weakness, syncope, and seizure. Weakness is characterized by a loss of energy and listlessness accompanied by a loss of muscle strength, paresis, or paralysis. It may be episodic or chronic. Syncope is a sudden, transient loss of consciousness caused by a decrease in cerebral blood flow and hypoxia or hypoglycemia. The causes of generalized muscle weakness and syncope are listed in Tables 5-1 and 5-2, respectively. Many of the causes that lead to hypoxemia, hypoglycemia, and generalized muscle weakness also cause syncope if cerebral function is impaired. If the cause of syncope is not terminated it may progress to sudden death. Known cardiovascular

causes of sudden death in the dog and cat are listed in Table 5-3.

PATHOPHYSIOLOGY

Generalized weakness is caused by factors primarily affecting muscle groups. Cardiovascular causes result in decreased cardiac output and poor peripheral blood flow to muscle. Generalized weakness due to cardiovascular causes is exacerbated by exercise or stress.

Metabolic causes of weakness include hypoglycemia and electrolyte imbalances. The nervous system and muscle require glucose for energy. With a gradual decline in serum glucose, weakness and depression occur. If the fall in blood glucose is rapid, syncope, seizure, or coma may occur. Hyperkalemia depresses cellular excitability and causes muscle weakness, bradycardia, and depressed reflexes. Hypokalemia and hypercalcemia also adversely affect muscle membrane excitability. Hypoadrenocorticism and deficiencies of cortisol and aldosterone may result in hypoglycemia and a decreased circulating blood volume, respectively, which contribute to

Table 5–1 *Causes of Weakness*

Cardiovascular causes	Sinus arrest, atrial standstill, sick sinus syndrome, atrial fibrillation, third-degree heart block, ventricular tachycardia
Rhythm disturbances	Sinus arrest, atrial standstill, sick sinus syndrome, atrial fibrillation, third-degree heart block, ventricular tachycardia
Cardiac abnormalities	Cardiomyopathy, congestive heart failure, cardiac tamponade, heartworm disease, bacterial endocarditis
Metabolic causes	Hypoglycemia, hypokalemia, hyperkalemia, hypocalcemia, hypercalcemia, acid-base abnormalities
Respiratory causes	Hypoxemia, cyanosis, pulmonary thromboembolism
Neurologic causes	Polymyositis, polyneuropathy, narcolepsy, myasthenia gravis, hepatic encephalopathy, botulism, tick paralysis, coonhound paralysis, spinal lesions, space-occupying central nervous system lesions
Drug-induced causes	Phenothiazines, barbiturates, digitalis, diuretics, diphenylhydantoin, prazosin
Drugs affecting neurotransmission	Phenothiazines, tetracyclines, organophosphates, carbamates, polymixins, aminoglycosides, phenytoin, quinidine sulfate, procainamide hydrochloride, propanolol
Endocrine causes	Hyperadrenocorticism, hypoadrenocorticism, hypothyroidism, diabetes mellitus, hypoparathyroidism, hyperparathyroidism
Other causes	Paraneoplastic syndrome, nutritional causes (obesity or cachexia), fever due to infectious disease, overexertion with exercise, heatstroke, hypothermia, anemia, psychogenic causes

hypotension and a lack of glucose for energy. Acid-base abnormalities may contribute to electrolyte changes (see Chapters 71 and 72).

Myasthenia gravis is characterized by a failure in neuromuscular transmission that is associated with a decrease in the number of available acetylcholine receptors at the neuromuscular junction. Clinically, it is recognized by weakness and fatigue associated with exercise. Signs are alleviated with the administration of the anticholinesterase edrophonium chloride (Tensilon Chloride) (0.5–5.0 mg IV). Polymyositis, polyneuropathies, and hepatic encephalopathy have also been associated with weakness. Polyneuropathies may be associated with endocrine diseases and result in decreased neuromuscular excitability. Hepatic encephalopathy is associated with impaired electrical and metabolic activity of the brain.

Drugs associated with weakness cause a decrease in cardiac output through alterations in stroke volume or heart rate and rhythm. Certain drugs also interfere with neuromuscular transmission. Drug-induced weakness has been recognized more often in humans. They may induce weakness by themselves, but are more often associated with prolonged weakness and respiratory depression in conjunction with general anesthesia and electrolyte or acid-base abnormalites. Subclinical myasthenia gravis may become apparent with the use of these agents (see Table 5-1).

Chronic debilitating diseases of the liver, kidney, gastrointestinal tract, or skin contribute to muscle weakness. Other chronic debilitating diseases include paraneoplastic syndromes, nutritional cachexia or obesity (Pickwickian syndrome), and chronic fever of infectious disease. Heatstroke or hypothermia may also be associated with weakness.

Syncope is associated with cardiovascular,

Table 5–2 *Causes of Syncope*

CARDIOVASCULAR CAUSES

RHYTHM DISTURBANCES
Sinus bradycardia, atrial standstill, atrial fibrillation, sick sinus syndrome, atrioventricular conduction defects, ventricular tachycardia

CARDIAC ABNORMALITIES
Aortic stenosis, pulmonic stenosis, hypertrophic cardiomyopathy, tetralogy of Fallot, patent ductus arteriosus, septal defects, cardiac tamponade, heartworm disease

VASCULAR ABNORMALITIES
Thromboembolic disease, vasovagal syncope, carotid sinus syndrome, glossopharyngeal neuralgia, vagovagal syncope (needle paracentesis), factors causing decreased venous return, hemorrhage, anticoagulant poisoning, excessive vomiting or diarrhea, hypoadrenocorticism, tussive syncope

METABOLIC CAUSES
Hypoglycemia (islet cell tumor, insulin overdose), acid-base abnormalities

RESPIRATORY CAUSES
Hyperventilation syndrome, pulmonary thromboembolism

NEUROLOGIC CAUSES
Cerebrovascular accident, brain tumor, encephalitis

DRUG-INDUCED CAUSES
Digitalis, phenothiazines, nitrates, propanolol, quinidine, prazosin, thiazides, furosemide

OTHER CAUSES
Anemia, polycythemia

Table 5–3 *Cardiovascular Causes of Sudden Death in Dogs and Cats*

Aortic stenosis (Newfoundland, boxer, German shepherd, golden retriever)
Hypertrophic cardiomyopathy (German shepherd, cats)
Congestive cardiomyopathy (dogs and cats)
Tetralogy of Fallot
Cardiac tamponade
Ventricular tachycardia
Sinus nodal disease and prolonged QT interval (dalmation)
His bundle degeneration (pug)
His bundle and atrioventricular degeneration (doberman)
Atrial tear (chronic mitral valvular insufficiency)

---

metabolic, respiratory, neurologic, or drug-induced diseases that lead to cerebral hypoxia or hypoglycemia. Cerebral blood flow depends on adequate cardiac output. Cardiac output is a function of stroke volume and heart rate and rhythm. Factors affecting stroke volume include preload or end diastolic volume, afterload or the resistance to ventricular outflow, and contractility. Factors decreasing venous return and end diastolic volume include hemorrhage, peripheral vasodilation, and excessive fluid loss from vomiting or diarrhea. Cardiac tamponade impairs ventricular filling, preload, and cardiac output. Severe hemorrhage associated with acute coumarin or indandione toxicity, or acute bleeding associated with splenic or hepatic hemangiosarcoma may also decrease venous return and cardiac output. Coughing leads to a marked increase in intrathoracic pressure and a decrease in venous return and cerebral blood flow.

Lesions obstructing ventricular outflow (aortic and pulmonic stenosis and severe heartworm) may be associated with syncope. Clinical signs may become apparent only with exercise and peripheral vasodilation, which, in conjunction with the decreased cardiac output, contribute to syncope.

Changes in heart rate or rhythm may be sufficient to affect cardiac output. Tachyarrhythmias, including atrial fibrillation and ventricular tachycardia, have been associated with syncope in the dog. Third-degree heart block is the most common example of an atrioventricular (AV) defect causing syncope.

Bradyarrhythmias are less often associated with syncope because latent AV junctional pacemakers continue to maintain an adequate ventricular heart rate. Sick sinus syndrome is a bradycardia–tachycardia rhythm disturbance that has been associated with syncope in the miniature schnauzer, boxer, dachshund, pug, other breeds of dog, and the cat.

Abnormal autonomic activity may lead to peripheral vasodilation, bradycardia, AV conduction block, and a fall in cardiac output and cerebral blood flow. Brachycephalic breeds appear to be predisposed. Vasovagal syncope associated with fright leads to intense vagal stimulation, bradycardia, peripheral vasodilation, and a fall in arterial blood pressure. Animals appear weak or confused, the respiratory rate and depth increases, and the pupils dilate. Postural hypotension is included in this category. Animals with postural hypotension suffer an acute fall in systolic and diastolic blood pressure and changes in heart rate upon rising. The condition may be a complication of diabetes mellitus, hypoadrenocorticism, or excessive diuretic, morphine, or phenothiazine use. With carotid sinus syndrome, fainting occurs with a sudden movement of the head or neck. It leads to stimulation of the baroreceptors, a fall in arterial blood pressure, and sinus arrest or AV block. Glossopharyngeal neuralgia should be considered in animals that faint with eating or drinking. Vagovagal syncope, leading to bradycardia, AV block, asystole, and possibly peripheral vasodilation, occurs with stimulation of vagal afferent fibers, which can be associated with visceral pain. Cases of transient collapse in small animals associated with needle paracentesis of the chest and abdomen may fit into this category.

Metabolic causes of syncope are most often associated with hypoglycemia. They include insulin-secreting tumors of the pancreas and insulin overdose.

Hyperventilation leads to a fall in the arterial P_{CO_2}, peripheral vasodilation, cerebral arterial vasoconstriction, and cerebral hypoxia. It occurs most often in hyperexcitable pets.

Syncope may occur secondary to decreased cerebral blood flow associated with intracranial tumors, intracranial hemorrhage, increased intracranial pressure, and encephalitis. Expanding intracranial lesions more often cause seizure activity.

Drug-induced causes of syncope lead to hypotension (acepromazine, prazosin, nitrates, propanolol, diuretics) or changes in cardiac rate or rhythm (digitalis, quinidine) and a decrease in cardiac output and cerebral blood flow (see Table 5-2).

CLINICAL SIGNS

A thorough history and complete physical examination will help differentiate weakness versus syncope. Weakness is characterized by chronic or episodic muscle weakness and fatigue. Recovery between episodes is slow and often incomplete. Weakness is not accompanied by a loss of consciousness.

Syncope may or may not be preceeded by periods of excitement. Animals become ataxic, fall unconscious, and appear relaxed, but may experience intense muscle activity, vocalization, and involuntary urination and defecation associated with cerebral hypoxia. Recovery is rapid and complete. Without direct clinical observation it may be difficult to differentiate syncope from seizure. Classically, seizures are preceded by an aura. The animal exhibits behavioral changes during this time. This phase may or may not be noticed by owners. The aura proceeds to the ictal phase, which is characterized by intense, involuntary tonic–clonic muscle activity, vocalization, urination, and defecation. The postictal period may include disorientation, confusion, and apparent blindness (see Chapter 53). Signs occur most often at rest or upon waking.

The clinical signs accompanying weakness and syncope can often be related to the cause. Cardiovascular disease may present with a history of cough, poor exercise tolerance, or fainting. Cardiac rate and rhythm abnormalities, diminished pulse amplitude, pulse deficits, murmurs, prolonged capillary refill time, and adventitial lung sounds may be noted on the physical examination. Pale mucous membranes may be indicative of anemia or poor peripheral perfusion.

Hypoglycemia associated with islet cell tumors characteristically presents with a history of episodic ataxia, weakness, muscle twitching, syncope, nervousness, depression, hyperactivity, seizure, polyphagia, or blindness. Signs may be precipitated by fasting, eating, excitement, or exercise.

Causes of acid-base and electrolyte abnormalities are addressed separately in this text (see Chapters 71 and 72).

Animals with myasthenia gravis prefer to lie down and are reluctant to move. With progressive exercise the stride is shortened, facial features droop, and the animal salivates. A weakened bark, regurgitation, and megaesophagus commonly accompany the disease. Signs are alleviated with rest. With polymyositis, weakness tends to be progressive and exacerbated by exercise.

Muscle trembling may be apparent following exercise. Muscles may be swollen and painful in the acute stages, or atrophic as the disease advances.

Polyneuropathies in small animals are most often associated with diabetes mellitus, hypoadrenocorticism, hyperadrenocorticism, hypothyroidism, or parathyroid disease. Most cases are associated with quadriparesis, quadriplegia, depressed spinal reflexes, and impairment of proprioception and pain. Diagnosis requires demonstration of the causative disease, electromyography, and peripheral nerve biopsy. Clinical signs of hepatic encephalopathy are varied and often paroxysmal. They may include depression, behavioral changes, seizures, ataxia, vomiting, diarrhea, polyuria or polydipsia, and intolerance to anesthesia or tranquilization. Clinical signs are often noted 1 to 3 hours after eating.

DIAGNOSTIC APPROACH

A minimum data base, including a complete blood count, serum biochemistry, electrolyte levels, urinalysis, electrocardiogram, and blood gas analysis, should be completed on all animals with a history of weakness or syncope (Table 5-4). Changes may not be apparent at rest. Serum electrolyte and glucose levels, an electrocardiogram, arterial blood gas analysis, and body temperature should be repeated following strenuous exercise. The history, findings on physical examination, and minimum data base should help categorize the likely cause.

The extended data base is directed to the apparent cause. Cardiovascular causes are pursued with chest radiographs, echocardiograms, and angiocardiograms. The clinician may attempt to unmask arrhythmias by physical or chemical stimulation of the autonomic nervous system. Direct digital carotid sinus massage or pupillary pressure for 1 to 2 minutes may augment vagal tone and induce bradyarrhythmias or heart block, although this technique has not been found to be very reliable in animals. Atropine (0.04 mg/kg IV) may be used to uncover pathologic tachyarrhythmias. A tentative diagnosis is made if a significant arrhythmia is provoked with the test.

Atropine can, however, induce atrial premature complexes, ventricular premature complexes, or second-degree heart block in normal animals. The test must be interpreted cautiously. A diagnosis can be confirmed only if the provoked arrhythmia and associated clinical signs are successfully managed medically.

The approach to metabolic and neurologic causes of weakness and syncope is listed in Table 5-4.

Table 5-4 *Diagnostic Approach to Patients with Weakness or Syncope*

	Tests and Possible Findings
MINIMUM DATA BASE	Complete blood count (anemia, infection)
	Serum biochemistry* (hypoglycemia; elevated urea, creatinine, creatine kinase; aspartate aminotransferase (AST); electrolyte abnormalities)
	Urinalysis (specific gravity)
	Electrocardiogram* (rate, rhythm, or conduction abnormalities)
	Arterial blood gas and acid-base*
EXTENDED DATA BASE	
Cardiovascular causes	Chest radiographs
	Heartworm testing
	Echocardiogram
	Angiocardiogram
	Physical and chemical manipulation of heart rate and rhythm
Metabolic causes	ACTH stimulation
	Dexamethasone suppression
	Thyrotropin stimulation
	Insulin-glucose ratio
	Parathyroid hormone levels
Neurologic causes	Cerebrospinal fluid tap
	Electroencephalogram
	Electromyogram
	Tensilon test
	Nerve biopsy
	Muscle biopsy
	Blood ammonia levels
	Ammonium tolerance test
	BSP retention test
	Serum bile acids
Other causes	Abdominal radiographs (tumor)
	Blood cultures (fever)

* *Before and after exercise*

MANAGEMENT AND PATIENT MONITORING

The management and monitoring of patients with weakness and syncope is directed at the primary cause, and can be found elsewhere in this text.

ADDITIONAL READING

Beckett SD, Branch CE, Robertson BT. Syncopal attacks and sudden death in dogs: Mechanisms and etiologies. Journal of the American Animal Hospital Association 1978; 14:378.

Ettinger SJ. Weakness and syncope. In: Ettinger SJ, ed. Textbook of veterinary internal medicine. Philadelphia: WB Saunders, 1983: 76.

Kelly MJ. Periodic weakness. Proceedings of the American Animal Hospital Association 1982: 159.

Lorenz MD. Episodic weakness: A diagnostic plan. Proceedings Amer Anim Hosp Assoc 1982: 145.

6

FEVER OF UNKNOWN ORIGIN

Dana G. Allen

Fever is the pathophysiologic increase in body temperature in response to infection, immune mediated-disease, neoplasia, or drug reaction. Fever of unknown origin is characterized by persistent, idiopathic fever 39.5°C (103°F) or higher, of at least 2 to 3 weeks' duration.

CAUSES

Causes of fever may be categorized as infectious, immune-mediated, neoplastic, and other. The reported causes of fever in veterinary medicine are listed in Table 6-1. Approximately 40% of cases have an infectious etiology, 20% are related to immune-mediated disease, 20% are neoplastic, 10% are due to other causes, and 10% remain undiagnosed (Feldman, Additional Reading).

According to Feldman, the most common cause of fever of an infectious etiology is bacterial endocarditis. In patients with bacteremia, *Escherichia coli* and *Staphylococcus aureus* account for more than 50% of the bacterial isolates. Common causes of bacteremia include bacterial endocarditis, discospondylitis, urinary tract infection, abscesses, and skin and wound infection. Fever is rare in animals with anaerobic bacteremia, especially those caused by clostridia. Bacteremias without primary organ involvement rarely pres-

ent with fever. In a report by Calvert (Additional Reading), bacterial endocarditis and discospondylitis accounted for 25% of all cases of bacteremia in dogs. *S. aureus, E. coli,* and β-hemolytic streptococci account for 90% of bacterial isolates in cases of bacterial endocarditis. *S. aureus* is the most often isolated bacterium in discospondylitis. Streptococci and *Brucella canis* are cultured less frequently. Bacterial endocarditis and discospondylitis are most often diagnosed in large male dogs. Bacteremia approaches 50% in critically ill dogs and cats. In cats with bacteremia, gram-negative bacilli (especially *Salmonella enteritidis*) and anaerobic bacteria are the most common bacterial isolates. Conditions predisposing to bacteremia include neoplasia, treatment with glucocorticoids or chemotherapeutic agents, diabetes mellitus, hyperadrenocorticism, renal or hepatic failure, neutropenia or defects in macrophage and neutrophil function, splenectomy, intravenous or urinary tract catheterization, and severe burns. Viral diseases are mostly self-limiting and rarely present with chronic fever.

Immunologic disease associated with fever may include systemic lupus erythematosis, rheumatoid arthritis, or polyarteritis nodosa. Fever is initiated by the production of interleukin-1 by sensitized lymphocytes or by the presence of anti-

Table 6–1 *Potential Causes of Fever in Small Animals*

INFECTIOUS CAUSES	**IMMUNE-MEDIATED CAUSES**

INFECTIOUS CAUSES

BACTERIAL
Endocarditis (*Staphylococcus aureus, Escherichia coli,*
  β-hemolytic streptococcus)
Discospondylitis (*S. aureus*)
Leptospirosis
Mycobacteriosis
Brucellosis
Nocardiosis
Actinomycosis
Borreliosis (Lyme disease)

VIRAL
Feline leukemia virus
Feline immunodeficiency virus
Feline infectious peritonitis
Feline panleukopenia
Feline upper respiratory disease (herpes virus, calicivirus,
  chlamydia)
Canine distemper
Canine infectious hepatitis

FUNGAL
Histoplasmosis
Blastomycosis
Coccidioidomycosis
Cryptococcosis

RICKETTSIAL
Infection with *Haemobartonella* organisms
Infection with *Ehrlichia* organisms
Rocky Mountain spotted fever

PROTOZOAN
Toxoplasmosis
Babesiosis
Cytauxzoonosis

METAZOAN
Dirofilariasis
Ectopic migrations

IMMUNE-MEDIATED CAUSES
Systemic lupus erythematosis
Immune-mediated polyarthritis
Polyarteritis nodosa
Autoimmune hemolytic anemia
Immune-mediated thrombocytopenia
Polymyositis

NEOPLASTIC CAUSES
Lymphosarcoma
Myeloproliferative disease
Plasma cell myeloma

OTHER CAUSES
Hyperthyroidism (older cats)
Nodular panniculitis
Hepatic cirrhosis
Drug reaction (aspirin, tetracyclines [cat], levamisole [cat], sul-
  fonamides, penicillins, amphotericin B, disophenol, quinidine,
  colchicine, bleomycin, novobiocin)
Pulmonary thromboembolism (heartworm)
Pheochromocytoma
Inflammatory bowel disease
Hyperlipemia
Pansteatitis (vitamin E deficiency in cats)

---

gen–antibody complexes, which may act as exogenous pyrogens. Systemic lupus erythematosis may cause fever secondary to immunosuppression, tissue necrosis, or injury, or fever may be a reaction to drug therapy (Greene, 1982, Additional Reading).

Tumors initiate fever through the production of endogenous pyrogen (interleukin-1) or secondary to necrosis, inflammation, or infection of the tumor. Hematopoietic neoplasia (lymphosarcoma), myeloproliferative disease, and plasma cell myeloma are the most common tumors associated with fever. The most common sites of localized neoplasia involve the skin, kidney, liver, bone, lymph nodes, stomach, and lungs. There is no association between fever and metastatic disease. Tumor breakdown associated with treatment may also be accompanied by fever.

Hyperthyroidism induces fever by increasing metabolic activity. In humans adrenal insufficiency and pheochromocytoma have also been associated with fever.

Drugs may interfere with thermoregulation and initiate fever. Paradoxically, aspirin in high doses may cause fever (Greene, 1982, Additional Reading).

PATHOPHYSIOLOGY

The hypothalamus regulates body temperature on the basis of information received from thermoreceptors in the skin and those in proximity to the hypothalamus itself. From this information body temperature is "set" and maintained by the production and conservation of heat or through heat loss. Body heat is generated by shivering, catabolizing fat, and increasing metabolism by increasing serum thyroxine and catecholamine concentrations. Heat is conserved through vasoconstriction, piloerection, seeking a warmer environment, and curling the body. Heat loss occurs primarily through evaporation and panting in the dog and cat. Control of body temperature is less effective in neonates owing to a lack of maturity of the hypothalamus.

Hyperthermia is defined as the elevation of body temperature above normal. Core body temperature increases, but the thermoregulatory "set point" does not. Dramatic elevations in body temperature (greater than 41°C or 106°F), termed *hyperpyrexia*, may occur. Hyperthermia is rarely associated with an infectious etiology. In most cases the acute increase in body temperature is caused by heat stroke, strenuous exercise, seizure, eclampsia, thyrotoxicosis, drug reaction, hypothalamic lesions, high ambient temperature and humidity, or malignant hyerthermia, including exercise-induced canine stress syndrome. In small animals heat stroke appears to be the most common cause of nonpyrogenic hyperthermia. Dehydration, tranquilization, anticholinergic agents, and inhalent anesthetics predispose to hyperthermia.

Fever is a specific form of hyperthermia in which the normal body temperature or "set point" is reset to a higher value. In small animals fever is classified as septic or remittent, chronic or sustained, and intermittent or undulant. Septic fever is characterized by daily increases in body temperature accompanied by periods of normal or even subnormal body temperature; it is associated with acute bacterial infections. Chronic fever is most often associated with bacterial endocarditis, discospondylitis, neoplasia, or lesions of the central nervous system. Intermittent fever is generally caused by persistent infectious processes, lymphosarcoma, immune-mediated disease, or brucellosis. Body temperatures rarely exceed 41°C (106°F) in cases with an infectious etiology. Body temperatures in this range are not deleterious to the animal in the short term. Body temperatures in excess of 43°C (109°F) are associated with a high degree of mortality.

True fever is initiated by exogenous pyrogens that cause tissue injury. Exogenous pyrogens include bacteria, endotoxins, viruses, fungi, protozoa, rickettsia, metazoa, antigen–antibody complexes, antigens associated with delayed hypersensitivity, neoplasia, vascular accidents, and physical agents. Bacterial endotoxins are the most potent exogenous pyrogens. Exogenous pyrogens do not affect body temperature directly. Exogenous pyrogens react with phagocytic leukocytes and lead to the increased production of endogenous pyrogen or interleukin-1, which directs an increased synthesis of prostaglandin, especially prostaglandin E_2 in the anterior hypothalamus. The increased prostaglandin levels reset the hypothalamus and maintain body temperature at a higher level (Fig. 6-1).

Other suspected mediators affecting the hypothalamic thermoregulatory center include cyclic adenosine monophosphate, monoamines, cholinergic agents, locally increased sodium:calcium ratios, and norepinephrine. Endogenous pyrogen is physically related to leukocyte endogenous mediator and leukocyte activating factor. Collectively these substances are referred to as interleukin-1. Leukocyte endogenous mediator lowers serum iron and zinc, impairs bacterial growth, promotes the synthesis of acute phase proteins, stimulates neutrophil release from the bone marrow, and causes fever. Lymphocyte activating factor stimulates T lymphocyte proliferation and antibody production in the presence of antigen. Most infectious diseases, immunologic reactions, and inflammatory processes induce mononuclear cell phagocytes to produce interleukin-1. Interleukin-1 activity is increased with fever. Phagocytic leukocytes, including neutrophils, monocytes, eosinophils, macrophages, and Kuppfer's cells, may be activated by infectious microorganisms, hypersensitivity, tissue necrosis, or immune-

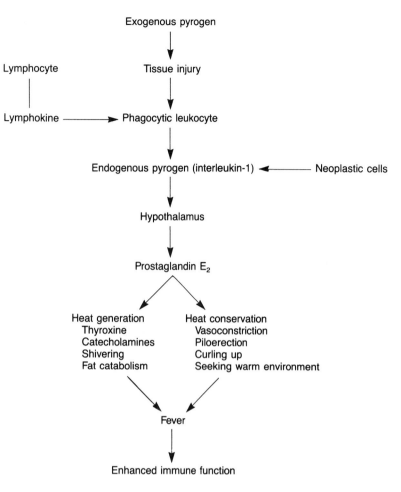

Figure 6–1. *Pathophysiology of fever.*

mediated disease to produce interleukin-1. Lymphocytes do not produce it, but do produce a lymphokine that stimulates macrophages to produce it. Some neoplastic cells can produce interleukin-1 directly.

Moderate fever, up to 41°C (106°F), can be beneficial to the body's defense against infection. Many microorganisms are more readily killed by temperatures associated with moderate fever. Moderate fever is associated with increased lyzosomal activity, lymphocyte transformation, antibody production, granulocyte mobility, and increased interferon activity. Survival rates are increased in puppies with herpesvirus infection if the ambient temperture is increased and the animals can maintain an increased body tempera-

ture. Enhanced immune mechanisms and a lack of tumor tolerance for heat contributes to increased neoplastic cell death in animals with concurrent fever.

Not all effects of fever are beneficial. Natural killer cell activity is decreased with fever. Prolonged fever is catabolic in nature and contributes to a sense of ill feeling, anorexia, and muscle wasting. The direct action of interleukin-1 on muscle results in an increase in prostaglandin E_2 production and protein degradation. Extremely high body temperatures (in excess of 43°C or 109°F—rarely seen with true fever) can contribute to disseminated intravascular coagulation and damage to the liver, kidney, and central nervous system.

CLINICAL SIGNS

Clinical signs are not specific. The increase in body temperature may be accompanied by an increase in the respiratory rate, heart rate, and urine specific gravity (in response to evaporation and the loss of body water), malaise, myalgia, fatigue, sleepiness, shivering, and anorexia. Initially, fever is accompanied by polydipsia and polyuria. Animals tend to drink less with chronic fever and often become dehydrated. Interleukin-1 induces increased sleep activity, which helps reduce metabolic demands and contributes to the defense and repair of the body. Chronic fever may be associated with depression, weakness, and weight loss. Clinical signs of a more definite nature are related to the specfic disease process (lameness associated with immune-mediated polyarthritis or hyperesthesia, stilted pelvic gait and hindlimb lameness associated with discospondylitis).

DIAGNOSTIC APPROACH

The diagnostic approach to animals with fever of unknown origin includes a complete history and physical examination followed by a minimum data base, including a complete blood count, serum biochemistry profile, and urinalysis (Table 6-2). Signalment is important. Older animals are predisposed to neoplasia. The history should include current vaccination status (canine distemper, canine hepatitis, feline panleukopenia, feline leukemia virus, feline calicivirus and herpesvirus), possible exposure to drugs and current medications (glucocorticoid treatment is a common contributing factor to bacteremia), travel to areas with endemic disease (deep mycoses, heartworm, infection with *Ehrlichia canis*, babesiosis), and diet (pansteatitis, vitamin E deficiency in cats).

The clinician should palpate all body areas, placing particular emphasis on lymph nodes, thyroid gland (cat), liver, spleen, kidneys, muscles, joints, and the umbilicus in young animals. Palpation is concluded with rectal examination of the prostate or vagina and cervix. Examination of

Table 6–2 *Diagnostic Approach to Fever of Unknown Origin—Minimum Data Base*

Test	What to Look For
Complete blood count	Anemia Leukocytosis Neoplastic cells
Serum biochemistry	Hypercalcemia (lymphosarcoma) Elevated thyroxine (older cats) Elevated creatine kinase, AST (muscle) Elevated ALT, AST, bilirubin, cholesterol, alkaline phosphatase (liver) Elevated blood urea nitrogen, creatinine (kidney) Elevated amylase, lipase (pancreas) Increased proteins (globulins)
Urinalysis	Red cells White cells Casts Bacteria Specific gravity

the ocular fundus may detect underlying infectious disease. Auscultation of the chest may reveal a murmur associated with bacterial endocarditis (see Chapter 22) or adventitial lung sounds associated with pneumonia (see Chapter 29). Temperature should be monitored every 4 to 6 hours to establish its pattern and its response to treatment.

A normochromic, normocytic nonresponsive anemia associated with sequestration of iron in the reticuloendothelial system is common in cases of chronic fever. Increased red cell sedimentation rates, corresponding to an increase in serum globulin and fibrinogen levels, are often noted. A marked neutrophilic leukocytosis may be indicative of bacterial infection or tissue necrosis (see Chapter 75). A left shift with toxic changes may precede granulocytosis. Toxic changes are more often documented with gram-negative bacteremia. Döhle's bodies are seen most often in cats; their presence is suggestive of severe infection. Most dogs with bacteremia have increased numbers of immature and segmented neutrophils and monocytes. Severe neutropenia or granulocytopenia occurs with severe, overwhelming bacterial infection, early viral disease, toxic or drug-induced causes, or bone marrow suppression (see Chapter 76). Lymphocytosis may be associated with viral disease, eosinophilia with parasitism or allergic disease, and monocytosis with granulomatous disease (brucellosis or the systemic mycoses) or subacute bacterial endocarditis. The complete blood count is usually normal in dogs with discospondylitis.

The biochemisty profile may help localize the disease process. Hypoglycemia is a variable occurrence with sepsis and bacteremia, but is more often noted with gram-negative infection or endotoxemia (see Chapter 77). Hypoglycemia resolves with resolution of the disease. Hyperglycemia has been observed in dogs with Rocky Mountain spotted fever and in cats under stress or with severe infection. Serum thyroxine levels are increased in cats with hyperthyroidism (see Chapter 61). Muscle enzymes are frequently elevated due to the catabolic nature of the disease. Intermittent fever, monocytosis, hypoalbuminemia, and increased serum alkaline phosphatase should alert the clinician to the possibility of bacteremia. Leukopenia, thrombocytopenia, and hypoglycemia have been observed in cases of overwhelming bacterial infection. Bacteriuria may be associated with bacteremia, bacterial endocarditis, or discospondylitis.

Further evaluation with an extended data base is called for if there is failure to resolve the fever and identify its cause (Table 6-3). The extended data base is organized into tests most appropriate to pursuing infectious, immune-mediated, or neoplastic causes. Infectious agents cause 30% to 40% of fevers. Approximately 80% of cases of bacterial endocarditis have positive blood cultures. Following aseptic preparation, three to four venous blood samples are drawn (there is no need to use different veins each time unless phlebitis is suspected) over a 24-hour period and cultured for aerobic and anaerobic bacteria. Drawing blood for blood culture during a febrile episode does not increase the likelihood of obtaining a positive culture in dogs with bacterial endocarditis. If, however, the source of bacteremia is extravascular, blood for culture should be drawn approximately 1 hour before the expected onset of fever. In these cases there is a delay between the influx of bacteria into the bloodstream and the onset of fever.

Table 6–3 *Extended Data Base for Animals with Fever of Unknown Origin*

Cause	Tests
Infectious	Blood, urine, joint, cerebrospinal fluid, bone marrow cytology and culture
	Echocardiography
	Prostatic wash
	Skeletal radiography
	Protein electrophoresis
	Serum titers (feline infectious peritonitis; Toxoplasma; deep mycoses; *Brucella, Coccidioides, Ehrlichia, Babesia, Leptospira*)
	Immunodiagnosis (feline leukemia virus, feline infectious peritonitis)
	Heartworm testing
	Cerebrospinal fluid analysis
Immune-mediated	Joint taps
	ANA titer
	LE prep
	Coomb's test
	Platelet factor 3 (PF3)
	Rheumatoid factor
Neoplastic	Chest and abdominal radiographs
	Abdominal ultrasound
	Fine needle biopsy of lesion
	Lymph node and bone marrow biopsy

Prior treatment of patients with antibiotics does not significantly affect the bacterial culture of blood, although the growth of the bacteria in culture may be slowed. If the blood is collected in an antimicrobial removal device (ARD, Marion Laboratories) antimicrobials are removed from blood specimens; this may permit earlier isolation of infective bacteria from patients pretreated with antibiotics. If the primary site of infection is not identified, the urine, prostatic fluid, joint fluid, and bone marrow should be reviewed cytologically and cultured for bacteria. If neurologic signs accompany the fever, cerebrospinal fluid aspiration should be performed (see Cerebrospinal Fluid Collection in Chapter 80). Echocardiography may help identify vegetative lesions associated with endocarditis. Discospondylitis most often involves the midthoracic spine, C-6–C-7 and L-7–S-1. Radiographic bony changes may take 4 to 6 weeks to become evident. Protein electrophoresis, serum titers, and immunodiagnostic testing for feline leukemia virus and feline immunodeficiency virus complete the approach to infectious disease (see Table 6-3; see Chapters 78 and 79).

If an infectious process cannot be identified and the animal is showing clinical signs consistent with immune-mediated disease (shifting leg lameness, intermittent fever, anemia, or thrombocytopenia), the following diagnostic tests should be considered: arthrocentesis, antinuclear antibody (ANA) titer, lupus erythematosus preparation (LE prep), rheumatoid factor, Coombs' test, and platelet factor 3. Several joints should be aspirated even if the animal is not apparently lame (see Arthrocentesis in Chapter 80). A marked increase in the number of nondegenerate neutrophils is highly suggestive of immune-mediated joint disease.

In older animals neoplasia is a common cause of fever. If the primary tumor is evident, fine needle or excisional biopsy should be completed. If a tumor is not evident, but neoplasia is suspect, radiographs (and where available, ultrasound) of the chest and abdomen should be completed. In many cases, fine needle aspiration of the lymph nodes (see Chapter 15) and bone marrow biopsy (see Bone Marrow Aspiration and Biopsy in Chapter 80) is required to locate and define the neoplastic process.

If the fever persists in spite of treatment and no cause can be found, it is wise to consider endoscopy and biopsy of the nasopharnyx, trachea, lung, esophagus, stomach, duodenum, colon, and large intestine even if there are no signs of specific organ involvement. As a last resort, exploratory laparotomy and biopsy of all major organs and lymph nodes may be considered. The chances of determining the cause of the fever with endoscopy or laparotomy in the absence of clinical signs suggestive of specific organ involvement are low, and in the case of laparotomy, potentially dangerous to the patient.

MANAGEMENT

The three classes of drugs most commonly used in the management of true fever are antipyretic agents, antibiotics, and corticosteroids. Antipyretic drugs are used only if fever is accompanied by anorexia and significant patient discomfort or if body temperature is excessively high and potentially deleterious (greater than 41°C or 106°F). These drugs lower the thermoregulatory "set point" and are therefore only of benefit in cases of true fever. Aspirin or the other nonsteroidal anti-inflammatory agents are indicated in animals with fever and concurrent joint destruction, muscle wasting, or myalgia. Animals with concurrent congestive heart failure may benefit from the relief that antipyretic agents offer.

The antipyretic of choice is aspirin (oral dose: 25–35 mg/kg every 8–24 hours in the dog and 12.5–25 mg/kg/day in the cat). Aspirin blocks interleukin-1-induced prostaglandin synthesis. It does not reduce interleukin-1 production or the increased amounts of sleep that accompany it. Higher doses are associated with an increased frequency of gastric irritation and bleeding. Side-effects may be minimized by giving the drug with food or by using buffered compounds (see Appendix).

Another common drug of choice is dipyrone (25 mg/kg three times daily IM, IV, or subcutaneously). Alternative drugs for use in the dog include acetaminophen, phenylbutazone, and flunixin. Acetaminophen (10–15 mg/kg every 8–24 hours) is as effective an antipyretic drug as aspirin. The drug is potentially hepatotoxic and should not be given to dogs with hepatic disease. In cats it readily causes methemaglobinemia and Heinz body formation (see Chapter 2). Flunixin (0.5–1 mg/kg IM, IV once only) is a potent antipyretic and analgesic for use in dogs. Phenylbutazone is associated with an increased incidence of gastric ulceration in dogs and cats and is not recommended in the management of fever. Similarly, indomethacin has been associated with hepatotoxicity in dogs and cats and fatal hemorrhagic gastrointestinal ulceration in dogs and cannot be recommended.

In cases of nonpyrogenic hyperthermia in which body temperatures exceed 41°C or 105°F, animals should be treated with cool water or alcohol baths, ice packs, cool water gastric lavage, and enemas, and kept in a cool environment or one equipped with a fan until the core body temperature has been lowered to about 39.4°C or 103°F.

If an infectious agent is found or if the laboratory data support it, antibiotics are the treatment of choice. Antibiotics should be chosen on the basis of culture and sensitivity. Clinical response should be evident within 48 hours. If not, the choice of antibiotic should be reconsidered. If the effects are beneficial, antibiotics should be continued for an additional 4 weeks. Most strains of *Staphylococcus aureus* are sensitive to cephalosporins, aminoglycosides, cloxacillin, erythromycin, and chloramphenicol. Most isolates of *Escherichia coli* are sensitive to gentamicin and cephalothin, but are resistant to ampicillin and chloramphenicol. β-Hemolytic streptocci are sensitive to penicillin, ampicillin, cephalosporins, and chloramphenicol. The antibiotic most useful against pseudomonas is gentamicin. Alternative drugs include third-generation cephalosporins, enrofloxacin, carbenicillin, and amikacin. Generally, cephalothin, gentamicin, erythromycin, and chloramphenicol are effective against gram-positive bacteremia, and gentamicin is effective against gram-negative bacteremia (Calvert, Additional Reading). Concurrent use of antipyretic drugs is discouraged so that clinical success of the antibiotic can be better judged. Antibiotics may be more effective than antipyretics in the presence of moderate fever.

Glucocorticoids decrease the amount of interleukin-1 released from monocytes and act centrally by decreasing the release of prostaglandin. They are indicated in animals with immune-mediated and neoplastic disease. The short-acting corticosteroids prednisone and prednisolone are preferred in the management of immune-mediated disease (2–4 mg/kg/day orally to start). It must be borne in mind that corticosteroids may mask or potentiate serious underlying infectious disease, and should only be used when infectious causes of fever have been eliminated or controlled.

PATIENT MONITORING

Appetite, mental alertness, and body temperature are monitored for response to therapy. Temperature is taken every 4 to 6 hours. If an infectious agent has been identified and treated, blood cultures are repeated during the course of therapy and 1 week following cessation of antibiotic therapy. Indwelling catheters should be removed and cultured. The most important factor affecting mortality in patients with bacteremia is the severity of the underlying condition. In a study by Dow and associates (Additional Reading) almost one half of the critically ill patients admitted to intensive care died within 1 week. Consequently, early recognition and treatment of signs indicative of bacteremia (abnormal body temperature, abnormal leukogram, shock) should reduce mortality associated with this disease. Complete blood counts should be monitored at least once weekly. Biochemistry profiles and serum titers should be repeated during the course of treatment. Thereafter the patient can be watched for signs of resurgence of the infection (loss of apetite, fever, or depression). Immune-mediated disease is monitored by repeating arthrocentesis, Coombs' test, or other tests as indicated. Joint cytology should return to normal with successful treatment of the disease (see Chapter 64).

ADDITIONAL READING

Calvert CA. Bacteremia in dogs: Diagnosis, treatment and prognosis. Compendium of Continuing Education 1986; 8:179.

Dow SW, Curtis CR, Jones RL, Wingfield WE. Bacterial culture of blood from critically ill dogs and cats: 100 cases (1985–1987). J Am Vet Med Assoc 1989; 195:113.

Dow SW, Jones RL. Bacteremia: Pathogenesis and diagnosis. Compendium of Continuing Education 1989; 11:432.

Drazner FH. Diagnostic appraoch to patients with prolonged febrile illness. Compendium of Continuing Education 1979; 1:753.

Feldman BF. Fever of undetermined origin. Compendium of Continuing Education 1980; 2:970.

Gilmore DR. Lumbosacral diskospondylitis in 21 dogs. Journal of the American Animal Hospital Association 1987; 23:57.

Greene CE. Fever. Proceedings of the American Animal Hospital Association 1982: 111.

Greene CE. Host–microbe interactions. In: Greene CE, ed. Clinical microbiology and infectious diseases of the dog and cat. Philadelphia: WB Saunders, 1984: 67.

Hirsh SC, Jang SS, Biberstein EL. Blood culture of the canine patient. J Am Vet Med Assoc 1984; 184:175.

McMillan FD. Fever: Pathophysiology and rational therapy. Compendium of Continuing Education 1985; 7:845.

7

WEIGHT LOSS AND WEIGHT GAIN

Doreen M. Houston

Weight loss is the result of insufficient calories present in the body to meet the animal's metabolic needs. A negative caloric balance exists. Weight loss is considered significant when a 10% decrease in normal body weight occurs unassociated with loss of body fluids. Weight loss of 30% to 50% of lean body mass is usually fatal. Emaciation is extreme weight loss due to severe undernutrition. Cachexia is a state of extreme ill health. Weight loss, anorexia, lethargy, and weakness are clinical manifestations of cachexia.

Obesity is the most common nutritional disorder in small animal practice. Obesity has been defined as a body weight 15% to 20% or more above the ideal body weight. Inability to palpate ribs suggests obesity. It has been estimated that anywhere from 25% to 66% of all dogs and 6% to 12% of pet cats are overweight. There is a higher incidence of obesity in pets belonging to obese and older people, and the incidence of obesity appears to increase with age. Cocker spaniels, beagles, dachshunds, Labrador retrievers, collies, and Cairn, Westhighland white, and Scottish terriers may be predisposed to obesity. Obesity is more common in female than male dogs and is about twice as prevalent in neutered than intact dogs of either sex.

Conditions that may be confused with obesity include generalized subcutaneous edema (see Chapter 10) or abdominal distension due to organomegaly, mass lesions, or fluid retention (see Chapter 11).

CAUSES

Weight Loss

There are three major categories responsible for weight loss in small animals (Fig. 7-1). Inadequate food intake (Table 7-1) may be due to dietary deficiency, oropharyngeal disease, nausea, vomiting, regurgitation, anorexia, or neurologic or psychologic factors. Causes of maldigestion and malabsorption are listed in Table 7-2. Excessive caloric expenditure may occur under certain physiologic conditions (pregnancy, lactation, heavy exercise, cold weather) and in diseases that increase metabolic rate or cause nutrient loss from the body (Table 7-3).

Weight Gain

Obesity is the result of the assimilation of food energy (calories) in excess of the animal's metabolic needs (Fig. 7-2). Excess energy is stored as fat. The causes of obesity are listed in Table 7-4.

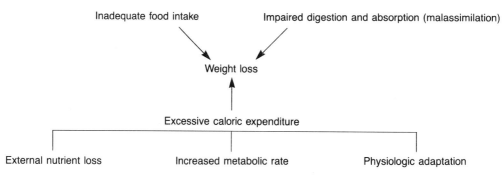

Figure 7–1. *Causes of weight loss.*

The most common cause of obesity in small animals is excess food intake relative to energy output in the form of exercise. Early (first 4–6 months of life in the dog) overfeeding results in adipocyte cell proliferation and predisposes the dog to obesity. Free choice feeding, feeding of highly palatable foods and table scraps, rewarding of positive behavior with food, and social competition for food may contribute to a weight

problem in the family pet. Physical inactivity in both humans and pets is a major factor in obesity.

Adipocyte numbers gradually increase with aging. This fact plus a reduction in basal metabolic rate (BMR) and physical activity leads to an increased incidence of obesity with age.

Food intake is under the control of the lateral appetite and ventromedial satiety center of the hypothalamus. Damage to the satiety center may result in a polyphagic animal and obesity.

Neutering influences obesity in several ways. Testosterone normally contributes to muscle protein formation through amino acid deposition. In the neutered male, the lack of testosterone allows more energy to be diverted to the formation of fat. In the female, follicle stimulating hormone stimulates food intake, while estrogen is thought to inhibit food intake. In the spayed female, estrogen levels are decreased while follicle stimulating hormone is increased. This may account, in part,

Table 7–1 *Causes of Inadequate Food Intake*

DIETARY DEFICIENCY

Being fed inadequate amount
Being fed poorly digestable diet
Protein–calorie imbalance

OROPHARYNGEAL DISEASE

Difficulty prehending food
Difficult or painful mastication or dysphagia (impairment of cranial nerve V, VII, IX, X, or XII)
Maxillary or mandibular fractures or dislocations
Tooth root abscess, foreign body, stomatitis, pharyngitis
Retrobulbar disease (abscess, tumor)
Myositis (temporal, mandibular, masseter muscles)
Tetanus
Esophagitis

NAUSEA, VOMITING, AND REGURGITATION

(see Chapters 35 and 36)

ANOREXIA

(see Chapter 8)

PSYCHOLOGICAL FACTORS

Stress
Environmental change
Anxiety
Fear

Table 7–2 *Causes of Impaired Digestion and Absorption (Malassimilation)*

MALDIGESTION

Exocrine pancreatic insufficiency
Bile salt deficiency
Brush border enzyme deficiencies

MALABSORPTION

Villous atrophy
Giardiasis
Infiltrative bowel diseases (lymphocytic–plasmocytic, eosinophilic, lymphoma)
Histoplasmosis
Ascites, portal hypertension
Effects of chemotherapy or radiation on gastrointestinal mucosa

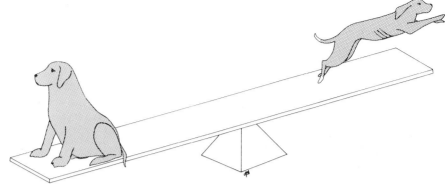

Figure 7–2. *Balance between energy intake and energy output. Weight gain results from an imbalance between energy intake (food) and energy output (exercise). The most common cause of weight gain in small animals is excessive food intake with inadequate exercise. Caloric intake exceeding the animal's metabolic needs is manifested as weight gain.*

for obesity in some spayed female dogs. Neutering also decreases roaming behavior, and inactivity in the face of unchanged caloric intake predisposes to obesity.

The decreased metabolic rate and lack of activity in the hypothyroid dog predispose it to obesity. Redistribution of body fat stores and muscle catabolism make animals with hyperadrenocorticism appear obese. Low blood glucose is a stimulus for an animal to eat; conse-

quently, dogs with islet cell tumors may gain excessive weight. Certain drugs (glucocorticoids, megestrol acetate, phenobarbital) are able to induce polyphagia, and if left unchecked, obesity may result.

Table 7–3 *Causes of Excessive Caloric Expenditure*

PHYSIOLOGIC FACTORS

Pregnancy
Lactation
Heavy exercise
Cold temperature

LOSS OF CALORIC NUTRIENTS (NUTRIENT LISTED IN PARENTHESES)

Diabetes mellitus (glucose)
Glomerular disease (protein)
Intestinal disease (protein)
Burns (protein)
Severe pyoderma (protein)
Chronic blood loss (protein)
Effusions (protein)
Vomiting (electrolytes, protein)
Diarrhea (electrolytes, protein)
Tumor—host competition for nutrients (selective nutrient uptake by tumor)

INCREASED METABOLIC RATE

Fever
Sepsis or infection
Neoplasia (pheochromocytoma, hyperthyroidism)
Congestive heart failure
Trauma

Table 7–4 *Causes of Obesity in Small Animals*

SOCIAL AND ENVIRONMENTAL FACTORS

Early overfeeding
Exposure to highly palatable foods
Physical inactivity
Degree of cortical activation (stress, emotional upset)

PHYSIOLOGIC FACTORS

Pregnancy
Altered responsiveness of medial satiety and lateral appetite center in hypothalamus

GENETIC PREDISPOSITION

Cocker spaniels, Labrador retrievers, collies, terriers (Cairn, WHW, Scottish), dachshunds, beagles

NEUROLOGIC FACTORS

Hypothalamic dysfunction or tumor
Pituitary dysfunction or tumor

HORMONAL FACTORS

Decreased estrogen in spayed female
Decreased testosterone in castrated male
Neutering; causing decreased physical activity
Hypothyroidism
Hyperadrenocorticism
Diabetes mellitus
Beta cell tumor (insulinoma)

DRUGS THAT INDUCE POLYPHAGIA

Glucocorticoids
Megestrol acetate (cats)
Anticonvulsant therapy (phenobarbital, primidone)

PATHOPHYSIOLOGY

Weight Loss

With weight loss of any cause there are insufficient calories to meet the metabolic needs of the animal. In the early stages of weight loss, the BMR may be decreased in an effort to conserve calories. Eventually, it increases. In a febrile state, the BMR increases 11% to 13% for every degree Celcius the body temperature rises, and protein (amino acid) needs increase by 10%. With time, there is depletion of body stores of fat and protein as amino acids are mobilized for gluconeogenesis in the liver. Mobilized amino acids are deaminated to make glucose, and the nitrogen is excreted as urea, creating a negative nitrogen balanace. During this phase there may be abnormalities in growth and tissue repair. Following the stage of tissue depletion, biochemical changes may become apparent. Total serum protein (predominantly albumin) falls, and clinical signs of hypoproteinemia may appear (loss of muscle mass, ascites). Vitamin and mineral deficiencies may be apparent. In contrast to the normal "starving" animal, whose BMR is initially decreased in an attempt to save calories, the cachectic cancer patient often has an increased BMR. This paradoxical increase in cellular energy consumption plus possible anorexia, concomitant fever, and sepsis results in a significant net caloric deficit. Inappetence and weight loss are common in animals with congestive heart failure (cardiac cachexia). Reasons for this include drugs depressing food intake (digitalis, captopril), drugs promoting loss of minerals (diuretics), inadequate perfusion of the gastrointestinal tract and liver, resulting in nutrient malabsorption and decreased production of albumin by the liver, and increased caloric demands with tachycardia and dyspnea.

Weight Gain

Regardless of predisposing causes, obesity is caused by prolonged caloric intake in excess of body needs. There are two recognized stages of obesity. In the initial or dynamic stage, energy intake exceeds that utilized in the form of exercise. In this period of positive energy balance, the surplus energy is deposited as fat.

During the second or "static" phase of obesity, dietary intake may actually be reduced, yet body weight is maintained. Decreased appetite is the result of the following factors:

1. Negative feedback to the appetite center from adipose stores
2. Increased plasma levels of insulin in obese individuals. Insulin is thought to act directly on the satiety center to decrease food intake.
3. A decrease in the meal-induced heat increment associated with feeding in the obese individual, and a subsequent increase in usable energy. As a consequence, less food needs to be consumed.

CLINICAL SIGNS

Weight Loss

Initially, the animal with weight loss may present with clinical signs in addition to the weight loss. The animal with diabetes mellitus may have polydipsia and polyuria; the cat with hyperthyroidism may have tachycardia and a gallop rhythm; the animal with malassimilation syndrome may present with diarrhea. Regardless of the underlying cause, with continuing weight loss clinical signs of malnutrition develop (Table 7-5).

With continued tissue depletion, body temperature and heart rate fall in an attempt to conserve calories. Once all tissue reserves are exhausted, severe depression, hypothermia, hypotension, and death occur.

The weight loss observed in animals with malignant disease (cancer cachexia) is usually associated with anorexia, vomiting, diarrhea, and/or severe organ dysfunction.

Weight Gain

Often owners are apparently unaware of a weight gain problem in their pet, and the animal is presented for a problem caused by obesity (Table 7-6).

Table 7–5 *Clinical Signs of Undernutrition*

Weight loss
Fatigue, irritability, mental depression
Weakness, exercise intolerance
Hypothermia
Bradycardia
Hypotension
Failure to grow
Poor wound healing, delayed convalescence
Anorexia, dehydration
Reduced muscle mass
Pallor (anemia)
Skin hemorrhages
Dry, inelastic, wrinkled skin
Dry, lusterless, brittle hair
Reproductive abnormalities
   Failure to cycle (female)
   Gonadal atrophy (male)
Periodontal disease
Edema or ascites (hypoproteinemia)
Increased susceptibility to infection, disease
Signs of mineral deficiency (e.g., zinc deficiency leads to
   anorexia, vomiting, decreased wound healing, and thinning of
   the haircoat)
Signs of vitamin deficiency (e.g., thiamine [vitamin B_1]
   deficiency leads to anorexia, paralysis, and ventroflexion of the
   neck in the cat)

Table 7–6 *Consequences of Obesity*

Organ System	Obesity Contributes to
General	Tendency for lethargy, irritability, fatigue, inactivity
	Increased risk of complications associated with anesthesia and surgery
Musculoskeletal	Intervertebral disk disease
	Arthritis
	Degenerative joint disease
	Rupture of anterior cruciate ligament
Cardiovascular	Myocardial hypoxia
	Myocardial fat deposits
	Increased cardiac workload (cor pulmonale)
	Arrhythmias
	Exercise intolerance
	Heart failure
Respiratory	Decreased lung compliance
	Decreased total and vital lung capacity
	Decreased expiratory reserve volume
	Hypoxemia
	Alveolar hypoventilation Pickwickian syndrome
	Dyspnea
Integumentary	Heat intolerance (due to insulating properties of excess subcutaneous fat)
Endocrine	Insulin resistance
	Glucose intolerance
	Increased risk of diabetes mellitus
	Increased risk of hypertension (possibly due to hyperinsulinemia)
Gastrointestinal	Hepatobiliary dysfunction (hepatic lipidosis in the cat)
	Possible increased risk of pancreatitis
	Increased risk of constipation and flatulence
Reproductive	Increased risk of dystocia
	Decreased reproductive efficiency
Immune	Increased susceptibility to infection (especially viral diseases)
	Increased risk of wound infection and dehiscence

Historically, obese animals may have fatigue, irritability, exercise intolerance, and various degrees of dyspnea. A clinical entity of alveolar hypoventilation, similar to the Pickwickian syndrome in humans, has been observed in dogs.

The simplest way to recognize obesity is by physical examination. Excess fat may accumulate over the thorax, abdomen, iliac crests (particularly in the dog), and ventral abdomen (particularly in the cat). Chest auscultation may reveal increased bronchovesicular sounds. Some obese dogs have concurrent tracheal collapse and a dry "honking" cough.

The animal may be tachypneic, dyspneic, or even cyanotic. On thoracic radiographs, the lung field may appear small and dense on inspiration. The cardiac silhouette may appear large, the mediastinum wide, and the diaphragm cranially displaced. On the electrogradiogram, some obese animals have smaller than expected QRS complexes (less than 0.5–0.7 mV). Blood gas abnormalities may include hypoxemia and hypercapnia.

DIAGNOSTIC APPROACH

Weight Loss

In general, most owners are aware of significant weight loss in their pet and present the animal with additional signs (polydipsia, anorexia, change in behavior). A thorough history and physical examination may suggest the organ system involved. A minimum data base and extended data base may be necessary (Fig. 7-3). With weight loss of unexplained origin the gastrointestinal tract (including liver and pancreas), lymph nodes, lung, and bone marrow should be carefully evaluated for suggestions of a neoplastic process.

Weight Gain

For the animal with weight gain, every attempt should be made to diagnose the underlying, predisposing cause(s). A thorough history and physical examination should be performed on each case. From the history, an assessment of the animal's diet should be made. How many times a day is the animal being fed, or is food always available? How much and what type of food is being

offered? What amount of protein and fat is in the diet? How often and what type of snacks does the pet receive? Are table foods part of the diet? Who feeds the pet? The type and amount of exercise the pet receives is also a vital part of the history in the obese animal. Results of a minimum data base and extended data base may be helpful in establishing an underlying endocrinologic cause for the obesity (hypothyroidism, hyperadrenocorticism, diabetes mellitus, insulinoma).

MANAGEMENT

Weight Loss

Therapy for weight loss is directed at correcting the underlying cause and reestablishing a positive caloric–nitrogen balance. For appetite stimulation, tube feeding, and parenteral alimentation, see Chapter 8.

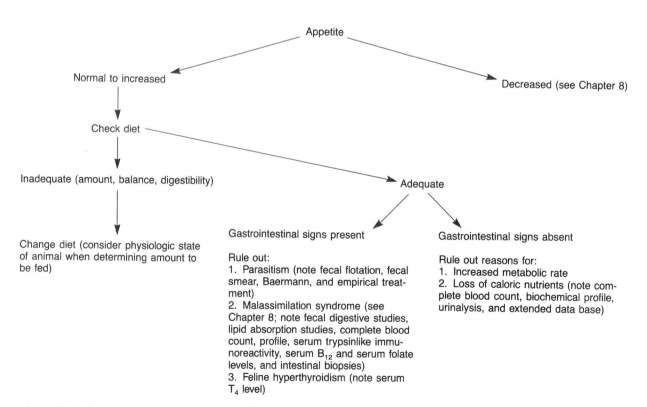

Figure 7–3. *Diagnostic approach to the patient with weight loss.*

Weight Gain

Therapy for weight gain is dependent on:

1. The successful identification and management of any underlying metabolic disease that may be contributing to the obesity
2. Setting up of a rational and proper dietary program
3. Excellent and continued rapport with the client
4. Total client compliance with dietary instructions

The greater the number of fat cells that develop during growth, the more difficult it is to lose weight and to maintain a lower body weight. Therefore, preventing obesity during growth is important. Once the animal becomes obese, a supervised weight reduction plan is needed.

Prior to instituting a weight reduction program, a complete physical and laboratory examination (complete blood count, biochemistry profile, urinalysis) should be performed. Any underlying disease contributing to the obesity or any disease occurring as a consequence of the obesity should be tended to.

There are five possible approaches to weight reduction: psychology, exercise, diet, surgery, and drugs (Table 7-7). At this time, surgery and drugs are not recommended. Providing psychologic support for the owner is critical. One should emphasize to the owner the deleterious effects of obesity (see Table 7-6) and stress that a successfully weight-reduced pet will be more active, alert, and healthy. A positive approach to weight reduction is important—emphasize that the animal can lose weight and you are willing to help see it happen!

Increasing exercise must be done with care, taking into account any underlying cardiopulmonary and musculoskeletal problems. Daily leash walks should be encouraged. As much as 10% of the total calories ingested can be utilized when moderate exercise (approximately 1 hour) is performed daily.

Treatment of obesity requires that caloric intake be less than caloric expenditure. Treatment of obesity by diet can be approached in one of two ways:

1. Moderate caloric restriction (providing 60% of canine and 70% of feline "optimal" weight maintenance energy requirements)
2. Total caloric restriction (starvation, dog only)

Moderate caloric restriction is the preferred method of weight reduction in small animals. The following steps are guidelines for a weight reduction program.

1. Weigh the dog or cat. Set a goal for weight reduction and estimate the time that will be needed to achieve that goal (Tables 7-8 and 7-9). Body weight decreases at a steady rate of 3% per week for the first 6 weeks, then about 2% per week after 8 weeks. Most animals will take 8 to 10 weeks to reach the desired body weight.
2. Decrease caloric intake to 60% (dog) or 70% (cat) of that required for maintenance of optimal body weight (not obese weight). For example calculations of amount of food to feed an obese dog or cat for weight reduction, see Tables 7-8 and 7-9. Calorie charts may be found in the nutrition textbooks listed under Additional Reading.
3. Choose an appropriate food for weight reduction. Feeding less of the dog or cat's regular diet (a diet not specifically formulated for weight reduction) may not work well because the lower food intake may not satisfy the animal's hunger sensation and because decreasing the amount fed may result in vitamin, mineral, or protein deficiencies. Feeding a commercially prepared weight-reducing diet that is low in fat and high in fiber (Table 7-10) is desirable for several reasons. The patient may continue to eat the same amount of food. Soluble carbohydrates and proteins provide fewer calories and elicit a more profound insulin response and a greater increase in metabolic rate than fat does. Meal-induced heat (the heat produced by the initial energy expended for food utilization) and a more sustained diet-induced thermogenesis, which occurs for several hours after a meal, is present with carbohydrate and protein ingestion but not with fat ingestion. Fiber (bulk) is an important satiety factor and reduces

Table 7–7 *Approaches to Weight Reduction*

Psychological: Need total client compliance
Exercise: Depends on medical condition
Diet: Change usually required (see text)
Surgery: Not recommended
Drugs: Not recommended. Do not use amphetamines to reduce appetite or thyroid hormone to increase metabolic rate. Dehydroepiandrosterone (DHEA) is a future possibility.

Table 7–8 *Calculation of Amount of Food to Feed a 25-kg Dog That Should Weigh 20 kg and Amount of Time Needed to Reach the Goal*

1. Determine the estimated maintenance energy requirement (MER)* for the obese dog's ideal adult weight:
   MER for dog = 2 ([30 × weight in kg] + 70)
   Obese dog weight = 25 kg
   Estimated ideal weight = 20 kg
   MER = 2[(30 × 20) + 70]
   = 1340 kcal/day
2. Determine daily energy intake for weight loss by moderate caloric restriction (60% for dog):
   MER = 1340 kcal/day
   MER × 0.60 = 840 kcal/day
3. Obtain the energy density of the diet to be fed for weight loss (see Table 7–10 or contact manufacturer for products not listed).
   Example: Canned canine (r/d)† = 260 kcal/15-oz can
4. Calculate the actual amount of food to feed each day for weight loss by dividing the daily energy intake for weight loss (step 2) by the energy density of the food (step 3):
   Daily energy intake for weight loss = 840 kcal/day
   Energy density of food = 260 kcal/can
   840 kcal/day ÷ 260 kcal/can = 3.2 cans/day
5. Divide the number of cans needed into two to four equal portions and feed two to four times/day.
6. Estimate time for weight loss to occur:
   Obese weight (25 kg) − ideal weight (20 kg) = excess body fat (5 kg)
   Excess body fat (5 kg) × 7700 kcal/kg‡ = total kcal excess (38,500 kcal)
   Estimated MER at ideal weight (1340 kcal) − kcal/day being ingested (840 kcal) = daily kcal deficit (500 kcal/day)
   Total kcal excess (38,500 kcal) ÷ the daily kcal deficit (500 kcal/day) = days required to reach ideal weight (73 days)

* MER represents the energy needed for nutrient digestion and absorption, normal physical activity, and temperature homeostasis. MER is measured in kcal metabolizable energy/day.
† Hill's Pet Products, Topeka, Kansas.
‡ The loss of 1 kg of adipose tissue requires an energy deficit of approximately 7700 kcal.
(Modified, with permission, from Lewis LD, Morris ML Jr, Hand MS. Small animal clinical nutrition III. Topeka: Mark Morris Assoc, 1987: 6–1.)

Table 7–9 *Calculation of Amount of Food to Feed a 7-kg Cat That Should Weigh 5 kg and Amount of Time Needed to Reach the Goal*

1. Determine the estimated maintenance energy requirement (MER)* for the obese cat's ideal adult weight:
   MER for cat = 1.4 ([30 × weight in kg] + 70)
   Obese cat weight = 7 kg
   Estimated ideal weight = 5 kg
   MER = 1.4 ([30 × 5] + 70)
   = 308 kcal/day
2. Determine daily energy intake for weight loss by moderate caloric restriction (70% for cat):
   MER = 308 kcal/day
   MER × 0.70 = 216 kcal/day
3. Obtain the energy density of the diet to be fed for weight loss (see Table 7–10 or contact manufacturer for products not listed).
   Example: Canned feline (r/d)† = 296 kcal/15-oz can
4. Calculate the actual amount of food to feed each day for weight loss by dividing the daily energy intake for weight loss (step 2) by the energy density of the food (step 3):
   Daily energy intake for weight loss = 216 kcal/day
   Energy density of food = 296 kcal/can
   216 kcal/day ÷ 296 kcal/can = 0.7 can/day
5. Divide 0.7 can into two to four equal portions and feed two to four times/day.
6. Estimate time for weight loss to occur:
   Obese weight (7 kg) − ideal weight (5 kg) = excess body fat (2 kg)
   Excess body fat (2 kg) × 7700 kcal/kg‡ = total kcal excess (15,400 kcal)
   Estimated MER at ideal weight (308 kcal) − kcal/day being ingested (216 kcal) = daily kcal deficit (92 kcal/day)
   Total kcal excess (15,400 kcal) ÷ the daily kcal deficit (92 kcal/day) = days required to reach ideal weight (167 days)

* MER represents the energy needed for nutrient digestion and absorption, normal physical activity, and temperature homeostasis. MER is measured in kcal metabolizable energy/day.
† Hill's Pet Products, Topeka, Kansas.
‡ The loss of 1 kg of adipose tissue requires an energy deficit of approximately 7700 kcal.
(Modified, with permission, from Lewis LD, Morris ML Jr, Hand MS. Small animal clinical nutrition III. Topeka: Mark Morris Assoc, 1987: 6–1.)

digestibility and availability of ingested energy nutrients. A high fiber, low calorie diet prolongs eating time and induces satiety at a lower caloric intake. Commercial and home-cooked reducing diets for the dog and cat are listed in Table 7-10.

4. Continue dietary management, either in the form of the diet used for weight loss or by using a diet that provides a fiber and fat content somewhere between that of a reducing diet and that of regular commercial food, for example, w/d (Hill's), Fit-n-Trim (Purina), Cycle 3 (Gaines), Alpo Lite (Alpo).

5. If the owner insists on giving snacks, recommend a cube of r/d (Hill's) or a nugget of dry r/d. Carrots (cooked) may be used as a treat. They provide 45 kilocalories per cup.

Total caloric restriction involves hospitalization and starvation. Water and vitamins are provided. This is not recommended in cats and should be used in dogs only when moderate caloric restriction has failed and the dog's condition warrants weight loss. For problems associated with total caloric restriction see Table 7-11.

Table 7–10 Pet Foods Intended for Management of Obesity

Diet	Form	Company	Fat (%)	Crude Fiber (%)	kcal ME/lb	kcal ME, % Below Average Commercial Diet	kcal/Can or Cup
FOR DOGS							
Canine r/d	Can	Hill's	7.0	25	1100	45.0	260/15-oz can
Canine r/d	Dry	Hill's	7.0	22	1150	36.1	200/cup
Canine w/d	Can	Hill's	12.1	13.2	1645	17.8	432/15-oz can
Canine w/d	Dry	Hill's	7.4	16.4	1429	20.6	220/cup
Canine low-fat homemade reducing diet			12.5	5.1	1614	19.3	
¼ lb cooked lean ground beef							
½ cup uncreamed cottage cheese							
2 cups carrots							
2 cups green beans							
1.5 tsp dicalcium phosphate							
Vitamin–mineral supplement							
Fit-N-Trim	Dry	Purina	8.7	9	1410	21.7	270/cup
Cycle 3	Can	Gaines	14	8	1647	17.6	357/14-oz can
Cycle 3	Dry	Gaines	10	5	1622	9.9	211/cup
FOR CATS							
Feline r/d	Can	Hill's	8.4	28.3	1340	31–43	296/15-oz can
Feline r/d	Dry	Hill's	8.2	18.5	1450	17	181/cup
Feline w/d	Can	Hill's	17	12	1635	15–30	211/cup
Feline low-fat homemade reducing diet			11.3	0.1	1950	0–18	
1.5 lb cooked liver, ground							
1 cup cooked rice							
1 tsp vegetable oil							
1 tsp calcium carbonate							
Vitamin–mineral supplement							

ME = metabolizable energy
(With permission from LD Lewis, ML Morris Jr, MS Hand. Small animal clinical nutrition III. Topeka: Mark Morris Assoc, 1987, 6-26.)

Dogs on total caloric restriction tend to exhibit less hunger after the first few days of the diet than dogs with partial caloric restriction. Expect 8% loss of body weight in the first week (primarily due to loss of water and sodium), 5% loss in the second week, and 3% to 4% loss thereafter. When the desired weight is achieved, introduce a maintenance diet gradually over 2 to 3 days. A 3% to 4% increase in weight is expected upon refeeding (largely due to sodium and water retention).

Table 7–11 Problems Associated with Total Caloric Restriction

Expense of hospitalization
Lack of owner compliance—obesity may recur once dog goes home
Diarrhea (during first 2 weeks of starvation)
Decreased urine production (particularly a problem in the older dog with compromised renal function)
Mild increase in circulating ketone bodies (not to be confused with diabetic ketoacidosis)
Magnesium depletion (predisposing to hyperirritability and convulsions)
Debatable effectiveness—weight loss in the form of adipose tissue is only 3% to 4% greater after 7 weeks of fasting than it is with 7 weeks of moderate caloric restriction

PATIENT MONITORING

The prognosis for the patient with weight loss depends on how quickly the underlying cause of the weight loss is identified and managed and how rapidly a positive caloric balance is reestablished in the body. Weight loss of 30% to 50% of lean body mass is usually fatal.

Weight gain predisposes the animal to other medical problems (see Table 7-6). The goal of weight reduction is slow, steady weight loss (1%–3% of total body weight per week). Once the desired weight is achieved, the animal should be weighed monthly. If the animal begins to regain weight, the amount being fed should be decreased by 10% or the animal should be placed back on a commercial reducing diet.

In the obese diabetic patient on a weight-reducing program, blood glucose should be monitored weekly, since insulin requirements are expected to decrease as weight decreases.

Prognosis for weight reduction is good if there is excellent owner acceptance and compliance with the program.

ADDITIONAL READING

Allen DG, Kruth SA. Obesity and the cardiopulmonary patient. In: Allen DG, Kruth SA, eds. Small animal cardiopulmonary medicine. Toronto: BC Decker, 1988: 137.

Anderson GL, Lewis LO. Obesity. In: Kirk RW, ed. Current veterinary therapy VII. Philadelphia: WB Saunders, 1980: 1034.

Brown SA. Obesity. In: Lorenz MD, Cornelius LM, eds. Small animal medical diagnosis. Philadelphia: JB Lippincott, 1987: 98.

Crow SE, Oliver J. Cancer cachexia. Compendium of Continuing Education 1981; 3:681.

Donoghue S, Kronfeld DS. A comparative medical approach to obesity. In: Pidgen G, ed. Proceedings of the 6th Annual Veterinary Medical Forum 1988: 705.

Fenner WR. Obesity and cachexia. In: Fenner WR, ed. Quick reference to veterinary medicine. Philadelphia: JB Lippincott, 1982: 355.

Hamlin RL, Buffington CA. Nutrition and the heart. Vet Clin North Am 1989; 19:527.

Hand MS, Armstrong PJ, Allen TA. Obesity: Occurrence, treatment and prevention. Vet Clin North Am 1989; 19:447.

Joshua JO. The obese dog and some clinical repercussions. Journal of Small Animal Practice 1970; 11:601.

Lewis LD, Morris ML, Hand MS. Small animal clinical nutrition III. Topeka: Mark Morris Assoc, 1987.

Lorenz MD. Weight loss. In: Lorenz MD, Cornelius LM, eds. Small animal medical diagnosis. Philadelphia: JB Lippincott, 1987: 90.

MacEwen EG. Hormonal approach for the treatment of obesity. In: Pidgen G, ed. Proceedings of the 6th Annual Veterinary Medical Forum 1988: 666.

MacEwen EG. Physiologic and metabolic aspects of obesity. In: Pidgen G, ed. Proc 6th Ann Vet Med Forum 1988: 663.

McKiernan BC. Lower respiratory tract diseases. In: Ettinger SJ, ed. Textbook of veterinary internal medicine. Philadelphia: WB Saunders, 1983: 760.

Nelson RW, Morrison WB, Lueus AG. Diencephalic syndrome secondary to intracranial astrocytoma in a dog. J Am Vet Med Assoc 1981; 179:1004.

Sheffy BE. Nutrition, infection and immunity. Compendium of Continuing Education 1985; 7:990.

Ward A. The fat-dog problem: How to solve it. Veterinary Medicine Small Animal Clinician 1984; 79:781.

8

ANOREXIA, POLYPHAGIA, AND PICA

Doreen M. Houston

Alterations in appetite are commonly encountered problems in veterinary practice. *Anorexia* occurs in a myriad of disease processes. It may be classified as complete or partial, sudden or gradual, pathologic, physiologic, or psychologic. Anorexia may also be classified as primary—if the disease process involves the appetite center of the hypothalamus, or secondary—if the disease process affects endocrine and neural control of hunger. Secondary anorexia is the major cause of anorexia in small animals. True anorexia must be differentiated from pseudoanorexia, a condition in which appetite is maintained but there is reluctance to eat due to oropharyngeal disease.

Polyphagia is the ingestion of food in excess of caloric requirements. In the dog and cat, polyphagia is usually the result of diseases that create either a negative caloric balance or an increased metabolic rate. Consequently, most cases of polyphagia are presented with other clinical signs.

Pica has been defined as the ingestion of unnatural objects. Coprophagy, the ingestion of feces, is perhaps the best known example of pica in the dog. Cats are less commonly afflicted with this behavioral abnormality.

CAUSES

Causes of anorexia are dealt with under the categories of pseudoanorexia (Table 8-1), primary anorexia (Table 8-2), and secondary anorexia (Table 8-3).

Causes of polyphagia are dealt with as physiologic, psychologic, or pathologic (Table 8-4).

The causes of pica in the dog and cat are speculative. They are listed in Table 8-5.

PATHOPHYSIOLOGY

Anorexia

The drive to eat is influenced by hunger (a physiologic state), appetite (the desire for food), and satiety (the lack of desire to eat because caloric needs have been satisfied).

Disorders or diseases that destroy or structurally inhibit the appetite center of the hypothalamus can result in complete anorexia.

Many diseases or disorders produce anorexia because they disturb the neurologic, endo-

Table 8–1 *Causes of Pseudoanorexia*

Neurologic disorder (difficulty prehending, masticating, or
swallowing food due to impairment of cranial nerve V, VII, IX,
X, or XII)
Disorder of the oral cavity (pharyngitis, stomatitis, tooth root
abscess, foreign body)
Retrobulbar disease (abscess, neoplasia)
Maxillary or mandibular fracture or dislocation
Myositis (temporomandibular, masseter muscles)
Tetanus (unable to open mouth)
Esophagitis
Blindness (unable to find food)

Table 8–2 *Possible Causes of Primary Anorexia*

Anosmia (sense of smell is especially important in cats)
Psychologic factors
  Stress
  Fear
  Anxiety
  Environmental change
  Unpalatable food
Neurologic dysfunction
  Hypothalamic disorder
  Intracranial pain
  Increased intracranial pressure due to edema or
    hydrocephalus

Table 8–3 *Causes of Secondary Anorexia*

Pain (any source)
Fever
Neoplasia
Infectious diseases
Abdominal organ disorders
  Enlargement
  Inflammation
  Neoplasia
Toxic agents
  Endogenous: metabolic waste products (e.g., urea, ammonia)
  Exogenous: drugs (e.g., erythromycin, doxorubicin), poisons
  (arsenic, detergents, mushrooms)
Endocrine disorders
  Hypoadrenocorticism
  Hypothyroidism
Other causes
  Congestive heart failure
  Hot weather
  Hypercalcemia

Table 8–4 *Causes of Polyphagia*

PHYSIOLOGIC (INCREASED METABOLIC DEMANDS)
Cold weather
Gestation
Lactation
Exercise

PSYCHOLOGIC
Overfeeding (e.g., due to recent change to more palatable food)

PATHOLOGIC
Primary polyphagia
  Destruction of satiety center due to neoplasia, trauma, or
    infection
Secondary polyphagia
  Increased metabolic rate (e.g., feline hyperthyroidism)
  Catabolic disorders (e.g., hyperadrenocorticism, diabetes
    mellitus, exocrine pancreatic insufficiency, malabsorption
    syndrome [lymphangiectasia], hypoglycemia, low calorie
    diet)
  Drug-induced (e.g., glucocorticoids, anticonvulsants,
    [phenobarbital, primidone], megestrol acetate)

Table 8–5 *Possible Causes of Pica*

PUPPIES
Teething discomfort
Exploratory behavior
Boredom
Lack of exercise
Hypophosphatemia (excessive calcium supplementation)
Esophageal dysphagia (vascular ring anomaly)
Intestinal parasitism
Improper diet (lack of adequate calories)

ADULT DOGS
Lack of exercise
Boredom
Lack of human contact
Sodium deficiency (e.g., hypoadrenocorticism, syndrome of
  inappropriate antidiuretic hormone)
Phosphorus deficiency (excessive dietary calcium
  supplementation)
Gastroenteritis (ingestion of grass)
Catabolic disease states (e.g., hyperadrenocorticism, diabetes
  mellitus)
Starvation (lack of caloric intake)

KITTENS
Wool chewing—lack of nursing time, possibly lanolin
  stimulation

ADULT CATS
Wool chewing—possibly hereditary in Siamese
Anemia
Catabolic disease states (e.g., hyperthyroidism)

crinologic, metabolic, or other mechanisms that control hunger, appetite, and satiety. Pain from any cause may inhibit neuronal stimulation of the appetite center. Pain may also produce a psychologic abnormality that inhibits the sensation of hunger. Inflammation of the liver, pancreas, stomach, bowel, kidneys, and peritoneum may produce anorexia via neural mechanisms that inhibit the appetite center (Fig. 8-1). This is a common cause of anorexia in small animals. Endogenous or exogenous toxins may directly inhibit the appetite center, may cause visceral organ inflammation, leading to inhibition of appetite, or may stimulate the chemoreceptor trigger zone in the medulla, creating a sensation of nausea and consequently anorexia (see Fig. 8-1). It is speculated that certain cancers in the dog and cat may produce peptides or nucleotides (*e.g.*, tryptophan) that inhibit feeding regulators.

Interleukin-1, a mediator released from mononuclear cells in infectious processes, is thought to be a factor in anorexia associated with sepsis.

If food intake remains low (regardless of the initiating cause of anorexia), compensatory measures occur in the body, sometimes with deleterious effects to the animal (Fig. 8-2).

Polyphagia

Polyphagia may be physiologic or pathologic in nature. Physiologic polyphagia is an appropriate response to cold weather, increased exercise, pregnancy, or lactation. It has been shown that

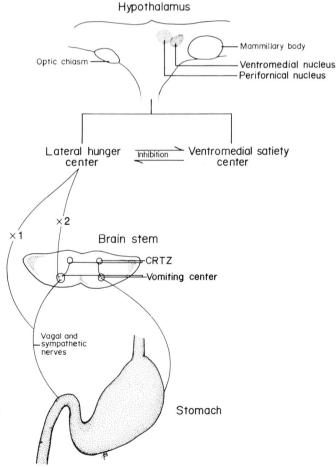

Figure 8–1. *Pathophysiology of secondary anorexia. X1: Inflammation, pain, or distension in the gastrointestinal tract, pancreas, liver, mesentery, peritoneum, and urinary tract can interfere with stimulation of the lateral hunger center by inhibiting vagal and sympathetic nerve input. X2: Bacterial toxins, metabolic disorders (e.g., uremia, acidosis), and drugs that create nausea (e.g., digitalis) can inhibit stimulation of the lateral appetite center directly or through input via the vomiting center and chemoreceptor trigger zone (CRTZ), which subsequently inhibits the appetite center.*

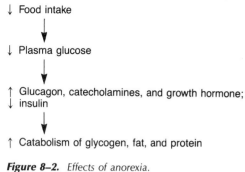

↓ Food intake

↓ Plasma glucose

↑ Glucagon, catecholamines, and growth hormone; ↓ insulin

↑ Catabolism of glycogen, fat, and protein

Energy produced not sufficient to meet energy demands

↓ Tissue repair
↓ Resistance to disease
↓ Body weight (see Chapter 7, Weight Loss and Weight Gain)

Figure 8–2. *Effects of anorexia.*

lowering environmental temperature from 15°C to 8.5°C results in approximately a 25% increase in caloric requirements to maintain body weight. With a moderate increase in exercise the animal will require about 40% more calories. A pregnant bitch requires 15% to 25% more calories during the last 3 to 4 weeks of gestation. During lactation, the bitch requires approximately one and a half times maintenance requirements in the first week of lactation, two times maintenance requirements in the second week, and three times maintenance requirements in the third week to the time of weaning.

Pathologic polyphagia may be primary or secondary. Primary polyphagic disorders (those that destroy the satiety center) are uncommon in small animals. In the normal animal, the accumulation of fat stores in the body tends to decrease feeding behavior (see Chapter 7). As the degree of adipose tissue increases, the rate of feeding decreases. Free fatty acids and other fat metabolites likely have a negative feedback regulatory effect on feeding. In the obese dog with primary polyphagia, a part of the feeding regulatory mechanism is likely lost or the response is blunted. Consequently, feeding continues despite the obvious accumulation of adipose tissue.

Secondary polyphagic disorders are common in small animals. Disorders such as feline hyperthyroidism cause inhibition of the satiety center and stimulation of the appetite center. Drugs such as glucocorticoids, anticonvulsants (phenobarbital, primidone), and megestrol acetate may directly stimulate the appetite center.

Pica

The pathophysiology of pica is speculative. Puppies with teething discomfort may chew on wood, shoes, socks, and so on to hasten tooth eruption and bring relief to swollen, painful gums. Exploratory behavior is normal in puppies and, with proper training, should last only a short time. Puppies with chronic esophageal dysphagia (vascular ring anomaly and megaesophagus) may have pica due to underlying malnutrition and vitamin or mineral deficiencies. Intestinal parasitism in the puppy may lead to malabsorption and pica. Puppies receiving an improper diet may develop pica as a response to caloric deficiencies.

Wool chewing in cats may be due to a lack of nursing time as kittens, and has been identified as a possible sex-linked, genetic defect in Siamese and Siamese-cross cats, becoming apparent between 5 and 6 months of age. Wool sucking can generalize to sucking of other fabrics.

Anemic cats and dogs will occasionally lick soil, litter, walls, or rusty objects, possibly as a result of deficiencies of iron or other minerals. Animals with sodium deficiency (*e.g.,* syndrome of inappropriate antidiuretic hormone secretion, Addison's disease) or phosphorus deficiency (*e.g.,* secondary to excessive calcium supplementation) may have behavioral changes, including pica.

Grass ingestion in dogs and cats results in vomiting, which may be therapeutic to an animal with gastroenteritis. It may also cause gastroenteritis.

Although ingestion of puppies' stools from

Table 8–6 *Diseases That May Lead to Coprophagy*

Exocrine pancreatic insufficiency
Intestinal parasitism
Feline hyperthyroidism
Diabetes mellitus
Hyperadrenocorticism
Malabsorption syndromes (e.g., lymphangiectasia)
Chronic esophageal dysphagia (e.g., vascular ring anomaly)

birth to approximately 3 weeks of age is considered normal behavior in the lactating bitch, coprophagy is otherwise abnormal. Coprophagy may occur secondary to dietary imbalance or to catabolic disease states in which the animal is not obtaining sufficient dietary calories to prevent malnutrition–starvation (Table 8-6).

Boredom, lack of exercise, and lack of human contact and discipline are likely leading causes of pica in the dog.

CLINICAL SIGNS

Anorexia

Animals that are anorectic for more than a few days may have potassium, zinc, vitamin B, or essential amino acid deficiencies. Potassium deficiency results in lethargy, weakness, and aggravation of the anorexia. Zinc deficiency decreases the sense of smell, contributing to the lack of desire to eat. Vitamin B deficiencies are a problem in the cat, especially because normal requirements are eight times higher than in the dog. Thiamine (vitamin B_1) deficiency in the cat results in ventral flexion of the neck, abnormal reflexes, and muscular weakness, which further contributes to the anorexia.

Arginine is an essential amino acid for both adult dogs and cats. It is a component of the urea cycle. With arginine deficiency, conversion of ammonia to urea is suppressed, allowing blood ammonia levels to rise to toxic levels. Clinical signs of arginine deficiency include hypersalivation, hyperesthesia, vomiting, ataxia, and muscular tremors. Some cases progress to coma and death.

If anorexia persists, nutritional depletion occurs (see Chapter 7). Physical examination may reveal a lack of subcutaneous fat and muscle wasting. Prolonged absence of food intake adversely effects all body systems. Weight loss of greater than 30% of lean body mass is often lethal.

Polyphagia

Because polyphagia is generally secondary to an underlying problem, the animal often presents with associated problems such as polydipsia, polyuria, alopecia, diarrhea, nervousness, or tachycardia, depending on the cause. Physical examination may reveal obesity, emaciation, or normal weight (see Chapter 7). Animals with malassimilation syndrome may have bulky, malformed stools.

Pica

Animals with pica often have no abnormal findings on physical examination. If the pica is due to a lack of sufficient caloric intake or catabolic disease, the animal may be thin or cachectic. Halitosis often accompanies coprophagy. There may be excessive wear of the teeth if the animal has been chewing rocks. If large amounts of dirt, sand, or wool have been swallowed, signs of gastroenteritis or gastrointestinal obstruction may be evident (vomiting, diarrhea, acute abdomen).

DIAGNOSTIC APPROACH

Anorexia

Since anorexia is a common sign of many diseases, the principal approach to the diagnosis is the identification and treatment of the underlying cause (Fig. 8-3). From the history one should determine if the diet has been changed to a less palatable food. The owner should be questioned as to whether the animal has had any apparent difficulty with vision. The animal should be offered food and watched to see if it sniffs the food. A

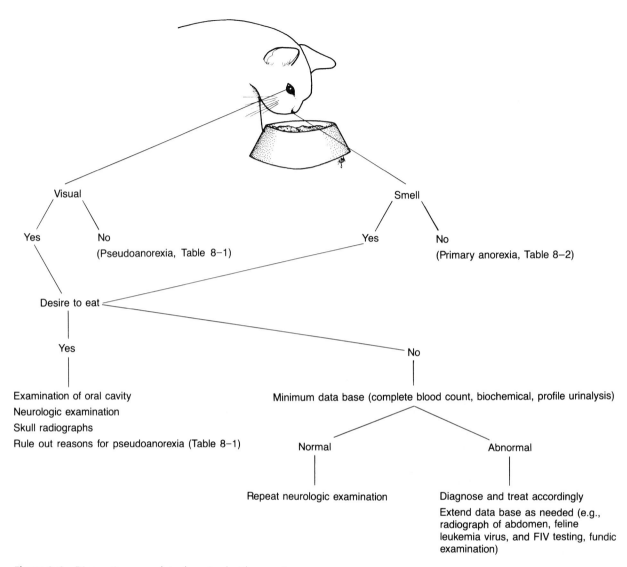

Figure 8–3. *Diagnostic approach to the animal with anorexia.*

complete physical examination should be performed. If no abnormalities of the head, oral cavity, or neck are detected, one should look for causes of secondary anorexia. A complete blood count, serum biochemistry profile, and urinalysis may be needed to rule out a variety of systemic, metabolic, and endocrinologic diseases that may be responsible for the anorexia. Depending on the results obtained, extension of the data base may be necessary (*e.g.,* radiography, laparotomy).

Polyphagia

The initial diagnostic step in the animal with polyphagia is to determine if the animal's weight has increased, decreased, or remained the same. If weight gain has occurred, the owner should be questioned carefully about drug therapy and diet (Table 8-7). A full neurologic and ophthalmologic examination should be performed if a hypothalamic tumor is suspected.

If weight loss has occurred, the clinician should look for evidence of caloric deficiency diseases (catabolic diseases) or disorders that result in an increased metabolic rate (Table 8-8).

A complete blood count, serum biochemistry profile, and urinalysis can help differentiate some causes of secondary polyphagia. Fecal digestive tests, lipid absorption studies, and results of trypsinlike immunoreactivity, serum B12, and serum folate measurements may be required to differentiate maldigestive disorders and intestinal malabsorption syndromes.

Pica

The diagnostic approach for an animal with pica includes a complete history and physical examination to help determine if the pica is strictly a behavioral problem or if an underlying metabolic

problem appears to exist. Dietary history should be carefully analyzed for any deficiencies. The owners should be questioned as to any change in the animal's environment (*e.g.*, addition to the family, change in the household, diet change). A minimum data base, including a complete blood count, serum biochemistry profile, urinalysis, and multiple fecal analyses (parasitology and fecal digestive studies) will help rule out underlying disease.

MANAGEMENT

The medical management of the patient with anorexia, polyphagia, or pica is usually directed toward the underlying primary disorder.

Anorexia

In the case of the anorectic patient, antipyretic, anti-inflammatory, analagesic, or antiemetic agents may be needed to reduce fever, pain, or gastrointestinal disturbances that cause or contribute to the anorexia.

Effective treatment of the anorectic patient also requires management of the nutritional status of the animal. Prolonged deficiency of certain amino acids, vitamins, and minerals may actually be more detrimental to the patient than the original cause of the anorexia.

Recent weight loss of greater than 10% of normal body weight (not caused by dehydration), restricted food intake for more than 3 days, and continuing nutrient losses (vomiting, diarrhea, cancer cachexia, burns, protein-losing enteropathy) are all indications for nutritional support. Before nutritional support is implemented, underlying fluid, acid-base, or electrolyte abnormalities should be corrected. Providing nutritional supplementation via the gastrointestinal tract is the preferred method except in patients with severe gastrointestinal disease (*e.g.*, vomiting, obstruction, pancreatitis). One of several approaches may be taken when enteral alimentation is indicated. If the oral cavity is normal, appetite may be stimulated or the animal may be force-fed (Table 8-9).

Table 8–7 *Causes of Polyphagia and Weight Gain*

DIET

Recent change to more palatable food

DRUGS

Excess glucocorticoids
Megestrol acetate
Anticonvulsant therapy (phenobarbital, primidone)

TUMORS

Hypothalamic tumor

Table 8–8 *Causes of Polyphagia and Weight Loss*

INCREASED METABOLIC RATE

Feline hyperthyroidism

CATABOLIC DISORDERS

Hyperadrenocorticism
Diabetes mellitus
Exocrine pancreatic insufficiency
Malabsorption syndrome (infiltrative bowel disease,
  lymphangiectasia)
Hypoglycemia (insulinoma, sepsis)
Low calorie diet

Table 8–9 *Oral Feeding*

METHODS TO STIMULATE APPETITE

GENERAL
Clean nose
Warm food (25.6°C to 39.4°C) to volatilize the odor
Sprinkle food lightly with garlic or onion powder
Feed food with strong odor (canned food, human baby food-strained meats)
Handfeed animal or stay with animal and encourage it to eat (pet animal)
Potassium supplementation (1 to 2 mEq/kg/day PO)
Zinc supplementation (1 to 2 mg/kg/day PO)
Vitamin B$_{12}$ supplementation (50 to 100 μg/day PO in cats; 100 to 200 μg/day PO in dogs)

DRUGS
Benzodiazepines (diazepam 0.05 to 0.4 mg/kg b.i.d. IV or oxazepam 2.5 mg PO per cat, flurazepam hydrochloride 0.2 to 0.4 mg/kg PO for 4 to 7 days in dogs and cats)
Cyproheptadine (4 mg/kg/day PO)
Prednisolone (0.25 to 0.5 mg/kg/day PO)
Stanozolol (1 to 2 mg b.i.d. PO or 25 to 50 mg IM weekly)
Nandrolone decanoate (5 mg/kg maximum or 200 mg/patient IM weekly)

FORCE-FEEDING METHODS

Place food on cat's paws to stimulate licking response
Place food into the pharyngeal area to stimulate the swallowing reflex
Use highly digestible, palatable, high-fat, and calorie-dense diets (c/d [Hill's], Clinical Care Liquid Diets (Pet-Ag Inc), human baby food strained meats such as chicken, lamb, veal, and beef)

In anorexic cats, benzodiazepines (diazepam, oxazepam, flurazepam) have been used successfully to stimulate appetite. Benzodiazepines stimulate eating by enhancing the inhibitory effect of τ-aminobutyric acid on serotonin. Under normal circumstances, serotonin is released from the medial hypothalamus and stimulates cholecystokinin release. Cholecystokinin inhibits endogenous opiates that normally stimulate eating. The benzodiazepines should not be used for more than 2 days to stimulate appetite.

Diazepam is most effective when given intravenously. The effect of intravenous diazepam is almost immediate and, consequently, food must be available at the time the drug is administered. Unlike the situation in normal animals, the appetite-stimulating properties of diazepam decrease with time in sick animals. Oxazepam is a more powerful appetite stimulant than diazepam, but its oral administration tends to make it less effective clinically. Flurazepam hydrochloride is also effective orally and has a longer duration of activity than diazepam and oxazepam. In severely ill or depressed animals, reduced dosages of the benzodiazepines should be used because of the sedative properties of the drugs.

Cyproheptadine and pizotyline are serotonin antagonists that have been shown, experimentally, to stimulate the appetite of cats but not dogs. Extreme excitability and aggression have been reported in approximately 20% of cats treated with cyproheptadine. Pizotyline is used to treat vascular headache in humans. No dose has been established for its use in the cat.

The specific mechanism of glucocorticoid stimulation of appetite is unknown; however, low doses in dogs and cats may be of some benefit. Anabolic steroids such as stanozolol and nandrolone decanoate have been used to stimulate appetite by providing a positive nitrogen balance. Prolonged use of oral anabolic steroids is not recommended, as hepatotoxicity may result. Although, experimentally, lithium, morphine sulfate, and phenobarbital can stimulate appetite in other species, they are not presently recommended for use in small animals for this purpose.

Human baby food meats may be used to stimulate appetite, but are not nutritionally balanced in vitamin or trace mineral content for the dog or cat and should not be used for more than 3 days.

If tube feeding (enteral nutrition) is required, one of several routes may be used: orogastric, nasoesophageal, pharyngostomy, or gastrostomy. For procedures, indications, and contraindications of the techniques see the appropriate section in Chapter 80. The goal of enteral nutrition in the anorectic patient is to provide caloric, protein, electrolyte, vitamin, and mineral requirements. An example of the calculations of appropriate nutritional requirements is given in Figure 8-4. Basal energy requirement (BER) is defined as the energy utilized by an animal lying down in a thermoneutral environment. Smaller animals have a higher energy requirement on a per kilogram basis because of the larger surface area : body weight ratio, and consequently have greater heat losses by radiation and convection.

1. Basal energy requirement (BER) = 30 × weight (kg) + 70
   30 × 20 kg + 70 = 670 kcal/day

2. Illness energy requirement (IER) = BER × 2
   670 kcal/day × 2 = 1340 kcal/day

3. Amount of feline p/d to be fed through tube = IER ÷ caloric density of p/d
   1340 kcal/day ÷ 0.8 kcal/ml = 1680 ml/day

4. 1680 ml/day divided into three feedings = 560 ml per feeding. In a 20-kg dog, 560 ml = 28 ml/kg, which is approximately 30% of normal gastric capacity and should be well tolerated.

5. Day 1: Give ⅓ the amount of blenderized diet needed (see Table 8–10) plus ⅔ water. Divide into three equal feedings. ⅓ (1680 ml of blenderized diet) + ⅔ (1680 ml of water) = 560 ml diet + 1120 ml water = 1680 ml of diluted diet/day

6. Day 2: Give ⅔ diet + ⅓ water divided into three equal feedings. ⅔ (1680 ml of blenderized diet) + ⅓ (1680 ml of water) = 1120 ml diet + 560 ml water

7. Day 3: Give 1680 ml undiluted diet divided into three equal feedings.

8. The dog should be offered unblended diet frequently to determine when voluntary eating begins and when the tube can be removed.

Figure 8–4. *Worksheet for calculation of nutritional requirements for enteral nutrition for a 20-kg dog with sepsis.*

The BER (kcal/day) is estimated to be 70 × body weight (kg) $^{0.75}$. For animals weighing more than 2 kg, BER may be estimated using the following formula:

$$BER (kcal/day) = 30 \times body\ weight\ (kg) + 70$$

Maintenance energy requirements (MER) represent the energy needed for nutrient digestion and absorption, normal physical activity, and temperature homeostasis. In the normal dog, MER is approximately two times BER. In the normal cat, MER is approximately 1.4 times BER. To determine the caloric needs of an ill patient, that is, the illness energy requirements (IER), an estimate of the effect of the disease process on energy expenditure must be made. The MER for mature hospitalized patients is approximately 1.25 × BER; the IER for a dog or cat undergoing major surgery or trauma is approximately 1.3 to 1.6 × BER; and for patients with severe infections, sepsis, or burns, the IER is approximately 1.5 to 2 × BER. To determine the amount of nutrients to feed the dog or cat, divide the calculated IER by the caloric density (metabolizable energy density) of the chosen food (Tables 8-10 and 8-11). Diets for tube feeding should supply all required nutrients without causing digestive disturbances and should supply requirements for specific organ disease. If canine or feline prescription diets are used for enteral nutrition, vitamin, mineral, or electrolyte supplemen-

Table 8–10 *Blenderized Tube Feeding Diet for Dogs and Cats**

½ can (224 g) Feline Prescription Diet p/d†
¾ cup (170 ml) water

Blend for 60 seconds at high speed. Strain twice through a kitchen strainer (approximately 1 mm mesh). Yields 390 ml. Administer an amount sufficient to meet the animal's energy needs. Divide the amount into two or three feedings per day.

	Analysis	
	As Fed	
	Dry Matter	
Moisture (%)	83	0
Protein (%)	7.4	44.2 or 33% of calories
Fat (%)	5.0	29.6 or 55% of calories
Carbohydrate (%)	2.8	17.0 or 12% of calories
Calcium (%)	0.19	1.1
Phosphorus (%)	0.13	0.8
Sodium (%)	0.10	0.6
Metabolizable energy	0.8 kcal/ml	7.76 kcal/g

* *Recommended for orogastric, nasogastric, pharyngostomy, or gastrostomy feeding (but not enterostomy). Administer through size 8 or larger French tubes that have an opening at the tip (end port). Additional ports on the sides are optional. Tubes with only side ports will plug with this diet. Failure to follow all instructions may result in plugging of the feeding tube. Straining removes particulates but has no effect on nutrient content.*
† *Use Feline, not Canine Prescription Diet p/d. Use of the canine diet results in a liquid that is too viscous for tube feeding.*
(With permission from LD Lewis, ML Morris Jr, MS Hand. Small animal clinical nutrition III. Topeka: Mark Morris Assoc, 1987, 5-29.)

Table 8–11 *Tube Feeding Diets for Dogs and Cats With Renal, Hepatic, or Gastrointestinal Disease*

Clinical Condition	Liquid Diet*	Metabolizable Energy Density† (kcal/ml)	Protein (g/500 ml)
CANINE			
renal failure	Canine k/d + water	0.62	9.5
Advanced renal failure	Canine u/d + water	0.66	6.4
Hepatic failure	Canine k/d + water	0.62	9.5
Gastrointestinal disease	Canine i/d + water	0.57	16.7
FELINE			
Fenal failure	Feline k/d + water	0.90	19.6
Hepatic failure	Feline k/d + water	0.90	19.6
Gastrointestinal disease	Feline c/d + water	0.62	27.5
Human Liquid Diets			
CANINE			
Renal failure	Travasorb Renal (Travenol)	1.35	11.5
Hepatic failure	Travasorb Hepatic (Travenol)	1.10	14.5
Gastrointestinal disease	Feed elemental diets		

* *For each diet, blend at high speed for 60 seconds ½ can (224 g) of Prescription Diet (Hill's) indicated plus 10 oz (282 ml) of water. Then strain the blended mixture twice through a 1-mm mesh strainer. The resulting liquid diet will pass through a size 8 or larger French tube. The tube must have an opening at the tip (end port). Additional side ports are optional.*
† *Administer an amount sufficient to meet the animal's energy needs. Divide this amount by the number of daily feedings recommended.*
(With permission from LD Lewis, ML Morris Jr, MS Hand. Small animal clinical nutrition III. Topeka: Mark Morris Assoc, 1987.)

tation is not necessary. Multiple small feedings, three or more times per day, are recommended, as some degree of gastric contraction and diminished digestive function is to be anticipated in the anorectic animal. The use of canned diets is preferred for enteral nutrition. These diets can be made into thin gruels and given to the animal through pharyngostomy and large-bore gastrostomy tubes (Chapter 80). Nasoesophageal (Chapter 80) and jujenostomy tube feeding is best accomplished with completely liquid diets (*e.g.,* Clinical Care Canine and Feline Liquid Diets). These veterinary products are better tolerated than those specifically formulated for humans (*e.g.,* Ensure and Osmalite). Ensure diets are highly osmolar and also need to be supplemented with additional protein. Vomiting, diarrhea, and abdominal cramping may occur with the use of this product.

If the gastrointestinal tract cannot be used for nutritional support, then intravenous feeding (parenteral nutrition) is required. This is a time-consuming and expensive endeavor and should be considered in the dog and cat only when one anticipates that there will be an inability to absorb enterally administered nutrients for longer than 3 to 5 days (*e.g.,* severe pancreatitis, intractable vomiting or diarrhea, small bowel resection). A central venous catheter (see Central Venous Pressure in Chapter 80) should be placed aseptically (feeding solutions are excellent media for microbial growth).

The three basic components of parenteral nutrition are amino acids, lipids, and dextrose. Solutions of amino acids and electrolytes are commercially available (Travasol With Electrolytes [Travenol Laboratories], Aminosyn [Abbott Hospital Products]). The basic solutions available contain all essential amino acids for dogs and cats with the exception of taurine. Taurine supplementation is recommended for cats requiring total parenteral nutrition (TPN) administration for longer than 7 days.

To provide some portion of the nonprotein calories and decrease the amount of dextrose required, lipids are used. They are an excellent concentrated energy source and supply essential fatty acids. Most of the commercially available products are isotonic and can be given through peripheral or central veins. Isotonic lipid emulsions may be given separately or mixed with the other components. Commercially available products contain soybean or sunflower oil, glycerol, and egg yolk phospholipids (Liposyn 10% and 20% [Abbott Hospital Products]). Lipid emulsions do not require a transition period for administration or a gradual reduction during termination.

Dextrose is used to provide a source of calories. Dextrose is inexpensive and compatible with most other solutions. If dextrose is used to provide all of the nonprotein calories, 25% of the anticipated amount is given initially and the administration rate is increased gradually over approximately 3 days. Hyperglycemia and hyperosmolality may occur if large volumes of concentrated dextrose solution are given without this transition period. Multivitamin additives may be combined with the TPN solution. Vitamin K should be given subcutaneously once weekly.

Example calculations of nutritional requirements for TPN in the dog and cat are presented in Figures 8-5 and 8-6. In meeting the calculated IER in the dog, 40% to 60% of the nonprotein calories are provided as lipid and the remainder as dextrose. In the cat, the protein calories are calculated and the result is subtracted from the IER (see Fig. 8-6). The remaining calories are provided as a 50 : 50 mixture of dextrose and lipid.

1. Basal energy requirement (BER) = 30 × weight (kg) + 70
   30 × 20 + 70 = 670 kcal/day

2. Illness energy requirement (IER) with sepsis = 1.5–2 × BER
   2 × 670 kcal/day = 1340 kcal/day (provide as nonprotein calories)

3. Protein requirement:
   4 g/kg in adult dogs
   6 g/kg in dogs with extraordinary protein loss
   1.5 g/kg in dogs with renal or hepatic failure

   4 g/kg × 20 kg = 80 g/day required

4. Volumes of nutrient solutions required:
   a. 8.5% amino acid solution = 85 mg protein/ml
      To supply 80 g of protein, approximately 941 ml is needed.
   b. 20% lipid solution = 2 kcal/ml
      To supply 40% to 60% of IER (1340 kcal × 50% = 670 kcal), 335 ml is needed (not for use in lipemic patient).
   c. 50% dextrose solution = 1.7 kcal/ml
      To supply 40% to 60% of IER (1340 kcal × 50% = 670 kcal), 394 ml is needed. Use 1/2 this volume on first day and increase to full volume on second day if no glucosuria is present.)

5. Total volume of TPN solution =
      941 ml of 8.5% amino acid solution
   + 335 ml of 20% lipid solution
   + 394 ml of 50% dextrose solution
   = 1670 ml
   Administer at approximately 70 ml/hour.

6. Electrolyte requirement: dependent on patient status and products selected

7. Vitamin requirement: Administer 0.5 mg/kg vitamin K subcutaneously on first day (10 mg) and weekly add 3 ml/10 kg day (6 ml) multivitamin to TPN solution. (Do not give more than 10 ml per day.)

Figure 8–5. *Worksheet for calculation of nutritional requirements for total parenteral nutrition (TPN) in a 20-kg dog with sepsis.*

1. Basal energy requirement (BER) = 30 × weight (kg) + 70
   30 × 5 kg + 70 = 220 kcal/day
2. Illness energy requirement (IER) = 1.4 × BER
   1.4 × 220 kcal/day = 308 kcal/day (provide as protein and nonprotein calories)
3. Protein requirement:
   6 g/kg in adult cats
   3.5 g/kg in cats with renal or hepatic failure

   6 g/kg × 5 kg = 30 g/day required
   Protein calories = 4 kcal/g = 120 kcal
   Nonprotein calories = IER − protein calories
   308 − 120 = 188 kcal
4. Volumes of nutrient solutions required:
   a. 8.5% amino acid solution = 85 mg protein/ml
      To supply 30 g of protein, 353 ml is needed.
   b. 20% lipid solution = 2 kcal/ml
      To supply 50% of nonprotein calories (i.e., 50% of 188 = 94 kcal), 47 ml is needed (not for use in lipemic cat).
   c. 50% dextrose solution = 1.7 kcal/ml
      To supply 50% of nonprotein calories (i.e., 50% of 188 = 94 kcal), approximately 55 ml is needed. Use ½ this volume on first day and increase to full volume on second day if no glucosuria is present.)
5. Total volume of TPN solution =
   353 ml of 8.5% amino acid solution
   + 47 ml of 20% lipid solution
   + 55 ml of 50% dextrose solution
   = 455 ml
   Administer at approximately 19 ml/hour.
6. Electrolyte requirement: dependent on patient status and products selected
7. Vitamin requirement: Administer 0.5 mg/kg vitamin K subcutaneously on first day (2.5 mg) and weekly add 3 ml/day multivitamin to TPN solution.

Figure 8–6. *Worksheet for calculation of nutritional requirements for total parenteral nutrition (TPN) in a mature 5-kg cat with vomiting.*

The amount of protein administered is adjusted according to disease conditions (*e.g.,* increase protein with burns, decrease protein with renal failure).

Total parenteral nutrition is best administered by constant infusion (intravenous infusion pump) over a 24-hour period. If this is not possible, TPN can be administered over a 15-hour period. In addition to TPN, fluid therapy may be necessary if there are ongoing losses due to vomiting or diarrhea. Fluids may be added to the TPN solution or may be administered through a peripheral catheter. When enteral intake has increased to provide greater than 50% of the IER, TPN may be discontinued. To avoid hypoglycemia, the rate of infusion may be gradually reduced over several hours or, alternatively, a 5% to 10% dextrose solution may be administered for a few hours after stopping TPN. Voluntary food consumption should be encouraged as soon as possible.

Polyphagia

The treatment of primary polyphagia is to restrict the diet in quantity and caloric density (see Chapter 7). The treatment of secondary polyphagia is management of the primary cause.

Pica

Management of the animal with pica depends on the etiology of the problem. If caloric intake is determined to be insufficient, dietary modification is recommended. If a malassimilation syndrome (*e.g.,* exocrine pancreatic insufficiency) is identified, the underlying cause should be treated accordingly. Internal parasitism, if present, should be treated. For some animals, alleviation of boredom by toys, a radio left on, increased exercise, and contact with the owner is needed to overcome the pica. If possible, the offending substance (wool, shoes) should be removed from the animal's environment. Behavioral modification may be needed (see Chapter 68).

If coprophagy is the problem, feces should be removed from the animal's environment as often as possible and litter pans should be cleaned and disinfected frequently. A balanced, highly digestible diet such as Hill's Prescription Diet i/d should be fed. Free-choice feeding may discourage coprophagy. If such measures fail to stop coprophagy, meat tenderizers may be lightly sprinkled on the food to give the stools a foul taste and discourage the habit.

There is no known treatment for the problem of wool chewing in Siamese cats.

PATIENT MONITORING

Anorexia

For patients receiving enteral nutrition, body weight, packed-cell volume, total protein, blood glucose, and urine glucose should be monitored daily. The patient should be monitored closely for signs of abdominal pain, vomiting, and diarrhea. Serum electrolytes should be monitored twice weekly. If hyperglycemia or glucosuria occur, the amount of calories fed should be decreased.

Patients requiring TPN are candidates for intensive care monitoring (emergency clinics or referral institutions). Vital signs (temperature, pulse, respiratory rate) and urine glucose should be monitored at least every 12 hours. If glucosuria occurs, the amount of dextrose should be reduced. If glucosuria persists, insulin therapy may be needed. Serum electrolytes, total serum protein, packed-cell volume, and body weight should be monitored daily. Although electrolyte abnormalities are uncommon during TPN administration, hypokalemia may develop since glucose and insulin accelerate intracellular movement of potassium. Potassium supplementation may be necessary. A complete blood cell count and biochemistry profile should be performed once or twice weekly throughout the duration of TPN. A mild elevation in blood urea nitrogen may be seen occasionally with TPN and is likely attributable to the amount of protein administered. Reduction in protein intake may be needed.

Serum lipemia is common during the first 48 hours of TPN administration. If lipemia persists longer than 72 hours, the calories provided by lipids should be decreased and replaced by dextrose calories.

Catheter malfunction (occlusion, disconnection, damage by chewing) is a common complication of TPN and is best avoided by close supervision. Other complications of TPN include sepsis and thrombosis, as well as intestinal atrophy. Catheter or TPN solution-related sepsis is a very serious complication of TPN and may be recognized early by pyrexia and clinical signs of phlebitis (swelling, heat, tenderness).

Patients receiving only TPN have hypoplastic and hypofunctional enterocytes and altered intestinal myoelectric activity. Enteral nutrition should be provided as early as possible to help avoid prolonged intestinal atrophy.

Polyphagia

See Chapter 7 for prognosis and monitoring of the patient on a weight-reducing program.

Pica

Long-term behavioral modification may be required for the animal with pica.

ADDITIONAL READING

Crowe DT Jr. Enteral nutrition for critically ill or injured patients. Parts I, II and III. Compendium of Continuing Education 1986; 8:603;719;826.

Donoghue S. Nutritional support of hospitalized patients. Vet Clin North Am 1989; 19:475.

Guyton AC. Dietary balances; Regulation of feeding; Obesity and starvation; Vitamins. In: Guyton AC. Textbook of medical physiology. Philadelphia: WB Saunders, 1986:861.

Houpt K. Ingestive behaviour problems of dogs and cats. Vet Clin North Am 1982; 12:683.

Legendre AM. Anorexia and polyphagia. In: Ettinger SJ, ed. Textbook of veterinary internal medicine. Philadelphia: WB Saunders, 1983: 139.

Lewis LD, Morris ML, Hand MS. Small animal clinical nutrition III. Topeka: Mark Morris Assoc, 1987; 1:1, 20; 3:2; 5:1; 7:51; 13:5.

Lippert AC, Armstrong PJ. Parenteral nutritional support. In: Kirk RW, ed. Current veterinary therapy X. Philadelphia: WB Saunders, 1989: 25.

Lorenz MD. Disturbances of food intake: Anorexia and polyphagia. In: Lorenz MD, Cornelius LM, eds. Small animal medical diagnosis. Philadelphia: JB Lippincott, 1987: 23, 63.

Macy DW, Ralston SL. Cause and control of decreased appetite. In: Kirk RW, ed. Current veterinary therapy X. Philadelphia: WB Saunders, 1989: 18.

Macy DW, Gasper PW. Diazepam-induced eating in anorectic cats. Journal of the American Animal Hospital Association 1985; 21:17.

Wheeler SL, McGuire BH. Enteral nutritional support. In: Kirk RW, ed. Current veterinary therapy X. Philadelphia: WB Saunders, 1989: 30.

William DA. New tests of pancreatic and small intestinal function. Compendium of Continuing Education 1987; 9:1167.

9

POLYURIA AND POLYDIPSIA

Dana G. Allen

The syndrome of polyuria and polydipsia represents one of the most common presenting complaints in small animal medicine. Although it may be caused by a number of disease states, a logical problem-orientated approach facilitates the approach and diagnosis of these cases.

CAUSES

Polyuria and polydipsia may be associated with diseases causing an osmotic diuresis, fluid therapy, conditions interfering with antidiuretic hormone (ADH) release or activity, or a loss of renal medullary tonicity. Table 9-1 lists the causes of polyuria and polydipsia (PUPD) in dogs and cats. Hardy (Additional Reading) categorized causes of (PUPD) into those associated with a water diuresis (urine specific gravity 1.001–1.007) and those associated with a solute diuresis (urine specific gravity 1.008–1.024). Characteristically, animals with disease causing a water diuresis have more severe PUPD. Primary polydipsia is a psychogenic disorder observed most often in hyperactive dogs that are rarely exercised or are exposed to some other form of stress. It is a rare

cause of PUPD in small animals. The mechanisms responsible for the initiation of PUPD are listed in Table 9-2.

PATHOPHYSIOLOGY

Normal hydration status is governed by the interaction of the hypothalamic thirst center, the secretion of ADH, a functional population of nephrons, and a hypertonic renal interstitium. To maintain normal homeostasis a balance between water intake and loss must be preserved. If too much water is retained, overhydration and edema will result. If too much water is lost from the body, dehydration occurs. Normal water intake in the dog and cat is approximately 60 to 70 ml/kg/day. Consumption of volumes in excess of 100 ml/kg/day is considered abnormal. Small dogs and cats may acquire sufficient daily water requirements from the consumption of food alone. Moist foods contain up to 70% water and dry foods up to 8% water.

Water intake is controlled by osmoreceptors that compose the thirst center in the hypothalamus. An increase in plasma osmolality, hy-

Table 9–1 *Causes of Polyuria and Polydipsia in Dogs and Cats*

WATER DIURESIS
(URINE SPECIFIC GRAVITY 1.001–1.007)

Pituitary diabetes insipidus
Renal tubular disease
Psychogenic polydipsia
Pyometra
Liver failure (rare)
Hypoadrenocorticism (rare)
Postobstructive diuresis (FUS)
Drugs: glucocorticoids, phenytoin, atropine, epinephrine

SOLUTE DIURESIS
(SPECIFIC GRAVITY 1.008–1.0024)

Primary renal disease
Pyelonephritis
Diabetes mellitus
Renal glycosuria
Liver failure
Hyperadrenocorticism
Hypoadrenocorticism
Hypercalcemia
Hypokalemia
Postobstructive diuresis (FUS)
Hyperthyroidism
Acromegaly
Drugs: progestins, mannitol, dextrose, furosemide
Salt supplementation

(Modified from Hardy RM. Disorders of water metabolism. In: Schaer M, ed. Vet Clin North Am 1982; 12:353.)

povolemia, hypernatremia, dryness of the mouth, and activation of the renin–angiotensin–aldosterone system stimulates these cells and initiates the sensation of thirst. Other factors that may stimulate the thirst center include fever, a fall in arterial blood pressure, pain, psychosis, and drugs (acetylcholine, barbiturates, morphine, cyclophosphamide, vincristine). Consumption of water, expansion of the extracellular fluid space, normalization of plasma osmolality, increased blood pressure, decreased body temperature, and a fullness of the gastrointestinal tract inhibit thirst (Grauer, Additional Reading).

Fluid is lost principally through urine. Normal urinary output in the dog and cat is approximately 20 to 44 ml/kg/day. Losses greater than 50 ml/kg/day are considered excessive. Fluid is also lost through the gastrointestinal and respiratory tracts. Losses here may be significant with severe vomiting, diarrhea, or panting. Urine volume is influenced by the action of ADH. Antidiuretic hormone is formed in the hypothalamus and stored in the posterior pituitary gland (Fig. 9-1). Osmoreceptors in the hypothalamus release ADH in response to increases in plasma osmolality. It is not known if these osmoreceptors are the same as

Table 9–2 *Mechanisms of Polyuria and Polydipsia*

Causal Condition	Mechanisms
Renal disease	Decreased population of nephrons leads to an increased glomerular flow per remaining nephron and a solute diuresis
	Lack of sodium and urea reabsorption leads to a fall in renal medullary tonicity
	Lack of tubular reabsorption of urea causes an osmotic diuresis
	Uremic toxins antagonize antidiuretic hormone (ADH)
Pyelonephritis	Bacteria induces tubular destruction
	Increased total renal blood flow promotes a fall in medullary tonicity
Diabetes mellitus	Osmotic diuresis occurs when serum glucose exceeds 180 mg/dl or 10.0 mmol/L
Diabetes insipidus	
Pituitary	Lack of sufficient ADH secretion
Nephrogenic	Response to ADH is absent
Psychogenic polydipsia	Extracellular fluid volume expansion inhibits ADH release and results in water diuresis
Hyperadrenocorticism	Glomerular filtration rate increases
	ADH release or action is impaired
	Renal tubular water reabsorption is inhibited
Hypoadrenocorticism	Loss of renal sodium results in a fall in medullary tonicity

(continued)

Table 9–2 (continued)

Causal Condition	Mechanisms
Hypercalcemia of malignancy	ADH renal receptors are damaged
	Tubules become mineralized
	Inactivation of sodium–potassium adenosine triphosphatase leads to decreased transport of sodium and chloride into the medullary interstitium, causing medullary tonicity to fall
	Inactivation of adenylate cyclase results in a decrease in renal tubular cyclic adenosine monophosphate
Pyometra	Infection with *Escherichia coli* causes endotoxic tubular damage
	Deposition of circulating immune complex causes glomerulonephritis
	Toxemia-induced interference with sodium and chloride reabsorption leads to a fall in medullary tonicity
Liver failure	Decreased urea production leads to a fall in medullary tonicity
	Metabolism of aldosterone, ammonia, or glucocorticoids is impaired
	Hypokalemia is sometimes associated with liver disease
Hyperthyroidism	Glomerular filtration rate increases, causing a subsequent decrease in medullary tonicity
Hypokalemia	Degeneration of renal tubular cells
	Decreased solute absorption leads to a fall in medullary tonicity
	Decreased intracellular potassium and water leads to intracellular dehydration and thirst
	Renin release is stimulated
	ADH activation of adenylate cyclase is impaired
	Release of ADH is disrupted
Postobstructive diuresis	Extracellular fluid volume expanded prior to relief of obstruction
	Impaired tubular ability to resorb water or sodium results in a water or osmotic diuresis
Dietary factors	Diets low in protein content may impair the concentrating ability of the kidney
Hypothermia	ADH release is inhibited
Acromegaly	Insulin antagonism causes hyperglycemia and an osmotic diuresis
Drug-induced causes Glucocorticoids, phenytoin, atropine, epinephrine	ADH release is inhibited
Barbiturates, tetracyclines, methoxyflurane, glucocorticoids, vinca alkaloids	Action of ADH on renal tubules is inhibited

those that initiate thirst; however, only a 2% increase in plasma osmolality is required to initiate the release of ADH. Much larger increases in plasma osmolality are required to stimulate thirst. Left atrial volume receptors and baroreceptors in the carotid sinus and aortic arch also initiate the release of ADH in response to a fall in circulating blood volume. Pain, trauma, and hypoxia also stimulate ADH release. Increases in cardiac output and circulating blood volume, hypothermia, emotional stress, phenytoin, atropine, glucocorticoids, and epinephrine inhibit the release of ADH.

Formation of a concentrated urine in response to ADH requires at least one third of the total functional nephron population and a hypertonic renal medullary interstitium. Antidiuretic hormone increases the permeability of the distal tu-

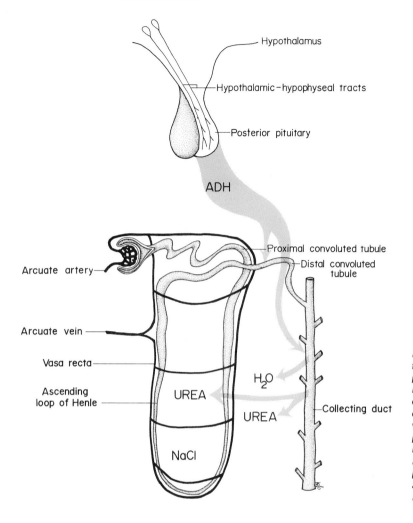

Figure 9–1. *Antidiuruetic hormone (ADH) is formed in the hypothalamus and stored in the posterior pituitary gland, where it is released in response to increases in plasma osmolality. Antidiuretic hormone increases the permeability of the distal convoluted tubules and collecting ducts to water and urea. The action of ADH depends on the presence of an adequate population of functional nephrons and a hypertonic medullary interstitium. Medullary tonicity is generated by the selective permeability of renal tubules to sodium, water, and urea and by the active transport of chloride. Hypertonicity is maintained by the vasa recta.*

bules and collecting ducts to water and urea through the activation of adenyl cyclase and the production of cyclic adenosine monophosphate. An absolute deficiency of ADH is termed pituitary or central diabetes insipidus (CDI). It has been associated with a congenital lack of ADH (rare), trauma, canine distemper, neoplasia, or vascular disease. Trauma to the head is the most common cause of transient or permanent CDI. Central diabetes insipidus is especially rare in the cat (Randolph and Jorgensen, Additional Reading). Partial CDI is associated with mild to moderate diuresis.

Nephrogenic diabetes insipidus (NDI) is the inability to concentrate urine in spite of adequate circulating levels of ADH. Primary or congenital NDI is rare in small animals. Secondary NDI may be due to chronic renal failure, pyelonephritis, hypercalcemia, hypokalemia, hyperadrenocorticism, hyperthyroidism, liver failure, or pyometra. Glucocorticoids and high serum calcium concentrations (hypercalcemia of malignancy) impair the production of cyclic adenosine monophosphate. Bacterial toxins (pyometra) compete with ADH for receptor sites on renal tubules. A lack of ADH leads to the formation of hypotonic urine. Kidneys still retain the ability to dilute urine. The collecting ducts remain permeable to water in the absence of ADH. In the presence of ADH, permeability is markedly increased. With partial ADH deficiency (partial diabetes insipidus), urine is isotonic or slightly hypertonic (475 mOsm/kg).

The effectiveness of ADH depends on the establishment of an osmotic gradient in renal tissue, which is formed by a hypertonic medullary interstitium and maintained by the vasa recta. Medullary tonicity develops as a result of selective permeability of renal tubules to sodium, water, and urea and as a result of the active transport of chloride. Urea accounts for at least half the medullary tonicity. Sodium and chloride also contribute. The loss of medullary tonicity may be the result of a lack of urea production associated with liver failure or a dietary lack of protein, which is rare. High renal blood flow impairs the ability of the kidney to resorb urea (hyperadrenocorticism, pyelonephritis, hyperthyroidism). Prolonged water and osmotic diuresis increases tubular flow rates and decreases the amount of urea and sodium reabsorption in the renal medulla. This is referred to as *medullary washout*. An osmotic gradient no longer exists and medullary tonicity approaches that of plasma. The loss of renal medullary sodium (hypoadrenocorticism) has also been associated with the impairment of renal concentrating ability.

Disease affecting the vasa recta may interfere with the function of countercurrent exchange and impair renal concentrating ability. Examples are hyperviscosity associated with polycythemia and hyperproteinemia, lymphatic obstruction caused by lymphosarcoma or lymphagiectasia, and systemic vasculitis associated with septicemia and systemic lupus erythematosus.

Significant impairment of the kidneys' ability to dilute or concentrate urine does not occur until more than two thirds of the total functional nephrons are destroyed. This results in an increased solute load per remaining nephron, an osmotic diuresis, an insensitivity to ADH, and an inability to concentrate urine. To excrete this excess solute load nephrons must excrete an increased volume of water. The urine remains isotonic. In this state the kidneys are less able to respond to rapid changes in hydration status. The inability to concentrate urine predisposes animals with renal failure to the rapid development of dehydration.

CLINICAL SIGNS

The clinician must differentiate PUPD from pollakiuria and urinary incontinence (see Chapter 42). Pollakiuria is an increased frequency of urination (not accompanied by increased volumes) often caused by urinary tract infection. Nocturia is one of the most common presenting complaints by owners with animals with PUPD. Polydipsia may be apparent along with the passage of large volumes of light-colored urine.

Other clinical signs reflect the initiating cause. Animals with hyperadrenocorticism may present with bilaterally symmetric alopecia, thin skin, muscle weakness, and polyphagia (see Chapter 59). Weakness, vomiting, diarrhea, and bradycardia are hallmarks of hypoadrenocorticism (see Chapter 60). Vomiting, diarrhea, jaundice, and weight loss often accompany liver disease (see Chapter 40). Generalized lymphadenopathy may signal lymphosarcoma (see Chapter 15). Hyperthyroidism is most often diagnosed in cats older than 8 years of age and is accompanied by polyphagia, voluminous stools, weight loss, hyperactivity, and a palpable thyroid mass(es) (see Chapter 61). Weight loss and polyphagia also occur with diabetes mellitus (see Chapter 58). Chronic renal disease is a debilitating disease characterized by weight loss, dehydration, vomiting, and anorexia (see Chapter 44). Dogs with primary renal disease lose the ability to concentrate urine and demonstrate clinical signs of polyuria before azotemia becomes apparent. Cats with azotemia, however, retain a considerable ability to concentrate urine (Ross and Finco, Additional Reading). Only one third of cats with chronic renal disease demonstrate PUPD, even though dehydration is common (DiBartola, Additional Reading). Pyometra occurs in intact females following whelping or during the metestrus or luteal phase of the estrus cycle. Anorexia, depression, fever, vomiting, and a vaginal discharge are characteristic (see Chapter 56).

DIAGNOSTIC APPROACH

Nocturia and PUPD in association with other clinical signs may direct the clinician to the likely cause of the problem (Fig. 9-2). If the physical

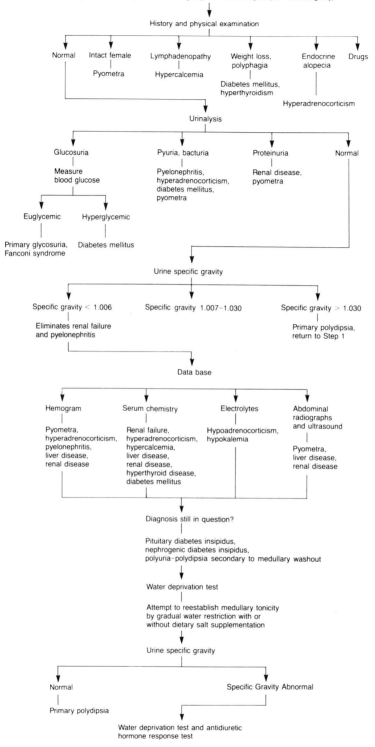

Figure 9–2. Diagnostic approach to animals with polyuria–polydipsia. (Modified from Feldman EC, Nelson RW. The differential diagnosis of polyuria and polydipsia. In: Feldman EC, Nelson RW, eds. Canine and feline endocrinology and reproduction. Philadelphia: WB Saunders, 1987: 7.)

examination is unremarkable and the urine is concentrated and does not contain glucose, a pathologic cause of PUPD is unlikely. In these cases animals are sent home and water consumption is monitored over a 7- to 10-day period, after which the patient is reevaluated. If these animals remain polydipsic at home, but can concentrate their urine and are not polydipsic under hospital observation, psychogenic polydipsia related to unknown stresses in the home environment must be considered. In these cases a change in the home environment, boredom, or hyperactivity are suspect. Most animals with chronic psychogenic polydipsia do not have concentrated urine.

Urine specific gravity less than 1.006 suggests that the kidney retains the ability to dilute urine; thus, renal failure or pyelonephritis would be unlikely causes of PUPD. In cases of renal disease, the ability to concentrate urine is lost before the ability to dilute urine. Consequently, low urine specific gravity signifies some degree of renal competence. If the urine specific gravity is consistently between 1.007 and 1.029 (dog) or 1.034 (cat) and the animal is azotemic, renal failure is present.

If the urine is glucosuric, the serum glucose should be evaluated. Diabetes mellitus is likely in animals with hyperglycemia and glucosuria, although in cats stress may also be the cause. Dogs with normoglycemia and glucosuria are likely to have canine Fanconilike syndrome or primary renal glucosuria. Dogs with Fanconilike syndrome have a renal tubular absorptive defect. Defective absorption of water, phosphorus, sodium, potassium, urea, and amino acids is generally present. The breed most commonly affected is the basenji. Clinical signs are generally not evident prior to middle age. Renal glucosuria in the absence of hyperglycemia may occur as a singular renal transport abnormality. It has been identified in various breeds of dogs and is an inherited defect in the Norwegian elkhound. Pyelonephritis, pyometra, or lower urinary tract infection secondary to hyperadrenocorticism or diabetes mellitus should be considered in animals with pyuria or bacteriuria. Animals with pyelonephritis may present with a "hunched up" appearance, fever, and lumbar pain. If the urinary sediment is normal and the urine specific gravity is low, the next step in the evaluation of the animal is the complete blood count and serum biochemistry profile.

The complete blood count and serum biochemistry profile help delineate the cause of PUPD (Table 9-3). An inflammatory leukogram may accompany pyometra or pyelonephritis. A stress leukogram is more consistent with hyperadrenocorticism. A nonresponsive anemia may be associated with chronic renal or liver disease. On the basis of the serum biochemistry profile and ACTH response test, renal failure, hyperadrenocorticsm, hypercalcemia, liver disease, diabetes mellitus, and hypokalemia can be differentiated. Animals with hypercalcemia most commonly suffer from lymphosarcoma. Other causes for hypercalcemia include parathyroid gland adenoma, myeloma, and carcinoma of the perianal and mammary glands. If the data are supportive of hepatic disease or pyometra, abdominal radiography and ultrasonography is indicated. The common laboratory findings and supportive tests of diseases causing PUPD are outlined in Table 9-3.

If the history and physical examination, complete blood count, serum biochemistry, and urinalysis do not render a diagnosis, CDI, NDI, primary (psychogenic) polydipsia, and severe medullary washout secondary to prolonged water and solute diuresis must be considered and a water deprivation test performed. Psychogenic polydipsia is diagnosed by eliminating other possible causes of PUPD and observing the response to the water deprivation test and treatment. Excessive drinking in animals with psychogenic polydipsia leads to a dilution of plasma osmolality. A plasma osmolality less than 290 mOsm/kg is suggestive of psychogenic polydipsia.

The water deprivation test creates a state of dehydration and an increase in plasma osmolality sufficient to stimulate the release of endogenous ADH. It assesses the integrity of the hypothalamic–pituitary–renal tubular and medullary axis. This test helps differentiate between CDI and NDI, and between psychogenic polydipsia and PUPD associated with medullary washout. Although the test is simple to complete, the results are often difficult to interpret because

Table 9–3 *Causes of Polyuria and Polydipsia and Common Laboratory Findings*

Cause	Complete Blood Count	Serum Chemistry	Other Tests
Diabetes insipidus	PCV N or I, TP N or I	SUN N or I, sodium and chloride N or I, urine/plasma osmolality <1	Water deprivation, ADH response
Psychogenic polydipsia	Normal	Serum osmolality N or D, urine/ plasma osmolality <1	Water deprivation, ADH response
Hyperadrenocorticism	Lymphopenia, eosinopenia, mature neutrophilia	ALT N or I, Alk Phos I, cholesterol I, glucose N or I, phosphorus D	ACTH response, dexamethasone suppression
Hypoadrenocorticism	Lymphocytosis, eosinophilia, PCV N, I, or D	SUN I, sodium N or D, potassium I, calcium N or I	ACTH response, ECG
Hypercalcemia	Usually normal	SUN N or I, creatinine N or I, calcium I, phosphorus N or D	Lymph node and bone marrow biopsy, chest, abdominal, and skeletal radiographs, PTH assay
Diabetes mellitus	PCV N or I	SUN N or I, ALT N or I, Alk Phos N or I, glucose I	Glucose tolerance
Liver disease	PCV N or D, TP N or D	SUN N or D, TP N or D, ALT I, Alk Phos I, Bilirubin I	BSP, blood ammonia, bile acids, abdominal radiographs, ultrasound, hepatic biopsy
Renal disease	PCV N or D	SUN I, creatinine I, phosphorus I, potassium N or I, metabolic acidosis	Sodium sulfanilate, PSP, creatinine clearance, radiographs, ultrasound, renal biopsy, urine analysis
Pyelonephritis	Leukocytosis	SUN N or I	Abdominal radiographs, renal ultrasound, renal biopsy, urinalysis and culture
Hyperthyroidism (cat)	Leukocytosis, eosinopenia, PCV N or I	ALT N or I, AST N or I, Alk Phos N or I, Serum T3 and T4 I	Electrocardiogram, echocardiogram, thyroid biopsy, thyroid imaging, T_3 suppression, TSH stimulation
Pyometra	Leukocytosis, nonresponsive anemia	TP I, SUN I, proteinuria	Abdominal radiographs and ultrasound, bacterial culture

PCV = packed-cell volume; TP = total protein; SUN = serum urea nitrogen; ALT = alanine aminotransferase; AST = aspartate aminotransferase; Alk Phos = alkaline phosphatase; ADH = antidiuretic hormone; N = normal; I = increased; D = decreased

many of the diseases that cause PUPD cause some degree of medullary washout. Until medullary tonicity is restored, these animals may not be able to adequately concentrate their urine in response to this test or to the administration of exogenous ADH.

At the start of the test the animal is weighed and baseline values are taken for urine specific gravity, urine osmolality, plasma osmolality, serum urea concentration, packed-cell volume, and total protein. Specific gravity is determined by the size, weight, and number of particles in a solution. Osmolality depends only on the number of particles in a solution and is a more accurate

assessment of plasma tonicity and renal concentrating ability than specific gravity.

An indwelling urinary catheter can be used for convenient urine collection. Aseptic technique and a closed collection system should be used to reduce the incidence of iatrogenic urinary tract infection. Water is withheld during the test. Some clinicians allow animals access to food during the test. However, some foods have a high water content and may prolong the duration of the test. Body weight, urine specific gravity or urine osmolality, and serum urea and osmolality are measured every other hour. The bladder should be emptied completely each time to prevent interference with the interpretation of subsequent samples. The test is ended when the animal concentrates urine greater than 1.029 (dog) or 1.034 (cat), there is a 5% loss in body weight, there is a less than 5% change in urine osmolality between two consecutive samples, or serum urea increases to a value greater than 30 mg/dl (10.7 mmol/L), or if animals become dehydrated or depressed. At the end of the test small volumes of water (10–20 ml/kg) are gradually reintroduced every half hour for 2 hours after the test is completed. If the patient is well at this time water may be given ad lib. Animals with diabetes insipidus or severe medullary washout may lose 5% of their body weight in 2 to 6 hours, whereas animals with psychogenic polydipsia may require more than 24 hours to lose that amount of weight.

The test should not be performed on animals that are initally dehydrated or azotemic. The inability to concentrate urine in the face of azotemia is indicative of renal impairment. Normal plasma osmolality in small animals is 280 to 310 mOsm/kg. A 1% to 2% increase (6 mOsm) is sufficient to stimulate the release of ADH. Consequently, animals that present with a plasma osmolality in the range of 315 to 320 mOsm/kg or higher already have sufficient stimulus for ADH release and are not candidates for this test. When the test is run, animals should be watched carefully for signs of dehydration. Changes in body weight and total protein are more accurate indices of hydration status than changes in skin pliability or changes in packed-cell volume. Animals with diabetes insipidus or severe medullary washout are predisposed to rapid dehydration and oliguric renal failure. Hypernatremia may occur in these animals if deprived of water, and may be characterized by lethargy, muscle weakness, twitching, seizure, coma, or death. Do not leave these animals unattended without water for extended periods.

Normal animals respond to water deprivation by producing smaller volumes of a more highly concentrated urine (specific gravity greater than 1.029 in the dog or 1.034 in the cat, corresponding to a urine osmolality of greater than 1100 mOsm/kg). Those with complete CDI or NDI are unable to concentrate urine in excess of 1.008 specific gravity (urine osmolality 290–310 mOsm/kg).

Following water deprivation, animals with partial diabetes insipidus or hyperadrenocorticism have urine specific gravities in the range of 1.008 to 1.019 (urine osmolality 300–1000 mOsm/kg), depending on the amount of ADH available and how well the kidney can respond to it. In some animals with partial diabetes insipidus, the urine specific gravity peaks before the end of the water deprivation test and then falls as ADH stores are exhausted.

The response of animals with psychogenic polydipsia depends on the severity of renal medullary washout. If washout is minimal, results are similar to normal animals. If washout is severe, results appear similar to animals with partial diabetes insipidus. If the urine specific gravity fails to exceed 1.029 (300 mOsm/kg) in the dog or 1.034 in the cat at the end of the test, CDI, NDI, psychogenic PD, or severe medullary washout must still be considered.

Many clinicians continue the water deprivation test with the administration of exogenous ADH (modified water deprivation test). However, the failure to respond to exogenous ADH at this time will not help rule out diabetes insipidus, psychogenic PD, or severe medullary washout. Prolonged PUPD is accompanied by some degree of medullary washout, which may interfere with the interpretation of the test. The reestablishment of medullary tonicity occurs within a 1- to 3-day period after fluid consumption has returned to normal. I therefore recommend that these animals return home on a gradually restricted water intake in an attempt to reestablish medullary hypertonicity. Water intake is gradually restricted (10% per day) over a 3- to 5-day period, but should never be less than the normal daily requirements of 70 ml/kg/day. The water deprivation test helps establish to what extent these animals can safely tolerate water restriction. At the end of this period the animals are reexamined. If the urine is concentrated on initial presentation, the diagnosis is psychogenic polydipsia. If the urine remains dilute, the water deprivation test is repeated. Exogenous ADH is given if the animals fail to concentrate their urine (modified water deprivation test).

The ADH response test is used to differentiate diabetes insipidus from severe medullary washout. Water is withheld and 2 to 5 units of aqueous vasopressin tannate (Pitressin [Parke-Davis]) is administered subcutaneously. Urine specific gravity and urine and plasma osmolality are measured every 30 minutes for a total of 90 minutes. The bladder is completely emptied each time. Alternatively, vasopressin tannate in oil (Pitressin Tannate in Oil [Parke-Davis]) is administered intramuscularly at 0.25 units/kg, not to exceed 5 units. In this case urine and plasma samples are taken 9 and 12 hours after the injection of pitressin tannate in oil. Animals with CDI respond to ADH by decreasing urine volume and increasing urine specific gravity (greater than 1.012) and urine osmolality (50%–800% over preinjection values). Urine specific gravity and osmolality do not change in animals with NDI. Urine specific gravity increases and urine osmolality may increase 10% to 50% following exogenous ADH administration in animals with hyperadrenocorticism or partial diabetes insipidus. Urine osmolality generally does not increase more than 10% following injection of ADH in animals with psychogenic polydipsia. The normal urine : plasma osmolality is 3 : 1. A urine : plasma osmolality greater than 3 : 1 may be normal or may be associated with psychogenic diabetes insipidus. A ratio less than 1.84 may be consistent with severe pituitary diabetes insipidus, and a ratio between 1.83 and 3 is suggestive of partial diabetes insipidus. These measurements, however, are inconsistent and are not recommended for the laboratory assessment of these patients.

The Hickey–Hare test differentiates between psychogenic polydipsia and diabetes insipidus. It is considered when the urine specific gravity remains low and the water deprivation test and ADH response test are inconclusive. Water is given by stomach intubation (20 ml/kg), and endogenous ADH release is stimulated by the intravenous administration of 2.5% sodium chloride at a rate of 0.25 ml/kg/min over a 45-minute period. Urine is collected every 15 minutes. In normal animals urine volume decreases and urine specific gravity and osmolality increase as the test proceeds. Animals with psychogenic polydipsia and severe medullary washout respond by producing decreasing volumes of urine of increasing concentration. In animals with diabetes insip-

idus no reduction in urine volume or increase in urine concentration occurs. Complications of the test include plasma hyperosmolality, with shaking, salivation, defecation, and seizure. The Hickey–Hare test is not routinely recommended because the water deprivation test is safer, easier to perform, and more accurate.

Radioimmunoassay for enodgenous ADH is not widely available on a commercial basis for small animals, but promises to greatly enhance the diagnostic procedure.

MANAGEMENT

Animals with CDI are managed with pitressin tannate (Pitressin) at a dosage of 2.5 to 5 units subcutaneously or intramuscularly until signs of polyuria return. The effect of the drug lasts 36 to 72 hours. An alternative is desmopressin acetate (DDAVP). The drug is available as a nasal spray and has an 8- to 20-hour duration of effect. In small animals it is best given as eye drops because intranasal administration often leads to sneezing and inadequate dosing. Two drops (0.1 ml of a 20-microunit solution) are placed into the subconjunctival sac once or twice daily. The drug is readministered when polyuria recurs. Desmopressin acetate is expensive.

Several agents may be useful in the management of partial diabetes insipidus. Chlorpropamide (Diabinase) is an oral hypoglycemic agent that potentiates the effects of ADH on renal tubules by increasing cyclic adenosine monophosphate levels and increasing the concentrating ability of the kidney. A dosage of 50 to 250 mg every 12 hours, depending on size, has been recommended. Clofibrate (Atromid-S) is a hypolipidemic drug that stimulates the hypothalamus to release ADH. Carbamazepine (Tegretol), an anticonvulsant, works in a similar manner. Dosages for clofibrate and carbamazepine are not available in the veterinary literature.

Congenital NDI is a rare disorder in small animals. Treatment includes the use of chlorothiazide (Diuril) and dietary salt restriction (Prescription Diet h/d [Hill's]). This regimen results in a decreased body sodium by a combination of decreased salt intake and increased loss. The kidney responds by increasing sodium and water resorption in the proximal tubules. Urine volume decreases by as much as 50% to 85%. Urine specific gravity does not change.

Psychogenic diabetes insipidus often responds to gradual water restriction alone. Water intake is reduced 10% per week over a 3- to 10-week period to a level consistent with normal water intake (70 ml/kg/day). Gradual water restriction prevents rapid dehydration and allows the reestablishment of renal medullary hypertonicity. Some animals with psychogenic polydipsia also benefit from the addition of oral sodium chloride (1 g/30 kg body weight b.i.d.) and oral sodium bicarbonate (0.6 g/kg body weight b.i.d.) over a 3- to 5-day period.

Treatment for secondary causes of PUPD is directed at the primary disorder (diabetes mellitus, hyperadrenocorticism).

PATIENT MONITORING

Animals with PUPD must be monitored for evidence of dehydration. Water must be available for animals with diabetes insipidus and severe medullary washout at all times. Failure to provide water may lead to dehydration, prerenal azotemia, hypernatremia, and oliguric renal failure. The prognosis for control of PUPD in cases of idiopathic or congenital CDI is good. Most animals respond to therapy. Those with acquired hypothalamic or pituitary lesions (tumors) have a grave prognosis, and progression of the disease is likely. Patients with NDI have a guarded to poor prognosis because these patients are especially prone to dehydration and secondary illness. The prognosis for patients with psychogenic polydipsia is excellent. These patients respond well to behavioral modification and water restriction, although relapses do occur.

ADDITIONAL READING

Allen TA, Wilke WL. Polyuria and polydipsia. In: Ford RB, ed. Clinical signs and diagnosis in small animal practice. New York: Churchill Livingstone, 1988: 55.

Barsanti JA. Polyuria and polydipsia. Proceedings of the American Animal Hospital Association 1982: 141.

Breitschwerdt EB. Clinical abnormalities of urine concentration and dilution. Compendium of Continuing Education 1981; 3:414.

Breitschwerdt EB, Verlander JW, Hribernik TN. Nephrogenic diabetes insipidus in three dogs. J Am Vet Med Assoc 1981; 179:235.

Bruyette DS, Nelson RW. How to approach the problems of polyuria and polydipsia. Vet Med 1986; 112.

Cotter SM. Polyuria and polydipsia. In: Ettinger SJ, ed. Textbook of veterinary internal medicine. Philadelphia: WB Saunders, 1983: 133.

DiBartola SP, Rutgers HC, Zack PM, Tarr MJ. Clinicopathologic findings associated with chronic renal disease in cats: 74 cases (1973–1984). J Am Vet Med Assoc 1987; 190:1196.

Feldman EC, Nelson RW. Diagnostic approach to polydipsia and polyuria. Vet Clin North Am 1989; 327.

Grauer GF. The differential diagnosis of polyuric–polydipsic disease. Compendium of Continuing Education 1981; 3:1079.

Hardy RM. Disorders of water metabolism. Vet Clin North Am 1982; 12:353

Randolph JF, Jorgensen LS. Selected feline endocrinopathies. Vet Clin North Am 1984; 14:1261.

Ross LA, Finco DR. Relationship of selected clinical renal function tests to glomerular filtration rate and renal blood flow in cats. Am J Vet Res 1981; 42:1704.

10

PERIPHERAL EDEMA

Dana G. Allen

The extravascular, extracellular spaces of the body are collectively called the interstitium. They constitute approximately 15% of total tissue by volume. The fluid in these spaces is called interstitial fluid. Edema is the accumulation of excess volumes of free fluid in the interstitial spaces of the body. Its distribution is categorized as general, focal, or regional (Olivier, Additional Reading). Generalized edema involves all four legs or areas of the trunk cranial and caudal to the diaphragm. Severe, whole body subcutaneous edema is referred to as anasarca. Regional edema appears symmetric and involves the head and neck or front legs (cranial) or the pelvic area and hind limbs (caudal). Focal edema appears asymmetric and involves a localized area of the body or a single limb.

CAUSES

Four basic pathologic mechanisms are responsible for the initiation of edema: increased hydrostatic pressure, increased capillary permeability, decreased plasma oncotic pressure, and lymphatic obstruction. The causes of these are listed in Table 10-1. Generalized edema in the presence of ascites is associated with right heart failure or pericardial effusion. Ascites may or may not accompany generalized edema in cases of hypoalbuminemia.

Regional edema occurs secondary to factors that cause increased hydrostatic pressure by the obstruction of venous or lymphatic drainage. Tumors compressing the cranial vena cava result in bilateral forelimb (cranial) edema. Thymoma, lymphoma, heartbase tumors, and right atrial hemangiosarcoma are potential causes. Similarly, pelvic masses causing compression or obstruction of the sublumbar iliac veins result in hindlimb (caudal) edema. Edema of the hindlimbs accompanied by ascites occurs with portal hypertension or compression of the caudal vena cava. Regional edema may also follow inflammation, infection, allergy, and increased capillary permeability. In the cat edema of the head has been associated with feline plague (*Yersinia pestis*), feline trypanosomiasis (*Trypanosoma brucei*), and the administration of acetaminophen. Clinically, catpox may be associated with edema of the head, neck, and distal extremities. In dogs, edema of the head has been recognized with hypothyroid disease (myxedema), the initial phases of juvenile pyoderma, anthrax, and allergic reactions to drugs, vaccines, or insect bites. Thrombosis of the cranial vena cava appears to be the most common cause of edema, affecting the head, neck, and forelimbs in the dog (cranial vena cava syndrome; see Chapter 16).

Table 10–1 *Mechanisms of Edema and Associated Causes*

Mechanisms	Associated Causes
Increased hydrostatic pressure	Congestive heart failure
	Pericardial effusion
	Tumors or thrombi obstructing vena cavae
	Arteriovenous fistula
	Overhydration
Increased capillary permeability	Immune-mediated vasculitis
	Inflammation
	Trauma
	Burns
Decreased plasma oncotic pressure	Liver failure
	Glomerular disease
	Protein-losing enteropathy
Lymphatic obstruction	Congenital factors
	Acquired factors
	Trauma
	Infection
	Tumor

Focal edema is a phenomenon that occurs most often in relation to increased capillary permeability, lymphatic and venous obstruction, or arteriovenous shunts.

PATHOPHYSIOLOGY

The interstitium is composed of a collagen and proteoglycan matrix. Collagen bundles provide tensile strength. Proteoglycan filaments fill the spaces between collagen bundles, forming a fine reticular network. Interstitial fluid is an ultrafiltrate of capillary plasma trapped within spaces among the proteoglycan filaments. Collectively, the proteoglycan filaments and interstitial fluid comprise tissue gel. Tissue gel prevents the formation of dependent edema and the spread of infection, and separates cells and capillaries for the efficient diffusion and excretion of nutrients and wastes. The extensive nature of the proteoglycan network limits fluid flow.

A very small amount of fluid (less than 1%) is not trapped in the proteoglycan network and can move freely through the interstitium. It forms a thin layer between the interstitial gel and adjacent cells, capillaries, and lymphatics. Free fluid and gel continually interchange by diffusion. If the amount of free fluid exceeds the expansile nature of the gel reticulum, edema results. The interstitial space can accommodate free fluid increases up to 30% of normal without the clinical appearance of edema. Up to this point the gel reticulum expands and pulls fluid into it, preventing frank edema. The freely mobile nature of this fluid becomes apparent if it is forcibly pushed away by digital pressure, forming a depression or pit in the affected tissue. It remains depressed for a few seconds to a minute or longer, until free fluid returns to fill the area once again.

The major mechanisms affecting the fate of interstitial free fluid include capillary hydrostatic pressure, plasma colloidal oncotic pressure, tissue colloidal oncotic pressure, interstitial fluid pressure, capillary permeability, and lymphatic drainage (Fig. 10-1). Several safeguards protect the body from early edema formation. Normal interstitital fluid pressure must increase from -6.5 to 0 mmHg before edema begins to appear. As the interstitial fluid pressure approaches zero, lymphatic flow increases dramatically and draws away the increased fluid volume. At the same time that it removes the excess fluid, it washes away interstitial protein, decreases interstitial colloidal osmotic pressure, and prevents the further drag of capillary fluid. To overcome these safety factors and cause edema, capillary hydrostatic pressure must double and plasma colloidal oncotic pressure must fall from 29 mmHg to below 10 mmHg, which corresponds to a serum albumin concentration of 1 to 1.5 g/dl (10 to 15 g/L).

The rate of capillary filtration is determined by the interaction of capillary hydrostatic pressure, capillary permeability, plasma oncotic pressure, and interstitial hydrostatic and oncotic pressure (Olivier, Additional Reading). As long as capillary filtration does not exceed lymphatic capacity, edema will not form. Lymphatic drainage is a function of the surface area and structural integrity of the lymphatic vessels and lymph nodes and the driving force that directs its flow. This driving force is governed by the interstitial hydrostatic pressure, the rhythmic contractile nature of the lymph vessels, and the hydrostatic pressure of the systemic veins into which it empties (Olivier, Additional Reading).

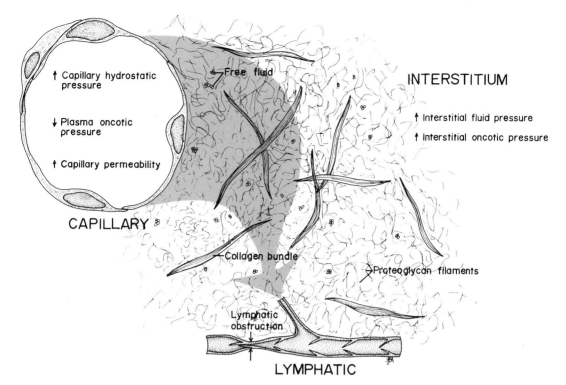

Figure 10–1. *Factors contributing to edema formation. Large arrow denotes normal direction of fluid flow.*

Edema most commonly occurs following increases in capillary hydrostatic pressure, decreases in plasma oncotic pressure, increases in capillary permeability, or lymphatic obstruction. Chronic edema stretches tissue spaces and facilitates further edema formation.

Increased Capillary Hydrostatic Pressure

Increased capillary pressure follows venous obstruction or arteriolar dilation. Increased venous hydrostatic pressure is most common with right heart failure, pericardial effusion, venous thrombosis, vascular compression, or arteriovenous shunts. Acute heart failure and cardiac tamponade are not associated with edema because in these cases peripheral capillary pressure actually falls.

With severe or chronic capillary hypertension, vascular endothelium is stretched, intercellular spaces enlarge, vascular permeability increases, and edema formation is exacerbated. Most fluid leaving capillaries is returned to the circulation by the venous system. Only 10% is returned by lymphatic drainage. Edema formation due to venous occlusion is often severe because the combination of increased capillary hydrostatic pressure, which favors increased capillary filtration, and venous obstruction overwhelm lymphatic drainage. Arteriovenous shunting of blood leads to increased venous fluid volume and pressure.

Decreased Plasma Colloidal Oncotic Pressure

The principal force tending to keep fluid within the vascular space is plasma colloidal oncotic pressure. Albumin accounts for most of the oncotic pressure (65%–70%). Globulin and fibrinogen account for the remaining 30% to 35%. Consequently, a fall in plasma oncotic pressure sufficient to cause edema is generally associated with the increased loss or decreased production of albumin. Increased loss occurs primarily through the gastrointestinal tract or kidney. Protein loss is related to the size of the intercellular space. Albumin is a smaller molecule than globulin and slips through the intercellular spaces more readily. With gastrointestinal tract disease both albumin and globulin are lost; they appear low on serum analysis. In kidney (glomerular) disease albumin is lost in the urine but globulin is not. Consequently, serum albumin concentrations are low and serum globulin concentrations are normal. Massive effusive disease (peritonitis, chronic hemorrhage) or severe burns may also cause significant protein loss. Decreased albumin production is a consequence of end-stage liver disease. It is an uncommon cause of hypoproteinemia because more than 85% of functional hepatic mass must be lost before albumin production is significantly impaired.

Increased Capillary Permeability

A small amount of free fluid and albumin normally filters into the interstitium and is returned to the circulation by lymphatic drainage. An increase in capillary permeability increases the rate at which plasma proteins can be effectively returned to the circulation by lymphatic drainage. This situation is exacerbated if lymphatic drainage is impeded by occlusive disease. Interstitial oncotic pressure increases and edema forms. Permeability changes may accompany inflammation and the release of vasoactive agents, including histamine, serotonin, kinins, prostaglandins, and proteolytic enzymes, or infection, trauma, and noxious agents.

Lymphatic Obstruction

Normally there is a slight pressure differential that favors the filtration of free fluid (plasma) from the capillaries into the interstitium, from which it is drained by the lymphatics. All areas of the body except the superficial skin, central nervous system, and bone have a well-developed lymphatic system. In the healthy animal lymphatic drainage keeps pace with the rate of capillary filtration. If capillary filtration overwhelms

lymphatic drainage, interstitial hydrostatic pressure increases, compresses lymph vessels, distorts the apposition of lymphatic valves, and further limits lymphatic drainage. The increased interstitial oncotic pressure augments capillary filtration and exacerbates edema formation. Lymphatic obstruction is classified as primary (congenital) or acquired. Primary lymphedema is a developmental abnormalitiy of the lymphatic system. Hereditary causes are often associated with poor formation of the proximal lymphatics in the region of the thigh, and hypoplasia or aplasia of the popliteal lymph nodes. Secondary causes of lymphedema lead to compression, occlusion, or structural change associated with infection, granulomatous disease, trauma, or neoplasia.

Other Causes

Hypothyroid disease is associated with an increase in the mucopolysaccharide content of the interstitial space. Fluid is absorbed by the mucopolysaccharide matrix and and becomes trapped. Because of its gelatinous consistency, myxedematous fluid is not mobile and cannot be pitted by digital palpation.

CLINICAL SIGNS

The affected skin of animals with edema appears tense, gelatinous, and rubbery, with poorly defined borders. The area may depress or pit with digital pressure. The ability to pit affected tissue is a reflection of the volume of free fluid present and its protein content. The greater the volume of free fluid and the higher its protein content, the more readily it will depress with digital pressure and remain depressed for a period of time.

The protein content adds to the viscosity of the fluid and may give some indication of the etiology of the edema. With chronic or severe increases in capillary hydrostatic pressure (congestive heart failure), protein content is high (4–5 g/dl or 40–50 g/L). Affected areas readily pit and remain depressed for some time following the release of digital pressure. Edema fluid associated with increased capillary permeability (inflammation) is also high in protein content and may exceed 10 g/dl or 100 g/L. Edema fluid associated with hypoproteinemia is low in protein content, does not readily pit with digital pressure, and recovers quickly. The cell content of such fluid is low. Coagulation of tissue protein in areas of infectious disease or trauma traps free fluid in the form of a gel ("brawny edema"). Cells in the affected area also tend to swell in response to the trauma, and the area will not pit.

Severe edema impairs peripheral perfusion and the diffusion and excretion of nutrients and waste products. Hypoxia, the release of vasoactive substances, and local acidosis contribute to cell dysfunction and death. Necrosis of the skin, subcutaneous tissue, and soft tissue follows. Lesions are more common in tissue with limited expansile capabilities (distal extremities) (Olivier, Additional Reading). Affected areas weep free fluid and are predisposed to secondary infection.

As fluid accumulates, body weight may increase; however, muscle mass is often decreased due to the cachexic nature of the inciting disease and the hypoproteinemia that accompanies it. Clinical signs often reflect the body system responsible for edema formation. Cough, dyspnea, poor exercise tolerance, and syncope are indicative of heart failure or pericardial effusion. On the physical examination jugular vein distention, tachycardia, and decreased pulse amplitude, along with cardiac murmurs or muffled heart sounds, may be apparent. Pleural effusion with or without ascites limits expansion of the lungs and contributes to dyspnea. Ascites precedes peripheral edema in cases of congestive heart failure or pericardial effusion. In cats the thorax can normally be compressed to some degree. If tumors occupy the mediastinal area, chest compressibility is markedly decreased.

Small arteriovenous shunts present as soft, painless swellings. A palpable thrill and a continuous murmur may be evident. Chronic edema, pain, lameness, and ulceration may accompany large fistulas. In severe cases gangrene may develop distal to the shunt (see Chapter 24).

Vomiting, diarrhea, and weight loss may indicate gastrointestinal disease or liver failure. Animals with protein-losing enteropathies commonly present with histories of small bowel diarrhea (see Chapter 37). Polyuria, polydipsia, anorexia, vomiting, weight loss, and anemia occur with chronic renal disease (see Chapter 44).

Primary lymphedema initially presents in young dogs as a transient limb edema that, with time, tends to progress. Secondary lymphedema is recognized as a recurrent limb edema that may be accompanied by pain, heat, swelling, and lameness associated with secondary lymphangitis. Ulceration, eczema, weeping, varicosities, and fat necrosis are more consistent with local venous stasis.

DIAGNOSTIC APPROACH

Patient signalment, the onset of edema formation, its duration, and whether or not it has relapsed are important historical facts. Other historical associations such as recent trauma, other illness, pain, or lameness may be important. A complete physical examination with emphasis on the cardiovascular, gastrointestinal, renal, and lymphatic system should be completed.

When edema is recognized in an animal it is categorized as general, regional, or focal (Fig 10-2). General edema associated with ascites may be related to right heart failure or pericardial effusion. In chronic cases the protein content of the edematous fluid is 2 to 4 g/dl (20–40 g/L) and devoid of cells. Chest radiography, electrocardiography, and central venous pressure measurement (see Central Venous Pressure in Chapter 80) will help confirm right heart changes. Mitral valvular insufficiency leading to congestive heart failure, pulmonic stenosis, congestive cardiomyopathy, and chronic, severe cases of heartworm should be be considered in the differential diagnosis. Cardiac ultrasonography is the most sensitive and least invasive tool for the diagnosis of pericardial effusion (see Chapter 23).

General edema in the absence of ascites is invariably secondary to hypoalbuminemia. Serum albumin concentrations must fall below 1 to 1.5 g/dl (10–15 g/L) before edema becomes clinically apparent. If right heart failure or portal hypertension accompanies hypoproteinemia, edema

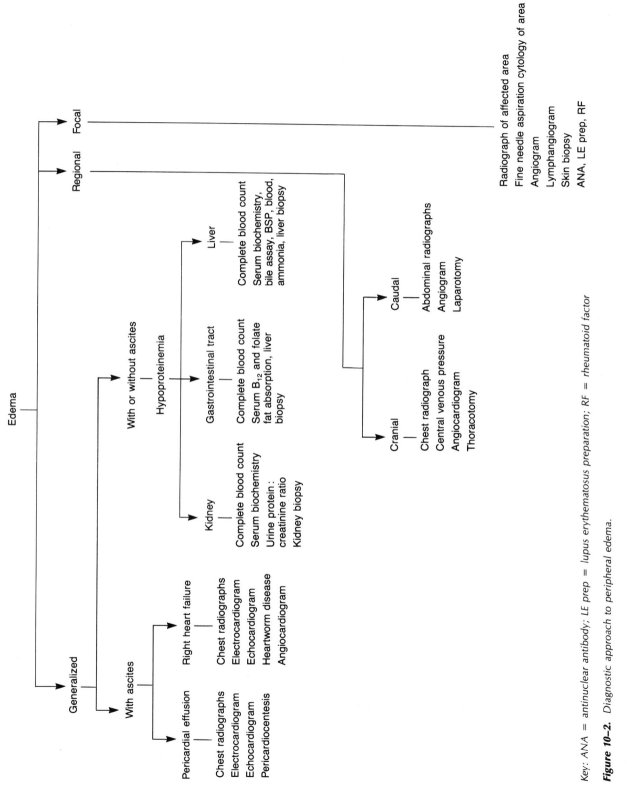

Edema

Generalized

With ascites

Pericardial effusion
Chest radiographs
Electrocardiogram
Echocardiogram
Pericardiocentesis

Right heart failure
Chest radiographs
Electrocardiogram
Echocardiogram
Heartworm disease
Angiocardiogram

With or without ascites

Hypoproteinemia

Kidney
Complete blood count
Serum biochemistry
Urine protein :
creatinine ratio
Kidney biopsy

Gastrointestinal tract
Complete blood count
Serum B₁₂ and folate
fat absorption, liver
biopsy

Liver
Complete blood count
Serum biochemistry,
bile assay, BSP, blood,
ammonia, liver biopsy

Regional

Cranial
Chest radiograph
Central venous pressure
Angiocardiogram
Thoracotomy

Caudal
Abdominal radiographs
Angiogram
Laparotomy

Focal

Radiograph of affected area
Fine needle aspiration cytology of area
Angiogram
Lymphangiogram
Skin biopsy
ANA, LE prep, RF

Key: ANA = antinuclear antibody; LE prep = lupus erythematosus preparation; RF = rheumatoid factor

Figure 10–2. *Diagnostic approach to peripheral edema.*

102

will form at serum albumin levels as high as 2 g/dl (20 g/L). The edema fluid is low in protein content (less than 2 g/dl or 20 g/L) and lacks cells. Renal or gastrointestinal tract protein loss or decreased hepatic production must be differentiated. With glomerular disease serum albumin concentrations fall. Serum globulin levels remain normal. Renal disease, including amyloidosis and nephrotic syndrome, are possible causes. Urine protein : creatinine ratios establish the extent of protein loss through the kidney (Center, Additional Reading). Increases in serum cholesterol are common. Renal biopsy may be needed to categorize the histologic type of disease and provide appropriate therapy (see Chapter 45 and Kidney Biopsy in Chapter 80). Gastrointestinal tract disease is characterized by the loss of serum albumin and globulin. Lymphagiectasia is the most common cause. Lymphopenia and fat malabsorption accompany the disease. Hypoalbuminemia is a late finding in liver disease. Serum globulin levels are normal or increased. A nonregenerative anemia may be present. Sulfobromophthalein sodium (BSP) excretion, serum ammonia levels, and bile assay may be completed to confirm decreased functional hepatic mass. Abdominal radiographs and ultrasound followed by hepatic biopsy (see Liver Biopsy in Chapter 80) confirm the diagnosis and may provide histologic evidence of its cause.

Regional edema is most often caused by mass lesions causing obstruction of the cranial or caudal vena cava or sublumbar iliac veins. Chest radiography and angiocardiography, followed by fine needle aspiration of the mass, is indicated to establish a diagnosis in cases with cranial edema. Thoracotomy may be required to gain access to the mass and determine if it is resectable. Rectal and deep pelvic palpation, and radiographs of the abdomen looking for changes in the size or shape of the kidneys and liver and displacement of organs by space-occupying masses is warranted in cases of caudal edema. If caudal edema is accompanied by ascites, portal hypertension should also be considered. Venography or lymphangiography may be required to confirm the presence of a vascular abnormality.

Focal edema is associated with local pathology of arteries, veins, or lymphatics. If the anastomotic area of a large arteriovenous shunt is oc-cluded, venous return is decreased and the heart rate falls (Branham's sign). Edema fluid due to vascular inflammation or injury is high in protein (greater than 4 g/dl or 40 g/L) and cellular content. Lymphedema is also high in protein content (greater than 4 g/dl or 40 g/L), but the cell content is low. Palpation of affected areas with evidence of pain, heat, and swelling are indicative of active inflammation. Radiography and fine needle biopsy of the tissue and associated lymph node(s) should follow. In animals in which an immune-mediated cause is suspect, a skin biopsy and immunologic studies, including antinuclear antibody, lupus erythematous (LE) prep, and rheumatoid factor, may be indicated. Lymphangiography or angiography is sometimes required to delineate the lesion. Lymphangiography is technically difficult to perform and interpret in the face of massive edema formation.

MANAGEMENT AND PATIENT MONITORING

The treatment of edema is directed at its primary cause. Capillary hypertension secondary to congestive heart failure is managed with a low salt diet and diuretic and vasodilator therapy (see Chapter 20). Pericardial effusion is drained by needle paracentesis (see Pericardiocentesis in Chapter 80) and, where indicated, is treated by pericardiectomy. Hypoalbuminemia is generally a grave prognostic sign. Renal, gastrointestinal tract, or hepatic disease leading to hypoalbuminemia is progressive and fatal. Supportive treatment involves plasma transfusion (10–20 ml/kg IV). Arteriovenous shunts are managed surgically. All arterial branches to the area are ligated and the shunt itself is removed. In large or chronically recurring fistulas, wide surgical excision or amputation of the limb may be required (Allen, Additional Reading). Disease causing capillary permeability changes may be treated with glucocorticoids or nonsteroidal anti-inflammatory agents. Treatment is based on evidence gathered from laboratory data. Treatment of primary lymphedema requires bandaging or surgical excision of subcutaneous and superficial fascia. The prognosis for curing the condition is guarded.

11

ASCITES

Dana G. Allen

Ascites is the accumulation of free fluid in the abdominal cavity. The fluid may be blood, bile, urine, chyle, transudates, or exudates. Although ascites itself rarely poses a significant clinical problem, it may be indicative of a more serious systemic disease.

CAUSES

Ascites secondary to transudates and modified transudates is most often associated with portal venous hypertension. Causes are classified as prehepatic (or presinusoidal), hepatic, and posthepatic (or postsinusoidal) (Fig. 11-1). Prehepatic causes are those diseases causing compression or obstruction of portal venous blood flow (portal vein thrombosis or stenosis) or intravascular or extravascular neoplasia. The most common cause of hepatic disease leading to ascites is portal venous hypertension secondary to hepatic fibrosis or cirrhosis. Chronic active hepatitis, diffuse hepatic fibrosis, cholangiohepatitis (cat), biliary obstruction, metastatic neoplasia, lipidosis, and hepatic vein thrombosis or intrahepatic atresia of branches of the hepatic vein are other possible causes. Although congenital portosystemic shunts increase portal venous blood flow, portal hypertension is rare and ascites does not form unless it is accompanied by hypo-albuminemia. Posthepatic causes of ascites include right heart failure, pericardial tamponade, constrictive pericarditis, intracardiac neoplasia, heartworm disease, and compression or obstruction of the caudal vena cava.

Exudative effusions are associated with inflammatory disease of the peritoneal cavity. Feline infectious peritonitis; peritonitis secondary to trauma, sepsis, pancreatitis, presence of bile, steatitis, rupture of the bowel, prostatic abscess, or pyometra; and irritation from products released by neoplasms are possible causes. Blood, chyle, and urine are also classified as exudates, but will be discussed separately.

The presence of blood in the abdomen is a grave prognostic sign. In older animals it most often occurs following rupture of a splenic tumor (hemangiosarcoma). This disease is especially common in the German shepherd. In other animals, bleeding disorders associated with anticoagulant toxicity (coumarins, indanediones), thrombocytopenia, or vascular trauma must be considered.

Abdominal chylous effusion is uncommon. It may be congenital and due to lymphangiectasia, or acquired and secondary to rupture of the cisterna chyli or invasion of lymphatics with neoplastic cells, as with lymphosarcoma or metastatic disease.

Rupture of the bladder may follow abdominal

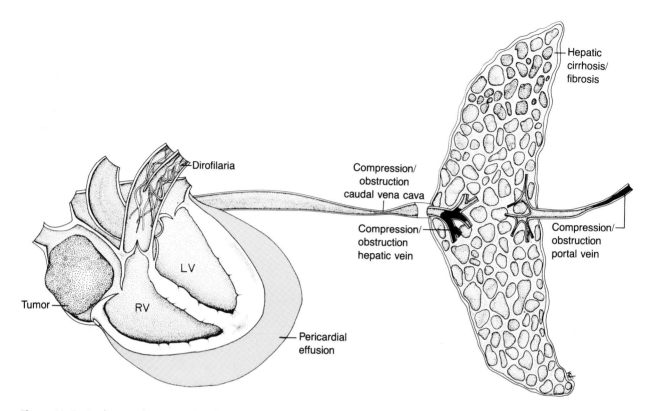

Figure 11–1. *Posthepatic, hepatic, and prehepatic factors contributing to portal hypertension and ascites.*

trauma. It occurs most commonly in male dogs struck by automobiles and in cats it may occur secondary to attempts to forcibly empty obstructed urinary bladders associated with feline lower urinary tract inflammation (see Chapter 48).

PATHOPHYSIOLOGY

Factors provoking ascites formation are increased portal venous hydrostastic pressure (modified transudate) and decreased plasma colloid osmotic pressure due to hypoalbuminemia (transudate). Portal hypertension develops with lesions that impair hepatic venous blood flow. Increased portal blood flow secondary to intrahepatic arteriovenous shunts is a less common cause. Portal hypertension leads to the formation of a high protein abdominal fluid derived from hepatic lymph (Greene, Additional Reading). Hepatic lymph is normally formed from the filtration of sinusoidal blood as it passes between endothelial cells and enters the space of Disse (Fig. 11-2). From the space of Disse, it enters lymphatics at the hepatic triads and empties into the cisterna chyli and thoracic duct. Hepatic venous stasis increases portal and sinusoidal blood pressure and increases the production of hepatic lymph. Fluid "weeps" from the surface of the liver and gravitates into the abdominal cavity. The high osmotic pressure of this fluid tends to draw additional fluid from the surfaces of the gut into the abdomen.

Portal hypertension is classified on the basis of the location of the inciting cause. Prehepatic causes associated with obstruction of the portal vein rarely lead to ascites. Prehepatic or presinusoidal portal hypertension leads to increased gastrointestinal capillary pressure and transient transudation of fluid from the serosa of the gut. Rapid collateral vessel development between the

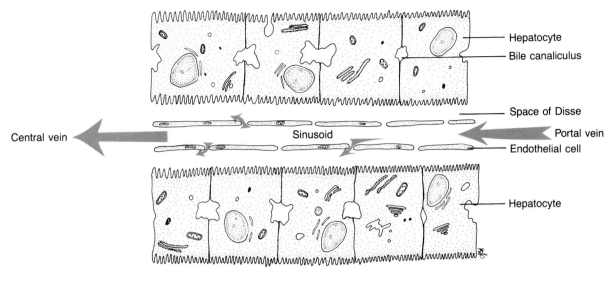

Figure 11–2. *Hepatic lymph is formed from the filtration of sinusoidal blood as it passes between endothelial cells and enters the space of Disse. From the space of Disse hepatic lymph enters lymphatics at the portal triad and empties into the cisterna chyli and the thoracic duct. Sinusoidal blood drains to the central vein and enters the hepatic vein and the caudal vena cava.*

portal vein and vena cava decreases capillary hydrostatic pressure and limits ascites formation. In addition, lymph flow from the gut increases dramatically and compensates for the increased portal pressure. Splenomegaly is uncommon because collateral vessel development facilitates splenic venous outflow. Ascites tends to form only if there is concurrent hypoalbuminemia. Subcutaneous edema, however, is more common with hypoproteinemia than ascites. The hypoproteinemia may be due to decreased dietary intake (rare), increased loss via the gastrointestinal tract or kidney, or decreased hepatic production. Serum albumin levels must fall below 1.5 g/dl (15 g/L) before edema or ascites occurs. In these cases the ascitic fluid is low in protein content (less than 2.5 g/dl or 25 g/L).

The most common cause of portal hypertension associated with liver disease is hepatic fibrosis or cirrhosis. Hepatic fibrosis and nodular regeneration associated with cirrhosis, hepatitis, neoplasia, and lipidosis impair hepatic venous blood flow and lead to portal and sinusoidal hypertension. Anastomosis between hepatic arterioles and the portal venous system augments portal hypertension. Portal hypertension in the

absence of sinusoidal hypertension rarely leads to the development of ascites.

Two theories have been postulated to explain the occurrence of ascites with liver disease. The traditional or "underfilling" theory contends that hypoalbuminemia and portal hypertension initiate the process. Ascites, hypoproteinemia, portal hypertension, and dilation of the splanchnic vascular bed lead to a fall in the circulating blood volume and a decrease in cardiac output and renal perfusion. The kidney responds by activating the renin–angiotensin–aldosterone system to promote water and sodium reabsorption. In addition, hepatic inactivation of aldosterone is impaired. The traditional theory is based on the assumption of a decreased circulating blood volume, which has not been documented. The traditional theory has been replaced by the overflow theory, which states that abnormal renal salt and water retention is the initiating event in the formation of ascites. This leads to the expansion of the extracellular fluid space and portal hypertension. With the subsequent development of hypoalbuminemia and portal hypertension, ascites forms. An increased sensitivity to aldosterone and a failure to release natriuretic factor in response to the increased extracellular volume have been implicated in the development of abnormal salt and water retention.

Posthepatic or postsinusoidal portal hypertension results in the formation of high protein ascites (greater than 2.5 g/dl or 25 g/L) derived from hepatic lymph. Blood flow in the caudal vena cava is impaired; this leads to portal hypertension.

Exudative effusions result from inflammatory disease and increased vascular permeability. Ascitic fluid is high in protein content (greater than 2.5 g/dl or 25 g/L). Septic or irritant substances initiate the inflammatory process. Blood is classified as an exudate. Its presence signifies vascular damage (neoplasia, trauma), thrombocytopenia, or factor deficiency (anticoagulant toxicity). Chylous effusion results from traumatic lymphatic rupture or blockage. Structural abnormalities associated with lymphangiectasia predispose to lymphatic leakage. Urine is a chemical irritant that incites peritoneal inflammation. Urine leakage follows rupture of the urinary tract, most commonly the bladder.

CLINICAL SIGNS

The presenting complaint is often that of a pendulous, enlarged abdomen. In humans, 500 ml or more of fluid must be present before ascites is clinically apparent. The onset of ascites may be acute, as with acute anticoagulant toxicity or rupture of the bladder, or more gradual, as with hypoalbuminemia or congestive heart failure. In many cases of hemangiosarcoma of the spleen or liver, intermittent episodes of weakness and collapse followed by spontaneous recovery can be related to hemorrhage from the neoplastic organ into the abdominal cavity and subsequent resorption of the abdominal blood. Ascites may be accompanied by pleural effusion and peripheral edema. Subcutaneous edema is present in many animals with hypoalbuminemia even in the absence of ascites. The presence of significant volumes of ascitic fluid limits excursions of the diaphragm and contributes to dyspnea, which, in the presence of concurrent pleural effusion, can be marked.

Weight gain in spite of a decreased appetite and loss of muscle mass may be related to the accumulation of significant volumes of abdominal fluid. In other cases weight loss predominates. Animals with chronic wasting disease are generally afflicted with diseases causing hypoproteinemia, (*e.g.*, protein-losing enteropathy or nephropathy), neoplasia, or cardiac disease. Hypoalbuminemia contributes to the cachexia associated with chronic liver disease. Lethargy and depression accompany the cachexic state.

Intrahepatic and prehepatic causes of portal hypertension are associated with shunting of blood around the liver. The liver no longer removes circulating toxins (*e.g.*, ammonia), and signs of hepatic encephalopathy may develop (see Chapter 40). The triad of icterus, hepatic encephalopathy, and ascites is strongly suggestive of cirrhosis.

Shunting of blood around the liver does not occur in cases of posthepatic portal hypertension because no gradient forms between the portal and systemic venous beds; thus hepatic encephalopathy is not seen.

Other clinical signs are related to specific organ involvement. Patients with cardiac disease or neoplasia of the liver or spleen present with decreased exercise tolerance, weakness, and collapse. Those with gastrointestinal disease leading to hypoproteinemia and ascites often present with chronic histories of small bowel diarrhea (see Chapter 37). Renal disease may be accompanied by polyuria, polydipsia, anorexia, vomiting, and diarrhea (see Chapters 43 and 44). A history of trauma should alert the clinician to the possibility of organ rupture. The ability to urinate is variable with rupture of the bladder and should not be considered a reliable indication of an intact bladder.

DIAGNOSTIC APPROACH

In the approach to the animal with abdominal distention, clinicians must initially determine if free fluid is present in the abdominal cavity (Fig. 11-3). In cases in which fluid is not detected, abdominal distention may be related to obesity, a gravid uterus, pyometra, gastric dilation, obsti-

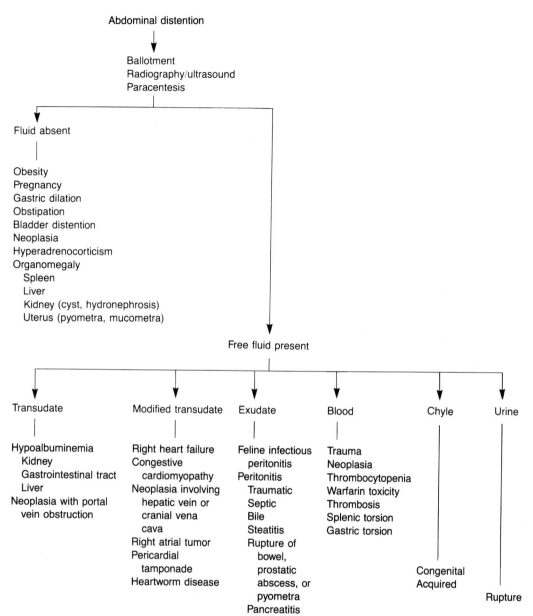

Figure 11–3. *Diagnostic approach to causes of abdominal enlargement.*

pation, a large atonic fluid-filled bladder, neoplasia of abdominal organ(s), hepatomegaly associated with passive venous congestion, splenomegaly associated with barbiturate use or torsion of the splenic pedicle, and renomegaly associated with cystic disease or hydronephrosis. Hyperadrenocorticism is accompanied by muscle laxity and the centrifugal redistribution of fat, which leads to abdomen enlargement.

The abdomen is palpated for organ enlargement and pain due to inflammatory disease and ballotted for the detection of fluid. In many cases the accumulation of abdominal fluid hinders adequate palaption of abdominal contents. To detect ascites, the palm of one hand is placed firmly on one side of the abdomen and the fingers of the other hand are used to percuss the opposite side of the abdomen and generate a palpable fluid wave. Ascites is confirmed by abdominal radiography or ultrasonography and paracentesis. Radiography is often limited by the loss of detail that accompanies ascites, but is useful prior to paracentesis for the detection of neoplastic disease, organomegaly, or trauma.

Passive venous congestion and hepatomegaly accompany posthepatic portal hypertension. Changes in liver shape accompany hepatic neoplastic disease. Microhepatica may be seen with hepatic cirrhosis, fibrosis, or congenital portovenous shunts. Liver size is normal with presinusoidal causes of portal hypertension. Abdominal ultrasonography is a safe, sensitive, non-invasive tool for the detection of abdominal fluid, neoplastic disease, and organ pathology. If fluid is detected, the most rewarding diagnostic procedure in the approach to animals with ascites is abdominal paracentesis. The technique is described in detail in Chapter 80.

Abdominal fluid is evaluated on the basis of its appearance, protein content, specific gravity, and cellular content (Table 11-1). Most clinicians initially approach the laboratory assessment of ascites on the basis of its physical appearance and protein content. Fluid is subsequently classified as transudate, modified transudate, exudate, chyle, blood, urine, or bile. The etiology of each fluid type can then be approached (see Fig. 11-3). Confirmation of the diagnosis can be established by completing additional tests, as outlined in Table 11-2.

Table 11–1 *Laboratory Assessment of Effusive Disease*

TRANSUDATE

APPEARANCE
Clear and colorless

PROTEIN CONTENT
<2.5 g/dl or 25 g/L

SPECIFIC GRAVITY
<1.018

CELLULAR CHARACTERISTICS
Cell counts <1000/µl, and include nondegenerate neutrophils and reactive mesothelial cells

OTHER
Serum albumin concentration is <1.5 g/dl (15 g/L) in cases secondary to hypoproteinemia.

MODIFIED TRANSUDATE

APPEARANCE
Red and pink or cloudy

PROTEIN CONTENT
2.5 to 5 g/dl or 25 to 50 g/L

SPECIFIC GRAVITY
>1.018

CELLULAR CHARACTERISTICS
Cell counts <5000/µl, and include red cells, nondegenerate neutrophils, mesothelial cells, macrophages, and occasional eosinophils (heartworm) and lymphocytes

EXUDATE

Nonseptic Exudate

APPEARANCE
White, pink, and cloudy

PROTEIN CONTENT
2.5 to 5 g/dl or 25 to 50 g/L

SPECIFIC GRAVITY
>1.018

CELLULAR CHARACTERISTICS
Cell counts 3000 to 50,000/µl or higher, and include nondegenerate neutrophils and variable numbers of macrophages, erythrocytes, and lymphocytes

OTHER
The exudate accompanying feline infectious peritonitis is characteristically viscid, yellow-green, and cloudy; it sometimes contains fibrin flecks.
Protein content is 3.8 to 8 g/dl (38–80 g/L).
Cell counts of 700 to 23,000/µl, and include nondegenerate neutrophils, with fewer macrophages.
Complete blood count: absolute neutrophilia with normal or low lymphocyte counts in many.

Septic Exudate

APPEARANCE
White, red, yellowish, and cloudy

PROTEIN CONTENT
2.5 to 5.5 g/dl or 25 to 55 g/L

SPECIFIC GRAVITY
>1.018

CELLULAR CHARACTERISTICS
Cell counts 3000 to 100,000/µl or higher, and include degenerate neutrophils and variable numbers of macrophages and intracellular or extracellular bacteria

OTHER
Foul odor

(continued)

Table 11–1 (continued)

Exudates due to infection with *Nocardia* and *Actinomyces* organisms may contain sulfur granules and gram-positive filamentous rods.

Ascitic fluid with levels of alkaline phosphatase greater than serum levels suggest intestinal trauma, ischemia, or leakage.

CHYLE

APPEARANCE

Pink, white, or opaque; straw- or tan-colored in fasting animals

PROTEIN CONTENT

2 to 6.5 g/dl or 20 to 65 g/L

SPECIFIC GRAVITY

1.012 to 1.037 or higher

CELLULAR CHARACTERISTICS

Cell counts <10,000/μl, and include small lymphocytes and variable numbers of nondegenerate neutrophils

OTHER

Forms a creamlike layer if refrigerated and allowed to stand
Fat droplets stain with Sudan III stain.
Clears when shaken with ether following alkalanization with two drops of 1 N sodium hydroxide
High triglyceride content and a low or normal cholesterol content compared with serum
Lymphopenia and hypoproteinemia may accompany the disease.

PSEUDOCHYLOUS EFFUSION

APPEARANCE

White

PROTEIN CONTENT

>2.5 g/dl or 25 g/L

SPECIFIC GRAVITY

1.009 to 1.035

OTHER

Milky appearance is due to the presence of lecithin–globulin complexes or cholesterol granules and is most commonly associated with feline cardiac disease, intrathoracic neoplasia, or infection.
Does not form a creamlike layer
Will not stain with Sudan III stain
Will not clear with ether
Triglyceride levels are normal but cholesterol content is higher than serum.

HEMORRHAGIC EFFUSIONS

APPEARANCE

Bloody, clear supernatant with red sediment

PROTEIN CONTENT

>3.0 g/dl or 30 g/L

SPECIFIC GRAVITY

Of no diagnostic value

CELLULAR CHARACTERISTICS

Packed-cell volume is similar to that of peripheral blood
Does not clot
Intact red blood cells and leukocytes similar to those of peripheral circulation

Platelets are not present unless bleeding has occurred within the previous 45 minutes.
With longer-standing effusions, macrophages with phagocytized red cells and hemosiderin are present.
Nucleated peripheral red blood cells may accompany hemangiosarcoma.

URINE

APPEARANCE

Clear or cloudy and pale yellow

PROTEIN CONTENT

>2.5 g/dl or 25 g/L

SPECIFIC GRAVITY

>1.018

CELLULAR CHARACTERISTICS

Cell counts 3000 to 50,000/μl or higher, and include nondegenerate neutrophils, macrophages, red cells, and lymphocytes

OTHER

If rupture has occurred within the preceding 24 hours the abdominal fluid will have a higher urea and creatinine content than serum.
Elevations in serum urea and creatinine, hyponatremia, hypochloremia, hyperkalemia, and metabolic acidosis frequently accompany the rupture.

BILE

APPEARANCE

Clear or cloudy and yellow

PROTEIN CONTENT

>2.5 g/dl or 25 g/L

SPECIFIC GRAVITY

>1.018

CELLULAR CHARACTERISTICS

Cell counts 3000 to 50,000/μl or higher, and include nondegenerate neutrophils, macrophages, red cells, and lymphocytes

OTHER

The presence of bilirubin can be confirmed with a urine dipstick or Icotest. In non-icteric animals the presence of bilirubin implies leakage from the biliary tree or proximal bowel.

PANCREATITIS

APPEARANCE

Variable

PROTEIN CONTENT

>2.5 g/dl or 25 g/L

SPECIFIC GRAVITY

>1.018

CELLULAR CHARACTERISTICS

Cell counts 3000 to 50,000/μl or higher, and include nongenerate neutrophils, macrophages, red cells, and lymphocytes

OTHER

Amylase content is higher than serum if acute pancreatitis is present.

Table 11–2 Additional Tests in the Approach to Animals with Ascites

Fluid Type	Association	Ancillary Tests
Transudate	Hypoproteinemia	
	Kidneys	CBC, serum biochemistry, urine protein:creatinine, kidney biopsy
	Gastrointestinal tract	CBC, serum biochemistry, serum B_{12} and folate, fat absorption, intestinal biopsy
	Liver	CBC, serum biochemistry, BSP retention, ammonia, bile acids, liver biopsy
Modified transudate	Cardiovascular	Chest radiographs, ECG, CVP, ultrasound, angiocardiogram, heartworm testing
Exudate	Feline infectious peritonitis	Serum globulin, serum titers
	Peritonitis	Radiographs, ultrasound, fluid analysis (see Table 11–1), bacterial/fungal culture of fluid
Blood	Coagulation abnormality	Abdominal radiographs or ultrasound, CBC, ACT or PT, PTT, FDP, clot retraction, platelet numbers
Chyle	Congenital, acquired	CBC, serum protein, lymphangiograms
Urine	Rupture	Radiographs, contrast cystograms, serum biochemistry, arterial blood-gas analysis

ACT = activated clotting time; CBC = complete blood count; CVP = central venous pressure; ECG = electrocardiogram; PT = prothrombin time; PTT = partial thromboplastin time; FDP = fibrin degradation products

High protein ascites (greater than 2.5 g/dl or 25 g/L) is associated with obstruction of blood flow from hepatic sinusoids, as with right heart failure, compressive lesions of the caudal vena cava, or hepatic vein (see Fig. 11-3). Low protein ascites occurs with hypoproteinemia (less than 2.5 g/dl or 25 g/L of transudate) or obstruction of presinusoidal blood flow due to hepatic arteriovenous fistula, portal fibrosis or neoplasia, portal vein atresia, or portal vein thrombosis. The protein content of ascitic fluid is initially high in hepatic cirrhosis. In time, portal hypertension is accompanied by the increased production of low protein ascites from intestinal lymph, and the protein level of the ascitic fluid varies. Neoplastic disease commonly leads to the formation of a high protein ascites, unless it is accompanied by impairment of blood flow to the liver (presinusoidal) and the increased production of low protein intestinal lymph.

In humans the ratio of albumin in serum to that in ascites is used to document the presence of portal hypertension and is considered more accurate in the approach to the diagnosis than the classification scheme of transudate vs. exudate (Rector, Additional Reading). In patients with portal hypertension associated with right heart failure, pericardial tamponade, restrictive pericarditis, and cirrhosis, the serum : ascites ratio is 1.1 g/dl (11 g/L). The ratio is less than 1.1 g/dl (11 g/L) in cases without portal hypertension. The usefulness of this ratio in veterinary medicine has yet to be determined.

MANAGEMENT

Treatment is directed at the cause of ascites formation. If animals are markedly uncomfortable or dyspneic, it may be necessary to remove ascitic fluid by abdominocentesis to promote patient relief. Abdominocentesis improves venous return, cardiac output, and renal blood flow, leading to improved diuresis. Rapid paracentesis does not cause immediate changes in blood pressure, heart rate, packed-cell volume, or serum electrolytes. Hypoproteinemia and hyponatremia may become apparent following abdominocentesis as ascitic fluid reforms. Complications of this procedure occur most often in patients with liver failure. Albumin depletion, peritonitis, hypovolemia, oliguria, and hepatic encephalopathy are possible, but uncommon, sequelae. If the ascitic fluid is high in protein, it can be collected aseptically and reinfused intravenously into those patients requiring repeated abdominocentesis.

If ascites is due to hypoproteinemia, intravenous plasma can be given (10–20 ml/kg IV); however, large volumes are required to cause any increase in serum protein levels, and the beneficial clinical effects are only temporary.

Sodium retention is a key factor in the initiation of ascites in liver disease and heart failure. Rest and sodium restriction result in spontaneous diuresis in 5% to 15% of humans with ascites. Ascites tends not to reform following paracentesis in animals with liver disease and heart failure if sodium intake is limited. Dietary salt restriction may be in the form of Prescription Diet h/d (Hill's). Alternatively, homemade diets can be substituted. Organ meats should be avoided; lean skeletal meats are preferred. In lieu of table salt, potassium chloride can be used to season foods.

Specific treatment of ascites due to liver disease includes dietary salt restriction and the potassium-sparing diuretic spironolactone (1–2 mg/kg b.i.d. orally). Diuresis may not be apparent for 3 to 4 days. If the animal fails to respond, the spironolactone dose can be doubled and the patient observed for an additional 3 to 4 days. Animals should be weighed daily. The gain or loss of 1 kg of body weight is equivalent to the gain or loss of 1 liter of fluid, assuming muscle mass has not changed. A gradual decrease in ascitic fluid is recommended and should not exceed more than 0.3 kg/day in a 20-kg dog (Grauer, Additional Reading).

If dietary salt restriction and diuretic use fails to improve the patient's condition, the potent loop diuretics furosemide (Lasix) or ethacrynic acid can be added to the regimen. Lasix is preferred and is given at a starting dose of 1 mg/kg b.i.d. orally. If diuresis is not achieved within 4 to 7 days, the dose can be doubled. Propanolol, a β-adrenergic blocking agent, has been used in humans to decrease portal pressure in patients with cirrhosis. The drug decreases cardiac output and induces peripheral vasoconstriction, leading to a decrease in portal venous pressure. To date its use in dogs has not been met with much success.

Animals refractory to medical therapy are potential candidates for surgery. The LeVeen peritoneovenous shunt is a unidirectional shunt that carries ascitic fluid from the abdominal cavity via a subcutaneous catheter into the jugular vein. The shunt is well tolerated by dogs. Alternatively, a portal systemic venous shunt can be surgically created.

Exudative causes of ascites, including blood, chyle, and urine, are managed according to the inciting disease. Laparotomy, closure of penetrating wounds, bacterial culture, and appropriate antibiotic treatment may be indicated in cases of peritonitis. Laparotomy, splenectomy, and biopsy of the liver and mesenteric lymph nodes follows the finding of abdominal blood in older animals. Chylous effusion is treated by the dietary restiction of fat and rest. Diets should be high in protein and carbohydrates and low in fat. Chicken, beef, eggs, and cottage cheese are excellent sources of protein, and rice is a good source of carbohydrate. If medical management is unsuccessful, surgical intervention may be required.

Although feline infectious peritonitis is a highly fatal disease, some cats undergo spontaneous remission. Successful treatment of cats has been reported only in those with mild clinical signs. The drugs used included prednisone or prednisolone and cyclophosphamide (Pedersen, Additional Reading).

PATIENT MONITORING

Ascites associated with hypoproteinemia, cardiac disease, and liver disease is frequently a grave prognostic sign. The inciting disease is progressive and fatal. Infection of the ascitic fluid with coliform bacteria may complicate liver failure. Care must be exercised with the use of diuretics to ensure that dehydration, azotemia, hypokalemia, metabolic alkalosis, and signs of hepatic encephalopathy do not accompany their use. Generalized peritonitis in the dog is most often associated with contamination from the gastrointestinal tract secondary to surgical wound dehiscence. Overall mortality approaches 70% (Hosgood, Additional Reading).

Non-neoplastic causes of hemoperitoneum can be successfully treated with removal of the inciting cause and medical management of the bleeding disorder (*e.g.,* vitamin K_1, fresh whole blood) (see Chapter 16). Dogs and cats with splenic hemangiosarcoma have a mean survival time of approximately 4 months regardless of therapy or the stage of disease (Brown et al; Scavelli et al, Additional Reading). Although spontaneous resolution of chylothorax has been reported, the prognosis for nontraumatic chylothorax is poor regardless of treatment regimen. The prognosis for the successful surgical management of chylothorax is also guarded. It is assumed that cases with chylous ascites would be similar. If rupture of the urinary bladder is not corrected, death may intervene within 48 to 72 hours. Rapid surgical correction of the rupture usually results in complete recovery.

ADDITIONAL READING

Brown NO, Patnaik AK, MacEwen G. Canine hemangiosarcoma: Retrospective analysis of 104 cases. J Am Vet Med Assoc 1985; 186:56.

Crowe DT, Lorenz MD, Hardie EM et al. Chronic peritoneal effusion due to partial caudal vena caval obstruction following blunt trauma: Diagnosis and successful surgical treatment. Journal of the American Animal Hospital Association 1984; 20:231.

Ettinger SJ. Ascites, peritonitis and other causes of abdominal enlargement. In: Ettinger SJ, ed. Textbook of veterinary internal medicine. Philadelphia: WB Saunders, 1983: 121.

Grauer GF, Nichols CE. Ascites, renal abnormalities and electrolyte and acid base disorders associated with liver disease. Vet Clin North Am 1985; 15:197.

Greene CE. Ascites: Diagnostic and therapeutic considerations. Compendium of Continuing Education 1979; 1:712.

Hardy RM. Diseases of the liver. In: Ettinger SJ, ed. Textbook of veterinary internal medicine. Philadelphia: WB Saunders, 1983: 1372.

Hosgood G, Salisbury K. Generalized peritonitis in dogs: 50 cases (1975–1986). J Am Vet Med Assoc 1988; 193:1448.

Johnson SE. Portal hypertension. Part I. Pathophysiology and clinical consequences. Compendium of Continuing Education 1987; 9:741.

Johnson SE. Portal hypertension. Part II. Clinical assessment and treatment. Compendium of Continuing Education 1987; 9:917.

Pedersen NC. Feline coronavirus infections. In: Greene CE, ed. Clinical microbiology and infectious diseases of the dog and cat. Philadelphia: WB Saunders, 1984: 514.

Prasse KW, Duncan JR. Laboratory diagnosis of pleural and peritoneal effusions. Vet Clin North Am 1976; 6:625.

Rector WG. An improved diagnostic approach to ascites. Arch Intern Med 1987; 147:215.

Scavelli TD, Patnaik AK, Mehlhaff CJ, Hayes AA. Hemangiosarcoma in the cat: Retrospective of 31 surgical cases. J Am Vet Med Assoc 1985; 187:817.

12

PAIN

Dana G. Allen

Pain is indicative of tissue trauma. It informs the animal that tissue injury has occurred and evasive action is necessary. It is also one of the earliest signs of systemic disease. The treatment of pain is often neglected in veterinary medicine because animals fail to communicate their discomfort in a manner we recognize. Close observation of a change in an animal's behavior may be the only indication of pain.

CAUSES

Pain may be generalized or localized to a specific body area. The common causes of pain in small animals are listed in Table 12-1. Although the list is extensive, it is by no means complete. Any disease provoking inflammation or ischemia may be accompanied by pain.

PATHOPHYSIOLOGY

Traumatic, chemical, mechanical, inflammatory, hypoxic, and thermal (greater than 45°C or 113°F) stimuli can initiate a sensation of pain. Although the perception of pain is similar between individuals, the tolerance to pain varies greatly. Tolerance to pain also varies within the same individual on different occasions. Anticipation, concentration on the situation, blood pressure, stress level, counterirritation, and emotional state affect the sensation to pain. Stress induces a relative state of analgesia and allows the animal to fight or flee from potentially dangerous situations.

Pain receptors, the nociceptive nerve endings located throughout the body, relay impulses to the spinal cord and substantia gelatinosa via the dorsal root ganglion. From the substantia gelatinosa the nerve fibers enter the lateral spinothalamic tract and ascend the spinal cord to the thalamic nuclei, from which they are directed to the somatic sensory area of the cerebral cortex (Fig. 12-1). Appropriate evasive motor reflex action may then occur.

Pain impulses from the head and face are carried to the brain by the trigeminal, facial, and vagus nerves. Mucous membrane pain is transmitted to the brain along these nerves and via the glossopharyneal nerve as well. Projected pain impulses are carried directly from the area where the stimulus was initiated. Referred pain describes pain felt in an area distant from the site in which it originated. Examples of referred pain are cervical disk disease referred to a forelimb, diaphragmatic pain referred to the neck and shoulder, stomach pain referred to the midthorax, and ureteral pain referred to the scrotum.

Three types of pain have been described. Cuta-

Table 12–1 *Common Causes of Pain in Small Animals*

ALL BODY SYSTEMS

Trauma
Neoplasia
Inflammation
Infection

GENERALIZED PAIN

Meningitis
Polyarthritis, polymyositis
Polyradiculoneuritis
Tetanus

SKIN AND SUBCUTANEOUS TISSUE PAIN

Pemphigus vulgaris or bullous pemphigoid
Toxic epidermal necrolysis
Erythema multiforme
Pannicullitis, steatitis
Abscess
Perianal fistulae, abscess
Foreign body

HEAD PAIN

Central nervous system disease, including hemorrhage and
  space-occupying lesions
Craniomandibular osteopathy
Eosinophilic myositis
Otitis externa

ORAL CAVITY PAIN

Tooth root abscess
Foreign body (e.g., porcupine quills)
Glossitis (e.g., "burr tongue," renal failure, pancreatitis,
  leptospirosis)
Tonsillitis
Retropharyngeal abscess
Feline upper respiratory viruses (herpesvirus, calicivirus)
Ingestion of toxic plants (e.g., dieffenbachia, philodendron,
  elephant ear)
Necrotizing ulcerative gingivitis
Insect bites or stings
Pemphigus vulgaris or bullous pemphigoid

NECK OR BACK PAIN

Cervical vertebral instability ("wobbler")
Atlantoaxial instability
Disk disease
Osteoarthritis
Diskospondylitis
Hypervitaminosis A (cat)
Myelitis, meningitis
Nerve root entrapment
Neoplasia affecting spinal cord (intradural, extradural,
  intramedullary)
Lumbosacral stenosis

CHEST PAIN

Pericarditis
Musculoskeletal pain
Tracheobronchitis
Pneumothorax
Pulmonary thromboembolism
Pleuritis

ABDOMINAL PAIN

INFLAMMATION

Hemorrhagic gastroenteritis
Feline panleukopenia
Canine parvovirus
Acute pancreatitis
Gastrointestinal ulceration

PERITONITIS

Gastrointestinal rupture
Urinary tract rupture
Biliary tree rupture
Hemoperitoneum
Acute pancreatitis
Ruptured abscess

OBSTRUCTION

Foreign body
Gastric dilation–volvulus
Intestinal volvulus
Intussusception
Incarceration of bowel in hernia or mesenteric tear
Stenosis or stricture
Vascular thrombosis of intestine

OTHER

Splenic torsion, rupture, or neoplasia
Pyelonephritis
Ureteral or urethral obstruction (FUS, urolith)
Torsion of retained testicle
Prostatitis
Hepatitis
Pelvic fracture
Hyperlipoproteinemia

LEG PAIN

Hypertrophic osteodystrophy
Panosteitis
Osteomyelitis
Osteochondritis
Hip dysplasia
Joint disease
Myositis
Vascular thrombosis
Nerve compression
Synovitis
Neoplasia

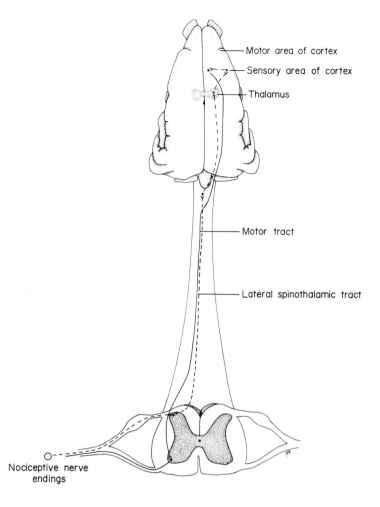

Motor area of cortex

Sensory area of cortex

Thalamus

Motor tract

Lateral spinothalamic tract

Nociceptive nerve endings

Figure 12–1. *Pain receptors (nociceptors) convey impulses to the spinal cord via the dorsal root ganglion. From here the impulses travel in the lateral spinothalamic tract to the thalamus and the sensory area of the cortex. Evasive reflex motor activity follows. (Modified from Chrisman CL. Problems in small animal neurology. Philadelphia: Lea & Febiger, 1982: 8.)*

neous or superficial pain is due to injury of the skin or subcutaneous tissue. Deep pain is dull, boring, and difficult to localize; an example is arthritic pain. Visceral pain is associated with stretching or distention of a viscus, muscular spasm, chemical or septic irritation, or ischemia. It too is difficult to localize. Gastric dilation and torsion and peritonitis are examples of problems that cause visceral pain.

Pain impulses activate *A* delta myelinated fibers and *C* unmyelineated fibers. The *A* fibers conduct pricking and sharp pain. The *C* fibers conduct burning or aching pain. When soft tissue is cut, the *A* fibers are activated first, and a sensation of sharp pain is transmitted to the brain. This is followed by a throbbing, dull ache carried to the brain along the slower-conducting *C* fibers. This phenomenon is referred to as "double pain."

Inflammation decreases the pain threshold. It is the principal factor initiating pain and maintaining its sensation. Inflammation, ischemia, trauma, and neoplasia result in the release of chemical mediators that cause pain, including histamine, serotonin, bradykinin, hydrogen ions, leukotrienes, prostaglandins, chemotoxins, Hageman factor, kallikrein, plasmin, complement, lysosomal products, substance P, and lymphokines. If ischemia is accompanied by exercise or increased metabolism, the onset of pain is faster and the intensity of pain is greater. Once the cause of ischemia is eliminated and blood flow returns, the sensation of pain decreases.

The gate-control theory is the most widely supported theory used to explain the mechanism of pain sensation. When large-diameter nonpain fibers (alpha *A* and *B*) are activated, they block stimulation from the slower-conducting pain fibers in the substantia gelatinosa. The substantia gelatinosa stimulates *T* cells, which in turn trigger the sensation of pain. This explains why rubbing an injured area helps decrease the intensity of pain. The character of pain felt depends on the strength and nature of the stimulus causing the pain, the activity of the animal preceding the pain, and the balance between the large and small fiber stimuli.

The brain further modifies the sensation of pain and governs the individual's reaction to it. β-Endorphins, found in the hypothalamus, thalamus, and anterior pituitary gland, are naturally occurring opioid analgesic agents. Enkephalins are similar substances found in the limbic system and pain pathways and in the intramural and sympathetic ganglia of the gastrointesintal tract. Collectively, the enkephalins and β-endorphins are called *endorphins*. Their effect is to create a state of emotional indifference to pain. In the spinal cord, endogenous opioids released under situations of stress inhibit the transmission of pain.

CLINICAL SIGNS

The clinical signs associated with acute pain include vocalization, tachycardia, panting, salivation, mydriasis, biting at the painful area, and self-mutilation, which may be manifested by licking, scratching, or chewing the affected area. Animals may appear timid or aggressive. They may be reluctant to move or may move slowly, guarding the painful area. Chronic pain such as that accompanying degenerative joint disease, skin disease, neoplasia, or periodontal disease contributes to weight loss, lethargy, groaning, whimpering, insomnia, anorexia, apathy, and aggressive behavior. Animals may appear restless. They constantly pace, get up, and lie down in an effort to find a comfortable position free of pain.

Specific clinical signs can be related to the area involved. Generalized pain is difficult to localize and may be associated with meningitis, polyarthritis, polymyositis, polyradiculoneuritis, or tetanus. Fever, general stiffness, neck pain, and cervical rigidity often accompany meningitis. Affected animals tend to turn their entire body as a unit rather than turning just the head and neck, and appear to be "walking on egg shells." Other central nervous system signs (*e.g.,* ataxia, weakness, seizure, visual deficits, changes in reflexes) may be apparent. Animals with painful lesions of the oral cavity may have halitosis, salivation, and difficulty eating and drinking. Palpation may elicit marked pain in the affected area. Weakness, pain, arching of the back, and ataxia may be reported with focal lesions of the thoracic or lumbar spinal column (disk disease, tumor, infection, vertebral fracture). Cervical disk disease is manifested as neck rigidity, reluctance to move, crying out with pain, and spasm of the cervical muscles (Gilmore, Additional Reading). Clinical signs due to chest pain, other than those from surgery, are rare in small animals. When present, chest pain may cause tachypnea. Abdominal pain can be acute and accompanied by vomiting and diarrhea, which may contain blood. The abdomen is tucked up, the abdominal muscles are rigid, and the back is arched. Animals often assume a "praying" position, with the chest lowered to the floor and the hind end raised. Signs of concurrent shock may occur with intestinal obstruction, hemoperitoneum, gastric dilation–volvulus, ruptured viscus, acute pancreatitis, intussusception, or intestinal volvulus. Anorectal pain due to perianal sacculitis, abscesses, fistulae, rectal stricture, tumor, or pseudocoprostasis may lead to constipation. Leg pain is noted by lameness or carrying of the affected limb, or, in some cases, self-mutilation of the limb.

DIAGNOSTIC APPROACH

Pain is initially classified as generalized and difficult to localize or localized and identified with a specific area. Sublumbar pain may occur with renal disease and pyelonephritis. Pain associated with pancreatitis can sometimes be localized to the cranial abdominal quadrant. The duration and associated clinical signs are noted. The history should document the events preceding the onset of pain (trauma, the ingestion of foreign bodies or toxins). The history is followed by a complete physical examination. Swelling, fever, and hyperemia accompany infection and inflammation. To ensure that the physical examination can be completed, the affected area should be palpated last. Abdominal organs are palpated for symmetry, distention, mass(es), and pain. Pain originating from the bowel tends to be difficult to localize. In addition to palpation, the abdomen is auscultated and ballotted. An abdomen devoid of sound may be associated with ileus and the presence of increased frequency; high-pitched sounds may be indicative of mechanical obstruction. Tympany often accompanies gastric dilation, and dullness denotes ascites or abdominal mass(es). A rectal examination looking for evidence of rectal pathology or pelvic fracture completes palpation of the abdomen.

The history and physical examination are followed by the minimum data base (Table 12-2). The complete blood count may give indication of infection. A degenerative left shift occurs with rupture of abdominal organs. An increase in the packed-cell volume accompanies hemorrhagic gastroenteritis. The serum biochemisty analysis may help localize the inciting cause of pain. Stress-induced hyperglycemia often accompanies acute pain. A urinalysis may contain red blood cells or leukocytes and bacteria if pyelonephritis is present (see Chapter 46). The minimum data base is followed by an extended data base. In cases in which the cause of abdominal pain cannot be established, radiography and abdominal ultrasonography are recommended. If these fail to clarify the etiology of the problem, abdominal paracentesis and lavage is indicated (see Abdominal Paracentesis and Lavage in Chapter 80). A barium study should be completed only if there is no evidence of gastrointestinal rupture.

Deep pain elicited by pinching of the toes is the last parameter to be lost with progressive spinal cord lesions (see Chapter 54). The expected progressive order of neural dysfunction due to compressive spinal cord leions is loss of conscious and subconscious proprioception, voluntary motor activity, superficial, and finally, deep pain sensation. If the order of functional loss varies from that listed, clinicians should consider inflammatory, degenerative, or vascular neurologic disease.

Table 12–2 *Diagnostic Approach to Pain in Small Animals*

MINIMUM DATA BASE
Complete blood count
Serum biochemistry
Urinalysis

EXTENDED DATA BASE
GENERALIZED PAIN
Cerebrospinal fluid analysis
Arthrocentesis
Muscle biopsy
SKIN AND SUBCUTANEOUS TISSUE PAIN
Skin biopsy
Immunofluorescence
HEAD PAIN
Neurologic and ophthalmologic examination
Cerebrospinal fluid analysis
Skull radiography
ORAL CAVITY PAIN
Skull radiography
Biopsy (muscle, mucous membranes, bone)
NECK OR BACK PAIN
Neurologic examination
Spinal radiography
Myelography
Lesional biospy
CHEST PAIN
Electrocardiography
Chest radiography
Cardiac ultrasonography
Transtracheal wash or pulmonary biopsy (including cytology and bacterial/fungal culture)
Arterial blood–gas analysis
ABDOMINAL PAIN
Repeated biochemical analysis
Abdominal radiography
Barium series
Abdominal ultrasound
Abdominal paracentesis and lavage (including cytology and bacterial/fungal culture)
Ejaculation or prostatic wash
Laparotomy and biopsy
LEG PAIN
Neurologic examination
Skeletal radiography
Arthrocentesis
Lesional biopsy
Muscle biopsy
Angiography
Electromyography

MANAGEMENT

The first goal of therapy is to identify and eliminate the cause of pain. Certain surgical procedures are invariably associated with a large degree of pain. Surgery of the ears or eyes, fracture repair, sternotomy, laminectomy, and vertebral disk repair are all considered painful procedures and warrant medical therapy regardless of whether or not the animal demonstrates obvious clinical discomfort. In some cases of disk disease, a certain level of discomfort is desired to encourage strict rest and allow healing to occur. In these animals oral diazepam may be used. Analgesics should never be substituted for appropriate diagnosis, specific treatment, and elimination of the primary disorder.

Two classes of analgesics are commonly used (Table 12-3). The mild analgesics are used for the treatment of mild to moderate pain, such as that accompanying degenerative joint disease. The analgesic effect is not enhanced by increasing the dose, nor is the effect augmented by the combination of two or more analgesics whose mode of

Table 12–3 Analgesic Agents for Use in Small Animals

Drug	Dosage Dog	Cat
MILD ANALGESIC AGENTS		
Acetaminophen	10 to 15 mg/kg t.i.d.–q.i.d.; PO	None (toxic)
Aspirin	10 mg/kg b.i.d.–t.i.d.; PO	10 mg/kg every 48 hours; PO
Flunixin meglumine	1 mg/kg s.i.d.; IV for 1 to 3 days	None
Phenylbutazone	10 mg/kg b.i.d.–t.i.d.; PO, IV	None
NARCOTIC ANALGESIC AGENTS		
Codeine	2 mg/kg q.i.d.; PO, SC	None
Meperidine	2 to 5 mg/kg every 1 to 2 hours; IM	Same as for dog
Methadone	0.11 to 0.55 mg/kg every 4 hours; IM	None
Morphine	0.25 to 1.25 mg/kg every 4 to 6 hours; IM, IV, SC	0.1 mg/kg every 6 to 7 hours; IM, SC
Oxymorphone	0.05 to 0.2 mg/kg every 6 hours; IM, IV, SC	0.01 mg/kg every 6 hours; IM, IV, SC
NARCOTIC ANTAGONISTS		
Butorphanol	0.1 to 0.2 mg/kg every 2 to 4 hours; IV *or* 0.2 to 0.4 mg/kg every 2 to 4 hours; IM, SC	Same as for dog
Nalorphine	1 mg/kg; IM, IV, SC	Same as for dog
Naloxone	0.01 to 0.04 mg/kg; IM, IV, SC	Same as for dog
Pentazocine	1.5 to 3.0 mg/kg every 2 to 3 hours; IM	0.75 to 1.5 mg/kg every 2 to 4 hours; IV

s.i.d. = once daily; b.i.d. = twice daily; t.i.d. = three times daily; q.i.d. = four times daily; IM = intramuscularly; IV = intravenously; PO = per os; SC = subcutaneously action is similar (*e.g.*, aspirin and acetaminophen). The combination of two analgesics with different modes of action, however, increases the analgesic effect significantly (*e.g.*, aspirin and codeine [Ascriptin with Codeine, Empirin with Codeine]). The mild analgesics are of no benefit in the treatment of acute or visceral pain.

Narcotics are effective in the management of severe pain. Unlike mild analgesics, the analgesic effects of narcotic agents are enhanced by an increase in dose. Narcotic analgesics increase sphincter tone and cause contraction of the biliary ducts. They should not be used in animals with biliary tract obstruction. Although morphine sulfate causes contraction of the pancreatic sphincter, which potentially impedes the flow of pancreatic secretions, it also decreases the production of pancreatic secretions. The benefits of reduced secretory activity and the control of pain may outweigh the disadvantage associated with increased sphincter tone when used in animals with pancreatitis (see Chapter 39). The initial emetic effect is transient and the antiemetic effect soon predominates. In case of accidental overdose, narcotic antagonists (nalorphine, naloxone) can be used. The duration of action of the antagonists is less than that of the narcotic itself. Consequently, animals must be monitored to assure that they do not regress into a state of narcosis. Other than naloxone, the narcotic antagonists also possess analgesic properties when used alone in patients not previously exposed to narcotic drugs. Their use, however, is limited by the occurrence of drowsiness, hallucination, anxiety, and insomnia. The indications and side-effects of these drugs can be found in Appendix II.

Stress and anxiety cause the release of endorphins and decrease the sensation of pain. The phenothiazines alleviate anxiety and enhance the sensation of pain and thus should be avoided. Although corticosteroids decrease inflammation and the release of factors that contribute to pain, they do not exert a direct analgesic effect and should not be substituted for the use of analgesics in pain control.

Local anesthesia is rarely used to provide analgesia other than for surgical procedures or skin biopsies. Topical anesthetics containing lidocaine are most often used to induce analgesia and decrease pruritis. They are otherwise of limited benefit, but may be used in conjunction with systemic analgesics in certain inflammatory skin conditions. It is important to note that methemoglobinemia has been induced in dogs and cats with the topical application of 5% benzocaine-containing cream on inflamed skin (see Chapter 2).

PATIENT MONITORING

Acute pain responds more readily to analgesic therapy than chronic pain. The prognosis is entirely dependent on the identification and elimination of the cause of the pain.

ADDITIONAL READING

Benson GJ, Thurmon JC. Species difference as a consideration in alleviation of animal pain and distress. J Am Vet Med Assoc 1987; 191:1227.

Carstens EE. Endogenous pain suppression mechanism. J Am Vet Med Assoc 1987; 191:1203.

Gilmore DR. Cervical pain in small animals: Differential diagnosis. Compendium of Continuing Education 1983; 5:953.

Haskins SC. Use of analgesics postoperatively and in a small animal intensive care setting. J Am Vet Med Assoc 1987; 191:1266.

Jenkins WL. Pharmacologic aspects of analgesic drugs in animals: An overview. J Amer Vet Med Assoc 1987; 191:1231

Kitchell RL. Problems in defining pain and peripheral mechanisms of pain. J Am Vet Med Assoc 1987; 191:1195

Potthoff A, Carithers RW. Pain and analgesia in dogs and cats. Compendium of Continuing Education 1989; 11:887.

Spinella JS, Markowitz H. Clinical recognition and anticipation of situations likely to induce suffering in animals. J Am Vet Med Assoc 1987; 191:1216.

Yoxall AT. Pain in small animals: Its recognition and control. Journal of Small Animal Practice 1978; 19:423.

13

CHRONIC COUGH

Dana G. Allen

Coughing is a protective mechanism that serves to clear the respiratory tract of foreign material. However, chronic cough perpetuates tracheobronchial irritation and can result in structural injury, including emphysema, pneumothorax, and pneumomediastinum. It may also propel bronchial secretions deep into the lower airways. Cough is often the first sign of cardiovascular, respiratory tract, or intrathoracic disease.

CAUSES

The trachea and bronchi are sensitive to irritation. Foreign material, gases, inflammation, structural abnormalities, or direct pressure predispose to coughing (Table 13-1). The Chihuahua, poodle, Yorkshire terrier, and Pomeranian are predisposed to tracheal collapse (Fig. 13-1) and concomitant bronchitis. This may be complicated by mitral valvular insufficiency and left atrial enlargement with compression of the left main stem bronchus (Fig 13-2). Boxers have a predilection for heartbase tumors and pulmonary neoplasia, and brachycephalic breeds in general are prone to upper airway obstruction. Cardiomyopathy is more common in the giant breeds of dog. Laryngeal paralysis may be congenital or acquired (see Chapter 14). The congenital form occurs in the Bouvier des Flandres, Siberian huskie, bull terrier, and Leonberger. Acquired forms of the disease have been reported in the Irish setter, Saint Bernard, golden retriever, Labrador retriever, German short-haired pointer, poodle, and terrier breeds. Interstitial pneumonia is not a common cause of cough. Metastatic pulmonary neoplasia is an uncommon cause of cough unless it is accompanied by secondary bacterial infection or causes compression of airways.

PATHOPHYSIOLOGY

Cough receptors are present in the larynx, pharynx, trachea, bronchi, and small airways. They are most numerous in the larynx, carina, and major lobar airways. There are none beyond the respiratory bronchioles. Mucosal irritation triggers bronchospasm, which is a postulated stimulus for initiation of the cough reflex in humans. Afferent impulses travel via the vagus and glossopharyngeal nerves to the cough center in the medulla. Efferent impulses travel down the vagal, phrenic, recurrent laryngeal, and spinal nerves to the larynx, diaphragm, intercostal muscles, and tracheobronchial tree to effect a cough.

There are three phases to the cough reflex. The

123

Table 13–1 *Respiratory Causes of Chronic Cough in Small Animals*

UPPER AIRWAY COUGH

Sinusitis
Pharyngitis, not including "reverse sneeze"
Tonsillitis
Upper airway obstruction
 Redundant soft palate
 Laryngeal paralysis, collapse, eversion of lateral ventricles
 Tracheal collapse, hypoplasia, obstruction, neoplasia, rupture
 Foreign body
Mediastinal tumors (lymphoma, thymoma, heart base tumor)
Esophageal disease accompanied by aspiration (myasthenia gravis, hypothyroidism, polymyositis)
Esophageal dilatation, diverticulation
Hilar lymphadenopathy (neoplasia, histoplasmosis, blastomycosis, coccidioidomycosis)
Left atrial enlargement with compression of left principle bronchus

LOWER AIRWAY COUGH

Bronchitis
 Infectious (*Bordetella bronchiseptica*, streptococci, *Escherichia coli*, pseudomonas, *Klebsiella pneumoniae*)
 Allergic (inhaled, parasitic disease, fungal infection, drug-induced)
 Irritant (smoke, dust, aerosol, noxious gases, foreign body)
Bronchiectasis
Parasitic lung disease
 Dog: *Filaroides* sp., *Crenosoma vulpis*
 Dog and cat: *Capillaria aerophila*, *Paragonimus kellicotti*, *Dirofilaria immitis*
 Cat: *Aelurostrongylus abstrusus*
Allergic lung disease (pulmonary infiltrate with eosinophils, feline asthma)
Pulmonary edema (cardiogenic and noncardiogenic)
Pneumonia
 Viral
  Dog: distemper, herpesvirus, reovirus, adenovirus, parainfluenza
  Cat: herpesvirus, calicivirus
 Bacterial (*Bordetella bronchiseptica*, *Streptococcus zooepidemicus*, *Staphylococcus aureus*, *Escherichia coli*, *Klebsiella* organisms, Pseudomonas)
 Mycotic (*Blastomyces dermatitidis*, *Histoplasma capsulatum*, *Coccidioides immitis*)
 Parasitic (*Filaroides milksi* and *F. hirthi*, *Aelurostrongylus abstrusus*, *Paragonimus kellicotti*, *Toxocara canis* and *T. cati*, *Strongyloides stercoralis*, *Ancylostoma caninum*, *Toxoplasma gondii*, *Pneumocystis carinii*)
Pulmonary neoplastic disease
Pulmonary hemorrhage
Pleural effusion

inspiratory phase is initiated by a deep inspiratory effort, which increases lung volume and elastic recoil for the expiratory effort. In between the inspiratory and expiratory phases is the compressive phase. This phase begins with closure of the glottis and contraction of the abdominal and in-tercostal muscles, which raises intrathoracic pressure. The expiratory phase starts with the sudden opening of the glottis and the release of air pressure from the lungs. The compression of the lungs collapses the noncartilagenous portions of the trachea and major bronchi and pushes secretions and foreign particles up the airway.

The aspiration reflex ("reverse sneeze") is not a true cough, but is often mistaken for one. It is characterized by spastic inspiratory efforts, gagging, and noisy nasal and pharyngeal sounds. It is thought to be associated with entrapment of the epiglottis in the glottis following mechanical stimulation of the nasopharynx. It has been reported in dogs and can be especially vigorous in cats.

The respiratory tract is lined by ciliated cells, epithelial goblet cells, and submucosal mucous glands. The epithelial goblet cells and submucosal mucous glands constantly secrete mucus. The presence of immunoglobulins and phagocytes in this secretion helps combat infection. Inflammation leads to an increase in the number and secretory activity of goblet cells and mucus production. The bronchial or tubuloacinar glands, under the control of the autonomic nervous system, also increase secretory activity in response to inflammation. Ciliary activity promotes the movement of foreign material to the oropharynx. Mucociliary transport is the most important protective clearance mechanism in the respiratory tract. Coughing becomes important when mucociliary clearance is impaired or is overwhelmed by excess secretions. Ciliary activity is impaired by smoke, allergens, dust, extremes in ambient temperature, and inflammatory disease. As respiratory secretions ascend the respiratory tree, they normally thicken. Adequate hydration and an intact cough reflex helps clear this material from the respiratory tract. If it remains there, it may become inspissated and predisposed to infection.

CLINICAL SIGNS

Cough is commonly characterized by the animal lowering its head, extending its neck, opening its mouth, and retching; sometimes this sequence ends with swallowing. Chronic coughing in-

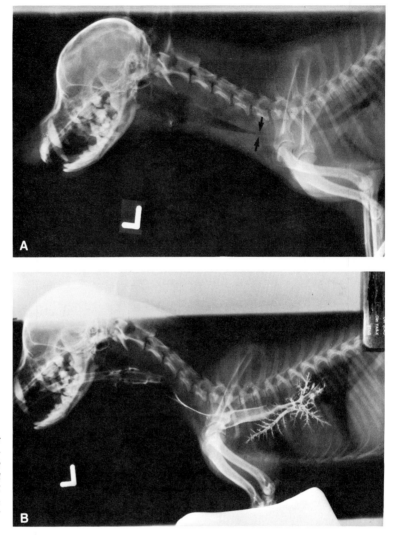

Figure 13–1. *Two-year-old male Yorkshire terrier with a history of chronic cough. (A) A plain radiograph demonstrates a narrowing of the trachea at the area of the thoracic inlet (arrows). (B) The narrowing becomes obvious following the use of radiographic contrast material. (Allen DG. Cough. In: Allen DG, Kruth SA, eds. Small animal cardiopulmonary medicine. Philadelphia: BC Decker, 1988: 25.)*

creases intrathoracic pressure, decreases venous return and cardiac output, and is physically tiring.

Weight loss may accompany heart failure, neoplasia, or chronic bronchopneumonia. Other clinical signs are related to the organ system involved. Animals with cardiovascular disease may present with decreased exercise tolerance and syncope. Abnormalities in cardiac rate or rhythm, murmurs, poor peripheral pulse, distended jugular veins, adventitial lung sounds, or ascites may accompany the disease (see Chapters 20 and 21). Stertorous inspiratory efforts are common in brachycephalic breeds with stenotic nares, redundant soft palate, and eversion of the lateral ventricles. Although not commonly associated with coughing, pleural effusion or pneumothorax may also present with dyspnea and rapid, shallow respirations. Tracheitis is often exacerbated by collars, excitement, and barking. Pneumonia may be accompanied by fever and lethargy. The onset of clinical signs is apt to be more acute with bacterial infectious disease and more gradual with fungal disease or heart failure. Skin lesions may be present with deep mycotic infection. Lameness may indicate hypertrophic pulmonary osteopathy and the presence of an intrathoracic mass. Regurgitation and aspiration of esophageal contents may signal esophageal dysfunction.

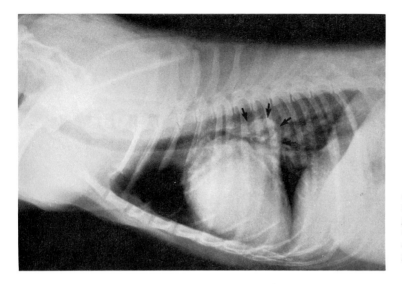

Figure 13–2. *Marked left atrial enlargement (arrows) causing collapse of the left main stem (principle) bronchus and a cough is apparent in this lateral radiograph. (Allen DG. Congestive heart failure. In: Allen DG, Kruth SA, eds. Small animal cardiopulmonary medicine. Philadelphia: BC Decker, 1988: 60.)*

DIAGNOSTIC APPROACH

The diagnostic approach to animals with chronic cough begins with a thorough history and complete physical examination; this is followed by a complete blood count, radiographs of the chest, fecal parasitology, and heartworm check. The goal of this approach is to separate the cause of cough into those diseases related to the cardiovascular system and those related to the respiratory system.

Travel to areas where endemic disease (heartworm, deep mycoses) is a concern, traveling to dog shows or field trials, and the kenneling of dogs predisposes to infectious disease. The vaccination history as it pertains to canine distemper, adenovirus, parainfluenza, bordetella, and feline calicivirus and herpesvirus is important, as is the use of heartworm prevention. Possible exposure to smoke, trauma, or foreign bodies (nasal and pharyngeal plant material) must also be considered. The onset, clinical course, and response to treatment should be evaluated. The history of a chronic cough responsive to antibiotics is suggestive of chronic obstructive pulmonary disease and bronchiectasis (Fig. 13-3).

The character of the cough may lend insight into its etiology and location within the respiratory tract. It is important to determine if the cough is productive or nonproductive. The productive cough contains mucus, purulent material, serous fluid, or blood, but often goes unrecognized by owners because the cough is often terminated by swallowing of the respiratory secretion. Soft, moist, productive coughs are associated with bronchiectasis, pulmonary edema, and some forms of pneumonia. The cough associated with bronchiectasis has been characterized as a rattling cough sometimes accompanied by a whistling noise. Harsh, dry, nonproductive coughs are associated with congestive heart failure, bronchitis, bronchial asthma, tonsillitis (rare), tracheal collapse, emphysema, pulmonary fibrosis, and some forms of pneumonia.

The cough associated with redundant soft palate, tracheal collapse, or eversion of the lateral ventricles is often only elicited by exercise or excitement. Chronic bronchitis is rare in dogs younger than than 5 years of age (see Chapter 28). Hemoptysis is uncommon in small animals, but has been reported with lungworm disease, heartworm disease, neoplasia, trauma, presence of a foreign body, bleeding tendencies, pulmonary abscess, fungal disease, and chronic bronchitis. A goose-honking cough in conjunction with bouts of dyspnea characterizes tracheal collapse, hypoplastic trachea, or collapse of the primary (principle) bronchi. It is elicited by excitement, tracheal pressure, eating, or drinking. Dry, nonproductive coughs are aggravated by exercise or exposure to

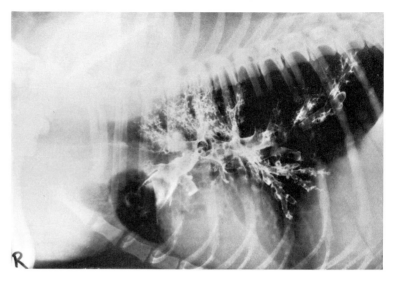

Figure 13–3. *Lateral radiograph of a 5-year-old male beagle with a history of chronic cough. Bronchial dilation is prominent and bronchial lumina are wider than normal and extend further into the peripheral lung field than normal. These changes are consistent with a diagnosis of bronchiecstatis. (Kruth SA. Chronic bronchitis in the dog. In: Allen DG, Kruth SA, eds. Small animal cardiopulmonary medicine. Philadelphia: BC Decker, 1988: 167.)*

cold air. The nonproductive cough may progress to a productive cough. The cough due to cardiac disease tends to be worse at night or when the animal is recumbent. Severe pneumonia, pulmonary edema, tracheal collapse, and psychogenic cough may also be nocturnal. The cough associated with chronic bronchitis or pneumonia is exacerbated by exercise and excitement and tends to be more serious during the day. Coughing following drinking or eating may also be due to laryngeal paralysis, esophageal disease with aspiration, cardiac disease, tracheitis, or tracheobronchitis. Coughing associated with inspiratory dyspnea is suggestive of upper airway pathology, pleural effusion, or restrictive lung disease. Expiratory dyspnea is indicative of lower airway disease (*e.g.*, asthma). The combination of inspiratory and expiratory dyspnea is seen with pulmonary edema and chronic bronchitis. Concurrent wheezing may occur with bronchiectasis and allergic respiratory disease. Adventitial lung sounds direct the clinician to disease of the lung.

Evaluation of the color of the mucous membranes, capillary refill time, heart rate and rhythm, peripheral circulation, pulse rate and amplitude, and heart and lung sounds completes examination of the cardiopulmonary system. The presence of a mediastinal mass may make the chest less compressible. This is most often documented in cats with mediastinal lymphoma. The

trachea is palpated from the base of the tongue to the thoracic inlet and is examined for pain, swelling, structural abnormalities, and the ease with which it can be collapsed or a cough elicited with digital pressure.

The oral cavity, pharynx, tonsils, tonsillar crypts, and glottis are assessed next. Pain, swelling, hyperemia, and the presence of abnormal secretions are recorded. Further examination of the glottis and trachea requires sedation or general anesthesia. A light plane of anesthesia is best to evaluate the passive inward movement of the vocal folds during inspiration that characterizes laryngeal paralysis. Examination of the ocular fundi may provide evidence for systemic disease (deep mycoses, canine distemper, lymphosarcoma). The physical examination is followed by thoracic radiographs (see Thoracic Radiography in Chapter 80). A complete blood count is included in the minimum data base (Table 13-2). Peripheral eosinophilia may be present with heartworm disease, lungworm disease, pulmonary infiltrate with eospinophils, allergic bronchitis, fungal pneumonia, chronic bacterial pneumonia, or feline asthma. Leukocytosis is suggestive of pneumonia.

At this point the clinician should be able to differentiate the cough as one associated with cardiovascular disease or with problems of the respiratory system. The extended data base,

Table 13–2 *Laboratory Approach to Animals with Chronic Cough*

MINIMUM DATA BASE

Complete blood count
Chest radiographs
Fecal Baermann (nematode larvae)
Fecal flotation (nematode ova)
Fecal sedimentation (fluke eggs)
Heartworm testing

EXTENDED DATA BASE

CARDIOVASCULAR SYSTEM
Electrocardiogram
Ultrasound

RESPIRATORY SYSTEM
Transtracheal wash
Endoscopy, cytology, bacterial culture
Fluoroscopy
Bronchography
Pulmonary biopsy
Thoracentesis
Serology (dirofilariasis, deep mycosis, toxoplasmosis, feline infectious periotonitis)
Arterial blood–gas analysis

EXTRAPULMONARY CAUSES
Barium series
Thoracentesis
Biopsy lesions

therefore, includes electrocardiography, cardiac ultrasonography, a transtracheal wash, endoscopy (see Chapter 80), cytology of the respiratory secretions, and, where indicated, fluoroscopy of the trachea (tracheal collapse), pulmonary biopsy, thoracentesis (see Thoracentesis and Insertion of Chest Tubes in Chapter 80), serology (see Chapter 79), and arterial blood gas analysis (see Chapter 71).

MANAGEMENT

The identification and elimination of the cause of the cough is the primary goal of therapy, but in many cases patient comfort and control of the cough are all that can be expected. Only control of the cough is discussed here. Specific therapies are discussed in their respective chapters. Obese animals with chronic cough benefit from weight reduction (see Chapter 7). Owners should be instructed to use harnesses in place of collars.

Strenuous exercise should be avoided until the cough is brought under control and the etiology of the problem is identified.

Adequate hydration is one of the most important forms of therapy in the management of the patient with chronic cough (Table 13-3). Moisture helps soothe inflamed mucous membranes and loosen and mobilize secretions so that they can be carried to the oropharynx and removed. Humidification of the environment is generally only beneficial to animals with problems involving the upper airway. Humidification can be accomplished at home by exposing animals to the steam of a bathroom shower for 15 to 30 minutes three to four or more times daily. Nebulization with 0.45% or 0.9% saline for a similar period of time can be accomplished in the hospital. Propylene glycol may improve the distribution of the mist in the airways. It also is antibacterial and possesses mucolytic properties. The drug may cause severe bronchospasm, and animals should be pretreated with bronchodilators (see Table 13-3). One to two milliters of 2% propylene glycol can be safely added to aerosol solutions. Animals weighing less than 5 kg are predisposed to overhydration with nebulization. Other potential adverse effects of nebulization include contamination and hyperthermia (due to an inability to dissipate heat while in a closed environment with high humidity and ambient temperature). Do not include antibiotics or mucolytic agents such as acetylcysteine (Mucomyst) in nebulization. They are ineffective and irritating and may induce bronchospasm. An exception to this may be the aerosol antibiotic treatment of infection with *Bordetella* organisms with gentamicin. Following aerosol treatment, percussion of the chest and mild exercise will help to loosen and mobilize secretions. This should be done for 5 to 10 minutes three to four or more times daily.

Expectorants help loosen respiratory tract secretions of the dry, nonproductive cough and facilitate their removal (see Table 13-3). Expectorants increase the production of a less viscous bronchial mucus by reflex stimulation of respiratory tract secretions through action on gastric receptors (saline expectorants, guaifenesin) or by the direct aerosol stimulation of the tra-

Table 13–3 *Therapeutic Modalities for Use in Patients With Chronic Cough*

EXPECTORANTS

Nebulization/humidification: 0.45% to 0.9% saline 15 to 30 minutes three to four or more times daily
Saline expectorants
   Ammonium chloride: 200 mg/kg t.i.d. PO (dog); 40 mg/kg t.i.d. PO (cat)
   Ammonium carbonate, calcium iodide, potassium iodide (Pima syrup); 2 to 5 ml every 4 to 6 hours PO (dog and cat)
Guaifenesin (dog) in combination with
   Theophylline: 1 capsule/20 to 30 kg b.i.d.–q.i.d. or 0.2 to 0.6 ml/kg b.i.d.–q.i.d. PO
   Oxtriphylline: 1 capsule/20 to 30 kg b.i.d.–q.i.d. or 0.2 to 0.6 ml/kg b.i.d.–q.i.d. PO
   Note: Guaifenesin may prolong activated clotting time and interfere with platelet function
Volatile oils (eucalyptis oil, pine oil, terpin hydrate)

ANTIHISTAMINES

Not recommended due to drying effect of respiratory secretions and impaired mucokinesis

ANTITUSSIVE AGENTS

Morphine sulfate: 0.1 mg/kg b.i.d.–q.i.d. SC (dog and cat)
Codeine (Robitussin A–C): 1 to 2 mg/kg every 4 to 8 hours PO (dog)
Hydrocodone bitartrate (Hycodan, Codone, Dicodid): 0.25 mg/kg b.i.d.–q.i.d. PO; not to exceed 0.5 to 1 mg/kg (dog)
Dextromethorphan: 1 to 2 mg/kg t.i.d.–q.i.d. PO (dog and cat)
Butorphanol (Torbutrol): 0.05 to 0.10 mg/kg b.i.d.–q.i.d. PO, SC (dog)
Noscapine (Vetinol): 0.5 to 1.0 mg/kg t.i.d.–q.i.d. PO (dog)

BRONCHODILATORS

Aminophylline: 10 mg/kg t.i.d.–q.i.d. PO, IM, IV (dog); 6.6 mg/kg b.i.d. PO (cat)
Theophylline (Theo-Dur, Theobid, Slo-bid): 20 mg/kg b.i.d. PO (dog); 4 mg/kg b.i.d.–t.i.d. PO (cat)
Oxtriphylline (Choledyl): 10 to 15 mg/kg t.i.d.–q.i.d. PO (dog and cat)
Ephedrine: 2 mg/kg t.i.d. PO (dog); 1 mg/kg t.i.d. PO (cat)
Isoproterenol hydrochloride (Isuprel elixir): 0.44 ml/kg b.i.d.–q.i.d. (dog)
Orciprenalin (Alupent, Metaprel): 0.5 mg/kg q.i.d. PO (dog)
Salbutamol: 2 mg t.i.d.–q.i.d. PO (dog; dose uncertain in small animals)
Atropine: Not recommended because it tends to increase the viscosity of secretions and impair their clearance from the respiratory tract

GLUCOCORTICOIDS

Prednisone
   Antiinflammatory dose: 0.5 to 1 mg/kg/day (dog); 1 to 2 mg/kg/day (cat)
   Immunosuppressive dose: 2 to 4 mg/kg/day (dog and cat)

b.i.d. = twice daily; t.i.d. = three times daily; q.i.d. = four times daily; IM = intramuscularly; IV = intravenously; PO = per os; SC = subcutaneously

cheobronchial glands (volatile oils). The iodides act by directly stimulating the bronchial glands through vagal reflexes. They are also said to possess mucolytic properties, potentiate natural proteases, and increase ciliary activity. The efficacy of expectorants, however, is questionable. They have not been shown to be effective in their ability to increase mucociliary clearance. Many human preparations combine expectorants with antitussive agents or bronchodilators (see Table 13-3). This practice is illogical. Once secretions are loosened, efforts should be made to facilitate their removal. Suppressing the cough reflex is not an effective way to accomplish this.

Antitussive agents are indicated for the nonproductive cough associated with pain and fatigue (see Table 13-3). The cough is a protective mechanism and should not be universally suppressed. Morphine sulfate, codeine, and hydrocodone are the most commonly used narcotic antitussives. Hydrocodone (Hycodan) is more potent than codeine in the suppression of cough. Dextromethorphan is a non-narcotic opioid with antitussive activity equal to that of codeine. Noscapine is a nonaddictive opium alkaloid comparable to codeine in its potency. Butorphanol tartrate is a narcotic antagonist and analgesic opioid that is 15 to 20 times more potent than codeine or dextromethorphan in the management of cough. Since bronchospasm may play a role in the initiation of the cough reflex, bronchodilatory drugs may be effective antitussive agents. One of the most commonly used drugs is aminophylline. Sustained release theophylline products (Theo-Dur, Theobid, Slo-Phyllin) are also currently available. These drugs permit less frequent dosing, improve client compliance, and better maintain adequate serum levels of the drug throughout the day. Isoperoterenol hydrochloride has also been suggested as a bronchodilator. It should not be used in animals with arrhythmias or in the advanced stages of heart failure.

Glucocorticoids are indicated in the allergic forms of respiratory disease. They may also be of use along with appropriate antifungal therapy in the management of severe fungal pneumonia accompanied by a severe inflammatory reaction.

Histamine contributes little to the pathogenesis of respiratory disease in small animals. The use of antihistamines is therefore questionable. In addition, antihistamines lead to drying of respiratory secretions and impair mucokinesis.

Guaifenesin is an expectorant generally used in combination with bronchodilators. The drug may prolong activated clotting time and interfere with platelet function; thus it should not be used in animals with bleeding tendencies.

The patient with aspiration reflex can be managed by pulling the tongue forward, compressing the chest, or forcing the animal to swallow water.

PATIENT MONITORING

Cough in many animals is incurable. The frequency and severity of each episode can often be controlled, but cure is unlikely with chronic bronchitis, bronchiectasis, and mitral valvular insuf-ficiency. Patients with aspiration reflex ("reverse sneeze") may resolve spontaneously or the problem may continue intermittently for years.

ADDITIONAL READING

Bonagura J. Approach to the patient with chronic cough and dyspnea. Proceedings of the American Animal Hospital Association 1980: 115.

Cornelius L. Pathophysiological mechanisms of problems in internal medicine: Coughing. Proceedings of the American Animal Hospital Association 1982: 147.

Legendre AM. Differential diagnosis of cough and dyspnea. Proceedings of the American Animal Hospital Association 1981: 193.

Roudebush P. Antitussive therapy in small companion animals. J Am Vet Med Assoc 1982; 180:1105.

Zenoble RD. Respiratory pharmacology and therapeutics. Compendium of Continuing Education 1980; 2:586.

14

DYSPNEA

Ned F. Kuehn
Philip Roudebush

Dyspnea, strictly defined, is the displeasing and distressful sensation of difficulty with breathing. It is a subjective phenomenon perceived by a patient. This sensation of breathlessness or shortness of breath is communicated by the patient to the physician. If the term *dyspnea* is to be used in veterinary medicine, an objective definition is required. A reasonable definition for dyspnea might be "an inappropriate degree of breathing effort as assessed by respiratory rate, rhythm, and character, and altered behavior (agitation, apprehension, restlessness) resulting from these changes in breathing effort." Another definition is simply "respiratory distress or difficulty." It is in the context of these two definitions that *dyspnea* is used in this chapter.

Dyspnea is a common sign associated with a wide variety of pulmonary and nonpulmonary diseases. Dyspnea may be recognized as being continuous, paroxysmal, or exertional. *Tachypnea* and *polypnea* refer to an increased rate of respiration, but do not imply distress or difficulty with respiration. Tachypnea and polypnea may be associated with dyspnea. As far as pulmonary diseases are concerned, dyspnea is a general symptom relating to many disorders of the upper and lower respiratory tracts. Abnormal breath sounds (stridor, snoring, wheezes, crackles) regularly ac-company dyspnea due to respiratory disease. The nature of respiratory distress exhibited by the animal (inspiratory or expiratory dyspnea or both) and physical examination findings can help the clinician determine the general category of pulmonary disease and the likely location of the problem.

CAUSES

The major categories of diseases causing dyspnea are disorders of the cardiac, hematologic, metabolic, respiratory, and central nervous systems (Fig. 14-1). The major causes of dyspnea resulting from respiratory diseases have been further clustered as obstructive, restrictive, or vascular diseases. Overlap occurs occasionally between these three categories. The typical causes for dyspnea are listed in Tables 14-1 and 14-2.

PATHOPHYSIOLOGY

Dyspnea may be a clinical sign associated with a number of respiratory and nonrespiratory diseases (see Tables 14-1 and 14-2). This discussion is confined to diseases of the respiratory system that may result in dyspnea.

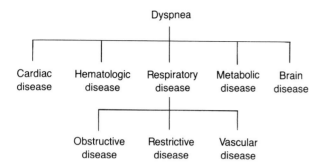

Figure 14–1. *Major categories of diseases causing dyspnea.*

Table 14–1 *Nonrespiratory Causes of Dyspnea*

CARDIAC

Low-output heart failure
Cyanotic heart disease
   Tetralogy of Fallot
   Reverse (right-to-left) patent ductus arteriosis
Shock
Severe cardiac arrhythmias
   Ventricular tachycardia
   Atrial fibrillation
   Other tachyarrhythmias

HEMATOLOGIC

Anemia (severe)
Methemaglobinemia

METABOLIC

Acidosis
   Diabetes (ketoacidosis)
   Uremia
   Other metabolic factors
Shock
Heat stroke

BRAIN (CENTRAL NERVOUS SYSTEM)

Head trauma
Central nervous system inflammatory diseases
Neoplasia

In addition to the three general pathophysiologic classifications of dyspnea due to respiratory disease (obstructive, restrictive, and vascular), a fourth is occasionally suggested: diffusion impairment respiratory diseases. However, these diseases, which result from reduced gas exchange by thickening of the alveolar or vascular walls or interstitium of the lung, are usually not severe enough to be a clinical problem.

Obstructive respiratory diseases are those that cause airflow (airway) obstruction. Obstruction to airflow may be endomural, as in the accumulation of mucus in the bronchioles with bronchitis or the impediment of airflow through the larynx associated with an elongated soft palate; mural, as in mucosal hyperplasia in chronic bronchitis or smooth muscle constriction in asthma; or extramural, as in dynamic compression of the airways in tracheal collapse or the impingement of a mass on the airways.

Restrictive respiratory diseases are those that limit expansion of the lungs either because of alterations in the lung parenchyma or because of diseases of the pleura, chest wall, or neuromuscular apparatus. These diseases are characterized by a small resting lung volume (reduced vital capacity) and normal airway resistance. Restrictive respiratory diseases in dogs and cats are most commonly due to limited expansion of the lungs resulting from diseases involving the pleural space (*e.g.*, pneumothorax, pleural effusion, thoracic wall tumors). Pulmonary fibrosis and interstitial pulmonary edema are examples of restrictive diseases that decrease compliance of the lungs. These diseases alter the elastic properties of the pulmonary interstitium, which reduces lung compliance and therefore impairs normal expansion of the lung. Finally, those diseases that reduce compliance of the chest wall (*e.g.*, scoliosis, rib tumors) and various neuromuscular diseases (*e.g.*, polyradiculoneuropathy, myasthenia gravis) also inhibit normal expansion of the lung.

Diseases that primarily affect the pulmonary vasculature generally cause dyspnea by virtue of perfusion–ventilation inequalities. For example, blood flow through the lobar arteries may become totally obstructed in dogs with advanced heartworm disease. This results in ventilated but nonperfused regions of the lung (wasted ventilation). Pulmonary parenchymal disease often occurs secondary to vascular disease in dirofilariasis. Perivascular edema and lung consolidation are not uncommon. When severe parenchymal disease is present, perfused but inadequately ventilated regions of lung are present. Massive pulmonary embolism, as may occur in hypercoagulable states or heartworm disease, occludes a pulmonary vessel and obstructs perfu-

Table 14–2 Respiratory Causes of Dyspnea

OBSTRUCTIVE DISEASE

EXTRATHORACIC DISEASE

Nose
  Stenotic nares
  Neoplasia
  Fungal granuloma
  Foreign body
  Trauma
  Epistaxis (blood clots)
Pharynx
  Elongated or edematous soft palate
  Pharyngeal edema
  Tonsilar enlargement or neoplasia
  Pharyngeal polyps (cats)
Larynx
  Laryngeal paralysis
  Laryngeal edema
  Laryngeal collapse
  Laryngospasm
  Allergic reaction (angioneurotic edema)
  Neoplasia
  Everted laryngeal saccules
  Foreign body
Trachea
  Cervical tracheal collapse
  Foreign body
  Neoplasia
  Stenosis
  Extraluminal compression (cervical mass)
  Traumatic rupture

INTRATHORACIC DISEASE

Trachea
  Thoracic tracheal collapse
  Foreign body
  Neoplasia
  Stenosis
  Extraluminal compression (mediastinal mass)
  Parasites
    Filaroides osleri
Principle bronchi
  Main stem (principle) bronchial collapse
  Foreign body
  Neoplasia
  Stenosis
  Extraluminal compression
    Hilar lymphadenopathy
    Heart base tumors
    Enlarged left atrium (chronic mitral valvular regurgitation)
  Parasites
    Filaroides osleri
Lower airways and pulmonary parenchyma
  Bronchial disease
    Chronic bronchitis (dogs)
    Bronchial asthma (cats)
Pulmonary edema
Pneumonia (viral, bacterial, fungal)
Parasitic pneumonitis
  Filaroides spp.
  Paragonimus kellicotti
Allergic or immune pneumonitis
Pulmonary hemorrhage
Inhalation pneumonia
Neoplasia

RESTRICTIVE DISEASE

Pneumothorax
Pleural effusions
Hernia
  Diaphragmatic hernia
  Peritoneal–pericardial diaphragmatic hernia
Anterior displacement of diaphragm
  Abdominal masses
Trauma
  Rib fractures
  Flail chest
Neoplasia
  Mediastinal neoplasia
  Neoplasia of the thoracic wall
Obesity
Neuromuscular diseases involving muscles of respiration
  Neuromuscular weakness
    Myasthenia gravis
    Polymyopathies
  Denervation
    Coonhound paralysis
Interstitial lung diseases
  Pulmonary fibrosis
  Pulmonary edema
  Interstitial pneumonias

VASCULAR DISEASE

Dirofilariasis
Pulmonary embolism

sion to a region of the lung. This also results in wasted ventilation.

The pathophysiologic classification of every respiratory disease that causes dyspnea into one of these three categories is not always possible. There are instances when a single disease process will overlap into two or all three of these categories. For example, the progression of events culminating in fulminant pulmonary edema involves an overlap between these categories. Once the forces causing net extravasation of fluid from the pulmonary veins exceed those responsible for fluid reabsorption, interstitial edema develops. A restrictive defect is first recognized by virtue of the altered elastic properties of the pulmonary interstitium caused by fluid accumulation. As edema continues to accumulate in the interstitium, there is eventual flooding of the alveoli and small airways. An obstructive defect emerges when the airways fill with fluid (including significant worsening of the patient's clinical condition).

The nature of respiratory distress may give a clue to functionally characterize the underlying pathophysiologic process. Dyspnea may be classified as inspiratory, expiratory, or both. With inspiratory dyspnea, more time during the respiratory cycle is spent on inspiration than expiration. The opposite occurs with expiratory dyspnea— that is, more time is spent on expiration than inspiration. Tachypnea is typically associated with either inspiratory or expiratory dyspnea. Combined inspiratory and expiratory dyspnea results when breathing effort is labored during both phases of the respiratory cycle.

Obstructive respiratory diseases cause either inspiratory or expiratory dyspnea, depending on the location of the impediment to airflow. Extrathoracic obstructions (above the level of the thoracic inlet) primarily cause inspiratory dyspnea, whereas intrathoracic obstructions (below the level of the thoracic inlet) primarily cause expiratory dyspnea. The internal diameter of the larynx and cervical trachea normally decreases slightly during inspiration. This normal dynamic compression of extrathoracic airways is a consequence of negative intraluminal pressures generated during inspiration. During expiration, the caliber of airways above the thoracic inlet typically increases slightly because of positive intra-

luminal pressure. The internal diameter of airways located inside the chest cavity normally decreases during expiration. This normal dynamic compression of airways within the chest is a consequence of increased intrathoracic pressure during expiration. The caliber of airways below the thoracic inlet normally increases slightly during inspiration. This occurs because radial traction by connective tissue surrounding the airways opens these structures during expansion of the lung. Obstructive lesions above or below the thoracic inlet accentuate the normal dynamic collapse of the airways because of the increased forces required to move air.

Collapsed trachea is a common problem in small breeds of dogs. Pathologic changes characteristic of this disease include a wide, flaccid dorsal tracheal membrane and flat, weak tracheal rings. The forces normally responsible for the slight dynamic compression of the trachea are accentuated in animals with collapsed trachea. Therefore, inspiratory dyspnea is typically associated with cervical tracheal collapse and expiratory dyspnea is typically associated with intrathoracic tracheal collapse. Principle bronchial collapse also occurs commonly and will typically result in expiratory dyspnea.

Fixed airway obstructions may occur either above or below the thoracic inlet. Animals with this type of obstruction typically present with both inspiratory and expiratory dyspnea. These lesions are fixed and relatively unchanged by the slight perturbation in airway diameter normally expected during the respiratory cycle. Combined cervical and thoracic tracheal collapse may mimic a fixed airway obstruction. Collapse of the cervical segment trachea during inspiration and collapse of the thoracic segment of the trachea during expiration will result in inspiratory and expiratory dyspnea, respectively.

Restrictive respiratory diseases are those that inhibit or restrict expansion of the lungs. With these diseases, breathing effort typically is accentuated during inspiration. A rapid, shallow breathing pattern (called restrictive breathing) may also be seen in animals with restrictive pulmonary disease. Orthopnea is also common.

Pulmonary vascular diseases can be associated with either inspiratory or mixed inspiratory and expiratory dyspnea.

The algorithm given in Figure 14-2 attempts to merge the three major pathophysiologic categories of dyspnea with clinical observations on the phase of major respiratory effort during breathing. The anatomic locations of diseases that may cause the observed pattern of breathing effort are also included.

CLINICAL SIGNS

Dyspnea is not always a symptom of disease. For example, dyspnea may be expected in an unconditioned animal after vigorous exercise. The clinician must decide whether the patient's symptoms of dyspnea are appropriate to the level of activity

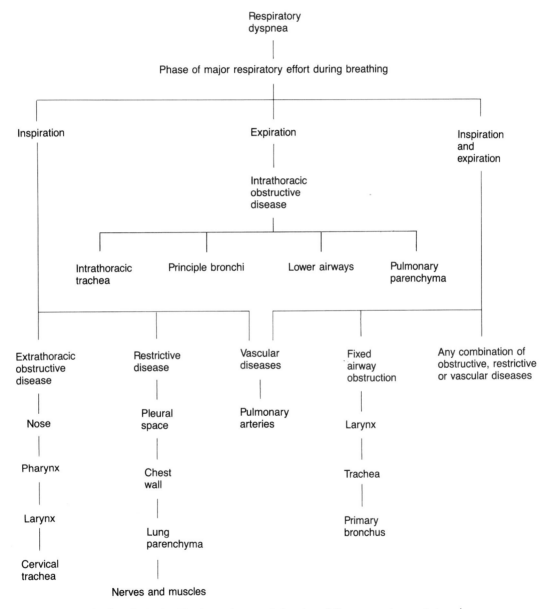

Figure 14–2. *Pathophysiologic classification and anatomic location of diseases causing respiratory dyspnea according to the phase of major respiratory effort during breathing.*

(normal) or not (abnormal). Also, the cause for dyspnea may not be primarily due to a disease of the respiratory system (see Fig. 14-1).

Those clinical signs and physical examination findings most often considered helpful in localization of the site of disease in patients with respiratory dyspnea are listed in Table 14-3.

DIAGNOSTIC APPROACH

Historic and physical examination findings may differentiate respiratory causes for dyspnea from nonrespiratory causes. An animal presented with dyspnea after being hit by a car may have rib fractures or pneumothorax, which suggest a respiratory cause; however, if the same animal is presented with fixed pupils, seizures, and stupor, dyspnea might be the result of extensive intracranial neurologic damage. An obtunded animal with dyspnea and a history of polydipsia and polyuria may have breathing difficulty secondary to the metabolic sequella of chronic renal failure or diabetic ketoacidosis. Pale mucous membranes might suggest either anemia or low cardiac output (*e.g.*, heart failure, shock) as causes for dyspnea (see Chapter 2). Ancillary procedures, such as blood tests (complete blood count, serum chemistry, urinalysis) and thorough cardiac or neurologic evaluation, are often needed to differentiate respiratory from nonrespiratory causes of dyspnea. This section is primarily concerned with respiratory causes for dyspnea.

Breed, in addition to age-related and regional prevalence for certain diseases, may be helpful in evaluating an animal with dyspnea due to respiratory disease. Viral upper or lower airway infections are common in young animals. Brachycephalic breeds commonly have several problems related to abnormal upper airway anatomy. Congenital laryngeal paralysis is seen repeatedly in certain breeds of dogs (Siberian husky, Bouvier des Flandres, bull terrier, Leonberger). Large breeds of dogs seem to develop acquired laryngeal paralysis more often than small breeds. Toy breeds of dogs commonly develop tracheal collapse. Diseases such as dirofilariasis, histoplasmosis (Mississippi River Valley), coccidioidomycosis (Southwestern United States), and infection with the parasite *Paragonimus kellicoti* (Great Lakes Region) are potential causes of dyspnea in a patient with lower respiratory tract disease.

Observation of the animal's respiratory pattern is suggested prior to the physical examination. The major phase of breathing effort during the respiratory cycle is often helpful in localizing the problem (see Fig. 14-2). Particular attention should be paid to the period and duration of breathing difficulty during the respiratory cycle.

The physical examination of patients with dyspnea should include inspection of the external nares for evidence of discharge and movement of the lateral alae. Observable or palpable evidence of trauma, deformities, or swellings of the head and muzzle, pharyngeal and cervical regions, and thoracic wall should be sought. The larynx and cervical trachea should be palpated for structural integrity and symmetry. The compressibility of the anterior thorax in cats should be evaluated, as it may be reduced with the presence of anterior mediastinal masses (*e.g.*, thymic lymphosarcoma). Finally, the chest should be palpated for evidence of chest wall disease (*e.g.*, rib fractures, thoracic wall tumor). A hand should be placed over the cardiac region to feel for palpable thrills that might suggest the presence of congenital or acquired heart disease (see Chapter 17).

Auscultation of the airways in the cervical and thoracic regions aids in the evaluation and localization of abnormal tracheobronchial and lung sounds. Auscultation should proceed systematically from the areas over the larynx to the peripheral lung fields. Normal breath sounds range from faint rustling sounds heard best in areas over the thorax away from the large airways to louder sounds of an extended frequency range heard best in locations over the large airways. Adventitious sounds are abnormal sounds superimposed upon breath sounds. The site of maximum intensity of an abnormal airway sound typically occurs at the location of disease. Methodical auscultation of the airways from over the larynx to the lung periphery can disclose the area of maximal adventitial sound intensity.

The two basic abnormal sounds are crackles (rales) and wheezes (ronchi). Crackles are short, explosive, nonmusical sounds. Wheezes, on the

Table 14–3 Localization of Clinical Signs for Respiratory Causes of Dyspnea

UPPER RESPIRATORY SIGNS

Nose
  Inspiratory dyspnea
  Snoring sounds (inspiratory)
  Open-mouth breathing
  Sneezing
  Nasal discharge
  Stenotic nares
  Swelling or tenderness of muzzle
Pharynx
  Inspiratory or expiratory dyspnea or both
  Snoring sounds (inspiratory or expiratory or both)
  Dysphagia
  Drooling
  Anorexia
  Tonsilar enlargement
  Mass lesions
  Cyanosis
Larynx
  Voice change
  Inspiratory or mixed inspiratory and expiratory dyspnea
  Stridor (inspiratory)
  Choking or gagging while eating or drinking
  Harsh cough
  Laryngeal sensitivity
  Abnormal laryngeal position or size
  Syncope
  Cyanosis

TRACHEA

Cervical trachea
  Inspiratory dyspnea
    Inspiratory and expiratory dyspnea (fixed obstruction)
  Stridor
    Inspiratory (tracheal collapse)
    Inspiratory and expiratory (fixed obstruction)
  Cough (generally nonproductive)
  Gagging
  Tracheal sensitivity
  Palpable architectural abnormalities
  Cyanosis
  Subcutaneous emphysema (trauma)
Intrathoracic trachea
  Expiratory dyspnea
    Inspiratory and expiratory dyspnea (fixed obstruction)
  Stridor (expiratory)
  Expiratory wheezes
  Coughing (generally nonproductive)
  Gagging
  Cervical tracheal sensitivity
  Cyanosis
Entire trachea
  Inspiratory and expiratory dyspnea
  Stridor (inspiratory and expiratory)
  Inspiratory and expiratory wheezes
  Cough (generally nonproductive)
  Gagging
  Tracheal sensitivity
  Cyanosis

LOWER RESPIRATORY SIGNS

Principle bronchi
  Expiratory dyspnea
    Inspiratory and expiratory dyspnea (fixed obstruction)
  Expiratory wheezes
    Inspiratory and expiratory wheezes (fixed obstruction)
  Coughing
  Gagging
  Cyanosis
Lower airways and pulmonary parenchyma
  Note: Highly variable depending on cause
  Cough (productive or nonproductive)
  Gagging
  Purulent nasal discharge (bronchopneumonia)
  Hemoptysis
  Syncope
  Cyanosis
  Fever
    Infectious diseases
    Noninfectious inflammatory diseases
  Obstructive disorders
    Expiratory dyspnea
    Expiratory wheezes
    Early inspiratory or early expiratory crackles
  Restrictive disorders
    Inspiratory dyspnea
    Restrictive breathing
    Late inspiratory crackles
    Orthopnea
    Muffled lung or heart sounds
    Pleural friction rub

other hand, are continuous musical sounds of variable pitch. *Stridor* is a term commonly used to convey a modified, harsh wheeze of the upper airways. Reference to crackles and wheezes is often modified by terms indicating the time of their occurrence during the respiratory cycle. Therefore, crackles or wheezes may be inspiratory, expiratory, or both. These modifiers may be refined further by the terms *early* or *late*, which indicate the specific time of occurrence of the adventitious sound during either the inspiratory or expiratory phase of the respiratory cycle (*e.g.*, early expiratory crackles).

Inspiratory wheezes and stridor are most often associated with extrathoracic airway obstructions. The site of maximal intensity for these sounds is over the laryngeal or pharyngeal region or at some point along the cervical trachea. Brachycephalic breeds commonly make stertorous sounds referable to abnormalities of the upper airway system. One should evaluate the entire nasal, pharyngeal, laryngeal, and upper tracheal region in these breeds for defects such as stenotic nares, elongated soft palate, everted laryngeal saccules, and hypoplastic trachea (English bulldog). Cervical tracheal collapse and laryngeal paralysis are other examples of diseases associated with inspiratory wheezes and stridor. A quick snapping sound also may be heard at end-inspiration in animals with cervical tracheal collapse.

Expiratory wheezes generally indicate intrathoracic airway obstruction. Examples of diseases causing expiratory wheezes are bronchitis, primary bronchial collapse, and intrathoracic tracheal collapse. A snapping sound is often heard at end-expiration in animals with either intrathoracic tracheal collapse or principle bronchial collapse.

Inspiratory and expiratory wheezes generally indicate fixed airway obstructions. These may be heard in animals with tracheal stenosis, intraluminal foreign bodies, mass lesions involving the trachea (Figs. 14-3 and 14-4), or airway compression and consolidation from diffuse lung tumors. Intrathoracic and extrathoracic tracheal collapse will also result in signs suggestive of a fixed airway obstruction. With combined intrathoracic and extrathoracic tracheal collapse, inspiratory wheezes will be heard with maximal intensity over the cervical tracheal region and expiratory wheezes will be heard with maximal intensity over the intrathoracic tracheal region. An endinspiratory and end-expiratory snapping sound also may be heard over the areas of the cervical and intrathoracic trachea, respectively.

Crackles are most often associated with lower respiratory tract diseases. Late inspiratory crackles may be heard in diseases such as pulmonary edema and interstitial pneumonia or pneumonitis, or in connection with lung, pleural, or

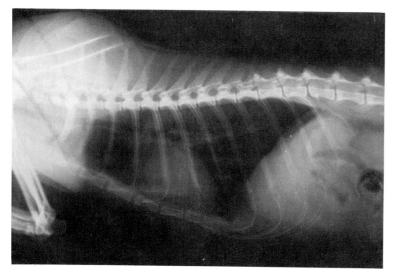

Figure 14–3. *Lateral radiograph of a 2-year-old female American shorthair cat, which presented with the chief complaint of a 6-month duration of mild inspiratory and expiratory wheezing during respiration. The referring veterinarian thought the cat had feline asthma; however, there was no clinical response to prednisolone and aminophylline. Notice the focal dorsal deviation to the luminal surface of the ventral border of the trachea just cranial to the cardiac silhouette (see Figure 14–4).*

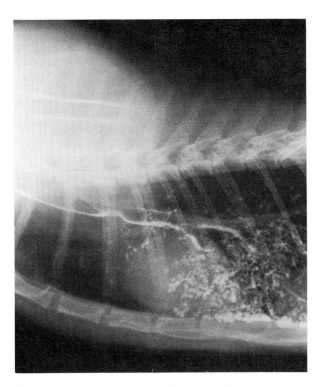

Figure 14–4. *Lateral thoracic radiograph of the same cat as in Figure 14–3 following positive contrast tracheobronchography. Notice the mass within the ventral wall of the trachea just cranial to the cardiac silhouette. This tracheal mass produced a fixed airway obstruction, which resulted in mild inspiratory and expiratory wheezing during respiration. A tissue diagnosis was not made because the owners declined further workup.*

chest tumors. Early inspiratory or early expiratory crackles are frequently associated with obstructive small airway diseases such as bronchopneumonia or the accumulation of tracheobronchial fluids occurring with advanced pulmonary edema.

When presented with a dyspneic patient, one should first determine whether the animal is exhibiting signs primarily referable to the upper respiratory tract (nasal–pharyngeal–laryngeal region), trachea, or lower respiratory tract. Diagnostic procedures indicated for each of these regions are outlined in Table 14-4. Many of these procedures require either heavy sedation or general anesthesia. It is imperative that full control of ventilation be established immediately upon induction of anesthesia and then maintained until the animal is fully awake.

MANAGEMENT

Any animal presented with dyspnea should be handled carefully because stress may worsen the clinical signs. Supplemental oxygen may be required prior to correction of the underlying cause. Management of some of the more common causes of dyspnea follows. For a discussion of management of pleural effusion, pulmonary edema, chronic bronchitis, pneumonia, and nasal obstruction and discharge see Chapters 27, 28, 29, 31, and 32.

Acute Airway Obstruction

Severe airway obstruction with prominent dyspnea and cyanosis requires immediate establishment of a patent airway. If the animal is conscious, supplemental oxygen should be given via a face mask. Depending on the condition of the patient, preparation for general anesthesia, intubation, and correction of the underlying problem may be indicated shortly after presentation. Angioneurotic edema of the larynx and substantial edematous swelling of the soft palate or tongue ordinarily respond to corticosteroids alone. If the animal is collapsed or unconscious, intubation with an endotracheal tube should be attempted. Foreign material and blood should be removed from the oropharynx and nasopharynx, if present. If intubation is not possible, as may be the case with severe upper airway obstruction, a tracheostomy should be performed promptly.

After control of the airways is established, oxygen therapy is instituted. Maintenance of body temperature and general supportive care, including intravenous fluids, antibiotics, corticosteroids, and bronchodilators, are instituted as indicated by the animal's underlying condition. Further diagnostic procedures may include radiography, laryngoscopy, tracheoscopy, or bronchoscopy if the underlying problem is not readily apparent. Correction of the fundamental problem should be attempted. This may include the removal of foreign bodies or tumors, repair of fractures or wounds, incision and drainage of abscesses, or correction of anatomic defects.

If a tracheostomy tube is placed, conscientious

Table 14–4 *Diagnostic Approach to Respiratory Causes of Dyspnea*

UPPER RESPIRATORY SIGNS

Nose (see Chapter 27)

Evaluation of external nares for evidence of stenosis

Radiographs—nasal series (requires general anesthesia) to reveal turbinate destruction (due to neoplasia, fungal disease, or a foreign body), trauma, or presence of a foreign body

Rhinoscopy for evaluation of turbinate anatomy or to perform biopsy, cytology, or culture (fungal)

Examination of nasopharyngeal region for foreign bodies, polyps (in cats), or tumors

Pharynx

Neurologic examination (note that further evaluation requires sedation or general anesthesia)

Examination of nasopharynx and oropharynx for foreign bodies, polyps (in cats), tumors, excessive pharyngeal tissue folds or edema, or soft palate elongation or thickening (edema)

Evaluation of tonsils to reveal abnormal size or shape (suggesting squamous cell carcinoma) or to perform biopsy

Surgical biopsy or removal of masses

Examination of regional lymph node to perform fine needle aspiration cytology or wedge biopsy

Radiographs to determine bone involvement (skull)—may be indicated if mass lesions are suspected

Larynx

Palpation of larynx to reveal pain, fractures of the hyoid apparatus, abnormality of size or position, or thyroid masses

Radiographs to reveal displacement of bony or cartilaginous structures, fractures or neoplasia of the hyoid apparatus, or masses

Laryngoscopy (requires light plane of general anesthesia) to:

Check for laryngeal paralysis (unilateral or bilateral). Paralysis may be present if the vocal cords do not abduct during inspiration or are immobile or in the paramedian position, if there is ventromedial displacement of the arytenoids, if the aryepiglottic folds are medially displaced, if the glottic lumen is small, or if there is evidence of chronic laryngitis (erythema and edema).

Evaluate relationship of soft palate to epiglottis. (Is the soft palate elongated or does it extend beyond the rostral edge of the epiglottis?)

Check for laryngeal collapse, evidenced by medial and ventral displacement of arytenoids and aryepiglottic folds, an obstructed glottic opening, everted saccules, and evidence of chronic laryngitis

Evaluate lumen of larynx. (Is there evidence of everted laryngeal saccules, masses such as tumors or polyps on excisional biopsy, or foreign bodies?)

In brachycephalic breeds

Examination of the entire upper respiratory system, including the:

Nose for stenotic external nares, a deformed nasal chamber, or a distorted turbinate structure

Pharynx for a misshapen pharynx, excessive tissue folds, an elongated and thickened soft palate, or infolding of the pharyngeal wall

Larynx for eversion of laryngeal saccules or laryngeal collapse

Trachea for hypoplasia (in the English bulldog)

TRACHEA

General

Radiographs to reveal trauma such as subcutaneous emphysema, displacement (due to external masses), foreign bodies, masses, or tracheal collapse (diagnosis is enhanced with fluoroscopy)

Inspiratory films to evaluate for cervical tracheal collapse

Expiratory films to evaluate for intrathoracic tracheal collapse or principle bronchial collapse

Chest films to evaluate for concurrent or underlying disease such as bronchitis, bronchiectasis, or pneumonia

Tracheoscopy to further evaluate for tracheal collapse, intraluminal masses, extraluminal compression, foreign bodies, stenosis, tracheal–esophageal fistula; to allow retrieval of foreign bodies; and to perform biopsy, cytology (including brush catheter and aspiration of fluids) or culture

LOWER RESPIRATORY SIGNS

General

Thoracic radiographs to evaluate lung pattern (bronchial, bronchointerstitial, or interstitial); to check for anterior mediastinal masses, neoplasia, and hilar lymphadenopathy; to allow cardiac evaluation, checking for heart enlargement; and to examine for pleural space disease such as pleural effusion, pneumothorax, diaphragmatic hernia, and masses

If bronchial or bronchoalveolar disease is suspected:

Transtracheal washing and aspiration to examine cytology and microbiology

Tracheobronchoscopy (flexible fiberoptic bronchoscope) to further evaluate for intraluminal bronchial masses, extraluminal compression of bronchi, and foreign bodies; to retrieve foreign bodies; and to perform biopsy, cytology (brush catheter and aspiration of fluids or bronchoalveolar lavage), or culture (biopsy specimens and fluids)

Transbronchial needle aspiration of extraluminal masses to examine cytology and culture

If diffuse pulmonary parenchymal disease is suspected:

Bronchoscopy and bronchoalveolar lavage to examine cytology and microbiology

Transtracheal aspiration

Transthoracic needle aspiration or biopsy or open lung biopsy (exploratory thoracotomy) to examine cytology, histopathology, and microbiology postoperative care is essential. Suction of the tracheostomy tube and proximal trachea using aseptic technique should be performed every 2 to 4 hours. Nebulization with saline solution is helpful in maintaining moisture in the airways (see Chapter 13). Normal hydration should also be maintained. Intravenous fluids should be given if the oral intake of liquids is contraindicated. A broad-spectrum antibiotic (*e.g.,* ampicillin) may be given while the tracheostomy tube is in place to prevent secondary infection. Body temperature should be determined every 1 to 4 hours and frequent (every 24 to 48 hours) radiographs of the thorax should be obtained to detect early signs of bronchopneumonia.

Removal of the tracheostomy tube is done only when the obstruction has been relieved and postoperative swelling has diminished. After withdrawal of the tracheostomy tube, the site is allowed to heal by second intention. The site should be cleaned daily until healing is accomplished.

Brachycephalic Upper Airway Syndrome

Brachycephalic breeds have several anatomic abnormalities that commonly result in airway obstruction. These abnormalities include stenotic nares, elongation of the soft palate, eversion of the lateral ventricles of the larynx, hypoplasia of the trachea (English bulldog), and laryngeal collapse.

The external nares should be evaluated for stenosis (occlusion) due to collapse of the lateral alar cartilages and overlying rhinarium. Surgical resection of the lateral alar cartilages is required for repair.

In brachycephalic breeds the soft palate is long in relation to the pharynx, so that the soft palate often ends up overlying the epiglottis. The palate also is often thickened and may mechanically obstruct the glottic opening. Surgical resection of the redundant tissue of the soft palate is required for correction of this problem. Circumstances requiring increased ventilatory effort by these animals, such as high ambient temperatures or strenuous exercise, may cause significant edema of the soft palate, pharyngeal, and laryngeal tissues. Corticosteroids (1 mg/kg of prednisolone once to twice daily) may be required to reduce

soft-tissue swelling before surgery is attempted. Corticosteroids and a cool environment generally alleviate the significant degree of dyspnea these patients often suffer.

Eversion of the laryngeal saccules is common in English bulldogs. Saccule eversion is believed to develop over time because of the excessive negative pressure in the pharynx and larynx developed by these dogs during inspiration. Everted saccules appear as a thin pink tissue that prolapses into the laryngeal lumen during inspiration. Correction of this problem requires sacculectomy.

Hypoplasia of the trachea results from inadequate growth of the tracheal rings. This also is commonly seen in English bulldogs. Since there is no specific correction for this problem, correction of specific anatomic defects in the nasal–pharyngeal–laryngeal region will facilitate breathing.

Laryngeal Paralysis

Laryngeal paralysis may be either acquired or congenital. Congenital laryngeal paralysis is typically bilateral, with clinical signs seen after 4 to 6 months of age. The breeds most often reported are the Bouvier des Flandres, bull terrier, and Siberian husky. Acquired laryngeal paralysis can be unilateral or bilateral, and is seen in both dogs and cats. Unilateral paralysis is usually the result of trauma to the recurrent laryngeal nerve, although tumors may occasionally be the cause. Acquired (idiopathic) laryngeal paralysis is generally bilateral, and may be the result of a neuropathy or polymyopathy.

Treatment requires a unilateral laryngectomy with removal of the vocal cord, arytenoid cartilage, and arytenoepiglottic fold. A modified castellated laryngofissure procedure is also reported to provide long-term relief of obstruction associated with bilateral laryngeal paralysis.

In our experience, some of the dogs presented with laryngeal paralysis also have dysphagia. The detection of abnormal electromyographic activity in laryngeal and skeletal muscles has suggested the cause to be a diffuse polymyopathy. Laryngeal and skeletal muscle biopsies, examined by specialized histochemical stains and direct immunofluoresence, have suggested an immune-mediated muscle disorder. Treatment with immunosupressive drugs (corticosteroids or cyclophosphamide or both) has resulted in resolution of clinical signs. The presence of additional neuromuscular abnormalities in patients with laryngeal paralysis should alert the clinician to a possible multiple-system disease.

Laryngeal Collapse

Laryngeal collapse generally occurs as the end-stage event in dogs with either brachycephalic airway syndrome or chronic airway obstruction due to laryngeal paralysis. This respiratory emergency often requires an immediate tracheostomy. Surgical treatment necessitates a partial laryngectomy with unilateral excision of the arytenoid cartilage and arytenoepiglottic fold. The long-term prognosis is fair to good for dogs with laryngeal collapse secondary to laryngeal paralysis, but poor for brachycephalic breeds with laryngeal collapse and multiple upper airway problems.

Nasopharyngeal Polyps

Nasopharyngeal polyps have been reported sporadically. They appear be a familial problem, and are often seen in related cats. The site of origin for these inflammatory (not neoplastic) growths is either the middle ear or auditory tube. Nasopharyngeal polyps cause respiratory distress by directly obstructing the upper airway. These polyps can be a predisposing factor for secondary bacterial rhinitis, sinusitis, or both. Either rhinitis or sinusitis may enhance upper airway obstruction. Complete surgical removal (including the base of the stalk) of these polyps is required for resolution of airway obstruction.

Tracheal and Principle Bronchial Collapse

Collapse of the main airways is a frustrating problem to manage. The cause for the problem is poorly understood; however, since the majority of cases involve the intrathoracic trachea and primary bronchi, chronic small airway disease may be the principal precipitating factor. Early expiratory closure or partial obstruction of the small airways will increase transtracheobronchial pressure. This increased pressure combined with cartilaginous malacia may lead to collapse of the tracheal rings. Repeated collapse of the trachea or bronchi during breathing produces chronic mechanical irritation to the mucosal surface of the airways. Airway irritation and inflammation, coughing, altered mucociliary clearance, chronic changes of the airway mucosa, excessive mucus production, and decreased mucus clearance with retention of mucus in the airways results from chronic collapse of the trachea or primary bronchi. The causes for cervical tracheal collapse are not clear. In certain circumstances, it may represent an extreme spectrum of cases beginning with those involving collapse of the intrathoracic airways.

Many small dogs also have chronic mitral regurgitation. It is important not to confuse the similar clinical signs of tracheal collapse with those associated with heart failure due to chronic mitral regurgitation. If a small-breed dog has a murmur compatible with mitral regurgitation, one cannot immediately assume that the patient's clinical signs are due to heart failure. In fact, they may be due to some other cause (such as tracheal collapse). It is crucial to obtain thoracic radiographs in these animals to differentiate these two diseases.

Treatment for tracheobronchial collapse is not curative. Weight control is extremely important, as many of these dogs are obese (see Chapter 7). Cervical, mediastinal, chest wall, and abdominal fat accumulations may impinge on the trachea and increase the effort required for breathing. The increase in breathing effort frequently encourages collapse. When coughing is severe, antitussives and corticosteroids may be of benefit. These drugs, however, should be used sparingly because retained secretions may become infected. Transtracheal wash and aspiration is suggested to collect material for cytologic evaluation and culture (see Transtracheal Wash in Chapter 80). Knowledge of an underlying or concurrent problem, such as bronchopneumonia or allergic bronchitis, can help in the management of these patients. Antibiotic therapy is indicated if culture results reveal an underlying bacterial infection.

General management should include the use of a harness rather than a collar, which will irritate the trachea when pulled against. Excessive excitement and exercise should also be avoided.

Surgical management of segmental tracheal collapse may benefit certain patients if done early in the course of disease. The reader is encouraged to review the article by Fingland (Additional Reading) for specifics if this procedure is contemplated.

Tracheal Stenosis

Tracheal stenosis is an unusual but serious cause of fixed airway obstruction (Figs. 14-5 and 14-6). Stenosis may occur secondary to endotracheal intubation, severe lacerations, chemical burns to the tracheal mucosa, foreign bodies, localized neoplasia, and, occasionally, undetermined causes. Treatment requires surgical resection of the stenotic section and reanastomosis of the severed tracheal segments.

Obstructive Small Airway Disease

Life-threatening bronchial obstruction occurs with acute fulminating bronchopneumonia, smoke inhalation, aspiration pneumonia, and

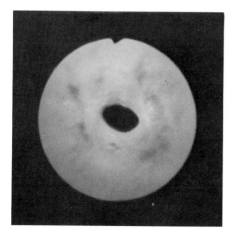

Figure 14–5. *View through a flexible fiberoptic bronchoscope of tracheal stenosis in a 6-month-old male miniature schnauzer. The clinical findings at the time of presentation were cyanosis and severe inspiratory and expiratory dyspnea.*

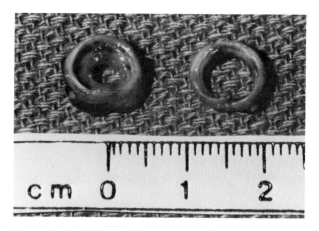

Figure 14–6. *A side-by-side comparison of the internal diameters of the stenotic segment of trachea removed from the schnauzer described in Figure 14–5 and a normal segment of trachea removed from the same dog. Surgical correction of the problem was successful. The clinical signs in this dog began several weeks after castration. Overinflation of an endotracheal tube placed at the time of surgery was suspected to be the cause of the stenosis.*

acute pulmonary edema. Oxygen therapy should be given by a face mask, nasal cannula, oxygen cage, or endotracheal tube. The patient should be evaluated for signs of shock and treated if necessary (see Chapter 4). If laryngospasm or upper airway obstruction occurs, a tracheostomy is indicated and positive pressure ventilation should be initiated. If possible, removal of aspirated material is recommended. Corticosteroids may be effective in the initial treatment of inhalation injuries. Bronchodilators are often beneficial in reversing associated bronchospasm and constriction. Antibiotic usage should be limited by culture and sensitivity results. Analgesics may be required to control extreme pain or distress in some patients (see Chapter 12). For specific therapy of bronchopneumonia and pulmonary edema, see Chapters 29 and 31.

Chronic small airway obstruction is a common cause of dyspnea in dogs with chronic bronchitis and in cats with bronchial asthma. See Chapters 28 and 30 for management of these problems.

Restrictive Diseases of the Pulmonary Parenchyma

Pulmonary edema and pneumonia are the most commonly occurring diseases of the pulmonary parenchmya that may result in reduced pulmonary compliance. Management of these two diseases is discussed in Chapters 29 and 31.

Pulmonary neoplasia and fibrosis may also cause restrictive lung disease. Pulmonary neoplasia can be the result of either primary or metastatic (secondary) tumors. When dyspnea is present, large areas of the pulmonary parenchyma are replaced by neoplastic tissue. Occasionally, dyspnea may also result from extraluminal obstruction of the principle bronchi due to hilar lymphadenopathy. Coughing is unusual in animals with metastatic tumors, except when secondary pulmonary infections are established or when there is extraluminal compression of airways. Advanced neoplasia may result in inspiratory and expiratory dyspnea provoked by neoplastic infiltration of the pulmonary interstitium and extraluminal compression of small airways by tumor foci. Definitive diagnosis requires the demonstration of tumor cells within the lung parenchyma. The method of treatment depends on the total tumor burden and type of tumor. The long-term prognosis is usually poor.

Pulmonary fibrosis is an uncommon pathologic consequence of a wide variety of inflammatory lung diseases. Generally, open lung biopsy is required for diagnosis. The prognosis for patients with pulmonary fibrosis is uniformly poor, with management consisting of symptomatic measures such as weight control and reduced activity.

Pneumothorax

Pneumothorax is the accumulation of free air in the pleural space. The pathophysiologic consequences are similar to those with pleural effusion. Trauma and wounds arising from bites or projectiles are the most common causes of pneumothorax. Spontaneous pneumothorax (not associated with trauma) occasionally develops from rupture of infarcted regions of the lung or bullous emphysematous or granulomatous lung lesions. Tension pneumothorax is a special condition occurring when a tear in lung parenchyma creates a one-way valve so that air is allowed to accumulate in the pleural space during inspiration but is not expelled during expiration. Intrapleural pressure often will increase rapidly. Pulmonary atelectasis and diminished venous return to the heart will bring about a rapidly deteriorating clinical situation in these patients.

Management of patients with pneumothorax is dependent on the degree of respiratory compromise and cause of air accumulation. Mild to moderate pneumothorax may be managed with cage rest, close clinical observation, and periodic radiographs of the chest to ensure that there is no progressive increase in free pleural air. A single aspiration of free air with a needle and syringe may be needed initially in some less severely affected patients. Persistent pneumothorax requiring periodic aspiration should be managed with an indwelling chest tube (see Thoracentesis and Insertion of Chest Tubes in Chapter 80).

If severe pneumothorax or tension pneumothorax is suspected, immediate thoracentesis is indicated. Placement of an indwelling chest tube followed by intermittent or continuous suction is required. Rarely, bilateral pneumothorax demands insertion of chest tubes in each side of the thorax.

The underlying cause should be determined as rapidly as possible and corrected (if indicated). Pneumothorax resulting from trauma usually resolves spontaneously; however, severe lacerations of the parenchyma and some cases of tension pneumothorax require surgical closure of rents in the lung tissue. Animals with recurrent spontaneous pneumothorax caused by periodic rupture of bullae may require either surgical excision of the lesions or pleurodesis for management of the problem.

Flail Chest

Flail chest occurs in the presence of both dorsal and ventral fractures in several sequential ribs. The chest wall in the area between the fractures is unstable and moves paradoxically with respiration (the flail segment moves inward during inspiration and outward during expiration). Flail chest is most often the result of automobile accidents or attacks by larger animals. Decreased ventilatory capacity and contusion of the underlying lung causes respiratory distress. Flail chest may also be accompanied by pneumothorax or hemothorax.

The animal should be placed in lateral recumbency with the flail segment on the down side. The need for evacuation of air or blood from the chest depends on their amounts. Surgical correction of the rib fractures is often required once the patient is stable.

PATIENT MONITORING

The severity of the underlying problem will largely dictate the frequency of checks on patient progress. Animals with brachycephalic upper airway syndrome or tracheal collapse require intermittent evaluation for evidence of worsening signs. Clients attempting to reduce the weight of obese animals with these problems need frequent support, particularly if they are also overweight or feel that treats are a necessary part of pet care (see Chapter 7). Animals having undergone surgical laryngoplasty for correction of laryngeal paralysis should be examined often to ensure that aspiration of food or water does not occur during eating or drinking. Owners of animals with recurrent spontaneous pneumothorax should be instructed to closely observe their animals and promptly report any evidence suggesting recurrence of the problem.

ADDITIONAL READING

Aron DN. Laryngeal paralysis. In: Kirk RW, Bonagura JD, eds. Current veterinary therapy X. Philadelphia: WB Saunders, 1989: 343.

Aron DN, Crowe DT. Upper airway obstruction: General principles and selected conditions in the dog and cat. Vet Clin North Am 1985; 15:891.

Berkwitt L, Berzon JL. Thoracic trauma: Newer concepts. Vet Clin North Am 1985; 15:1031.

Ettinger SJ. Dyspnea and tachypnea. In: Ettinger SJ, ed. Textbook of veterinary internal medicine. Philadelphia: WB Saunders, 1983: 97.

Fingland RB. Tracheal collapse. In: Kirk RW, Bonagura JD, eds. Current veterinary therapy X. Philadelphia: WB Saunders, 1989: 353.

Hribernik T. Respiratory distress or difficulty. In: Ford RB, ed. Clinical signs and diagnosis in small animal practice. New York: Churchill Livingstone, 1988: 221.

Leonard HC. Tracheal collapse. In: Kirk RW, ed. Current veterinary therapy IX. Philadelphia: WB Saunders, 1986: 303.

Vaden S, Ford RB. Medical management of upper respiratory tract disease. In: Kirk RW, Bonagura JD, eds. Current veterinary therapy X. Philadelphia: WB Saunders, 1989: 337.

Venkervan Haagen AJ. Laryngeal diseases of dogs and cats. In: Kirk RW, ed. Current veterinary therapy IX. Philadelphia: WB Saunders, 1986: 265.

15

LYMPHADENOPATHY AND SPLENOMEGALY

Alan S. Hammer
C. Guillermo Couto

LYMPHADENOPATHY

Lymphadenopathy is a common response of the immune and reticuloendothelial systems to various antigenic stimuli. It may also occur as a result of infiltrative diseases (neoplasia) or an inflammatory process (lymphadenitis). Thus lymphadenopathy is a common finding in many disease states and may be the only abnormal finding in some patients with nonspecific signs such as lethargy, anorexia, or fever. A logical approach to lymphadenopathy is more likely to result in a complete evaluation of the patient.

Lymphadenopathy can be defined as an enlargement or change in the consistency of a lymph node. The involved nodes may be solitary, regional, or generalized. The distribution of the lymphadenopathy may aid in establishing its possible causes (Table 15-1). Other findings regarding the lymph nodes can aid in determining the cause of the lymphadenopathy. A soft consistency to the node usually indicates abscessation, necrosis, or hemorrhage. Heat and pain may accompany acute inflammation or metastatic neoplasia. A firmer than normal consistency is asso-

ciated with hyperplasia, inflammation, and infiltrative processes such as lymphoma or other neoplastic infiltrates.

Causes

The causes of lymphadenopathy are numerous; they can be grouped according to the histologic or cytologic changes in the affected lymph nodes. Table 15-2 classifies the causes of lymphadenopathy as reactive or hyperplastic, and neoplastic. Further classification is possible based on the cytologic features of the lymphadenitis (*i.e.*, suppurative, granulomatous, pyogranulomatous, or eosinophilic), the etiology (see Table 15-2), or the distribution of the lymphadenopathy (solitary, regional, or generalized) (see Table 15-1).

Pathophysiology

Histologically, lymph nodes are composed of a capsule, subcapsular spaces, a cortical area, a paracortical area, and a medulla (Fig. 15-1). Anti-

Table 15–1 *Distribution of Lymphadenopathy by Etiology*

	Solitary/Regional	**Thoracic**	**Abdominal**	**Generalized**
Bacterial	Corynebacteria *Yersinia* Actinomycetes *Nocardia* Mycobacteria Streptococci Staphylococci *Borrelia*	Actinomycetes *Nocardia* Mycobacteria	Actinomycetes Mycobacteria	Brucella Bacterial endocarditis *Borrelia*
Mycotic	*Cryptococcus* *Sporothrix* *Zygomyces*	*Histoplasma* Blastomyces Coccidioides	*Histoplasma* Coccidioides Zygomyces	*Histoplasma* Blastomyces *Coccidioides* *Cryptococcus*
Rickettsial				*Ehrlichia canis* *Rickettsia rickettsii* *Neorickettsia helminthoeca*
Parasitic	*Demodex*			*Demodex* Trypanosoma Leishmania
Viral		Feline infectious peritonitis	Feline infectious peritonitis	Feline infectious peritonitis Feline leukemia virus Feline immunodeficiency virus
Noninfectious non-neoplastic	Localized inflammation			Vaccinations Arthritis (rheumatoid arthritis, polyarthritis) Systemic lupus erythematosus Hypereosinophilic syndrome (cat) HES Idiopathic
Neoplastic	Melanoma Mammary carcinoma Squamous carcinoma Fibrosarcoma Osteosarcoma Mast cell tumor	Mammary carcinoma Melanoma Lung carcinoma Fibrosarcoma Osteosarcoma	Perirectal carcinoma Prostatic carcinoma Bladder carcinoma Intestinal carcinoma Mast cell tumor	Lymphoma Leukemias Malignant histiocytosis

(Hammer AS, Couto CG. Lymphadenopathy. In: Fenner WR. Quick reference to veterinary medicine, 2nd ed. Philadelphia: JB Lippincott, in press.)

genic particles delivered to the node by afferent lymphatics are filtered through the subcapsular, trabecular, and medullary sinuses. In this way, the macrophages lining these sinuses can phagocytize the particles and present them to the lymphoid cells.

The cortex is comprised primarily of B lymphocytes arranged in lymphoid follicles. These follicles are divided into primary and secondary follicles. Primary follicles are composed of small lymphocytes, while secondary follicles have central clusters of immature lymphocytes and macrophages. The pale central areas of the secondary follicles are referred to as germinal centers. The paracortical area surrounds the primary and secondary follicles and is composed primarily of T lymphocytes. More centrally located in the node are the medullary cords, which lie between the reticuloendothelial sinuses and may be packed with plasma cells during an immune response.

Table 15–2 Etiologies of Lymphadenopathy

**REACTIVE OR HYPERPLASTIC LYMPHADENOPATHY
AND LYMPHADENITIS**

INFECTIOUS

Bacterial
  Corynebacteria sp. (dog, cat)
  Brucella canis (dog)
  Yersinia pseudotuberculosis subspecies *pestis* (cat)
  Actinomyces (dog, cat)
  Nocardia (dog, cat)
  Mycobacteria (dog, cat)
  Localized bacterial infection (periodontal disease, abscess,
    pyoderma) (dog, cat)
  Streptococci (puppy and kitten strangles) (dog, cat)
  Staphylococci (dog, cat)
  Borrelia burgdorferi (dog)
Mycotic
  Histoplasma capsulatum (dog, cat)
  Blastomyces dermatitidis (dog, cat)
  Coccidioides immitis (dog, cat)
  Cryptococcus neoformans (cat, dog)
  Sporothrix schenckii (dog, cat)
  Candida sp (dog, cat)
  Phaeohyphomyces sp (dog, cat)
  Zygomyces sp (dog, cat)
Algal
  Prototheca sp (dog, cat)
Rickettsial
  Ehrlichia canis (dog)
  Neorickettsia helminthoeca (dog)
  Rickettsia rickettsii (dog)
Parasitic
  Demodex sp (dog, cat)
  Trypanosoma cruzi (dog)
  Babesia canis (dog)
  Leishmania donovani (dog)
  Hepatozoon canis (dog)
  Toxoplasma gondii (dog, cat)
Viral
  Infectious canine hepatitis
  Canine herpesvirus
  Canine viral enteritides
  Feline leukemia virus
  Feline infectious peritonitis
  Feline immunodeficiency virus

NONINFECTIOUS

Postvaccinal (dog, cat)
Immune-mediated
  Rheumatoid arthritis (dog)
  Polyarthritis (dog, cat)
  Systemic lupus erythematosus (dog, cat)
Localized inflammation (dog, cat)
Non-neoplastic mast cell infiltrate (dog, cat)
Eosinophilic granuloma complex (cat)
Hypereosinophilic syndrome (cat)
Idiopathic
  Distinctive peripheral lymph node hyperplasia secondary to
    retrovirus infection (cat)
  Maine coon cat lymphadenopathy
  Plexiform vascularization of lymph nodes (cat)

NEOPLASTIC LYMPHADENOPATHY

HEMATOPOIETIC NEOPLASMS

Lymphoma (dog, cat)
Malignant histiocytosis (dog)
Leukemias
  Acute lymphoblastic (dog, cat)
  Chronic lymphocytic (dog)
  Myelogenous (dog, cat)
  Monocytic (dog, cat)
  Erythroleukemic (dog, cat)
  Megakaryocytic (dog, cat)
Multiple myeloma (dog, cat)
Mast cell neoplasia (dog, cat)

METASTATIC NEOPLASMS

Malignant melanoma (dog, cat)
Mammary adenocarcinoma (dog, cat)
Squamous cell carcinoma (dog, cat)
Perirectal adenocarcinoma (dog, cat)
Prostatic adenocarcinoma (dog)
Primary lung carcinoma (dog, cat)
Fibrosarcoma (dog, cat)
Osteosarcoma (dog, cat)
Others (dog, cat)

(Hammer AS, Couto CG. Lymphadenopathy. In: Fenner WR. Quick reference to veterinary medicine, 2nd ed. Philadelphia: JB Lippincott, in press.)

Since lymph flows from the medullary to the hilar region, where the efferent lymphatics are located, the various lymphocyte products are carried into the circulation in this way. The majority of circulating lymphocytes are T cells, which enter the bloodstream through the postcapillary venules in the lymph node. It is this recirculating lymphocyte pool that accounts for much of the plasticity of response of the immune system.

The lymph nodes and the anatomic areas they drain in the dog and cat are listed in Table 15-3. The lymphatic pathways listed are the most common ones, but structures are not limited to drainage only through these pathways. The lymph nodes most easily palpated in the dog and cat are the mandibular, prescapular, axillary, superficial inguinal, and popliteal nodes.

Lymphadenopathy occurs as a result of excess numbers of normal or abnormal cells within the node. The cell type involved is usually helpful in

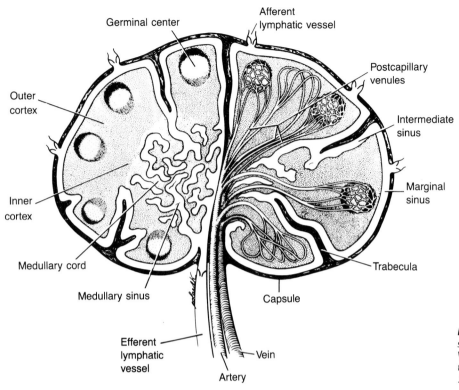

Germinal center

Afferent
lymphatic vessel

Postcapillary
venules

Outer
cortex

Intermediate
sinus

Inner
cortex

Marginal
sinus

Medullary cord

Trabecula

Medullary sinus

Capsule

Efferent
lymphatic
vessel

Vein

Artery

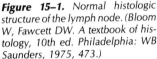

Figure 15–1. Normal histologic structure of the lymph node. (Bloom W, Fawcett DW. A textbook of histology, 10th ed. Philadelphia: WB Saunders, 1975, 473.)

defining the type of lymph node pathology in response to specific agents (Fig. 15-2). If normal lymphoreticular cells proliferate in a node, the term *reactive lymphadenopathy* is used. This occurs in response to infectious and immunologic stimuli and is characterized by an increase in the number of large lymphocytes, lymphoblasts, plasma cells, and macrophages; occasionally, neutrophils can also be seen. This type of reaction can be observed following vaccinations especially in younger animals. If polymorphonuclear leukocytes, eosinophils, or macrophages (or epithelioid cells) predominate in the lymph node infiltrate, then the term *lymphadenitis* is used. The lymphadenitis may be suppurative if neutrophils predominate, as in moist juvenile pyoderma (puppy strangles); granulomatous if macrophages are the predominant cell, as seen in some fungal infections or diseases caused by higher bacteria (*e.g.,* histoplasmosis, mycobacteriosis); or pyogranulomatous if both neutrophils and macrophages are present, as is classically seen in feline infectious peritonitis and blastomycosis. A

form of eosinophilic infiltrate (eosinophilic lymphadenitis) occurs in the hypereosinophilic syndrome of cats.

Clinical Signs

The history may aid in raising or lowering the suspicion for specific diseases in patients with lymphadenopathy. Geographic location or recent travel history may alert the clinician to certain infectious diseases (Fig. 15-3). For example, infection with *Yersinia pseudotuberculosis* subsp. *pestis* in cats is most commonly reported in the western United States, where it is endemic as sylvatic plague, and certain fungal diseases (*e.g.,* coccidioidomycosis, histoplasmosis, blastomycosis) are associated with particular geographic regions.

A history of recent vaccination may suggest that the modified-live viral vaccine is the cause of mild generalized lymphadenopathy (especially in a younger animal). An owner presenting a cat with lymphadenopathy must be questioned con-

Table 15–3 *Anatomic Location of Lymph Nodes and Drainage Patterns*

Lymph Node	Structures Drained
Parotid	Eyelids and associated glands, external ear, parotid gland
Mandibular	All portions of head not drained by parotid lymph node, including oral cavity
Medial and lateral retropharyngeal	Parotid and mandibular lymph nodes, muscles of head and neck, paranasal sinuses, nasal cavity, hyoid apparatus, larynx, pharynx, oral cavity
Superficial cervical (prescapular)	Caudal portion of head, lateral surface of neck, thoracic limb
Deep cervical	Larynx, trachea, esophagus, thyroid
Axillary	Thoracic wall, thoracic limb, cranial end of mammary chain
Sternal	Diaphragm, mediastinum, pleura, thoracic wall, cranial end of mammary chain, pectoral muscles
Mediastinal	Sternal, tracheobronchial, and cervical lymph nodes, mediastinum, esophagus, heart, aorta, vertebrae
Tracheobronchial	Lungs, bronchi, esophagus, trachea, heart, mediastinum
Lumbar/aortic	Lumbar vertebrae, adrenal glands, urogenital system
Medial iliac (sublumbar)	Pelvis, pelvic limb, urogenital system, caudal digestive tract, inguinal lymph nodes
Hypogastric	Thigh, pelvis, pelvic viscera, tail, lumbar region
Deep inguinal	Pelvic limb
Hepatic	Stomach, duodenum, pancreas, liver
Splenic	Esophagus, stomach, pancreas, spleen, liver, omentum, diaphragm
Cranial mesenteric	Jejunum, ileum, pancreas
Colic	Ileum, cecum, colon
Gastric	Esophagus, stomach, liver, diaphragm, peritoneum
Pancreaticoduodenal	Duodenum, pancreas, omentum
Popliteal	Pelvic limb
Femoral	Medial side of the pelvic limb
Superficial inguinal	Ventral abdominal wall, caudal mammary chain, prepuce, scrotum, pelvic limb

(Hammer AS, Couto CG. Lymphadenopathy. In: Fenner WR. *Quick reference to veterinary medicine*, 2nd ed. Philadelphia: JB Lippincott, in press.)

cerning the cat's feline leukemia virus (FeLV) and feline immunodeficiency virus (FIV) status, when the cat was last tested, and whether the cat is mostly outdoors. The time of year at which the animal presents with lymphadenopathy must be considered with regard to the possibility of seasonal diseases such as Rocky Mountain spotted fever, which is primarily seen during spring and summer. Finally, the owners should be fully questioned about other coexistent signs such as cough, dyspnea, vomiting, diarrhea, fever, lameness, weakness, polydipsia and polyuria, or anorexia.

The physical examination should be primarily directed toward the hemolymphatic system, but a thorough general examination of the animal should still be performed. The clinician should note the distribution of lymphadenopathy, the consistency of the nodes, and the presence of heat or pain. The liver and spleen should be carefully palpated to determine their relative size, shape,

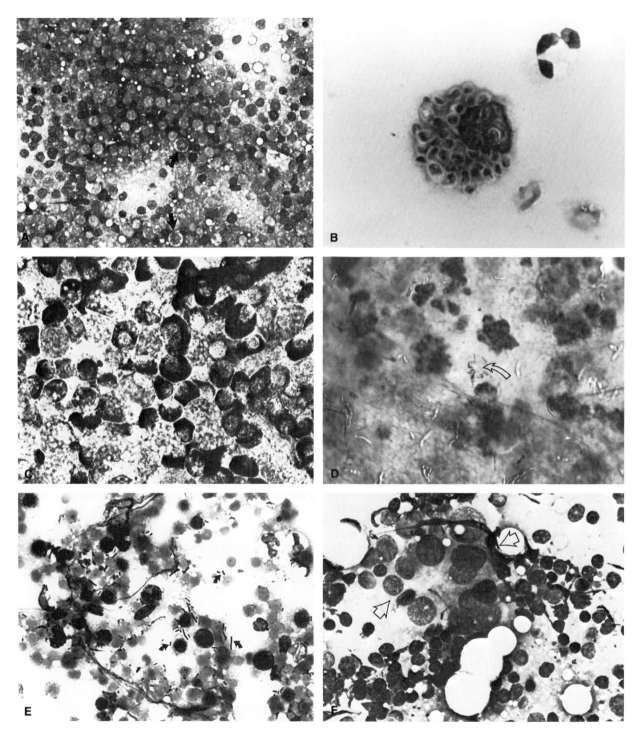

Figure 15–2. Cytologic findings in lymph nodes. (A) Canine lymphoma. Note mitotic figures at arrows. (B) Macrophage from lymph node with intracellular Histoplasma capsulatum. (C) Well-differentiated mast cell tumor in lymph node. (D) Lymph node aspirate revealing mycobacteria (arrow) (acid-fast stain). (E) Bacterial lymphadenitis. Note bacterial organisms at arrows. (F) Fine-needle aspirate of mandibular lymph node revealing metastatic nasal carcinoma (arrows).

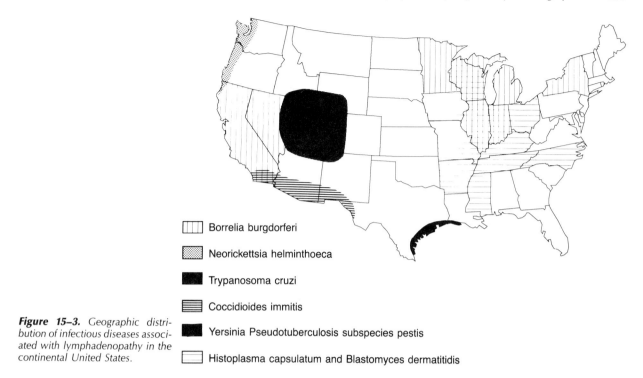

Borrelia burgdorferi

Neorickettsia helminthoeca

Trypanosoma cruzi

Coccidioides immitis

Yersinia Pseudotuberculosis subspecies pestis

Histoplasma capsulatum and Blastomyces dermatitidis

Figure 15–3. Geographic distribution of infectious diseases associated with lymphadenopathy in the continental United States.

and consistency. In many dogs and cats, the severity of skin disease or past history of skin disease should be evaluated, as skin disease is a common cause for generalized lymphadenopathy (dermatopathic lymphadenopathy). While examining the oral cavity, any sign of pallor should be noted. The presence of periodontal disease or gingivitis may explain mild to moderate mandibular lymphadenopathy. A misdiagnosis of lymphadenopathy may be made with the observance of fat (especially in the prescapular and popliteal regions) or the mistaking of the mammary gland for the superficial inguinal lymph node or of the salivary glands for the mandibular lymph nodes. Solitary lymphadenopathy should prompt the clinician to initiate a closer examination of the area drained by the node for infection, inflammation, or neoplasia (see Table 15-3). Table 15-4 lists some of the clinical signs and physical findings in patients with lymphadenopathy.

Diagnostic Approach

The approach to the patient with lymphadenopathy is directed to a large extent by the patient's history and clinical findings, including the re-

sults of general screening tests (*e.g.*, complete blood count, serum biochemistry profile) and the observance of cytologic or histopathologic changes in the affected lymph node.

Hematologic findings in patients with lymphadenopathy vary from specific (*e.g.*, leukemia with circulating blasts) to nonspecific (*e.g.*, anemia, leukocytosis) changes (see Chapters 73 and 75 respectively). Anemia accompanying lymphadenopathy is commonly nonregenerative and may be due to chronic disease in inflammatory,

Table 15–4 Clinical Signs and Physical Findings in Dogs and Cats With Lymphadenopathy

Lymph nodes enlarged, painful, fixed to underlying tissue, firm, or irregular
Cough
Fever
Lameness
Polydipsia and polyuria
Weakness
Vomiting
Diarrhea
Splenomegaly
Hepatomegaly
Pallor
Local ulcerations or masses

infectious, or neoplastic disorders. The anemia associated with FeLV infection is usually nonregenerative and may be macrocytic due to dyserythropoiesis; it may also result from myelophthisis secondary to lymphoproliferative or myeloproliferative diseases. Hemoparasites usually result in a strongly regenerative anemia (except for chronic canine ehrlichiosis). Leukocytosis is common in patients with lymphadenopathy and is usually an inflammatory neutrophilia with a mild left shift and monocytosis. In leukemic patients, circulating blasts are usually detected in the blood smear; however, in dogs with chronic lymphocytic leukemia, mature lymphocytosis constitutes the main change in the leukogram. Lymphadenopathy in association with thrombocytopenia may be seen in canine ehrlichiosis, Rocky Mountain spotted fever, FeLV infection, sepsis, leukemias, lymphomas, and systemic lupus erythematosus. Bone marrow aspiration is indicated for further evaluation of patients with leukemia or cytopenias and lymphadenopathy (see Bone Marrow Aspiration and Biopsy in Chapter 80).

Two serum biochemistry findings of particular interest in patients with lymphadenopathy are hypercalcemia and hyperglobulinemia. Lymphoma is the disease most commonly associated with hypercalcemia and generalized lymphadenopathy in the dog; hypercalcemia is rare in cats (see Chapter 72). However, multiple myeloma and blastomycosis may also result in generalized lymphadenopathy with hypercalcemia. Other neoplasms may result in solitary or regional lymphadenopathy and hypercalcemia (apocrine gland adenocarcinoma, fibrosarcoma, thyroid carcinoma). Hyperglobulinemia may be due to monoclonal or polyclonal gammopathies (see Chapter 78). If a monoclonal gammopathy is detected in the serum of a dog, multiple myeloma, lymphoma, chronic lymphocytic leukemia, leishmaniasis, or ehrlichiosis should be suspected; in cats monoclonal gammopathies are usually associated with lymphomas and multiple myeloma. Differential diagnoses in patients with polyclonal gammopathies include mycotic infections, feline infectious peritonitis, lymphoma, and ehrlichiosis.

Radiographic evaluation of patients with lymphadenopathy may reveal sternal or hilar involvement, mediastinal masses, hepatosplenomegaly, or iliac (sublumbar) lymphadenopathy with ventral deviation of the colon. Further evaluation of the abdomen with ultrasonography may reveal hepatic or splenic changes, as well as mesenteric, iliac, or aortic lymphadenopathy. Table 15-5 summarizes the laboratory and radiographic assessment of patients with lymphadenopathy.

The most often indicated diagnostic procedure in patients with lymphadenopathy is percutaneous fine needle aspiration of the affected node. This procedure allows for cytologic classification of the lymphadenopathy as reactive, hyperplastic, or inflammatory (lymphadenitis), or as infiltrative (see Table 15-2). The technique and choice of lymph nodes is important in order to obtain a diagnostic specimen. Since soft nodes often have necrotic or hemorrhagic centers, they should not be aspirated in a patient with generalized lymphadenopathy. The mandibular nodes often have a component of reactive lymphadenopathy secondary to concurrent periodontal disease; this may also impair cytologic interpretation.

The skin overlying peripheral lymph nodes is not usually clipped and scrubbed; aspiration of intracavitary lymph nodes requires surgical preparation. A 12- or 20-ml syringe, a 25- or 22-

Table 15–5 *Laboratory and Radiographic Evaluation of the Patient With Lymphadenopathy*

Test	Abnormalities
Complete blood count	Anemia (regenerative or nonregenerative) Lymphocytosis Circulating blasts Thrombocytopenia Leukocytosis
Serum biochemistry	Hypercalcemia Hyperglobulinemia
Radiographs	Sternal lymphadenopathy Mediastinal lymphadenopathy Metastatic pulmonary disease Mycotic pulmonary infiltrate patterns Hepatosplenomegaly
Ultrasonography	Mesenteric, iliac, or aortic lymphadenopathy Hepatic and splenic architectural changes

gauge needle, coverslips, and stain are required (Fig. 15-4). The needle is inserted into the lymph node, and 10 to 15 ml of negative pressure is applied two to three times. The needle is redirected several times to thoroughly sample the node. Negative pressure must be released prior to withdrawing the needle, or the cells will be aspirated from the hub of the needle into the barrel of the syringe and lost for examination. The needle is then removed, the syringe filled with air, and the cells in the hub expelled onto coverslips for pull–smear preparation and staining. The amount of material contained within the needle hub is usually sufficient for six to eight slide preparations. The use of an aspiration gun such as Aspir Gun (Everest Co.) allows for greater control of the needle tip and better cytologic results.

While there are innumerable stains available for cytology, three major types are in common use. Wright's stain is probably the best; however, it requires quality control standards and is probably best for commercial laboratories with large numbers of cytologic specimens. There are several modified Wright's stains available as kits (*e.g.,* Diff-Quick, Dade Diagnostics) that are more reproducible and easier to use. Lastly, new methylene blue used as a wet mount on a dried smear can be used for cytology. It gives different qualitative results and complements the Wright's or modified Wright's stains. New methylene blue is not a permanent stain.

The normal lymph node is comprised of 80% to 90% small lymphocytes with occasional macrophages, large lymphocytes, and plasma cells (see Fig. 15-2). Reactive lymph nodes have a higher number of large lymphocytes and immunoblasts, more plasma cells, occasional neutrophils, and mast cells. Lymphadenitis can be classified as suppurative if neutrophils predominate, granulomatous if macrophages are the dominant cell, pyogranulomatous if there is a mixed population of macrophages and neutrophils, and eosinophilic if eosinophils predominate. Neoplastic cells that infiltrate lymph nodes can be classified as hemolymphatic or metastatic solid neoplasms. Often there is little or no lymphoid tissue observed if the tumor has completely replaced the lymph node. Lymphomas are usually characterized by a monomorphic population of large, immature lymphoid cells with a high nuclear : cytoplasmic ratio, multiple nucleoli, vacuolization, and a basophilic cytoplasm. Other lymphoproliferative diseases (especially acute lymphoblastic leukemia) involving the lymph node can look similar to lymphomas. Further evaluation of peripheral blood and bone marrow may be required to confirm the diagnosis (Table 15-6).

When cytologic evaluation of the lymph node is nondiagnostic, an alternative procedure is to perform a biopsy for histopathologic evaluation. The biopsy procedure may be excisional, incisional, or

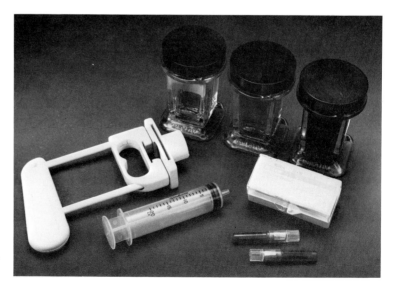

Figure 15–4. *Aspiration gun and equipment for fine needle aspiration cytology.*

Table 15–6 *Clinical Features of Lymphoproliferative Disorders*

	ALL	CLL	LSA	MM
Lymphadenopathy	+	+ +	+ + +	+
Hyperglobulinemia	+/−	+/+ +	+	+ + +
Systemic signs	+ + +	+/−	+/−	+ +
Cytopenias	+ + +	+/−	+/−	+/+ +
Circulating blasts	+ + +	+ +*	+/−	+/−
Hepatosplenomegaly	+ +	+ +	+ +	+ +
Hypercalcemia	−	−	+ +	+ +
Abnormal bone marrow cytology	+ + +	+ +	+/−	+ +

* Circulating leukemic cells appear as mature lymphocytes
ALL = acute lymphoblastic leukemia; CLL = chronic lymphocytic leukemia; LSA = lymphoma; MM = multiple myeloma; + = present; − = not present

needle (ABC Needle, Monoject) biopsy. An excisional biopsy yields the most tissue for evaluation but is the most invasive of the three procedures. An incisional lymph node biopsy is only slightly less invasive. Before placing the tissue in formalin, the node or node section should be incised longitudinally for impression smears for cytology and to allow for better fixation. A needle biopsy is the least invasive procedure but is the most likely to miss a focal lesion or yield insufficient tissue to adequately evaluate lymph node architecture. The core of tissue from a needle biopsy should also be gently rolled on a slide for cytologic evaluation before placing the tissue in formalin.

In diffficult cases determining the cause of lymphadenopathy may require an active integration of clinical and laboratory information. Certain general principles may be of assistance in assessing these cases. Solitary lymphadenopathy necessitates an extensive examination of the region drained by the node for inflammation, infection, or neoplasia. Occasionally a metastatic neoplasm can be larger than the primary tumor. An example is the massive popliteal lymphadenopathy secondary to metastases from some digital squamous carcinomas. Massive (5–10 times normal size), generalized lymphadenopathy in an otherwise relatively normal patient should lead one to suspect lymphoma. In systemically ill animals with lymphadenopathy one should search for one of the many infectious or inflammatory etiologies listed in Table 15-2 or for acute leukemias. If the history or physical examination warrant it, serologic tests for various infectious agents (*e.g.*, brucellosis, histoplasmosis, blastomycosis, ehrlichiosis) should be performed. Necrotic lymph nodes should be cultured not only for typical microorganisms (*e.g.*, *Escherichia coli*, staphylococci, streptococci), but also for atypical organisms such as *Nocardia* organisms, actinomyces, other fungal organisms, and mycobacteria. Finally, the lymphadenopathy may be only one manifestation of the disease process. Many diseases require integration of the lymph node cytologic findings with the complete blood count, physical examination, and signalment. Examples include the hypereosinophilic syndrome in cats and chronic lymphocytic leukemia in dogs. A diagrammatic perspective of the approach to patients with lymphadenopathy is shown in Figure 15-5.

Management and Patient Monitoring

The management and prognosis of lymphadenopathy depends on the etiology. The remainder of this section will discuss lymphoma in the dog and cat and several of the recently described idiopathic lymphadenopathies of cats.

Canine Lymphoma

Lymphoma (malignant lymphoma, lymphosarcoma) is a lymphoid neoplasm arising in solid tissues (*e.g.*, lymph nodes, liver, spleen, skin, intestines, central nervous system). Lymphomas represent 7% to 9% of all malignant neoplasms in the dog. There are four traditional anatomic forms of presentation. Lymphomas that are primarily associated with the lymph nodes are termed multicentric. Multicentric lymphoma is the most common form in the dog, representing more than 80% of all cases. Alimentary lymphomas may present with solitary or diffuse gastrointestinal involvement, and the mesenteric lymph nodes, liver, and spleen can also be affected. Alimentary lymphomas comprise approximately 7% of all canine lymphomas. The mediastinal form involves the cranial mediastinal lymph

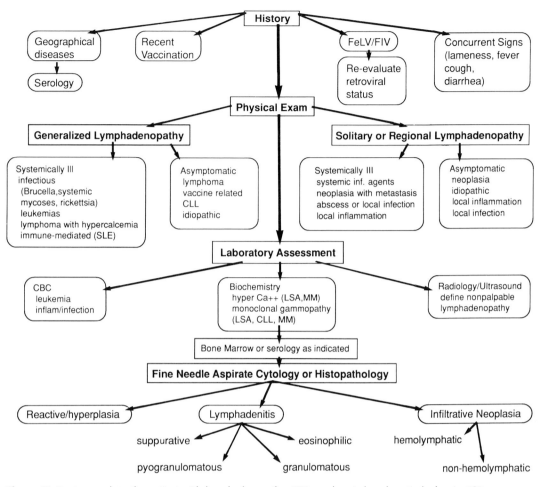

Figure 15–5. *Approach to the patient with lymphadenopathy. (CLL = chronic lymphocytic leukemia; LSA = lymphoma; MM = multiple myeloma; SLE = systemic lupus erythematosus)*

nodes and may result in pleural effusion. This form represents only 2% to 3% of all canine lymphomas. Those lymphomas primarily involving nonlymphatic tissues (*e.g.*, ocular, cutaneous, central nervous system, renal) are often called extranodal lymphomas; extranodal lymphoma represents 7% of all canine lymphoma. The clinician should also be aware of the variety of clinical syndromes that may be associated with lymphomas (*e.g.*, hypercalcemia, thrombocytopenia, coagulopathy, monoclonal gammopathy, hemolytic anemia, and myelophthisis).

The minimum database for patients with suspected or confirmed lymphoma should include a complete blood count, serum biochemisty profile, urinalysis, and cytologic or histopathologic evaluation of the lesion. Radiographs of the thorax and abdomen may be warranted. A bone marrow aspiration is necessary for complete staging and to evaluate cytopenias. Lymphoid leukemia must be differentiated from lymphoma with circulating blast cells. This is a difficult distinction to make, as both forms can have nodal, bone marrow, and peripheral blood involvement. A clinical judgment must be based on the physical examination, blood smear, and complete blood count, and a bone marrow evaluation (see Table 15-6). The lymphomas have more solid tissue involvement with less circulating neoplastic cells; the leukemic form originates in the bone marrow and is involved primarily in hematopoietic organs (marrow and spleen) and secondarily in lymph nodes and other tissues. The acute lymphoid leukemias have a poorer prognosis than the lymphomas.

Clinical staging of lymphomas can be performed in all cases for accurate recording of the patient's status. Table 15-7 gives the criteria for staging based on World Health Organization (WHO) protocol. All extranodal lymphomas are classified as stage V, although this classification is inconsistent with the prognosis of a solitary extranodal lymphoma—for example, solitary cutaneous lymphoma has a better prognosis than stage V multicentric lymphoma. The stages are subclassified as *a* or *b* based on whether the patient is asymptomatic (a) or symptomatic (b).

Untreated dogs with lymphoma survive approximately 3 to 6 weeks from the time of diagnosis. The mean survival times of dogs with lymphoma treated with several chemotherapy protocols are shown in Figure 15-6. While the decision as to which protocol to use should theoretically be based solely on length of survival, it may actually depend on the clinician's ability to obtain, administer, and monitor the side-effects

Table 15–7 *World Health Organization Clinical Staging of Canine and Feline Lymphoma*

Anatomic type
  a. Multicentric
  b. Alimentary
  c. Mediastinal
  d. Miscellaneous

Stage (to include anatomic type)
  I. Involvement limited to a single node or lymphoid tissue in a single organ*
  II. Involvement of lymph nodes in a regional area
  III. Generalized lymph node involvement
  IV. Generalized lymph node involvement plus liver or spleen involvement (Stages I to III)
  V. Manifestation in the blood and involvement of bone marrow or other organ systems (Stages I to IV)

Subclassification of stage:
  A. Without systemic signs
  B. With systemic signs

* *Excluding bone marrow*

of chemotherapy and the owner's ability to comply with the protocol in terms of financial and time requirements. The preferred protocol for initial therapy of lymphoma patients at the Veterinary Teaching Hospital–Ohio State University (VTH-OSU) is the COAP protocol with LMP maintenance therapy (Table 15-8). This protocol is

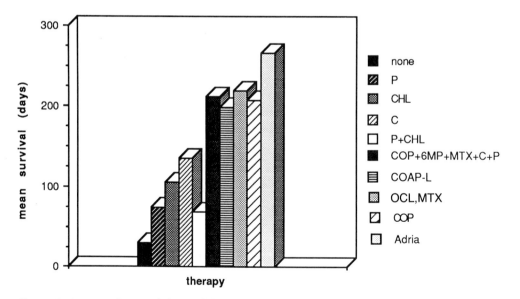

Figure 15–6. *Survival times of dogs with lymphoma treated with various chemotherapy protocols. P = prednisone; CHL = chlorambucil; C = cyclophosphamide; O = oncovin (Vincristine); 6MP = 6-mercaptopurine; MTX = methotrexate; A = cytosine arabinoside; L = L-asparaginase; Adria = doxorubicin (Adriamycin) (Modified from Couto CG. Canine lymphomas: Something old, something new. Compend Cont Ed 1985; 7:291.)*

Table 15–8 COAP-LMP Protocol for Induction of Remission in Patients with Lymphoma

CANINE

C Cyclophosphamide (Cytoxan) 50 mg/m² PO every 48 hours for 8 weeks
O Vincristine (Oncovin) 0.5 mg/m² IV weekly for 8 weeks
A Cytosine arabinoside (Cytosar) 100 mg/m²/day divided b.i.d. subcutaneously for the first 4 days of the first week (can be given as a continuous IV drip for the first 24 to 48 hours)
P Prednisone 50 mg/m² PO s.i.d. for the first week, then 25 mg/m² PO every 48 hours

FELINE

C Cyclophosphamide (Cytoxan) 50 mg/m² PO every 48 hours for 6 weeks
O Vincristine (Oncovin) 0.5 mg/m² IV weekly for 6 weeks
A Cytosine arabinoside (Cytosar) 100 mg/m²/day divided b.i.d. subcutaneously for the first 2 days of the first week (can be given as a continuous IV drip for the first 12 to 24 hours)
P Prednisone 50 mg/m² PO s.i.d. for the first week, then 25 mg/m² PO every 48 hours

MAINTENANCE (CANINE AND FELINE)

L Chlorambucil (Leukeran) 20 mg/m² PO every 2 weeks
M Methotrexate 2.5 mg/m² PO twice weekly
P Prednisone 25 mg/m² PO every 48 hours

m² = square meters of body surface

Table 15–9 Rescue Protocols for Patients With Lymphoma

CANINE

1. Doxorubicin (Adriamycin) 30 mg/m² IV and DTIC (dacarbazine) 1000 mg/m² IV every 3 weeks for 9 weeks
2. Vincristine (Oncovin) 0.75 to 1.0 mg/m² IV every 2 weeks alternated with cyclophosphamide (Cytoxan) 200 to 300 mg/m² IV every 2 weeks
3. COAP plus ʟ-asparaginase (Elspar) 10,000 to 20,000 iu/m² subcutaneously once

FELINE

1. Doxorubicin (Adriamycin) 20 mg/m² IV every 3 weeks for 9 weeks
2. COAP plus ʟ-asparaginase (Elspar) 10,000 to 20,000 iu/m² subcutaneously once

COAP = cyclophosphamide (Cytoxan), vincristine (Oncovin), cytosine arabinoside (Cytosar), and prednisone

simple to administer, relatively inexpensive, and has minimal side-effects. Complete remission is achieved in 80% to 85% of the cases and, on the average, lasts 5 to 6 months. By not using doxorubicin hydrochloride in the initial induction protocol, this drug can be used in subsequent "rescue" protocols. A negative prognostic factor appears to be the prior treatment with corticosteroids, since this usually shortens survival times. The presence of hypercalcemia has also been associated with lower median survival times (112 days) when compared to normocalcemic controls (190 days).

It is important for the clinician and the owner to realize that a cure is rarely achieved and that the patient will be receiving chemotherapy for the remainder of its life. If relapses occur, they can be managed with further rescue chemotherapy protocols (Table 15-9); however, the duration of second remissions is usually shorter than the initial ones. In general, the patient's quality of life is good and owners are impressed with the efficacy and overall lack of toxicity of chemotherapy in their pets.

The clinician should be aware of potential complications and toxicities associated with chemotherapy that may occasionally arise. The COAP-LMP protocol has been designed so that drug toxicities are minimized. Cyclophosphamide (Cytoxan) at the dosage used (50 mg/m² per os every 48 hours) has minimal myelosuppressive effects, although it may cause gastroenteritis. However, using this drug beyond the 8-week induction period increases the risk for sterile hemorrhagic cystitis. If hemorrhagic cystitis does occur, discontinue the drug, flush the bladder with cold saline, and place the patient on prophylactic antibiotics; this will usually suffice to alleviate the cystitis.

The dosage of vincristine used in this protocol usually causes only mild myelosuppression. A common complication of vincristine therapy is the severe perivascular sloughing that results if extravasation occurs. For this reason, a clean venipuncture must be achieved. A butterfly or teflon-coated over-the-needle catheter is used. If extravasation occurs, flush 20 to 60 ml of saline (to which 5 to 10 mg of dexamethasone sodium phosphate has been added) through the same catheter. Infiltration of the site may need to be repeated the next day; cold packing the area may help reduce the side-effects.

Cytosine arabinoside (Cytosar-U) is used only

during the first 4 days of the 8-week induction period. This drug results in moderate myelosuppression 7 to 10 days following administration. If there is significant bone marrow involvement by the lymphoma, the myelosuppression may be severe. Lastly, prednisone is used. The side-effects associated with chronic glucocorticoid administration are well known and include immunosuppression, Cushingoid syndrome, hepatic changes, and enterocolitis.

In addition to the side-effects discussed above, all chemotherapeutic agents have the potential to induce pancreatitis. Another complication that may appear during the induction period is acute tumor lysis syndrome (ATLS). This occurs when a sensitive tumor such as lymphoma treated with multiple-agent chemotherapy causes massive tumor cell death. The patient develops depression, vomiting, and diarrhea. Hyperkalemia, hyperphosphatemia, hypocalcemia, hyperuricemia, ketoacidosis, and azotemia may be seen. Deaths have occurred secondary to ATLS. The mechanism is thought to be an overwhelming burden of cellular metabolites on the kidney. Patients with concurrent renal disease appear to be particularly susceptible to developing ATLS. Since this occurs shortly after the initiation of chemotherapy, the initial response is to blame the drugs and halt treatment. The proper response is to take supportive measures and place the patient on intravenous fluids until the metabolic derangements resolve.

Maintenance therapy for dogs with lymphoma at VTH-OSU consists of oral chlorambucil (Leukeran) pulse-dosed at 20 mg/m^2 every 2 weeks, methotrexate 2.5 mg/m^2 twice weekly orally, and prednisone at 25 mg/m^2 orally every other day. If nausea, anorexia, or vomiting occur and cannot be controlled with antiemetics, the methotrexate should be discontinued, as this is usually the offending drug.

Feline Lymphoma

Lymphomas are the most common hemolymphatic neoplasm in cats; the majority of lymphomas in cats are induced by FeLV. Lymphoma in the cat may present in a number of anatomic forms (*e.g.*, mediastinal, alimentary, multicentric, miscella-

neous) (Table 15-10). The frequency with which the various forms present varies with geographic location. This may be due to differing genetic populations of cats, differing strains of virus, or differing classification schemes.

Clinical evaluation of the cat with lymphoma is similar to that in the dog, with the notable exception that retroviral assays (FeLV) should be employed. A staging protocol similar to that in the dog is used (see Table 15-7). Many investigators feel that the anatomic classification is a more useful prognostic factor. The untreated survival time varies based on the anatomic form of lymphoma, but, overall, is short (3–6 weeks). As in the dog, a number of treatment protocols have been devised (Fig. 15-7).

The protocol used at VTH-OSU is COAP (see Table 15-8). It is similar to the COAP protocol used in dogs with two major exceptions. First, cytosine arabinoside is used for 2 days only; second, the entire induction period lasts 6 weeks rather than 8 weeks. COAP results in similar survival times when compared to other protocols. Maintenance therapy consists of chlorambucil, methotrexate, and prednisone at the same dose as in dogs. Rescue protocols for refractory or relapsed lymphomas are given in Table 15-9.

Several prognostic factors in cats with lymphoma have been identified in one study (Mooney et al, 1989, Additional Reading). Stage of disease (WHO classification, see Table 15-7) was found to be significantly related to survival. Median survival time for cats with stage I and II lymphomas was 7.6 months, for stage III lymphomas was 3.16

Table 15–10 *Anatomic Forms of Lymphoma in the Cat*

Anatomic Form	Prevalence*	FeLV$^+$	Average Age of Onset
Mediastinal	18% to 48%	80%	2 to 3 years
Alimentary	15% to 45%	30%	8 years
Multicentric	18% to 43%	80%	4 years
Miscellaneous	<10%		Variable
Ocular		Most	
Renal		50%	
Central nervous system		Most	
Cutaneous		None	

* *Varies greatly with geographical location*
FeLV$^+$ = feline leukemia virus-positive

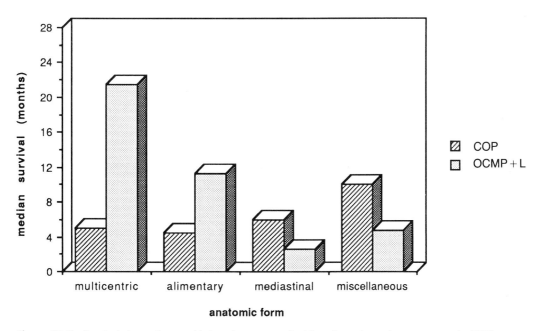

Figure 15–7. *Survival times of cats with lymphoma treated with various chemotherapy protocols. (COP = Cyclophosphamide, oncovin (Vincristine), and prednisone, OCMP + L = Oncovin (Vincristine), cyclophosphamide, methotrexate, prednisone, and L-asparaginase)*

months, and for stages IV and V lymphomas was 2.57 months. Feline leukemia virus status was also found to relate to survival, with FeLV-negative cats having a higher median survival time than FeLV-positive cats (7 vs. 3.5 months). Overall, survival times in cats with lymphoma are shorter than for the canine counterpart.

Idiopathic Lymphadenopathies in Cats

Several lymphadenopathy syndromes of unknown pathogenesis have recently been reported in cats. The first is referred to as distinctive peripheral lymph node hyperplasia, and is similar to that seen in cats with experimental FeLV infection. Most affected cats had circulating FeLV p27 antigen. Clinical signs included fever, lethargy, anorexia, and vomiting. A significant number of cats were anemic, and several were neutropenic.

Another report describes young cats with marked generalized lymphadenopathy clinically and histologically resembling lymphoma. Half of the cats reported were Maine coon cats, and all of the cats tested for FeLV viremia were negative. Several histopathologic features of lymphoma

were present, including loss of normal nodal architecture and a uniform population of cells in the paracortical areas. However, other features present were not compatible with malignancy, including active germinal centers and a mixed population of cells in the sinuses. Except for a cat that was euthanized on presentation, the other cats had resolution of the lymphadenopathy and were alive 12 to 84 months after the diagnosis, indicating a very distinctive entity from lymphoma.

Plexiform vascularization of solitary cervical or inguinal nodes in cats has been described. There was replacement of interfollicular pulp by a plexiform proliferation of small capillary-sized vascular channels, and lymphoid atrophy. The cats were asymptomatic at the time of presentation, and surgical removal of the affected nodes resulted in an uneventful recovery in most cats.

Feline Immunodeficiency Virus

Lymphadenopathy has been reported in association with infection with FIV. The incidence of lymphadenopathy ranged from 8% to 11% in several serologic surveys. Due to the viral-induced immunodeficiency, the lymphadenopathy may in part be caused by secondary infections. Experimentally, lymphadenopathy is seen in the initial stages of infection, along with fever and neutropenia. The lymphadenopathy may be of longer duration (2–9 months) than that induced by FeLV in the initial stages of infection. Histologically, the lymph node changes induced by FIV are both hyperplastic and dysplastic, whereas the changes induced by FeLV are mainly hyperplastic.

SPLENOMEGALY

The spleen is the single largest reticuloendothelial organ in the body. It has numerous functions, including extramedullary hematopoiesis in the fetus (and occasionally in the adult), blood filtration, phagocytosis, mediation of immune response, and serving as a blood reservoir. The finding of splenomegaly or a splenic mass on physical examination is a signal for concern and needs to be further investigated.

Causes

Splenomegaly can be divided into focal splenomegaly (*i.e.*, masses; more common in dogs) and diffuse splenomegaly (more common in cats). Splenic masses can be further divided into neoplastic and non-neoplastic. Diffuse splenomegaly can be classified based on the pathogenesis into inflammation, lymphoreticular hyperplasia, congestion, or infiltration. Table 15-11 lists causes of splenomegaly in small animals.

Pathophysiology

The spleen lies in the left cranial quadrant of the abdomen, but its location varies with body configuration and stomach volume. Histologically, the spleen consists of a fibromuscular capsule with trabeculae, white pulp, and red pulp (Fig. 15-8). The fibromuscular capsule is partially comprised of smooth muscle and is capable of contraction. Barbiturate anesthesia induces muscle relaxation and results in a physiologic splenomegaly. The white pulp is composed of lymphocytes and reticuloendothelial cells surrounding the arteries and arterioles (periarterial lymphatic sheath). Zones rich in T and B lymphocytes can be found within the white pulp (lymphoid nodules). The red pulp is composed of arterial capillaries, venous vessels, and a reticulum filled with macrophages and blood. The central arteries of the white pulp terminate in arterial capillaries that deliver blood to the red pulp reticulum. Once arteries enter the red pulp, they loose the periarterial lymphatic sheath and are surrounded by a sheath of macrophages and reticulum (periarteriolar macrophage sheath). The endothelial cells of the terminal arterial capillaries are separated by gaps that allow blood cells, particles, and plasma to pass into the red pulp reticulum. These red pulp reticular spaces comprise an intermediate circulation between the arterial and venous vessels.

Anatomic and functional differences in the venous vessels in the red pulp comprise one of the major differences between canine and feline spleens. In dogs, the venous vessels consist of an anastomosing system of closed, blunt venous sinuses that terminate by converging to form major veins. The endothelial structures are incompletely covered by rings of basement membrane and reticular cells. In order to leave the spleen, blood cells must squeeze between adjacent endothelial cells and enter the venous sinus lumen. The canine spleen is termed a sinusal spleen.

In contrast, red pulp venules in the cat are open-ended and have large apertures between endothelial cells, through which the erythrocytes may pass without any deformity in shape. Cat spleens are considered to be nonsinusal.

The spleen is one of the major hematopoietic organs during fetal development. In the adult dog and cat, the spleen may again initiate hematopoietic activity; this is termed extramedullary hematopoiesis. It may occur with diseases of the bone marrow (*e.g.*, leukemia, hypoplasia, myelofibrosis) or splenic disorders (*e.g.*, splenitis, neoplasia), or when the peripheral utilization or destruction of cells outstrips the bone marrow's ability to meet the demand (leukocytosis of pyometra, immune-mediated hemolytic anemia). Extramedullary hematopoiesis results in a leukoerythroblastic reaction (the presence of im-

Table 15–11 *Classification of Splenomegaly*

DIFFUSE SPLENOMEGALY	FOCAL SPLENOMEGALY (SPLENIC MASSES)
INFLAMMATORY SPLENOMEGALY	*NEOPLASTIC SPLENOMEGALY*
Suppurative splenitis	Hemangioma (dog)
Bacterial endocarditis (dog, cat)	Hemangiosarcoma (dog)
Septicemia (dog, cat)	Fibrosarcoma (dog)
Splenic torsion (dog)	Leiomyosarcoma (dog)
Toxoplasmosis (dog, cat)	Lymphoma (dog, cat)
Infectious canine hepatitis	Other metastatic neoplasia (dog, cat)
Necrotizing splenitis	*NON-NEOPLASTIC SPLENOMEGALY*
Splenic torsion (dog)	Hematoma (dog)
Infectious canine hepatitis	Abscess (dog, cat)
Salmonellosis (dog, cat)	
Eosinophilic splenitis	
Eosinophilic enteritis (dog, cat)	
Hypereosinophilic syndrome (cat)	
Lymphoplasmacytic splenitis	
Infection with *Ehrlichia canis* (dog)	
Pyometra (dog, cat)	
Brucellosis (dog)	
Hemobartonellosis (dog, cat)	
Granulomatous splenitis	
Histoplasmosis (dog, cat)	
Mycobacteriosis (dog, cat)	
Leishmaniasis (dog)	
Pyogranulomatous splenitis	
Blastomycosis (dog, cat)	
Sporotrichosis (dog)	
Feline infectious peritonitis	
HYPERPLASTIC SPLENOMEGALY	
Bacterial endocarditis (dog, cat)	
Brucellosis (dog)	
Discospondylitis (dog)	
Systemic lupus erythematosus (dog)	
Hemolytic disorders (dog, cat)	
CONGESTIVE SPLENOMEGALY	
Drug-induced splenomegaly (acepromazine, barbiturates) (dog, cat)	
Portal hypertension (dog, cat)	
Splenic torsion (dog, cat)	
INFILTRATIVE SPLENOMEGALY	
Neoplastic splenomegaly	
Acute and chronic leukemias (dog, cat)	
Systemic mastocytosis (dog, cat)	
Malignant histiocytosis (dog)	
Lymphoma (dog, cat)	
Multiple myeloma (dog, cat)	
Non-neoplastic splenomegaly	
Extramedullary hematopoiesis	
Amyloidosis	

(Modified from Couto CG. Diseases of the lymph nodes and the spleen. In: Ettinger S, ed. Textbook of veterinary internal medicine, 3rd ed. Philadelphia: WB Saunders, in press.)

mature red and white cell precursors in the peripheral blood), probably because the factors inhibiting the release of immature cells from the marrow are not operative at extramedullary sites.

The spleen's unique vascular arrangement allows for biologic filtration of cells and particles by the reticuloendothelium. The major difference between sinusal (dog) and nonsinusal (cat) spleens lies in their ability to "pit" cytoplasmic inclusions. Rigid cytoplasmic inclusions (*e.g.*, Heinz bodies, hemoparasites, nuclear remnants)

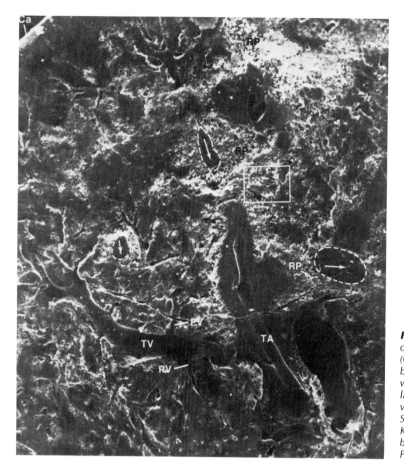

Figure 15–8. *Scanning electron micrograph demonstrating normal splenic architecture (75×). (Ca = capsule; RP = red pulp; areas enclosed by broken lines = periarterial lymphatic sheath or white pulp; arrows = central artery; TA = trabecular artery; TV = trabecular vein; PV = red pulp veins.) (From Tissues and Organs: A Text–Atlas of Scanning Electron Microscopy. By Richard G. Kessel and Randy H. Kardon. Copyright © 1979 by W.H. Freeman and Company. Reprinted with Permission.)*

or poorly deformable cells (*e.g.*, spherocytes, acanthocytes) are removed as the erythrocytes squeeze through the endothelial slits in sinusal spleens. Splenomegaly results in an enhanced filtering ability secondary to a translocation of a greater number of erythrocytes to the red pulp.

Canine and feline spleens have a great capacity to store blood (10%–20% of the total blood volume). Barbiturates and tranquilizers may induce pooling of blood in the enlarged spleen (up to 30% of total blood volume). In addition to acting as an erythrocyte reservoir, the normal spleen may store (sequester) 30% of the total platelet mass. Therefore, splenectomy usually results in a physiologic thrombocytosis.

The immunologic functions of the spleen include phagocytosis (immunoglobulin M, tuftsin, and properdin synthesis) and protection from hemoparasitemia. Immunosuppression resulting in

fatal sepsis was seen in only four of 130 dogs undergoing splenectomy. Each of these four dogs was splenectomized for immune hemolytic anemia and was undergoing aggressive immunosuppressive therapy at the time. Another study indicating the immunologic importance of the spleen involved dogs with osteosarcoma treated with amputation and a biologic response modifier, with or without splenectomy. Those dogs treated with amputation, biologic response modifier, and splenectomy did poorly (experiencing earlier metastasis when compared to the nonsplenectomized group), indicating the role the spleen plays in immune surveillance.

Splenomegaly can be categorized as diffuse or focal. Diffuse splenomegaly appears to be more common in the cat. It is further divided into four categories based on the cells present (inflammatory, lymphoreticular hyperplasia, congestion, and infiltrative diseases). Diffuse inflammatory splenomegaly can be suppurative (*e.g.*, septicemia), necrotizing (*e.g.*, splenic torsion), eosinophilic (*e.g.*, hypereosinophilic syndrome of cats), lymphoplasmacytic (*e.g.*, ehrlichiosis), granulomatous (*e.g.*, histoplasmosis), or pyogranulomatous (*e.g.*, blastomycosis). Lymphoreticular hyperplasia or "work hypertrophy" may be seen in hemolytic anemias. Congestion is seen with drug-induced splenomegaly, right-sided congestive heart failure, and splenic torsion. The infiltrative splenomegalies are associated with neoplastic diseases such as acute and chronic leukemias, myelomas, lymphomas, systemic mastocytosis, and malignant histiocytosis, and non-neoplastic conditions such as amyloidosis and extramedullary hematopoiesis.

Splenic masses or localized splenomegalies are more common in dogs than cats. Splenic masses can be classified as neoplastic or non-neoplastic. Neoplastic masses primarily include hemangiosarcomas and hemangiomas, and much less frequently, fibrosarcomas, leiomyosarcomas, spindle cell sarcomas, and lymphomas. Hematomas and abscesses comprise the majority of non-neoplastic splenic masses.

Clinical Signs

The clinical signs in dogs and cats with splenomegaly or splenic masses are often nonspecific, and in general are more directly related to the primary disease than to the splenic enlargement. Signs in dogs with splenomegaly or splenic masses include anorexia, weakness, fever, weight loss, abdominal distension, vomiting, diarrhea, pigmenturia, abdominal pain, and polydipsia and polyuria (Table 15-12). The polydipsia and polyuria may be due to psychogenic factors due to pain or distension of splenic stretch receptors. Pigmenturia may result from hemolysis and renal excretion of hemoglobin or bilirubin. Collapse, weakness, sudden intracavitary bleeding, and pallor may be present if splenic rupture occurs.

The physical examination in patients with splenomegaly should be directed toward differentiating diffuse splenomegaly from splenic masses

Table 15–12 *Clinical Signs Associated With Splenomegaly*

Anorexia	Diarrhea
Weakness	Pigmenturia
Fever	Abdominal pain
Weight loss	Polydipsia and polyuria
Abdominal distension	Pale mucous membranes
Vomiting	Collapse

and toward detecting coexisting findings. The physical characteristics of the spleen (size, surface characteristics) and location within the abdominal cavity should be noted. Coexisting findings may aid in the diagnostic process. These findings include subcutaneous masses (*e.g.*, mast cell tumor, hemangiosarcoma); pallor, petechiae, and ecchymoses (*e.g.*, hematopoietic neoplasia, hemangiosarcoma, disseminated intravascular coagulation); lymphadenopathy and hepatomegaly (*e.g.*, lymphoma, multiple myeloma, leukemia); fever (*e.g.*, infectious diseases); and the presence of ascites, heart murmur, jugular vein distension, or hepatomegaly (right-sided congestive heart failure, heartworm disease, portal hypertension).

Diagnostic Approach

Several tests are indicated in the patient with splenomegaly (complete blood count, serum biochemistry profile, urinalysis); however, it should first be determined if the splenomegaly is focal or diffuse. Figure 15-9 illustrates one possible approach to patients with splenomegaly. Often palpation of the spleen alone will determine if the splenomgaly is focal or diffuse, but other means of splenic imaging, including abdominal radiography and ultrasonography, should be used to confirm this presumptive finding. Abdominal radiographs usually determine that the mass palpated is indeed the spleen. However, very large abdominal masses or the presence of abdominal fluid can obliterate normal abdominal detail, making the spleen difficult to visualize. Abdominal ultrasonography is a very effective means of evaluating the splenic architecture. The presence of abdominal fluid actually enhances the imaging

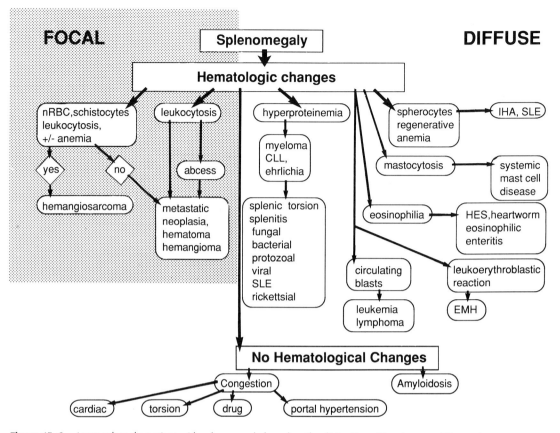

Figure 15–9. *Approach to the patient with splenomegaly based on the distinction of focal versus diffuse spleno-megaly. (CLL = chronic lymphocytic leukemia; IHA = immune-mediated hemolytic anemia; SLE = systemic lupus erythematosus; HES = hypereosinophilic syndrome; EMH = extramedullary hematopoiesis)*

capabilities of this modality. Ultrasonography may reveal the presence of fluid, splenic size and contour, and splenic echogenicity when compared to other organs (*e.g.,* liver and kidneys), and enables differentiation between diffuse and focal splenic lesions. Ultrasonography may reveal marked distension of the splenic vessels, which occurs in splenic torsions and in posthepatic portal hypertension. The two most common patterns of ultrasonographic splenic changes are normal to decreased echogenicity without parenchymal changes, as observed in congestive splenomegaly and diffuse infiltrative disorders, and focal parenchymal abnormalities such as hematomas, abscesses, or neoplasia (Fig. 15-10). Recently, radionucleide imaging using technetium 99m sulfur colloid has been used to visualize the spleen and to indirectly evaluate splenic function.

The spleen can exert a marked influence on the hemogram. The three patterns of hematologic changes associated with splenic disorders are leukoerythroblastic reactions, hypersplenism, and hyposplenism (Table 15-13). Leukoerythroblastic reactions have already been discussed; hypersplenism results from increased reticuloendothelial activity and is rare, while hyposplenism is common and results in hematologic changes similar to those seen in splenectomized patients. Hyposplenism occurs secondary to splenic torsion, infiltrative processes, and suppurative or necrotic splenitis.

Other tests to evaluate the patient with splenomegaly include echocardiography to identify right atrial masses (hemangiosarcoma) and thoracic radiographs to evaluate the pulmonary parenchyma for metastatic or fungal disease (see

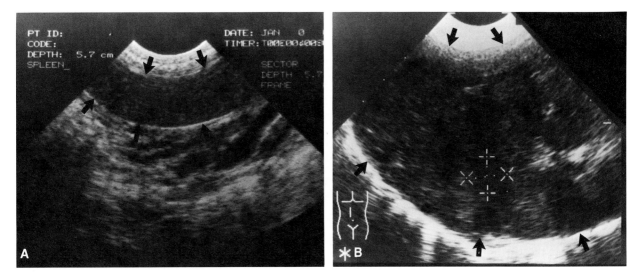

Figure 15–10. (A) Ultrasound demonstrating diffuse splenomegaly in a patient with lymphoma (arrows demarcate spleen). (B) Ultrasound demonstrating focal splenomegaly in a patient with hemangiosarcoma (small arrows demarcate spleen; ultrasound cursors indicate hemangiosarcoma).

Echocardiography and Thoracic Radiography in Chapter 80). Table 15-14 summarizes the clinical assessment of a patient with splenomegaly.

The final etiologic diagnosis in dogs and cats with splenomegaly usually requires cytologic or histopathologic evaluation of the enlarged spleen. Fine needle aspiration of the spleen is a safe, reli-

able, and cost-effective method to evaluate the spleen. The procedure for fine needle aspiration is to have the patient lie in right lateral or dorsal recumbency. The area to be aspirated is identified, shaved, and surgically prepared. Phenothiazine and barbiturate tranquilization should be avoided, as the resulting splenic congestion usu-

Table 15–13 Hematologic Changes in Patients With Splenomegaly

LEUKOERYTHROBLASTIC REACTIONS

Immature neutrophils
Nucleated red blood cells

HYPERSPLENISM

Neutropenia
Regenerative anemia
Thrombocytopenia
Bicytopenias
Pancytopenia

HYPOSPLENISM

Nucleated red blood cells
Target cells
Thrombocytosis
Acanthocytes
Howell–Jolly bodies
Reticulocytosis

Table 15–14 Clinical Assessment of the Patient With Splenomegaly

Test	Abnormality
Complete blood count	Anemia, neutropenia, thrombocytopenia, leukocytosis, eosinophilia, circulating blasts, leukoerythroblastosis, spherocytes
Biochemical profile	Hyperproteinemia, hypercalcemia
Urinalysis	Pigmenturia
Radiography	Splenomegaly, abdominal fluid, abnormal location of the spleen within the abdomen, gas density in spleen, other abdominal masses or organomegaly
Abdominal ultrasonography	Diffuse splenomegaly, hyperechoic or hypoechoic focal splenic masses, hyperechoic or hypoechoic nodules, changes in other organs
Echocardiography	Right atrial mass

ally results in a blood-diluted specimen. The spleen is manually isolated and aspirated in a manner similar to that described for lymph nodes, and pull smears are made using coverslips. The patient is observed for 3 to 6 hours following the procedure for potential intracavitary bleeding.

In a recent series of 33 dogs and cats with splenomegaly, no complications associated with splenic aspiration were detected even in patients with splenic masses, thrombocytopenia, and other coagulopathies. The most common cytologic diagnoses were extramedullary hematopoiesis and hematopoietic neoplasia.

If cytology is inconclusive or in conflict with the other clinicopathologic data, the clinician must decide whether or not to perform an exploratory celiotomy and, possibly, a splenectomy. This provides tissue for histopathology and information regarding the gross morphology of the spleen and other abdominal organs. However, diagnoses based on gross disease alone may be misleading. Hematomas and hemangiomas are difficult to differentiate from hemangiosarcoma grossly, and can be accompanied by hepatic nodular hyperplasia (which may be mistaken for metastatic foci). Euthanasia based on gross morphologic impressions should be avoided. Splenectomy is recommended for splenic torsion, splenic rupture, splenic masses, and symptomatic splenomegaly. Splenectomy is controversial in immune-mediated blood disorders, lymphomas, and leukemia. The bone marrow should be eval-

uated prior to considering splenectomy in patients with cytopenias and splenomegaly. If the marrow is hypoplastic or aplastic, the spleen may be the primary source of circulating blood cells and should not be removed. The underlying causes for 130 canine splenectomies were recently reviewed and are depicted in Figure 15-11.

Management and Patient Monitoring

The management and prognosis of the patient with splenomegaly depend on the diagnosis. Lymphomas have been discussed previously in this chapter. The remaining discussion will center on the most common cause of splenomegaly in the dog, hemangiosarcoma.

Hemangiosarcoma

Endothelial neoplasia is one of the most common underlying causes for splenomegaly resulting in splenectomy in the dog (see Fig. 15-11). The prevalence of hemangiosarcoma is 0.3% to 2%, and it comprises approximately 7% of all canine malignancies. Male dogs and German shepherd dogs are at high risk for the development of hemangiosarcoma. Figure 15-12 depicts the sites of origin of hemangiosarcoma in 181 dogs compiled from three studies. Since splenic hemangiosarcoma represents the greatest single site, the remaining discussion will center on splenic hemangiosarcoma.

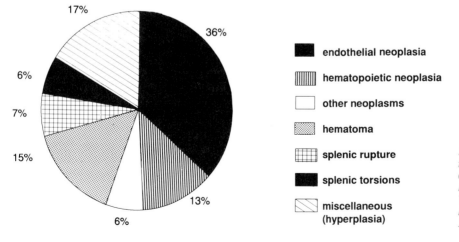

Figure 15–11. *Underlying causes for 130 splenectomies in the dog. (Couto CG. Diseases of the lymph nodes and the spleen. In: Ettinger S. Textbook of veterinary internal medicine, 3rd ed. Philadelphia: WB Saunders, in press.)*

- ■ endothelial neoplasia
- ▥ hematopoietic neoplasia
- ☐ other neoplasms
- ▦ hematoma
- ▦ splenic rupture
- ■ splenic torsions
- ▨ miscellaneous (hyperplasia)

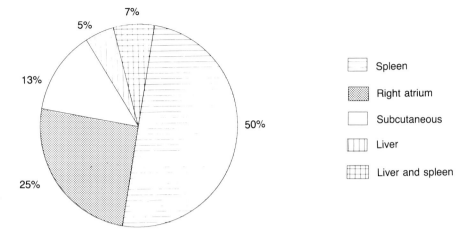

Figure 15–12. Anatomic forms of presentation for hemangiosarcoma in the dog.

Clinical signs and physical findings in dogs with splenic hemangiosarcoma include weakness, depression, collapse, pale mucous membranes, splenic enlargement, and abdominal distention. The finding of free blood in the abdomen is highly suggestive of ruptured hemangiosarcoma. Cytologic evaluation of effusions is rarely diagnostic. Fine needle aspiration of solid neoplasms yields diagnostic information in approximately 50% of the patients. The diagnosis of hemangiosarcoma is confirmed by histopathology and must never be based solely on the gross appearance of the spleen at surgery, as hemangiomas and hematomas look similar. Hematologic findings include regenerative anemia, nucleated erythrocytes, fragmented erythrocytes, and a neutrophilic leukocytosis. Serum biochemical changes are secondary to dehydration, hypovolemic shock, and organ involvement by the tumor. Immediate therapy for a patient with ruptured splenic hemangiosarcoma is to stabilize the patient and to remove the tumor to stop the bleeding.

Surgical resection (splenectomy) has been the major treatment modality for splenic hemangiosarcoma in the dog, but median survival times have been short (19–65 days). Dogs with splenic hemangiosarcoma and hemoperitoneum apparently have a worse prognosis than do dogs with a nonruptured splenic hemangiosarcoma (median survival 17 days vs. 121 days) (Prymak et al, Additional Reading).

The poor prognosis associated with hemangio-sarcoma appears to be due not only to the aggressive biologic behavior of the tumor, but also to the cardiac arrhythmias (see Chapter 18) and hemostatic abnormalities (disseminated intravascular coagulation; see Chapter 16) commonly associated with this neoplasm. Various adjuvant chemotherapy and chemoimmunotherapy protocols evaluated in the past appear to have some efficacy in the postoperative management of dogs with hemangiosarcoma (Fig. 15-13).

The VAC chemotherapy protocol is used at VTH-OSU following surgical cytoreduction in dogs with hemangiosarcoma. Median survival of six patients with splenic hemangiosarcoma was 145 days. The VAC protocol consists of diphenhydramine (Benadryl) 2.2 mg/kg intramuscularly given 20 minutes before treatment in an attempt to prevent anaphylactoid reactions from doxorubicin; doxorubicin (Adriamycin) 30 mg/m² intravenously (diluted to a concentration of 0.5 mg/ml in 0.9% sodium chloride and administered over 20–30 minutes) on day 1; cyclophosphamide (Cytoxan) 100 to 150 mg/m² intravenously (diluted to a concentration of 10 mg/ml in sterile water and administered over 10 minutes) on day 1; and vincristine (Oncovin) 0.75 mg/m² intravenously (diluted to a concentration of 0.25 mg/ml in normal saline and administered as a bolus) on days 8 and 15. The cycle is repeated every 21 days. We attempt to administer five cycles of chemotherapy.

Cardiotoxicity is monitored by means of M-mode echocardiography and electrocardiogra-

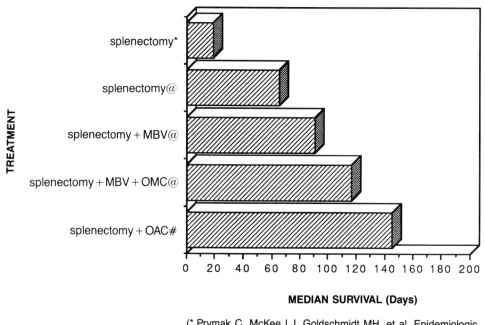

MEDIAN SURVIVAL (Days)

(* Prymak C, McKee LJ, Goldschmidt MH, et al. Epidemiologic, clinical, pathologic, and prognostic characteristics of splenic hemangiosarcoma and splenic hematoma in dogs: 217 cases (1985). J Am Vet Med Assoc 1988; 193:706;

@ Brown NO, Patnait AK, MacEwe EG. Canine hemangiosarcoma: Retrospective analysis of 104 cases. J Am Vet Med Assoc 1985; 186:56;

Hammer AS, Couto CG. Lymphadenopathy. In: Fenner WR. Quick reference to veterinary medicine, 2nd ed. Philadelphia: JB Lippincott, in press.)

Figure 15–13. *Median survival times for dogs with splenic hemangiosarcoma. (MBV = mixed bacterial vaccine; OMC = oncovin [Vincristine], methotrexate, and cyclophosphamide; OAC = oncovin [Vincristine], doxorubicin [Adriamycin], and cyclophosphamide)*

phy performed before institution of therapy and every third cycle. Doxorubicin is discontinued if signs of cardiotoxicity (*e.g.*, arrhythmias, decreased fractional shortening) occur. Complete blood counts are performed weekly while receiving VAC therapy. Chemotherapy is postponed if the neutrophil count is less than 2000 cells per microliter (2 × 109 per liter) or if severe gastroenteritis occurs. If repeated episodes of severe neutropenia or gastroenteritis occur, the doses of doxorubicin are either divided into weekly administrations of 10 mg/m² or decreased by 30%; the dose of cyclophosphamide is also decreased by 30%. If the neutropenia or gastroenteritis is associated with vincristine administration, the dose is decreased by 30%.

Most toxicities associated with VAC chemotherapy are not life-threatening. Neutropenia is the most common complication. The use of a sulfadiazine–trimethoprim combination prophylactically has been proposed to decrease febrile events. There are marginal decreases in the packed-cell volume over time, and no significant thrombocytopenia. In fact, the platelet count often rises as therapy progresses, possibly due to vincristine-induced thrombocytosis or lack of microangiopathic platelet consumption by the tumor. The development of cardiotoxicity is another important toxicity. Myocardial dysfunction may develop at doses well below the suggested cardiotoxic cumulative dose of doxorubicin of 240 mg/m². Other side-effects of doxorubicin include perivascular necrosis if extravasation occurs, alopecia, hyperpigmentation, and gastroenterocolitis. Hemorrhagic enterocolitis can be controlled with the use of bismuth subsalicylate. The side-effects of vincristine and cyclophosphamide were discussed previously.

ADDITIONAL READING

Brown NO, Patnaik AK, MacEwen EG. Canine hemangiosarcoma: Retrospective analysis of 104 cases. J Am Vet Med Assoc 1985; 186:56.

Carter RF, Harris CK, Withrow SJ et al. Chemotherapy of canine lymphoma with histopathological correlation: Doxorubicin alone compared to COP as first treatment regime. Journal of the American Animal Hospital Association 1987; 23:587.

Cotter SM. Treatment of lymphoma and leukemia with cyclophosphamide, vincristine, and prednisone: II. Treatment of cats. Journal of the American Animal Hospital Association 1983; 19:166.

Couto CG. Canine lymphomas: Something old, something new. Compendium of Continuing Education 1985; 7:291.

Couto CG. Diseases of the lymph nodes and the spleen. In: Ettinger S, ed. Textbook of veterinary internal medicine, 3rd ed. Philadelphia: WB Saunders, 1989:2225.

Couto CG. Oncology. In: Sherding RS, ed. The cat: Diseases and clinical management. New York: Churchill Livingstone, 1989.

Greene CE. Clinical microbiology and infectious diseases of the dog and cat. Philadelphia: WB Saunders, 1984:356.

Hammer AS, Couto CG. Lymphadenopathy. In: Fenner WR, ed. Quick reference to veterinary medicine, 2nd ed. Philadelphia: JB Lippincott, in press.

Hammer AS, Couto CG, Filppi J et al. Efficacy and toxicity of VAC chemotherapy (vincristine, doxorubicin, cyclophosphamide) in dogs with hemangiosarcoma. Journal of Veterinary Internal Medicine, in press.

Ishida T, Washizu T, Toriyabe K et al. Feline immunodeficiency virus infection in cats of Japan. J Am Vet Med Assoc 1989; 194:221.

Jeglum KA, Whereat A, Young K. Chemotherapy of lymphoma in 75 cats. J Am Vet Med Assoc 1983; 190:174.

Lucke YM, Davies JD, Wood CM et al. Plexiform vascularization of lymph nodes: An unusual but distinctive lymphadenopathy in cats. J Comp Pathol 1987; 97:109.

MacEwen EG, Hayes AA, Matus RE et al. Evaluation of some prognostic factors for advanced multicentric lymphosarcoma in the dog: 146 cases (1978–1981). J Am Vet Med Assoc 1987; 190:564.

Mooney SC, Hayes AA, MacEwen EG et al. Treatment and prognostic factors in lymphoma in cats: 103 cases (1977–1981). J Am Vet Med Assoc 1989; 194:696.

Mooney SC, Patnaik AK, Hayes AA et al. Generalized lymphadenopathy resembling lymphoma in cats: Six cases (1972–1976). J Am Vet Med Assoc 1987; 190:897.

Moore FM, Emerson WE, Cotter SM et al. Distinctive peripheral lymph node hyperplasia of young cats. Vet Pathol 1986; 23:386.

Prymak C, McKee LJ, Goldschmidt MH et al. Epidemiologic, clinical, pathologic, and prognostic characteristics of splenic hemangiosarcoma and splenic hematoma in dogs: 217 cases (1985). J Am Vet Med Assoc 1988; 193:706.

Weller RE, Theilen GH, Madewell BR. Chemotherapeutic responses in dogs with lymphosarcoma and hypercalcemia. J Am Vet Med Assoc 1982; 181:891.

Yamamoto JK, Hansen H, Ho EW et al. Epidemiologic and clinical aspects of feline immunodeficiency virus infection in cats from the continental United States and Canada and possible mode of transmission. J Am Vet Med Assoc 1989; 194:213.

Yamamoto JK, Sparger E, Ho EW et al. Pathogenesis of experimentally induced feline immunodeficiency virus infection in cats. Am J Vet Res 1988; 49:1246.

16

DISORDERS OF HEMOSTASIS AND PRINCIPLES OF TRANSFUSION THERAPY

Alan S. Hammer
C. Guillermo Couto

DISORDERS OF HEMOSTASIS

Defects in hemostasis arise in a variety of clinical situations. They represent an obvious difficulty to the surgeon. Bleeding disorders are a primary reason that clients seek emergency care. The internist is constantly beset by a variety of disorders associated with hemorrhagic and thrombotic tendencies. As veterinarians' knowledge of primary diseases and ability for therapeutic intervention increase, patient management is often limited by secondary disorders such as hemostatic abnormalities. Rapid recognition and intervention in cases in which imbalance of the hemostatic system has occurred is necessary by all primary care clinicians.

CAUSES

A wide variety of disorders can upset the hemostatic balance; many of these are listed in Table 16-1. Spontaneous bleeding can be the result of vascular disorders, quantitative and qualitative platelet disorders, and hereditary and acquired coagulation disorders. Hemostatic abnormalities can also result in excessive clotting (thrombosis).

PATHOPHYSIOLOGY

When dealing with disorders of the hemostatic system, one wonders why normal patients do not bleed to death or, alternatively, why the blood does not suddenly clot. Descriptions of the normal checks and balances operating in hemostasis fill literally hundreds of books. Fortunately, only a small fraction of this system need be kept in mind for proper management of most clinical cases. Figure 16-1 illustrates some important concepts of hemostasis.

Hemostasis involves three main components: the vessel wall, platelets, and humoral factors. Primary hemostasis involves the initial interactions between the vessel wall and platelets, cul-

Table 16–1 *Classification of Hemostatic Disorders in Dogs and Cats*

PRIMARY HEMOSTATIC DISORDERS

VASCULAR DISORDERS
Vasculitis (dog, cat)
Hyperadrenocorticism (dog)
Ehlers–Danlos syndrome (dog, cat)

QUANTITATIVE PLATELET DISORDERS (THROMBOCYTOPENIA)
Due to decreased platelet production
 Immune-mediated megakaryocytic hypoplasia (dog, cat)
 Idiopathic bone marrow aplasia (dog, cat)
 Drug-induced megakaryocytic hypoplasia (estrogen) (dog)
 Myeloproliferative disorder (dog, cat)
 Multiple myeloma (dog, cat)
 Bone marrow lymphoma (dog, cat)
 Cyclic thrombocytopenia (dog)
 Myelofibrosis (dog, cat)
 Metastatic bone marrow neoplasms (dog, cat)
Due to increased platelet destruction and sequestration
 Immune-mediated thrombocytopenia (as with immune-mediated thrombocytopenia, systemic lupus erythematosus, or immune-mediated hemolytic anemia) (dog, cat)
 Live viral vaccine-induced thrombocytopenia (dog)
 Drug-induced thrombocytopenia (see Table 16–2) (dog, cat)
 Microangiopathy (dog)
 Disseminated intravascular coagulation (dog, cat)
 Vasculitis (dog, cat)
 Splenomegaly (dog, cat)
 Splenic torsion (dog)
 Endotoxemia (dog, cat)
 Acute hepatic necrosis (dog, cat)
 Neoplasia (immune-mediated, microangiopathy) (dog, cat)

QUALITATIVE PLATELET DISORDERS
Hereditary
 von Willebrand's disease (dog, cat)
 Canine thrombasthenic thrombopathia (otterhounds)
 Canine thrombopathia (basset hounds, foxhounds)
Acquired
 Drug-induced disorders (see Table 16–2) (dog, cat)
 Disorders secondary to disease states such as myeloproliferative disorders, systemic lupus erythematosus, renal disease, liver disease, or dysproteinemias (dog, cat)

SECONDARY HEMOSTATIC DISORDERS

CONGENITAL COAGULATION DEFECTS
Factor I: hypofibrinogenemia and afibrinogenemia (St. Bernards and borzois)
Factor II: hypoprothrombinemia (boxers)
Factor VII: hypoproconvertinemia (beagles and malamutes)
Factor VIII: hemophilia A (dog, cat)
Factor IX: hemophilia B (dog, cat)
Factor X: Stuart–Prower factor deficiency (cocker spaniels)
Factor XI: hemophila C (English springer spaniels, Great Pyrenees, Kerry blue terrier)
Factor XII: Hageman factor deficiency (dog, cat)

ACQUIRED COAGULATION DISORDERS
Liver disease due to decreased production of factors or qualitative disorders (dog, cat)
Vitamin K antagonism (dog, cat)

MIXED HEMOSTATIC DISORDERS

Disseminated intravascular coagulation due to neoplasia, sepsis, feline infectious peritonitis, leptospirosis, dirofilariasis, babesiosis, pancreatitis, shock, heat stroke, idiopathic hyperaldosteronism, acute hepatic necrosis, gastric torsion syndrome, or trauma (dog, cat)

THROMBOTIC DISORDERS

Antithrombin III deficiency (dog, cat)
Nephrotic syndrome
Disseminated intravascular coagulation
Liver disease
Heparin-induced
Protein-losing enteropathy

---

minating in a primary hemostatic plug, which is short-lived and unstable. Following injury, sympathetic-mediated vasoconstriction occurs to slow blood flow and limit blood loss. Vasoconstriction can be prolonged by thromboxane A_2 release from aggregated platelets. Exposure of the subendothelial components results in platelet adherence with assistance from von Willebrand's factor (vWF : Ag or VIIIR : AG). Following adherence, platelets release bioactive factors (*e.g.*, adenosine diphosphate, serotonin, histamine) to recruit more platelets for aggregation. Other changes occurring in the aggregated platelets include release of platelet factor 3 (a surface glycoprotein important in the common pathway for secondary hemostasis as a site for enzymatic reactions) and synthesis of thromboxane A_2 (responsible for vasoconstriction and platelet aggregation).

Secondary hemostasis involves the humoral factors, and results in the formation of a fibrin clot, which is long-lived and stable. The synthesis of fibrin is the result of a carefully controlled cascade of enzymatic reactions that is capable of

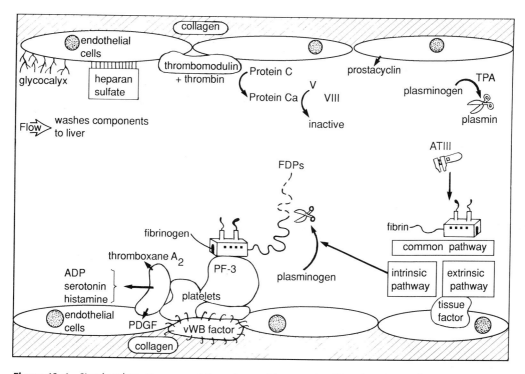

Figure 16–1. *Simple schematic representation of normal hemostasis with active plasmin depicted as scissors, antithrombin III (ATIII) depicted as a monkey wrench, and the combined factors V, X, prothrombin, and calcium represented as a fibrin-synthesizing factory. (TPA = tissue plasminogen activator; FDP = fibrin degradation products; PF-3 = platelet factor 3; ADP = adenosine diphosphate; vWB = von Willebrand's; PDGF = platelet-derived growth factor)*

amplifying the initial event. The end result is a microfactory complex for fibrin synthesis deposited on platelet surfaces (see Fig. 16-1). The liver is responsible for synthesis of most of the coagulation factors, including antithrombin III (AT III) and proteins C and S but excluding factor VIII, calcium, and vWF. Vitamin K is necessary for modification of glutamic acid residues in factors II, VII, IX, and X and proteins C and S by the hepatocytes following protein synthesis. There are two traditional mechanisms for activation of factor X (the common pathway): the intrinsic and extrinsic pathways (Fig. 16-2). As research into coagulation continues, the distinction between these pathways becomes blurred. Activation of the extrinsic pathway begins with the release of tissue thromboplastin from damaged endothelium, damaged tissues, or hemolyzed red blood cells (RBCs), converting factor VII to the active serine protease, which in turn activates factor X. The tissue thromboplastin–factor VII

complex is also capable of activating factor IX of the intrinsic system.

The contact phase of the intrinsic pathway involves factors XII and XI, which activate the intrinsic pathway through factors IX and VIII. The fibrinolytic, kinin, and complement systems are also activated by contact phase reactants. Factors VIII and IX then activate factor X and inititate the common pathway.

The common pathway results in the deposition of a fibrin synthesizing "factory" complex that is comprised of factors Va, Xa, prothrombin, and calcium. (The *a* following the factor indicates that this is the active form.) Thrombin acts on fibrinogen to form fibrin monomers, which polymerize to form a delicate gel. Factor XIII crosslinks and stabilizes the gel. (See Figures 16-1 and 16-2 for a schematic illustration of the clotting cascade and specific tests of the hemostatic system.)

Just as there are complex mechanisms to con-

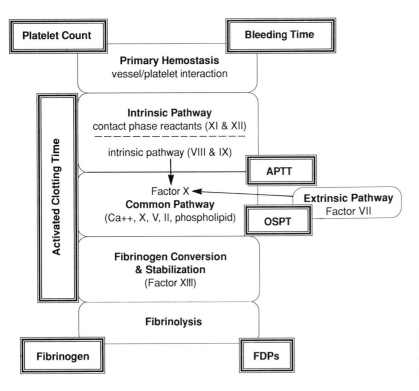

Figure 16–2. *Schematic illustration of laboratory evaluation of hemostasis. (APTT = activated partial thromboplastin time; OSPT = one-stage prothrombin time; FDP = fibrin degradation products)*

trol hemorrhage, there must obviously be mechanisms to prevent inappropriate activation of the hemostatic system. At the vessel surface level, heparan sulfate and glycocalyx repel platelets; endothelial cells also synthesize prostacyclin (PGI₂), which inhibits platelet aggregation. Thrombomodulin is also present at the endothelial surface and can inhibit thrombin. The thrombomodulin–thrombin complex activates protein C (a vitamin K-dependent zymogen) to a protease, which in conjunction with another vitamin K-dependent protein, protein S, specifically inactivates the accelerating factors of coagulation, factors V and VIII. Another element in controlling hemostasis is blood flow. Adequate flow dilutes coagulation factors in situ and washes the activated components to the liver, where they are metabolized.

Specific inhibitors of the coagulation cascade probably represent one of the main controls of hemostasis. Antithrombin III is a potent factor (see Fig. 16-1) capable of shutting down the fibrin-synthesizing factory complex on the platelet surface. The liver is the primary site of synthesis of AT III. Antithrombin III inhibits factors II, IX, X, XI, and XII. Antithrombin III is markedly (2,000- to 10,000-fold) potentiated by heparin of either endogenous or exogenous origin. Antithrombin III is depleted by its inhibitory interaction with the various coagulation factors. Lack of AT III plays a major role in some hemostatic disorders, such as disseminated intravascular coagulation (DIC), and in the thromboembolic disease seen in patients with nephrotic syndrome and protein-losing enteropathy. Other inhibitory serum proteins include alpha₂-macroglobulin, alpha₁-antitrypsin, and C1 esterase inhibitor.

The final phase of hemostasis is fibrinolysis. The inactive plasminogen is converted to plasmin by tissue plasminogen activator and the intrinsic pathway. Plasmin cleaves fibrin, fibrinogen, and factors V and VIII. Usually plasminogen is incorporated within the clot, so dissolution occurs from within as well as from the surface of the clot. Alpha₂-antiplasmin circulates to inhibit free plasmin and to prevent systemic fibrinolytic activity. The fibrinogen and fibrin fragments released during the fibrinolytic process are termed fibrin degradation products (FDPs). Fibrin degradation products are capable of decreasing platelet plug formation, fibrin polymerization, and thrombin activity, thus acting as potent anticoagulants.

Pathologic processes can disrupt normal hemostasis at several levels. At the primary hemostatic level, vascular defects are uncommon but may include congenital disorders such as Ehlers–Danlos syndrome or acquired diseases such as hyperadrenocorticism and immune-mediated vasculitis. The most common cause of spontaneous bleeding in dogs and cats is thrombocytopenia, which is also a primary hemostatic defect. Thrombocytopenia may arise from decreased platelet production or from increased platelet destruction and sequestration (see Table 16-1). Diseases in which patients have normal platelet numbers but decreased platelet function include von Willebrand's disease and other congenital platelet defects. Acquired platelet dysfunctions can be associated with the administration of certain drugs (Table 16-2), myeloproliferative disorders, uremia, and multiple myeloma.

Disruption of secondary hemostasis can occur at the intrinsic, extrinsic, or common pathways, either singly or in combination. There can be deficiencies in specific factors, such as factor VIII (hemophilia A) or factor IX (hemophilia B), or deficiencies in several factors, as is seen in liver disease and DIC, among others. Loss of inhibitory factors such as AT III due to glomerulonephritis, protein-losing enteropathy, liver disease, DIC, or heparin therapy may also lead to severe hemosta-

tic disorders characterized predominantly by thromboembolism. Qualitative disorders of the coagulation factors are induced by liver disease or, more frequently, by vitamin K antagonists. These antagonists include warfarin and its second-generation derivative, brodifacoum, and the indanedione anticoagulants diphacinone and chlorophacinone. By inhibiting carboxylation of glutamic acid residues on factors II, VII, IX, and X and proteins C and S, marked abnormalities of hemostasis occur.

Disseminated intravascular coagulation is a multifactorial disease resulting in inappropriate activation of the clotting process. It represents the most common bleeding disorder affecting both the primary and secondary hemostatic systems. A variety of conditions are associated with DIC (*e.g.*, neoplasia, sepsis, canine infectious hepatitis, feline infectious peritonitis, acute pancreatitis, shock, immune-mediated hemolytic anemia, heat stroke, severe tissue damage, acute hepatitis). Disseminated intravascular coagulation also results in activation of the fibrinolytic process, producing increased serum concentrations of FDPs that compound the hemostatic abnormalities.

CLINICAL SIGNS

The signalment (age, breed, sex) of a patient with a bleeding disorder can be helpful in raising the index of suspicion for hereditary defects. For example, hemophilia A should be included in the differential diagnosis for a young, male German shepherd pup presenting with spontaneous hemarthrosis and deep hematomas. Important information to obtain from the owner includes any history of spontaneous bleeding disorders (*e.g.*, prolonged bleeding during elective surgeries; past bleeding episodes; bleeding disorders in the dam, sire, or littermates; and perinatal mortality in the litter). Extensive questioning about access to rodenticides, including storage of rodenticides and agricultural or municipal rodent control programs is necessary, as most cases of ingestion of rodenticides occur without the owner's knowledge. Travel to areas endemic to *Ehrlichia* or exposure to ticks is also important to ascertain. If

Table 16–2 *Drugs That May Adversely Affect Platelet Function*

Aspirin	Dipyridamole
Phenylbutazone	Caffeine
Ibuprofen	Gentamicin
Indomethacin	Antihistamines
Theophylline	Procaine hydrochloride
Heparins	Halothane
Dextrans	Penicillin
Phenothiazines	Carbenicillin
Moxolactam disodium (and	Ticarcillin disodium
other third-generation	Ampicillin
cephalosporins)	Sulfonamides
Cytosine arabinoside	Propranolol
Prostaglandin I$_2$	Lidocaine
Isoprenaline	Estrogen

the past medical history is not available, a detailed inquiry should be made regarding any past immune-mediated disorders, neoplasms, or liver or kidney disorders, and past or present administration of drugs. Recent live viral vaccination (especially with those vaccines containing modified-live canine distemper virus) may suppress the primary hemostatic response (cause thrombocytopenia) for 3 to 10 days and should also be noted.

In general, several groups of patients should be evaluated for abnormalities of the hemostatic system: symptomatic patients with obvious (or not so obvious) clinical signs related to bleeding, patients having medical conditions or receiving drugs that predispose them to hemostatic abnormalities, and surgical patients in which hemostatic abnormalities are suspected. Table 16-3 summarizes some of the clinical features that are useful in differentiating vascular or platelet abnormalities from coagulation factor abnormalities in patients with spontaneous bleeding. The initial physical examination may be helpful in differentiating primary from secondary hemostatic defects. Primary hemostatic disorders result in petechiation, ecchymoses, and superficial mucosal bleeding (*e.g.*, melena, epistaxis, hematuria), whereas secondary hemostatic disorders result in hematomas, deep muscular and cavitary hemorrhages, and delayed bleeding from venipuncture sites.

Conditions predisposing patients to hemostatic failure include sepsis, shock, uremia, solid neoplasms, lymphoproliferative and myeloproliferative diseases, heartworm disease, hemolytic anemia, pancreatitis, hyperadrenocorticism, anticoagulant therapy, blood transfusions, and various drugs, including nonsteroidal anti-inflammatory agents, antibiotics, anesthetic agents, anticoagulants, gold salts, dapsone, estrogens,

and antineoplastic agents, among others. Diagnosis of these diseases or use of these drugs should direct the physical examination and laboratory evaluation toward the early recognition and correction of hemostatic abnormalities.

Diagnostic Approach

The first step in evaluating a patient with a bleeding disorder is recognition of the predisposing condition or signs of a current problem. This is best accomplished by a thorough clinical history and physical examination, as discussed previously. Often, the diagnosis of a primary vs. secondary hemostatic disorder can be tentatively made at this point. Next, samples must be collected in order to confirm and better define the bleeding disorder. Proper collection of these samples prior to instituting therapy is important to prevent misleading results. This includes an atraumatic venipuncture to prevent tissue factors from contaminating the sample and invalidating the results (the activated partial thromboplastin time [APTT] is particularly sensitive); collection into citrated siliconized glass or plastic tubes (except for FDP determinations); and use of the proper blood : citrate ratio (1 part of 3.8% citrate to 9 parts blood). A hemostasis panel can be used to screen for abnormalities and often is sufficient to diagnose the specific condition (Table 16-4). This panel should include RBC morphology, platelet count, bleeding time, fibrinogen concentration, APTT, one-stage prothrombin time (OSPT), and FDPs.

The presence of schistocytes (fragmented RBCs) in blood smears usually indicates microangiopathic hemolysis (Fig. 16-3). Abnormalities in the microvasculature may result from DIC or

Table 16–3 *Clinical Features of Primary and Secondary Bleeding Disorders*

PRIMARY BLEEDING DISORDERS *PLATELET OR VASCULAR ABNORMALITIES*	SECONDARY BLEEDING DISORDERS *COAGULATION ABNORMALITIES*
Petechiae and ecchymoses common	Petechiae and ecchymoses rare
Hematomas rare	Hematomas common
Bleeding at mucous membranes	Bleeding into muscles, joints, and body
Bleeding from multiple sites	cavities

Table 16–4 Laboratory Evaluation of Bleeding Patients

	OSPT	APTT	ACT	BT	PLT	FDP
Thrombocytopenia	N	N	N	P	D	No
Platelet dysfunction	N	N	N	P	N	No
Vitamin K deficiency	P	P	P	N	N	No
Hemophilia	N	P	P	N	N	No
Disseminated intravascular coagulation	P	P	P	P	D	Yes

P = prolonged; N = normal; D = decreased or shortened; OSPT = one-stage prothrombin time; APTT = activated partial thromboplastin time; ACT = activated coagulation time; BT = bleeding time; PLT = platelets; FDP = fibrin degradation products

microvascular changes in neoplastic tissues (hemangiosarcoma). Red blood cells are sliced by the fibrin strands or the abnormal neoplastic endothelial cells, and the fragments reseal. Schistocytes are not exclusively seen in microangiopathic hemolysis and can be seen in Heinz-body hemolytic anemia, hyposplenism or asplenia, iron deficiency anemia, heartworm disease, and structural defects of the heart and great vessels.

The platelet count can also be estimated from examination of the blood smear. A monolayer field (RBCs close together and half of the cells touching) is examined under a 1000× oil immersion lens. Normal numbers of platelets are 11 to 25 per field in dogs and 11 to 29 per field in cats. Each platelet in the monolayer field represents approximately 15,000 platelets per microliter

$(15 \times 10^9/L)$ of peripheral blood (Fig. 16-4). Since clumping of platelets may lead to artificially low numbers, it is important to scan the feathered edge of the smear to detect platelet clumps. More accurate platelet counts can be obtained using quantitative automated or manual methods. Platelet numbers in cats are best determined by manual means.

Bleeding time is a test of the primary hemostatic system and is the most readily available test for vessel and platelet function. Bleeding time is subject to wide variations in technique. In an attempt to standardize this useful procedure, we use a commercial bleeding time template (Surgicutt [International Technidyne Corporation]) and create a wound of standard width and depth on the buccal mucosa (Fig. 16-5). The blood welling up from the incision is blotted away with a

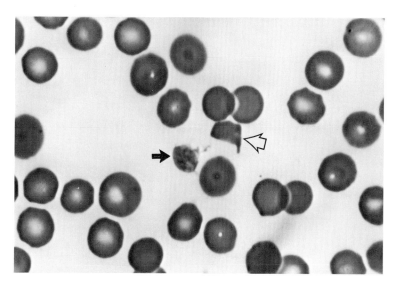

Figure 16–3. Fragmented red blood cell (schistocyte) is shown at large arrow. Macroplatelet is shown at small arrow.

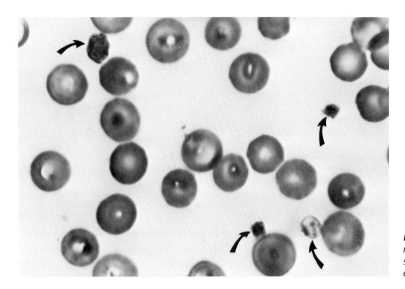

Figure 16–4. *Estimation of platelet count from monolayer field on blood smear. Each platelet represents 15,000 platelets/μL (small arrows). Actual count was 68,000 platelets/μL.*

tissue (being careful not to touch the wound) and the time to cessation of bleeding is noted. For dogs, the normal bleeding time is 2.6 ± 0.5 minutes. For this procedure, cats are lightly sedated with ketamine hydrochloride (18.3 mg/kg) and acepromazine (0.18 mg/kg) intramuscularly; the normal bleeding time is 1.9 ± 0.5 minutes. Nail bed bleeding time also evaluates primary hemostasis. This test is performed by cutting the nail back to the quick with a nail trimmer and observing the time required for cessation of bleeding. The bleeding time in normal dogs using this tech-

nique is 2 to 8 minutes. Platelet aggregation in response to low concentrations of aggregating agents is a more sophisticated test of platelet function, and is usually available only at referral and specialty hospitals. Another test of platelet function is observation of clot retraction due to contraction by platelet thrombosthenin. This test may be affected by low fibrinogen concentration.

The APTT evaluates the intrinsic and common coagulation systems (all coagulation factors except VII). Prolongation of the APTT can be caused by contact phase defects (factors XI or XII defi-

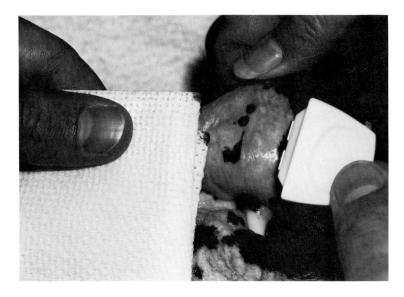

Figure 16–5. *Buccal mucosal bleeding time is performed by incising the buccal mucosa in a uniform manner and observing the time required for cessation of bleeding.*

ciencies where clinical bleeding is unlikely), factor VIII or IX deficiencies (bleeding is commonly seen), common pathway deficiencies (factors II, V, and X), and heparin therapy. Any given factor must be decreased to approximately 30% of normal concentration before prolongation occurs.

The OSPT evaluates the extrinsic and common systems and is prolonged by factor VII deficiencies (*e.g.*, congenital liver disease, vitamin K deficiency). Common pathway defects also result in prolongation of the OSPT, but heparin therapy usually does not. In both the APTT and OSPT, prolongations of more than 25% of the control should be considered abnormal.

Plasmin's action on fibrinogen and fibrin results in the release of various cleavage fragments, termed fibrinogen or fibrin degradation products (FDPs). These can be measured using commercial kits with latex particles coated with anti-FDP antibody (Thrombo-Wellcotest [Burroughs Wellcome]). It is our experience that minor elevations of FDPs occur in many disease states and are not always indicative of DIC. In general, FDPs greater than 10 g/ml are suggestive of pathologic fibrinolysis.

Fibrinogen (factor I) is the only coagulation factor that can be directly assayed. It is usually measured by the difference in protein concentration between heated and unheated plasma using a refractometer. Heating plasma at 56°C for 3 minutes precipitates fibrinogen. Decreases in fibrinogen concentrations may result from advanced liver disease or DIC. Hyperfibrinogenemia is usually associated with chronic DIC, renal disease, or inflammatory conditions.

Several tests that can be performed in an emergency situation are helpful in rapidly classifying most bleeding patients (see Table 16-4). The first of these, evaluating the blood smear for platelet numbers and RBC abnormalities, has already been discussed. In-office tests of the intrinsic system include the activated clotting time (ACT) and the Lee–White clotting time. To perform the ACT, 2 ml of blood is added to diatomaceous earth in a glass tube to activate the clotting sequence (Becton-Dickinson, tube #6522). The sample is incubated at 37°C for 60 seconds and then evaluated every 5 seconds until clotting occurs. Normal clotting times are 60 to 90 seconds. Prolonga-

tion may occur from intrinsic or common pathway defects and severe hypofibrogenemia. It should be noted that mini-dose heparin therapy for DIC (10 IU/kg) does not prolong the ACT. The Lee–White clotting time evaluates the time required for clot formation to occur when blood is placed in a plain glass tube (reference range 6–7.5 minutes in the dog and 8 minutes in the cat). Observation of blood left in plastic syringes may lead to falsely prolonged clotting time due to the lack of activation of the contact phase reactants by the plastic. The buccal mucosal bleeding time can also be used if platelet dysfunction is suspected. Lastly, the Thrombo-Wellcotest for FDPs is a simple, rapid test that can be very helpful in identifying DIC if the FDP concentration is markedly elevated.

Depending on the results of the initial hemostasis screen, specific factor assays and other special laboratory tests may be required. If special tests are contemplated, discussions with the laboratory regarding sample type, volume, and transportation should take place prior to obtaining it. Virtually all of the clotting factors, as well as AT III and vWF, can be assayed.

Figure 16-6 shows a flow chart for the approach to the bleeding patient. With a complete blood count, platelet count, biochemistry profile, and hemostasis screen, most bleeding disorders can be rapidly identified. Thrombocytopenia can occasionally present a diagnostic difficulty. A more indepth diagnostic approach to thrombocytopenia is given in Figure 16-7.

Management and Patient Monitoring

Emergency management of a patient with a bleeding disorder is directed first at physically stopping or slowing the flow of blood—if possible, and second, at collecting blood samples before instituting therapy. The patient should be handled as atraumatically as possible, minimizing the number of venipunctures. Most patients with bleeding disorders have a deficiency or dysfunction of one or more components of the hemostatic system, which fresh whole blood can usually correct. Occasionally, the use of whole blood is contraindicated, as in the case of Evans's syndrome

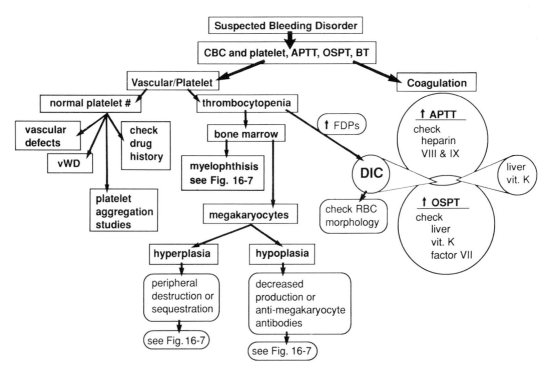

Figure 16–6. *Approach to the patient with a bleeding disorder. (CBC = complete blood count; APTT = activated partial thromboplastin time; OSPT = one-stage prothrombin time; BT = bleeding time; FDP = fibrin degradation products; DIC = disseminated intravascular coagulation; vWD = von Willebrand's disease; RBC = red blood cell)*

(concurrent immune-mediated thrombocytopenia and immune-mediated hemolytic anemia), in which the transfused RBCs may rapidly lyse, adding to the disease process. Therefore, if time permits, determining the specific factor needed is better than blindly administering whole blood (see Principles of Transfusion Therapy at the end of this chapter).

Thrombocytopathia

Thrombocytopathias (platelet dysfunction syndromes) are often difficult to recognize. Thrombocytopathias are either congenital or acquired. Congenital platelet function defects have been identified in the otterhound, bassett hound, and fox hound. Management of these disorders involves recognition of the problem and transfusion with fresh functional platelets, stoppage of the administration of the offending drug, or treatment of the underlying disease. Clinical signs in

dogs and cats with thrombocytopathia are the same as with other primary hemostatic disorders (*e.g.*, petechiae, ecchymoses, mucosal bleeding).

Another hereditary thrombocytopathia, von Willebrand's disease (vWD), probably constitutes the most common hereditary bleeding disorder in animals. Von Willebrand's factor is a 270,000-dalton glycoprotein subunit that polymerizes into variable-sized multimers and has a circulating half-life of approximately 12 hours. This large complex acts as a bridge between damaged endothelium and platelets to initiate primary hemostatic plug formation. In the dog, vWF appears to be synthesized mainly by endothelial cells. In humans, vWD constitutes a heterogenous group of diseases with varying clinical signs. This also appears to be the case in dogs. Deficiencies of vWF have been identified in more than 30 breeds of dogs. In addition to its bridging action, vWF acts to stabilize factor VIII in the plasma. Physiologic or pathologic increases in vWF have been

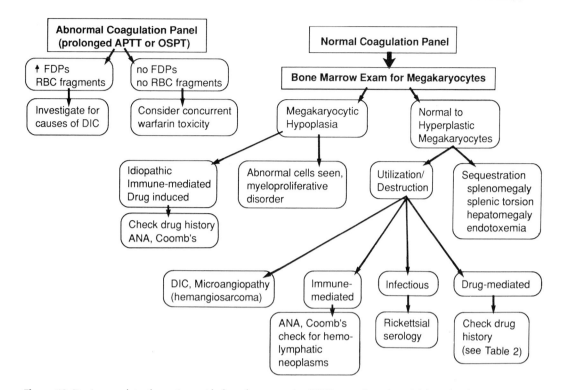

Figure 16–7. *Approach to the patient with thrombocytopenia. (APTT = activated partial thromboplastin time; OSPT = one-stage prothrombin time; FDP = fibrin degradation products; RBC = red blood cell; DIC = disseminated intravascular coagulation; ANA = antinuclear antibody)*

identified following whelping, liver disease, endotoxemia, and administration of desmopressin acetate (DDAVP, a synthetic vasopressin analog) in the dog. Laboratory identification of vWF deficiency requires electroimmunoassay; however, a presumptive clinical diagnosis may be obtained by performing a buccal mucosal bleeding time. Seven doberman pinschers with vWD thus evaluated had mean buccal mucosal bleeding times of 10.7 ± 3.7 minutes (control: 2.6 ± 0.5 minutes). Hemorrhagic crises in these patients are best managed by administering blood products or cryoprecipitate. Occasionally, desmopressin acetate has been administered to blood donor dogs 30 minutes prior to phlebotomy to raise the vWF levels. Studies of desmopressin acetate administration to clinically bleeding doberman pinschers with vWD indicate that 1 μg/kg subcutaneously or intravenously may decrease or halt excessive intra- or postoperative hemorrhage. The effects of

desmopressin acetate, however, last only 2 to 3 hours, and refractoriness can develop quickly. Levothyroxine (0.04 mg/kg) has also been used in the management of dogs with hypothyroidism, vWD, and problems of platelet dysfunction. The drug is reported to cause a more substantial and sustained increase in vWF and platelet adhesiveness than desmopressin acetate.

Drug-induced thrombocytopathias can be classified into those induced by drugs that block adenosine diphosphate binding sites, raise platelet cyclic adenosine monophosphate, and affect prostaglandin synthesis, and those induced by drugs that interfere with membrane actions. Table 16-2 lists drugs that are known or suspected to cause platelet dysfunction. Abnormal platelet function can also be seen in association with renal and liver disorders and in primary bone marrow diseases such as myeloproliferative diseases and myelodysplastic syndromes. Dysproteinemias can decrease platelet function by coating the membrane surfaces. Patients with multiple myeloma may have significant primary bleeding disorders due to both thrombocytopenia and thrombocytopathia.

Thrombocytopenia

Thrombocytopenia is the most common acquired bleeding disorder in the dog. Clinical signs of primary bleeding disorders (*e.g.*, petechiae, hematuria, epistaxis) do not occur until the platelet count is less than 25,000 per microliter (25×10^9 per liter), although bleeding may occur at higher platelet counts if thrombocytopathia or a coagulopathy are concurrently present. There are regional differences in the causes of thrombocytopenia; for example, immune-mediated thrombocytopenia is by far the most common cause in Ohio, while rickettsial diseases are reportedly the most common etiology in Texas.

The approach to the thrombocytopenic patient can be difficult due to the variety of conditions that can cause low platelet counts (see Table 16-1). When evaluating such patients, it is important to proceed in a logical but expeditious manner (see Fig. 16-7). The first step is to determine whether the hemostatic disorder is limited to a primary defect or if there are concurrent secondary hemostatic abnormalities present. If the coagulation panel is otherwise normal, the next step is to evaluate the status of platelet production. This is best accomplished by performing bone marrow aspiration or biopsy (see Bone Marrow Aspiration and Biopsy in Chapter 80). Decreased platelet production may be associated with megakaryocyte hypoplasia secondary to myeloproliferative diseases, immune-mediated causes, or drug-induced hypoplasia. Normal to increased numbers of megakaryocytes are suggestive of adequate platelet production with increased sequestration or peripheral destruction. Sequestration may occur secondary to hepatosplenomegaly or increased platelet margination associated with endotoxemia or vasculitis. Increased destruction or utilization of platelets may be due to microangiopathy (*e.g.*, DIC, hemangiosarcoma), immune-mediated disorders (*e.g.*, immune-mediated thrombocytopenia, systemic lupus erythematosus), infectious causes (ehrlichiosis, infectious cyclic thrombocytopenia, Rocky Mountain spotted fever, feline leukemia virus), or drug-induced thrombocytopenia, among others.

Immune-Mediated Thrombocytopenia

Immune-mediated thrombocytopenia is a common cause of bleeding in dogs but is rare in cats. It primarily affects middle-aged female dogs, with toy breeds and Old English sheepdogs being overrepresented. As a primary bleeding disorder, its clinical signs include petechiae, ecchymoses, and superficial bleeding. The complete blood count in patients with immune-mediated thrombocytopenia is characterized by thrombocytopenia with or without anemia (depending on the degree of spontaneous bleeding); leukocytosis with a left shift may be present. Bone marrow cytology is usually characterized by megakaryocytic hyperplasia, although in rare instances megakaryocytic hypoplasia may be present; occasionally, large numbers of free megakaryocytic nuclei are seen. When immune-mediated hemolytic anemia is associated with immune-mediated thrombocytopenia (Evans's syndrome), a Coombs' positive, regenerative anemia with spherocytosis is present. In addition to the thrombocytopenia, the bleeding time is the only other laboratory test that provides abnormal results (*i.e.*, ACT, APTT, OSPT, FDPs, and fibrinogen concentration are normal).

Since currently there are no laboratory tests to reliably diagnose immune-mediated thrombocytopenia, other diagnoses should be excluded before establishing this diagnosis. Conditions to be excluded include canine ehrlichiosis, drug-induced thrombocytopenia, and infectious cyclic thrombocytopenia. When the index of suspicion for immune-mediated thrombocytopenia is high, a therapeutic trial with immunosuppressive doses of corticosteroids (equivalent to 2–4 mg/kg/day of prednisone) should be instituted. In general, responses are seen within 48 to 96 hours. Fresh whole blood is administered as needed to maintain oxygen-carrying capacity. In addition to immunosuppressive doses of corticosteroids, cyclophosphamide (as a single dose of 200–300 mg/m^2 IV) can be used for induction of remission.

Azathioprine (Imuran) at a dose of 50 mg/m² orally every 24 to 48 hours is also indicated to maintain remission; in some dogs, azathioprine is better tolerated for chronic administration than corticosteroids. Vincristine sulfate has been used at a dose of 0.3 to 0.5 mg/m² to stimulate platelet production. Danazol, an androgenic steroid, at doses of 5 mg/kg orally every 12 hours has received recent attention as a potential therapy for humans and dogs with immune-mediated thrombocytopenia. Splenectomy may be useful in the management of dogs with relapsing episodes of immune-mediated thrombocytopenia (Jans, Additional Reading).

Vitamin K Deficiency

Small animals with vitamin K deficiency usually have ingested vitamin K antagonists such as warfarin and diphacinone or their derivatives, brodifacoum and bromadiolone. If ingestion has just occurred, induction of vomiting may remove the bulk of the product. Due to the pharmacokinetics of the newer antagonists, it is often necessary to administer vitamin K for several weeks to prevent problems. If the ingestion of anticoagulant rodenticides is questionable and there are no clinical signs suggestive of coagulopathies (*e.g.*, hematomas, hemothorax, hemoabdomen), the OSPT may be evaluated to identify subclinical or preclinical disease. Factor VII is the shortest-lived vitamin K-dependent protein (half-life of 4–6 hours), so prolongation of the OSPT is usually the first laboratory abnormality before clinical signs become evident. Newer laboratory tests for proteins induced by vitamin K absence (PIVKA) may soon become commercially available and will aid in early diagnosis of rodenticide toxicity.

Most animals with vitamin K deficiency present with acute collapse and no history of rodenticide ingestion. These animals usually have clinical signs of secondary bleeding disorders (*e.g.*, hemoabdomen, hemothorax, hematomas, deep muscular hemorrhages), pale mucous membranes, anemia that is usually regenerative if sufficient time has elapsed, and hypoproteinemia that normalizes with resolution of internal hemorrhage. These animals are "walking time bombs" and must be handled gingerly to prevent

further hemorrhage. Even with proper handling, sudden death may occur due to acute central nervous system or pericardial hemorrhage. Management of these patients may require immediate whole fresh blood transfusions, as parenteral vitamin K therapy may take approximately 12 hours to take effect. In severely vitamin K-depleted animals, it may take up to 48 hours for the OSPT to return to reference ranges and the clinical bleeding to cease.

Therapeutic vitamin K is available in several forms, with phytonadione (vitamin K₁) being the most effective. Menadione (vitamin K₃) is less expensive but is also apparently a far less effective antidote. It should never be used as the sole antidote in a rodenticide-intoxicated animal. Phytonadione is available for oral or parenteral use. Intravenous administration is not recommended due to the risk of anaphylaxis. Also, intramuscular injections in a dog with a coagulopathy may result in hematoma formation. If the patient is not hypoperfused (in shock), we prefer to administer phytonadione subcutaneously using a 25-gauge needle at a loading dose of 5 mg/kg, followed in 8 hours by 2.5 mg/kg, divided, subcutaneously three times daily. If the patient is stable and is not vomiting after the first injection, the drug may be given orally at 2.5 mg/kg, divided, three times daily. There is recent evidence that oral phytonadione loading doses may be as effective as the parenteral form. Absorption is best if given with fatty meals; animals with cholestatic or malabsorptive syndromes may require continued subcutaneous injections. Since there is a delay in the onset of action, if immediate therapy is needed it is better to administer whole blood or fresh frozen plasma to replenish the missing clotting factors. Ideally, in critical cases the OSPT should be monitored every 8 hours until it normalizes.

If the anticoagulant is known to be warfarin or another first-generation hydroxycoumarin, 1 week of oral phytonadione therapy is usually sufficient. However, if the poison is not known or if it is indandione or any of the second-generation anticoagulants, oral phytonadione must be given for a prolonged time (3 weeks) (Table 16-5). Patients must be examined and the OSPT repeated within 48 to 72 hours of cessation of phytonadione ther-

Table 16–5 *Management of Rodenticide Intoxication*

KNOWN IMMEDIATE INGESTION; NO CLINICAL SIGNS

Induce vomiting with apomorphine hydrochloride (dogs only, place tablet in conjuctiva of eye and remove when vomiting occurs) or xylazine (in cats, 0.1 mg/kg IM)
Perform gastric lavage
Administer vitamin K_1 orally (2.5 mg/kg divided t.i.d.)
Evaluate one-stage prothrombin time

SUSPECTED INGESTION

Evaluate one-stage prothrombin time
Evaluate proteins induced by vitamin K absence
Institute 3 weeks of vitamin K_1 (2.5 mg/kg divided t.i.d. orally)

CLINICAL BLEEDING DISORDER

Evaluate one-stage prothrombin time
Handle gently; give oxygen
Tap hemothorax or hemopericardium only if necessary to stabilize
Perform transfusion
Administer parenteral and oral vitamin K_1 (5 mg/kg subcutaneously followed by 2.5 mg/kg divided t.i.d. orally)

apy. If the OSPT is still prolonged at that point in time, therapy should be reinstituted for another 2 weeks and the OSPT again determined within 2 days of cessation of therapy.

Other causes of vitamin K deficiency include cholestatic or malabsorptive syndromes with subsequent poor uptake of vitamin K, and long-term second- and third-generation cephalosporin administration. Certain cephalosporins, such as moxalactam, can decrease gut bacterial production of vitamin K and also directly inhibit phytonadione metabolism in the liver.

Congenital Coagulopathies

A deficiency in almost every factor has been described in small animals (see Table 16-1). Many defects cause only mild coagulopathies, while in others severe clinical bleeding is common. Hemophilia A (factor VIII deficiency) is one of the more severe congenital coagulopathies. Factor VIII is a glycoprotein with a molecular weight of 300,000 daltons. It circulates in the plasma in tight association with VIIIR : AG (von Willebrand factor). Factor VIII is produced primarily by endothelial cells and has a half-life of 6 to 14 hours. Hemophilia A can be mild, moderate, or severe, and signs may include prolonged bleeding from the umbilical cord, excessive gingival bleeding at teething, hemarthroses, and hematomas, along with other signs of secondary bleeding disorders. Hemophilia A is a sex-linked recessive disorder and has been reported in many breeds of dogs and in domestic cats. Immunization with live viral vaccines may exacerbate mild bleeding disorders. Patients with hemophilia A can form the primary hemostatic plug, so the bleeding time is normal; however, the plug is unstable and the secondary hemostatic plug is defective, resulting in delayed bleeding from venipunctures. Therapy for acute crises involves administration of fresh or fresh frozen plasma or plasma cryoprecipitate.

Suspicion of hemophilia A can be based on clinical history and signs and on a prolonged APTT with a normal OSPT. However, hemophilia B and factor XI and XII deficiencies cannot be excluded until specific factor determination has been performed.

Following diagnosis of a congenital coagulation disorder, the veterinarian is obliged to inform the owner or breeder of the genetic nature of the disease. Unfortunately, due to the broad range of normal values, it is difficult to accurately identify carrier animals by a testing program.

Hemophilia B or factor IX deficiency is another congenital coagulopathy with variable clinical severity. It is also a sex-linked recessive disorder. Factor IX is a 60,000-dalton glycoprotein with a half-life of 18 to 36 hours that is synthesized in the liver. The APTT is usually prolonged (but the OSPT is normal); therapy involves factor IX replacement of fresh whole blood or fresh frozen plasma. Breeds affected include the Alaskan malamute, black and tan coonhound, Cairn terrier, cocker spaniel, Labrador retriever, Scottish terrier, Saint Bernard, and British shorthair cat.

Deficiencies of factors XI and XII (the contact phase of the intrinsic pathway) result in few or no clinical signs of bleeding. Patients with factor XI deficiencies may have minor bleeding episodes or persistent bleeding following surgery. Both defects can cause prolongation of the APTT and are inherited in an autosomal recessive manner. Again, specific factor assays are needed to diagnose the disorder. Breeds with factor XI deficiency include the Kerry blue terrier, English springer spaniel, and Great Pyrenees. Factor XII deficiencies have been reported in domestic cats and miniature poodles. Interestingly, in birds, reptiles, and some marine mammals, factor XII deficiency is a normal physiologic phenomenon.

Another uncommon congenital coagulopathy causing few clinical signs is factor VII deficiency. The condition usually results in isolated prolongation of the OSPT. It has been reported in beagles and Alaskan malamutes.

Renal Disease

Two major hemostatic syndromes are recognized in animals with renal disease: uremic thrombocytopathia and thromboembolic events associated with glomerulonephropathy. Of the two syndromes, sudden development of thromboembolism is of greater clinical significance.

The nephrotic syndrome is characterized by hypercholesterolemia, hypoalbuminemia, edema, and proteinuria, and is usually seen in patients with renal amyloidosis and glomerulonephritis (see Chapter 45). In a study of 52 dogs with renal amyloidosis, 20 dogs had clinical signs of thrombosis (*e.g.*, dyspnea secondary to pulmonary thromboembolism). Loss of AT III in the urine is thought to represent the major pathogenesis of thrombosis in these patients, although dehydration, hemoconcentration, and endothelial damage may add to the risk of thrombosis. Some researchers consider dogs with a 50% decrease in AT III to be at high risk for thrombosis.

Due to the devastating effects of thromboembolism, it is important to identify the patient at risk in order to institute prophylaxis. Therapeutic intervention in patients with severe proteinuria includes aspirin or heparin administration. Aspirin is commonly used in our practice to decrease platelet aggregation and to minimize the development of thrombosis. The recommended oral dose is 10 to 25 mg/kg twice daily in dogs and 25 mg/kg twice weekly in cats. Aspirin is an irreversible cyclooxygenase inhibitor, but its effect on platelet thromboxane A_2 production is greater than the effects on endothelial cell prostaglandin production due to the fact that endothelial cells can synthesize more cyclooxygenase to replace that inhibited by aspirin. Platelets, as anucleated cells, do not have that ability. Use of prostaglan-

din inhibitors is not without its detrimental effects. In addition to the known ulcerogenic effects, prostaglandin inhibitors can precipitate acute renal crises by inhibiting normal vasodilatory prostaglandin production within the kidney. In the normal patient this is usually of little consequence, but in a patient with underlying renal disease and subjected to volume depletion, it can lead to severe consequences. Therefore, concurrent use of potent loop diuretics should be carefully monitored in these patients.

If more aggressive therapy for overt thromboembolism is needed, heparin is recommended. Heparin can be administered subcutaneously and does not cause gastric ulceration. It should not be given intramuscularly, as deep local hemorrhages may occur. Heparin enhances AT III activity 2,000- to 10,000-fold, but also causes consumption of AT III. We use low-dose heparin (150–250 IU/kg) in severely proteinuric patients two to three times daily subcutaneously. A pretreatment ACT or APTT should be obtained in order to establish a baseline value. Therapy is aimed at prolonging the ACT or APTT from 2 to 2.5 times the baseline. Heparin has the added advantage that a specific antidote, protamine sulfate, can be used if undue hemorrhage should occur. For every 100 IU of heparin administered in the last dose, 1 mg of protamine sulfate should be given slowly intravenously (over 60 minutes) as a 1% solution. Protamine sulfate should be used with caution in dogs, as it may cause anaphylactic reactions. Since heparin may cause gradual declines in AT III levels in a patient already deficient in this factor, the administration of fresh whole blood or fresh plasma may be necessary in severely proteinuric patients to replenish AT III. It is because of this lowering of AT III during heparin therapy that sudden cessation of heparin therapy may induce a hypercoagulable state. To avoid this, the dose of heparin should be gradually reduced over 24 hours and another anticoagulant agent, such as aspirin, should be given or fresh AT III administered.

Once thromboembolism has occurred, treatment must be directed toward supporting the patient and slowing thrombus formation through the use of anticoagulants (*e.g.*, aspirin, low-dose heparin). Efforts at clot lysis by administration of thrombolytic drugs such as streptokinase and urokinase have not been successful. A new agent, recombinant tissue plasminogen activator, shows some promise in clot lysis; however, significant side-effects must be overcome and further clinical trials performed before it can be adopted for general use.

A platelet dysfunction syndrome, uremic thrombocytopathia, has been recognized in uremic patients; however, it is usually of little clinical importance. It is thought that an imbalance in prostaglandin synthesis occurs when excessive amounts of prostacyclin are present. Alternatively, accumulation of metabolites of phenylalanine, tyrosine, or the hepatic urea cycle may decrease endothelial–VIIIR : AG interactions. In one study, buccal mucosal bleeding times in dogs with severe azotemia (serum urea nitrogen greater than 124 mg/dl or 44 nmol/L) were prolonged, with a mean of 12.6 ± 6 minutes.

Liver Disease

The liver represents not only the major source for synthesis of clotting factors, but also a vast endothelial surface where vasculitis, platelet aggregation, and activation of the clotting cascade may occur. More than 60% of dogs with liver disease have abnormal hemostasis; however, only 2% have clinical evidence of bleeding. In acute hepatic inflammation and necrosis, significant vasculitis and endothelial damage may occur, resulting in thrombocytopenia due to local aggregation or consumption of platelets. If liver damage continues, thrombocytopathia and coagulopathies may compound the picture. If the hepatic injury is severe, DIC may occur. If bleeding disorders are present in a patient with liver disease, extrahepatic causes (*e.g.*, DIC, microangiopathy, immune-mediated thrombocytopenia, vitamin K deficiency) should be eliminated before concluding that the liver is primarily responsible for the coagulopathy. Management is directed at treating the underlying cause of the hepatic disorder and supporting the hemostatic system (*e.g.*, blood component therapy, mini-dose heparin).

Disseminated Intravascular Coagulation

Disseminated intravascular coagulation represents the most common mixed (primary and secondary) bleeding disorder in dogs (and possibly in cats). It can be triggered by a wide variety of diseases and is associated with a high mortality rate. Often, it is a preterminal event in a life-threatening illness.

By definition, DIC is the intravascular activation of the components of the hemostatic system with resultant microcirculatory thromboembolism and attendant organ failure; paradoxically, DIC is usually associated with excessive bleeding. There are numerous causes of DIC in animals; however, most cases of spontaneous DIC are multifactorial in nature. Mechanistically, three pathways are postulated to initiate the intravascular coagulation (Fig. 16-8). Realistically, this is an

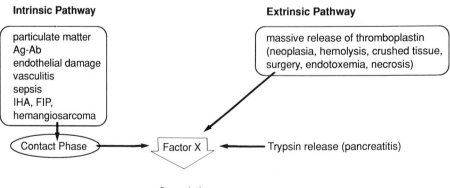

Figure 16–8. Mechanisms that initiate intravascular coagulation.

artifactual distinction, as few diseases utilize one pathway exclusively to initiate DIC. The initial phase of DIC results in microcirculatory disturbances and may affect many organs (*e.g.,* brain, lungs, liver, kidneys, intestines). Platelet consumption begins at this point and results in thrombocytopenia. Depending on the degree of activation of coagulation factors, the resulting DIC may be chronic or acute.

The increased activation of the hemostatic system results in elevated plasma concentrations of circulating activated thrombin and plasmin. The reticuloendothelial system is overwhelmed by particulate matter, FDPs, and inactivated coagulation factors, and cannot adequately clear the thrombin and plasmin from the circulation. If functional hyposplenism is present due to splenic neoplasia, the reticuloendothelial system is further incapacitated. Splenic hemangiosarcoma is a prime example of a disease that can both initiate and promote DIC through its abnormal vasculature and decreased splenic function. The activated, circulating thrombin and plasmin enzymes result in degradation and consumption of coagulation factors, which in turn lead to the hemorrhagic state often associated with systemic DIC. As plasmin-induced fibrinolysis occurs, FDPs are produced that further add to the coagulopathy by inhibiting the platelet function and increasing the burden on the reticuloendothelial system. The patient has now progressed from microcirculatory thromboembolism and fibrinolysis to systemic inactivation of coagulation factors, thrombocytopenia, and thrombocytopathia.

Circulating plasmin and thrombin play a pivotal role in the progression of DIC from a local to a systemic disease. Secondary "enhancers" promote the progression of DIC. These include low AT III (*e.g.,* liver disease, nephrotic syndrome, DIC itself, asparaginase therapy), acidosis and hypoxia (inhibition of AT III, increased endothelial damage), circulatory stasis or collapse, and a poorly functioning reticuloendothelial system.

Clinical signs of DIC can vary from organ failure due to thromboembolic events (*e.g.,* renal and liver failure, neurologic signs, pulmonary thromboembolism, intestinal infarcts) to hemorrhages (petechiation, ecchymosis, delayed bleeding from venipuncture sites, epistaxis, gastrointestinal hemorrhages, hematoma formation). The diagnosis of acute DIC is usually easily made, but the diagnosis of chronic DIC may be more difficult. All of the clinical and laboratory findings must be evaluated in order to establish a diagnosis. Platelet numbers and fibrinogen concentrations are greatly decreased in acute DIC, but can be elevated in chronic DIC due to compensatory overproduction. The APTT and OSPT may or may not be prolonged. A high concentration of circulating FDPs is probably the most specific test for diagnosing DIC. However, significant liver disease may falsely elevate the FDPs due to poor clearance. Finally, a negative FDP test does not necessarily eliminate DIC from consideration. Schistocytes in the blood smear constitute a significant finding but are also not specific for DIC. The AT III concentration is usually low in DIC due to consumption, although it may also be low in other disease states (*e.g.,* nephrotic syndrome). In general, the diagnosis of DIC may be entertained when thrombocytopenia, prolonged APTT or OSPT, and elevated FDP concentrations or schistocytes are found.

There is no "magic bullet" with which to treat DIC. The single most important step in the treatment of DIC is to attempt to treat or remove the underlying cause. Correcting any of the secondary "enhancers" of DIC also plays a vital role. The major treatable complication in most patients with DIC is hemorrhage. Transfusion therapy may be necessary to replenish RBCs, platelets, coagulation factors, and AT III. The use of minidose heparin (10–20 IU/kg three times daily subcutaneously) appears to offer a possible mode of therapy in DIC by enhancing AT III activity. Minidose heparin does not prolong the ACT or APTT and allows for reliable monitoring of the coagulopathy. If plasma is to be administered to replenish AT III, a dose of heparin can be added to it and incubated at 37°C for 30 minutes prior to administration. Adequate administration of fluids, correction of acid-base imbalances, and hypoxia are all additional measures to attempt to slow or halt DIC. The use of aspirin in DIC remains controversial; it is currently not in wide use except in chronic DIC. Finally, if sepsis or shock are the cause of DIC, a single dose of cortico-steroids may be indicated.

PRINCIPLES OF TRANSFUSION THERAPY

Indications

Transfusion of whole blood or blood components (*e.g.*, packed red blood cells, platelet-rich plasma, or plasma) is indicated in several clinical situations; however, this form of therapy should not be misused. The most common indication for whole blood transfusion is the need to restore oxygen-carrying capacity secondary to anemia. Anemias may occur due to blood loss, chronic inflammation, hemolysis, or other causes. Transfusion of the patient with immune-mediated hemolytic anemia is performed only if clinically necessary in a life-threatening situation, as life-threatening acceleration of hemolysis is possible (see Chapter 73). Table 16-6 gives the indications for transfu-

sion and the appropriate blood components to be used.

Blood components are less commonly used to correct hypoproteinemia. Hypoalbuminemia may be due to decreased production (hepatic) or increased loss (renal or intestinal). Protein concentrates are the ideal replacement; however, they are not readily available for veterinary use. Fresh or frozen plasma at a dose of 10 to 20 ml/kg is, therefore, the next logical treatment for patients with hypoproteinemia. Volume overloading should be avoided. One should ascertain that the infused plasma has a sufficiently high albumin concentration to be of benefit. Marked continuous protein loss may make replacement therapy unsuccessful.

Coagulation factor deficiencies resulting in hemorrhage can be corrected with fresh whole blood or, more ideally, with fresh or fresh frozen plasma. Life-threatening bleeding from thrombocytopenia may be temporarily halted with transfusion therapy. Whole blood replaces the lost erythrocytes, but large quantities are needed to

Table 16–6 *Indications for Transfusion*

	Fresh Whole Blood	Packed Red Blood Cells	Fresh or Fresh Frozen Plasma	Platelet Rich Plasma
ANEMIAS				
Hemolytic anemia	+/−	+	−	−
Blood loss	+	+	−	−
Chronic renal disease	+/−*	+	−*	−
Chronic inflammation	+/−	+	−	−
Pure red cell aplasia	+/−	+	−	−
BLEEDING DISORDERS				
Thrombocytopenia	+†	−	−	+
Thrombocytopathia	+	−	−	+
Hemophilia	+	−	+	−
Vitamin K deficiency	+	−	+	−
Disseminated intravascular coagulation	+‡	−	+‡	−
HYPOPROTEINEMIA				
Renal, liver, gastrointestinal	−	−	+§	−
Blood loss	+	+	+§	−

* *Fresh blood or plasma may be indicated in antithrombin III deficiency.*
† *Whole blood may be contraindicated in Evan's syndrome (immune-mediated hemolytic anemia and thrombocytopenia).*
‡ *Mini-dose heparin may be incubated with blood or plasma prior to administration.*
§ *Does not need to be fresh or fresh-frozen plasma.*
+ = *may be used;* − = *do not use*

significantly raise the platelet count. Platelet-rich plasma, if available, is superior in this respect.

Blood Donors

Blood donor dogs should weigh more than 25 kg, be in good physical condition, and have a packed-cell volume greater than 40% (0.40 L/L). Female donors should be spayed to eliminate fluctuations in platelet number and function secondary to serum estrogen concentrations. Immunizations should be up-to-date; however, one should realize that thrombocytopenia may occur 5 to 10 days following modified-live viral vaccination. Routine fecal examinations should be performed. Canine blood donors should ideally be blood group DEA 1.1, 1.2 (formerly blood group A), and 7 negative. DEA 1.1 and 1.2 are the most likely to cause transfusion reactions. At VTH-OSU, greyhounds are the preferred donors because of their docile nature, lean build with ready access for venipuncture, high packed-cell volume, and low occurrence rate of DEA 1.1, 1.2, and 7.

Canine donors should be evaluated for infection with the following: *Ehrlichia canis, Babesia canis, Hemobartonella canis, Dirofilaria immitis, Brucella canis,* and possibly *Trypanosoma cruzi*. At VTH-OSU, all donors are splenectomized to facilitate identification of hemoparasites and increase the blood yield in each collection.

Blood donor cats should weigh more than 5 kg and have a packed-cell volume greater than 35% (0.35 L/L). Females should be spayed. While blood group antigens exist on cat erythrocytes (A, B, and AB), routine typing of donor cats is not performed due to the lack of available reagents. Cats tested in the United States have almost exclusively been A positive; the incidence of B positive cats varies greatly from region to region (in Australia, 26% of tested cats were B positive). Donor cats should be negative for feline infectious peritonitis, feline leukemia virus, feline immunodeficiency virus, and infection with *Hemobartonella felis* and *Toxoplasma gondii*. Routine fecal examinations should also be performed for intestinal parasites. Both donor dogs and cats should be maintained on a high-quality nutritional plane,

including iron and vitamin supplements (*e.g.,* Felobits, Vi-Sorbits).

Blood Collection

The jugular vein is the preferred site for repeated phlebotomy. The donor may be sedated or anesthetized if necessary; ketamine (20–30 mg intramuscularly) is routinely given to all cats for bleeding. The venipuncture site is surgically prepared. For dogs, a closed collection set is used (Blood Collection Set [Abbott Laboratories]) (Fig. 16-9) and the blood is collected into a plastic bag with anticoagulant (Acid Citrate Dextrose [ACD] Solution or Citrate Phosphate Dextrose [CPD]). The bag is gently swirled during collection to enhance mixing. In the cat, 10 ml of ACD (ACD Evacuated Blood Collection Bottles [Diamond Laboratories]) is drawn into a 60-ml syringe. Using a 19-gauge butterfly catheter, 50 ml of blood is drawn into the same 60-ml syringe (Fig. 16-10). This will result in the same anticoagulant : blood ratio as stored blood. If blood is to be transfused within 24 hours, 250 units of heparin drawn into 2 ml of saline per 50 ml of blood may be used as an alternative anticoagulant.

Dogs may donate 22 ml/kg every 10 to 14 days. Cats may donate 50 ml every 14 days.

Blood Storage

If the blood is not used immediately, it should be stored at 4°C. The oxygen-releasing capacity (based on 2,3-diphosphoglycerate concentrations) of canine erythrocytes decreases within 2 weeks of collection if stored in ACD. Blood collected in CPD retains its oxygen-carrying capacity for 4 weeks. All whole blood and packed cells must be discarded after 4 weeks of storage. Any blood that was warmed to room temperature cannot be placed back into storage and must be discarded due to the risk of bacterial contamination. At VTH-OSU, feline blood is not stored; only fresh whole blood is administered.

Stored blood nearing its expiration date requires a significant metabolic effort on the part

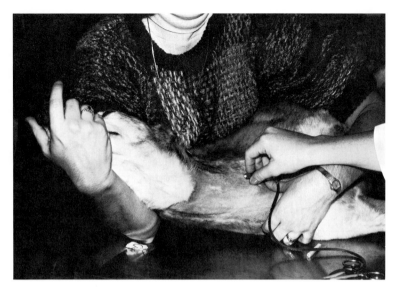

Figure 16–9. *Blood collection in a dog using a closed collection system.*

of the recipient to "recharge" the transfused erythrocytes. This effort may have significant negative impact on the severely debilitated patient and may warrant the use of fresh blood rather than stored blood. In addition, stored blood or RBCs should not be used in patients with severe liver disease or portosystemic shunts, since the increased ammonia content in stored RBCs may worsen signs of hepatic encephalopathy.

Crossmatching

Crossmatching is an alternative to blood typing of in-house donors; it can be used in patients that have a history of past transfusions or for patients that will require multiple transfusions. Crossmatching detects many incompatibilities, but does not guarantee complete compatibility. Table 16-7 describes the procedure for major and minor crossmatching.

Blood Administration

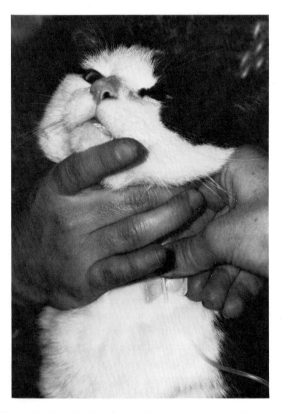

Figure 16–10. *Blood collection in a cat using a butterfly catheter and a 60-ml syringe with anticoagulant.*

Refrigerated blood should be warmed to room or body temperature prior to or during administration. Excessive heat should be avoided, as fi-

Table 16–7 *Crossmatching Procedure*

1. Collect 2 ml of blood from donor and recipient in EDTA tubes.
2. Centrifuge samples at 3000 G for 1 minute. Remove and retain plasma.
3. Resuspend red blood cells in saline; centrifuge, and discard supernatant. Repeat three times.
4. Prepare a 2% red blood cell suspension composed of 0.02 ml of washed red blood cells and 0.98 ml of saline.
5. Major crossmatch:
    two drops of donor red blood cell suspension
    two drops of recipient plasma
6. Minor crossmatch:
    two drops of recipient red blood cell suspension
    two drops of donor plasma
7. Negative control:
    two drops of donor red blood cell suspension
    two drops of donor plasma
8. Incubate major, minor, and control samples at 25°C for 30 minutes.
9. Centrifuge all tubes at 3000 G for 1 minute.
10. Agglutination is a positive test.

brinogen precipitation or autoagglutination may occur. The administration set should have a filter in place (Blood Administration Set [Travenol Laboratories]) to remove clots and other particulate matter (*e.g.,* platelet aggregates). The blood is usually administered via the cephalic, saphenous, or jugular veins. However, in small patients, neonates, or patients with poor peripheral circulation, intraosseous infusion may be performed. To administer intraosseous fluids, the skin over the femur is surgically prepared, and the skin and periosteum of the femoral trochanteric fossa are anesthetized with 1% lidocaine. A bone marrow aspiration needle (16- to 18-gauge) is placed into the marrow cavity parallel to the shaft of the femur (see Bone Marrow Aspiration and Biopsy in Chapter 80). Suction with a 10-ml syringe should yield marrow elements (fat, spicules, and blood), confirming the correct placement of the needle. The blood is administered through a standard blood administration set.

The recommended rate of administration is variable, but should not exceed 22 ml/kg/day. Patients with cardiac failure may not be able to tolerate more than 5 ml/kg/day. A single unit of blood should not be exposed to room temperature during administration for longer than 4 to 6 hours to prevent bacterial contamination. If necessary, two smaller volumes of blood can be administered in succession. Blood should never be administered with lactated Ringer's injection due to the risk of calcium chelation with citrate and consequent clot formation. Normal saline (0.9% sodium chloride) should be used.

A simple rule of thumb for the expected increase in the recipient's packed-cell volume is that 2.2 ml/kg of transfused blood will raise the packed-cell volume by 1% (0.01 L/L) if the donor has approximately a 40% packed-cell volume (PCV; 0.4 L/L). A more precise manner to calculate the volume of blood required is given in the following formula:

$$\text{Volume of blood required} = \text{recipient weight (kg)} \times 90 \text{ (dog) or } 70 \text{ (cat)}$$
$$\times \frac{\text{desired PCV} - \text{recipient PCV}}{\text{PCV of donor}}$$

Complications of Transfusion

Complications arising from transfusion can be divided into those that are immunologically mediated and those that are of nonimmunologic origin. The immune-mediated reactions include urticaria, hemolysis, and fever. Nonimmune-mediated reactions include fever due to improperly stored blood, circulatory overload, citrate intoxication, disease transmission, and the metabolic burden associated with the transfusion of aged blood. Signs of immediate immune-mediated hemolysis occur within minutes and include tremors, emesis, fever, and hemoglobinuria. Delayed hemolytic reactions are more common and are manifested primarily as an unexpected decline in the packed-cell volume following transfusion. Circulatory overload may be seen as vomiting, dyspnea, or coughing. Citrate intoxication occurs when the infusion rate is too fast or the liver is not able to metabolize the citrate. Signs of citrate intoxication are related to hypocalcemia, and include tremors and cardiac arrhythmias (see Chapter 72). If signs of a transfusion reaction are recognized, the transfusion must be slowed or halted.

ADDITIONAL READING

Badylak SF, Van Vleet JF. Alterations of prothrombin time and activated partial thromboplastin time in dogs with hepatic disease. Am J Vet Res 1981; 42:2053.

Davenport DJ, Breitschwerdt EB, Carakostas MC. Platelet disorders in the dog and cat. Part I: Physiology and pathogenesis. Compendium of Continuing Education 1982; 4:762.

Davenport DJ, Breitschwerdt EB, Carakostas MC. Platelet disorders in the dog and cat. Part II: Diagnosis and management. Compendium of Continuing Education 1982; 4:788.

Dodds JW. Inherited bleeding disorders. Canine Practice 1978; 5:49.

Feldman BF. Coagulopathies in small animals. J Am Vet Med Assoc 1981; 179:559.

Jans HE, Armstrong J, Price GS. Therapy of immune-mediated thrombocytopenia. A retrospective study of 15 dogs. Journal of American College of Veterinary Internal Medicine. 1990; 4:4.

Jergens AE, Turrentine MA, Kraus KH, Johnson GS. Buccal mucosa bleeding times of healthy dogs and of dogs in various pathologic states, including thrombocytopenia, uremia, and von Willebrand's disease. Am J Vet Res 1987; 48:1337.

Meric SM. Drugs used for disorders of coagulation. Vet Clin North Am 1988; 18:1217.

Mount ME, Woody BJ, Murphy MJ. The anticoagulant rodenticides. In: Kirk RW, ed. Current veterinary therapy IX. Philadelphia: WB Saunders, 1986: 156.

Otto CM, McCall-Kaufman G, Crowe DT. Intraosseous infusion of fluids and therapeutics. Compendium of Continuing Education 1989; 11:421.

Pichler ME, Turnwald GH. Blood transfusion in the dog and cat. Part I: Physiology, collection, storage, and indications for whole blood therapy. Compendium of Continuing Education 1985; 7:64.

Rebar AH, Boon GD. An approach to the diagnosis of bleeding disorders in the dog. Journal of the American Animal Hospital Association 1981; 17:227.

Turnwald GH, Pichler ME. Blood transfusion in dogs and cats. Part II: Administration, adverse effects, and component therapy. Compendium of Continuing Education 1985; 7:115–126.

Veterinary Clinics of North America 1988; 18:1 (entire issue devoted to hemostasis).

Weiss DJ. Uniform evaluation and semiquantitative reporting of hematologic data in veterinary laboratories. Vet Clin Pathol 1988; 13:27.

Williams DA, Maggio-Price L. Canine idiopathic thrombocytopenia: Clinical observations and long-term follow-up in 54 cases. J Am Vet Med Assoc 1984; 185:660.

THE CARDIOVASCULAR SYSTEM

3

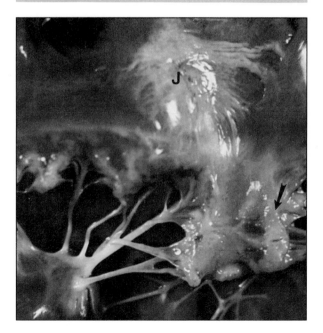

17

ABNORMAL HEART SOUNDS

Clarke E. Atkins
Patti S. Snyder

Heart sounds are produced by valve movements and the resultant vibrations in the heart, vascular walls, and blood columns. In the normal dog and cat, heart sounds that are typically audible include S_1 ("lub") and S_2 ("dub") (Fig. 17-1). S_1, which is associated with closure of the atrioventricular (mitral and tricuspid) valves, is louder, longer, and of lower pitch than S_2, and is best heard over the valve regions indicated in Figure 17-2. S_1 becomes louder with exercise, excitement, or anemia. It becomes less intense with bradycardia or first-degree heart block. The intensity of S_1 is variable in cases with atrial fibrillation, atrial or ventricular premature beats, or marked sinus arrhythmia. S_2 coincides with semilunar (aortic and pulmonic) valve closure and is best heard over the valve locations indicated in Figure 17-2. The intensity of S_2 may increase with pulmonic stenosis, heartworm disease, hyperthyroidism, or pulmonary or systemic hypertension. The intensity is decreased in cardiogenic shock. In normal dogs and cats, S_3 (produced by vibrations associated with rapid ventricular filling) and S_4 (produced by atrial systole) are not audible (see Fig. 17-1). These sounds, termed *cardiac gallops*, are, however, detectable in certain disease states.

Abnormal heart sounds offer the veterinarian an indication of the presence of cardiac disease, as well as specific information as to the underlying diagnosis. In some, but not all, instances, abnormal heart sounds give some indication of the severity of the underlying lesion. Careful auscultation, along with information obtained from the remainder of the physical examination, history, and ancillary diagnostic procedures, provides the means by which a specific diagnosis of cardiac disease is made. It should be kept in mind that, in some instances (*e.g.*, anemia), abnormal cardiac sounds do not represent organic heart disease.

Ideally, auscultation of the heart should be performed in a quiet room, with a standing, cooperative patient. Usually the more dramatic heart sounds are evaluated after listening to the more subtle respiratory sounds. A stethoscope is placed over each heart valve (see Fig. 17-2) in turn, as well as over the carotid arteries and other areas of interest. The stethoscope's diaphragm is pressed

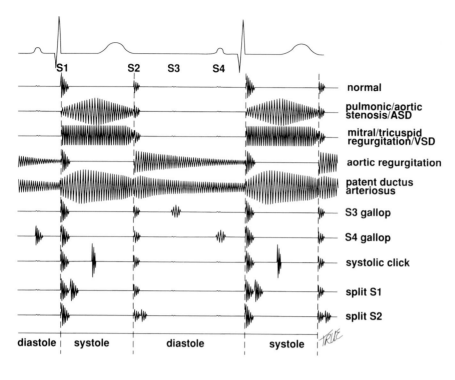

Figure 17–1. Cardiac cycle with electrocardiographic and phonocardiographic events schematized. Both normal and abnormal sounds are included. See text for detailed descriptions. (ASD = atrial septal defect; VSD = ventricular septal defect)

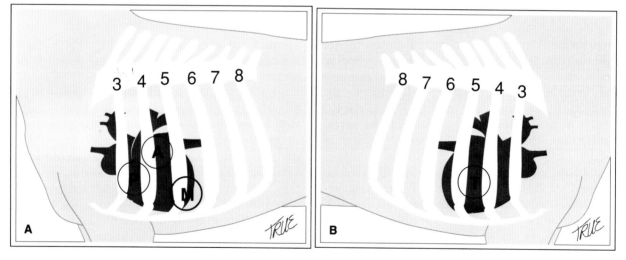

Figure 17–2. Location of sites for stethoscope head placement during auscultation of specific valves of the canine heart from the left (A) and right (B) sides. (P = pulmonic, A = aortic, M = mitral, and T = tricuspid valve areas)

firmly to the thorax to maximize high frequency sounds, while the bell portion is lightly applied, maximizing low frequency sounds such as cardiac gallops.

Auscultation is but one portion of the cardiac examination. Palpation of the femoral pulse provides additional information as to pulse quality and strength and, hence, blood pressure and tissue perfusion. Simultaneous auscultation and pulse palpation aids in the detection of pulse variability and deficits, indicating arrhythmias. Information on tissue perfusion, presence of cyanosis, the state of hydration, and the status of the erythron can be obtained by examination of the mucous membranes. The finding of peripheral venous distension or the presence of ascites is compatible with right heart failure. Auscultation of the respiratory tract may reveal adventitious lung sounds compatible with pulmonary edema of left heart failure or concurrent respiratory disease. Thoracic malformation, cardiac hyperkinesis and enlargement, precordial thrill (palpable murmur), or abnormal cardiac position may be revealed by thoracic palpation, while thoracic percussion is employed to detect pleural effusion.

CAUSES, PATHOPHYSIOLOGY, AND CLINICAL SIGNS

Abnormal heart sounds are divided into several categories: murmurs, abnormal splitting of heart sounds, gallops (audible S_3 or S_4), clicks, friction rubs, audible arrhythmias, and muffled heart sounds. Of these, only cardiac gallops and friction rubs are consistently associated with heart disease.

Murmurs

Heart murmurs (see Fig. 17-1) result when turbulence is produced within the heart or vessels by abnormalities in size of vascular or valve orifices, abnormal communications, and alterations in blood velocity and viscosity. The intensity of a murmur is not a reliable indication of the severity of the causative lesion. Specific causes include valvular incompetence or stenosis, abnormal vascular or cardiac chamber communications, anemia, fever, and anxiety.

Murmurs, which may be innocent (associated with alterations in blood flow, but not with organic cardiac disease) or pathologic (associated with cardiac disease), are classified by their location, duration, timing within the cardiac cycle, intensity, and character. Murmurs may be systolic (occurring during systole—between S_1 and S_2) or diastolic (occurring during diastole—between S_2 and S_1), and are described as continuous or holo- (or pan-), early, mid-, and late systolic or

diastolic (see Fig. 17-1). The intensity of heart murmurs is graded on a scale of I to VI as described by Ettinger (Table 17-1). The pitch of the murmur, described as high, low, or mixed frequency, may help to identify the underlying disorder. An important diagnostic clue, especially in the instance of congenital heart disease, is the further characterization of murmurs according to their quality. Regurgitant murmurs are rectangular or plateau-shaped, and ejection murmurs are diamond-shaped or crescendo–decrescendo in nature (see Fig. 17-1). A cardiologist's description of a murmur might read: "a grade V, holosystolic, mixed frequency, regurgitant murmur, most audible over the fifth left intercostal space (mitral valve region)."

Systolic regurgitant murmurs are associated with mitral and tricuspid insufficiency and ventricular septal defects (Fig. 17-3). Systolic ejection murmurs suggest pulmonic or aortic stenosis or atrial septal defect. Continuous murmurs are produced by arteriovenous connections (patent ductus arteriosus or arteriovenous fistulae) (see Fig. 17-3). Diastolic murmurs, which are uncommonly encountered, are associated with semilunar valvular insufficiency or atrioventricular valvular stenosis (see Fig. 17-1). Noncontinuous, systolic–diastolic murmurs are most often associated with vegetative endocarditis (see Chapter 22).

Innocent murmurs, characterized by low intensity (lower than grade III) and short duration, are relatively common in young dogs (younger than 6–12 months), and must be distinguished from the murmurs of congenital heart disease. These innocent or functional murmurs, due to

Table 17–1 *Grading of Murmurs Using Ettinger's Method*

Grade	Diagnostic Criteria
I	Murmur is barely audible
II	Murmur is very soft, but definitely audible
III	Murmur is easily audible, but of low intensity
IV	Murmur is of moderate intensity with no thrill
V	Murmur is loud and associated with precordial thrill
VI	Murmur is very loud and is audible with the stethoscope removed from the thorax

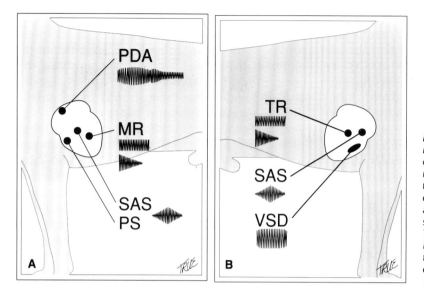

Figure 17–3. *Typical sites of the point of maximal intensity and the phonocardiographic configurations for the most common canine murmurs. (A) Left hemithorax. (B) Right hemithorax. See text Chapters 19 and 20 for more detailed explanation. (PDA = patent ductus arteriosus; MR = mitral regurgitation; SAS = subaortic stenosis; PS = pulmonic stenosis; TR = tricuspid regurgitation; VSD = ventricular septal defect) (Modified with permission from Bonagura JD. In: Quick reference to veterinary medicine. Philadelphia: JB Lippincott, 1982, 19.)*

turbulent flow in the great vessels during ventricular ejection, often change in character or disappear when the patient's position is altered. Such murmurs usually do not persist into adulthood. Likewise, the murmurs of anemia (packed-cell volume less than 20%, or 0.20 L/L), fever, anxiety, or pregnancy are not associated with structural cardiac disease and have been termed *physiologic murmurs.*

Split Heart Sounds

Either the first (S_1) or second (S_2) heart sound may be split, producing two nearly simultaneous sounds, similar in quality to the single sound from which they arose ("lub-lub dub" or "lub dub-dub" for split S_1 or S_2, respectively). Splitting of the first heart sound is produced by asynchronous closure of the atrioventricular valves. While it is considered to be normal in large breed dogs, it may be associated with ventricular conduction disturbances, ventricular pacing, or arrhythmias (see Fig. 17-1). Splitting of the second heart sound occurs when the semilunar valves close asynchronously (see Fig. 17-1). Normally, the aortic valve closes slightly before the pulmonic valve. Splitting of S_2 is most frequently associated with delayed closure of the pulmonic valve, as is seen in pulmonary hypertension (usually due to heartworm disease), pulmonic stenosis, or right bundle branch block, or in normal dogs, during inspiration. It is occasionally observed with early closure of the aortic valve in states of diminished left ventricular output. Paradoxical splitting of S_2 results when significant prolongation of left ventricular conduction and/or ejection time (left bundle branch block, subaortic stenosis, systemic hypertension, or severe left ventricular hypertrophy) delays closure of the aortic valve until after pulmonic valve closure.

Cardiac Gallops

Cardiac gallops or gallop rhythms, consisting of a series of sounds reminiscent of a galloping horse, are composed of S_1, S_2, and S_3 or S_4 ("lub dub thud"); the extra sound is of low frequency and may be difficult to hear. Cardiac gallops occur when S_3 (protodiastolic gallop), S_4 (presystolic gallop), or a combination of S_3 and S_4 (summation gallop) is abnormally accentuated (see Fig. 17-1). S_3 gallops are produced when blood rushes into an incompletely emptied ventricle during rapid ventricular filling (*e.g.,* in mitral insufficiency or dilated cardiomyopathy), while S_4 gallops result when a noncompliant ventricle (*e.g.,* hypertrophic cardiomyopathy) receives blood during atrial systole. Cardiac gallops are considered to be pathologic in dogs and cats, and are often associated with a poor prognosis.

Systolic Clicks

Systolic clicks are abnormal, usually midsystolic, high frequency sounds associated with mitral valve prolapse in humans. They are thought to be a preregurgitant phenomenon in dogs (see Fig. 17-1).

Sounds Associated With Pericardial Disease

Friction rubs, associated with pericarditis and rarely heard in small animals, are "scratchy" biphasic or triphasic sounds audible during portions of both systole and diastole. They occur when inflamed and roughened pericardial and epicardial surfaces contact each other.

A pericardial bump, variable in its number of components and intensity, accompanies early diastolic ventricular filling in the presence of restrictive pericarditis. It occurs when the rapidly filling ventricles are suddenly restricted by the limiting pericardium.

Muffled Heart Sounds

Attenuation or muffling of normal heart sounds may be an important indicator of thoracic disease. Disorders associated with muffled heart sounds include pericardial and pleural effusion, diaphragmatic hernias, thoracic neoplasia, obesity, and hypothyroidism.

Audible Arrhythmias

Certain arrhythmias, such as sinus arrhythmia and atrial fibrillation, are virtually diagnostic upon cardiac auscultation when the femoral pulse is palpated concurrently. Sinus arrhythmia is "regularly irregular" without pulse deficits, and changes in rate are usually associated with respiration. Atrial fibrillation is characterized as being "irregularly irregular," with marked variability in the intensity of S_1, variable pulse strength, and frequent pulse deficits. Unifocal ventricular tachycardia is typically regular, and the pulses, although often weak, are palpable and without deficits. Supraventricular (atrial or junctional) tachycardia tends to be very rapid, but is difficult to distinguish from sinus and ventricular tachycardia without electrocardiographic evaluation (see Chapter 18). Isolated supraventricular and ventricular ectopic beats produce early, abnormal heart sounds (often only S_1 is heard), followed by a pause and a typically weak or nonexistent pulse. With sinus bradycardia or second- and third-degree heart block, the rate is slow and there is no pulse deficit. Audible sounds may emanate from junctional or ventricular escape beats. In the case of first- and second-degree atrioventricular block, S_4 (atrial systole) can occasionally be heard.

DIAGNOSTIC APPROACH AND MANAGEMENT

The diagnostic approach to the finding of cardiac auscultatory abnormalities varies with the abnormality, the accompanying clinical picture, and the client's wishes. The finding of a supposedly innocent murmur in a healthy pup requires no more than a follow-up examination at the next vaccination appointment, whereas the finding of a systolic–diastolic murmur in a dog with fever, joint pain, and dyspnea may require a complete cardiologic and medical workup, blood cultures, and hospitalization (Fig. 17-4).

If the abnormal heart sound(s) cannot be accurately characterized, its exact character can often be determined by obtaining a phonocardiogram (see Fig. 17-1). This procedure, although not routinely available in private practice, may be necessary to determine the exact timing or character of a murmur and the type of gallop, or in distinguishing, for example, whether a subtle sound is a gallop, split sound, or systolic click. Phonocardiography is particularly useful in small animal

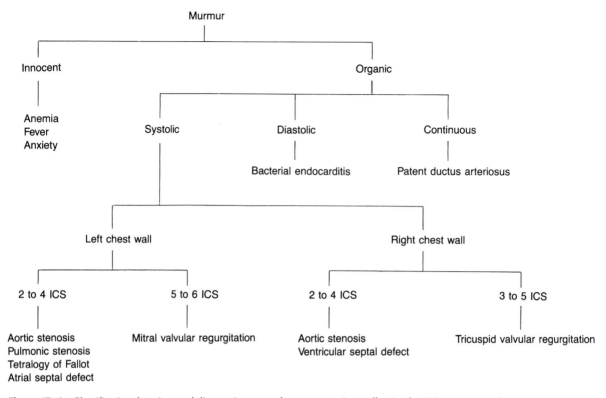

Figure 17–4. *Classification, location, and diagnostic approach to murmurs in small animals. (ICS = intercostal space) (Allen DG. Murmurs and abnormal heart sounds. Allen DG, Kruth SA, eds. Small animal cardiopulmonary medicine. Philadelphia: BC Decker, 1988: 13.)*

practice where such factors as uncooperative patients, rapid heart rates, and panting or purring decrease the sensitivity and accuracy of cardiac auscultation. In our clinic an electronic digital stethoscope (DSP 200 [International Acoustics]), which allows the murmur to be recorded and replayed at one half speed, is also employed in cases in which the character of a murmur or exact nature of an abnormal heart sound is difficult to accurately assess.

Once abnormal sounds have been identified, the goal is to determine the presence, severity, and exact nature of underlying cardiac disease. This is accomplished by performing the following procedures, when indicated: thoracic radiography, electrocardiography, extended electrocardiographic (Holter) monitoring, echocardiography with or without Doppler studies, blood gas analysis, and cardiac catheterization (selective or nonselective) with oximetry, pressure measurement, and angiography. The indications for such procedures and the expected results are explored in greater detail in subsequent chapters.

PATIENT MONITORING

Depending on the diagnosis, the patient's condition, and the prognosis, a follow-up schedule is established. This timing is variable, but may require no more frequent visits than the yearly vaccination appointment. Patients with more severe afflictions (those with impending heart failure, heart failure, or potentially life-threatening arrhythmias) obviously require more frequent reevaluation. It should be emphasized that if the nature of an abnormal heart sound or the resultant diagnosis is unclear, referral to a specialist with the expertise and specialized equipment to effect a more in-depth examination and evaluation is advisable.

ADDITIONAL READING

Allen DG. Heart murmurs and abnormal heart sounds. In: Allen DG, Kruth SA, eds. Small animal cardiopulmonary medicine. Philadelphia: BC Decker, 1988: 13.

Bonagura JD, Berkwitt L. Cardiovascular and pulmonary disorders. In: Fenner WR, ed. Quick reference to veterinary medicine. Philadelphia: JB Lippincott, 1982: 3.

Ettinger SJ, Suter PF. Heart sounds and phonocardiography. In: Canine cardiology. Philadelphia: WB Saunders, 1970: 12.

Ettinger, SJ. Canine heart sounds (audio tape). Evsco Pharmaceuticals, 1987.

Gompf, RE. The clinical approach to heart disease: History and physical examination. In: Fox PR, ed. Canine and feline cardiology. New York: Churchill Livingstone, 1988: 29.

18

CARDIAC ARRHYTHMIAS AND ELECTROCARDIOGRAPHIC ENLARGEMENT PATTERNS

John E. Rush
Clarke E. Atkins

Electrocardiography is an invaluable tool in the investigation of cardiovascular diseases, providing insight into the sequence of electrical activation of the heart and allowing the clinician to make inferences about many clinically important phenomena. Changes in the surface electrocardiogram (ECG) may indicate serum electrolyte abnormalities (see Chapter 72), myocardial hypoxia, or impaired myocardial perfusion. Certain other electrocardiographic findings are indicative of cardiac chamber enlargement. Lastly, the ECG is the definitive diagnostic tool for cardiac arrhythmias. This chapter will review the normal ECG and will describe several frequently encountered electrocardiographic changes in dogs and cats.

The surface ECG is a record of the sum of the electrical potentials generated by the heart during the cardiac cycle. This electrical activity is transmitted through the body to electrodes placed on the skin. The ECG displays and records this electrical activity, allowing the clinician to determine heart rate and cardiac rhythm, and to make inferences about cardiac chamber size. It is important to recognize that abnormalities in the surface ECG result not only from abnormal cardiac activation, but from changes in cardiac position within the thoracic cavity, differences in conduction of the electrical impulse through body tissues, improper connection of the electrodes to the patient, and improper adjustment of the electrocardiographic recording device.

The veterinary practitioner has many options available to aid in obtaining and interpreting ECGs. Good quality electrocardiographs are available at prices that are cost-effective for most busy veterinary practices. Transtelephonic ECG transmission and interpretation are also available at reasonable cost. Computer-assisted ECG recording and interpretation can also be obtained. The person best suited to interpret the ECG and decide how the ECG findings relate to the case is the person who has evaluated the patient.

An ECG is indicated in any animal suspected of having cardiac disease, and should be obtained in any animal with heart failure, cardiac murmur or gallop, radiographic evidence of cardiovascular disease, or indication of cardiac arrhythmias on auscultation. Furthermore, an ECG may be useful in animals with syncope, cyanosis, suspected electrolyte imbalance or acid-base disorders, and as part of the preanesthetic screening procedure in geriatric animals. The ECG can also be used to evaluate cardiac responses to drug therapy and to screen for drug toxicity.

Following a brief synopsis of the normal ECG, this chapter will consider two major categories of electrocardiographic abnormalities: cardiac arrhythmias and morphologic abnormalities of P-QRS-T complexes. The reader who desires further review of basic cardiac physiology or anatomy or of the principles of electrocardiography is referred to the sources listed in the Additional Reading section.

THE NORMAL ELECTROCARDIOGRAM

An appreciation of the normal ECG is a prerequisite for proper interpretation of abnormal ECGs. The activation process of the heart leads to se-quential activation of the atria and ventricles, with the normal pacemaker impulse originating in the sinoatrial (SA) node (Fig. 18-1). The SA node firing rate is altered to meet the demands for increases or decreases in cardiac output. This impulse is simultaneously conducted to the atrioventricular (AV) node through atrial specialized fibers and throughout the atria by cell-to-cell conduction. Depolarization of atrial muscle produces the electrocardiographic P wave and atrial contraction. The impulse is then conducted slowly through the AV node toward the ventricle. This delay (and atrial depolarization), indicated by the P-R interval on the ECG, is important, allowing atrial contraction to precede ventricular activation, thereby coordinating cardiac activity and maximizing stroke volume. The impulse exits the AV node and is conducted quickly through the bundle of His to the left and right bundle branches; the left bundle branch divides into the left anterior fascicle and the left posterior fascicle. The Purkinje fibers, located at the termination of the bundle branches, conduct the impulse to the ventricular myocardium. The myocardium is activated in an endocardial-to-epicardial and an apical-to-basilar direction. Ventricular depolarization produces the QRS complex on the surface ECG and is followed by ventricular contraction. Ventricular repolarization is the final event,

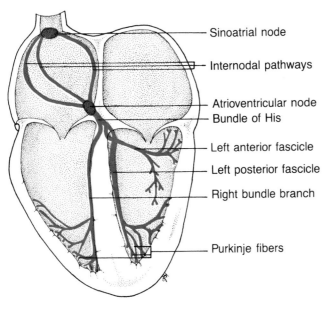

Sinoatrial node

Internodal pathways

Atrioventricular node
Bundle of His

Left anterior fascicle

Left posterior fascicle

Right bundle branch

Purkinje fibers

Figure 18–1. Schematic diagram of the heart and conduction system. The impulse, which normally originates in the sinoatrial node, travels through the internodal pathways to the atrioventricular node. After a delay in conduction through the atrioventricular node, the impulse rapidly travels through the bundle of His and bundle branches to Purkinje fibers, leading to ventricular depolarization.

and is recognized as the electrocardiographic T wave.

There is a great deal of variability in the normal canine and feline ECG. When reading an ECG, one should refrain from overinterpretation of findings at the upper or lower limits of the normal range. Similarly, an ECG that is within the limits of normal (Table 18-1) does not preclude the possibility of cardiac disease. Many cardiac changes, such as right ventricular enlargement, may not be reflected on the ECG until they are advanced.

CARDIAC ARRHYTHMIAS

An arrhythmia can be defined as an abnormality in the rate, regularity, site of origin, or conduction of the cardiac impulse such that the normal sequence of atrial and ventricular activation is altered. Cardiac arrhythmias are frequently encountered, and the veterinarian must be prepared to determine their nature and severity. Although arrhythmias may be initiated by a variety of mechanisms, successful management is not usually dependent on identification of the cellular basis. Some arrhythmias do not require therapy, and many arrhythmias can be effectively managed without the use of antiarrhythmic drugs. An appreciation of the potential causes of arrhythmias, the clinical signs that may result, and the potential sequelae is important for successful management.

Etiologies for arrhythmias can be divided into primary cardiac and extracardiac causes. Primary cardiac causes include cardiomyopathy, endocardiosis, cardiac neoplasia, myocarditis, en-

Table 18–1 *Normal Electrocardiographic Parameters in the Dog and Cat*

Lead II, 50 mm/sec, 1 cm = 1 mV		
Parameter	**Dog**	**Cat**
Heart rate	70 to 160 beats/min for adult Up to 180 beats/min for toy breeds Up to 220 beats/min for puppies	160 to 240 beats/min Mean: 197 beats/min
Rhythm	Normal sinus rhythm Sinus arrhythmia Wandering SA pacemaker	Normal sinus rhythm Sinus tachycardia (physiologic reaction to excitement)
Measurements		
P wave	Width: max 0.04 sec (2 boxes) Height: max 0.4 mV (4 boxes)	Width: max 0.04 sec (2 boxes) Height: max 0.2 mV (2 boxes)
PR interval	Width: 0.06 to 0.13 sec (3 to 6½ boxes)	Width: 0.05 to 0.09 sec (2½ to 4½ boxes)
QRS complex	Width: max 0.05 sec (2½ boxes) in small breeds; max 0.06 sec (3 boxes) in large breeds	Width: max 0.04 sec (2 boxes)
	Height of R wave:* max 3 mV (30 boxes) in large breeds; max 2.5 mV (25 boxes) in small breeds	Height of R wave: max 0.9 mV (9 boxes)
	Depth of S wave: max 0.35 mV	
ST segment	Depression: max 0.2 mV (2 boxes) Elevation: max 0.15 mV (1½ boxes)	No depression or elevation greater than 0.1 mV
T wave	Can be positive, negative, or biphasic Amplitude: max one fourth the amplitude of the R wave	Can be positive, negative, or biphasic; is most often positive Amplitude: max 0.3 mV (3 boxes)
QT interval	Width: 0.15 to 0.25 sec (7½ to 12½ boxes) at normal heart rate; varies with heart rate (faster rates have shorter QT intervals)	Width: 0.12 to 0.18 sec (6 to 9 boxes) at normal heart rate (range is 0.07 to 0.2 sec, 3½ to 10 boxes); varies with heart rate (faster rates have shorter QT intervals)
Electrical axis (frontal plane)	+40 to +100	0 to +160

* *Not valid for thin, deep-chested dogs under 2 years of age.*

docarditis, myocardial trauma, ischemic heart disease, congenital cardiac malformations—including ventricular preexcitation, and other conduction disorders. Extracardiac causes include hypoxia, electrolyte imbalances (see Chapter 72), acid-base disturbances (see Chapter 71), and a variety of neurologic disorders. Many endocrine and metabolic diseases, such as hyperthyroidism (see Chapter 61), gastric torsion (see Chapter 36), renal failure (see Chapters 43 and 44), and pancreatitis (see Chapter 39) are also known to lead to arrhythmia formation. Cardiac arrhythmias are also commonly observed as a result of drugs such as digitalis, anesthetic agents, sympathomimetics, and diuretics (see Tables 18-3, 18-4, 18-6, 18-7, and 18-8). Identification of potential causes for an arrhythmia is an important step in determining the appropriate therapy. Many arrhythmias resulting from secondary causes may not require therapy if the underlying cause can be removed or treated.

Clinical Signs

The clinical manifestations of arrhythmias may include syncope (see Chapter 5), muscular weakness, posterior paresis (see Chapter 54), heart failure (see Chapter 20), or death. A syncopal event typically results in collapse and loss of consciousness, and possibly in involuntary urination. Animals may appear to struggle or paddle when they try to stand up after the event, but tonic–clonic limb activity and facial chewing actions are usually absent. Syncopal episodes are of short duration, and the animal is usually reported to have normal mentation before and shortly after the episode. Syncope is often associated with exercise or excitement. Muscular weakness or posterior paresis resulting from arrhythmias may be intermittent with paroxysmal arrhythmias or sustained with persistent or frequent arrhythmias, especially if myocardial failure accompanies the rhythm disturbance. Finally, cardiac arrhythmias may result in heart failure. Sustained tachyarrhythmias frequently exacerbate congestive heart failure, leading to acute decompensation. A common example is the development or worsening of heart failure associated with the onset of atrial fibrillation. Animals known to have certain

arrhythmias, such as sustained ventricular tachycardia, are thought to be at increased risk for sudden death; it is generally believed that ventricular tachycardia leads to ventricular fibrillation, the ultimately lethal dysrhythmia.

Diagnostic Approach

It is important for each individual to develop a standardized approach to the evaluation of ECGs. The following method is used in our clinical practice and has also proved useful in training students (Table 18-2). Initially, a general inspection of the ECG is performed to look for trends or gross abnormalities. The second task is to determine the heart rate and whether the rate is normal, bradycardic, or tachycardic. If the atrial rate and ventricular rate are different, both rates are calculated. Following calculation of heart rate, one should determine if there are P waves for each QRS complex, whether each QRS complex has a P wave, and if they are related (consistent temporal relationship between P and QRS complexes). Next it is important to look for the presence of premature depolarizations. If premature complexes are present, one must decide whether they are supraventricular or ventricular in origin. The sixth step is to determine if there are any pauses in the rhythm. If pauses are present, one first determines the reason and then identifies the site of origin of the impulse that ends the pause. Finally, the electrocardiographic findings are summarized as the ECG diagnosis.

Table 18–2 *Electrocardiographic Evaluation of Arrhythmias in Small Animals*

1. General inspection of the electrocardiogram
2. Determine the heart rate. Is it normal or is there bradycardia or tachycardia?
3. Note whether there are P waves for every QRS complex. Are they temporally related?
4. Note whether there is a QRS complex for every P wave. Are they temporally related?
5. Identify premature complexes. Are they supraventricular or ventricular?
6. Identify pauses in the rhythm. What caused the pause? What ends the pause?
7. Summarize the electrocardiographic diagosis.

MORPHOLOGIC ABNORMALITIES OF THE P-QRS-T COMPLEXES

Sinus Rhythms

Rhythms originating from the sinus node are termed *sinus rhythms*. The term *normal sinus rhythm* includes rhythms whose rates fall within the normal range for the species (Fig. 18-2; see Table 18-1). The firing rate of the sinus node is controlled by the balance of prevailing sympathetic and parasympathetic tone. Increased sympathetic tone increases the heart rate and enhanced parasympathetic tone decreases it. Sinus rhythms exceeding the upper limit of normal are termed *sinus tachycardia;* those that are slower than the established normal lower limit are referred to as *sinus bradycardia* (Table 18-3, see Fig. 18-2).

Sinus Tachycardia

Sinus tachycardia (see Table 18-3 and Fig. 18-2) is associated with a variety of physiologic and pathologic situations. Physiologic responses that cause sinus tachycardia, such as fear, pain, excitement, and exercise, are normal and rarely need to be treated. Sedation or tranquilization (*e.g.,* diazepam or acetylpromazine for anxiety, butorphanol or morphine sulfate for pain) may be appropriate in some instances. Antiarrhythmic drug therapy is inappropriate for most of the pathologic conditions that lead to sinus tachycardia, including fever, shock, and anemia. Specific therapy with digitalis or beta-blockade is, however, sometimes indicated for sinus tachcardia that persists in spite of specific therapy for hyperthyroidism or heart failure. A large number of drugs can cause sinus tachycardia (see Table 18-3), either as a desirable response or as a side-effect. A vagal maneuver, performed either by carotid sinus massage or by ocular pressure, will usually result in a transient slowing of the heart rate.

Sinus Bradycardia

Sinus bradycardia (see Table 18-3 and Fig. 18-2) may also result from both physiologic and pathologic conditions. Sinus bradycardia is observed in normal large-breed and well-conditioned dogs at rest. It can also result from increases in vagal tone associated with ocular or carotid sinus pressure (vagally mediated), increases in cerebrospinal fluid pressure, gastrointestinal and respiratory disorders, and hypothermia. Some drugs and toxins cause sinus bradycardia, and in the critically ill or anesthetized patient may be a sign of impending cardiac arrest. Treatment is indicated if the decrease in heart rate is associated with

Table 18–3 *Sinus Rhythms*

Rhythm	Associated Conditions	Therapy
Sinus tachycardia	Physiologic: exercise, fear, pain Pathologic: fever, shock, hypotension, anemia, congestive heart failure, hyperthyroidism, infection Drugs: sympathomimetics, parasympatholytics, vasodilators, theophylline	None, tranquilizer or analgesic(s) Treat underlying cause: propranolol, metoprolol, atenolol, or digitalis
Sinus bradycardia	Physiologic: normal young dogs, athletic dogs Pathologic: severe systemic diseases, anesthesia, forerunner of cardiac arrest, central nervous system lesion, intoxicants, hypothermia, hypothyroidism, increased ocular or cerebrospinal fluid pressure Drugs: tranquilizers, anesthetics, digitalis, beta-blockade, calcium channel blockade	None Treat underlying cause: atropine, glycopyrrolate, epinephrine, isoproterenol, dopamine, or right atrial pacing
Sinus arrhythmia	Physiologic: normal, athletic dogs Pathologic: gastrointestinal or respiratory disease Drugs: digitalis	None, treat underlying cause

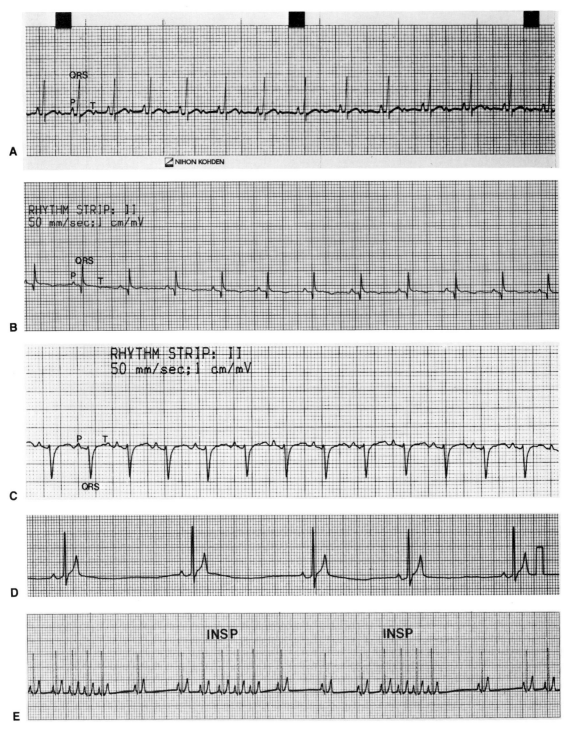

Figure 18–2. Examples of sinus rhythms. (A) Normal sinus rhythm in a dog. The heart rate is 120 beats/min. Recorded at 25 mm/sec, 1 cm/mV. (B) Normal sinus rhythm in a cat. The heart rate is 190 beats/min. Recorded at 50 mm/sec, 1 cm/mV. (C) Sinus tachycardia in a cat with hyperthyroidism. The heart rate is 260 beats/min. Recorded at 25 mm/sec, 1 cm/mV. The QRS complex has a deep S wave due to a left anterior fascicular block (see Fig. 18-7) (D) Sinus bradycardia in a sleeping dog, obtained from a Holter monitor recording. The heart rate is 35 beats/min. Recorded at 25 mm/sec, 1 cm/mV. (E) Pronounced sinus arrhythmia with periods of sinus pause in a dog. Note the increase in heart rate during inspiration. Recorded at 12.5 mm/sec, 1 cm/mV.

clinical evidence of inadequate cardiac output, such as syncope, weakness, impending arrest, anesthesia, or heart failure. Potential therapies include parasympatholytic drugs, sympathomimetic drugs, and right atrial pacing. Anticholinergics, such as atropine or glycopyrrolate, are indicated when high vagal tone is suspected, while sympathomimetic drugs, including isoproterenol, epinephrine, or dopamine, may be more useful in the critically ill patient or when atropine is ineffective. Right atrial pacing is usually reserved for patients with sinus bradycardia that is refractory to drugs.

Sinus Arrhythmia

Sinus arrhythmia (see Table 18-3 and Fig. 18-2) is defined as a rhythmic speeding and slowing of the sinus rhythm such that the variability of the R-R interval is greater than 10%. It is often associated with a wandering pacemaker (see Abnormalities in P Wave Morphology in Table 18-9). When sinus arrhythmia is linked to the respiratory cycle (when the rate increases with inspiration and slows on expiration) it is termed *respiratory sinus arrhythmia*. This phasic speeding and slowing, which results from the effects of waxing and waning vagal tone on the sinus node, is normal in dogs and is most frequently noted in young, athletic individuals. It is also frequently observed in patients with upper airway obstruction or chronic respiratory disease. Sinus arrhythmia is infrequent in patients with congestive heart failure. Sinus arrhythmia is an abnormal and infrequent finding in cats, and when observed is often associated with respiratory disease or digitalis use.

Premature Depolarizations and Tachyarrhythmias

Premature depolarizations are defined as impulses having a shorter R-R or P-P interval than the underlying rhythm. Premature depolarizations can also be described as extrasystoles, premature complexes, premature contractions or beats (the term *premature beats* is correct only if accompanied by mechanical activity), and premature impulses. The use of ECG calipers can be helpful in identification of premature beats. Premature complexes may be described as isolated or as occurring in couplets (two), triplets or salvos (three), or paroxysms (more than three), or as nonsustained tachycardias (more than three beats but less than 30 seconds in duration) or sustained tachycardias (more than 30 seconds in duration).

It is important not only to identify premature depolarizations, but to determine their site of origin so that appropriate therapy can be administered. Supraventricular premature complexes (originating in the atria or AV junctional region) are usually normal or very similar in configuration to the QRS-T complexes that make up the underlying supraventricular rhythm. A premature P wave (termed P′) may be identified in association with the premature complex. It often has a different configuration than the normal P waves. Ventricular premature complexes are usually wider and taller and have a markedly different configuration (bizarre appearance) when compared to the normal complexes. The T wave is often large and in the opposite direction from the abnormal complex. The normal shelf in the ST segment, typically present in complexes of supraventricular origin, is frequently absent.

Supraventricular Premature Depolarizations

Supraventricular premature depolarizations (Table 18-4, Fig. 18-3) can be divided into those that originate from ectopic foci within the atrium (atrial premature depolarizations) and those that originate from the AV junctional tissue (junctional premature depolarizations). Specific criteria exist to discriminate between atrial and junctional premature complexes, such as the presence and direction of the P′ wave (typically negative in junctional complexes) and the P′-R duration, but clinical management is similar for both types of premature beats. For this discussion, atrial and junctional premature complexes will be considered together as *supraventricular premature depolarizations* and treated identically. See the Additional Reading section for sources that address further differentiation of atrial and AV junctional premature complexes.

Premature depolarizations are identified as su-

Table 18–4 *Premature Depolarizations and Tachyarrhythmias*

Rhythm	Associated Conditions	Therapy*
Supraventricular premature beats and supraventricular tachycardia	Atrial enlargement, atrial tumor, electrolyte abnormality, digitalis intoxication, anesthesia	None, vagal maneuver, digitalis, atenolol, propranolol, metoprolol, diltiazem, verapamil
Atrial fibrillation	Same as above, especially atrial enlargement with dilated cardiomyopathy, chronic valvular disease, congenital disease, trauma, heartworm in dogs, hypertrophic cardiomyopathy in cats	Digitalis followed by propranolol, atenolol, metoprolol, or diltiazem. Quinidine if minimal or no atrial enlargement
Ventricular premature beats or ventricular tachycardia	Myocardial disease, pericardial disease, valvular disease, congenital disease, myocardial trauma, electrolyte abnormality, hypoxia, anemia, uremia, gastric dilatation–volvulus, pyometra, acidosis, pancreatitis	None, lidocaine, procainamide, quinidine, propranolol, metoprolol, mexiletine, tocainide

* In each instance, the underlying cause should be treated.

praventricular in origin when they have the following characteristics. The underlying rhythm, which is usually sinus in origin, is interrupted by one or more premature complexes that have a QRS-T morphology that is identical or very similar to the normal (sinus) complexes. A premature P' wave, often with a different configuration than the normal P wave and in or near the preceding T wave, may be identified. The P'-R duration is highly variable, depending on the site of origin of the ectopic impulse; it may be longer or shorter than the normal P-R interval, and the P' wave may be superimposed on or even follow the QRS complex. For isolated supraventricular premature complexes, the sinus node is usually depolarized by the premature impulse, causing the sinus node to be reset. This resetting results in a pause in the rhythm that is less than would be expected if the sinus node had continued to fire at the normal rate. Therefore the pause, termed a *noncompensatory pause*, is less than two normal R-R intervals.

Supraventricular premature depolarizations are associated with atrial enlargement, atrial neoplasms, digitalis intoxication, anesthetics, and electrolyte or acid-base abnormalities. Isolated supraventricular complexes rarely require specific therapy unless they are very frequent or result in clinical symptoms (*e.g.*, syncope). Therapy is usually directed at the underlying cause. If specific therapy is required, digitalis, β-blockers (*e.g.*, propranolol, atenolol, or metoprolol), or calcium channel blockers (*e.g.*, verapamil or diltiazem) are employed. Digitalis derivatives should be used when supraventricular premature complexes are accompanied by congestive heart failure. While β-blockers or calcium channel blockers are also effective, they have negative inotropic effects and should be used with caution in animals with congestive heart failure. Calcium channel blockers, in particular verapamil, are ideally used in patients known to have good myocardial function determined by clinical or echocardiographic examination.

Supraventricular Tachycardias

Supraventricular tachycardias (see Table 18-4 and Fig. 18-3) are runs or paroxysms of ectopic beats, three or more in number, that originate from the atrial or AV junctional tissue. Supraventricular tachycardias are usually regular and can occur at extremely high rates, sometimes in excess of 350 beats per minute (see Fig. 18-3). Variable degrees of AV block can accompany rapid supraventricular tachycardias. Sustained supraventricular tachycardia must be differentiated from sinus tachycardia because, unlike sinus tachycardia, supraventricular tachycardias usually require specific therapy. The P' wave morphology is often abnormal. In contrast to sinus tachycardia, a vagal maneuver may abruptly terminate supraventricular tachycardias. In addition, atrial tachycardia is associated with cardiac disease and usually occurs at faster rates.

Asymptomatic paroxysmal supraventricular tachycardias are usually treated with oral formulations of the same antiarrhythmic drugs described for isolated supraventricular complexes. Rapid or sustained supraventricular tachycardia can be a life-threatening condition requiring immediate therapeutic intervention. A logical progression for treatment begins with a vagal maneuver. A vagal maneuver is performed by firm ocular or carotid sinus massage. Carotid sinus massage is performed with the patient's neck extended and turned slightly away from the side to be massaged. The bifurcation of the artery, found at the edge of the trachea just caudal to the angle of the jaw, is then compressed against the transverse processes of the vertebral bodies and massaged in a cranial-to-caudal direction. If this procedure proves ineffective, intravenous digitalization is employed when the arrhythmia is accompanied by heart failure. If myocardial function is preserved, then intravenous propranolol or verapamil may be used. Sequential administration of β-blockers and calcium channel blockers is generally avoided, as the negative inotropic effects of these drugs may be additive. If sustained supraventricular arrhythmia is severe or refractory to drug therapy, electrical cardioversion may be the next step if an ECG-synchronized defibrillator is available. Lidocaine and procainamide are occasionally effective. If other drugs or equipment are unavailable, a brisk thump to the chest may terminate supraventricular tachycardia.

Atrial Flutter

Atrial flutter (see Fig. 18-3) is an uncommon rhythm disturbance in veterinary patients. When it does occur it is often the forerunner of atrial fibrillation. In some cases, atrial flutter cannot be distinguished from fibrillation and the rhythm is described as atrial flutter–fibrillation. The typical characteristics of atrial flutter are extremely rapid (more than 300 beats per minute) P or flut-

ter waves, which give the baseline a sawtooth appearance (see Fig. 18-3). Physiologic block of some of the flutter waves in the AV node is common and results in a ventricular rate that is slower than the atrial rate. Conduction through the AV node to the ventricle may follow a pattern expressed as *2 : 1 or 3 : 1 AV conduction.* The QRS configuration is usually normal.

Atrial flutter is associated with the same conditions that cause other atrial arrhythmias, except that atrial enlargement is usually present. A vagal maneuver followed by digitalis administration is the therapy of choice. Other therapies include cardioversion, calcium channel blockers, propranolol, and quinidine. If atrial flutter is converted, then oral therapy with quinidine or propranolol may prevent recurrence. If atrial flutter degenerates to atrial fibrillation, the animal should be treated as described below.

Atrial Fibrillation

Atrial fibrillation (see Table 18-4 and Fig. 18-3), a common arrhythmia in dogs, is less frequently observed in cats. In atrial fibrillation, the atria are activated in a totally chaotic manner, and are unable to effectively pump blood to the ventricles. The rapid, chaotic electrical activity in the atria results in irregular conduction through the AV node, with rapid and irregular ventricular activation.

The following ECG findings are observed in animals with atrial fibrillation (see Fig. 18-3). The baseline of the ECG lacks discrete P waves and has either fine or coarse oscillations termed *f* or *fibrillation waves.* The QRS complexes are usually normal in configuration, and may vary slightly in amplitude, especially at rapid heart rates. The QRS complexes occur in an "irregularly irregular" manner; in other words, there is no pattern to the irregularity. The ventricular rate is usually quite rapid (200–280 beats per minute in dogs, faster in cats) in untreated cases. The irregularity of the ventricular response is less apparent at very rapid heart rates.

The same conditions that are associated with supraventricular premature depolarizations can lead to atrial fibrillation. Severe atrial dilation

(text continues on page 216)

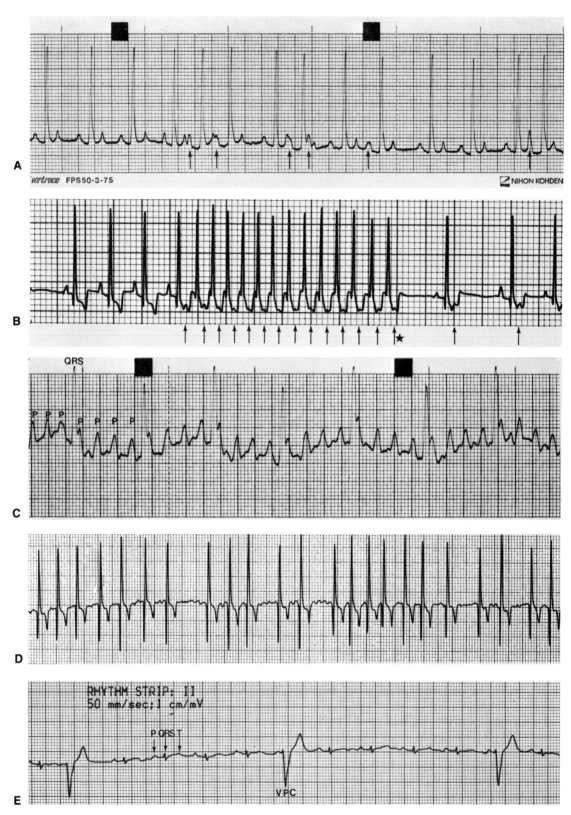

A

vertrace FPS50-3-75   NIHON KOHDEN

B

QRS

P P P   P P P P

C

D

RHYTHM STRIP: II
50 mm/sec; 1 cm/mV

P QRS T

VPC

E

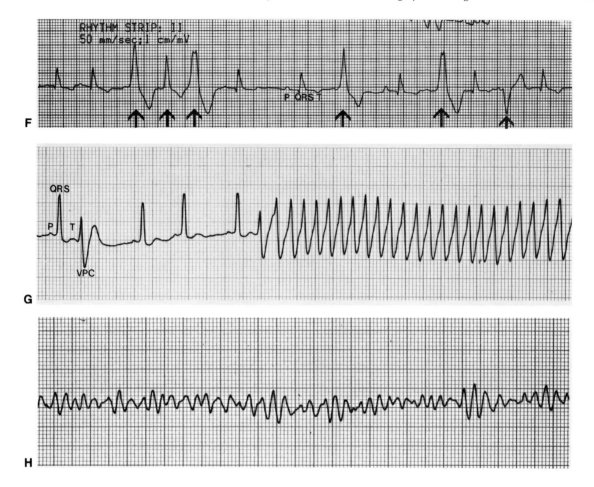

Figure 18–3. Examples of premature depolarizations and tachyarrhythmias. (A) Frequent supraventricular premature depolarizations recorded from a dog with aortic insufficiency and marked left atrial and ventricular enlargement. This supraventricular arrhythmia was atrial in origin (atrial premature depolarizations), evidenced by the upright P' (arrows) and normal P–R interval. The premature complexes have the same configuration as the normal sinus beats. In this example, many of the premature P' waves are buried within the T wave of the previous complex. The fourth arrow indicates a nonconducted P'. The R wave in lead II is greater than 2.5 mV, which is compatible with left ventricular enlargement. Recorded at 25 mm/sec, 1 cm/mV. (B) Paroxysmal supraventricular tachycardia in a dog. A P' is buried in the T wave of the fourth QRS complex (first arrow), initiating a paroxysm of reentrant atrial tachycardia at a rate of 300 beats/min. The tachycardia ends when conduction of the P' in the T wave of the 17th QRS complex (star) is blocked, probably at the AV node. A P' is noted throughout the tachycardia and a nonconducted P' is also present in the T waves of the QRS complexes following the tachycardia (arrows) recorded at 12.5 mm/sec and 0.5 cm/mV. (C) Atrial flutter with 4 : 1 conduction in a dog with severe mitral insufficiency. The atrial rate is in excess of 500 beats/min and the ventricular rate is 140 beats/min. Recorded at 50 mm/sec, 1 cm/mV. (D) Atrial fibrillation in a dog with cardiomyopathy.The heart rate is approximately 200 beats/min. The rhythm is irregular, there are no P waves, and fibrillation waves are present in the baseline. A slight beat-to-beat variation in QRS amplitude is present. Recorded at 25 mm/sec, 1 cm/mV. (E) Ventricular premature depolarizations (VPC) in a cat with hypertrophic cardiomyopathy. Sinus rhythm is interrupted by isolated, unifocal VPCs. Recorded at 50 mm/sec, 1 cm/mV. (F) Ventricular arrhythmias in a boxer with cardiomyopathy. Sinus rhythm is interrupted by a short run of ventricular tachycardia and frequent, multiform VPCs (arrows). Recorded at 50 mm/sec, 1 cm/mV. (G) Ventricular tachycardia and the R on T phenomenon in a dog. The second VPC, occurring during the T wave of the previous QRS complex, results in ventricular tachycardia. Recorded at 25 mm/sec, 1 cm/mV. (H) Ventricular fibrillation in a dog during cardiopulmonary arrest. Note the rapid, irregular, chaotic oscillations of the tracing. Recorded at 25 mm/sec, 1 cm/mV. (Rush JE, Keene BK. ECG of the month. J Am Vet Med Assoc 1989; 194:52.)

from dilated cardiomyopathy, chronic valvular disease, and severe congenital heart disease are the most common causes in the dog. Atrial dilation due to hypertrophic cardiomyopathy is the most common cause in the cat. Atrial fibrillation is less commonly observed in association with trauma, anesthesia, digitalis intoxication, and hypothyroidism.

Treatment of atrial fibrillation is complicated by the occurrence of severe atrial dilation in most animals. Even when atrial fibrillation can be converted to normal sinus rhythm, recurrence within a few days is frequent. Therefore, while quinidine and calcium channel blockers may result in conversion to normal sinus rhythm, these therapies are usually reserved for animals without coexisting atrial dilation. Animals without concurrent atrial dilation are initially treated with quinidine for 48 to 72 hours. If atrial fibrillation persists, then the animal can be treated conventionally (with digitalis, β-blockers, or calcium channel blockers) or cardioversion can be attempted using an ECG-synchronized defibrillator. If quinidine or cardioversion are successful in converting the patient to normal sinus rhythm, then quinidine is usually continued for several months to help prevent reversion to atrial fibrillation. In animals with atrial dilation, the aim of therapy is to slow the ventricular response to atrial fibrillation to less than 160 beats per minute. Digitalis is initiated and the heart rate is reevaluated in 2 to 7 days. If serum digitalis levels are adequate and the rate is not reduced to 160 beats per minute or less in the dog or 200 beats per minute or less in the cat, a β-blocker or calcium channel blocker can be added to the drug regimen. Caution is advised when these agents are employed in animals with myocardial failure or severe congestive heart failure because negative inotropic effects of these drugs have the potential to exacerbate or worsen heart failure. The prognosis for dogs with atrial fibrillation is guarded; although some giant breed dogs may live longer than 2 years with atrial fibrillation, many die within the first year of diagnosis.

Ventricular Premature Complexes

Ventricular premature complexes (see Table 18-4 and Fig. 18-3), the most common arrhythmia en-countered in the dog, result from spontaneous depolarization of the ventricular Purkinje system or myocardium. The impulses are conducted cell to cell rather than through the normal conduction pathways, accounting for the unusual morphologic appearance of ventricular extrasystoles (see Fig. 18-3). Ventricular premature depolarizations are identified by their prematurity, excessive width and height, and abnormal or bizarre configuration in comparison to the normal complexes. The normal ST segment shelf is frequently absent, and the T wave is usually large and opposite in polarity to the premature QRS complex.

There is no cause-and-effect relationship between ventricular premature depolarizations and P waves that may be observed near them. The impulse generated by a ventricular premature depolarization rarely penetrates the AV node in the retrograde direction. Therefore, the SA node is usually not depolarized and continues to fire at a regular rate. The interruption in rhythm caused by the ventricular extrasystole (compensatory pause) is equal to or longer than two normal R-R intervals. On occasion, especially at slow heart rates, a ventricular premature depolarization can be interpolated between two sinus complexes so that no pause is observed.

A ventricular extrasystole may occur approximately simultaneously with a sinus-conducted beat, resulting in fusion of the two impulses. These fusion beats have a variable appearance that is intermediate between the sinus-conducted impulse and the ventricular premature complex.

Ventricular Tachycardia

Ventricular premature depolarizations may be isolated, in pairs, or in paroxysms or runs of ventricular tachycardia (see Table 18-4 and Fig. 18-3). When ventricular premature complexes alternate with normal sinus complexes in a 1 : 1 ratio the rhythm is termed *ventricular bigeminy*. Frequent or sustained ventricular arrhythmias are more likely to result in clinical signs of weakness, syncope, or sudden death (see Chapter 5). Therapy for severe arrhythmias should be more aggressive than therapy for infrequent, isolated ventricular depolarizations.

Etiologies for ventricular arrhythmias may be divided into primary cardiac and noncardiac causes. Primary cardiac causes include congenital heart disease, cardiomyopathy, valvular diseases, myocarditis, pericardial diseases, and cardiac neoplasia. Noncardiac causes of ventricular arrhythmias include electrolyte or acid-base imbalance, hypoxia or ischemia, gastric dilation and volvulus, pancreatitis, toxins, drugs, or anesthetics, and central nervous system disease. Isolated, infrequent ventricular premature depolarizations may be noted in normal individuals.

Therapy should be directed toward the underlying cause and then, if necessary, toward the arrhythmia itself. Ventricular arrhythmias producing clinical signs of episodic weakness, collapse, or syncope should be aggressively treated. When ventricular extrasystoles have more than one morphologic appearance they are termed *multiform.* Multiform ventricular extrasystoles are thought to originate from differing foci within the ventricle, suggesting a multifocal disease process. Ventricular extrasystoles may also be treated based on the knowledge that these arrhythmias may progress to a lethal ventricular rhythm. Although not always based on scientific data, specific indications for the treatment of ventricular arrhythmias have been established (Table 18-5).

The drug of choice for symptomatic ventricular tachycardia in the dog is intravenous lidocaine at a dose of 1 to 2 mg/kg. This bolus dose may be repeated until a total dose of 4 mg/kg has been given. If the arrhythmia is unaffected by the initial use of lidocaine then another antiarrhythmic drug should be selected. If lidocaine proves effective, then a continuous-rate infusion of lidocaine is initiated at 40 to 80 ug/kg/min. Procainamide can also be administered intravenously as a bolus followed by continuous infusion for immediate treatment of ventricular tachycardia. If the animal is not symptomatic for the arrhythmia and if life-threatening ventricular arrhythmias do not appear to be imminent, oral antiarrhythmic therapy is usually preferred. Procainamide or quinidine are commonly used as initial therapies. If these drugs are ineffective or only partially effective, a β-blocker such as propranolol may be added to the regimen. The combination of a class I antiarrhythmic (lidocaine, procainamide, or quinidine) with a β-blocker or an analgesic (butorphanol or morphine) has proved to be useful in the management of ventricular arrhythmias resulting from traumatic myocarditis. Alternatively, therapy may be changed to include one of the newer antiarrhythmic drugs, such as mexiletine or tocainide (see Appendix II). Phenytoin may be useful for ventricular arrhythmias resulting from digitalis intoxication.

The therapeutic options for treatment of ventricular arrhythmias in the cat are more limited, and specific criteria indicating when ventricular antiarrhythmics should be administered are lacking. Lidocaine has a pronounced neurotoxicity in the cat, so must be used with caution and at a greatly reduced dose. β-Blockers, such as propranolol, may be useful for ventricular arrhythmias in the cat, but caution is advised, given the drug's negative inotropic effects, if congestive heart failure accompanies the arrhythmia. Procainamide has been administered to some cats with ventricular arrhythmias (one fourth of a 250-mg capsule orally three times daily), although reports of efficacy or toxicity are not available. Cats appear to tolerate ventricular arrhythmias better than dogs, and the occurrence of ventricular flutter or fibrillation is less frequent. Therefore, with the exception of sustained ventricular tachycardia, any underlying predisposing factors (*e.g.*, heart failure, digitalis intoxication, electrolyte abnormalities, treatable myocardial diseases) are treated first, followed by reevaluation of the arrhythmia. For sustained or severe ventricular tachycardia requiring immediate treatment, either lidocaine (0.25–0.5 mg/kg IV)

Table 18–5 *Ventricular Arrhythmias Requiring Treatment in Dogs*

Isolated ventricular premature depolarizations at a rate greater than 20/minute

Ventricular bigeminy, frequent couplets or triplets, or sustained ventricular tachycardia

Multiform ventricular premature complexes, suggesting multiple foci of origin

Clinical signs of weakness or syncope resulting from ventricular ectopic activity

Close coupling of the ventricular premature complex to the T wave of the preceding QRS complex, termed "R on T" phenomenon. Premature depolarizations during this vulnerable period of the cardiac cycle may cause ventricular tachycardia or ventricular fibrillation.

Ventricular arrhythmias in breeds susceptible to sudden death (*e.g.*, Doberman pinschers)

or procainamide (3–6 mg/kg IV or 6–10 mg/kg intramuscularly) can be administered.

After drug therapy has been initiated, the clinician must decide whether it has been effective. A desirable end-point would be total elimination of ventricular ectopic activity. While this may be achieved in some patients, many will continue to have some ventricular extrasystoles. A more realistic goal may be elimination of clinical signs and elimination of the more severe ventricular arrhythmias that are associated with sudden death.

Finally, one must decide on the duration of antiarrhythmic therapy in each patient. Animals with primary underlying heart disease that cannot be cured may remain on antiarrhythmic therapy for life. Animals with arrhythmias resulting from trauma, metabolic diseases, or acid-base imbalance may require therapy for several days or several weeks. When the decision is made to discontinue therapy, these animals should be closely monitored for recurrence of the arrhythmia.

Ventricular Flutter and Ventricular Fibrillation

Ventricular flutter and ventricular fibrillation (see Fig. 18-3) are terminal arrhythmias that lead to cardiac arrest. Ventricular fibrillation, frequently preceded by ventricular tachycardia, occurs as the terminal event for a variety of diseases, including some anesthetic "accidents." The electrical activation and subsequent contraction of the heart occurs in a totally disorganized fashion with ventricular fibrillation. Cardiac output falls dramatically, and rapid intervention is required before hypoxia and acidosis lead to irreversible cellular damage in the heart, brain, and other tissues.

Ventricular flutter is characterized by very rapid, rhythmic ventricular flutter waves that have a sine wave appearance. Ventricular fibrillation is recognized by rapid, irregular, unorganized deflections on the ECG. P waves, QRS complexes, and T waves are not detectable (see Fig. 18-3). Ventricular fibrillation can be classified as coarse or fine. Coarse fibrillation has deflections of higher amplitude and may be easier to convert by a defibrillatory shock than fine fibrillation. A witnessed episode of ventricular fibrillation should be treated with an immediate defibrillatory shock. When ventricular fibrillation is not observed, but is recognized during the course of cardiac resuscitation, the "A-B-C-D-E" of resuscitation should be followed (see Tilley, Additional Reading), including DC shock. Chemical defibrillation has been reported using bretylium tosylate or a combination of potassium chloride (1 mEg/kg IV) and acetylcholine chloride (6 mg/kg IV). Bretylium tosylate appears to be ineffective as a defibrillatory agent in the dog.

Failure of Impulse Formation

Sinus Arrest and Sinoatrial Block

Sinus arrest (Table 18-6, Fig. 18-4) is present when the sinus node fails to fire for a time duration of two P-P intervals or longer. If this finding occurs in a regular manner, such that the pause is exactly two or three times the normal P-P intervals, SA block is thought to be present (the impulse is blocked before exiting the SA node). The

Table 18–6 *Failure of Impulse Formation*

Rhythm	Associated Conditions	Therapy
Sinus arrest	Sick sinus syndrome, high vagal tone or vagal stimulation, digitalis intoxication, sinus nodal or other myocardial disease, electrolyte imbalance	None, atropine, glycopyrrolate, isoproterenol, pacemaker
Atrial standstill	Permanent: English springer spaniel cardiomyopathy Temporary: hyperkalemia, Addison's disease, acute renal failure, potassium infusion, potassium-sparing diuretics	Pacemaker, treat congestive heart failure if present Treat underlying cause: fluids, bicarbonate, and insulin and dextrose

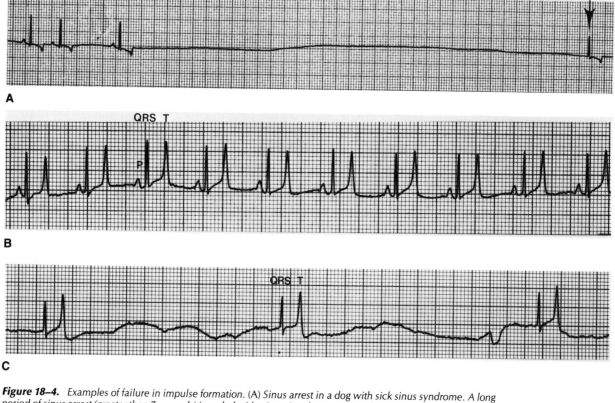

Figure 18–4. *Examples of failure in impulse formation. (A) Sinus arrest in a dog with sick sinus syndrome. A long period of sinus arrest (greater than 7 seconds) is ended with a junctional escape complex (arrow). (B) Early effects of hyperkalemia on the ECG of a dog with hypoadrenocorticism. Note the tall, peaked T waves. The heart rate is 100 beats/min. Recorded at 25 mm/sec, 1 cm/mV. (C) Atrial standstill in a dog with severe hyperkalemia. P waves are absent, the heart rate is slow (30 beats/min), and T waves are tall and peaked. The serum potassium level was 8.7 mEq/L. Recorded at 25 mm/sec, 1 cm/mV.*

pauses that result from sinus arrest or SA block can result in clinical signs of weakness, syncope, or, rarely, sudden death if subsidiary pacemakers fail to fire (sick sinus syndrome). The period of arrest may be followed by a sinus impulse or an escape complex (see below). Sinus arrest may occur with disease of the sinus node or secondary to conditions that cause high vagal tone. It may also be observed as an incidental finding in brachycephalic dog breeds or as a pathologic finding with myocardial disease, digitalis intoxication, electrolyte disturbances, or sick sinus syndrome.

When clinical signs or hemodynamic embarrassment result from sinus arrest, therapy is indicated. Initial therapy, when possible, should be directed at the underlying disease (*e.g.*, high vagal tone, digitalis intoxication). Specific therapy for sinus arrest may include anticholinergic drugs or isoproterenol hydrochloride. When sinus arrest is associated with sick sinus syndrome and is unresponsive to oral anticholinergics such as propantheline, implantation of a pacemaker is indicated.

Atrial Standstill

Atrial standstill (see Table 18-6 and Fig. 18-4) results from a total absence of atrial activity. This rhythm is characterized by an absence of P waves and the presence of an escape rhythm (see below), which usually has a supraventricular configuration (see Fig. 18-4). Atrial standstill may be transient or persistent. Transient atrial standstill may result from hyperkalemia or severe digitalis intoxication. Persistent atrial standstill has been reported as part of a muscular dystrophy complex in English springer spaniels.

The electrocardiographic features of hyperkalemia (usually associated with urinary obstruction or Addison's disease) typically progress in severity as serum potassium levels rise. The initial findings include repolarization changes, causing tall and peaked T waves. Progressive elevation of serum potassium leads to bradycardia; prolonged P wave, P-R interval, and QRS duration; and decreased P wave and QRS amplitude. As the serum potassium level rises above approximately 8 mEq/L (8 mmol/L), P waves disappear and atrial standstill (sinoventricular rhythm) is present. Further elevations in serum potassium concentration lead to progressive QRS widening and eventual cardiac arrest. Hyperkalemia is treated by administration of hypokalemic fluid, sodium bicarbonate, and insulin with dextrose in emergency situations. Calcium gluconate can also be used to counteract the effects of hyperkalemia on the heart if other therapies are ineffective (see Chapter 72). The underlying cause for the development of hyperkalemia should be corrected.

Escape Rhythms

An escape rhythm can occur only when the normal cardiac pacemaker (usually the SA node) stops or slows to a rate less than that of a subsidiary automatic pacemaker. The subsidiary pacemakers (AV nodal or junctional tissue and the Purkinje fibers in the ventricle) function as a rescue mechanism during severe bradycardia. For this reason, escape rhythms should never be suppressed! The tissue with the fastest rate of automaticity after the SA node is the junctional tissue, with an intrinsic rate of 40 to 60 beats per minute. Junctional escape complexes (Table 18-7, see Fig. 18-4) are identified as QRS complexes of normal configuration that occur after a pause in the rhythm. Junctional complexes frequently have a retrogradely conducted P' (often negative) that occurs before, within, or after the QRS complex. Junctional escape rhythms that are faster than 60 beats per minute are termed *enhanced* or *accelerated junctional rhythms*.

Ventricular escape rhythms (see Table 18-7 and Fig. 18-5) are slow, and the escape beat follows a pause in the normal rhythm. The ventricular escape originates from automatic tissues within the ventricle (Purkinje fibers). The QRS complex is wide and bizarre, identical to the configuration described for ventricular premature complexes. The rate of the ventricular escape rhythm is usually less than 40 beats per minute. No cause-and-effect relationship exists between the P waves and the ventricular escape rhythm. If junctional or ventricular escape rhythms continue uninterrupted, the resulting rhythm is usually very regular. Occasionally, ventricular arrhythmias may accompany escape rhythms; however, antiarrhythmic therapy should never be administered unless a pacemaker has first been implanted.

Escape rhythms are never a primary diagnosis; they always result from an abnormality in impulse generation or conduction. Treatment should be directed at the underlying disorder (*e.g.*, complete AV block, sick sinus syndrome, digitalis intoxication). Some improvement may result after administration of atropine, glycopyrrolate, terbutaline, or isoproterenol. Right atrial pacing or permanent pacemaker implantation may be required, depending on the underlying disorder of impulse generation or conduction.

Table 18–7 *Escape Rhythms*

Rhythm	Associated Conditions	Therapy
Junctional or ventricular escape complex	Sinus arrest, sinus bradycardia, complete atrioventricular block, digitalis intoxication, sick sinus syndrome	Treat underlying cause: atropine, glycopyrrolate, dopamine, terbutaline, isoproterenol, or pacemaker

Atrioventricular Conduction Disturbances

The normal sequence of cardiac activation includes slowed conduction through the AV node, allowing sequential activation of the atria and then the ventricles. A variety of factors may alter conduction through the AV node, including enhanced vagal tone, drugs, and structural disease of the AV node. If AV conduction delays are present, an understanding of the severity of block, the physiologic significance, and the likelihood of progression to more serious AV block is useful in determining proper management.

First-degree AV block (Table 18-8, Fig. 18-5) is simply a delay in conduction across the AV node. The physiologic significance is minimal, yet recognition of a mild conduction delay is useful in that drugs that would further compromise AV conduction may be avoided.

Second-degree AV block (see Table 18-8 and Fig. 18-5) results when not all sinus impulses are conducted to the ventricle. It is recognized by the presence of some P waves that are not causally associated with QRS complexes. The remainder of the P waves and QRS complexes have a normal temporal and causal relationship to each other. Second-degree AV block is classified as either type I (Wenckebach) or type II. The former, which occurs when the P-R interval is progressively prolonged until a P wave is blocked, is associated with normal P waves and QRS complex configurations. It may be normal in young dogs, and is frequently associated with high vagal tone and digitalis intoxication.

Type II second-degree AV block is defined by the presence of P waves that are intermittently or regularly blocked, although the P-R interval remains constant in the normal P-QRS-T complexes. The QRS complex may be prolonged and associated with ventricular conduction disturbances; however, the P waves are usually normal. Type II second-degree AV block is more frequently associated with structural disease of the AV node, and affected patients, especially those with ventricular conduction disturbances, may be at risk of developing complete heart block. Symptomatic animals may be treated with anticholinergics, sympathomimetics, or pacemaker implantation.

Third-degree AV block (see Table 18-8 and Fig. 18-5) or complete heart block occurs when all of the impulses generated by the sinus node are blocked at the AV node or bundle branches. There is no relationship between the P waves and the QRS complexes, and the ventricular rate is typically slower than the atrial rate. The QRS complexes represent either AV junctional or ventricular escape beats. Complete heart block may result in weakness, syncope, congestive heart failure, or sudden death. Associated conditions include bacterial endocarditis, idiopathic fibrosis of the AV node, infiltrative cardiomyopathy, cardiac neoplasia, and Lyme myocarditis (infection with *Borrelia burgdorferi*). Drug therapy (anticholinergic agents or adrenergic agonists, such as pro-

Table 18–8 *Atrioventricular (AV) Conduction Disturbances*

Rhythm	Associated Conditions	Therapy
First-degree AV block	High vagal tone, old age, digitalis intoxication, beta-blockade, electrolyte imbalance	None
Second-degree AV block		
Type I	High vagal tone, digitalis intoxication, electrolyte imbalance, xylazine anesthesia	None, treat underlying cause, atropine or glycopyrrolate for anesthetic cases
Type II	Structural AV nodal disease, drug intoxications	Atropine, glycopyrrolate, isoproterenol, pacemaker
Third-degree AV block	Structural AV nodal disease, infiltrative cardiomyopathy, cardiac neoplasia, digitalis intoxication, bacterial endocarditis, hypertrophic cardiomyopathy (cat)	Pacemaker, isoproterenol, terbutaline, propantheline, atropine

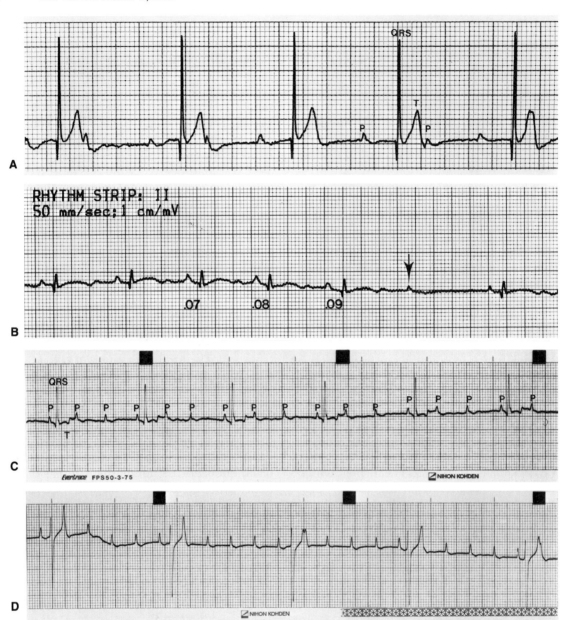

Figure 18–5. Examples of arterioventricular (AV) conduction disturbances. (A) First- and second-degree AV block in a dog. The P–R interval is prolonged at 0.26 seconds. Blocked P waves are found buried within or following each T wave. Recorded at 25 mm/sec, 1 cm/mV. (B) Second-degree AV block, Mobitz type I in a cat. The P–R interval is progressively prolonged until a P wave is blocked (arrow). Recorded at 50 mm/sec, 1 cm/mV. (C) High-grade (Mobitz type II) second-degree AV block in a dog. The P–R interval is constant, but two P waves are blocked for every P wave that is conducted through the AV node. Recorded at 25 mm/sec, 1 cm/mV. (D) Third-degree AV block with ventricular escape complexes in a dog. The atrial rate is 160 beats/min and the ventricular rate is 40 beats/min. There is no cause-and-effect relationship between the P waves and the QRS complexes. Recorded at 25 mm/sec, 1 cm/mV.

pantheline or terbutaline, respectively) is rarely effective. Permanent pacemaker implantation is indicated for long-term management.

MORPHOLOGIC CHANGES IN P-QRS-T DEFLECTIONS

Many factors may alter the morphology of the P-QRS-T deflections on the ECG. The surface ECG is a recording of the summation of the electrical activity of the heart from electrodes placed on the skin. Any alterations in the electrical activity of the heart, or in the transmission of this electrical activity to the skin electrodes, can result in morphologic abnormalities of the recorded deflections. Certain disease states lead to specific changes in P-QRS-T complexes. Although most veterinary ECG texts list criteria for cardiac enlargement patterns and other morphologic abnormalities, the user must already suspect a certain disease process in order to effectively use the information. With the approach presented here,

the reader can determine the abnormality that is present on the ECG in question and then follow through Tables 18-9 and 18-10 to arrive at a diagnosis. Alternatively, if one wants to determine whether electrocardiographic evidence of a specific pathologic condition is present (*e.g.*, ventricular enlargement), the necessary information is available in Table 18-10.

Measurement of the duration of the P wave, P-R interval, QRS complex, or QT interval is required for proper use of these tables. The time duration of each small box is 0.02 seconds when the ECG is recorded at 50 mm/sec (Fig. 18-6), and 0.04 seconds when recorded at 25 mm/sec.

Evaluation of the mean electrical axis is also important in evaluation of ventricular enlargement patterns and bundle branch blocks. The mean electrical axis can be calculated using the lead systems in the frontal plane, leads I, II, III, aVR, aVL, and aVF. One method is to determine which lead has the greatest positive deflection and pick that lead as the mean electrical axis. Using Figure 18-7 as an example, the tallest R

Table 18–9 *Abnormalities in P-QRS-T Complexes*

Finding/Criteria	Associations and Approach
ABNORMALITIES IN P WAVE MORPHOLOGY	
PROLONGED P WAVE DURATION; P-MITRALE–LEFT ATRIAL ENLARGEMENT (SEE FIG. 18–6)	
Dog: P wave >0.04 sec; +/− notched P wave	Chronic valvular disease, cardiomyopathy, congenital heart disease
Cat: P wave >0.04 sec	Cardiomyopathy, congenital heart disease
INCREASED P WAVE AMPLITUDE; P-PULMONALE–RIGHT ATRIAL ENLARGEMENT (SEE FIG. 18–6)	
Dog: P wave >0.4 mV	Chronic respiratory disease, collapsing trachea, tricuspid dysplasia or severe tricuspid insufficiency
Cat: P wave >0.2 mV	Tricuspid dysplasia, chronic respiratory disease; may also be observed with severe left atrial enlargement and hypertrophic cardiomyopathy
DECREASED OR VARIABLE P WAVE AMPLITUDE	
Dog and cat: No values estabished for small P waves	Variation of normal may be seen with hyperkalemia (see atrial standstill) (see Fig. 18–4C). P waves of variable height and configuration are seen with wandering pacemaker. Look for supraventricular premature beats if variable P wave height is seen with irregular QRS intervals or premature complexes.
ABNORMALITIES IN QRS MORPHOLOGY	
TALL R WAVES	
Dog: R wave >2.5 mV in leads II, III, aVF, or V_2 (CV_6LL); R wave >3 mV in large breeds Cat: R wave >0.9 mV in lead II or >1 mV in lead V_2	Measure QRS duration and mean electrical axis; evaluate ST segment and T wave. Suspect left ventricular enlargement or left bundle branch block (see Table 18-10).

(continued)

Table 18–9 (continued)

Finding/Criteria	Associations and Approach
DEEP S WAVES IN LEADS II, III, aVF, OR V$_2$ (CV$_6$LL) Dog: S waves in lead II >0.35 mV; S wave in lead V$_2$ >0.8 mV Cat: S waves in leads II, III, or aVF >0.5 mV or S waves in lead V$_2$ >0.7 mV	Measure QRS duration and mean electrical axis; evaluate ST segment and T wave. Suspect right ventricular enlargement or right bundle branch block if right axis shift; suspect left anterior fascicular block or concentric left ventricular hypertrophy if left axis shift (see Table 18-10).
DEEP Q WAVES IN LEADS II, III, OR aVF No well-established values. In lead II, Q waves in dogs >1 mV and >0.5 mV in cats is probably abnormal.	May be normal in doberman pinschers and deep-chested breeds; may indicate right ventricular enlargement (see Table 18-10) or septal hypertrophy. Is suggestive of biventricular enlargement if seen in association with left ventricular enlargement.
PROLONGED QRS DURATION Dog: QRS >0.05 sec in small and medium breeds; QRS >0.06 sec in large breeds. QRS >0.08 sec suggests bundle branch block. Cat: QRS duration >0.04 sec. QRS >0.06 sec suggests bundle branch block.	Measure mean electrical axis; look for tall R waves or deep S waves. If right axis shift, suspect right ventricular enlargement or right bundle branch block; if normal axis or left axis shift, suspect left ventricular enlargement or left bundle branch block (see Table 18-10).
ABNORMAL MEAN ELECTRICAL AXIS (MEA) Dog: MEA < +40 = left axis shift; MEA > +100 = right axis shift Cat: MEA <0 = left axis shift; MEA > +160 = right axis shift	If right axis shift suspect right ventricular enlargement or right bundle branch block (see Table 18-10). If left axis shift suspect left ventricular enlargement, left bundle branch block, or left anterior fascicular block (see Table 18-10).
SMALL (LOW-VOLTAGE) QRS COMPLEXES (SEE FIG. 23–5) Dog: QRS <0.5 mV in leads I, II, III, and aVF or QRS <1 mV in all chest and limb leads Cat: No established criteria	Pericardial effusion, pleural effusion, obesity, hypothyroidism, pneumothorax, incorrect standardization of the electrocardiograph, poor lead-to-skin contact
ELECTRICAL ALTERNATION OF THE QRS COMPLEXES (SEE FIG. 23–5) Dog and cat: Regular beat-to-beat variation (every other complex, every third complex) in P, QRS, or T wave configuration	Pericardial effusion, supraventricular arrhythmias, alternating bundle branch block—should not be confused with electrocardiographic changes resulting from respiration

ABNORMALITIES IN ST SEGMENT AND T WAVE MORPHOLOGY

ST SEGMENT DEPRESSION OR ELEVATION Dog: Elevated >0.15 mV or depressed >0.2 mV from T-P baseline Cat: Elevated or depressed greater than 0.1 mV from T-P baseline	May be a variation of normal in some animals. Elevation may be observed with hypoxia, infarction, epicarditis, and pericarditis. Depression may be observed with infarction, ischemia, ventricular enlargement, tachycardia, conduction disturbance, digitalis therapy, electrolyte imbalance, or cardiac trauma.
QT INTERVAL CHANGES Dog: QT interval <0.15 sec or >0.25 sec Cat: QT interval <0.12 sec or >0.18 sec	QT interval may be prolonged with hypocalcemia, hypothermia, hypokalemia, quinidine or procainamide therapy, central nervous system disorders, and ventricular hypertrophy or conduction disorders. QT interval may be shortened with hypercalcemia, digitalis therapy, or hyperkalemia.
T WAVE CHANGES T waves may normally be positive, negative, or biphasic. Change in T wave polarity on comparison with a previous electrocardiogram suggests abnormality. Dog: T wave usually not greater than 25% of the height of the QRS complex. Cat: T wave not greater than 0.3 mV in lead II	Abnormalities in T wave height or a switch in T wave polarity may occur with hypoxia, ventricular enlargement or abnormal conduction, severe metabolic disorders, and some drug therapies. Hyperkalemia may cause T waves to be peaked (see Fig. 18-4); hypokalemia may cause small, biphasic T waves. Most T wave changes are nonspecific in dogs and cats.

Table 18–10 *Ventricular Enlargement Patterns and Bundle Branch Blocks*

Criteria	Associations

RIGHT VENTRICULAR ENLARGEMENT PATTERN (SEE FIG. 19–8)
Dog: Any three of the following:
  1. S waves in leads I, II, III, and aVF
  2. S wave in lead II >0.35 mV
  3. S wave in lead I >0.5 mV
  4. S wave in lead V_2 >0.08 mV
  5. S wave in lead V_4 >0.07 mV
  6. Right axis shift
  7. R wave : S wave ratio in lead V_4 <0.87 mV
  8. W-shaped QRS in V_{10}
  9. Positive T wave V_{10} (except in Chihuahuas)
Cat: S wave in leads I, II, III, and aVF (especially S wave >0.5 mV), right axis shift, S waves in leads V_2 or V_4 >0.7 mV
	Congenital heart defects such as pulmonic stenosis, tetralogy of Fallot, other defects with right-to-left shunting, heartworm disease, cor pulmonale, chronic respiratory diseases, chronic tricuspid valve insufficiency, and pulmonary embolism. Less commonly observed in cats. In both dogs and cats, the electrocardiogram may be insensitive to mild or moderate right ventricular enlargement.

RIGHT BUNDLE BRANCH BLOCK Criteria similar to those for right ventricular enlargement, especially right axis shift and S waves in leads I, II, III, and aVF, with additional finding of terminal R wave in right-sided chest leads and prolonged QRS duration Dog: QRS duration >0.07 sec Cat: QRS duration >0.06 sec	Occasionally observed in normal dogs, but can result from congenital heart disease, cardiac neoplasia, cardiac trauma or surgery, myocarditis, or as an intermittent conduction block with some tachyarrhythmias
LEFT VENTRICULAR ENLARGEMENT (SEE FIG. 19–5) Dog: Normal axis or left axis shift, R waves >2.5 mV in leads II, III, aVF, or V_2 (except in young, deep-chested dogs) or >3 mV in lead V_4, normal or prolonged QRS duration, ST segment coving, tall T wave Cat: Normal or left axis shift, R waves >0.9 mV in lead II or R wave >1 mV in lead V_4, ST segment coving, T wave >0.3 mV in lead II	Congenital defects such as patent ductus arteriosus, ventricular septal defect, and aortic stenosis; mitral or aortic valve insufficiency; dilated cardiomyopathy in dogs and cats. Hypertrophic cardiomyopathy, anemia, systemic hypertension, and hyperthyroidism in cats
LEFT BUNDLE BRANCH BLOCK Dog and cat: Criteria similar to those for left ventricular enlargement, with positive QRS in leads I, II, III, and aVF and QRS duration >0.07 sec	Usually associated with severe myocardial or bundle branch disease; may be seen in ischemic heart disease or after cardiac trauma or surgery
LEFT ANTERIOR FASCICULAR BLOCK (OR CONCENTRIC LEFT VENTRICULAR HYPERTROPHY, ESPECIALLY IN CATS) (SEE FIG. 18–7) Dog and cat: Deep S waves in leads II, III, and aVF, small q wave and tall R wave in leads I and aVL, marked left axis shift, QRS duration normal or slightly prolonged	Hypertrophic or restrictive cardiomyopathy; causes of concentric left ventricular hypertrophy such as systemic arterial hypertension, and aortic stenosis, hyperkalemia, cardiac trauma or surgery

wave is in lead aVL, making the axis − 30 degrees. A second method that is more precise is to find the lead with an equal deflection above and below the baseline (determine the isoelectric lead, aVR in Fig. 18-7), and evaluate the lead that is perpendicular (90 degrees) to the isoelectric lead (lead III in this example). The mean electrical axis is calculated by determining the direction of the majority of the QRS complex in the perpendicular lead. If the perpendicular lead is mostly positive (tall R wave), then the axis is toward the lead; if the QRS complex is mostly negative (large S wave), then the mean electrical axis is away from this lead. In Figure 18-7, the deep S wave in lead III indicates that the axis is away from lead III. It would be calculated as − 60 degrees. Both methods indicate a left axis shift for the example in Figure 18-7. The final method to determine the electrical axis is to plot leads I and III; however, this method is time-consuming and is rarely required in clinical practice.

Table 18-9 is used to help determine causes or disease associations when specific morphologic abnormalities are detected in P-QRS-T com-

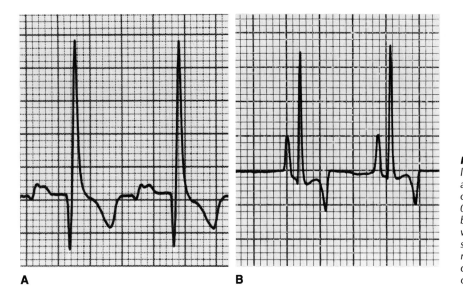

A   **B**

Figure 18–6. Examples of atrial enlargement patterns. (A) P–mitrale or left atrial enlargement pattern in a dog with cardiomyopathy. The P wave duration, 0.06 seconds, is prolonged (three boxes, each box = 0.02 sec) and the P wave is notched. Recorded at 50 mm/sec, 1 cm/mV. (B) P–pulmonale or right atrial enlargement pattern in a dog. The P wave is 0.5 mV tall. Recorded at 25 mm/sec, 1 cm/mV.

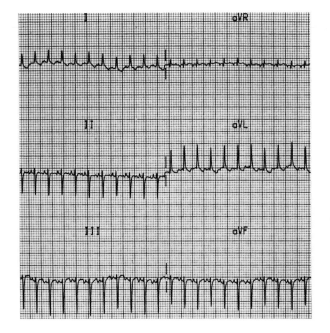

Figure 18–7. Example of left axis shift in a cat with hyperthyroidism. The mean electrical axis is shifted to the left (−60 degrees). Deep S waves are noted in leads II, III, and aVF, and a qR pattern is present in leads aVL and I. This pattern is common in cats with concentric left ventricular hypertrophy or left anterior fascicular block.

plexes. In some cases (ventricular enlargement patterns and bundle branch blocks) the reader is directed to Table 18-10 for final electrocardiographic diagnosis and disease associations.

If ventricular enlargement or bundle branch block is suspected based on information from Table 18-9 or from other clinical information, Table 18-10 is used to determine the specific enlargement pattern or ventricular conduction abnormality and its disease associations.

ADDITIONAL READING

Edwards NJ. Bolton's handbook of canine and feline electrocardiography. Philadelphia: WB Saunders, 1987.

Harpster NK. The cardiovascular system. In: Holzworth J, ed. Diseases of the cat: Medicine and surgery. Philadelphia: WB Saunders, 1987: 831.

Miller MS, Tilley LP. Electrocardiography. In: Fox PR, ed. Canine and feline cardiology. New York: Churchill Livingstone, 1988: 43.

Tilley LP. Essentials of canine and feline electrocardiography. Philadelphia: Lea and Febiger, 1985.

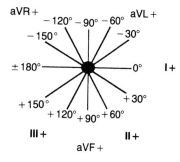

19

CONGENITAL HEART DISEASE

John E. Rush, Clarke E. Atkins

Congenital heart defects, the most common and important heart diseases observed in young dogs and cats, often present a significant diagnostic challenge. Identification of the type of defect and its functional significance is essential for accurate prognosis and appropriate therapy. A knowledge of the potential causes of cardiac murmurs in dogs and cats, their modes of inheritance, and possible treatment of the common congenital defects is useful in advising both the pet owner and breeder. Table 19-1 lists the common congenital defects in dogs and cats in approximate order of frequency.

The earliest indication of cardiac malformation is usually auscultation of a cardiac murmur. When a murmur is auscultated, the owner should be asked whether cardiac abnormalities have been discovered in littermates or other related animals. The animal's exercise capacity, growth rate, or size in relation to its littermates may provide some indication of the severity of the defect. Loud murmurs of long duration are usually the result of cardiac malformation and should always be investigated. The intensity (loudness) of a murmur, however, is not an accurate indication of the severity of the defect. Murmurs of softer intensity may be physiologic in origin (innocent murmurs) or they may result from anemia or a congenital cardiac defect. Factors that con-

tribute to the presence of innocent murmurs in young animals include a lower hematocrit, thinner and less muscular chest wall, and less fat deposition around the thorax and heart.

In addition to cardiac and pulmonary auscultation, the physical examination should include palpation of the precordium to find the site of the apex beat and determine if the murmur is associated with a palpable thrill. Palpation of femoral arterial pulse quality and observation of the jugular veins for distention or pulsation will assist in establishing any pathophysiologic changes resulting from cardiac malformation. The abdomen should be palpated for hepatomegaly or ascites, and mucous membrane color and capillary refill time should be carefully evaluated.

Congenital heart defects may result from hereditary factors, environmental factors, or a combination of the two. In some animals it is likely that a genetic predisposition for a defect is combined with exposure to an environmental factor, which leads to development of a congenital cardiac defect. Environmental factors that may contribute to the formation of congenital cardiac defects include drugs, toxins, and certain infectious agents. The majority of congenital defects in dogs and cats are thought to result, at least in part, from hereditary factors. Although a hereditary

Table 19–1 *Common Congenital Cardiac Defects in Dogs and Cats*

CANINE CARDIOVASCULAR ANOMALY

Patent ductus arteriosus
Pulmonic stenosis
Aortic stenosis
Ventricular septal defect
Vascular ring anomaly
Atrial septal defect
Tetralogy of Fallot
Atrioventricular valve malformations

FELINE CARDIOVASCULAR ANOMALY

Atrioventricular valve malformations
Ventricular septal defect
Patent ductus arteriosus
Endocardial fibroelastosis
Vascular ring anomaly
Aortic stenosis
Tetralogy of Fallot
Atrial septal defect
Pulmonic stenosis

component has not been proven for each cardiac defect, breed predisposition frequently argues strongly for a genetic influence. Many defects are reported to be transmitted in a polygenic fashion that allows some offspring to carry genes for the defect without demonstrating clinical disease. This variable phenotypic expression with gradations of severity makes genetic counseling more difficult.

Our approach is to assume that all congenital heart diseases may have a hereditary (genetic) component. This approach is quite conservative, but diminishes the chance of propagating hereditary defects. Based on this assumption, it is safest to advise not only that the affected animal not be bred, but that the littermates, dam, and sire be restrained from breeding as well. Some breeders may find these recommendations too stringent, or they may believe that some of the animals have enough desirable traits to risk a repeat breeding. In these cases, a more practical approach is to suggest that only the affected animal be restrained from breeding, preferably by neutering. New owners of littermates that have been examined and found to be free of murmurs should be advised of the affected animal. Breedings involving littermates, future breedings between the dam and sire, or outbreedings using either the

dam or sire should be carefully scrutinized for the presence of animals with similar or different congenital cardiac defects. If congenital defects appear in these subsequent breedings, one can then strongly advise against future breeding of these animals.

When a murmur is auscultated in a young dog or cat, the general approach is to determine if the murmur is innocent or if it represents congenital heart disease. Innocent murmurs are typically systolic, of short duration, and of low intensity (grade III or less). Some innocent murmurs may be described as having a musical character. The localization of innocent murmurs may be over the aortic or pulmonic valve. These murmurs frequently change in character or disappear completely with changes in the animal's body position. Innocent murmurs become softer as the animal ages and usually disappear by 12 months of age.

Based on the findings of a murmur that is loud, occupies a substantial portion of the cardiac cycle, is not altered with changes in body position, or is associated with evidence of cardiac dysfunction, diagnostic testing for congenital heart disease is initiated. The cardiovascular workup includes a physical examination, thoracic radiographs, and an electrocardiogram (ECG), plus possibly an echocardiogram, nonselective angiography (see Nonselective Angiocardiography in Chapter 80), selective cardiac catheterization, or other specialized tests to determine the severity of the defect and the specific diagnosis (Fig. 19-1). Once the specific diagnosis and severity are established the owner can be advised as to the potential outcome for the animal, possible therapies, and whether the animal should be restrained from breeding.

Although it is ideal to make a specific diagnosis in every case, it is not always possible, based on financial limitations or limitations in equipment or expertise. In these instances, one must pursue the diagnosis within these limitations and make some assessment as to the severity of the lesion. In some cases, it is adequate to determine only whether the defect is mild or severe, giving the owner some prognostic information. This can often be achieved with only thoracic radiographs and electrocardiography. In certain cases, for ex-

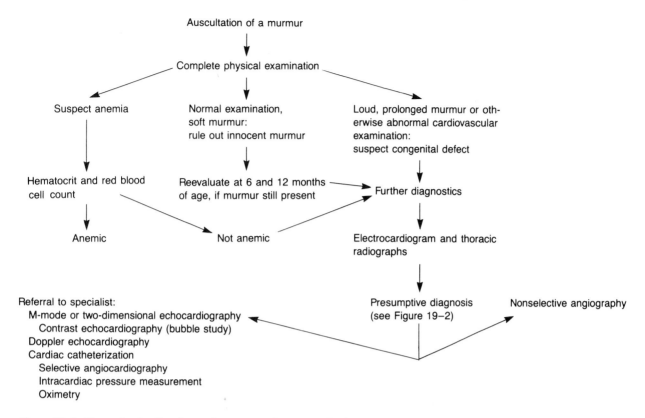

Figure 19–1 Diagnostic algorithm for cardiac murmurs in young animals.

ample patent ductus arteriosus, a definitive diagnosis can usually be made with these procedures alone. Certain information that is available without specialized procedures provides an inexpensive source of information to the practicing veterinarian. Specifically, knowledge of breed and gender predisposition for each defect, pulse character, presence or absence of cyanosis, and location and character of the murmur(s) expected with each defect is useful. It is emphasized that a more definitive workup is ideal so that potential surgical intervention might be employed.

Cardiac auscultation provides the greatest information relative to cost and risk. However, auscultation is a learned technique, compounded by the fact that animals may be uncooperative, making auscultation potentially a frustrating and unrewarding experience. Since most practitioners can readily determine whether the murmur is loudest on the right or left side of the thorax, a simplistic algorithm is provided to aid in the di-

agnosis of congenital heart disease (Fig. 19-2). After it is determined whether the murmur is loudest on the left or right side, the clinician must determine the portion of the cardiac cycle that the murmur occupies (systolic, diastolic, both, or continuous) and the quality or shape of the murmur (ejection or crescendo–decrescendo vs. regurgitant or plateau-shaped). Thoracic radiographs and electrocardiography are then utilized to determine if the left or right side of the heart is enlarged and if the pulmonary vasculature has normal, decreased, or increased circulation. As one can see from looking at the algorithm, a presumptive diagnosis can be made at this point. Referral to a cardiologist is often indicated to confirm the diagnosis, determine the hemodynamic severity of the lesion, and determine whether surgical correction is possible or indicated.

Referral may be required to obtain echocardiography, cardiac catheterization, or the advan-

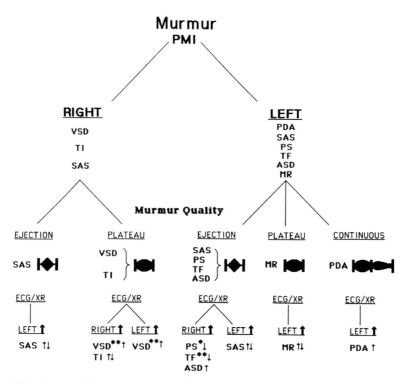

* 65% of cases of PS are interpreted as having undercirculation.
** Radiographic and electrocardiographic findings with VSD are quite variable and may be normal or show evidence of right- or left-sided heart enlargement, depending on the location and size of the defect. TF may be differentiated from PS based on the finding of cyanosis and polycythemia in many cases.

Figure 19–2 *Diagnostic algorithm for common congenital cardiac defects. Using this algorithm, the murmur's point of maximal intensity is located (right or left hemithorax); the exact location (intercostal space) is also useful (see text in this chapter and Chapter 17). The quality of the murmur is determined next, followed by a determination of which side of the heart is enlarged using electrocardiography and thoracic radiography. Pulmonary circulation (over- or undercirculation) is also helpful in making a final distinction when more than one diagnostic possibility exists in the final tier. A presumptive diagnosis can be made in most cases using this algorithm in combination with breed, gender, exact murmur location, specific radiographic findings, and frequency of occurrence. It is emphasized that this algorithm provides only a presumptive diagnosis and that more sophisticated studies may be necessary to provide a definitive diagnosis, prognosis, and indication for surgery. (PMI = point of maximal intensity; VSD = ventricular septal defect; TI = tricuspid insufficiency; SAS = subaortic stenosis; PS = pulmonic stenosis; PDA = patent ductus arteriosus; TF = tetralogy of Fallot; ASD = atrial septal defect; MR = mitral regurgitation; ECG/XR = electrocardiographic and radiographic findings; RIGHT ↑ = right heart enlargement; LEFT ↑ = left heart enlargement; ↑ = pulmonary overcirculation; ↓ = pulmonary undercirculation; ↑↓ = normal pulmonary circulation)*

tage of the specialist's opinion. Doppler echocardiography (see Echocardiography in Chapter 80) is particularly useful in evaluating animals with congenital heart disease. Selective cardiac catheterization is indicated in some cases to perform selective angiography or to obtain direct measurement of intracardiac pressures and blood oximetry. Selective angiocardiography is indicated to document most cardiac defects in large-breed dogs or in animals in which the diagnosis is still in question after noninvasive diagnostic tests. Measurement of intracardiac pressures allows documentation of the hemodynamic severity of the lesion (gradients across stenotic valves). This hemodynamic information can be used to formulate a more accurate prognosis and allows the clinician to make judgments on the need for therapeutic interventions. Measurement of blood oxygen content (oximetry) allows identification of left-to-right or right-to-left shunting defects and provides a quantitative assessment of the degree of shunting and the need for surgery.

PATENT DUCTUS ARTERIOSUS

Causes

During fetal life, blood returning to the heart either passes through the foramen ovale to the left atrium or is pumped through the right ventricle to the pulmonary artery. Because the pressure through the pulmonary vascular circuit is high during fetal life, blood pumped into the pulmonary artery is shunted through the ductus arteriosus to the aorta, preventing unneeded pulmonary circulation. At the time of birth, the pressure through the pulmonary circuit drops dramatically with expansion of the lungs, and the pressure in the systemic circuit rises. This results in a reversal of blood flow through the ductus arteriosus so that blood now flows from the aorta to the pulmonary artery. This reversal in blood flow, an inhibition of prostaglandin synthesis, and a local increase in PO_2 results in vasoconstriction of the ductus, with functional closure normally completed by 72 hours post partum in dogs and cats. Failure of ductal closure results in patency (patent ductus arteriosus [PDA]) and in the permanent connection from the aorta to the pulmonary artery (Fig. 19-3). A polygenic mode of inheritance has been proven in the poodle.

Pathophysiology

In most animals with PDA, the pulmonary vascular resistance is normal (lower than systemic vascular resistance) and blood flows continuously from the aorta to the pulmonary artery through the ductus arteriosus. This continuous, turbulent

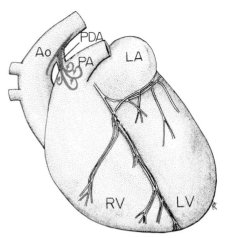

Figure 19–3 Diagram of patent ductus arteriosus (PDA). Blood flows from the enlarged aorta (Ao) through the PDA to the pulmonary artery (PA). Arrows indicate turbulent blood flow, which contributes to enlargement of the main pulmonary artery. The left ventricle (LV) and left atrium (LA) are typically enlarged, and biventricular enlargement may be noted in some cases. (RV = right ventricle) (Allen DG. Congenital cardiac defects. In: Allen DG, Kruth SA, eds. Small animal cardiopulmonary medicine. Philadelphia: BC Decker, 1988: 86.)

blood flow produces a continuous cardiac murmur. This left-to-right shunt increases blood flow through the proximal aorta, pulmonary vasculature, left atrium, and left ventricle, producing enlargement of the left atrium and ventricle as well as pulmonary overcirculation. Mitral regurgitation frequently develops, probably secondary to left ventricular dilation and stretching of the mitral valve annulus. Volume overloading of the left heart results in increased filling pressures to the left atrium and left ventricle. Pulmonary edema may occur as a result of left ventricular failure. Right ventricular enlargement is uncommon, but may develop with large shunts.

Animals with PDA have unusually wide arterial pulse pressures. The peak systolic arterial pressure is normal or elevated due to an increased stroke volume (blood entering the pulmonary artery courses through the lungs and reenters the left heart), but the arterial diastolic blood pressure rapidly drops as blood "runs off" into the low-pressure pulmonary artery. This causes the bounding or waterhammer pulse characteristic of PDA.

If the high pulmonary vascular resistance present in the fetus fails to regress, or if pulmonary arteries develop muscular hypertrophy in response to voluminous, high-pressure blood flow through the pulmonary vasculature, pulmonary hypertension will result, leading to bidirectional or right-to-left shunting through the ductus. A right-to-left PDA often causes differential cyanosis; the head is supplied with oxygenated blood but the aorta, distal to the site of the ductus, carries oxygen-desaturated venous blood. The elevated pulmonary arterial pressure, which equals or exceeds the systemic arterial pressure, places an increased load on the right ventricle and may cause right heart failure. Arterial thromboembolism is another complication associated with a right-to-left PDA.

Clinical Signs

Patent ductus arteriosus is most common in female purebred dogs, and while a genetic basis for the defect has only been proved in the poodle, several other breeds of dogs, including Pomeranians, collies, Chihuahuas, Maltese, Shetland sheepdogs, German shepherds, cocker spaniels, and Irish setters, are predisposed. Siamese cats may be predisposed to PDA. Animals with PDA may be presented for evaluation of poor growth, exercise intolerance, or respiratory distress. Approximately 25% of dogs with PDA are presented with signs of congestive heart failure, while a small number of dogs live for several years without apparent clinical signs. The latter dogs likely have a small ductus with minimal hemodynamic change. Patent ductus arteriosus is usually found as an isolated defect.

The hallmark finding on physical examination of animals with PDA is a continuous murmur, loudest at the left heart base and peaking in intensity near the time of the second heart sound. The systolic component of the murmur radiates well and may be auscultated over the entire thorax. However, the diastolic component may be missed in some animals if one fails to listen carefully at the left base. A systolic, regurgitant murmur, due to mitral insufficiency, may accompany the continuous murmur. The pulse character is strong and sharp, then rapidly drops off due to diastolic runoff of blood into the pulmonary artery. If left heart failure is present, the animal may be tachy-pneic or dyspneic, and pulmonary crackles may be noted.

In animals with pulmonary hypertension and right-to-left PDA, the murmur is attenuated and the diastolic component of the murmur is absent. A loud second heart sound may be heard at the left base. Cyanosis may be observed; it is usually more pronounced in the caudal mucous membranes (differential cyanosis). In some advanced cases, the right ventricle may fail, leading to jugular venous distention and other signs of right heart failure.

Diagnostic Approach

Thoracic radiographs (see Thoracic Radiography in Chapter 80) usually demonstrate marked left ventricular and left atrial enlargement; an elongated heart is most evident on the ventrodorsal view (Fig. 19-4). Pulmonary overcirculation is indicated by enlargement of the pulmonary arteries and veins in addition to an increased interstitial pattern throughout the lungs. The ventrodorsal radiographic view variably demonstrates three "bumps" at the left cranial aspect of the heart. The bumps represent dilation of the descending aorta ("ductus bump") at the 1 o'clock position, enlargement of the main pulmonary artery (2 o'clock), and left auricular enlargement (3 o'clock). If heart failure is present, interstitial or alveolar pulmonary edema may be present.

The ECG frequently shows high-amplitude QRS complexes in leads II and aVF, with prolonged QRS duration, ST segment slurring or depression, and large T waves indicative of left ventricular enlargement (Fig. 19-5). Left atrial enlargement may result in prolongation of the P wave duration (P-mitrale). Sinus tachycardia is frequently noted in dogs with congestive heart failure. Ventricular or supraventricular arrhythmias may be observed. Atrial fibrillation is common in dogs with marked left atrial enlargement.

The diagnosis can usually be confirmed on the basis of the continuous murmur and typical ECG and radiographic findings. Echocardiographic findings (see Echocardiography in Chapter 80) supportive of the diagnosis include left atrial and ventricular enlargement and prominent aortic root motion, with the ductus rarely being visu-

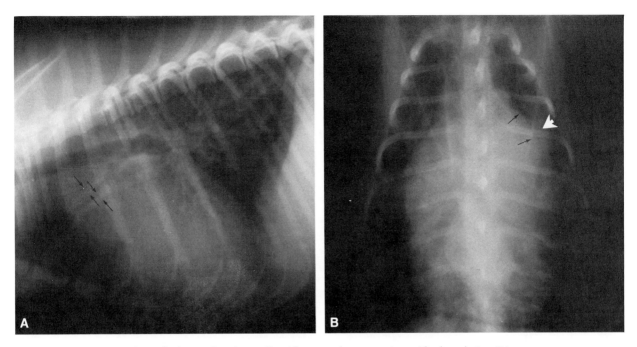

Figure 19–4 *Thoracic radiographs from a female poodle with patent ductus arteriosus. The lateral view (A) demonstrates left ventricular and left atrial enlargement, evidenced by a tall heart with tracheal elevation. Pulmonary overcirculation is noted in the caudal lung lobes, and both the artery (upper pair of arrows) and vein (lower pair of arrows) to the cranial lung lobe are enlarged. The ventrodorsal projection (B) demonstrates the typically elongated heart with the dilation of the descending aorta (ductus bump) at the site of the patent ductus arteriosus (small black arrows). The enlarged pulmonary artery segment is noted at the 2 o'clock position (white arrow).*

alized. Cardiac catheterization is reserved for animals in which the findings suggest pulmonary hypertension or other concomitant congenital cardiac defects. Animals with right-to-left PDA have markedly different findings: the ECG often demonstrates a right ventricular enlargement pattern, and thoracic radiographs document biventricular enlargement. The triad of bumps may be replaced by an aneurysmal dilation in the descending aorta and dilated or tortuous pulmonary arteries. The lung fields appear hypovascular, and right ventricular hypertrophy is evident on echocardiographic examination.

Management

The treatment of choice for animals with PDA is early surgical ligation of the ductus, preferably before 4 months of age. The natural history of dogs with uncorrected PDA is poor, with a 60% to 70% mortality rate in the first year of life. Surgery

should be performed by a surgeon experienced with the procedure, since surgical skill is strongly correlated with success.

If congestive heart failure is present, stabilization prior to surgery is required. Medical therapy is similar to that described for mitral regurgitation in Chapter 20, and includes cage rest, a low sodium diet, diuretics, oxygen therapy, vasodilators, and antiarrhythmics as indicated.

When PDA is complicated by pulmonary hypertension and right-to-left shunting, surgical ligation of the ductus is contraindicated. The ductus provides a "pop-off valve," and ligation of the ductus may lead to fatal increases in pulmonary arterial pressure.

Patient Monitoring

Surgical ligation of the PDA in young animals is usually curative. Young animals with secondary mitral insufficiency from mitral valve annulus

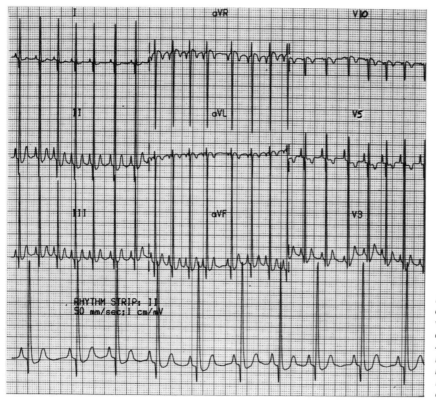

Figure 19–5 Electrocardiogram from a dog with patent ductus arteriosus. A left ventricular enlargement pattern is present with tall R waves in leads II (R wave = 4.5 mV), III, aVF, and V3. Upper leads (I, II, III, aVR, aVL, aVF, V3, V5, and V10) are recorded at 25 mm/sec, 1 cm/1 mV. The lead II rhythm strip at the bottom is recorded at 50 mm/sec and 1 cm/mV.

stretching have the opportunity to "grow into" their mitral valve. A postsurgical murmur of mitral insufficiency is fairly common; these animals should be monitored for regression or progression of the murmur. Animals with long-standing congestive heart failure prior to surgery or surgical correction after 1 year of age may succumb to heart failure. These patients usually require long-term drug therapy and dietary sodium restriction to control the signs of congestive failure. Animals with right-to-left PDA may live comfortably for several months to a few years before developing clinical signs of weakness, right heart failure, respiratory difficulties, or arterial thromboembolism.

PULMONIC STENOSIS

Causes

Pulmonic stenosis may be due to valvular dysplasia, subvalvular stenosis, or, rarely, supravalvular stenosis (Fig. 19-6). Valvular stenosis is most

common in dogs and is recognized by the finding of thickened, malformed valves, which are often fused at the commissures. Bicuspid or single dome-shaped valves with a small orifice are also recognized. The valve annulus may be hypoplastic. Subvalvular stenosis, which may accompany valvular stenosis or occur as an isolated lesion, is manifested as a thick fibrous ridge of tissue below the valve in the right ventricular outflow tract. Both valvular dysplasia and subvalvular pulmonic stenosis can be exacerbated by ventricular myocardial hypertrophy in the infundibular region of the right ventricular outflow tract. Isolated pulmonic stenosis is rare in the cat; however, pulmonic stenosis is observed in combination with other defects, such as tetralogy of Fallot.

Pathophysiology

Normally the right ventricular systolic pressure is equal to the pulmonary arterial systolic pressure. Pulmonic stenosis places resistance on the

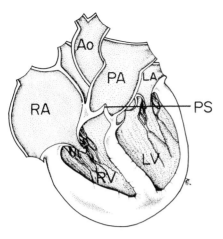

Figure 19–6 *Diagram of valvular pulmonic stenosis (PS). Right ventricular (RV) muscular hypertrophy and poststenotic dilation of the pulmonary artery (PA) are evident. The right atrium (RA) enlarges secondary to tricuspid insufficiency or right ventricular failure. (Ao = aorta; LV = left ventricle) (Allen DG. Congenital cardiac defects. In: Allen DG, Kruth SA, eds. Small animal cardiopulmonary medicine. Philadelphia: BC Decker, 1988: 88.)*

right ventricle such that it must generate pressures greater than normal to maintain cardiac output across the narrowed pulmonary outflow tract. In response to this pressure overload, the right ventricle concentrically hypertrophies to generate the required pressure. Excessive infundibular hypertrophy may result in an additional dynamic obstruction. Secondary right atrial enlargement may develop.

Forward heart failure in pulmonic stenosis occurs when the right ventricle is unable to pump a sufficient volume of blood through the lungs to the left ventricle. The left ventricle is deprived of adequate preload and is unable to increase cardiac output in response to exercise or excitement. Syncope results when the heart fails to maintain adequate blood flow to the brain, and muscular weakness or fatigue occur when the heart is unable to supply working skeletal muscles with sufficient blood (see Chapter 5). While right ventricular myocardial failure may occur with isolated severe stenosis, concurrent volume overload from tricuspid regurgitation or pulmonic valve insufficiency may contribute to the development of right heart failure. Sodium and water are retained in response to inadequate renal perfusion, leading to signs of congestive heart failure.

Clinical Signs

Several breeds of dogs are recognized as being predisposed to pulmonic stenosis, including the English bulldog, schnauzer, beagle, Chihuahua, terrier, cocker spaniel, and Samoyed. Many dogs have a mild degree of pulmonic stenosis, and most of these dogs remain asymptomatic. Dogs with moderate or severe stenosis may be presented for abdominal distention due to right ventricular failure, exercise intolerance, or syncope. Dogs with severe pulmonic stenosis may be stunted in size compared to littermates. In symptomatic dogs, signs typically develop during the first 3 years of life.

Physical examination reveals the presence of a prominent systolic murmur with a point of maximal intensity at the left cardiac base (second or third intercostal space). The murmur is typically a loud, harsh, ejection (crescendo–decrescendo) murmur, and frequently has a thrill. A second murmur of regurgitant quality may be auscultated on the right hemithorax in dogs with tricuspid insufficiency. The cardiac apex beat may be strongest on the right hemithorax. Mucous membrane color and pulse quality at rest are normal in dogs with mild to moderate stenosis; however, those with critical stenosis may have pallor and weak pulse quality, especially after exercise. Signs of right ventricular failure include hepatomegaly, ascites, pleural effusion, and jugular venous distention or pulsation.

Diagnostic Approach

Thoracic radiographs frequently demonstrate some evidence of right ventricular enlargement, with a poststenotic dilation of the main pulmonary artery evident on the ventrodorsal radiographic projection at the 2 o'clock position (Fig. 19-7). Right atrial enlargement may be present, and an enlarged caudal vena cava may be noted if right heart failure is present or imminent. Pulmonary vasculature is usually otherwise normal, although in some cases apparent hypovascularity is noted.

The ECG is often normal with mild stenosis, but electrocardiographic criteria of right ven-

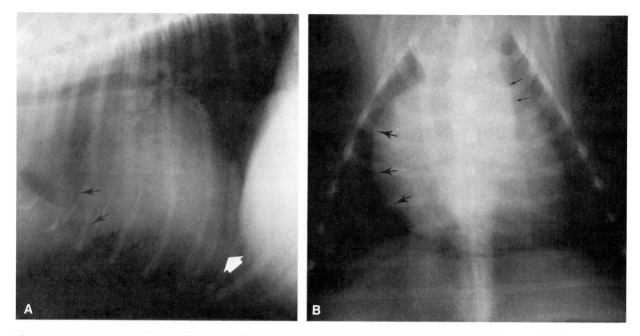

Figure 19–7 *Thoracic radiographs from a 1-year-old male schnauzer with pulmonic stenosis. The lateral view (A) demonstrates right ventricular enlargement with a prominent cranial border of the heart (black arrows), increased sternal contact, and elevation of the apex of the heart from the sternum (white arrow). Right heart enlargement is confirmed on the ventrodorsal projection (B) with the right border of the cardiac silhouette extending further than normal toward the chest wall (large black arrows). A poststenotic dilation of the main pulmonary artery is observed at the 2 o'clock position (small black arrows).*

tricular enlargement or a right axis shift are usually present with more severe pulmonic stenosis (Fig. 19-8). Electrocardiographic evidence of right atrial enlargement (P-pulmonale) is less frequently recorded. Ventricular arrhythmias may occur; supraventricular arrhythmias are more common in dogs with significant right atrial enlargement.

The echocardiogram (see Echocardiography in Chapter 80) reliably identifies compensatory right ventricular hypertrophy, and the poststenotic dilatation of the pulmonary artery can frequently be appreciated. The pulmonary outflow tract may appear narrowed; it is accompanied by thickened valve leaflets or abnormal valve excursion in animals with valvular stenosis. The interventricular septum is hypertrophied and may move toward the right ventricle during systole (paradoxical septal motion). Doppler echocardiography can be used to document turbulent blood flow in the main pulmonary artery, and in

many cases will provide an accurate estimate of the pressure gradient across the pulmonic valve.

Both selective and nonselective angiocardiography (see Nonselective Angiocardiography in Chapter 80) are useful for documentation of right ventricular hypertrophy and poststenotic dilatation. Selective right ventricular angiocardiography is frequently required to differentiate between valvular and subvalvular pulmonic stenosis (Fig. 19-9), especially if the right atrium is enlarged. While the diagnosis can be established in many dogs without selective cardiac catheterization, the severity of the defect (pressure gradient) cannot be documented without catheterization or Doppler echocardiography. Selective cardiac catheterization documents right ventricular systolic hypertension and allows for grading of the severity of disease based on the pressure gradient across the stenosis. Mild pulmonic stenosis in dogs is defined as a gradient of 10 to 50 mmHg; moderate gradients are between 50 and

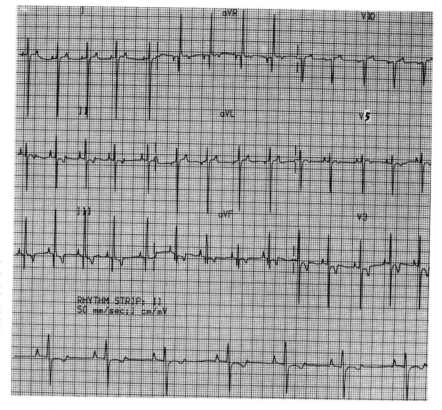

Figure 19–8 *Electrocardiogram obtained from a dog with pulmonic stenosis. A right ventricular enlargement pattern is present, demonstrated by deep S waves in leads I, II, V3, and V5 and a tall R wave in aVR. There is a right axis shift with a mean electrical axis of + 160. The T wave is positive in V10. Upper leads (I, II, III, aVR, aVL, aVF, V3, V5, and V10) are recorded at 25 mm/sec and 1 cm/mV; the lead II rhythm strip at the bottom is recorded at 50 mm/sec and 1 cm/mV.*

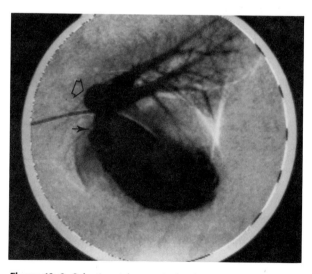

Figure 19–9 *Selective right ventricular digital subtraction angiocardiogram (lateral view) from the same dog in Figure 19–7. Valvular pulmonic stenosis is noted where the dye column is severely narrowed (black arrow). Right ventricular enlargement, mild tricuspid regurgitation, and the poststenotic dilation of the pulmonary artery (open arrow) are also observed.*

100 mmHg, and severe gradients for pulmonic stenosis are those in excess of 100 mmHg. Similar criteria for mild, moderate, or severe pulmonic stenosis in the cat are not available.

Management

Dogs with mild pulmonic stenosis do not require therapy. Animals that have clinical signs and those with moderate to severe stenosis are candidates for balloon valvuloplasty or surgery. Medical therapy is limited to antiarrhythmic drugs, judicious use of diuretics, and a low salt diet to control signs of congestive heart failure.

Balloon valvuloplasty is a relatively new technique that has proven effective in some dogs with valvular pulmonic stenosis. A specially designed catheter with an inflatable balloon is passed through the pulmonic valve such that the center of the balloon is at the site of the valve. The balloon is expanded to tear open the commisures of the valve and relieve the stenosis (Fig. 19-10). Initial results suggest that not all dogs will benefit from the procedure, but the dramatic reduction in the pressure gradient observed in some animals and the decreased risk of balloon valvuloplasty as compared to some surgical techniques makes this an attractive therapeutic option.

Several surgical procedures have been developed, including bistoury and valvotomy techniques to surgically enlarge the pulmonic valve. Patch graft techniques, using either the pericardium or a synthetic patch material, can be used to

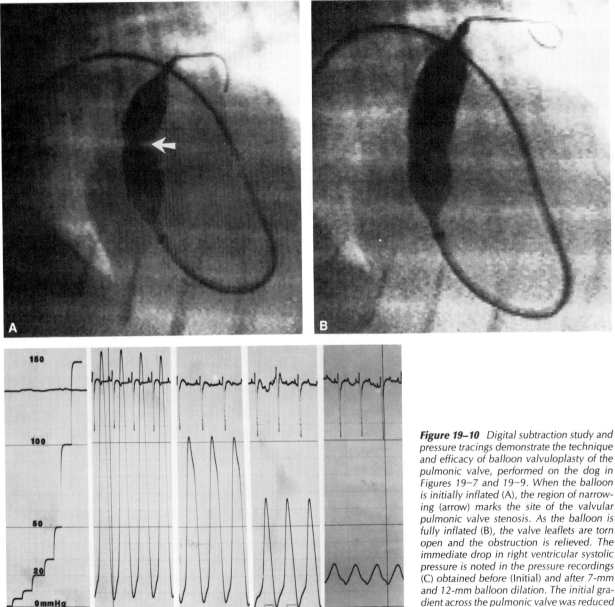

Figure 19–10 *Digital subtraction study and pressure tracings demonstrate the technique and efficacy of balloon valvuloplasty of the pulmonic valve, performed on the dog in Figures 19–7 and 19–9. When the balloon is initially inflated (A), the region of narrowing (arrow) marks the site of the valvular pulmonic valve stenosis. As the balloon is fully inflated (B), the valve leaflets are torn open and the obstruction is relieved. The immediate drop in right ventricular systolic pressure is noted in the pressure recordings (C) obtained before (Initial) and after 7-mm and 12-mm balloon dilation. The initial gradient across the pulmonic valve was reduced from 125 mmHg to 40 mmHg. (PA = pulmonary artery pressure)*

enlarge the entire pulmonic outflow region. The appropriate technique is selected for each animal based on the type and location of the stenosis (valvular, subvalvular, or both). The defect must therefore be fully characterized prior to surgery. Effective surgery results in a significant decrease in the gradient across the pulmonic valve. The efficacy of surgery and the incidence of complications is, in part, dependent on the surgeon's skill.

Patient Monitoring

Dogs with mild pulmonic stenosis are unlikely to suffer debilitation or substantial reduction in life expectancy. Untreated dogs with severe stenosis and clinical signs rarely live beyond 4 years of age. If balloon valvuloplasty or surgery is successful in reducing the pressure gradient to less than 50 mmHg, the animal may be able to lead a nearly normal life. Young animals with mild or moderately severe pulmonic stenosis should be periodically reevaluated, as the severity of the gradient and cardiac lesions may worsen with age.

AORTIC STENOSIS

Causes

Aortic stenosis may result from narrowing at the subvalvular, valvular, or, rarely, supravalvular locations in the aortic outflow tract. Subvalvular aortic stenosis, present in more than 90% of affected dogs, is evident as a deposition of a thick band or ridge of fibrous connective tissue in the aortic outflow tract just below the valve (Fig. 19-11). Valvular stenosis results from valvular dysplasia with thickened or fused leaflets. All forms of aortic stenosis have been observed in the cat, although the defect is less commonly encountered than in the dog. Aortic stenosis has been proven to be transmitted genetically in the Newfoundland dog.

Pathophysiology

Because aortic stenosis causes obstruction to ventricular outflow, the left ventricle must develop a greater than normal systolic pressure to maintain

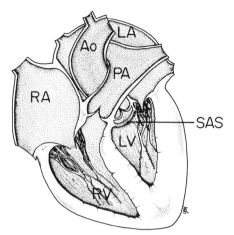

Figure 19–11 Diagram of subvalvular aortic stenosis (SAS). A thick ridge of fibrous tissue is present in the outflow region of the left ventricle (LV). Marked thickening of the left ventricular wall and a poststenotic dilation of the aorta (Ao) accompany the defect. Left atrial (LA) enlargement is present in some cases. (RA = right atrium; RV = right ventricle; PA = pulmonary artery) (Allen DG. Congenital cardiac defects. In: Allen DG, Kruth SA, eds. Small animal cardiopulmonary medicine. Philadelphia: BC Decker, 1988: 89.)

normal stroke volume. Concentric left ventricular hypertrophy results from this pressure overload, and turbulent blood flow, generated by the stenosis, causes a murmur and poststenotic dilation distal to the site of obstruction. With advanced disease and left ventricular failure, the left ventricular end diastolic pressure rises, leading to left atrial enlargement and, eventually, pulmonary edema. Mitral or aortic insufficiency may accompany and complicate aortic stenosis. Cats may be more likely than dogs to develop pulmonary edema.

While left ventricular failure is a potential sequela of aortic stenosis, the more common pathophysiologic problems in dogs result from an inability to increase cardiac output in response to exercise and compromised myocardial perfusion. Aortic stenosis limits the ability of the left ventricle to increase stroke volume in response to increased tissue demands, so increases in cardiac output result largely from increases in heart rate. If the ventricle is unable to meet the increased tissue demands, then muscular weakness, exercise intolerance, or syncope results (see Chapter 5). Ventricular hypertrophy, combined with increased heart rate, results in an increased myocardial oxygen demand. Unfortunately, elevated intraventricular and intramyocardial pressures limit the coronary arterial blood flow during systole, and tachycardia shortens diastole. Thus myocardial oxygen demand increases while coronary artery perfusion decreases, leading to left ventricular endocardial ischemia. Myocardial ischemia leads to myocardial depression, decreased myocardial compliance, and increased risk for arrhythmia. All of these factors may contribute to sudden death, which is occasionally observed in dogs with aortic stenosis.

Clinical Signs

Several breeds of dogs, including German shepherds, boxers, Newfoundlands, golden retrievers, rottweilers, and German shorthair pointers, are predisposed to aortic stenosis. There are no proven breed predispositions for the cat. Many dogs with mild aortic stenosis remain asymptomatic, while dogs with moderate to severe aortic stenosis may remain asymptomatic or may be presented for syncope, weakness, stunted growth, or exercise intolerance. Signs may be progressive. If left ventricular failure occurs, dyspnea and cough may be noted. One of the most common sequelae of aortic stenosis in dogs is sudden death during a period of physical exertion or excitement, most likely caused by an arrhythmia resulting from subendocardial ischemia.

Physical examination reveals the presence of a systolic ejection (crescendo–decrescendo) murmur, which is often easily auscultated on both sides of the thorax. The point of maximal intensity is typically at the left heart base, usually at the third or fourth intercostal space. The murmur may be equally loud at the right heart base, and may radiate to the thoracic inlet and up the carotid arteries. A thrill often accompanies loud murmurs, and a prominent left apical impulse may be noted on precordial palpation. Femoral pulses in severely affected animals are weak and are described as slow-rising. Left heart failure, when present, causes tachypnea, dyspnea, and pulmonary crackles. Arrhythmias and pulse deficits are noted in some animals.

Diagnostic Approach

Thoracic radiographs may demonstrate left ventricular enlargement, but the concentric nature of the hypertrophy can be difficult to detect radiographically. The poststenotic dilatation of the aorta is, however, a frequent radiographic finding, and appears as an increased density cranial to the heart on both lateral and ventrodorsal projections (Fig. 19-12). In advanced cases, left atrial enlargement and evidence of congestive heart failure may be observed.

Electrocardiographic findings with aortic stenosis vary with the severity of the stenosis; the ECG is normal in mild cases. Increased QRS amplitude or duration reflect left ventricular enlargement. Abnormalities in the ST segment or T wave may be noted; significant ST segment depression is suggestive of myocardial ischemia. An ECG following provocative exercise testing that demonstrates ST segment depression or ventricular arrhythmias is compatible with exertional myocardial ischemia, which may result in episodic weakness and be a harbinger of sudden death.

The echocardiogram is useful in demonstration of both valvular and subvalvular aortic stenosis. Poststenotic dilation of the aorta, left ventricular hypertrophy, and a small left ventricular end-systolic cavity are supportive of the diagnosis. Two-dimensional echocardiography may demonstrate an echodense ridge or band of tissue in the left ventricular outflow tract in dogs with subvalvular stenosis, or abnormal valvular anatomy or motion in the case of valvular stenosis. Doppler echocardiography can be used to demonstrate turbulent blood flow in the ascending aorta and to estimate the pressure gradient across the aortic valve.

Cardiac catheterization, with measurement of the pressure gradient across the aortic valve, is still the best method to determine the hemodynamic severity of the lesion. Mild stenosis is defined by a gradient of 10 to 40 mmHg, moderate stenosis by a 40 to 80 mmHg gradient, and severe stenosis by a gradient in excess of 80 mmHg. Dogs with minor pathologic changes and corresponding soft murmurs may not have a measurable gradient across the stenosis during anesthesia.

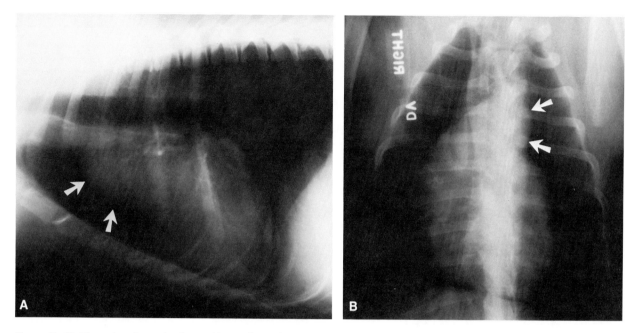

Figure 19-12 *Thoracic radiographs obtained from a dog with aortic stenosis. A marked poststenotic dilation of the aorta (arrows) is observed cranial to the heart on both the lateral (A) and dorsoventral (B) views. The left ventricular hypertrophy is concentric and is not radiographically apparent in every case.*

Selective angiocardiography documents the valvular and subvalvular anatomy, left ventricular hypertrophy, and poststenotic dilation. A supravalvular contrast injection is frequently performed to check for aortic insufficiency.

Management

Due to the high incidence of complications, a high surgical mortality, and the need for cardiopulmonary bypass techniques, surgical correction of subaortic stenosis has been little used. Animals that are candidates for surgical therapy are those with remarkable clinical signs, severe arrhythmias, and electrocardiographic evidence of ischemia, and those with gradients in excess of 80 mmHg that are thought to be at risk for sudden death.

Balloon valvuloplasty is of questionable value in dogs with subvalvular aortic stenosis, as the balloon appears to be incapable of consistently stretching the fibrous tissue ring. This technique may prove to be useful in animals with isolated valvular aortic stenosis. Propranolol or other β-blockers have been used to reduce the myocardial oxygen demand and diminish the risk of arrhythmic death. It is unknown whether β-blockers actually reduce the risk of sudden death or disease progression, but their use is probably indicated in dogs with severe stenosis or ventricular arrhythmias. If ventricular arrhythmias are not effectively controlled with β-blockers, other ventricular antiarrhythmics should be added (*e.g.*, procainamide, quinidine). Because positive inotropes (*e.g.*, digitalis, dobutamine) may exacerbate dysfunction associated with subvalvular stenosis and increase myocardial oxygen demand, and because vasodilators may cause hypotension, both types of drugs are generally contraindicated.

Patient Monitoring

Dogs with mild aortic stenosis (gradient less than 40 mmHg) usually remain asymptomatic and do not require therapy. Dogs with moderate stenosis may live for several years, or may die suddenly. Periodic reevaluations should be performed in these animals to monitor radiographic progression, arrhythmias, and ST segment abnormalities. Dogs with severe stenosis may die suddenly or may develop congestive heart failure, the latter being most common in dogs with concurrent aortic insufficiency, mitral insufficiency, or atrial fibrillation. Aortic stenosis may predispose dogs to aortic valve endocarditis, therefore prophylactic antibiotics (*e.g.*, penicillin for dental procedures, ampicillin and gentamicin for genitourinary or gastrointestinal surgery) are indicated for procedures associated with bacteremia. Cats with aortic stenosis frequently develop heart failure or sudden death, and many die before reaching 1 year of age.

VENTRICULAR SEPTAL DEFECT

Causes

A ventricular septal defect (VSD) results from malformation of the interventricular septum and allows communication between the left and right ventricles (Fig. 19-13). A VSD may occur anywhere in the interventricular septum, although the most common site is in the membranous portion below the aortic valve, under the septal tricuspid leaflet. Defects are found less frequently in the lower muscular portion of the septum. A VSD may occur alone or in combination with other congenital defects, such as tetralogy of Fallot or the endocardial cushion defect. The endocardial cushion defect is comprised of a high VSD, a low (ostium primum) atrial septal defect, and an abnormally developed mitral or tricuspid valve.

Pathophysiology

The hemodynamic consequences of a VSD depend on the size of the defect and the pulmonary vascular resistance. Small defects usually result in minimal hemodynamic changes; therefore, clinical signs are usually observed only in animals with large defects. In most circumstances, the left ventricular systolic pressure exceeds that

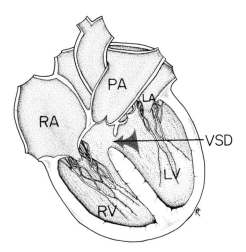

Figure 19–13 *Diagram of a ventricular septal defect (VSD). The arrow indicates the direction of blood flow through the defect with a left-to-right shunting VSD. Left atrial (LA) enlargement, left ventricular (LV) or biventricular enlargement, and dilation of the main pulmonary artery (PA) segment may occur with a VSD of significant size. (RV = right ventricle; RA = right atrium) (Allen DG. Congenital cardiac defects. In: Allen DG, Kruth SA, eds. Small animal cardiopulmonary medicine. Philadelphia: BC Decker, 1988: 91.)*

of the right, producing a left-to-right shunt. Because most VSDs are located high in the ventricular septum, the shunted blood is ejected directly into the right ventricular outflow tract. This results in overcirculation of blood in the pulmonary vasculature, left atrium, and left ventricle, with minimal hypertrophy of the right ventricle. The left ventricle hypertrophies eccentrically to accommodate the volume overload. Congestive heart failure results when the left ventricle is unable to accommodate this increased blood volume. Dogs with large VSDs and heart failure usually develop pulmonary edema, while cats are more prone to the development of biventricular failure with pulmonary edema, pleural effusion, and, less frequently, ascites. In some animals, the missing septal tissue may include the supporting structure for one of the aortic valve leaflets, leading to aortic insufficiency and deleterious additional volume overload to the left ventricle.

If the VSD is very large, the ventricular systolic pressures tend to equilibrate, right ventricular hypertrophy ensues, and the pulmonary vasculature is subjected to high pressures and increased blood volume, which may contribute to the development of pulmonary hypertension. If the right ventricular pressure equals or exceeds the pressure in the left ventricle, then bidirectional blood flow or right-to-left shunting will occur. Pulmonary hypertension with a right-to-left shunting VSD is called Eisenmenger's syndrome. Blood flowing from right to left results in systemic arterial oxygen desaturation, cyanosis, and polycythemia. Neurologic abnormalities (depression, focal neurologic deficits, or seizures) may result from cerebrovascular accidents or brain abscess caused by paradoxical embolism (venous thrombi or bacteria not filtered by the lung), or from severe polycythemia.

Clinical Signs

Ventricular septal defect is one of the most common congenital heart defects in cats, occurring either as an isolated defect or as a component of the endocardial cushion defect. While VSD is also a common canine congenital cardiac defect, the only breeds thought to be at increased risk are keeshonds and English bulldogs.

Presenting complaints with left-to-right VSD depend on the severity of the accompanying hemodynamic changes. Small defects rarely result in clinical signs other than a murmur, while animals with larger VSDs and congestive heart failure may present for weakness, coughing, and respiratory distress. Dogs with pulmonary hypertension and Eisenmenger's syndrome are typically presented for exercise intolerance, episodes of weakness, syncope, or seizures.

The typical cardiac murmur is a harsh, holosystolic murmur auscultated loudest at the right cranial sternal border. The murmur is quite variable in character, and may be described as plateau, crescendo, or crescendo–decrescendo. Other murmurs may be present, including a flow murmur of relative pulmonic stenosis, produced when a large volume of shunted blood is pumped across a normal pulmonic valve. Animals with endocardial cushion defect may also have murmurs of mitral or tricuspid insufficiency. If VSD is complicated by aortic insufficiency, a diastolic murmur may be auscultated. In animals with a right-to-left or bidirectional shunting VSD, the murmur may be soft or absent and the second heart sound may be loud or split.

Arterial pulses are usually normal, but tend to be brisk with large defects and weak with congestive heart failure. Jugular venous distention or pulsation are usually absent, unless VSD is complicated by pulmonary hypertension or biventricular failure. Cyanosis is usually present in cases of right-to-left shunting and may be exacerbated with exercise.

Diagnostic Approach

Thoracic radiographs are often normal, but may demonstrate left atrial and ventricular enlargement, pulmonary overcirculation, and variable right ventricular enlargement. Pulmonary edema is observed in cases with congestive heart failure. Right ventricular enlargement with enlarged, tortuous pulmonary arteries is a common radiographic finding in animals with pulmonary hypertension and right-to-left shunting.

The ECG is normal with small ventricular septal defects, while animals with larger defects may have electrocardiographic evidence of left atrial or ventricular enlargement. Additional electrocardiographic abnormalities reported from animals with VSD include conduction disturbances such as right bundle branch block and ventricular or supraventricular arrhythmias. Electrocardiographic criteria for right ventricular enlargement are usually present only in those animals with pulmonary hypertension or very large defects.

Typical echocardiographic findings include left atrial enlargement and a hyperdynamic, dilated left ventricle. When the VSD is large enough (usually 1 cm or greater) it can be visualized as an echolucent region in the ventricular septum, usually just below the aortic valve (Fig. 19-14). Contrast echocardiography (bubble study) can be performed, using intravenous saline injection to demonstrate bidirection or right-to-left shunting. Doppler studies can be used to confirm and identify the direction of blood flow through the defect.

Selective cardiac catheterization is indicated if the diagnosis is in question after initial diagnostic tests, if pulmonary hypertension is suspected,

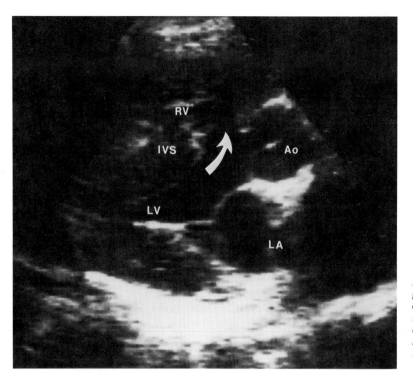

Figure 19–14 *Two-dimensional echocardiogram from a dog with a large ventricular septal defect (VSD) in the typical position, high in the interventricular septum. The white arrow indicates the site and direction of blood flow through a left-to-right VSD. (RV = right ventricular cavity; LV = left ventricular cavity; Ao = aorta; LA = left atrium; IVS = interventricular septum)*

or if surgical therapy is being considered as a therapeutic option. Selective angiography is useful to confirm the diagnosis, demonstrate the direction of shunting, and establish the functional integrity of the aortic valve. Oximetry data, obtained during cardiac catheterization, can be used to calculate the magnitude of the shunt. The size of the shunt is usually expressed as a ratio of the blood flowing through the pulmonary and systemic circulations. If the flow through the pulmonary circuit is greater than or equal to 2.5 times the systemic circulation, the animal is at risk of developing pulmonary vascular disease or heart failure, and surgical therapy is recommended.

Management

Animals that are asymptomatic, have minimal cardiomegaly and no evidence of congestive heart failure, or have pulmonary blood flow less than two times the systemic flow probably do not require surgical therapy. Those that have clinical signs of failure may respond well to symptomatic medical therapy with low sodium diets, diuretics, and arterial vasodilators. Therapeutic options in animals with right-to-left shunts are limited to exercise restriction, periodic phlebotomy to keep the hematocrit below 60% (0.60 L/L) if neurologic signs are manifest, and low-dose aspirin therapy (5–7 mg/kg/day orally) to reduce the risk of systemic thromboembolism.

Surgical therapy should be considered if clinical signs are present or if shunt flow is great. Such treatment may involve palliative surgery or anatomic correction of the defect. Anatomic closure of a VSD requires open heart surgery, which is not feasible at most institutions because of the cost of maintaining needed equipment and personnel. Pulmonary artery banding, a palliative technique, increases pulmonary vascular resistance, decreasing the magnitude of the left-to-right shunt. If the pulmonary artery band is applied too tightly or if the animal outgrows the band, then right-to-left shunting may result. Surgical therapy is not indicated for dogs with pulmonary hypertension and right-to-left shunting.

Patient Monitoring

The natural history of animals with VSD depends on the severity of hemodynamic alterations. Dogs and cats with small defects remain asymptomatic and live normal lives. In fact, in some animals with small defects, especially of the muscular septum, spontaneous closure of the defect may occur during the first 2 years of life. Asymptomatic animals should be reevaluated on a yearly basis for progression of cardiac enlargement or development of congestive failure. Animals with large defects often develop signs of congestive heart failure during the first 18 months of life. Patients with pulmonary hypertension and right-to-left shunting have a poor prognosis for long-term survival.

ATRIAL SEPTAL DEFECT

Causes

Malformation of the atrial septum permits abnormal blood flow between the left and right atria. The ostium primum defect results from failure of formation of atrial tissue low in the atrial septum. Ostium primum defects are limited ventrally by the ventricular septum or annulus of the atrioventricular valves. The ostium secundum defect (high atrial septal defect [ASD]) is located in the middle of the atrial septum and results from failure of normal septation at the site of the oval fossa of heart. Isolated ASDs are uncommon in dogs and cats, and are observed more frequently in association with other congenital heart defects, such as endocardial cushion defect, pulmonic stenosis, and tricuspid dysplasia.

Pathophysiology

The ostium primum and ostium secundum defects, located in different positions and probably resulting from different embryologic mechanisms, have similar pathophysiologic consequences. If the remainder of the cardiovascular structures are normal, then left atrial pressures exceed right atrial pressures and blood is shunted from the left atrium, through the defect, to the right atrium. Blood flow is increased through the circuit formed by the right atrium, right ventricle, pulmonary vasculature, and left atrium. Animals with small defects are unlikely to develop clinical signs. The magnitude of the shunt depends on the size of the defect and the diastolic compliance of each ventricle. Because ASD places a volume overload on the right heart, large defects result in right atrial and ventricular dilation.

Accompanying pulmonic stenosis, tricuspid dysplasia, or right ventricular failure may produce elevation of the right atrial pressure. These conditions may lead to reversal of the direction of the shunt. As deoxygenated blood flows from the right atrium to the left atrium, systemic arterial oxygen desaturation results. In contrast to VSD and PDA, ASDs rarely result in obstructive pulmonary vascular disease and pulmonary hypertension in dogs and cats. Atrial septal defect is also observed as a component of the endocardial cushion defect.

Clinical Signs

The breeds recognized as being predisposed to ASDs include boxers, Samoyeds, Doberman pinschers, and Old English sheepdogs. Atrial septal defects rarely lead to clinical signs; however, large ASDs result in exercise intolerance, respiratory distress, or syncope, and may predispose animals to lower respiratory tract infections. When ASD is present in combination with conditions that produce right-to-left shunting, cyanosis, weakness, and arterial thromboembolism may be observed.

There is no murmur generated by the flow of blood through an ASD. If the defect is large, murmurs of relative tricuspid stenosis or relative pulmonic stenosis may be auscultated. The murmur of tricuspid stenosis is a low-intensity, rumbling diastolic murmur. The systolic flow murmur of relative pulmonic stenosis (increased blood flow across a normal pulmonic valve) is heard at the left heart base over the pulmonic valve. Fixed splitting of the second heart sound is a classic auscultatory finding with ASD.

Diagnostic Approach

Thoracic radiographs are usually normal with small, isolated ASD, while larger defects are associated with enlargement of the right atrium and ventricle, pulmonary overcirculation, and variable degrees of left atrial enlargement. The ECG is usually normal, although a right ventricular enlargement pattern may occur in large shunts.

The most useful noninvasive diagnostic technique for ASD is echocardiography. If the defect is sufficiently large, an echolucent space will be visualized in the atrial septum. Several echocardiographic planes should be used to document the presence of the ASD, as "dropout" of the atrial septum can be observed as an artifact in normal animals. Contrast or Doppler echocardiography may be useful in documenting right-to-left or bidirectional blood flow across the atrial septum.

Cardiac catheterization is the most reliable method for documentation of the presence of ASD. Oximetry data will document the presence, direction, and magnitude of shunt flow, while selective angiocardiographic studies from pulmonary arterial injections or after passage of the catheter through the defect will also demonstrate the ASD and the direction of blood flow.

Management

Most dogs with ASD remain asymptomatic and require no specific therapy. Dogs with signs of congestive heart failure can be managed with medical therapy, including exercise restriction, low sodium diets, diuretics, and, potentially, vasodilators. Surgical correction of the ASD usually requires cardiopulmonary bypass techniques. Palliative procedures such as pulmonary artery banding may lead to elevation of right atrial pressure and cause reversal of blood flow. If right-to-left shunting is present, aspirin therapy may be indicated to reduce the risk of thromboembolic disease.

Patient Monitoring

The majority of dogs with small ASDs remain asymptomatic. In fact, in many animals with a small ASD the malformation goes unrecognized. Animals with very large defects may develop heart failure within the first few years of life. When ASD is present in association with other defects, the degree of hemodynamic disturbance caused by the combination of the two defects will determine the clinical course.

ATRIOVENTRICULAR VALVE MALFORMATIONS

Causes

Congenital mitral and tricuspid malformations may result in insufficiency, stenosis, or both. Atrioventricular valvular insufficiency is the most common sequela to malformation. Valve leaflets may be thickened or fused, and abnormal (short and thick or long and thin) chordae tendineae may be observed. In addition, the papillary muscles may be malpositioned, incompletely developed, or absent; malpositioning of the papillary muscles on the ventricular wall has been frequently described.

Pathophysiology

Atrioventricular valvular insufficiency places a volume overload on the affected ventricle. The pathophysiology of congestive heart failure with congenital atrioventricular insufficiency is similar to that described for acquired chronic valvular disease (see Chapter 20). With each beat, the ventricle must eject blood forward through the semilunar valve. This is in addition to the volume of blood ejected backward through the malformed atrioventricular valve. If the mitral valve is affected, the left ventricle will hypertrophy in an eccentric fashion and the left atrium will be dilated. Left ventricular failure due to mitral valve malformation leads to pulmonary edema. Tricuspid dysplasia will result in right ventricular eccentric hypertrophy, and often in dramatic increases in right atrial size. When tricuspid dysplasia causes right heart failure, the animal may develop ascites or pleural effusion.

Animals with atrioventricular valve stenosis have impaired ventricular filling, with the potential for elevations in atrial pressures and congestive heart failure. Severe atrial dilation can result from either valvular insufficiency or stenosis, predisposing to atrial arrhythmias. Atrial tachyarrhythmias, which shorten diastole and the time available for ventricular filling, are particularly detrimental to animals with atrioventricular valve stenosis.

Clinical Signs

Mitral and tricuspid valve dysplasia have been suggested as the most common congenital cardiac defects in the cat. Large-breed dogs, especially the Great Dane, German shepherd, Labrador retriever, and weimaraner, may be predisposed to atrioventricular valve dysplasia.

Dogs with atrioventricular valve dysplasia often develop clinical signs at an early age, including weight loss, exercise intolerance, dyspnea, or coughing. Tricuspid dysplasia may lead to abdominal distention from ascites, or dyspnea from pleural effusion. Episodic weakness or syncope may result from cardiac arrhythmias with disease of either valve. While some cats are severely affected at a young age, a few cats live for many years with no evidence of cardiac dysfunction. These cats likely have less severe malformations.

It is likely that some adult cats with mitral valve murmurs actually have congenital mitral valve malformation. Cats with mitral valve malformation may develop pulmonary edema or biventricular failure, as well as systemic arterial embolism.

Physical examination usually reveals a pansystolic murmur over the affected valve. Animals with mitral dysplasia have typical left apical regurgitant murmurs that may radiate dorsally toward the mitral valve. Dyspnea, tachypnea, and pulmonary crackles are present in animals with congestive heart failure. In dogs with tricuspid dysplasia, the murmur is loudest on the right hemithorax over the third to fifth intercostal space. Jugular distention or pulsations, as well as hepatomegaly or ascites, are frequently observed.

Diagnostic Approach

Animals with mitral insufficiency have radiographic evidence of left atrial and ventricular enlargement (Fig. 19-15). Pulmonary venous distention and pulmonary edema are observed with heart failure in the dog; cats tend to develop biventricular failure. Electrocardiographic find-

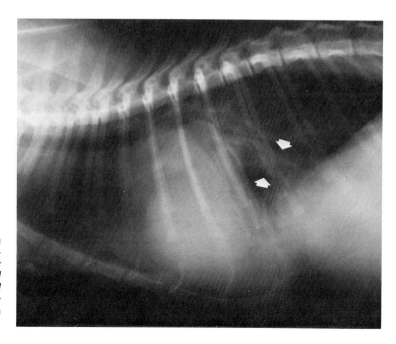

Figure 19–15 Thoracic radiograph from a 6-month-old cat with mitral and tricuspid valve dysplasia. The lateral view demonstrates left ventricular enlargement, severe left atrial enlargement, and marked tracheal elevation. This cat had developed biventricular failure, evidenced by both pulmonary edema and an enlarged caudal vena cava (arrows) and hepatomegaly.

ings may include P-mitrale, left ventricular enlargement pattern, and supraventricular arrhythmias. The abnormal morphology of the mitral valve leaflets, chordae tendineae, or papillary muscles, or left atrial and ventricular enlargement may be appreciated with echocardiography. Angiocardiography or Doppler studies are employed to document atrioventricular valvular regurgitation.

Tricuspid dysplasia results in right ventricular enlargement; it may cause severe right atrial enlargement, enlarged caudal vena cava, hepatomegaly, ascites, and pleural effusion. The ECG frequently demonstrates right ventricular or right atrial enlargement patterns in dogs. The abnormal tricuspid valve apparatus, as well as right atrial and right ventricular enlargement, can often be visualized by two-dimensional echocardiography. Cardiac catheterization will reveal normal oximetry, elevated right atrial pressures, and tricuspid regurgitation on selective right ventricular angiocardiography.

Management

Animals with atrioventricular valve malformations are usually managed with medical therapy alone (see Chapter 20). Exercise restriction, low sodium diets, diuretics, digitalis, and vasodilators can all be employed to treat the heart failure. Arterial vasodilators may be particularly helpful in mitral dysplasia, in which they are thought to reduce the degree of mitral regurgitation and increase forward blood flow. Digitalis is usually employed in animals that are refractory to diuretics and vasodilators, that appear, by echocardiography, to have diminished myocardial function, or that have atrial tachyarrhythmias. Additional antiarrhythmics should be employed as needed.

Patient Monitoring

Animals without congestive heart failure and with minimal cardiomegaly, especially cats, may lead a nearly normal life, free of disease for several years. These animals should be reevaluated at least on a yearly basis to monitor for disease progression. The prognosis for animals with congestive heart failure is guarded, although some animals can be effectively managed with medical therapy. In spite of this, the disease is usually progressive, and survival longer than a few years is uncommon.

TETRALOGY OF FALLOT

Causes

Tetralogy of Fallot is defined as a cardiac defect with four pathologic findings:

1. Pulmonic stenosis
2. A high VSD
3. Dextroposition of the aorta such that it overrides the interventricular septum
4. Secondary right ventricular hypertrophy (Fig. 19-16).

A genetic predisposition for a spectrum of conotruncal abnormalities, including tetralogy of

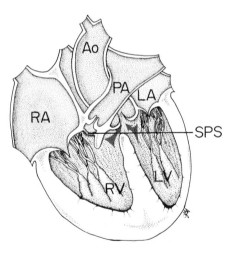

Figure 19-16 *Diagram of tetralogy of Fallot. Right ventricular (RV) hypertrophy, valvular and subvalvular pulmonic stenosis (SPS), a ventricular septal defect, and a dextropositioned aorta (Ao) that overrides both ventricles comprise the defect in this figure. Arrows indicate that the aorta receives blood flow from both the left and right ventricles. The pulmonary artery (PA), because it receives less blood, is smaller than normal. (RA = right atrium; LV = left ventricle; LA = left atrium) (Allen DG. Congenital cardiac defects. In: Allen DG, Kruth SA, eds. Small animal cardiopulmonary medicine. Philadelphia: BC Decker, 1988: 93.)*

Fallot, has been documented in the keeshond breed. The English bulldog is also predisposed.

Pathophysiology

The obstruction to pulmonary outflow forces the right ventricle to develop increased systolic pressures. Blood typically shunts from right to left at the level of the VSD, and, in addition, the overriding aorta receives blood from both ventricles. Resultant arterial oxygen desaturation leads to cyanosis and increases in red blood cell mass. Clinical signs usually result from arrhythmias, systemic hypoxemia, or complications of polycythemia. Hypoxemia results in exercise intolerance and dyspnea, while polycythemia can produce hyperviscosity and red blood cell sludging in small vessels and may lead to cerebrovascular accident. An additional sequela of tetralogy of Fallot is systemic embolism, because thrombi, normally filtered by the lungs, freely cross the VSD to the systemic circulation. Congestive heart failure is uncommon in animals with tetralogy of Fallot.

Clinical Signs

Tetralogy of Fallot is a relatively common defect in the cat. Affected dogs and cats may be presented for exertional weakness or dyspnea, cyanosis, stunting, or syncope. Most animals are cyanotic at the time of examination, and the cyanosis may worsen with exercise or excitement. A murmur of pulmonic stenosis is heard best at the left heart base, and a second murmur (VSD), is loudest at the right cranial sternal border. The murmurs may be attenuated in animals with polycythemia, severe pulmonic stenosis, or minimal blood flow through the VSD.

Diagnostic Approach

Thoracic radiography may demonstrate right ventricular hypertrophy; however, some animals with tetralogy of Fallot have nearly normal cardiac size radiographically. Pulmonary undercir-

culation, evident by decreased vascular marking, and a poststenotic dilatation of the main pulmonary artery may be observed. In other animals, the main pulmonary artery remains small, compatible with pulmonary undercirculation. Evidence of right ventricular failure (*e.g.*, pleural effusion, ascites) is typically absent. Most cyanotic animals with tetralogy of Fallot have electrocardiographic evidence of right ventricular enlargement.

Polycythemia is a common finding in animals with tetralogy of Fallot; the hematocrit may be higher than 75% (0.75 L/L) in some animals. Blood gas analysis documents hypoxemia.

The echocardiogram can be very useful in documenting tetralogy of Fallot. The VSD is typically evident high on the septum, just below the aortic valve; right ventricular hypertrophy and abnormalities in the pulmonic valve or pulmonary outflow tract may also be imaged. Dextroposition of the aorta is difficult to appreciate in some cases. Contrast echocardiography will demonstrate right-to-left blood flow across the VSD with the appearance of microbubbles in the ascending aorta. Cardiac catheterization is required in some animals to rule out Eisenmenger's syndrome (pulmonary hypertension) and other complex cardiovascular malformations. Cardiac catheterization is definitely indicated if surgical therapy is contemplated.

Management

Animals that are not cyanotic and that have mild pulmonic stenosis may be managed conservatively. Low-dose aspirin therapy is indicated in all patients to reduce the likelihood of venous-to-arterial thromboembolism. Polycythemia, present in more severely affected animals, increases the risk of thromboembolism and can result in compromised cerebral perfusion due to increased blood viscosity. Periodic phlebotomy is indicated in polycythemic animals to maintain a hematocrit near 60% (0.60 L/L). β-Blockers (*e.g.*, propranolol) are advocated in animals with tetralogy of Fallot for several reasons. Nonselective β-blockade decreases heart rate and myocardial contractility. The latter may diminish additional pulmonary outflow obstruction posed by infundibular hypertrophy. Additionally, nonselective β-blockers increase systemic vascular resistance, which decreases right-to-left shunting.

Surgical therapy is indicated in most cyanotic animals; however, it is difficult and requires performance of a cardiopulmonary bypass. Several palliative surgical procedures appear to be useful. They involve anastomosis of a systemic artery (either the aorta or a subclavian artery) to the pulmonary artery, thereby increasing pulmonary blood flow.

Patient Monitoring

Acyanotic animals with mild pulmonic stenosis should be frequently reevaluated for disease progression, including hypoxemia, arrhythmias, pulmonary hypertension, and polycythemia. Periodic reevaluation and phlebotomy is often required in polycythemic patients. Animals that have had successful surgical palliative procedures may remain comfortable for several years. Cyanotic animals with clinical signs of disease that do not have surgery have a guarded to poor prognosis. Most die by 2 years of age.

ADDITIONAL CARDIOVASCULAR DEFECTS

Many other congenital defects have been reported in dogs and cats. Some of these defects are combinations or variations of the above cardiovascular malformations, whereas others involve malposition of the great vessels or failure in development of cardiac chambers. These defects are frequently referred to as *complex congenital defects*. It is likely that many complex congenital cardiac defects in animals are lethal within the first few hours of life, and go unrecognized. In addition to combinations of the above defects, a few other malformations of the heart and great vessels are observed in companion animals, including endocardial fibroelastosis and vascular ring anomalies.

Endocardial fibroelastosis has been reported as a congenital disease in Burmese and Siamese cats. Typical findings with endocardial fibroelastosis are dilation of the left atrium and left ventricle, with dramatic thickening of the endocardium. Grossly, the endocardium is diffusely white in color and firm to the touch. Affected animals develop congestive heart failure, usually accompanied by pulmonary edema, by 2 to 4 months of age. The prognosis for survival is poor.

A large number of vascular ring anomalies have been reported in dogs and cats. Vascular ring anomalies result from abnormal embryologic development of the aortic arches. Associated clinical signs are referable to the gastrointestinal tract, and include regurgitation.

ADDITIONAL READINGS

Bonagura, JD. Congenital heart disease. In: Ettinger SJ, ed. Textbook of veterinary internal medicine. Philadelphia: WB Saunders, 1989: 976.

Bright J, Jennings J. Percutaneous balloon valvuloplasty for treatment of pulmonic stenosis in a dog. J Am Vet Med Assoc 1987; 191:995.

Fingland R, Bonagura J. Pulmonic stensis in the dog: 29 cases (1975–1984). J Am Vet Med Assoc 1986; 189:218.

Fox PR. Congenital feline heart disease. In: Fox PR, ed. Canine and feline cardiology. New York: Churchill Livingstone, 1988: 391.

Levitt L, Fowler JD, Schuh JCL. Aortic stenosis in the dog: A review of 12 cases. Journal of the American Animal Hospital Association 1989; 25:357.

Olivier NB. Congenital heart disease in dogs. In: Fox PR, ed. Canine and feline cardiology. New York: Churchill Livingstone, 1988: 357.

Ringwald RJ, Bonagura JD. Tetralogy of Fallot in the dog: Clinical findings in 13 cases. Journal of the American Animal Hospital Association 1988; 24:33.

20

ATRIOVENTRICULAR VALVULAR INSUFFICIENCY

Clarke E. Atkins

Acquired insufficiency or incompetence of the heart valves represents an important group of acquired canine cardiac disorders. Valve anatomy and function can be affected directly or indirectly by a variety of diseases, including parasitic (heartworm disease), neoplastic (intracardiac tumors), degenerative (endocardiosis and cardiomyopathy), traumatic, and inflammatory (vegetative endocarditis) disorders, which may produce incompetence. Endocardiosis, particularly in the small breeds, is the most prevalent and clinically significant of these disorders. Although endocardiosis may affect any of the cardiac valves, the atrioventricular valves are those typically involved. Mitral valvular endocardiosis and insufficiency is most commonly encountered, frequently leading to clinically apparent dysfunction and heart failure.

Although the cat can be affected with acquired atrioventricular valvular incompetence, this appears to be an infrequent cause of heart failure in the adult cat. Signs and therapy are similar to those of the dog and, hence, no specific discussion of the cat will be presented here. For a more in-depth discussion of this disease in the cat, see the Additional Reading section.

CAUSES

Valvular endocardiosis (myxomatosis, fibrosis, or chronic valvular disease) is of unknown etiology. It is known to affect males more often than females (1.5 : 1), to predominantly affect small and toy breeds, and to progress with advancing age. A similar degenerative process in human heart valves is thought to be due to a primary defect in collagen production (dyscollagenosis). In a survey of canine necropsy specimens, Buchanan (Additional Reading) showed that the mitral valve was affected alone in 62% of cases, and together with the tricuspid valve in 33% of cases; the tricuspid valve was affected alone in only 1% of cases. Murmurs of chronic valvular disease are recognized in 10% of middle-aged dogs, increasing to approximately 33% in aged dogs. Although heart murmurs of mitral insufficiency may be apparent in the middle years, florid left or biventricular failure is unusual before the age of 8 to 10 years.

This degenerative process begins with the formation of mucopolysaccharide (glycosaminoglycan) in the subendothelial portion of the valve leaflets. Initially, this produces valvular thicken-

251

ing with discrete nodules and opacities. With progression, the affected valve becomes irregularly thickened, with coalescence of the lesions producing large, plaquelike nodules. In time, the valves become grossly distorted with contracture of valve cusps; this deformity is further complicated as the free edge of the valve cusp rolls toward the mural attachment (Fig. 20-1). Histologically, affected valves show mucopolysaccharide deposition, edema, hemorrhage, fibrosis, and calcification. There is no inflammatory component to this condition. The chorda tendineae cordis are likewise affected, becoming thickened, lengthened, and fragile. In long-standing cases, the ventricular myocardium, particularly the papillary muscles, is affected with arteriosclerosis of small (intramural) coronary arteries, and areas of resultant myocardial necrosis and fibrosis are demonstrable.

PATHOPHYSIOLOGY

The mitral valve apparatus is made up of a group of interdependent structures, including the mitral valve leaflets with their fibrous point of attachment and fulcrum (the mitral valve annulus); the chordae tendineae, which hold valve leaflets in apposition, preventing eversion; the left atrium; and the left ventricular wall and papillary muscles. The ultimate result of the degenera-

tive process described above is stiff, deformed valve leaflets, which, because of thickening and contracture, fail to coapt normally, resulting in systolic regurgitation of blood through the incompetent valve. The amount of regurgitant flow is small early in the course of the disease, but, as the disease progresses, an increasing percentage of cardiac output is ejected into the left atrium. Effective (forward) cardiac output falls, left atrial pressure rises, and the left atrium and mitral valve annulus enlarge. This distortion of the left atrium and mitral valve annulus, along with the described changes in the chordae tendineae, potentiate existing valve leaflet dysfunction, increasing the size of the mitral valve orifice and regurgitant fraction, and further reducing forward (aortic) cardiac output. With the drop in forward cardiac output, neurohumoral compensatory mechanisms cause fluid retention and peripheral vasoconstriction. While helping to maintain cardiac output and blood pressure early on, these processes ultimately increase afterload (resistance of ventricular emptying), cardiovascular volume (thereby producing signs of congestion), and cardiac work. Thus, a vicious cycle begins, with mitral insufficiency resulting in cardiovascular abnormalities and adaptations, which lead to further mitral regurgitation. The resultant chronic volume overload is not well tolerated by the left ventricle. In some cases, cardiac output is further lowered with the development of dimin-

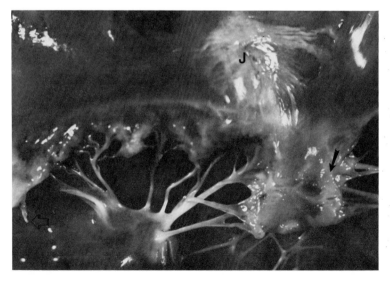

Figure 20-1 *Heart of a dog with mitral valvular endocardiosis (arrow) and a ruptured chorda (open arrow). Note the regurgitant jet lesion (J) in the left atrium. (Published with permission. Keene BW. Chronic valvular disease in the dog. In Fox PR, ed. Canine and feline cardiology. New York: Churchill Livingstone, 1988: 409.)*

ished contractility, due in part to left ventricular fibrosis.

Falling cardiac output may produce signs of forward heart failure and poor tissue perfusion, including exercise intolerance, syncope, and prerenal azotemia. The rise in left atrial and, hence, pulmonary venous pressure associated with large mitral regurgitant volume produces venous congestion (backward failure) and ultimately interstitial and alveolar pulmonary edema (left heart failure; Table 20-1). Prolonged left heart failure can lead to right heart failure with systemic venous congestion, hepatosplenomegaly, ascites, or hydrothorax, especially when tricuspid insufficiency is also present (see Table 20-1).

Other complications of mitral insufficiency include cardiac arrhythmias, rupture of the chordae tendineae, tearing of the left atrium, and, rarely, vegetative endocarditis (see Table 20-1). Arrhythmias, such as sinus tachycardia, atrial premature complexes, supraventricular tachycardia, atrial fibrillation, ventricular premature complexes, and ventricular tachycardia, may further reduce cardiac output. The sudden onset of an arrhythmia can precipitate or worsen signs of

heart failure or cause syncope as cerebral blood flow abruptly falls. Rupture of the chordae tendineae, depending on the chorda involved, often increases the intensity of the murmur and the regurgitant volume, and may cause acute and catastrophic decompensation (see Fig. 20-1). Tearing of the stretched and pressurized left atrium produces acute pericardial tamponade and acute, often terminal, decompensation (Fig. 20-2). Vegetative endocarditis is discussed in Chapter 22.

CLINICAL SIGNS

The earliest sign of valvular insufficiency is a midsystolic click or an early, low-intensity, mixed-frequency systolic murmur (Figs. 20-3, 20-4), heard loudest at the left fifth intercostal space at the apex. As the disease progresses, the murmur becomes longer in duration, ultimately becoming holosystolic (Fig. 20-5). The murmur of mitral regurgitation typically antedates by years the onset of clinical signs.

As left heart failure ensues, classical signs such as orthopnea, dyspnea, cough, reduced exercise tolerance, syncope, anorexia, and weight loss may be observed (see Table 20-1). The cough associated with heart failure has been ascribed to edema of the bronchial walls and excessive mucus production as bronchial veins, which empty into the left atrium, become congested; pressure produced by the enlarged heart (particularly the left atrium) on airways or the recurrent laryngeal nerve; the pressure of interstitial edema on airways; and edematous froth in the airways. The cough is typically deep and resonant; it is often worse in the morning and evening hours and after exertion. A cough associated with heart disease is often due to underlying respiratory disease. Other physical findings can include audible arrhythmias, cardiac gallop (typically S_3), respiratory crackles (rales) and dyspnea associated with pulmonary edema, ashen or cyanotic mucous membranes with prolonged capillary refill time, cold extremities, weak pulses, and pulse deficits. Pink froth may be evident in the nostrils and oropharynx terminally.

Right heart failure may complicate the clinical picture of left heart failure due to mitral insuffi-

Table 20–1 *Mitral Insufficiency: Recognized Clinical Consequences and Their Potential Manifestations*

Consequence	Manifestations
Left heart failure	Dyspnea, cough, orthopnea, exercise intolerance, syncope, depression, weakness, anorexia, weight loss
Right heart failure (uncommon)	Systemic venous distension, ascites, hydrothorax, depression, weakness, anorexia, weight loss
Myocardial failure	Worsening of signs of heart failure, refractoriness to therapy
Rupture of chordae tendineae	Acute decompensation of left heart failure, death
Torn left atrium	Acute decompensation with signs of forward heart failure and possibly right heart failure, death
Vegetative endocarditis (rarely complicates endocardiosis)	Left heart failure, sepsis
Arrhythmias	Worsening of signs, syncope, weakness, death

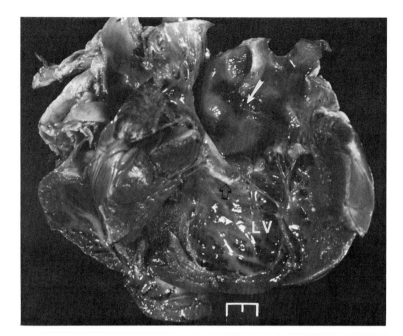

Figure 20–2 *Heart of dog demonstrating endocardiosis of mitral valve (open arrow) and a tear in the left atrium (white arrow). (LV = left ventricle) (Photograph courtesy of Dr. James Cooley, University of Wisconsin)*

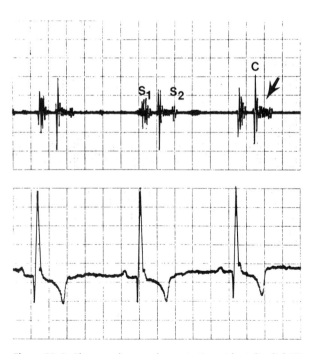

Figure 20–3 *Phonocardiogram demonstrating midsystolic click (C) and late systolic murmur (arrow). This is thought to represent pre-regurgitant phenomenon in the dog. The electrocardiogram is normal except for notching of the R wave.*

ciency. This is variably manifested by systemic venous congestion, hepatosplenomegaly, ascites, hydrothorax (with or without dyspnea), syncope, anorexia, weight loss, and diminished exercise tolerance (see Table 20-1). Again, mucous membrane color may be ashen with prolonged capillary refill time, pulses are characteristically weak, possibly with deficits, and a murmur of tricuspid regurgitation may be audible at the fourth right intercostal space at the level of the costochondral junction. The latter determination is not always easy, as the the murmur of mitral regurgitation may radiate well to the right hemithorax.

Dogs with ruptured chordae tendineae, particularly primary chordae of the anterior mitral valve leaflet, are presented with a sudden onset or worsening of the signs of left heart failure. The murmur is loud, often having increased in intensity, and is typically accompanied by a precordial thrill and cardiac gallop.

Acute tamponade with decompensation is the hallmark of a torn or ruptured left atria. The signs are those of heart failure, with ashen mucous membranes, weak pulses, generalized weakness, and depression. However, there is not fulminating pulmonary edema, because hemopericardium

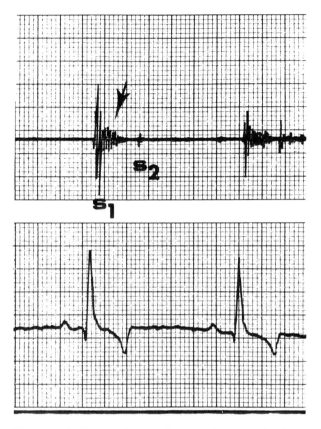

Figure 20–4 *Phonocardiogram demonstrating an early decrescendo murmur (arrow) typical of early mitral regurgitation. On the electrocardiogram, the QRS complex is prolonged, suggesting left ventricular enlargement or conduction abnormality.*

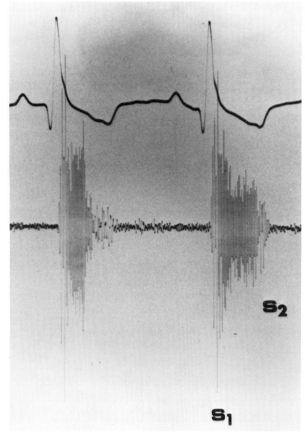

Figure 20–5 *Phonocardiogram illustrating a pansystolic murmur of advanced mitral regurgitation.*

produces tamponade that diminishes cardiac inflow, thus unloading the pulmonary vasculature. Most signs are related to diminished tissue perfusion (low output or forward failure), but may also reflect backward (congestive) right heart failure, evident as jugular venous distention, hepatosplenomegaly, and, potentially, ascites.

Table 20–2 *Functional Classification of Heart Disease and Failure in the Dog*

Class I	No clinical manifestation
Class II	Cough or decreased exercise tolerance only with extreme exertion
Class III	Cough, orthopnea, reduced exercise tolerance, ascites, hydrothorax, syncope
Class IV	Signs of class III with the addition of dyspnea at rest

The phases of heart disease and failure have been adapted for the dog after the classification of the New York Heart Association (Table 20-2). Although this classification scheme has limitations for use in humans and animals, it still has merit for illustration of the progression of the signs of heart failure and as an instructional scaffold for demonstrating therapeutic strategy.

DIAGNOSTIC APPROACH

The diagnosis of mitral insufficiency is relatively straightforward because of the typical murmur, age, and breeds affected. The task of determining whether the patient is in heart failure and what role cardiac disease plays in the dog's symptomatology is more difficult. This can be particularly problematic in discerning the role of cardiac disease, if any, in small-breed dogs suffering from chronic cough. The cause of the cough may actually be primary respiratory disease with or without left heart failure. This is even more vexing because heart disease due to mitral insufficiency is progressive, thus its contribution to the cough is ever changing and must be periodically reassessed. Table 20-3 outlines features useful for differentiating patients with cough due to respiratory disease from those with cough due to heart failure.

Another important, but difficult, determination is whether dogs with mitral insufficiency are afflicted with myocardial failure. In other words, is the problem of mitral regurgitation compounded by muscle dysfunction? Although the majority (80%) of dogs with primary valvular disease (endocardiosis) and heart failure do not appear to have myocardial failure, this determination is important as one criterion used in making the therapeutic decision of whether to employ

positive inotropic therapy in a given patient. Assessment of myocardial function in this setting is confounded by alterations in loading conditions (increased preload, reduced afterload) associated with mitral insufficiency, which invalidate commonly used isovolumic (pre-ejection period, dP/dt) and ejection phase (fractional shortening) indices of myocardial performance. This problem is partially obviated by methods described later in the section on Echocardiography.

The electrocardiographic findings in mitral insufficiency are nonspecific and, unless an arrhythmia is present, are not of great diagnostic utility. In fact, the electrocardiogram (ECG) (see Electrocardiography in Chapter 80) is frequently normal (see Fig. 20-3). The usefulness of the ECG can be enhanced by serial evaluations. The ECG can be used as an aid in distinguishing cardiac from respiratory causes for chronic cough (see Table 20-3).

Typically, the ECG demonstrates tachycardia if failure is present. The mean electrical axis is

Table 20–3 *Historical and Clinical Findings That May Aid in Differentiation of Cough Due to Mitral Insufficiency From Cough Due to Chronic Respiratory Disease**

Heart Failure	Respiratory Disease	Heart Failure and Respiratory Disease
Weight loss	Often obese	Weight loss, obesity, or neither
Cough worse at night; may be accompanied by frothy, pink nasal discharge or sputum	Cough with exercise; may be accompanied by mucopurulent nasal discharge or sputum	Variable
Dyspnea variable; often worse at night	Usually not dyspneic	Variable
Murmur	With or without murmur	Murmur
Respiratory crackles or no ALS	Respiratory crackles, wheezes, or no ALS	Respiratory crackles, wheezes, or no ALS
Sinus tachycardia or other arrhythmias	Normal to slow heart rate with exaggerated sinus arrhythmia	Variable heart rate
P-mitrale or LVE on ECG	P-pulmonale or RVE on ECG	Variable ECG chamber enlargement patterns
Pulmonary edema, left atrial enlargement on radiographs	No pulmonary edema, left atrial enlargement mild or absent on radiographs	Variable pulmonary edema, left atrial enlargement on radiographs
No airway collapse or bronchial infiltrate on radiographs	Airway collapse or bronchial/parenchymal infiltrate on radiographs	Airway collapse or bronchial/parenchymal infiltrate on radiographs
Normal respiratory cytology	Abnormal respiratory cytology	Abnormal respiratory cytology
Normal or stress leukogram	Variable inflammatory leukogram	Variable leukogram findings
Diuretic responsive	Diuretic unresponsive	Partially diuretic responsive

* *Each finding need not be present in all cases.*
ALS = adventitious lung sounds; ECG = electrocardiogram; LVE = left ventricular enlargement; RVE = right ventricular enlargement

usually within normal limits. Widening of P waves (greater than 40 msec, with or without notching), a specific, but insensitive, indicator of left atrial enlargement, is detected in 30% of cases (Fig. 20-6). Lombard and Spencer (Additonal Reading) have shown that left ventricular enlargement patterns (see Chapter 18) were inconsistent, having been observed in only 55% of cases, and did not correlate well with echocardiographic and radiographic evidence of left ventricular enlargement. In the case of tearing of the left atrium with pericardial tamponade, ECG complex amplitude may actually be diminished.

Thoracic radiography is useful in diagnosing cardiomegaly and impending (pulmonary venous congestion) or florid heart failure, in determining specific cardiac chamber size, and in detecting the presence of concurrent respiratory disease (see Thoracic Radiography in Chapter 80). In addition, radiographs are helpful in evaluating the efficacy of therapeutic interventions. It must be kept in mind that the radiographic changes associated with mitral insufficiency occur gradually, and that serial examinations often amplify the value of this procedure.

Radiographs early in the disease course are unremarkable, but with time and worsening of mitral regurgitation, left heart enlargement becomes apparent. Left atrial enlargement is an early and relatively consistent sign. Enlargement of the left atrium and its auricle (the latter is visible between 1 and 3 o'clock on the dorsoventral projection; see Thoracic Radiography in Chapter 80) is indicated by a flattening of the caudal cardiac border, elevation of the caudal trachea and main stem bronchi (particularly the left) on the lateral projection, and a radiodense mass between the main stem bronchi on the dorsoventral projection. Left ventricular enlargement is evident in an increasing convexity and rounding of the left border of the cardiac silhouette on both radiographic views (Fig. 20-7).

The combined enlargement of the left atrium and ventricle results in a reduction of the angle of trachea to the vertebral column, as well as a loss of the caudal waist of the heart. The enlarged heart occupies a greater than normal portion of the thoracic cavity.

As heart failure ensues, the left atrium enlarges further, and the hilar pulmonary veins become more radiodense, together producing a left atrial "mass," which extends dorsal and caudal to the tracheal carina. Pulmonary venous congestion is indicated by enlargement of the apical pulmonary vein to a size larger than the proximal one third of the fourth rib, or to a size larger than the apical pulmonary artery (Fig. 20-8). Florid left heart failure is diagnosed when hilar interstitial density or diffuse alveolar densities are identified (Fig. 20-9).

With rupture of a primary chorda, severe cardiac decompensation can occur with fulminant pulmonary edema and minimal to moderate left atrial enlargement, as the left atrium has had little time to stretch in compensation. With left atrial tearing and tamponade, the heart may lose some of its contour, but usually the round cardiac silhouette typical of pericardial effusion does not

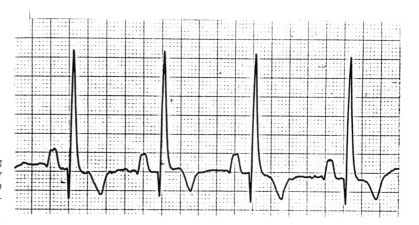

Figure 20–6 *Electrocardiogram demonstrating P–pulmonale, P–mitrale, and left ventricular enlargement (tall R wave, wide QRS complex) in a dog with mitral regurgitation and cardiomegaly.*

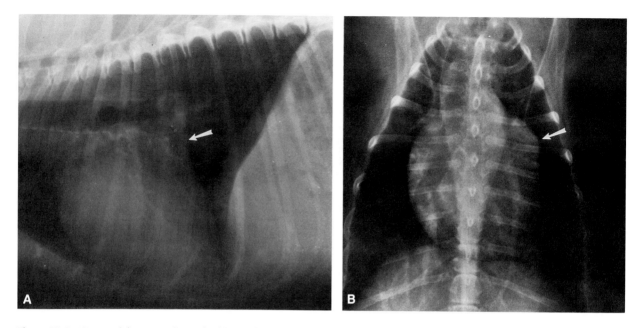

Figure 20–7 *(A) Lateral thoracic radiograph of dog with compensated mitral regurgitation. Note mild to moderate cardiac enlargement, particularly in the left atrium (arrow). There is no pulmonary venous congestion or pulmonary edema. (B) Ventrodorsal view demonstrating mild cardiomegaly and left auricular enlargement (arrow). See text for more detailed explanation of radiographic findings.*

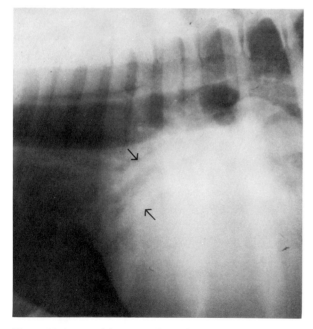

Figure 20–8 *Lateral thoracic radiograph of a dog with impending pulmonary edema due to left heart failure. Note that although the apical pulmonary vein (lower arrow) is no larger than the proximal one third of the fourth rib, it is larger than the apical pulmonary artery (upper arrow).*

develop because of the rapidity of onset. With secondary right heart failure, ascites and caudal vena caval enlargement may be visualized.

In general terms, although the echocardiogram can be used to diagnose myocardial dysfunction (pump or muscle failure), it does not diagnose heart failure (see Echocardiography in Chapter 80). More specifically, it cannot diagnose mitral regurgitation and, because of factors mentioned above, it is limited in its ability to diagnose myocardial failure as a complication of mitral regurgitation. Two-dimensional and M-mode echocardiography are, however, the most accurate determinants of specific cardiac chamber enlargement. Therefore, both are useful in confirming cardiac changes compatible with mitral insufficiency. Echocardiographic findings with mitral insufficiency include left atrial and ventricular enlargement and, typically, exuberant left ventricular septal and posterior wall motion (Fig. 20-10). In addition, thickening of valve leaflets may be recognized. Abnormal valve leaflet motion in the case of ruptured chordae, and the pericardial fluid associated with left atrial tears

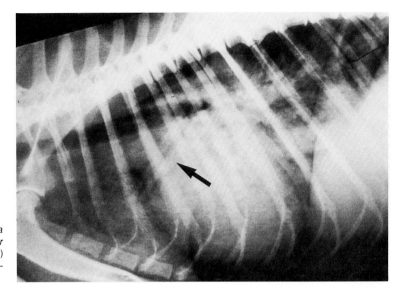

Figure 20–9 *Lateral thoracic radiograph from a dog in florid left heart failure due to mitral valvular insufficiency. Note the large pulmonary vein (arrow) and diffuse alveolar lung density, suggestive of pulmonary edema.*

Figure 20–10 *An M-mode echocardiogram from a 10-kg dog with mitral regurgitation and left heart failure, showing the left ventricle (LV), mitral valve (M), aortic root (AO), valve (open arrow), and left atrium (LA). (Panel A) The large end-diastolic volume index (128 ml), hyperdynamic left ventricle (fractional shortening = 54%), and end-systolic volume index (13 ml), suggest volume overloading and adequate myocardial function. (Panel B) The E point septal separation (arrow) is normal, suggesting normal left ventricular function. (Panel C) The ratio of the left atrium to the aortic root dimension is 1.4, indicating left atrial enlargement. (S = septum; LP = left ventricular posterior wall; M = anterior mitral valve leaflet; open arrow = aortic valve)*

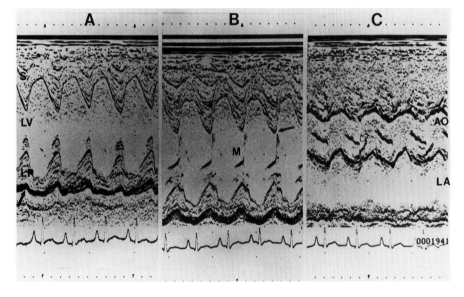

can both be visualized with echocardiography (Fig. 20-11).

Kittleson and associates (Additional Reading) suggest that a left ventricular end-diastolic volume index (end-diastolic dimension^3 divided by body surface area) greater than 100 ml/m^2 is diagnostic of volume overloading. Because of changes in loading conditions, measurement of fractional shortening tends to overestimate myocardial function in patients with mitral regurgitation (see Fig. 20-10). An attempt can be made to correct for this by calculation of left ventricular end-systolic volume index (end-systolic dimension^3 divided by body surface area), which provides an estimate of left ventricular contractility minimally influenced by loading conditions. A value greater than 30 ml/m^2 indicates myocardial failure. More simply, a fractional shortening that is normal or subnormal, when associated with significant mitral regurgitation, suggests diminished myocardial function.

When right heart failure is present, the evalua-

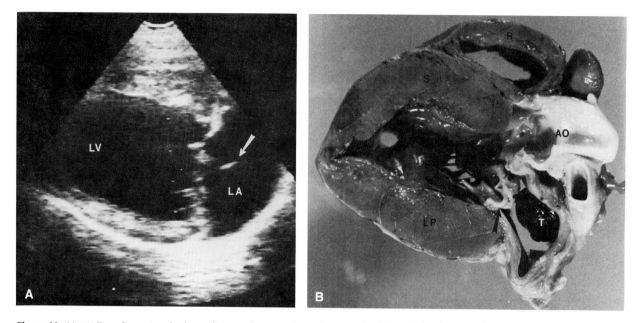

Figure 20–11   (A) Two-dimensional echocardiogram demonstrating left ventricular (LV) and left atrial (LA) enlargement and flailed anterior mitral valve leaflet with prolapse into the left atrium (arrow). (B) Heart of same dog, cut in echocardiographic plane, approximately 10 months later, demonstrating ruptured chorda tendineae, prolapse of mitral valve (arrow), and a clinically silent left atrial ball thrombus (T). (R = right ventricular wall; S = interventricular system; AO = aorta; LP = left ventricular posterior wall) (Photograph courtesy of Dr. Lisa Miller, University of Wisconsin)

tion of thoracic or ascitic fluid (see Thoracentesis and Insertion of Chest Tubes, and Abdominal Paracentesis and Lavage in Chapter 80) will help to rule out other potential causes for its accumulation. Typically, the fluid associated with heart failure is a modified transudate. The analysis of arterial blood gas concentration will confirm hypoxemia and metabolic acidosis when present. The cause of hypoxemia is reduced pulmonary oxygen diffusion or ventilation perfusion mismatching. The cause of metabolic acidosis is diminished tissue perfusion and resultant excess lactic acid accumulation. Venous blood gas analysis provides similar information about acid-base status, but little information about the ability of the lungs to oxygenate blood (Chapter 71). Venous Po_2 declines as blood stagnates in the tissues when cardiac output is subnormal. A Pvo_2 of less than 30 mmHg (normal = 40 mmHg), unless severe arterial hypoxemia exists, indicates forward heart failure and can be used as an adjunct for evaluation of the need for vasodilator therapy.

With serial Pvo_2 measurements, the efficacy of such therapy can be determined. When a dog in heart failure is presented, a complete blood count, modified Knott test, serum chemistry and electrolyte panel, and urinalysis should be obtained and evaluated to rule out concurrent disease processes and for use as a baseline for future evaluations after institution of therapy. Chronic heart failure may modestly raise liver enzymes, while diuretic therapy may result in hypokalemia, metabolic alkalosis, and azotemia.

Differential diagnoses for the murmur of endocardiosis with mitral regurgitation include dilated or hypertrophic cardiomyopathy with secondary mitral insufficiency, bacterial endocarditis, tricuspid insufficiency, congenital heart disease, and innocent murmurs, such as those produced by anemia. Heart failure must be differentiated from primary respiratory disease (see Table 20-3) such as bronchitis, airway collapse, pneumonia, neoplasia, and degenerative disease; from pleural diseases with effusion; from anemia and metabolic acidosis; and from other causes of heart failure such as cardiomyopathy, congenital disease, and valvular endocarditis.

MANAGEMENT

The overall therapeutic objective is to to enhance both the quality and the duration of life for the symptomatic dog with mitral insufficiency. It should be determined whether failure exists, the nature of its clinical manifestations (forward, backward, or both; Table 20-4), whether myocardial failure is present, and whether cardiac rhythm disturbances, respiratory disease, or right heart failure complicate the clinical picture. Therapeutic goals for heart failure, and more specifically, failure associated with mitral insufficiency, are detailed in Table 20-5. A time sequence for employment of various therapeutic modalities is put forth in Table 20-6, and dosages are provided in Table 20-7.

Several basic areas of cardiac function can be addressed with therapy (see Table 20-5). These include severity of mitral regurgitation, myocardial contractility, loading conditions, and cardiac rate and rhythm. An effort is made to optimize each of these determinants of forward cardiac output. In addition, precipitating causes of heart failure, such as sodium-loading and exercise, should be minimized. Animals should be treated according to the problem(s) with which they are presented; that is, those with clinical signs of poor forward blood flow (poor exercise tolerance) are treated with arterial vasodilators (*e.g.*, hydralazine, captopril, or enalapril), while those with pulmonary edema are treated with preload-reducing agents (*e.g.*, furosemide, nitroglycerin, captopril, or enalapril) (see Tables 20-5 and 20-7).

Reduction of Mitral Regurgitation

Surgical correction of valvular dysfunction, although theoretically very appealing, is impractical. Mitral regurgitant volume can, however, be reduced with a variety of therapeutic agents, including cardiac glycosides and other positive inotropic drugs, diuretics, and vasodilators, each of which reduces cardiac size or afterload, thereby diminishing regurgitant fraction.

Positive Inotropic Therapy

Myocardial function is thought to be unaffected in the majority of dogs with symptomatic mitral insufficiency, emphasizing the fact that heart failure can, and often does, exist without concurrent myocardial failure. The use of cardiac glycosides (digitalis) is controversial. Because of potential intoxication, many clinicians feel that they should be employed only when echocardiographic evidence of myocardial failure exists, in cases refractory to other therapy, or when right heart failure or supraventricular tachyarrhythmias arise (atrial fibrillation, atrial tachycardia, or frequent atrial premature complexes; see Table 20-7). Glycosides can also be used to optimize heart rate, with a goal of no more than 150 beats per minute in the clinic or less than 120 beats per

(text continues on page 264)

Table 20–4 *Clinical Signs and Treatment for Forward (Low Output) and Backward (Congestive) Heart Failure Due to Any Cause*

	Signs	**Treatment**
Low output (forward) heart failure	Azotemia, weakness, exercise intolerance, venous hypoxemia, syncope	Afterload reduction, inotropic support, exercise restriction, fluid therapy
Congestive (backward) heart failure	Fluid accumulation, venous distension, cough, dyspnea, arterial hypoxemia, exercise intolerance	Preload reduction (diuretics, salt restriction, venodilation), afterload reduction, inotropic support, exercise restriction

Table 20–5 *Principles of Therapy for Heart Failure due to Mitral Insufficiency*

Therapeutic Goal	Treatment
Reduce cardiac workload	Exercise restriction Weight loss Cardiovascular volume reduction* Vasodilators
Reduce mitral regurgitation	Arterial vasodilators Possibly digitalis Cardiovascular volume reduction
Maintain adequate cardiac output	Vasodilators (arterial or mixed) Digitalis Dobutamine Cardiovascular volume expansion†
Reduce venous pressure	Salt restriction Diuretics Vasodilators (venous or mixed)
Improve exercise capacity	Vasodilators (arterial or mixed) Bronchodilators Cough suppressants Treatment of heart failure
Control arrhythmias	Antiarrhythmic drugs Avoidance of hypokalemia Avoidance of digitalis intoxication
Alleviate pleural and abdominal effusion	Diuretics Thoracentesis Abdominal paracentesis Vasodilators (captopril, enalapril) Treatment of heart failure
Avoid complications	Prevention of fluid and electrolyte imbalance Avoidance of drug intoxication Management of extracardiac disorders
Reduce clinical signs	Successful management of heart failure

* Using diuretics, salt restriction
† Using fluid therapy
(Modified with permission from Keene BW, Bonagura JD. Valvular heart disease. In: Kirk RW, ed. Current veterinary therapy VIII. Philadelphia: WB Saunders, 1983: 311.)

Table 20–6 *Schema Based on Functional Class of Heart Disease (see Table 20–2) for Therapy of Heart Failure Due to Mitral Insufficiency*

Treatment	Functional Class		
	II	III	IV
Exercise restriction	Yes	Yes	Yes
Salt restriction	Moderate	Yes	Yes
Diuretics	Yes (late class II)	Yes	Yes
Digitalis	No	No*	Yes (late class IV)*
Vasodilators†	No	Yes (late class III)	Yes
Other inotropic drugs	No	No	Yes (late class IV)‡

* Digitalis may be indicated earlier when myocardial failure or supraventricular arrhythmias are recognized. Glycosides may also be used to optimize heart rate in the absence of arrhythmias. The use of cardiac glucosides in the treatment of heart failure remains controversial.
† The selection of vasodilators depends on the predominance of signs. Each type of vasodilator may be beneficial when congestive signs predominate; when forward failure signs predominate, arterial or mixed vasodilators are preferred. In time, vasodilators will likely be used even earlier in the course of the progression of heart failure.
‡ Dobutamine may be used in critical class IV patients that are unresponsive to other therapy.

Table 20–7 *Medical Management of Factors Contributing to Signs and Complications of Heart Failure in Dogs*

Factor	Management	Agent and Dosage
Fluid retention	Salt restriction	Hill's h/d
Increased preload	Diuresis	Furosemide 1 to 4 mg/kg s.i.d.–t.i.d. IV, IM, SC, or PO
		Hydrochlorothiazide 2 to 4 mg/kg b.i.d. PO
		Chlorthiazide 20 to 40 mg/kg b.i.d. PO
		Spironolactone 2 to 4 mg/kg b.i.d. PO
		Triamterene 2 to 4 mg/kg/day PO
	Venodilation	Nitroglycerin 2% ointment $1/8$ to 2 inch t.i.d.–q.i.d. topically
		Captopril 0.5 to 2 mg/kg t.i.d. PO
		Enalapril 0.5 mg/kg s.i.d.–b.i.d. PO
		Prazosin 1 mg t.i.d. if <15 kg; 2 mg t.i.d. if >15 kg
		Sodium nitroprusside 1 to 5 μg/kg/min IV
Increased afterload	Arterial vasodilation	Hydralazine 1 to 3 mg/kg b.i.d. PO
		Captopril 0.5 to 2 mg/kg t.i.d. PO
		Enalapril 0.5 mg/kg s.i.d.–b.i.d. PO
		Prazosin 1 mg t.i.d. PO if <15 kg; 2 mg t.i.d. if >15 kg PO
		Sodium nitroprusside 1 to 5 μg/kg/min IV
Diminished contactility*	Positive inotropic support	Digoxin 0.005 to 0.01 mg/kg or 0.22 mg/m² body surface area b.i.d. PO for maintenance. Rapid oral: 0.01 mg/kg b.i.d. to 0.02 mg/kg t.i.d. for 1 day, then to maintenance. Rapid IV: 0.01 to 0.02 mg/kg given one half IV immediately and one fourth IV at 30- to 60-minute intervals p.r.n.
		Digitoxin 0.01 to 0.03 mg/kg t.i.d. PO. Rapid IV: 0.01 to 0.03 mg/kg, given one half IV immediately and one fourth IV at 30- to 60-minute intervals p.r.n.
		Dobutamine 2.5 to 20 μg/kg/min IV for <72 hours
		Dopamine 2 to 10 μg/kg/min IV for <72 hours
		Amrinone 1 to 3 mg/kg IV followed by 10 to 100 μg/kg/min
		Milrinone† 0.5 to 1.0 mg/kg b.i.d. PO
Abnormal heart rate		
Bradyarrhythmia		Atropine sulfate 0.1 to 0.2 mg/kg SC or IM
		Glycopyrrolate 0.05 to 0.01 mg/kg SC or IM
		Dopamine 2 to 10 μg/kg/min IV for <72 hours
		Terbutaline 1.25 to 2.5 mg b.i.d.–t.i.d. PO
		Pacemaker implantation
Supraventricular tachycardia		Digoxin: Same as above
		Digitoxin: Same as above
		Propranolol 5 to 40 mg t.i.d. PO; 0.1 to 0.3 mg/kg IV slowly
		Verapamil‡ 1 to 5 mg/kg t.i.d. PO; 0.05 to 0.25 mg/kg IV slowly
		Diltiazem‡ 1.5 mg/kg t.i.d. PO
Ventricular tachycardia		Lidocaine 2 to 4 mg/kg IV; repeat up to 8 mg/kg over 20 minutes
		Procainamide 5 to 15 mg/kg t.i.d.–q.i.d. PO; 5 to 10 mg/kg IV
		Quinidine 5 to 15 mg/kg q.i.d. PO
		Propranolol 5 to 40 mg t.i.d. PO; 0.1 to 0.3 mg/kg IV
		Tocainide 5 to 10 mg/kg t.i.d. PO

* *In most instances of mitral insufficiency, positive inotropic support is unnecessary; see text for explanation.*
† *Not commercially available at the time of this writing.*
‡ *Calcium channel blockers (verapamil and diltiazem) should be used with extreme caution in patients in heart failure.*
s.i.d. = once daily; b.i.d. = twice daily; t.i.d. = three times daily; q.i.d. = four times daily; IM = intramuscularly; IV = intravenously; SC = subcutaneously; PO = per os

minute at home. Under these circumstances, oral chronotropic and inotropic support is provided by the use of cardiac glycosides, such as digoxin or, less frequently, digitoxin. Glycosides are generally avoided in the face of ruptured chordae, diastolic failure associated with torn left atria and tamponade, and ventricular arrhythmias, and are contraindicated in digitalis intoxication. Parenteral inotropic drugs, such as dobutamine, dopamine hydrochloride, amrinone, and milrinone, are usually not indicated in mitral regurgitation because of the low incidence of myocardial failure, but may be useful in critical, refractory cases, especially when demonstrable myocardial failure exists (see Tables 20-5, 20-6, and 20-7). In addition, by altering ventricular geometry, positive inotropic agents may diminish the regurgitant fraction by reducing the size of the valve orifice.

Off-loading Therapy

Congestive signs (venous congestion or backward failure; see Table 20-4) can frequently be reduced or eliminated by the use of off-loading therapies, such as low salt diet, diuretics, and vasodilators. Of these, cardiac output is enhanced only with arterial vasodilation (see Tables 20-5 and 20-7). Care must be taken because overzealous use of off-loading therapy may reduce filling pressure and cardiac output excessively, thus aggravating signs of forward failure.

It is well documented that clearance of a salt load in dogs with heart failure is dramatically diminished and that, although serum sodium concentrations are normal, total body sodium is increased. This sodium retention leads to fluid retention, which, while useful in the acute state of low cardiac output, is ultimately harmful in chronic heart failure, producing signs of congestion. Dietary sodium restriction is, therefore, one of the primary methods for reducing signs of congestive (backward) heart failure. Heavily salted foods should be avoided, even prior to the onset of signs (Class I). Along with exercise restriction and diuretic therapy, rigorous sodium restriction (less than 12 mg/kg sodium daily) is instituted at the onset of signs of heart failure (see Table 20-6), preferably by feeding a balanced, commercially available low-salt diet (Hill's Prescription diet h/d). Low salt diets can also be prepared by the owner (see Lewis, Additional Reading).

The diuretics most frequently used include the loop diuretic furosemide, the thiazides, and, in cases complicated by hypokalemia, the potassium-sparing diuretics spironolactone and triamterene (see Table 20-7). Various combinations of diuretics, for instance, a thiazide and furosemide, may be utilized to enhance their efficacy and reduce untoward side-effects. Diuretics are utilized at the lowest dose that alleviates signs of congestion and are instituted relatively early in the disease course (see Table 20-6). Restriction of water intake may be necessary in some dogs that drink excessively, which effectively negates diuretic therapy. This measure should be employed only in dogs with adequate renal function. Restriction to 45 to 60 ml/kg body weight is advised under these circumstances. Careful monitoring of body weight and hydration status is mandatory. Potential complications to diuretic therapy include inappetance, dehydration, azotemia, hypokalemia, and acid-base disturbances.

The exact role and method for use of vasodilators is not yet defined. They are thought to be effective, and, although generally recommended for use when other modalities fail (see Table 20-6), will undoubtedly receive more attention for use earlier in the course of heart failure. For example, animals presented with a cough due to left atrial enlargement causing compression of the left main stem bronchus may benefit from the use of an arterial vasodilator (*e.g.*, hydralazine) and nothing more.

Vasodilators that predominantly affect preload (venodilators; see Table 20-7) include nitroglycerin and isosorbide dinitrate, each acting directly to relax venous smooth muscle. These drugs are effective only in alleviating congestive signs (*e.g.*, pulmonary edema) and do not improve cardiac output. They are less apt to produce symptomatic hypotension than arterial or mixed vasodilators.

Arterial vasodilators (see Table 20-7), by enhancing ventricular emptying and lowering end-diastolic left ventricular pressures, will improve cardiac output and reduce regurgitant volume with amelioration of cough caused by impingement of the left atrium on the bronchial tree. Therefore, similar to mixed vasodilators but unlike venodilators and diuretics, these drugs are effective at improving cardiac output and reducing congestive signs. Hydralazine is a direct-acting, afterload-reducing (arterial) vasodilator that ideally is titrated for each patient, using an increase in central Pvo_2 or a reduction in arterial blood pressure as the determinant of therapeutic success.

Mixed vasodilators (see Table 20-7), which dilate both arterioles and veins, include captopril, and enalapril, angiotensin-converting enzyme inhibitors; prazosin, an α-blocker; and sodium nitroprusside, which acts directly on vascular smooth muscle. Captopril and enalapril, in addition to dilating arterioles and veins, will theoretically effect diminished fluid retention and potassium wasting by reducing aldosterone and angiotensin II concentrations. Doses of captopril greater than 2 mg/kg three times daily have been associated with renal failure. Sodium nitroprusside can be administered only intravenously, and, because of its potency, arterial blood pressure should be monitored when it is employed. Undesirable side-effects associated with vasodilator therapy include gastrointestinal upset and hypotension, the latter being manifested by somnolence, weakness, or syncope. Hydralazine, in particular, may also result in reflex tachycardia.

Miscellaneous therapies (see Tables 20-5 and 20-7) employed in the management of symptomatic mitral regurgitation include thoracentesis and abdominal paracentesis when right heart failure complicates left heart failure (see Thoracentesis and Insertion of Chest Tubes and Abdominal Paracentesis and Lavage in Chapter 80). Potassium chloride is infrequently required, but its administration may benefit dogs with poor appetites and requiring high doses of diuretics, or those with arrhythmias unresponsive to therapy. Hypokalemia, which can precipitate arrhythmias and digitalis intoxication, can be treated or prevented by offering foods high in potassium, such as bananas, citrus fruits, dates, and Brazil nuts. Judicious use of fluid therapy (5% dextrose in water, supplemented with 30 mEq potassium chloride per liter and administered at approx-

imately 1 ml/kg/hour) is indicated in some dogs showing poor tissue perfusion or dehydration. Monitoring of congestive signs and possibly central venous pressure (see Central Venous Pressure in Chapter 80) is imperative when fluid therapy is employed. Class IV heart failure may dictate the use of cage rest, 40% to 50% oxygen by mask, nasal tube, or oxygen cage, and morphine sulfate for its sedative and potential inotropic and venodilatory benefits. Cough suppressants and bronchodilators, such as aminophylline, theophylline, and terbutaline, are usually not employed in the treatment of respiratory signs associated with heart failure. These products may, however, be quite useful in palliation of intractable cough, or when primary respiratory disease complicates cardiac disease (see Chapter 13). Control of supraventricular and ventricular arrhythmias will improve cardiac output by increasing filling time and by normalizing the sequence of ventricular depolarization, thereby being an important adjunct to therapy of mitral insufficiency (see Chapter 18).

Treatment for Complications of Mitral Insufficiency

Ruptured Chordae Tendineae

The therapy for rupture of chordae tendineae is similar to that discussed above with the aggressive use of parenteral furosemide (1–4 mg/kg IV or intramuscularly, once to three times daily) and oxygen therapy, coupled with a combination of topically applied nitroglycerin (2% ointment, $1/8$–2 inch three or four times daily, topically for 24 hours, then alternating treatment 12 hours on, 12 hours off) and hydralazine (1–3 mg/kg orally twice daily) or the use of a mixed vasodilator such as sodium nitroprusside (1–5 μg/kg/min IV, only with hemodynamic monitoring), captopril (0.5–2 mg/kg orally three times daily), or enalapril (0.5 mg/kg once or twice daily, orally). In this instance, digoxin is not indicated as a positive inotrope, as it may actually increase the regurgitant fraction. It may, however, be useful if supraventricular arrhythmias (*e.g.*, atrial fibrillation) are present. Morphine (0.1–0.25 mg/kg subcutaneously) may also be administered for its sedative and off-loading potential.

Atrial Tears

Acute cardiac decompensation associated with tears in the left atrium is due to rapidly developing pericardial effusion with tamponade. The resultant diastolic failure is a relative contraindication to digitalization in dogs not already receiving digitalis, because it may further impair ventricular filling. Pericardiocentesis (see Pericardiocentesis in Chapter 80) may be life-saving, but should be reserved for cases in which death is feared to be imminent, as further hemorrhage may follow this procedure. Less severely affected animals will recompensate with cage rest and continued therapy for the underlying mitral insufficiency. Vasodilation is of questionable value and, while controversial, volume expansion or positive inotropic support with dobutamine have been advocated in humans as interim therapy prior to surgery.

Refractory Phase IV Patients

In acute situations, treatment for these patients is similar to that described for acute chorda rupture, with the exception that digoxin is added to the regime, as it is assumed that such patients have developed myocardial failure (see Tables 20-6 and 20-7). In some instances, dobutamine (2.5–20 μg/kg/min IV) may be administered for its inotropic benefit. Treatment is typically initiated at lower doses and titrated upward, based on clinical response. Once stabilized, conventional therapy, including digoxin, is continued. Often, reeducation of the client about the importance of salt and exercise restriction and the institution of combination diuretic therapy (a thiazide coupled with furosemide) may be helpful.

Right Heart Failure

Fluid accumulation with right heart failure may be eliminated or diminished by digitalization, the use of diuretics, salt restriction, thoracentesis or abdominal pericentesis, and the use of vasodilators (see Table 20-7). Captopril and enalapril, in particular, has shown promise in cases of refractory ascites.

Each of these complications to mitral insufficiency carries a poor to grave prognosis for long-term survival. Short-term recompensation is certainly possible in many instances, however.

PATIENT MONITORING

The prognosis for mitral insufficiency varies with the stage of its development. Early, asymptomatic mitral insufficiency carries a good prognosis, with dogs usually surviving many years. Owners presenting a dog for examination with a recent onset of signs of cardiac failure should be given a guarded prognosis with estimated survival of 1 year. The prognosis for complications of mitral insufficiency (chorda rupture, atrial tears, and so on) is poor.

Follow-up visits should be established based on the severity of the dog's signs and the client's interest in providing the input of time, effort, and money into caring for such a patient. Asymptomatic dogs with murmurs need only be reevaluated at the yearly vaccination appointment. Baseline radiographic and electrocardiographic evaluation is generally advisable. Symptomatic dogs should be evaluated as needed to maintain compensation, but should be seen no less often than at 3- to 6-month intervals. Dogs with severe signs of failure, cardiac arrhythmias, or other complications may require more frequent office visits.

During follow-up visits, the presence and character of cough, dyspnea, ability to exercise, and general demeanor should be carefully evaluated. Body weight is monitored to assure that the patient's condition is not deteriorating further and to assess hydration. Evaluation of skin turgor, mucous membranes, blood urea nitrogen, and packed-cell volume and serum total protein allow crude approximations of the state of hydration. Heart failure patients are intentionally kept in a state of mild dehydration (azotemic, packed-cell volume greater than 45%–50% or 0.45–0.50 L/L, total serum protein greater than 7.5 g/dl or 75 g/L). Serum electrolyte concentrations (sodium and potassium) are periodically measured, especially in dogs afflicted with arrhythmias or digitalis intoxication. One week after institution of digoxin therapy, serum digoxin concentrations are evaluated (8 hours postadministration). Desirable levels are between 0.8 and 2 ng/ml or 1.3 and 2.6 nmol/L. Dose adjustments can be made using this value and the dog's clinical response, as well as the presence of physical and electrocardiographic signs of digitalis intoxication.

Once heart failure has been diagnosed, thoracic radiographs are obtained at 6-month intervals, or more frequently if necessary, to follow changes in cardiac size, to observe impending heart failure, and to evaluate the respiratory tract. Electrocardiography, utilized to evaluate heart rate and to detect arrhythmias, should be routinely performed. Echocardiograms are useful in evaluating left atrial and ventricular size, ventricular function, and the presence of pericardial effusion.

ADDITIONAL READING

Buchanan JW. Chronic valvular disease (endocardiosis) in dogs. Adv Vet Sci Comp Med 1979; 21:75.

Ettinger SK. Valvular heart disease. In: Ettinger SJ, ed. Textbook of veterinary internal medicine. Philadelphia: WB Saunders, 1983: 959.

Harpster NK. The cardiovascular system. In: Holzworth J, ed. Diseases of the cat. Philadelphia: WB Saunders, 1987: 820.

Harpster NK. Chronic valvular–myocardial heart disease in dogs. In: Kirk RW, ed. Current veterinary therapy V. Philadelphia: WB Saunders, 1974: 282.

Keene BW. Chronic valvular disease in the dog. In: Fox PR, ed. Canine and feline cardiology. New York: Churchill Livingstone, 1988: 409.

Keene BW, Bonagura JD. Valvular heart disease. In: Kirk RW, ed. Current veterinary therapy VIII. Philadelphia: WB Saunders, 1983: 311.

Keene BW, Rush JE. Therapy of heart failure. In: Ettinger SJ, ed. Textbook of veterinary internal medicine. Philadelphia: WB Saunders, 1989: 939.

Kittleson MD, Eyster GE, Knowlen GG et al. Myocardial function in small dogs with chronic mitral regurgitation. J Am Vet Med Assoc 1984; 184:455.

Lewis LD, Morris Jr ML, Hand MS. Heart failure. In: Small animal clinical nutrition III. Topeka: Mark Morris Associates, 1987: 11–1.

Liu SK, Tashijan RJ, Patnaik AK. Congestive heart failure in the cat. J Am Vet Med Assoc 1970; 156:1319.

Lombard CW, Spencer CP. Correlation of radiographic, echocardiographic, and electrocardiographic signs of left heart enlargement in dogs with mitral regurgitation. Veterinary Radiology 1985; 26:89.

Sisson D. Acquired valvular heart disease in dogs and cats. In: Bonagura JW, ed. Contemporary issues in small animal practice. Vol 7: Cardiology. New York: Churchill Livingstone, 1987: 59.

Whitney JC. Observations on the effect of age on the severity of heart valve lesions in the dog. Journal of Small Animal Practice 1974; 15:511.

21

CARDIOMYOPATHY

Clarke E. Atkins, Patti S. Snyder

As defined by some authors, the term *cardiomyopathy* refers only to primary heart muscle disorders with no known cause. Here *cardiomyopathy* will refer to primary (idiopathic) or secondary myocardial dysfunction in the absence of primary valvular or congenital heart disease. Such disorders affect both dogs and cats, producing serious cardiac dysfunction and heart failure. Although there are numerous etiologies and manifestations of cardiomyopathy, two forms are clinically important and recognized in both the dog and cat: dilated and hypertrophic cardiomyopathies (Fig. 21-1).

Dilated cardiomyopathy (DC), also termed *congestive* or *dilatative cardiomyopathy*, when idiopathic, carries a poor to grave prognosis. This disorder is characterized by biventricular myocardial failure (diminished contractility). The result is systolic failure, although diastolic dysfunction coexists and may precede systolic dysfunction.

In contrast, hypertrophic cardiomyopathy (HC), rare in the dog but common in the cat, is characterized by extreme concentric left ventricular hypertrophy, resulting in a noncompliant ventricle with a small lumen. Diminished left ventricular filling results in diastolic failure.

Restrictive (RC) or intermediate cardiomyopathy has been described in the cat. It is characterized by fibrous infiltration of the ventricular wall and endocardium, producing diastolic failure and variable signs common to both DC and HC. Another form of cardiomyopathy, characterized by excessive left ventricular moderator bands and biventricular failure, has been described in a small number of cats. This may represent a congenital defect. See the Additional Reading section for in-depth discussion of this disorder.

At this time, no idiopathic cardiomyopathy is known to be curable. In these cases, treatment is palliative. Recent breakthroughs in the understanding of DC in both dogs and cats provide hope that correction of certain biochemical or nutritional factors may provide a cure or even prevent the development of these disorders.

CANINE DILATED CARDIOMYOPATHY

Causes

Although the cause of DC in the dog is generally unknown, Keene and associates (Additional Reading) have recently demonstrated a deficiency in myocardial carnitine concentration in approximately one half of dogs with DC, and improvement in cardiac function and signs with car-

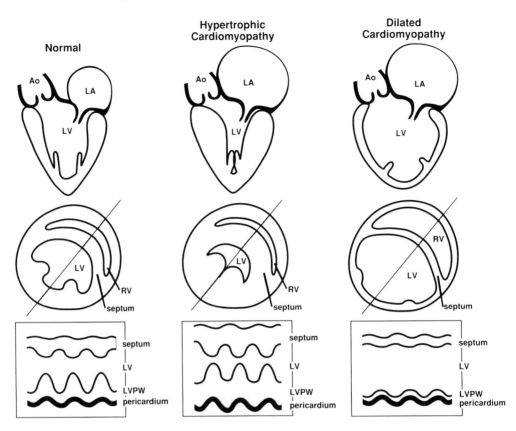

Figure 21–1 *Schematic representations of normal, hypertrophic cardiomyopathic, and dilated cardiomyopathic anatomy in long axis, short axis, and M-mode echocardiographic perspectives. Note the dilated LA, concentrically hypertrophied LV, unaffected RV, and hyperdynamic left ventricular echocardiographic function in the hypertrophic cardiomyopathic heart. Note the dilated (eccentrically hypertrophied) LA, LV, and RV, as well as the hypokinetic LV echocardiographic motion in the dilated cardiomyopathic heart. (Line through short axis view of heart represents M-mode echo beam (cursor); LVPW = left ventricular posterior wall; Ao = aortic outflow tract; LV = left ventricle; RV = right ventricle; LA = left atrium)*

nitine supplementation in a subset population. Alternatively, dogs may suffer from DC as a sequela to myocarditis caused by parvovirus, *Trypanosoma cruzi* (Chagas' disease), and possibly other organisms (*Borrelia burgdorferi*, distemper virus, and *Toxoplasma gondii*). Other causes may include ischemia, atherosclerotic intramural coronary artery infarction, toxins (gossypol poisoning), immune-mediated disorders, and the administration of drugs such as doxorubicin. Endocrinopathies have also been associated with poor cardiac performance. While its exact role is uncertain, hypothyroidism has been associated with DC, and diabetes mellitus has been shown to produce mild, clinically insignificant cardiac dysfunction in dogs. Infiltrative disorders, such

as neoplasia, glycogen storage diseases, and amyloidosis, can also produce myocardial dysfunction and failure. Nevertheless, in most cases an etiology cannot be determined. A familial tendency in giant breeds (Great Dane, Irish wolfhound, Saint Bernard), German shepherds, Irish setters, greyhounds, boxer dogs, English springer spaniels ("silent atrium syndrome"), English cocker spaniels, and particularly Doberman pinschers, suggests a genetic predisposition. The lack of consistent histologic evidence of severe myocardial disease, and the recognition of DC associated with plasma taurine deficiency (cats) and myocardial carnitine deficiency (humans, dogs), suggest that the underlying cause(s) may be subcellular and metabolic in nature.

Pathophysiology

Lesions of DC include generalized cardiac dilatation (eccentric hypertrophy), myocardial necrosis and fibrosis, interstitial edema, and myocardial fiber thinning. Certain breed differences are apparent. For example, English springer spaniels show marked thinning of the atrial myocardium and severe atrioventricular valve incompetence, English cocker spaniels are described as having features of both DC and HC (although in our experience, DC with biventricular failure has been the rule), while Doberman pinschers and boxer dogs may exhibit disproportionate involvement of the left heart, more severe histologic lesions, including inflammation and myointimal proliferation of small coronary arteries, and mitral valvular endocardiosis.

The final common pathway for DC, regardless of cause, is myocardial systolic failure (Fig. 21-2). In addition, diastolic dysfunction (failure of the heart to relax and fill normally) has been recognized in human and canine DC. Tricuspid or mitral valvular incompetence may develop secondary to geometric alterations in the relationship of affected atria, ventricles, papillary muscles, and chordae tendineae. Atrial and ventricular tachyarrhythmias, possibly due to myocardial stretching, infiltration, and ischemia, contribute to short-term dysfunction by shortening diastole, thereby limiting filling time and coronary perfusion, as well as by altering the route of ventricular depolarization. Tachyarrhythmias may precipitate heart failure or hasten the long-term deterioration of cardiac function by increasing myocardial work. In English springer spaniels, conduction disturbances, such as complete heart block, produce bradycardia and diminish an already suboptimal cardiac output.

In summary, systolic failure complicated by diastolic dysfunction, arrhythmias, and secondary mitral valvular incompetence all contribute to a fall in cardiac output. Compensatory mechanisms (tachycardia, fluid retention, increased afterload, and myocardial hypertrophy), as described for mitral valvular disease (see Chapter 20), are activated and, while potentially beneficial in increasing cardiac output and maintaining blood pressure early, ultimately cause deterioration in cardiac performance and the development of heart failure. Heart failure may be manifested by signs of low output (forward) or congestive (backward) failure, as well as right or left heart failure (see Chapter 20).

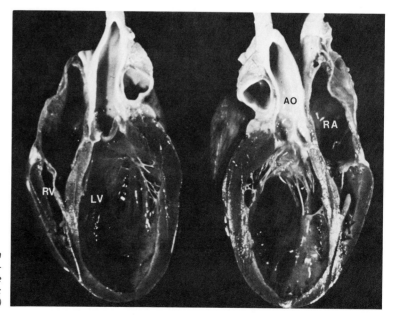

Figure 21-2 *Sections through heart of Doberman pinscher with dilated cardiomyopathy. Note biventricular and atrial enlargement and the relative thinning of ventricular walls. (RV = right ventricle; LV = left ventricle; AO = aorta; RA = right atrium)*

Clinical Signs

The incidence of DC appears to be increasing. In most practices, DC is second only to mitral valvular disease as a cause of heart failure in dogs. A male predisposition is known to exist, and the age of onset is generally between 4 and 8 years, regardless of breed. However, cases of DC have been documented in dogs younger than 1 and older than 15 years of age.

The clinical presentation of dogs with DC varies widely. Affected dogs may be diagnosed while asymptomatic, or may be presented moribund in phase IV heart disease (see Table 20-2). Historical and physical findings are tabulated in Table 21-1. Clinical findings vary from breed to breed (Table 21-2). Approximately one third of affected boxer dogs are discovered by the presence of clinically silent arrhythmias, one third are presented for syncope, and one third exhibit heart failure. Doberman pinschers typically exhibit left heart failure with a high incidence of ventricular arrhythmias. English springer spaniels most often suffer from syncope due to bradyarrhythmias with or without concurrent left or biventricular failure. Unlike giant breed dogs, these breeds are uncommonly affected with atrial fibrillation. The typical cardiomyopathic giant breed dog is in atrial fibrillation, either asymptomatic or demonstrating signs of right or left heart failure.

Physical examination may reveal signs of right and left heart failure (see Table 21-1), including dyspnea, ashen or cyanotic mucosa, prolonged capillary refill time, ascites, tachycardia, and weak or deficient pulses. Auscultatory findings may include pulmonary crackles, cardiac gallops (typically S_3), murmurs of atrioventricular valvular competence, and evidence of premature beats.

Table 21–1 *Abnormal Historical and Physical Findings in Canine and Feline Dilated Cardiomyopathy*

HISTORICAL FINDINGS

Anorexia
Weight loss (often severe in dog)
Exercise intolerance
Weakness
Lethargy
Tachypnea or dyspnea
Orthopnea
Cough (dog)
Emesis (cat)
Abdominal distention (dog)
Syncope
Signs of thromboembolism (cat)
Sudden death

PHYSICAL FINDINGS

Hypothermia
Depression
Weight loss or dehydration
Tachycardia or bradycardia
Weak, irregular, deficient, or absent (cat) pulses
Cold gums and extremities
Prolonged capillary refill time
Ashen or cyanotic mucosa
Jugular venous distention or pulsation
Diminished strength of cardiac apex beat
Pleural effusion
Ascites (dog)
Hepatosplenomegaly (dog)
Dyspnea
Pulmonary crackles (less common in cat)
Muffled heart or lung sounds (less common in dog)
Heart murmur
Cardiac gallop
Cardiac arrhythmias

Diagnostic Approach

Because of the typical age and breeds affected, the diagnosis of DC is usually straightforward, particularly when arrhythmias are present. However, to exclude other diseases and to determine the severity of cardiac dysfunction, the presence of heart failure, and the exact nature of arrhythmias, more extensive diagnostic evaluation is usually necessary. This is frequently best performed at a referral clinic.

The electrocardiogram is abnormal in the majority of cases of DC. Abnormalities include left ventricular (tall R, wide QRS) and left atrial (wide P) enlargement patterns, as well as ST segment depression, sinus tachycardia, and supraventricular and ventricular arrhythmias (Fig. 21-3). As suggested above, the frequency and type of arrhythmia varies with breed. More than 80% of giant breed dogs with DC are afflicted with atrial fibrillation (see Fig. 21-3A), while English springer spaniels and boxer dogs are infrequently affected. Hill and Calvert (Additional Reading)

Table 21–2 *Clinical Features of Dog Breeds Affected with Dilated Cardiomyopathy*

Clinical* Features	Large or Giant Breeds (Classic Form)	Doberman Pinscher	Boxer	English Cocker Spaniel	English Springer Spaniel
Age					
Average	4 to 6 yr	6.5 yr	8 yr	5 to 6 yr	27 mo
Range	6 mo to 14 yr	2.5 to 14.5 yr	6 mo to 15 yr	10 mo to 9 yr	10 mo to 5 yr
Sex predominance	Male	Male	None	None	Possibly female
Electrocardiography	AF (80%), LVE, VPC	Sinus rhythm, LVE, LBBB, AF (20%)	VPC, AF (2% to 11%)	Tall R waves, deep Q waves in leads II and aVF, APC, SVT, AF (10%), 2° AV block	3° or 2° AV block, silent atrium (PAS), tall R waves
Radiography	Generalized cardiomegaly, biventricular heart failure	LAE, acute or severe pulmonary edema, pleural effusion mild or uncommon	Normal or cardiomegaly	Generalized cardiomegaly, pulmonary edema	Generalized cardiomegaly, LAE, pulmonary edema
Echocardiography	Ventricular and atrial dilatation, reduced FS	Ventricular and atrial dilatation, reduced FS	Possible ventricular dilatation, possible FS depression	LV dilatation (usually), one fourth with normal fractional shortening	LVE, LAE, reduced FS
Other	Ascites (20%)	Cardiogenic shock common during CHF, systolic murmur (20%), syncope (10% to 50%), cardiac gallop (60%), ascites (10% to 20%)	Clinical category I: Asymptomatic with arrhythmias II: Syncope with arrhythmias III: CHF with arrhythmias Arrhythmias often refractory, systolic murmur (50%), ascites (10%), cardiac gallop (10%)	Chronic AV valvular disease (endocardiosis) common, long asymptomatic period common, syncope (up to 50%), systolic murmur (50% to 100%)	Syncope, CHF, systolic murmur
Prognosis	Six-month surival (25% to 40%), some survive more than 24 mo	Grave, most die within 6 to 8 wk	Category I: 2 yr II: 1 to 2 yr III: <6 mo, sudden death possible	Guarded, most die within 1 yr	Guarded, may survive 6 to 12 mo with pacemaker

* Much overlap occurs between findings, and breed characteristics should not be considered pathognomonic.
APC = atrial premature complex; VPC = ventricular premature complex; AF = atrial fibrillation; AV = atrioventricular; CHF = congestive heart failure; FS = fractional shortening; LAE = left atrial enlargement; LBBB = left bundle branch block (QRS >0.07 sec in upright lead II or aVF); LVE = left ventricular enlagement; PAS = persistent atrial standstill; SVT = supraventricular tachycardia)
(Modified with permission from Fox PR. Canine myocardial disease. In: Fox PR, ed. Canine and Feline Cardiology. New York: Churchill Livingstone, 1988: 467.)

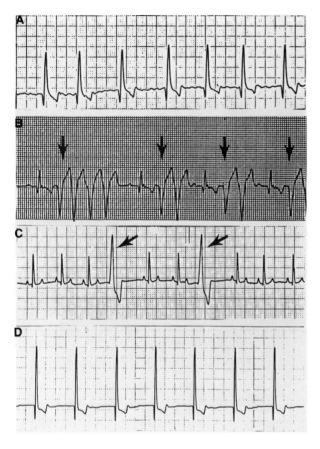

Figure 21–3 *Electrocardiograms from dogs with various forms of cardiomyopathy. (A) Atrial fibrillation, typical of cardiomyopathy in giant breeds and less frequently observed in other breeds. (B) Ventricular premature complexes (arrows) and unsustained ventricular tachycardia in a Doberman pinscher with dilated cardiomyopathy. These premature complexes are conducted in a right bundle branch pattern, suggesting origination in the left ventricle. (C) Right ventricular (conducted with a left bundle branch pattern) premature complexes (arrows) punctuating sinus rhythm. These are typical of dilated cardiomyopathy in boxer dogs. (D) Absent P wave in the electrocardiogram from a young English springer spaniel with silent atrium cardiomyopathy. There is inadequate atrial tissue to produce a P wave on the surface electrocardiogram. These dogs frequently demonstrate atrioventricular conduction abnormalities as well.*

reported atrial fibrillation in 67% of 9 and 19% of 39 Doberman pinschers with DC, respectively. In these same studies, 0% and 92% of the same dogs were documented as having ventricular arrhythmias (see Fig. 21-3B). The differences in the findings of these studies may reflect variable population subsets or, perhaps, the evolution of the disease process over time. Our experience suggests that the Doberman pinscher is frequently

afflicted with ventricular arrhythmias, often resulting in sudden death (Fig. 21-4). Ventricular arrhythmias are recognized in a high percentage (greater than 70%) of boxer dogs with DC and are believed to be responsible for syncopal episodes. These ventricular premature complexes and tachycardia are frequently conducted in a left bundle branch block morphology, suggesting origination in the right ventricle (see Fig. 21-3C). Dogs with silent atrium syndrome may demonstrate complete or advanced second-degree heart block, or an absence of P waves on the electrocardiogram (see Fig. 21-3D), while other arrhythmias are uncommon.

While radiographic findings may support the suspicion of DC, changes are frequently not dramatic, especially in the absence of heart failure. In addition, the radiographic findings do not necessarily correlate well with clinical signs and prognosis. Cardiomegaly ranges from mild to severe and typically involves all chambers. The left heart, particularly the left atrium, is often selectively enlarged in the boxer and Doberman pinscher breeds. English springer spaniels may develop significant left atrial enlargement, presumably because of profound mitral regurgitation into a thin-walled atrium (Fig. 21-5).

With right heart failure, pleural effusion and enlargement of the caudal vena cava and liver may be detected. If left heart failure is present, the development of left atrial and pulmonary venous engorgement is followed by interstitial and, subsequently, alveolar pulmonary edema (Fig. 21-6).

The echocardiogram (Chapter 82) is extremely beneficial in confirming the diagnosis of DC and determining its severity, as well as in ruling in or out such disorders as vegetative endocarditis or pericardial effusion. Typical echocardiographic findings (Fig. 21-7; see Fig. 21-1) include asynchrony of the interventricular septum and left ventricular wall, diminished shortening fraction, atrial and ventricular enlargement, increased E-point septal separation, diminished aortic root motion, and alterations of systolic time intervals and their derivatives. The echocardiogram may be normal or near normal early in the disease course, even when arrhythmias are present.

(text continues on page 277)

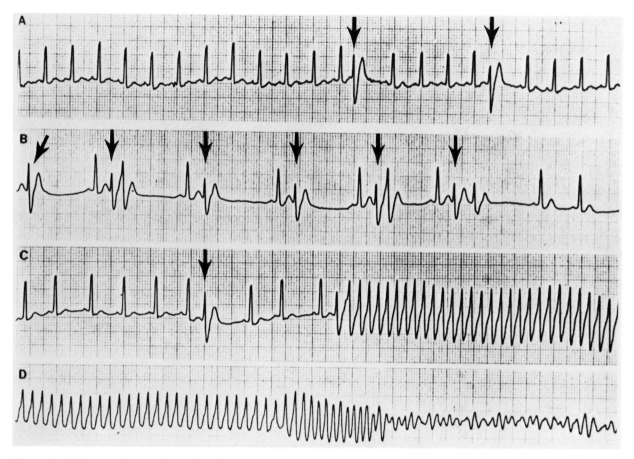

Figure 21–4 Electrocardiogram obtained with 24-hour (Holter) monitoring, demonstrating sinus rhythm with ventricular premature complexes (A, B; arrows). These premature complexes occur very early (R on T phenomenon), resulting in ventricular tachycardia and later fibrillation (C, D). This is a documented case of sudden "electrical" death, common in Doberman pinschers with dilated cardiomyopathy. (Rush JE, Keene BW. ECG of the month. J Am Vet Med Assoc 1988; 194:52. Published with permission.)

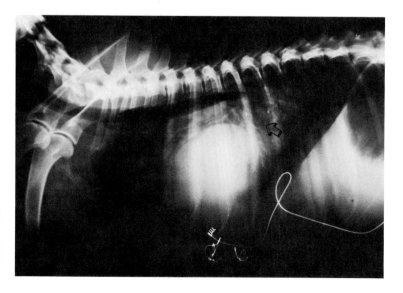

Figure 21–5 Lateral thoracic radiograph demonstrating generalized cardiomegaly and tremendous left atrial enlargement (arrow) in an English springer spaniel with silent atrium dilated cardiomyopathy. The electrode represents the lead wire from a pacemaker, used to treat third-degree atrioventricular block in this dog.

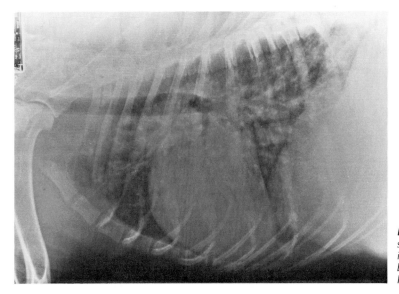

Figure 21–6 Lateral thoracic radiograph demonstrating mild to moderate cardiomegaly and patchy interstitial and alveolar pulmonary edema in a Doberman pinscher with left heart failure due to dilated cardiomyopathy.

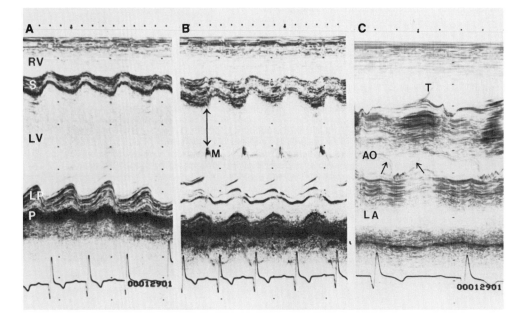

Figure 21–7 (A) M-mode echocardiogram from an English cocker spaniel demonstrating left and right ventricular enlargement and hypokinesis, (B) increased E-point septal separation (arrow), and (C) increased preejection period (time from the onset of QRS complex until aortic valve opening) and shortened left ventricular ejection period (time from opening to closing of aortic valve). (RV = right ventricle; S = septum; LV = left ventricle; LP = left ventricular posterior wall; P = pericardium; M = mitral valve; T = tricuspid valve; AO = aortic root; LA = left atrium)

Calvert (Additional Reading) has reported that increased E-point septal separation (see Fig. 21-7) is an early and sensitive indicator of cardiac dysfunction in Doberman pinschers afflicted with DC. In our experience, dogs with very poor myocardial function (fractional shortening less than 10%) have poorer prognoses for long term survival.

Laboratory abnormalities may include elevation in liver enzyme activity (serum alanine, aspartate aminotransferase, and alkaline phosphatase) and azotemia. Thoracic and abdominal effusions are typically characterized as modified transudates. Serum electrolytes should be evaluated, particularly in the face of poorly responsive cardiac arrhythmias or with intensive diuresis. The measurement of central venous pressure (see Central Venous Pressure in Chapter 80) may be useful in determining a cardiac cause for ascites, quantitatively complementing jugular vein examination. In addition, serial measurement allows monitoring of fluid therapy in cardiac patients. Thyroid function should be evaluated, as there is a known correlation between hypothyroidism and DC. We have observed atrial fibrillation and subclinical cardiac dysfunction associated with hypothyroidism that resolved with thyroid supplementation. Serologic antibody titers for borreliosis and toxoplasmosis may also be indicated in some cases of DC. In addition, Keene and associates (Additional Reading) demonstrated the utility of endomyocardial biopsy in the histologic, ultrastructural, and biochemical evaluation of dogs with DC. This procedure requires use of a referral center, but may provide useful information as to the underlying cause and potential therapy of DC.

Certain other disorders must be differentiated from DC; signalment, clinical signs, physical findings, laboratory tests, electrocardiography, radiography, echocardiography, cardiac catheterization, and angiocardiography (see Nonselective Angiocardiography in Chapter 80) are all used to this end. Cardiac diseases that must be excluded include primary valvular degeneration, vegetative endocarditis, heartworm disease, pericardial disease, congenital heart disease, liver failure, hypoalbuminemia (due to hepatic, intestinal, or renal disease), abdominal or thoracic neoplasia, primary pulmonary or pleural disease, hydrothorax, chylothorax, pyothorax, pulmonary embolism, and disorders that might cause weakness or signs mimicking syncope, such as hypoadrenocorticism and neuromuscular diseases, respectively.

Management

Treatment goals for heart failure include reduction of cardiac work, improvement of cardiac output (thereby minimizing signs of low output and congestive heart failure), and normalizing heart rate and rhythm (Table 21-3). More specifically, improving contractility and optimizing loading conditions and heart rate will frequently improve the quality and duration of life. These goals are accomplished by the judicious use of inotropic, off-loading, antiarrhythmic, and, in some cases, fluid therapies. Drug doses are listed in Table 20-7 and the Appendix. The sequence in which these drugs are administered differs somewhat from that used in the treatment of mitral regurgitation (Table 21-4).

Since DC is often detected before the onset of heart failure, early therapeutic management may require nothing more than gradual sodium and exercise restriction. If arrhythmias, with or without syncope, are detected, antiarrhythmic drugs may also be employed (see Chapter 18). With the development of more severe signs of cardiac dysfunction, more aggressive therapy is needed (see Tables 21-3, 21-4, and 21-5).

Inotropic Support

Digitalis glycosides (digoxin, digitoxin, and ouabain) are the drugs most frequently used for their positive inotropic and negative chronotropic effects. Unfortunately, the cardiac glycosides are relatively weak inotropes, producing demonstrable improvement in less than 50% of dogs with DC. The strongest indications for the use of digitalis are myocardial failure and atrial fibrillation, signs frequently observed alone or in combination in DC. Digoxin, the glycoside most commonly used, is rarely administered intravenously (see Table 20-7). Rapid oral digitaliza-

Table 21–3 Canine Dilated Cardiomyopathy: Therapeutic Goals and Methods Used to Accomplish Them

Therapeutic Goal	Agents Employed
Reduce cardiac work	Digitalis, beta-blockade, calcium channel blockade, antiarrhythmic agents, exercise restriction, afterload reduction (nitroprusside, hydralazine, captopril, enalapril, prazosin)
Improve cardiac output	Digitalis, milrinone, dobutamine, fluids (5% dextrose in water), afterload reduction
Alleviate signs of congestive heart failure	Diuretics, sodium restriction, preload reduction (nitroglycerin, nitroprusside, captopril, enalapril, prazosin), oxygen, thoracentesis
Optimize heart rate and rhythm	Digitalis, lidocaine, procainamide, beta-blockade, calcium channel blockade, pacemaker

Table 21–4 Schema and Sequence for the Management of Dilated Canine Cardiomyopathy (Myocardial Failure), Based on the New York Heart Association's Functional Classification of Heart Disease (see Table 20–2)

Treatment	Functional Class		
	II	III	IV
Salt restriction	Moderate	Yes	Yes
Diuretics	Yes (late II)	Yes	Yes
Digitalis	Yes	Yes	Yes
Vasodilators*	No	Yes (late III)	Yes
Other inotropic agents**	No	No	Yes (late IV)

* The selection of vasodilators depends on the predominance of signs. Venodilators may be beneficial when congestive signs predominate; when signs of low output predominate, arterial or mixed vasodilators are preferred. In time, vasodilators will likely be used even earlier in the course of the progression of heart failure.
** Dobutamine may be used in critical class IV patients that are unresponsive to other therapy.

tion (0.01–0.02 mg/kg three times on day 1 only, then to maintenance), however, may be indicated in cases in which inotropic or chronotropic needs are urgent, or prior to dobutamine infusion in cases with atrial fibrillation. More often, slow oral digitalization (see Table 20-7 and Appendix I) is adequate, with digitalization determined by the presence of clinical improvement, slowing of the heart rate, PR interval prolongation (to 120 msec or prolongation by 20 msec), or steady state (after 5 days of therapy) serum digoxin concentrations of approximately 1 to 2 ng/ml (1.3–2.6 nmol/L) 6 to 10 hours after drug administration (or digitoxin levels 15–35 ng/ml 6–8 hours after treatment).

Digitalis has a narrow therapeutic window. Signs of intoxication include anorexia, vomiting, diarrhea, arrhythmias, and central nervous system depression. Such findings in a dog on digitalis therapy should prompt interruption of treatment and, ideally, the measurement of serum digoxin concentrations. Digitalis is contraindicated in the face of severe ventricular arrhythmias and is used with caution in the face of isolated ventricular premature complexes. In the latter instance, slowing the heart rate and improving cardiac output frequently diminishes or abolishes such arrhythmias. Digitalis glycosides can be used in conjunction with newer inotropic agents.

Table 21–5 *Emergency Treatment, Based on Signs of Phase IV Heart Disease Due to Canine Dilated Cardiomyopathy**

Sign	Treatment
Dyspnea	Parenteral furosemide
	Thoracentesis
	Oxygen
	Bronchodilator (aminophylline or theophylline)
Anxiety	Morphine
	Acetylpromazine
Sinus tachycardia	Digitalis
	Treat heart failure
Arrhythmia	
Supraventricular	Digitalis (often with propranolol or diltiazem)†
Ventricular	Lidocaine, procainamide, or propranolol
Myocardial failure and low output signs	Digoxin, dobutamine, or amrinone (or milrinone)
	Afterload reduction (hydralazine, captopril, enalapril, prazosin, nitroprusside)
Congestive signs	Parenteral furosemide
	Thoracentesis (or abdominal paracentesis)
	Digitalis, dobutamine, or amrinone (or milrinone)
	Preload reduction (nitroglycerin,** captopril, enalapril, prazosin, or nitroprusside)
Cardiogenic shock	Digitalis, dobutamine, or amrinone (or milrinone)
	Fluids (5% dextrose in water with potassium chloride, IV)

* *Dosages are provided in Table 20–7 and Appendix I.*
† *Used in conjunction with digitalis when necessary for further negative chronotropic effect*
** *After first 24 hours, used in a "16 hours on, 8 hours off" regimen.*

The newer catecholamines, dopamine and dobutamine, provide superior inotropic support as compared to digitalis with less potential for arrhythmias, tachycardia, and vasoconstriction than with the older catecholamines, such as epinephrine and isoproterenol. Disadvantages include their short half-life and lack of an oral formulation, potential for arrhythmias and sinus tachycardia, tachyphylaxis due to receptor downregulation—limiting efficacy to 2 to 3 days, and expense. Experimental data from normal dogs in our laboratory suggest that dobutamine produces improvement in diastolic as well as systolic function, and that reductions in left ventricular afterload can be achieved with little increase in heart rate. Dobutamine, predominantly a β_1-adrenergic agonist, is the preferred agent and is indicated in refractory phase IV heart failure, in instances of extremely poor myocardial function, and in cardiogenic shock. Clinical experience in humans and dogs suggests that dobutamine improves cardiac performance in these circumstances.

Bipyridine phosphodiesterase inhibitors (amrinone and milrinone) represent a new group of potent positive inotropic agents that also has arterial vasodilatory properties. Milrinone, not commercially available at the time of this writing, appears to be superior to amrinone in that it will be marketed in an oral and intravenous form, while amrinone can only be administered intravenously. Kittleson, Pipers, and associates (Additional Reading) demonstrated positive responses in cardiac performance and clinical improvement after the administration of milrinone to dogs with DC. Disadvantages to this group of drugs include cost, potential arrhythmogenesis, and positive chronotropy. The exact role for phosphodiesterase inhibitors in the management of DC remains to be determined.

Off-loading Therapy

Congestive signs (venous congestion or backward failure) can frequently be reduced or eliminated by the use of off-loading therapies (see Table 20-7), such as a sodium-restricted diet, diuretics (furosemide, thiazides, potassium-sparing diuretics), and vasodilators (nitroglycerin, hydralazine, captopril, enalapril, prazosin). Of these, cardiac output is enhanced only with arterial vasodilation. Care must be taken because overzealous use of off-loading therapy may produce excessive reduction in filling pressures and, therefore, cardiac output, thus aggravating signs of forward failure with or without hypotension (see Table 20-4).

It is well documented that clearance of a sodium load in dogs with heart failure is dramatically diminished and that, although serum sodium concentrations are normal, total body sodium is increased. This sodium retention leads to fluid retention, which, while useful in the acute state of low cardiac output, is ultimately harmful in chronic heart failure, producing signs of congestion. Dietary sodium restriction is, therefore, one of the primary methods for reducing signs of congestive (backward) heart failure. Heavily salted foods should be avoided, even prior to onset of signs (Class I). Along with exercise restriction and diuretic therapy, rigorous sodium restriction (less than 12 mg/kg of sodium daily) is instituted at the onset of signs of heart failure (see Table 21-4), preferably by feeding a balanced, commercially available, sodium-restricted diet (Hill's Prescription Diet h/d). Alternatively, sodium-restricted diets can be prepared by the owner (Lewis and associates, Additional Reading).

The diuretics most frequently used include the loop diuretic furosemide, thiazides, and, in cases complicated by hypokalemia, the potassium-sparing diuretics spironolactone and triamterene. Various combinations of diuretics, for example, a thiazide and furosemide, may be utilized to enhance their efficacy and reduce untoward side-effects. Diuretics are utilized at the lowest dose that alleviates signs of congestion. Restriction of water intake may be necessary in some dogs that drink excessively, which effectively negates diuretic therapy. This measure should be employed only in dogs with adequate renal function. Restriction to 45 to 55 ml/kg per day is advised under these circumstances. Careful monitoring of body weight and hydration status is mandatory. Whenever diuresis is employed, and particularly when therapy is aggressive, patients should be monitored for the development of dehydration and prerenal azotemia, electrolyte imbalances (hypokalemia), and acid-base disturbances. Parenteral furosemide (2–4 mg/kg IV or IM) is frequently life-saving in fulminant pulmonary edema associated with congestive heart failure.

The exact choice, role, and method for use of vasodilators is not yet defined. Although they are generally employed when other modalities fail (see Table 21-4), vasodilators will undoubtedly receive future attention for use earlier in the course of heart failure. Those vasodilators that predominantly affect preload (venodilators) include nitroglycerin and isosorbide dinitrate, each acting directly to relax venous smooth muscle. Because they act primarily on veins, these drugs are effective only in alleviating congestive signs. They do not improve cardiac output, and are less apt to produce symptomatic hypotension than arterial or mixed vasodilators.

Arterial vasodilators (*e.g.*, hydralazine) by enhancing ventricular emptying and lowering end-diastolic left ventricular pressures, improve cardiac output and reduce atrial regurgitant volume and size, thereby ameliorating the cough produced by impingement of the left atrium on the bronchial tree. Therefore, similar to mixed vasodilators but unlike venodilators and diuretics, these drugs are effective both at improving cardiac output and reducing congestive signs. Hydralazine is a direct-acting afterload-reducing (arterial) vasodilator. It is ideally titrated for each patient, using an increase in central or jugular venous Pvo_2 (to greater than 30 mmHg) or a reduction in arterial blood pressure as determinants of therapeutic success.

Mixed vasodilators, which dilate both arteries and veins, include the angiotensin-converting enzyme inhibitors captopril and enalapril; prazosin, an α-adrenergic blocking agent; and sodium nitroprusside, which acts directly on vascular smooth muscle. Captopril and enalapril, in addition to dilating arterioles and veins, will theoretically effect diminished fluid retention and potassium wasting by reducing aldosterone and angiotensin II concentrations. Doses of captopril greater than 2 mg/kg three times daily may result in renal damage. Sodium nitroprusside can be administered only intravenously, and, because of its potency, arterial blood pressure should be monitored when it is employed. This drug has been shown to be effective in the treatment of fulminant cardiac failure associated with DC when administered concurrently with dobutamine. Undesirable side-effects associated with vasodilator therapy include gastrointestinal upset and hypotension, the latter being manifested by somnolence, weakness, or syncope. Hydralazine, in particular, may also result in reflex tachycardia.

Antiarrhythmic Therapy

An important consideration in the successful management of DC is the control of arrhythmias, described in detail in Chapter 18 (also see Table 21-5). Specifically, atrial fibrillation is treated with digoxin, and if the heart rate has not decreased adequately (to 100–150 beats per minute) in 2 to 3 days, β-blocking agents (*e.g.*, propranolol, atenolol, or metoprolol) are employed to further reduce the heart rate. Digoxin, when used alone, is successful in less than 25% of cases, but a reduction to 150 to 160 beats per minute or less is possible in the majority of cases with the addition of β-blockade. β-Blockade is probably indicated in all cases of DC because it has been shown to increase longevity in humans with DC; however, the negative inotropic potential of these drugs dictates that they be used with caution and, generally, only in conjunction with digitalis. Recent work suggests that the calcium channel blocker diltiazem may be superior to β-blockade in lowering the heart rate in atrial fibrillation. Calcium channel blockers should be used with caution with digoxin because of the potential for each to effect atrioventricular conduction. In addition, verapamil will increase digoxin concentration, predisposing to intoxication.

Ventricular arrhythmias are typically treated with lidocaine, procainamide, or propranolol. If an arrhythmia develops while digoxin is being administered, glycoside therapy should be interrupted and reevaluated. In silent atrium syndrome, pacemaker implantation is an effective method of improving cardiac output and ameliorating syncopal episodes due to bradyarrhythmias.

Miscellaneous Therapy

Miscellaneous therapies employed in the management of heart failure due to DC include thoracentesis and abdominal paracentesis when bi-

ventricular failure exists (see Chapter 80). Hypokalemia, which can precipitate arrhythmias and digitalis intoxication, can be treated or prevented by offering foods high in potassium, such as bananas, citrus fruits, dates, and Brazil nuts. Potassium chloride is infrequently required, but its administration may benefit dogs with poor appetites and those requiring high doses of diuretics. Judicious use of fluid therapy (5% dextrose in water supplemented with 30 mEq per liter of potassium chloride and administered at approximately 1 ml/kg/hour) is indicated in some dogs showing poor tissue perfusion and dehydration. Sodium-containing fluids (0.9% sodium chloride and lactated Ringer's injection) should be avoided; monitoring of congestive signs, and possibly central venous pressure, is imperative when fluid therapy is employed. Class IV heart failure may dictate the use of cage rest, 40% to 50% oxygen by mask or oxygen cage, and morphine for its sedative and potential inotropic and venodilatory benefits (see Table 21-5). Cough suppressants and bronchodilators, such as hydrocodone, aminophylline, theophylline, and terbutaline, are usually not employed in the treatment of respiratory signs associated with heart failure. These products may, however, be quite useful in palliation of intractable cough or when primary respiratory disease complicates cardiac disease.

Dietary carnitine supplementation has been shown to be of therapeutic benefit in a family of dogs with proven myocardial carnitine deficiency. While this exciting discovery holds promise, the exact role of carnitine therapy in the management of DC remains to be determined. Thyroid supplementation should be provided to dogs with proven hypothyroidism and DC. Systemic thromboembolism may occur, but it is infrequent and, therefore, anticoagulative therapy is generally not recommended in the dog with DC. However, if blood flow is particularly sluggish, if left atrial enlargement is extensive, or if evidence of thrombosis or embolism exists, aspirin therapy is advisable (0.5 mg/kg twice daily to 5 mg/kg once daily). Lastly, before and after release from the hospital, exercise restriction is an important aspect of patient management.

Patient Monitoring

The prognosis for DC is guarded to poor, with the overall mean life expectancy generally accepted at approximately 6 months. Giant breed dogs with DC may live substantially longer—up to 2 to 3 years in some instances, while the Doberman pinscher has a mean survival period of less than 3 months (ranging up to 1 year) after diagnosis. English springer spaniels with silent atrium cardiomyopathy have survived 6 to 12 months in our experience, while the English cocker spaniel is reported to have a life expectancy ranging from less than 2 weeks to more than 2 years. Harpster (Additional Reading) reports that boxers with cardiomyopathy survive approximately 6 months after the onset of heart failure, 1 year after the onset of cardiac syncope, and 2 years when diagnosed prior to the onset of symptoms.

The prognosis, expense, burden of treatment (often with a plethora of drugs), patient quality of life, and necessity of frequent clinical reevaluation should be carefully discussed with the owner prior to embarking on the treatment of a dog with DC. The use of referral centers for patient stabilization and diagnostic, prognostic, and therapeutic aid should be considered; follow-up care can frequently be provided by the primary care clinician.

Reevaluations are established based on the severity of the dog's signs and the client's interest in providing the input of time, effort, and money required in caring for such a patient. Asymptomatic dogs need only be examined at 3- to 6-month intervals. Symptomatic dogs should be evaluated as needed to maintain compensation, but should be seen no less often than at 3-month intervals. Dogs with severe signs of heart failure, cardiac arrhythmias, or other complications may require frequent office visits.

During follow-up visits, the presence and character of cough, dyspnea, exercise capacity, and general demeanor should be carefully evaluated. Body weight is monitored to assure that the patient's condition is not deteriorating further and to assess the state of hydration. Evaluation of skin turgor, mucous membranes, blood urea nitrogen, packed-cell volume, and total serum protein concentration allows crude approximations of the state of hydration. Patients with heart failure are intentionally kept in a state of mild dehydration (mildly azotemic, packed-cell volume 45%–50% [0.45–0.50 L/L], total serum protein greater than 7.5 g/dl [75 g/L]). Serum electrolyte concentrations (sodium and potassium) are periodically measured, especially in dogs afflicted with arrhythmias or past digitalis intoxication, both of which may be precipitated by hypokalemia. One week after institution of digoxin therapy, serum digoxin concentrations are evaluated (8 hours following administration). Desirable levels are between 1 and 2 ng/ml (1.3–2.6 nmol/L). Dosage adjustments can be made using this value, the dog's clinical response, and the presence of historical, physical, and electrocardiographic signs of digitalis intoxication.

Once heart failure has been diagnosed, thoracic radiographs are obtained at 6-month intervals, or more frequently if necessary, to follow changes in cardiac size, to check for recurrence of heart failure, and to evaluate the respiratory tract. Electrocardiography, used to evaluate heart rate and to detect arrhythmias, should be performed routinely. Echocardiograms are useful in evaluating left atrial and ventricular size, ventricular function, and the presence of pericardial effusion.

CANINE HYPERTROPHIC CARDIOMYOPATHY

Causes and Pathophysiology

While relatively common in humans and the cat, HC has been described in only a small number of dogs. Males appear to be predisposed, but all age groups are affected. Heredity is known to play an etiologic role in human HC and, while German shepherd dogs have been overrepresented in clinical reports—suggesting a familial (breed) predisposition, the etiology of canine HC remains unknown.

The underlying lesion consists of marked concentric hypertrophy of the left ventricle with compensatory left atrial enlargement (see Fig.

21-1) in the absence of an underlying cause such as aortic outflow obstruction (*e.g.*, aortic stenosis), hyperthyroidism, or systemic hypertension. Myocardial hypertrophy, fibrosis, and possibly cellular disorganization result in impaired ventricular filling, termed *diastolic failure* (decreased distensibility or compliance and prolonged or incomplete relaxation). Myocardial ischemia, due to the development of a large, relatively underperfused heart muscle, further impairs diastolic function. The end result is a small left ventricular lumen with a thickened, stiff, noncompliant ventricular wall, producing elevated ventricular end-diastolic, atrial, and pulmonary venous pressures. This is variably complicated by obstruction of left ventricular outflow by asymmetric septal hypertrophy and abnormal mitral valve motion, as well as by secondary mitral regurgitation, tachycardia, and cardiac arrhythmias. The ventricle is typically hyperdynamic and ejection fraction is usually high, although because of poor ventricular filling stroke volume is decreased. Clinical signs are produced by resultant diastolic left heart failure or by arrhythmias originating from the distended left atrium or the pathologically hypertrophied, fibrotic, and relatively underperfused left ventricle.

Clinical Signs

Manifestations reported in dogs with HC include unexpected death in asymptomatic dogs, particularly during anesthesia, reduced exercise tolerance, tachypnea, cough, and syncope. Fox (Additional Reading) reports that affected dogs may exhibit signs of right heart failure as well. Physical examination is often unrewarding, but may reveal a murmur, gallop, midsystolic click, arrhythmia, or pulmonary crackles.

Diagnostic Approach

The diagnosis of HC is typically made at necropsy or after echocardiographic examination. Suspicion of HC, based on clinical signs, is confirmed by the finding of left ventricular hypertrophy in the absence of an underlying cause such as sub-

aortic stenosis, hyperthyroidism, or systemic hypertension.

Electrocardiographic findings have included ventricular arrhythmias and first- and third-degree atrioventricular block. Interestingly, while common in humans and the cat, left ventricular enlargement patterns have been rarely described in the dog. Radiographic evidence of HC is subtle, but may include mild left atrial and ventricular enlargement, pulmonary venous congestion and edema, and pleural effusion.

Echocardiography provides the most useful noninvasive means of obtaining a diagnosis of HC. Reported echocardiographic findings (see Fig. 21-1) include thickened left ventricular and septal walls, asymmetric septal thickening, diminished left ventricular luminal size, enlarged left atrial dimension, systolic anterior mitral valve motion, and early closure and systolic flutter of the aortic valve. Similar anatomic abnormalities can be demonstrated with cardiac catheterization and angiocardiography (see Nonselective Angiocardiography in Chapter 80). Left ventricular end-diastolic pressure elevation and a pressure gradient from the left ventricle to the aorta is detected in some cases. Pathologic manifestations of HC substantiate echocardiograpic and angiographic findings, and include an increased heart weight : body weight ratio, hypertrophy of the interventricular septum and left ventricular free wall, a small left ventricular lumen, left atrial enlargement, and a fibrous plaque on the anterior mitral valve leaflet and the septum due to mutual contact. In the dog, histologic findings have been inconsistent, although myofiber disarray has been described.

Management and Patient Monitoring

Humans and cats afflicted with HC may live for years after diagnosis, even if heart failure has occurred. Because there is little information on the treatment of canine HC, recommendations are based on those of humans and the cat. Treatment should include either β-adrenergic or calcium channel (*e.g.*, verapamil or diltiazem) blockade. Because sudden death has been associated with exertion, exercise restriction should be employed. In addition, moderate salt restriction is enforced, even if the diagnosis is made prior to the onset of signs. The therapy for heart failure due to HC should also include salt and exercise restriction. Positive inotropic drugs are contraindicated because they may increase left ventricular end-diastolic pressure and the aortic pressure gradient. Concern over increasing the pressure gradient across the aortic valve has also resulted in recommendations against the use of arterial vasodilators and aggressive diuresis when obstruction to aortic outflow is present or expected. In the face of left heart failure, diuretics and venodilators may be employed. Arrhythmias are managed as described in Chapter 18. Although relatively contraindicated, digoxin's negative chronotropic effects may be useful in cases of atrial fibrillation with a rapid ventricular response, when β- and calcium channel blockade have failed to adequately reduce the heart rate.

Treatment as described above may prolong life, possibly delay progression of the disease, and prevent heart failure and sudden death due to arrhythmias. Nevertheless, owners should be carefully apprised of the possibility of sudden death and given a guarded prognosis.

FELINE DILATED CARDIOMYOPATHY

Causes and Pathophysiology

Cardiomyopathies represent a relatively more important cause of cardiac disease in the cat than in the dog, comprising nearly 10% of all feline necropsies in one study (Liu, 1977, Additional Reading). In this same study, congenital disease had a relative frequency of only one fifth that of dogs, and acquired valvular disease was uncommon. Because the relative prevalence of DC, HC, and RC seem to be in constant flux, with geographic influence as well, firm statements about the relative incidence are impossible. Of these cardiomyopathies, DC has traditionally carried the gravest prognosis.

Cats of all ages are afflicted with DC, with a mean age of onset of approximately 7 years. Although all breeds are affected, Siamese, Burmese, and Abyssinian cats may be predisposed.

There is no obvious gender predisposition for feline DC.

Previously considered to be primary or idiopathic, a large percentage of feline DC is now known to be nutritional in origin. Recent work by Pion and associates (Additional Reading) demonstrated a relationship between low plasma taurine concentrations and feline DC. It seems clear, based on the findings of low plasma taurine concentrations in cats with DC that were fed a taurine-deficient diet, the dramatic clinical response to taurine supplementation, and the ability to experimentally produce cardiac dysfunction in cats fed a taurine-deficient diet, that the relationship between plasma taurine deficiency and DC is causal. Early evidence suggests that primary DC (unrelated to taurine deficiency) still does exist, even after adequate taurine supplementation of commercial diets. Nevertheless, the overall incidence of DC has plummeted. Other causes of secondary DC include end-stage thyrotoxic heart disease and, possibly, HC. Many other potential causes exist, including viral, fungal, bacterial, protozoan, toxic, and ischemic insults to the myocardium.

The heart in DC is eccentrically hypertrophied, with relatively thin walls, enlarged atrial and ventricular chambers, and flattened papillary muscles (Fig. 21-8). Histologic evidence of myocyte thinning with accumulation of extracellular edema and fibrosis is also noted. The pathophysiology of cardiac decompensation is similar to that described for canine DC, the primary defect being depressed global ventricular contractile performance, secondary atrial and ventricular enlargement (eccentric hypertrophy), and atrioventricular valvular incompetence (see Fig. 21-1). The end result is diminished tissue perfusion, fluid retention, afterload elevation, compensatory tachycardia (often absent in the cat with DC), arrhythmias, and elevated ventricular end-diastolic pressures. Since both ventricles are affected, signs of left and right forward and congestive heart failure are observed. Most of the signs manifested by cats with DC are those of right congestive heart failure (pleural effusion) and low cardiac output (cold extremities, hypothermia, azotemia, weakness). Cats with cardiomyopathy are prone to the development of systemic arterial

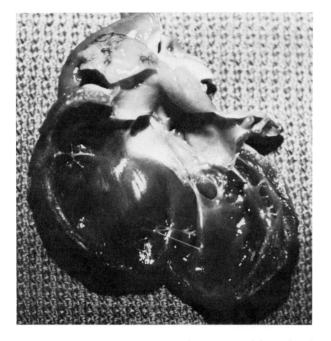

Figure 21–8 *Postmortem specimen demonstrating left atrial and ventricular enlargement in a cat with dilated cardiomyopathy. Note the relative absence of papillary muscles.*

embolization (SAE), which can precipitate heart failure, worsening the prognosis (see Chapter 24).

Clinical Signs

Cats affected with DC typically have a subacute (1- to 3-day) onset of signs unless failure is precipitated by the stress of SAE. Historical findings (see Table 21-1) most often include lethargy, anorexia, dyspnea, or unexpected death. In the presence of SAE, rear or front leg lameness, paresis, or paralysis may be noted. Emesis, ascites, and syncope have been uncommonly described. Although ascites is frequently suggested as a sign of DC, Harpster (Additional Reading) reported ascites in only 3% of 31 cats with DC. Cough is not a typical finding of cardiac failure of any cause in cats.

Physical examination (see Table 21-1) reveals a dyspneic, dehydrated, hypothermic, and depressed patient. The heart rate varies from subnormal to increased. The extremities are cold and the mucous membranes ashen with prolonged capillary refill time. Thoracic auscultation fre-

quently allows appreciation of a systolic murmur (left apical) or diastolic gallop (S_3), muffling of heart and lung sounds by pleural effusion, and, uncommonly, pulmonary crackles produced by pulmonary edema. Significant effusion can be suggested by thoracic percussion. The pulses are generally weak (absent with SAE), and arrhythmias may be detected. Abdominal ballotment and palpation may infrequently disclose evidence of ascites and hepatosplenomegaly.

Diagnostic Approach

The majority of cats with DC have some electrocardiographic abnormality (Fig. 21-9). The heart rate is less than 150 beats per minute in approximately 10% and less than 200 beats per minute in 50% of cases. Harpster (Additional Reading) reports that 71% of affected cats have wide QRS complexes, 19% have P-mitrale, 16% have conduction disturbances, and 61% have arrhythmias (predominantly ventricular). Tall R waves are noted less than 50% of the time.

Radiographic findings in DC include a globoid, markedly enlarged heart, which is often obscured by pleural effusion (Fig. 21-10). If signs of right heart failure predominate, caudal vena caval and hepatic enlargement, as well as ascites, may be evident. Nonselective angiocardiography (see Chapter 80), while useful in making a diagnosis, may be dangerous in cats with extreme cardiac dysfunction. Findings include slow circulation time, dilatation of all four cardiac chambers, flattening of left ventricular papillary muscles, and a small aorta, reflecting diminished cardiac output. Distinction of types of cardiomyopathy using radiology alone, or even in conjunction with electrocardiographic and clinical findings, can be misleading.

Echocardiography offers the most accurate, sensitive, and safest means of making a definitive diagnosis of DC. Findings are similar to those described for the dog, and include left ventricular hypokinesis, global cardiac chamber enlargement, and relatively thin left ventricular and interventricular septal walls (Fig. 21-11; see Fig. 21-1).

Laboratory findings in cats with DC may in-

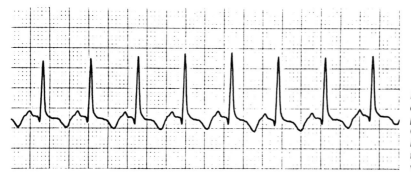

Figure 21–9 Electrocardiogram typifying feline dilated cardiomyopathy. Tachycardia (240 beats per minute), tall R waves (1.7 mV), and wide QRS complexes (60 msec) are noted. The rapid heart rate is compatible with anxiety or heart failure, while the other parameters suggest left ventricular enlargement.

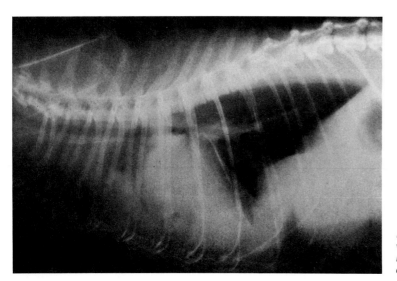

Figure 21–10 Lateral thoracic radiograph of a cat with heart failure secondary to dilated cardiomyopathy. Note cardiac enlargement and presence of pleural effusion.

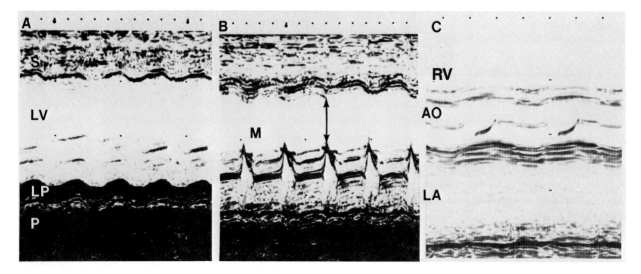

Figure 21–11 M-mode echocardiogram obtained from a cat with dilated cardiomyopathy. (A) Note left ventricular enlargement and hypokinesis, (arrow, B) increased E-point septal separation and (C) enlarged left atrium : aortic root ratio and hypodynamic aortic root movement. (RV = right ventricle; S = septum; LV = left ventricle; LP = left ventricular posterior wall; P = pericardium; M = mitral valve; AO = aortic root; LA = left atrium)

clude a modified thoracic transudate, elevated central venous pressure, elevation in liver enzyme activity (serum alanine aminotransferase in approximately 50% of cases), prolonged sulfobromphthalein (BSP) retention, subnormal plasma taurine concentrations, prerenal azotemia, and stress-induced hyperglycemia. In addition, when SAE is present, typical findings of disseminated intravascular coagulation, and increased serum creatine kinase, lactic dehydrogenase, and aspartate aminotransferase activities may be detected. Because hyperthyroidism can produce cardiac dysfunction, serum T4 concentrations should be measured in all aged (older than 5 years) cats with heart failure (see Chapter 61).

Other diagnoses that should be considered include chylothorax, primary or metastatic thoracic neoplasia (especially mediastinal lymphosarcoma), pyothorax, feline infectious peritonitis, hydrothorax, ascites due to hypoalbuminemia, heartworm disease, primary respiratory disease, thoracic trauma or hemorrhagic diathesis, and diaphragmatic hernia. Cardiac disorders that might be confused with DC are other cardiomyopathies (including hypertensive and thyrotoxic heart disease), high output failure due to anemia or arteriovenous fistula, congenital heart disease, vegetative endocarditis, and noninfectious acquired valvular disease.

Management

The treatment goals for feline DC are similar to those described for the dog (see Table 21-3), although the means by which these goals are attained is somewhat different. Most cats are presented in phase IV heart disease, often in cardiogenic shock. The challenge of maintaining life through the first 24 to 72 hours is difficult in such instances. Emergency therapy is outlined in Table 21-5; certain differences, applicable to the cat, are discussed below.

Emergency Care

In the cat with cardiogenic shock and dyspnea, excessive handling and stress should be avoided. Cage rest, preferably in a heated oxygen cage

(40% oxygen) should be employed before or after (if necessary as a lifesaving measure) thoracentesis. Digoxin and taurine (250–500 mg twice daily) should be administered and, in some instances, intravenous fluid therapy (5% dextrose in water with 30 mEq of potassium chloride per liter at 1 ml/kg/hour) is beneficial. Indications for fluid therapy include cardiogenic shock (see Chapter 4) and dehydration. Monitoring of central venous pressure (see Chapter 80) may be helpful, but if the installation of a central venous pressure line is too stressful to the patient, it should be forgone. Because congestive signs can generally be alleviated with thoracentesis, and because cardiac output is further imperiled by reduction in preload, vasodilators and aggressive diuresis are avoided. An exception is the case in which dyspnea due to pulmonary edema persists after pleural effusion has been removed.

Inotropic Support

Cardiac glycosides are indicated in feline DC; studies in our laboratory have demonstrated their efficacy in cats with DC. Digoxin has been shown to be beneficial in cats with heart failure due to DC that are receiving taurine supplementation. Typically, digoxin is administered at oral maintenance doses (0.01 mg/kg/48 hours, reduced to 0.007 mg/kg/48 hours when furosemide, aspirin, and a salt-restricted diet are used concurrently), but it has been used intravenously in the face of cardiogenic shock. The presence of heart failure does not dictate further lowering of digoxin dosage. Digoxin may be administered as a fraction of a tablet or, more accurately, as an elixir; we prefer to first try the latter, finding that many cats accept this formulation. Because of individual variation, serum digoxin concentrations should be evaluated at steady state (1–2 weeks after beginning treatment), ideally falling between 1 to 2 ng/ml (1.3–2.6 nmol/L). Data from our laboratory suggest that samples drawn 8 hours after drug administration correlate very well with mean serum digoxin concentrations when digoxin is administered on an every other day regime.

Although dobutamine is theoretically useful in the treatment of DC, its results in cats have been disappointing, with seizures and vomition being common complications. Milrinone has not yet been evaluated in the cat.

Off-loading Therapy

As stated above, preload reduction with diuretics and vasodilators may further reduce cardiac output in cardiogenic shock due to DC. For this reason we avoid their use unless there is compelling evidence for their need, utilizing thoracentesis as a safer and more effective alternative (see Thoracentesis and Insertion of Chest Tubes in Chapter 80). Furosemide, however, can be administered chronically after stabilization, at the lowest dosage resulting in alleviation of signs. Furosemide (1–4 mg/kg once to three times daily orally or parenterally) should be accompanied by the provision of a sodium-restricted diet (Hill's Feline Prescription Diet h/d). Selective afterload reduction (hydralazine) may improve cardiac output, but can also produce significant hypotension in this setting. Vasodilators do have an indication in chronic treatment of heart failure due to DC; however, since the advent and success of taurine supplementation, their use is often unnecessary.

Antiarrhythmic Therapy

Frequently, digoxin administration and control of heart failure alleviates arrhythmias; if not, propranolol, lidocaine, procainamide, or quinidine (listed in order of preference) may be employed. Propranolol is the antiarrhythmic drug of choice for cats because of the prevalence of adverse reactions to other commonly used ventricular antiarrhythmic agents. It is indicated for both supraventricular and ventricular arrhythmias. The use of the other antiarrhythmic drugs is controversial and may be associated with hypotension and, with lidocaine, seizures. The routine use of propranolol cannot be advocated in cats with DC and sinus rhythm because of its negative inotropic effect, the infrequency of sustained ventricular and supraventricular arrhythmias, and its potential to increase afterload by causing peripheral vasoconstriction. The presence of significant ventricular arrhythmia is a relative contraindication to the use of digoxin, and it should be employed cautiously in this setting.

Miscellaneous Therapy

Taurine (250–500 mg orally twice daily) should be administered to all cats with DC, regardless of whether taurine deficiency is proved. The mortality in cats with DC is markedly reduced with taurine supplementation. Although echocardiographic evidence of improved myocardial function is inapparent prior to 3 to 6 weeks of therapy, clinical response suggests an earlier benefit. Oxygen therapy, supplemental heat, and intravenous fluid administration (5% dextrose in water with potassium chloride added) may be indicated. Prevention of SAE is attempted with anticoagulative therapy, typically aspirin (1¼ grain every 72 hours), which is used for its ability to suppress formation of platelet-generated thromboxane. Specific therapy for SAE is discussed in Chapter 24.

Patient Monitoring

The prognosis for feline DC has traditionally been poor to grave, with approximately an 85% mortality rate. However, with taurine supplementation mortality has been reduced to approximately 30% to 50%. The prognosis for nontaurine-deficient DC (*e.g.*, thyrotoxic DC) remains poor. Responsive cats will return quickly to normal activity, but will have echocardiographic evidence of diminished cardiac function for months (Fig. 21-12). Ultimately, radiographic and echocardiographic abnormalities resolve. At that time, cardiac therapy, including taurine supplementation (assuming adequate dietary intake), can be discontinued.

FELINE HYPERTROPHIC CARDIOMYOPATHY

Causes and Pathophysiology

Hypertrophic cardiomyopathy is the most prevalent feline cardiac disorder, its relative importance having increased with the decline in the incidence of DC. It is a disease of middle-aged cats (average 5–7 years), but all ages are affected.

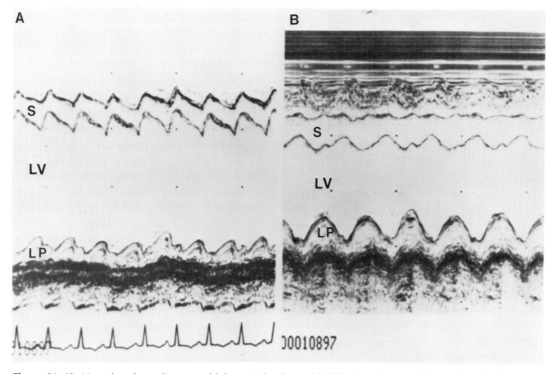

Figure 21–12 *M-mode echocardiograms of left ventricle of cat with dilated cardiomyopathy associated with taurine deficiency before (A) and 12 months after continued taurine supplementation (B). Note the decrease in heart rate and left ventricular (LV) dimensions and the improved septal (S) and left ventricular posterior wall (LP) motion with therapy. Prior to therapy, LV diastolic and systolic dimensions were 2.5 and 2 cm, respectively, with a shortening fraction of 20% (normal is greater than 35% to 40%). After therapy, LV diastolic and systolic dimensions were 1.8 and 1.2 cm, respectively, with a shortening fraction of 33%.*

There is a male predisposition, with a nearly 90% male incidence in one study. In humans there is an important hereditary predisposition for HC in 55% of cases. In humans this disorder may be congenital or acquired, and probably represents a group of diseases. Although the etiology of feline HC is unknown, the Persian cat has appeared to be predisposed in some case series, suggesting a genetic influence. As is the case with systemic hypertension, hyperthyroidism (see Chapter 61), and aortic stenosis, HC is associated with marked left ventricular hypertrophy, but in this instance no underlying cause can be identified.

Cardiac lesions are similar to those described for the dog, with severe left ventricular concentric hypertrophy and secondary left atrial dilatation being the hallmarks (Fig. 21-13; see Fig. 21-1). Asymmetric septal hypertrophy, present in the majority of dogs and humans with HC, is present in only 30% of cats with HC. Histologic cardiac myofiber disarray is reported in 27% of affected cats and only in those with asymmetric septal hypertrophy. Other histologic features of feline HC include myocardial and endocardial fibrosis and narrowed coronary arteries (Liu, 1977, Additional Reading). Dynamic aortic outflow obstruction, secondary mitral insufficiency, myocardial ischemia, and SAE may complicate this syndrome.

The left heart is predominantly affected, and clinical signs manifest as sudden death or, more commonly, left heart failure, due to diastolic dysfunction. The pathophysiologic mechanisms of diastolic failure are identical to those described in the dog, while systolic function is usually adequate or enhanced. The onset of left heart failure is typically acute and often associated with a stressful event (Fig. 21-14). Lord and associates (Additional Reading) demonstrated an elevated resting left ventricular end-diastolic pressure

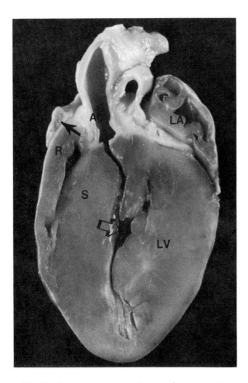

Figure 21–13 *Postmortem specimen demonstrating cardiac changes of feline hypertrophic cardiomyopathy. The enlarged left atrium (LA) is contrasted with the normal right atrium (arrow). The left ventricular posterior (LV) and septal (S) walls are severely hypertrophied, while the right ventricular wall (R) is spared. Note the small left ventricular lumen (open arrow). (AO = aorta) (Photograph courtesy of Dr. James Cooley, University of Wisconsin)*

(LVEDP) in feline HC. With the administration of isoproterenol, which mimics endogenous, stress-related sympathoadrenal activity, the LVEDP pressure doubled. Left ventricular end-diastolic pressure is indicative of pressures in the left atrium and pulmonary veins, which reflect the tendency for the development of pulmonary edema. In addition, during stressful situations acceleration of the heart rate reduces cardiac filling time and myocardial perfusion. The former further diminishes cardiac volume and the latter results in relative myocardial ischemia in a rapidly beating heart with high oxygen needs, thereby aggravating diastolic dysfunction. Stressful incidents, such as a car ride, restraint for an electrocardiogram, or confrontation with a dog, or an embolic event may precipitate left heart failure and pulmonary edema.

Clinical Signs

With the aid of electrocardiography, thoracic radiographs, and echocardiography, a high percentage of cases of HC are diagnosed prior to the onset of symptomatology (Table 21-6). Suspicion is raised when the attending clinician discovers a murmur, gallop, or arrhythmia. At the other end

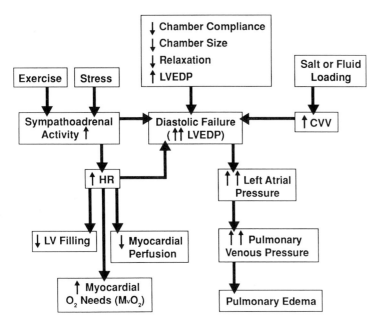

Figure 21–14 *Schematic diagram demonstrating precipitory mechanisms of heart failure in hypertrophic cardiomyopathy. The left ventricles (LV) of affected hearts are small-chambered and noncompliant, relax slowly or incompletely, and have elevated resting end-diastolic pressures (LVEDP). Stressful events produce sympathoadrenal discharge with sinus tachycardia. This increases myocardial oxygen needs, and, by shortening diastole, further impairs LV filling and limits myocardial perfusion. Resultant myocardial ischemia aggravates already suboptimal myocardial relaxation, the end result being further elevation of LVEDP. This pressure increase is reflected to the left atrium and pulmonary veins; increased pulmonary venous hydrostatic pressure, if sufficient, results in pulmonary edema. Alternatively, or in conjunction, salt or fluid loading can increase cardiovascular volume (CVV), producing left heart failure by elevating pulmonary venous pressures, as the noncompliant LV cannot accommodate this volume load. (HR = heart rate)*

Table 21–6 *Abnormal Historical and Physical Findings in Feline Hypertrophic Cardiomyopathy*

HISTORICAL FINDINGS

Periods of dyspnea
Acute onset of dyspnea or signs of embolism; or asymptomatic
Emesis
Sudden death

PHYSICAL FINDINGS

Dyspnea
Tachypnea
Anxiety
Ashen (or cyanotic) cool mucous membranes
Prolonged capillary refill time
Pulmonary crackles
Normal or muffled heart sounds
Normal or accentuated cardiac apex beat
Murmur
Cardiac gallop (S₄)
Auscultable arrhythmias
Normal pulse, pulse deficits (arrhythmias), or absence of femoral pulses (with saddle thrombus)

hypertrophy, such as hyperthyroidism, systemic hypertension, and aortic stenosis, must also be ruled out.

The electrocardiogram is abnormal in 35% to 70% of cases, and can provide useful diagnostic information. Many electrocardiographic findings are not specific. Left axis deviation and left anterior fascicular block (Fig. 21-15) are strongly suggestive of HC, but also may be recognized in RC, hyperkalemia, hyperthyroidism, and, rarely, DC. Other electrocardiographic abnormalities include P-mitrale and P-pulmonale (10% and 20%, respectively), tall R waves (40%), wide QRS complexes (35%), conduction disturbances (50%, including left axis deviation in 25% and left anterior fascicular block in 15%), and arrhythmias (55%, usually ventricular in origin).

of the spectrum, cats may die unexpectedly with no prior signs. The most common clinical sign is the sudden onset of dyspnea, with or without evidence of SAE (the prevalence of dyspnea was 16% in clinical studies and 48% in autopsy studies). Physical examination typically reveals a well-fleshed, dyspneic cat with audible pulmonary crackles, murmur (50% of cases)—typically loudest at the left apex, gallop (40%, usually S₄), or arrhythmia (25%–40% of cases). Heart sounds may be muffled. The oral mucosa is ashen and the pulses normal, weak, or absent (SAE), the apex beat may be hyperdynamic, and the liver may be palpably enlarged. Cats with HC are generally not hypothermic, a characteristic that is useful in differentiation from DC (see Table 21-1).

Diagnostic Approach

The diagnosis of HC is not difficult, but does require special testing to confirm clinical suspicions. Without the aid of echocardiography, DC and RC can be difficult to distinguish from HC. This distinction is especially important in the case of DC, because it requires an entirely different therapeutic approach and prognosis. Other disorders that produce left ventricular and septal

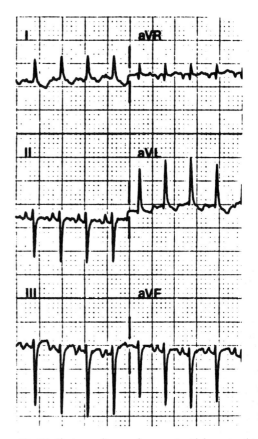

Figure 21–15 *Electrocardiogram from a cat with hypertrophic cardiomyopathy demonstrating changes compatible with left anterior fascicular block (S₂, S₃, aVF, R₁, aVL, and left axis deviation). This finding may also be recognized in normal cats and in those with hyperthyroidism or hyperkalemia.*

Thoracic radiographic findings suggestive of HC include cardiomegaly with a prominent left ventricle and atrium, and pulmonary congestion or edema (Fig. 21-16). In the ventrodorsal projection, the heart may appear "valentine-shaped," reflecting the concentric ventricular hypertrophy and enlarged left auricle (Fig. 21-17). Additionally, the apex is often shifted to the right.

On the lateral view the heart is enlarged, with increased sternal contact, left atrial prominence, left ventricular convexity, and a prominent caudal cardiac waist (see Fig. 21-16). Pleural effusion may be noted in 25% to 33% of cases in heart failure, but is usually of much less volume than that noted in DC.

Nonselective angiocardiography (see Chapter

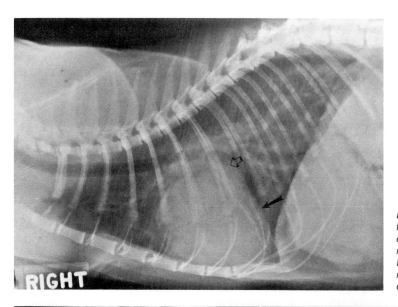

Figure 21–16 *Lateral thoracic radiograph obtained from a cat in left heart failure due to hypertrophic cardiomyopathy. Note increased lung density (pulmonary edema), most prominent in caudal lung lobes; generalized cardiomegaly; left atrial enlargement (open arrow); and rounded left ventricular caudal border (arrow).*

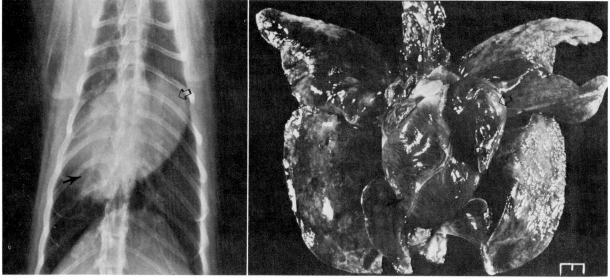

Figure 21–17 *Ventrodorsal radiograph accompanying necropsy specimen from a cat with hypertrophic cardiomyopathy. Note rightward shift of apex (arrows), left auricular enlargement (open arrows), and classical "valentine" appearance of the feline hypertrophic myopathic heart. (Necropsy photograph courtesy of Dr. James Cooley, University of Wisconsin.)*

80) is of less risk in HC than in DC. This procedure typically reveals normal or enhanced circulation, pulmonary venous tortuosity, left atrial enlargement, a small left ventricular lumen, thickening of the left ventricular wall, and papillary muscle enlargement. The diagnosis of SAE (saddle thrombus) can be confirmed by the finding of an abrupt termination of the dye column in the aorta at its trifurcation.

Nonselective angiocardiography is extremely useful for distinguishing HC from DC, but, because of overlap of echocardiographic reference values, differentiation of normal from asymptomatic HC and HC from RC may be difficult. Concentric left ventricular hypertrophy and left atrial enlargement are features useful in confirming the diagnosis of HC (see Fig. 21-1). Cardiac function is normal to exaggerated due to diminished afterload and possibly to hypercontractility. Systolic anterior mitral valve motion may be evident, suggesting dynamic aortic outflow obstruction. If present, asymmetric septal hypertrophy, left atrial thrombi, pleural effusion, or pericardial effusion may be evident.

In the case of sudden death, the diagnosis is made at necropsy by disclosure of typical gross and histologic cardiac pathology. Other laboratory findings, with the exception of hypotaurinemia, are similar to that described for feline DC. Differential diagnoses are also similar, with the addition of restrictive pericarditis and emphasis of systemic hypertensive and hypertrophic thyrotoxic heart disease.

Management

The treatment of HC is different from that of DC and entails the goals of reducing LVEDP, abolishing sinus tachycardia and other arrhythmias, improving myocardial oxygenation, and alleviating and preventing pulmonary edema (Table 21-7). Positive inotropic agents are not needed and are generally contraindicated because they may increase LVEDP and aggravate outflow obstruction. The latter precaution should be exercised in the use of arterial vasodilators and, to a lesser degree, preload reducing agents (diuretics and mixed vasodilators or venodilators). These concerns are discussed under the topic of canine HC.

Off-loading Therapy

Diuretic therapy is indicated to eliminate pulmonary edema. Furosemide is the diuretic of choice in emergencies because it reduces LVEDP and, hence, left atrial and pulmonary venous pressures through diuresis and venodilation. In the emergency situation, treatment with parenteral furosemide (2–4 mg/kg IV or IM) is accompanied by the use of topical nitroglycerin ($^1/_8$–$^1/_4$ inch three–four times daily) and oxygen supplementation (40%). Nitroglycerin's effect is maintained after the first 24 hours only if used in a "16 hours on and 8 hours off" regimen. Although furosemide diuresis is usually successful, the addition of supplemental diuretic agents (*e.g.*, thiazides) and possibly vasodilators (*e.g.*, captopril) is indicated in refractory cases or when secondary right heart failure ensues. Chronic furosemide therapy is maintained at the lowest possible dose, usually 1.0–4.0 mg/kg orally one to three times daily.

β-*Adrenergic and Calcium Channel Blockade*

Drugs that enhance ventricular relaxation and slow the heart include the β-adrenergic (*e.g.*, metoprolol, propranolol) and calcium channel (*e.g.*, verapamil and diltiazem) blockers. Such therapy is indicated in treatment of the diastolic failure of HC. β-Blockers may improve diastolic compliance directly or may merely enhance ventricular filling by reducing heart rate and improving myocardial oxygenation. Traditionally, propranolol has been administered orally after stabilization (24–36 hours after institution of diuretic therapy at 2.5–5 mg two to three times daily) to reduce and prevent elevations in LVEDP, to lower systolic pressure gradients and myocardial oxygen requirements, to prevent stress-induced tachycardia, and to reduce resting heart rate, as well as for its antiarrhythmic effects. When arrhythmias are present, this drug may be initiated earlier in the disease course.

Table 21–7 *Feline Dilated and Hypertrophic Cardiomyopathies: Treatment Goals, With Agents and Methods Used to Accomplish Them*

Dilated Cardiomyopathy

Therapeutic Goal	Agents Employed
Reduce cardiac work	Digitalis (0.007 mg/kg every 48 hours, PO), exercise restriction (venodilators, nitroglycerin at ¼ to ⅛ inch t.i.d.)*
Improve cardiac output	Digitalis, fluids (5% dextrose in water)†
Alleviate signs of congestive heart failure	Thoracentesis, possibly diuretics,‡ sodium restriction
Optimize heart rate and rhythm	Digitalis, specific antiarrhythmic therapy, depending on rate and rhythm
Miscellaneous	Taurine (250 to 500 mg b.i.d., PO), supplemental heat, oxygen, aspirin (1¼ grains every 72 hours, PO), treat thromboembolism

Hypertrophic Cardiomyopathy

Therapeutic Goal	Agents Employed
Improve diastolic function and cardiac output	Calcium channel blockade (diltiazem at 3 mg t.i.d., PO), beta-blockade (propranolol, metoprolol)
Alleviate signs of congestive heart failure	Diuretics (furosemide at 1 to 4 mg/kg s.i.d.–t.i.d., PO, SC, IM, IV), venodilators, sodium restriction, calcium channel (or beta) blockade
Optimize heart rate and rhythm and reduce cardiac work	Calcium channel blockade, beta-blockade, exercise restriction
Miscellaneous	Oxygen, aspirin, sedation (acetylpromazine), treat thromboembolism

* *Although afterload reduction is theoretically indicated, such therapy is questionable in the face of cardiogenic shock, the typical presentation of cats with dilated cardiomyopathy. Recommendations for arterial vasodilation in chronic therapy have not been forthcoming. For these reasons, we generally avoid such therapy in cats with dilated cardiomyopathy, particularly in those with dramatic response to taurine supplementation and conventional therapy.*
† *Although dobutamine and dopamine are theoretically indicated in cats with severe heart failure due to dilated cardiomyopathy, their efficacy has not been established.*
‡ *Diuretics should be used cautiously, if at all, in the cat presented in cardiogenic shock due to dilated cardiomyopathy.*

Calcium channel blocking agents have been effective in human HC by reducing heart rate, myocardial oxygen consumption, and diastolic dysfunction. In addition to directly enhancing myocardial relaxation, these drugs dilate peripheral and coronary arteries. Recently, Bright and Golden (Additional Reading) demonstrated the utility of diltiazem (3 mg orally three times daily) in the treatment feline HC, including those cases refractory to propranolol. Unfortunately, current packaging for human use makes accurate feline dosing of diltiazem difficult.

Antiarrhythmic Therapy

Drugs other than those described above should be used sparingly and with caution (see section on feline DC). Digoxin, while generally contraindicated in HC, may be used when supraventricular arrhythmias are refractory to calcium channel and β-adrenergic blocking agents.

Miscellaneous Therapy

Other therapies, including oxygen, aspirin, home confinement, and salt restriction, should be instituted as needed and as described for DC. Taurine supplementation is not necessary in the treatment of HC. In asymptomatic cats with HC we advise home confinement, moderate salt restriction, propranolol and/or diltiazem, and aspirin indefinitely.

Patient Monitoring

Cats with asymptomatic HC should be evaluated at 6- to 12-month intervals, while those with symptoms should ideally be seen no less frequently than every 3 months. The prognosis for HC is guarded to good, with many cats surviving for years. Refinement of calcium channel blocking therapy may further enhance survival. The prognosis worsens with the development of right heart failure, arrhythmias, and SAE.

RESTRICTIVE CARDIOMYOPATHY

Causes and Pathophysiology

Restrictive cardiomyopathy, also termed *intermediate cardiomyopathy*, is less common than DC and HC, comprising 15% of 73 consecutive cases of feline cardiomyopathy described by Harpster (Additional Reading). The relative prevalence of RC will likely rise as DC becomes less common. It is a disease of middle to old age (average 11 years), but cats of all ages have been affected. There is no obvious breed or gender predisposition.

The cause of RC is unknown, but it is characterized by diastolic failure secondary to severe endocardial and myocardial fibrosis (Fig. 21-18). Fibrosis is accompanied by patchy areas of myocyte atrophy, necrosis, and inflammation. Myxomatous changes in the mitral valve have also been described. There is neither the extreme concentric hypertrophy of HC nor the eccentric hypertrophy of DC, but the heart weight:body weight ratio is increased and moderate left atrial dilatation is recognized.

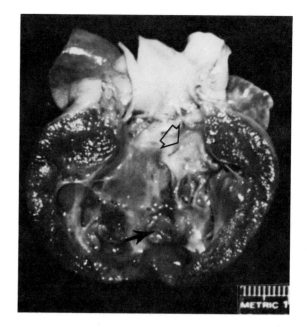

Figure 21–18 *Heart from cat with restrictive cardiomyopathy. The thickened endocardial surface is evident* (open arrow) *and a mural vegetation* (arrow) *can also be seen.*

The end result, diastolic failure, has similarities to restrictive pericarditis in that there is a physical restriction to cardiac filling, thereby reducing diastolic volume and cardiac output. Systolic function too may be somewhat compromised. Complications include arrhythmias, mitral insufficiency, and SAE. Cardiac dysfunction culminates in left, right, or biventricular failure, manifested variably by pulmonary edema, pleural or pericardial effusion, and ascites.

Clinical Signs

The onset is acute or subacute, often preceded by illness of several days' duration. Prodromal signs include lethargy, weakness, anorexia, weight loss, and, rarely, vomiting and cough. The acute presentation is for dyspnea with or without SAE. Physical examination variably reveals hypothermia, dyspnea, muffled thoracic sounds, pulmonary crackles, left- or right-sided murmurs (20%), gallops (25%), arrhythmias, ashen mucous membranes with prolonged capillary refill time, weak or absent pulses, and hepatomegaly with ascites.

Diagnostic Approach

Differentiation of RC from other forms of cardiomyopathy, particularly HC, is difficult. Fortunately, because therapy is not different between the two syndromes, this distinction is less important. Other differential diagnoses are similar to those of HC and DC.

The electrocardiogram is abnormal in 30% to 70% of cases, with arrhythmias identified in 7 of 11 cases in one report. Prolongation of the P wave and QRS complex and conduction disturbances are also common. Thoracic radiography discloses pulmonary edema or pleural effusion, generalized cardiomegaly with particular prominence of the left atrium, hepatomegaly, and ascites. A globoid heart is produced when a large amount of pericardial effusion is present. Nonselective angiocardiography (see Chapter 80) has been suggested as the best method for diagnosing RC. It reveals enlargement of the left atrium, encroachment on and filling defects of the left ventricle, enlarged, tortuous pulmonary veins, and, occasionally, left atrial thrombi. Echocardiography may demonstrate left and right ventricular and septal hypertrophy with asymmetry of the ventricular lumen, abnormal intraluminal echodensities, enlarged left atrium—occasionally with a thrombus, diminished papillary muscle size, mildly depressed left ventricular function, increased echogenicity of the endocardium, and pericardial effusion.

Management and Patient Monitoring

Therapy for heart failure due to RC is not uniformly successful, nor is a treatment protocol well established. Pleural effusion may be life-threatening and, if clinically warranted, should be removed by thoracentesis. Furosemide and nitroglycerin are used to combat pulmonary edema. Mixed or arterial vasodilators may be utilized in unresponsive cases. Although digoxin has been advocated, it would seem to be of little value unless severe myocardial dysfunction or unresponsive supraventricular arrhythmia is documented. Arrhythmias are treated as previously described (see Chapter 18). Salt and exercise restriction and aspirin should also be employed.

The long-term prognosis for cats with RC is guarded to poor. The prognosis worsens when cardiogenic shock, arrhythmias, SAE, or biventricular failure complicate the picture.

ADDITIONAL READING

Atkins CE, Snyder PS, Keene BW. The effect of aspirin, furosemide, and commercial low salt diet on digoxin kinetics in normal cats. J Am Vet Med Assoc 1987; 193:1264.

Atkins CE, Snyder PS, Keene BW, Rush JE. The effect of compensated heart failure on digoxin pharmacokinetics in cats. J Am Vet Med Assoc, 1989; 195:945.

Atkins CE, Snyder PS, Keene BW et al. Efficacy of digoxin in the treatment of feline dilated cardiomyopathy. J Am Vet Med Assoc, in press.

Bright JM, Golden AL. The use of calcium channel blockers in cats with hypertrophic cardiomyopathy (abstr). Proc Sixth Ann Intern Med Forum 1988: 184.

Calvert CA. Dilated (congestive) cardiomyopathy in Doberman pinschers. Compendium of Continuing Education 1986; 6:417.

Fox PR. Canine myocardial disease. In: Fox PR, ed. Canine and feline cardiology. New York: Churchill Livingstone, 1988: 467.

Fox PR. Feline myocardial disease. In: Fox PR, ed. Canine and feline cardiology. New York: Churchill Livingstone, 1988: 435.

Harpster NK. The cardiovascular system. In: Holzworth J, ed. Diseases of the cat. Philadelphia: WB Saunders, 1987: 820.

Hill BL. Canine idiopathic congestive cardiomyopathy. Compendium of Continuing Education 1981; 3:615.

Keene BW, Panciera DL, Regitz V et al. Carnitine-linked defects of myocardial metabolism in canine dilated cardiomyopathy (abstr). Proc Fourth Ann Intern Med Forum 1986: 54.

Keene BW, Rush JE. Therapy of heart failure. In: Ettinger SJ, ed. Veterinary internal medicine, 3rd ed. Philadelphia: WB Saunders, 1989: 939.

Kittleson MD, Eyster GE, Knowlen GG et al. Effect of digoxin administration in dogs with idiopathic congestive cardiomyopathy. J Am Vet Med Assoc 1985; 186:162.

Kittleson MD, Pipers FS, Knauer KW et al. Echocardiographic and clinical effects of milrinone in dogs with myocardial failure. Am J Vet Res 1985; 46:1659.

Lewis LD, Morris ML, Hand MS. Heart failure. In: Small animal clinical nutrition, 3rd ed. Topeka: Mark Morris Associates, 1989; 11:1.

Liu SK. Pathology of feline heart diseases. Vet Clin North Am [Small Anim Pract] 1977; 7:323.

Liu SK, Fox PR, Tilley LP. Excessive moderator bands in the left ventricle of 21 cats. J Am Vet Med Assoc 1982; 180:1215.

Liu SK, Tashjian RJ, Patnaik AK. Congestive heart failure in the cat. J Am Vet Med Assoc 1970; 156:1319.

Lord PF, Wood A, Tilley LP et al. Radiographic and hemodynamic evaluation of cardiomyopathy and thromboembolism in the cat. Am J Vet Res 1974; 164:154.

Pion PD, Kittleson MD, Rogers QR, Morris JG. Myocardial failure in cats associated with low plasma taurine: A reversible cardiomyopathy. Science 1987; 237:764.

Rush JE, Keene BW. ECG of the month. J Am Vet Med Assoc 1988; 194:52.

Staaden RV. Cardiomyopathy of English cocker spaniels. J Am Vet Med Assoc 1981; 178:1289.

Tilley LP. Persistent atrial standstill ("silent atrium"). In: Tilley, LP, ed. Essentials of canine and feline electrocardiography, 2nd ed. Philadelphia: Lea & Febiger, 1985: 164.

22

BACTERIAL ENDOCARDITIS

Clarke E. Atkins

Bacterial endocarditis represents a relatively uncommon, but clinically devastating syndrome in small animal patients. Bacterial infection may affect both the heart valves and the mural endocardium, producing both cardiac and extracardiac manifestations. Affected dogs are typically large (average greater than 30 kg), male (70%), and older than 4 years of age. German shepherds and dogs with congenital heart disease have been suggested as being at increased risk. The incidence, based on postmortem studies, has ranged from less than 1% to more than 6%. The cat also develops bacterial endocarditis, but as is the case with heart disease in general, the frequency is less than that of the dog. In both dogs and cats, the mitral and aortic valves are most often affected. In five studies involving 187 dogs, the left side was affected alone in 79% and mural lesions were present in only 8% of cases. The mitral valve was involved in 67%, the aortic in 23%, and both in 15%; the tricuspid was involved in 10%, and the pulmonic in less than 1% of dogs with bacterial endocarditis (Figs. 22-1 and 22-2). More than one valve may be affected (there were two affected valves in 27% and three affected valves in 8% of 40 necropsied cases).

CAUSES

Bacterial colonization of the endocardium, and particularly the heart valves, usually affects animals predisposed by dental and other "septic" surgical procedures, indwelling catheters, immunosuppressive therapy, infections of the skin or genitourinary tract, cellulitis or abscessation, neoplasia, severe gingivitis, and parturition. The prostate gland appears to be a frequent source of infection in male dogs. Even though most dogs that develop vegetative endocarditis do not have preexisting congenital or acquired heart disease, dogs with congenital subaortic stenosis and ventricular septal defects are thought to be at increased risk. The incidence of bacterial endocarditis is no greater in dogs with than without valvular endocardiosis.

More than two thirds of canine cases of bacterial endocarditis are caused by *Staphylococcus aureus*, streptococci, and *Escherichia coli*. Other causative organisms include *Corynebacterium pyogenes, Clostridium perfringens, Enterobacter* organisms, protei, enterococci, *Pseudomonas aeruginosa, Klebsiella* organisms, *Serratia marcescens*, and *Erysipelothrix rhusiopathiae*. The of-

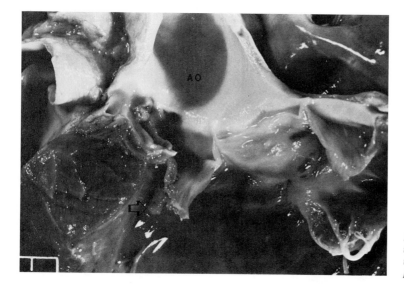

Figure 22–1 *Aortic vegetation (open arrow) and torn aortic valve cusp due to staphylococcal infection. (AO = aorta) (Photograph courtesy of Dr. James Cooley, University of Wisconsin.)*

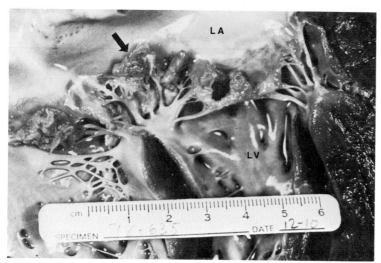

Figure 22–2 *Mitral valvular vegetations (arrow) in dog with vegetative endocarditis. The mitral valve leaflet was also torn. (LA = left atrium; LV = left ventricle) (Photograph courtesy of Dr. Richard Dubielzig, University of Wisconsin.)*

fending organism frequently reflects the site by which the bacteria gained access to the bloodstream (*e.g., Escherichia coli* from the bowel or urinary tract, *Staphylococcus aureus* from the skin). Excluding those associated with discospondylitis, Calvert and Greene (Additional Reading) report that 60% of canine bacteremias involve gram-positive and 40% involve gram-negative organisms. Little information is available for bacterial endocarditis in cats, but offending organisms are generally similar to those reported for the dog.

PATHOPHYSIOLOGY

Bacterial endocarditis is classified as being either acute or subacute. The acute form, usually caused by virulent organisms, tends to have a rapid, fulminant course. Subacute bacterial endocarditis, which carries a better prognosis, results from less virulent bacteria or results when virulent bacterial infections are treated early and aggressively. The pathogeneses for these two forms of endocarditis are different.

Acute Bacterial Endocarditis

In more than 50% of human cases of acute bacterial endocarditis, previously normal heart valves represent the site of infection. Even small numbers of highly invasive organisms, such as *Staphyloccus aureus* and β-hemolytic streptococci, are capable of colonizing normal valves during transient bacteremia. Pathogen-induced ulcerations of valve endothelium allow collagen exposure and platelet aggregation. Bacteria and leukocytes are entrapped within the resultant platelet–fibrin thrombus. Ultimately, necrosis of the valve stroma with alteration of valvular anatomy and function results.

Subacute Bacterial Endocarditis

Four mechanisms are thought to be important in the development of subacute bacterial endocarditis: valvular damage due to "jetting" of blood from a high to a low pressure chamber, presence of a sterile platelet–fibrin thrombus, bacteremia, and high agglutinating–antibody titer for the offending organism. As blood flows over a malformed valve, a "whipping" effect is produced, promoting platelet deposition followed by local fibrin formation and a platelet–fibrin clot. During subsequent bacteremia, bacterial colonization of damaged valves occurs, with the end result being the development of a vegetative lesion containing bacteria, platelets, and leukocytes, eventually leading to necrosis, fibrosis, calcification, and further deterioration of valve function. Circulating antibodies, particularly agglutinins, may contribute to the development of endocarditis by allowing conglutination of bacteria within the platelet–fibrin thrombus, promoting their subsequent multiplication.

The progression of acute and subacute bacterial endocarditis is similar from this point on. Growth and organization of valvular vegetations may result in distortion, ulceration, tearing, and fenestration of the leaflet(s), abscessation of the aortic root, spread to other leaflets or valves, and rupture of chordae tendineae, thereby severely complicating some cases. The ultimate clinical features of bacterial endocarditis are variably produced by cardiac dysfunction, sepsis, septic embolization, and immune-mediated complications.

When valvular vegetations lead to valvular dysfunction, incompetence and, less frequently, stenosis are the result. Insufficiency of the mitral and aortic valves reduces forward blood flow, causing volume overloading of the left heart with resultant left heart failure (pulmonary congestion and edema). Arrhythmias, coronary artery embolization, and torn chordae or leaflets hasten cardiac decompensation. Sudden death, probably due to arrhythmias or massive embolization, was observed in 8% of 45 canine cases of bacterial endocarditis.

Septic embolization is detected in 15% to 50% of cases and involves primarily the kidneys, spleen, central nervous system, and joints, variably producing signs of sepsis, abscessation, pain, infarction, and organ dysfunction. Emboli associated with bacterial endocarditis are typically small, most frequently involving the kidneys and spleen, with resultant abdominal tenderness and microscopic hematuria (Fig. 22-3). Larger emboli may cause disastrous results (*e.g.*, myocardial infarction or stroke) if the coronary or cerebral arteries are affected. Cats suffering from systemic bacterial embolization demonstrate similar consequences, but, in addition, may develop obstructive thromboembolization of the aortic trifurcation ("saddle thrombus"). With septic embolization, especially in staphylococcal infections, abscessation of the liver, spleen, brain, heart, and kidney may be observed. Signs attendant to this phenomenon are related to sepsis, pain, and specific organ dysfunction. In addition, immune complexes are deposited in joints (polyarthritis) and glomeruli (glomerulonephritis), producing pain in the former and proteinuria and potentially renal failure in the latter (see Chapters 45 and 64).

Anemia is associated with bacterial endocarditis (Table 22-1). This anemia, typically low-grade and normocytic and normochromic, is thought to be due to bone marrow suppression by chronic infection in some cases, as well as by hemolysis in more acute infections. In cases of

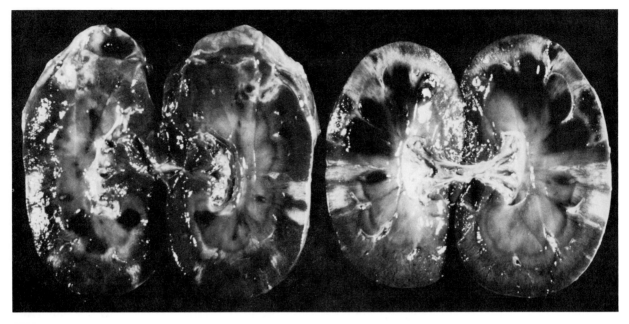

Figure 22–3 *Kidneys from a dog with staphylococcal aortic vegetative endocarditis and left heart failure. Note acute (dark) and chronic (light) renal infarcts. (Photograph courtesy of Dr. James Cooley, University of Wisconsin.)*

gram-negative endocarditis, disseminated intravascular coagulation is a common complication, substantially worsening the prognosis.

Clinical Signs

Cardiovascular findings include a newly recognized murmur in the majority of cases (see Table 22-1), typically a systolic murmur of mitral regurgitation. However, a "to and fro" (systolic–diastolic) murmur of aortic insufficiency and relative or preexistent congenital stenosis (Fig. 22-4) is noted in many cases of aortic valvular endocarditis (see Fig 17-3 for location of murmurs). The latter finding is highly suggestive of bacterial endocarditis in dogs and cats. Signs of left heart failure, which are more frequently recognized with aortic than mitral valvular endocarditis, include tachycardia, dyspnea, tachypnea, and pulmonary crackles. Syncope is sometimes associated with diminished cardiac output, tachyarrhythmias, or conduction disturbances (see Chapter 5). With heart failure, pulses tend to be weak; water-hammer or "BB-shot" pulses indicate aortic insufficiency. Cardiac gallops suggest heart failure, while pulse deficits are associated

with ventricular or supraventricular arrhythmias. Mucous membrane color is sometimes observed to be pale or ashen, reflecting anemia and poor tissue perfusion, respectively, and capillary refill time is typically prolonged.

Table 22–1 *Clinical Manifestations of Bacterial Endocarditis From Six Studies Involving 184 Canine Cases*

	Number Cases	Percent
Murmur	110/155	71
Fever	118/184	64
Lameness	62/158	39
Arrhythmia	46/152	30
Heart failure	17/91	19
Anemia	53/95	56
Hypoglycemia	26/116	22
Leukocytosis	94/114	83
Left shift	8/24	33
Monocytosis	70/83	84
Azotemia	28/91	31
Positive blood culture	73/101	72
Positive urine sediment*	10/18	56
Positive ANA	2/9	22
Survivors	17/70	24

* *Hematuria, proteinuria, or pyuria*

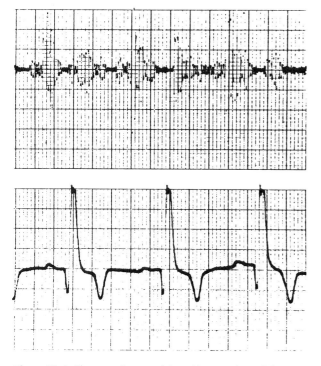

Figure 22–4 *Phonocardiogram of dog with corynebacterial vegetative endocarditis, demonstrating a "to and fro" systolic and diastolic murmur of aortic insufficiency and relative stenosis. The electrocardiogram demonstrates prolongation of the QRS duration (80 msec), suggesting left ventricular enlargement or left bundle branch block.*

Noncardiac manifestations of vegetative endocarditis, related to sepsis, embolization, or immune-mediated disease, include anorexia, fever, depression, weight loss, lameness, signs of gastrointestinal and renal disease, visual impairment, and central nervous system dysfunction (see Table 22-1). Physical examination may reveal joint pain (typically one joint with embolization from bacterial vegetations or multiple joints with immune-mediated disease), fever, pale mucous membranes (occasionally with petechiation), retinal hemorrhage or exudation, splenomegaly, and discomfort upon palpation of embolized, infected, or infarcted viscera (sublumbar pain with renal embolization and infarction).

DIAGNOSTIC APPROACH

While the history and physical findings are suggestive, many cases of bacterial endocarditis go unrecognized until postmortem examination. The finding of a new systolic–diastolic murmur in a dog with heart failure, fever, and joint pain is adequate to make a presumptive diagnosis. Cases in which a murmur was known to antedate the development of signs or in which no murmur is detected (29%) present a greater diagnostic challenge. In such instances, a high index of suspicion is necessary. Ancillary tests such as a complete blood count, serum biochemistry profile, urinalysis, prostatic fluid evaluation (see Prostatic Massage, Urethral Brush Technique, and Ejaculation in Chapter 80), abdominal ultrasonography, radiography, cerebrospinal fluid analysis and culture (see Cerebrospinal Fluid Collection in Chapter 80), arthrocentesis (Chapter 80) antinuclear antibody detection, biopsy, and echocardiography (see Chapter 80) are useful in ruling out or rendering less likely the differential diagnoses. These diagnoses include neoplasia, immune-mediated disease, other septic conditions (discospondylitis, pyelonephritis, prostatitis, meningoencephalitis, and bacteremia or septicemia without endocarditis), immune-mediated disorders, and primary heart disease (feline cardiomyopathy with embolization, canine dilated cardiomyopathy, or noninfectious valvular disease). Specific culturing can be used to rule out fungal endocarditis, an entity uncommonly encountered in dogs and cats.

A presumptive diagnosis of bacterial endocarditis is supported by the typical, but variable, hematologic findings of leukocytosis, left shift, monocytosis, normocytic and normochromic anemia, and thrombocytopenia (see Table 22-1). Supportive evidence is provided by the finding of azotemia, proteinuria, abnormal urine sediment, increased serum alkaline phosphatase and alanine aminotransferase activities, hypoglycemia, hyperglobulinemia, and hypoalbuminemia (see Table 22-1).

Thoracic radiographs may aid in diagnosing or excluding other diseases that mimic bacterial endocarditis; however, they are frequently noncontributory. Cardiac enlargement with evidence of pulmonary congestion or edema may be observed, but these changes, while compatible with heart failure due to bacterial endocarditis, are nonspecific (Fig. 22-5). Electrocardiographic findings, although also nonspecific, may be sup-

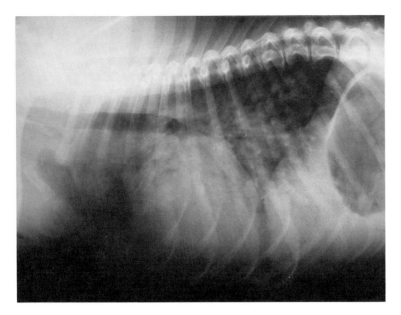

Figure 22–5 *Lateral thoracic radiograph demonstrating diffuse alveolar density of pulmonary edema in a boxer dog with aortic valvular vegetation, aortic insufficiency, and congestive heart failure.*

portive of the diagnosis in that left atrial and ventricular enlargement patterns, conduction disturbances, and supraventricular and ventricular premature complexes are often noted. Echocardiographic evaluation of affected dogs can provide valuable supportive information, as valvular lesions may appear as echodense masses on the mitral or aortic valves, both on two-dimensional (Figs. 22-6 and 22-7) and M-mode studies. Such findings require a relatively large vegetation (greater than 3 mm) and worsen the prognosis. Left atrial and ventricular enlargement is evident if heart failure is present or impending. Abnormal aortic valvular motion and mitral valve shuddering may be detected on M-mode echocardiograms obtained from patients with aortic insufficiency (Fig. 22-8).

The diagnosis of bacterial endocarditis is strongly supported by the finding of positive blood cultures. This is possible in more than two thirds of canine cases (see Table 22-1). Studies in humans have shown that the likelihood of obtaining a positive culture improves with multiple sampling, approaching 100% if three or more samples are cultured in a 24-hour period. Culture should precede antibiotic therapy when possible; if not, antibiotics should be discontinued for several days prior to culturing, when clinically advisable. Bacteriologic isolation and deter-

mination of antibiotic sensitivity allows the identification of not only a specific etiologic agent, but also the antibiotics to which it is susceptible. The skin is aseptically prepared and three samples are obtained, preferably at intervals of no less than 1 hour and from two or more sites over a 24-hour period. Samples are placed in

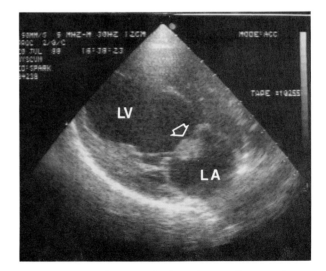

Figure 22–6 *Two-dimensional echocardiogram demonstrating anterior mitral valve vegetation (arrow). (LA = left atrium; LV = left ventricle) (Photograph courtesy of Dr. N. Sydney Moise, Cornell University.)*

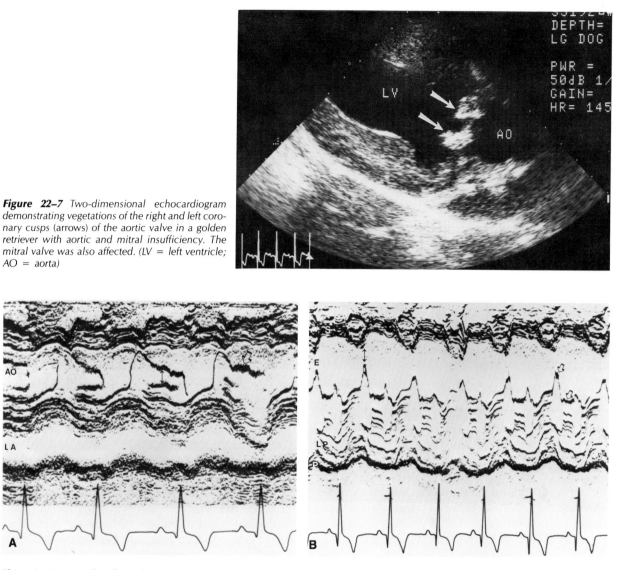

Figure 22–7 *Two-dimensional echocardiogram demonstrating vegetations of the right and left coronary cusps (arrows) of the aortic valve in a golden retriever with aortic and mitral insufficiency. The mitral valve was also affected. (LV = left ventricle; AO = aorta)*

Figure 22–8 *M-mode echocardiograms obtained from dog depicted in Figures 22–1 and 22–4. (A) Note that the aortic valve cusps do not coapt normally during diastole (two-directional arrow), suggesting that the left coronary cusp is torn. Also, the affected and the unaffected valve cusps (open arrow) are shuddering. (B) There is increased E-point septal separation (two-directional arrow), indicating left ventricular enlargement or diminished left ventricular function and mild diastolic mitral valve shuddering (open arrows), suggesting aortic insufficiency. (AO = aortic root; LA = left atrium; S = interventricular septum; E = mitral valve E-point; LP = left ventricular posterior wall; P = pericardium)*

specially designed commercial tubes and cultured for aerobic and anaerobic organisms. As much blood as is feasible (usually 5–20 ml, depending on the size and condition of the patient) is obtained to maximize the chances of isolating an organism.

MANAGEMENT

Early diagnosis and antibiotic therapy are essential in eradicating infection as well as minimizing damage to heart valves. Therapeutic goals (Table 22-2) are to eliminate infection while supporting

Table 22–2 *General Therapeutic Goals for the Management of Bacterial Endocarditis*

1. Identify and determine source and antimicrobial sensitivity of infective organism
2. Eradicate organism from:
   - Heart
   - Primary source
   - Secondary site(s)
3. Support patient during therapy, minimizing secondary disease
   - Institute fluid therapy
   - Correct, prevent hypoglycemia
4. Specifically or symptomatically treat secondary disease(s), including:
   - Renal disease or failure
   - Heart failure
   - Central nervous system embolism
   - Musculoskeletal disease
   - Anemia
   - Coagulopathy (disseminated intravascular coagulation)

life and minimizing sequelae to endocarditis. Owners should be apprised as to the guarded to poor prognosis and the likelihood of prolonged and expensive therapy. If possible, the source of infection (*e.g.*, gingivitis, prostatic abscess) is identified and eradicated.

Aggressive therapy with bactericidal antibiotics, ideally chosen on the basis of culture and sensitivity determination, are administered intravenously and at high doses for 7 to 14 days and followed by parenteral or oral antibiotic therapy for an additional 4 to 6 weeks. Selection of an antibiotic should take into consideration its spectrum, cost, toxicity, and ability to penetrate fibrin. In the event that a culture cannot be obtained or if the culture is negative or is pending, antibiotics are chosen based on the best overall likelihood of success, assuming the presence of the most common bacterial isolates. Calvert has shown that cephalosporins, gentamicin (or amikacin), and chloramphenicol are most frequently indicated by sensitivity testing for gram-positive bacteria, while gentamicin (or amikacin) and cephalosporins are usually best suited for gram-negative organisms. The quinolones (norfloxacin, ciprofloxacin, and enrofloxacin) hold promise as orally available antibiotics with efficacy against gram-negative bacteria and staphylococci. Anaerobic infections, suspected when bacterial endocarditis complicates deep abscesses or granu-

lomas, osteomyelitis, gingival disease, or septic arthritis or pleuritis, are sensitive in vitro to penicillin, ampicillin, cephalosporins, clindamycin, chloramphenicol, metronidazole, and trimethoprim-sulfa. A combination of gentamicin or amikacin and either penicillin, ampicillin, or a cephalosporin is recommended when specific identification and sensitivity determination are lacking (Table 22-3). Nephrotoxic antibiotics, such as gentamicin and amikacin, should be used with caution in the face of renal involvement, and corticosteroids are contraindicated in the treatment of bacterial endocarditis.

Therapy aimed at organs involved secondarily is usually symptomatic. The treatment of heart failure should entail diuresis with furosemide, often parenterally in fulminant cases, as well as other off-loading agents, such as nitroglycerin paste or patches, hydralazine, or a mixed vasodilator such as captropril or enalapril. Positive inotropic support (*e.g.*, digoxin, dobutamine, or dopamine) is generally not indicated unless concurrent myocardial failure is suspected. Oxygen therapy may be useful in the face of life-threatening pulmonary edema, and morphine is administered for its sedative effects in instances where severe dyspnea produces apprehension, contributory to the patient's decompensation and discomfort. Antiarrhythmic therapy or even pacemaker therapy may be indicated if serious arrhythmias or conduction disturbances exist. Salt and exercise restriction are instituted during the acute and convalescent phases of heart failure. Anticoagulation therapy has not been shown to be of benefit in the treatment of bacterial endocarditis.

If renal failure follows renal embolization, intravenous fluids, along with the antibiotic(s) least likely to be nephrotoxic, are administered to ensure adequate hydration and promote renal perfusion. Fluid therapy must be administered with caution when heart failure is present or impending. In this difficult situation, 5% dextrose in water with potassium chloride supplementation is the fluid of choice. As in all septic conditions, the potential for life-threatening hypoglycemia exists; blood glucose concentration should be monitored. Analgesics and nonsteroidal anti-inflammatory agents, such as aspirin, are indicated for pain and inflammation associated with arthropa-

Table 22–3 *Common Bacterial Isolates From Dogs With Bacterial Endocarditis and the Antibiotics Most Likely to be Useful in Their Treatment**

Organism	Antibiotics Likely to be Useful in Treatment
Gram-negative	
Escherichia coli	Gentamicin, cephalosporins
Klebsiella organisms	Cephalosporins, gentamicin, amikacin, quinolines
Pseudomonas	Gentamicin, amikacin, quinolones
Gram-positive	
Staphylococcus aureus	Gentamicin, amikacin, cephalosporins, chloramphenicol, quinolones
Streptococci	Penicillin, cephalosporins, ampicillin
Anaerobes	Penicillin, ampicillin, cephalosporins, clindamycin, chloramphenicol, metronidazole, trimethoprim-sulfa
Negative culture	Amikacin or gentamicin with amoxicillin or a cephalosporin

* Bacterial isolation and sensitivity determnation should be performed.

thies (see Chapters 63 and 64). The therapy for disseminated intravascular coagulation is discussed in Chapter 16.

While there are no specific guidelines for the prophylaxis of bacterial endocarditis in animals, the recommendations put forth by the American Heart Association for humans are useful. Prior to dental or other potentially septic procedures, penicillin or ampicillin is administered, by any route, 1 hour prior to and 6 hours after surgery. Since Calvert (1982, Additional Reading) has shown that 33% of bacterial isolates from dogs with endocarditis are *Staphylococcus aureus*, which is frequently resistant to penicillin and ampicillin (82% and 73%, respectively), cephalosporins may be a better choice when this organism is of concern. It is generally felt that animals with preexistent cardiac disease require greater attention in this regard, particularly those with subaortic stenosis and ventricular septal defects. In these high risk patients, ampicillin (50 mg/kg) and gentamicin (1.5 mg/kg) are administered IM or IV 30 minutes prior to and 8 hours after the procedure. When genitourinary or gastrointestinal tract surgery is contemplated, the American Heart Association advises the use of a similar regime of gentamicin and ampicillin. Regardless of drug or dosage, I prefer to continue oral antibiotic therapy for a minimum of 5 days after the procedure and do not advocate routine antimicrobial prophylaxis prior to uncompli-

cated dentistries in low risk patients, such as those with endocardiosis.

PATIENT MONITORING

As is indicated in Table 22-1, the prognosis is poor for bacterial endocarditis, with an overall survival rate of less than 25%. It is apparent that gram-negative sepsis, embolic complications, renal failure, or heart failure worsen the prognosis. Additionally, delays in the institution of therapy or failure to address complicating disorders, such as cardiac arrhythmias, disseminated intravascular coagulation, hypoglycemia, renal failure, and fluid, electrolyte, and acid-base disturbances, further diminishes the chances of survival. In 17 dogs (from three studies) with endocarditis and heart failure, only three survived. Calvert (1982, Additional Reading) reported that none of six dogs with renal failure complicating bacterial endocarditis survived.

Patients with bacterial endocarditis should be hospitalized, if at all possible, for the initial treatment period of 7 to 14 days. After release, the body temperature should be monitored twice daily at home during and after prolonged antibiotic therapy. Periodic complete blood counts may disclose early recrudescence and allow the attending clinician to monitor anemia; microscopic hematuria may also be indicative of disease recurrence. Ideally, blood cultures should be obtained and the patient examined weekly for 1 month after discontinuation of therapy.

Dogs with bacterial endocarditis may be presented in heart failure, may develop heart failure during treatment, or may develop heart failure after elimination of infection. Therefore, after release from the hospital dogs should be periodically monitored as to cardiac function. The electrocardiogram is used to identify developing rhythm and conduction disturbances, while echocardiograms and thoracic radiographs are helpful in identifying progression of cardiac enlargement, dysfunction, and failure. Once present, heart failure is monitored as needed, based on its severity and response to therapy. Chronic therapy for heart failure is similar to that described for mitral valvular incompetence (see Chapter 20). Follow-up evaluation and treatment for other organ failure or dysfunction is described in appropriate sections of this book.

ADDITIONAL READING

Anderson CA, Dubielzig R. Vegetative endocarditis in dogs. Journal of the American Animal Hospital Association 1984; 20:149.

Calvert C. Valvular bacterial endocarditis in the dog. J Am Vet Med Assoc 1982; 180:1080.

Calvert CA. Endocarditis and bacteremia. In: Fox PR, ed. Canine and feline cardiology. New York: Churchill Livingstone, 1988: 419.

Calvert CA, Greene CE. Cardiovascular infections. In: Greene CE, ed. Clinical microbiology and infectious diseases of the dog and cat. Philadelphia: WB Saunders, 1984: 220.

Calvert CA, Greene CE, Hardie EM. Cardiovascular infections in dogs: Epizootiology, clinical manifestations, and prognosis. J Am Vet Med Assoc 1985; 187:612.

Drasner FH. Bacterial endocarditis in the dog. Compendium of Continuing Education 1979; 1:918.

Ellison GW, King RR, Mays M. Medical and surgical management of multiple organ infarctions secondary to bacterial endocarditis in a dog. J Am Vet Med Assoc 1988; 193:1289.

Gompf RE. Bacterial endocarditis. Proceedings of the 9th Annual Kal Kan Symposium 1985: 73.

Harpster NK. The cardiovascular system. In: Holzworth J, ed. Diseases of the cat. Philadelphia: WB Saunders, 1987: 820.

Hirsch DC, Jang SS, Biberstein EL. Blood culture of the canine patient. J Am Vet Med Assoc 1984; 184:175.

Liu SK. Pathology of feline heart disease. Vet Clin North Am [Small Anim Pract] 1977; 7:323.

Sisson D, Thomas WP. Endocarditis of the aortic valve in the dog. J Am Vet Med Assoc 1984; 184:570.

23

PERICARDIAL DISEASE
John E. Rush, Clarke E. Atkins

The pericardium and pericardial space are involved in a variety of disease processes, and the hemodynamic changes resulting from pericardial disease may be dramatic and life-threatening. Pericardial disease can be a diagnostic challenge, as affected animals frequently lack a cardiac murmur and the clinical signs may be nonspecific. The prevalence of clinically significant pericardial disease, usually involving effusion, has been estimated to be 1% of canine cardiovascular disease; it is less common in the cat. Fortunately, pericardial disease can often be effectively managed by medical or surgical therapy.

CAUSES

Congenital Pericardial Diseases

A variety of congenital pericardial abnormalities have been reported in the dog and cat. These include partial or complete absence of the pericardial sac (usually asymptomatic), pericardial cysts, and peritoneopericardial diaphragmatic hernia. Of these, only peritoneopericardial diaphragmatic hernia is a frequent cause of clinical disease. The persistent communication between the pericardial cavity and the abdomen allows

herniation of abdominal organs into the pericardial cavity. Abdominal organs most frequently herniated include the liver, gall bladder, small intestine, stomach, spleen, and omentum. Sternal deformities or pectus excavatum may accompany peritoneopericardial diaphragmatic hernia; the weimaraner breed appears to be predisposed.

Animals with peritoneopericardial diaphragmatic hernia may remain asymptomatic or may develop clinical signs referable to the gastrointestinal tract (*e.g.,* vomiting, anorexia, weight loss, or diarrhea), respiratory system (*e.g.,* dyspnea or cough), or cardiovascular system (*e.g.,* shock, collapse, or signs of cardiac tamponade). Physical examination reveals muffled or absent heart sounds, displaced precordial impulse, or sternal deformity. Large hernias may result in a relative absence of palpable organs on abdominal palpation. Heart failure is generally not associated with peritoneopericardial diaphragmatic hernia.

Thoracic radiographs are a valuable diagnostic technique and often demonstrate peritoneopericardial diaphragmatic hernia as an incidental finding (Fig. 23-1). The cardiac silhouette is dramatically enlarged and the trachea is usually elevated. The caudal border of the heart overlaps the diaphragm on both radiographic views. Ab-

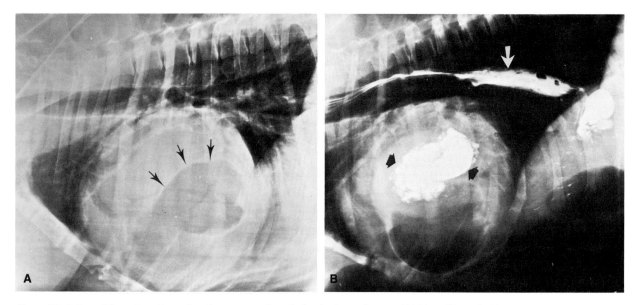

Figure 23–1 *Lateral thoracic radiograph and upper gastrointestinal series from a 2-year-old Irish wolfhound with a peritoneopericardial diaphragmatic hernia and a 5-day history of vomiting and collapse. (A) The lateral thoracic radiograph demonstrates dramatic enlargement of the cardiac silhouette. The large gas density (arrows) within the pericardial sac is air within the stomach. (B) The upper gastrointestinal series documents the peritoneopericardial diaphragmatic hernia. Contrast media is present in the esophagus (white arrow) and within the stomach (black arrows), located inside the pericardial sac. The stomach, spleen, omentum, two liver lobes, and a portion of the small intestines were found during surgery to be herniated into the pericardial sac.*

normal gaseous or fat densities may overlie the heart. Survey abdominal radiographs may demonstrate absence or malposition of cranial abdominal structures, while the electrocardiogram variably reveals low amplitude QRS complexes or deviation of the mean electrical axis as a result of malposition of the heart within the thorax. While additional diagnostic tests may include an upper gastrointestinal barium series (see Fig. 23-1), fluoroscopy, nonselective angiocardiography, and negative or positive contrast peritoneography, the preferred diagnostic test is echocardiography (Fig. 23-2), due to its accuracy and noninvasive nature. The recommended therapy is surgical repair. Animals with uncomplicated peritoneopericardial diaphragmatic hernia have a good prognosis for resolution of clinical signs following surgery.

Acquired Pericardial Diseases

There are two major pathologic processes that may affect the pericardium: pericardial effusion and constrictive pericarditis. Most animals with

pericardial disease have pericardial effusion; constrictive pericarditis is rarely recognized. The causes of pericardial pathology differ for dogs and cats (Table 23-1).

The two conditions most commonly associated with pericardial effusion in the dog are cardiac neoplasia and idiopathic pericardial effusion. The cardiac tumors most frequently reported are hemangiosarcoma (also known as angiosarcoma and hemangioendothelioma) originating in the right atrial wall or atrial appendage (Fig. 23-3) and heart base tumors (chemodectoma, aortic body tumor, thyroid carcinoma). Idiopathic pericardial effusion has also been described as benign pericardial effusion and idiopathic hemorrhagic pericardial effusion. The term *benign pericardial effusion* is misleading, as life-threatening cardiac tamponade is a very real potential sequela; in addition, the effusions are not universally hemorrhagic. Therefore, the preferred name for this condition is *idiopathic pericardial effusion.* Thickening of the parietal pericardium and epicardium with fibrosis and mild inflammation are the predominant histologic features of idiopathic peri-

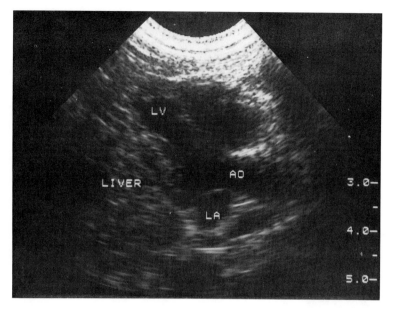

Figure 23–2 Two-dimensional echocardiogram, right intercostal long axis view from a cat with peritoneopericardial diaphragmatic hernia. The liver is in contact with the left ventricle (LV) and left atrium (LA). Both the heart and the liver are within the pericardial sac. (AO = aorta)

Table 23–1 Diseases Associated With Pericardial Effusion in Dogs and Cats

Disease Category*	Dogs	Cats
Neoplasia	Hemangiosarcoma	Lymphosarcoma
	Heart-based tumor	Metastatic carcinoma
	Mesothelioma	Metastatic hemangio-
	Thyroid carcinoma	sarcoma
	Metastatic neoplasia	Mesothelioma
Inflammation	Idiopathic pericardial effusion	Unknown
Cardiac failure	Cardiomyopathy	Cardiomyopathy
	Chronic valvular disease	Congenital defects
	Congenital defects	Hyperthyroidism
Cardiac rupture	Left atrial tear	Trauma
	Trauma	Left atrial tear
	Cardiac catheterization	Cardiac catheterization
	Endomyocardial biopsy	
Infections		
Viral	Canine distemper virus	Feline infectious peritonitis
Bacterial	*Actinomyces*	Systemic bacterial
	Nocardia	infections
	Leptospirosa	Pasteurella
Fungal	Infection with *Coccidioides immitis*	
Protozoan		Toxoplasmosis
Metabolic disease	Hypoproteinemia	Hyperthyroidism
		Hypoproteinemia
Coagulopathies	Anticoagulant toxicity	Anticoagulant toxicity
	Other coagulopathies	Other coagulopathies

* Listed in approximate order of frequency for the dog

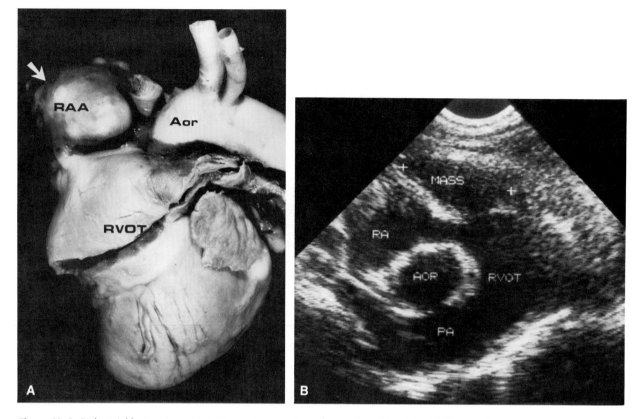

Figure 23–3 *Right atrial hemangiosarcoma. (A) Necropsy specimen from a dog with a right atrial hemangiosarcoma. The tumor (white arrow) is in a typical location at the cranial aspect of the heart, in the right atrial appendage (RAA). (B) Two-dimensional echocardiogram, right intercostal long axis view from a dog with right atrial hemangiosarcoma. The majority of the tumor (MASS) is outside the right atrium (RA) and lies within the pericardial space. (Aor = aorta; RVOT = right ventricular outflow tract, PA = pulmonary artery) (Courtesy of Dr. Matthew Miller, Texas A&M University.)*

cardial effusion. Other diseases associated with pericardial effusion in dogs include infectious pericarditis, uremia, trauma, left atrial tears, and metastatic neoplasia.

While cardiac tamponade is rarely recognized in the cat, the pericardial cavity may be affected in a variety of disease situations (see Table 23-1). Pericardial effusion has been reported in association with feline infectious peritonitis, congestive heart failure, renal failure, metastatic neoplasia, coagulopathies, and bacterial pericarditis. Primary cardiac tumors resulting in pericardial effusion are uncommon in the cat and there are no reports of idiopathic pericardial effusion in cats.

Constrictive pericarditis is an uncommon disease resulting from thickening and fibrosis of the pericardial sac, sometimes with adherence to the epicardial surface. Although constrictive pericarditis has been associated with pericardial foreign bodies, infection, and neoplasia, and is a possible sequela of idiopathic pericardial effusion in the dog, the etiology is usually unclear. Constrictive pericarditis is very rare in the cat.

PATHOPHYSIOLOGY

The pericardial sac is composed of two layers: the fibrous outer layer and the inner serous layer. The fibrous pericardium, which has both elastic and fibrous properties, is attached to the great vessels at the base of the heart. The heart invaginates the serous pericardium such that one surface is adherent to the heart (the visceral layer), becoming the epicardium, and the other is adherent to the fibrous pericardium (the parietal layer). The pericardial cavity, between the two layers of the serous pericardium, normally contains a small amount (0.5–2.5 ml) of a clear, serous fluid, which lubricates the epicardial surface. Additional functions of the pericardial sac include protection of the heart from infectious processes, prevention from acute overfilling, and maintainance of equality of right and left ventricular stroke volumes.

Pericardial effusion, defined as excessive fluid accumulation within the pericardial cavity, may be clinically silent or may result in life-threatening cardiac tamponade. In clinically apparent disease, fluid develops within the pericardial space and the elastic limit, or stretching capacity, of the pericardial sac is exceeded. At this point, the pressure in the pericardial cavity, normally equal to intrapleural pressure, begins to rise and is transmitted to the structures within. As pericardial pressure exceeds the cardiac filling pressures, diastolic filling is impaired (cardiac tamponade). If severe enough, this causes increased venous pressures and ultimately congestive heart failure. Signs of right-sided congestive heart failure (*e.g.*, ascites, hepatomegaly, jugular venous distention) predominate with chronic pericardial disease because right-heart filling pressures are lower than those of the left heart. As pericardial pressure increases, the left heart receives an inadequate supply of blood, and signs of forward or low output heart failure (*e.g.*, reduced exercise tolerance, syncope, hypotension, azotemia) result. Signs of forward heart failure usually predominate with acute pericardial effusion because inadequate time has elapsed for compensatory mechanisms to result in fluid retention.

The development of clinical signs depends on the pericardial fluid volume, the rate of fluid accumulation, and the physical properties of the pericardial sac. The pericardial sac can more readily adapt to slowly developing effusions by stretching, and as a result, chronic pericardial effusions often have very large volumes (greater than 1 L in the dog). Effusions that develop acutely (*e.g.*, effusion due to trauma, left atrial tear, or a bleeding neoplasm) may result in dramatic clinical signs with only a small volume of effusion (50–100 ml in the dog). In these cases, the elastic limit of the pericardium is quickly exceeded, resulting in rapid pressure elevations within the pericardial space. This explains why some dogs may have severe clinical signs with small effusions, while other dogs with chronic, voluminous effusions may remain relatively symptom-free.

Constrictive pericardial disease also results in impaired diastolic filling, but by a slightly different mechanism. The pericardium is extremely thickened, noncompliant, and frequently adherent to the surface of the heart (although a small volume of effusion may be present). In contrast to pericardial effusion in which cardiac filling is impaired throughout diastole, early diastolic filling in constrictive pericarditis is normal. Once the limit of the restrictive, fibrotic pericardium is reached, the ventricular pressure rises rapidly, equaling atrial pressure and abruptly stopping cardiac filling. The result is right-sided congestive heart failure.

CLINICAL SIGNS

Idiopathic hemorrhagic pericardial effusion occurs most frequently in male dogs of medium and large breeds with an age range of 1 to 14 years (average 6 years). Golden retrievers, German shepherds, Great Danes, and Saint Bernards appear to be overrepresented. Large-breed dogs of middle to old age are predisposed to neoplastic effusions, with the German shepherd and Golden retriever predisposed to both right atrial hemangiosarcoma and idiopathic pericardial effusion. Boxers, bulldogs, and Boston terriers have been reported to be predisposed to the development of heart base tumors.

Historical findings (Table 23-2) of pericardial disease include lethargy, weakness, exercise intolerance, weight loss, abdominal distention, syncope, and tachypnea. Dogs presented with torn left atria usually have a history of mitral insufficiency with acute decompensation (*e.g.*, weakness, collapse, pallor, or worsening of heart failure). Other acutely developing effusions likewise produce acute decompensation with weakness and collapse.

Table 23–2 *Clinical Signs Frequently Associated With Pericardial Disease*

HISTORICAL FINDINGS

Lethargy
Weakness
Exercise intolerance
Abdominal distention
Syncope
Tachypnea
Cough

PHYSICAL FINDINGS

Tachypnea
Dyspnea
Mucous membrane pallor
Prolonged capillary refill time
Diminished precordial impulse
Muffled heart sounds
Pericardial friction rub
Jugular venous distention
Tachycardia
Weak pulse
Arrhythmias
Pulsus paradoxus
Hepatomegaly or splenomegaly
Positive hepatojugular reflex
Ascites

Physical examination findings with chronic disease (see Table 23-2) typically include muffled heart sounds, pericardial friction rub (an uncommon finding in small animals), jugular venous distention, weight loss, ascites, hepatosplenomegaly, pleural effusion, pallor, sinus tachycardia, and arrhythmias. In more acutely developing cases, collapse, pallor, and hypotension are recognized.

Constrictive pericarditis is uncommon, usually occurring in medium to large breed, middle-aged dogs. Clinical signs usually reflect right heart failure and are similar to those of chronic pericardial effusion. Heart sounds are often muffled, with additional abnormal auscultatory findings (*e.g.*, gallops, murmurs, midsystolic clicks); the mid-diastolic pericardial knock described in humans, caused by the abrupt cessation of diastolic filling, is infrequently reported in the dog.

DIAGNOSTIC APPROACH

Results of routine laboratory tests are unlikely to provide the definitive diagnosis for animals with pericardial disease. Dogs with pericardial effusion

or constrictive pericarditis may have hypoproteinemia, anemia, or a neutrophilic leukocytosis. Nonspecific changes in the serum biochemistry profile may include elevated hepatic enzymes secondary to right heart failure, and mild azotemia if renal perfusion is compromised. Dogs with hemangiosarcoma may be more likely to have anemia, circulating nucleated red blood cells, and schistocytes. Affected cats may have high titers to feline infectious peritonitis virus, and cats with lymphosarcoma may test positive for feline leukemia virus. The results of fluid analysis of abdominal or thoracic effusions usually indicates a modified transudate, compatible with heart failure. Animals with acutely developing effusions typically exhibit a nearly normal cardiac silhouette or one suggestive of mitral regurgitation, while long-standing pericardial disease results in stretching of the fibrous component of the pericardial sac and radiographic evidence of severe globoid cardiomegaly with loss of cardiac chamber definition (Fig. 23-4). Enlargement of the caudal vena cava is variably noted, and pleural effusion may interfere with evaluation of the cardiac silhouette. Dogs with heart base tumors may have an increased soft-tissue density at the heart base or tracheal displacement. Differential diagnosis for these radiographic findings should include primary myocardial disease, mitral insufficiency, and congenital defects (especially tricuspid insufficiency). Cats frequently demonstrate moderate cardiomegaly.

A number of electrocardiographic changes have been reported in dogs and cats with pericardial disease, including diminished QRS amplitude, electrical alternans, and abnormalities in the ST segment (Fig. 23-5). Small QRS complexes, defined in the dog as QRS in all leads less than 1 mV, are frequently observed with pericardial disease. Low-amplitude QRS complexes are difficult to define in the cat; however, the finding of extremely small QRS complexes (less than 0.15 mV) in all leads or complexes that are significantly smaller than those from previous examinations is compatible with pericardial disease. P-mitrale and ST segment elevation have also been reported in dogs with pericardial effusion. Electrical alternans is defined as the regular variation in QRS size or morphology (every second or third complex) that results from swinging of the

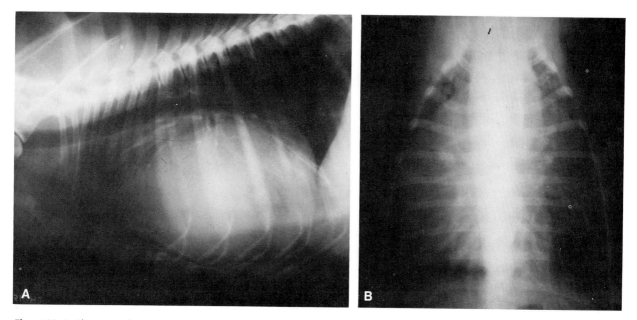

Figure 23–4 Thoracic radiographs from a dog with long-standing pericardial effusion due to idiopathic pericardial effusion. Both the lateral (A) and dorsoventral (B) views demonstrate the markedly enlarged, globoid-shaped cardiac silhouette.

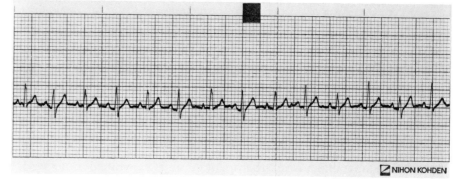

Figure 23–5 Electrocardiographic features of pericardial effusion in the dog. Low-voltage QRS complexes (voltages were less than 1 mV in all leads) and electrical alternation of the QRS complexes is apparent. Electrocardiogram was recorded at 25 mm/sec, 1 cm/mV.

heart within the fluid-filled pericardial cavity. Although electrical alternans is not observed in every case (it is more common with large effusions), its presence is highly suggestive of pericardial effusion. Normal sinus rhythm or sinus tachycardia are common rhythm diagnoses, but ventricular or supraventricular arrhythmias may be recorded.

Measurement of central venous pressure, an easy and probably underutilized technique for measuring right-sided cardiac filling pressures, is particularly useful for determining whether ascites is due to cardiac dysfunction (see Chapter 80). The central venous pressure is usually less than 5 cm of water; ascitic patients with right heart failure due to pericardial disease will usually have measurements in excess of 10 to 15 cm of water.

Echocardiography, the most sensitive and specific means for detection of pericardial effusion, demonstrates an echo-free space between the myocardium and the pericardium (Fig. 23-6). This space is observed circumferentially with two-dimensional echocardiography, and the heart may be noted to swing to and fro within the pericardial sac. Diastolic right atrial and ventricular collapse suggests cardiac tamponade.

Two-dimensional echocardiography may also

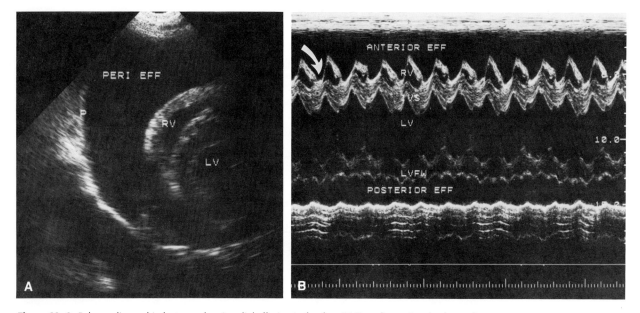

Figure 23–6 *Echocardiographic features of pericardial effusion in the dog. (A) Two-dimensional echocardiogram, right intercostal short axis view demonstrates the echo-free space between the pericardium (P) and the cardiac chambers. (LV = left ventricular cavity; RV = right ventricular cavity; PERI EFF = pericardial effusion) (B) M-mode echocardiogram at the level of the ventricles from the same dog demonstrates an echo-free space both above (anterior effusion) and below (posterior effusion) the heart. The posterior motion of the right ventricular wall during diastole (arrow), also termed diastolic collapse of the right ventricle (RV), can be observed on both M-mode and two-dimensional echocardiograms and is an indication of cardiac tamponade. (RV = right ventricular cavity; LV = left ventricular cavity; LVFW = left ventricular free wall; IVS = interventricular septum; EFF = effusion)*

provide more specific etiologic information in selected cases of pericardial disease. In dogs with cardiac neoplasia or other mass lesions, the masses can be imaged directly (Fig. 23-7) and the location of the mass can often be identified (*e.g.,* right atrium or heart base). This localization provides important diagnostic, therapeutic, and prognostic information. Additionally, the lack of an identifiable mass (after careful imaging from both right and left sides) is suggestive of idiopathic pericardial effusion. Two-dimensional echocardiography may also provide a definitive diagnosis in dogs or cats with peritoneopericardial diaphragmatic hernia or in cats with underlying cardiomyopathy.

Pericardiocentesis can be performed with minimal risk and is the preferred therapy for cardiac tamponade, providing prompt relief of clinical signs. Pericardiocentesis can be performed when pericardial effusion has been diagnosed by echocardiography, or may be used to confirm the diagnosis when pericardial effusion is suspected

based on historical, physical, electrocardiographic, and radiographic findings. The decision whether to perform pericardiocentesis is difficult in cases of confirmed or suspected active pericardial hemorrhage. If stable, the patient should be carefully monitored and pericardiocentesis avoided or delayed. If death due to tamponade is imminent, pericardiocentesis must be performed with the realization that further hemorrhage may occur and that iatrogenic tears in the pericardium may permit exsanguination into the thoracic cavity.

Mild sedation or traquilization may be required in anxious or refractory patients. Pericardiocentesis (see Chapter 80) is performed with the patient in left lateral or sternal recumbency. The right hemithorax is clipped and aseptically prepared between the third and eighth intercostal space, from the sternum to just above the costochondral junction. Lidocaine is infiltrated into the skin and intercostal muscles at the fourth or fifth intercostal space. A variety of catheters can

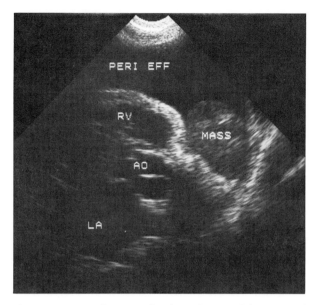

Figure 23–7 Two-dimensional echocardiogram, left intercostal long axis/oblique view of a dog with pericardial effusion (PERI EFF) secondary to a heart base tumor (MASS). The tumor was attached to the root of the aorta (AO) and bulged into the pericardial cavity. (LA = left atrium, RV = right ventricular outflow tract)

be used to tap the pericardial space, although we prefer over-the-needle catheters. The catheters must be long enough to reach the pericardial space (at least 5 cm) and must have a large enough diameter to easily remove fluid, usually 16-gauge. The catheter is attached to polyethylene tubing, a three-way stopcock, and a large (30- to 60-ml) syringe. With the patient attached to an electrocardiograph for continuous electrocardiographic monitoring, the catheter and needle are cautiously advanced through the skin and intercostal muscles toward the heart. Gentle suction is applied to the syringe, and, once pericardial fluid is obtained, the catheter is advanced over the needle into the pericardial sac. As much fluid as possible is removed.

Complications of pericardiocentesis include coronary artery laceration, ventricular arrhythmias, and exsanguination in cases of active intrapericardial hemorrhage. The risk of coronary artery laceration is reduced by tapping from the right hemithorax. Ventricular arrhythmias result from contact of the catheter or needle with the myocardium. If ventricular arrhythmias are observed, the needle or catheter should be retracted a short distance. Life-threatening hemorrhage into the pleural space is an uncommon complication. Its occurrence can be detected by frequent evaluation of total protein, packed-cell volume, capillary refill time, mucous membrane color, and femoral pulse rate and quality. The attending clinician should be prepared to provide emergency care in the form of intravenous fluid administration and whole blood transfusions or emergency thoracotomy.

A portion of the sample obtained by pericardiocentesis should be submitted for fluid analysis and cytologic evaluation, and another portion of the sample saved for culture and sensitivity testing if indicated from cytologic examination. The fluid can be classified as a transudate, exudate, or hemorrhagic effusion. Transudates may result from congestive heart failure, hypoalbuminemia, or peritoneopericardial diaphragmatic hernias, while exudates are observed with viral, bacterial, or fungal infections. The vast majority of dogs with pericardial effusion have a sterile, noninflammatory hemorrhagic effusion, compatible with either neoplasia or idiopathic pericardial effusion. Cytologic evaluation of hemorrhagic pericardial effusates usually fails to discriminate between hemangiosarcoma, heart base tumors, and idiopathic pericardial effusion. There is significant overlap of the protein content, red cell count, and nucleated cell count for these three diseases. In addition, reactive mesothelial cells, which have many characteristics in common with neoplastic cells, are present in all three diseases. Therefore, while fluid evaluation is valuable in the diagnosis of bacterial or fungal pericarditis, the etiology of the pericardial effusion in dogs is rarely proven by fluid analysis alone.

Because most effusions in the dog are grossly hemorrhagic, concern may arise as to whether the fluid obtained is from the heart or the pericardial space. Pericardial fluid of chronic nature rarely clots, the packed-cell volume is usually different from that of the peripheral blood, and xanthochromia is frequently noted in the supernatant after centrifugation. Frank blood, particularly if it clots and has a packed-cell volume similar to that of peripheral blood, suggests active, acute pericardial hemorrhage; it is difficult to differentiate from cardiac puncture.

Contrast pneumopericardiography may be used in an attempt to find a cause for the effusion (Fig. 23-8), although this technique is more invasive and is diagnostically inferior to two-dimensional echocardiography for identification of mass lesions. Following pericardiocentesis, with the catheter in the pericardial sac, a volume of either carbon dioxide or room air equal to two thirds of the removed volume of effusion is introduced into the pericardial sac. Right lateral, left lateral, dorsoventral, and ventrodorsal radiographic views are then obtained. The lateral views are the most informative, and the dorsoventral radiographic view will outline structures at the base of the heart better than the ventrodorsal projection. A successful study depends on adequate fluid removal and gas infusion, multiple radiographic views, and a thorough knowledge of the radiographic anatomy. The gas should be removed and the catheter retrieved after the procedure.

Angiocardiography (see Chapter 80) is rarely indicated to diagnose pericardial disease, although cranial caval venography may reveal the presence of heart base tumors. The presence of pericardial effusion is suggested by elevation of the cardiac chambers from the sternum and increased distance from the pericardial shadow to the endocardial surface, outlined by contrast material. Additional potential angiographic findings include the presence of a filling defect within the heart caused by an intracardiac tumor (typically within the auricular wall), the vascular blush of a heart base tumor, or displacement of normal cardiac structures by a mass lesion.

Dogs with constrictive pericarditis have minimal pericardial effusion, and as a result, thoracic radiographs are usually normal or demonstrate only mild to moderate cardiomegaly. Pleural effusion and caudal vena cava distention may be evident, while pericardial calcification is an unusual finding. Small QRS complexes can be observed on the electrocardiogram, although P-mitrale is more consistently reported. The rhythm is usually sinus in origin and may be complicated by supraventricular arrhythmias. While echocardiographic findings in dogs or cats with constrictive pericardial disease are not available, findings reported in humans include pericardial thickening and abnormal diastolic motion to the left ventricular wall, interventricular septum, and mitral valve. Selective cardiac catheterization and exploratory thoracotomy are probably the best diagnostic tools for documentation of constrictive pericarditis in cases highly suggestive of it. Restrictive pericarditis is a difficult diagnosis; this disease should be suspected when evidence of right heart failure is accompanied by normal thoracic radiographs and the lack of physical findings of heart disease.

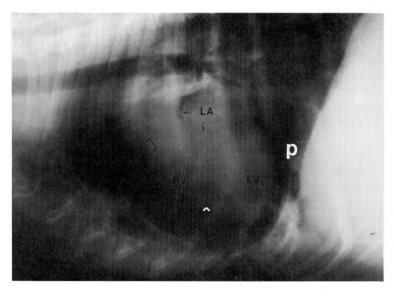

Figure 23–8 Pneumopericardiographic right lateral view of the anatomy in the dog. Small black arrows indicate the extent of the left auricular appendage, larger black arrows outline the cranial extent of the aorta, open arrow points to the right auricular appendage, and the white arrowhead points to the interventricular sulcus. (LA = left atrium; LV = left ventricle; RV = right ventricle; P = pericardium) (Courtesy of Dr. Lawrence J. Kleine, Tufts University.)

MANAGEMENT AND PATIENT MONITORING

General Therapy for Pericardial Effusion

The management of animals with pericardial disease will vary greatly, depending on the underlying disorder and the pathophysiologic consequences. Pericardial effusions associated with systemic or metabolic disease processes (*e.g.,* hypoproteinemia, renal failure, congestive heart failure, peritoneopericardial diaphragmatic hernia) will usually resolve with correction of the underlying disease. The initial therapy for animals with substantial pericardial effusion and tamponade is pericardiocentesis. All animals with cardiac tamponade and without active hemorrhage require pericardiocentesis. The issue of pericardiocentesis in the face of active pericardial hemorrhage was discussed under the section Diagnostic Approach. There is no medical therapy that takes the place of or provides the immediate and specific therapeutic benefit of pericardiocentesis. Repeated pericardiocentesis is preferred to excessive diuretic or other medical therapy. The pericardial space has limited venous and lymphatic drainage, and inflammation accompanying the disease further impedes fluid escape; therefore, diuretic therapy will not benefit these patients by reducing the volume of pericardial effusion.

Most animals with pericardial effusion have normal myocardial function; therefore, digitalization is not indicated unless clinically significant supraventricular tachyarrhythmias accompany the pericardial effusion. Afterload-reducing agents (arteriolar vasodilators) should be avoided, as hypotension frequently accompanies cardiac tamponade. In chronic right-sided heart failure due to pericardial effusion, low sodium diets (Hill's Prescription Diet h/d, k/d) are indicated. Diuretics and venous vasodilators should be used cautiously or avoided because overzealous preload reduction will further decrease cardiac output, leading to azotemia, hypotension, and weakness. No medical therapy will reduce fluid accumulation as quickly or effectively as pericardiocentesis.

Therapy for Specific Disease Processes

Idiopathic Pericardial Effusion

Dogs suspected of having idiopathic pericardial effusion should be initially managed in a conservative fashion. Approximately 50% of dogs will respond to one or two therapeutic pericardiocenteses. The remaining dogs will have recurrence several days to several years after pericardiocentesis. Some anecdotal reports suggest that pericardiocentesis in combination with anti-inflammatory drugs, such as antiprostaglandins and either oral or intrapericardial corticosteroids, may be valuable, although there are no controlled studies to document this.

Dogs that require frequent or repeated pericardiocentesis may benefit from surgical therapy. We believe that it is reasonable to recommend pericardiectomy on the first or second recurrence of pericardial effusion. Subtotal pericardiectomy below the phrenic nerve is the surgical procedure of choice, and many dogs remain asymptomatic afterwards. Surgical formation of a pericardial window has met with less than satisfactory results. A small percentage of dogs may develop recurrent hemorrhagic pleural effusion after subtotal pericardiectomy and require repeated thoracentesis. Dogs that respond to pericardiocentesis and those that remain asymptomatic after pericardiectomy have a good prognosis for a normal life expectancy.

Cardiac Mass Lesions

Animals that are identified as having mass lesions may undergo surgery or be managed with repeated pericardiocentesis. The prognosis for surgery depends largely on the nature of the mass. Pericardial cysts or abscesses may be surgically resectable, while pericardial granulomas are usually fungal in origin, and treatment should be directed at the underlying agent. Primary cardiac neoplasms have variable prognoses based on location, size, presence of metastasis, and tumor type.

If metastasis is noted at the time of surgery, the prognosis for long-term survival is poor and further surgery is generally to no avail. Small masses may be resectable, but are found in the minority of cases. Hemangiosarcoma is typically incurable, and surgical attempts to remove the mass are associated with a high postoperative mortality. This type of tumor tends to bleed, with possible exsanguination into the thoracic cavity after pericardiectomy. Heart base tumors, though slower growing and less likely to metastasize, are difficult or impossible to excise. However, pericardiectomy is frequently useful to relieve clinical signs of cardiac tamponade, with comfortable survival for several months to years. Cats with lymphosarcoma involving the pericardial sac may be placed on chemotherapeutic protocols, although a favorable response to chemotherapy with this form of lymphosarcoma has not been well documented.

Surgical therapy may be elected in dogs with no evidence of a mass. Potential advantages of early surgery include discovery of small resectable tumors not previously identified, the ability to perform therapeutic pericardiectomy after a negative exploratory procedure, and the opportunity to perform biopsy of the pericardial sac.

Viral, Bacterial, or Fungal Pericarditis

Antibiotic therapy for infectious pericarditis should be dictated by the results of bacterial or fungal culture and determination of sensitivity. Aggressive therapy might include intravenous antibiotics, intrapericardial antibiotics, and placement of an indwelling pericardial catheter for continuous drainage or intermittent lavage and antibiotic instillation. Infectious pericarditis often results in marked fibrous tissue deposition and constrictive pericarditis. Cats with feline infectious pericarditis virus often have other organ systems affected, and specific antiviral therapy is unavailable. Infectious pericarditis carries a guarded to poor prognosis.

Pericardial Hemorrhage

Pericardial hemorrhage represents the exception to the rule that pericardiocentesis is always indicated with cardiac tamponade. If tamponade is life-threatening, pericardiocentesis is performed with the realization that further pericardial hemorrhage may result in reoccurrence of tamponade or exsanguination into the thorax. If the latter occurs, whole blood transfusions or emergency thoracotomy to repair the site of hemorrhage are indicated. If hemorrhagic diathesis (*e.g.,* anticoagulant intoxication) produces life-threatening tamponade, pericardiocentesis and specific therapy (*e.g.,* vitamin K_1) are indicated (see Chapter 16).

When pericardial hemorrhage is associated with less severe compromise in cardiac function, conservative management such as cage rest, gentle expansion of the central venous volume with intravenous fluids to maintain cardiac output, and careful patient monitoring is advised. Many such patients will stabilize as a fibrin clot forms over the rent in the heart chamber or as specific anticoagulant therapy is administered. If cardiac function declines, pericardiocentesis, as described above, is performed. The long-term prognosis for pericardial hemorrhage varies with the cause, being poor with torn left atria or bleeding tumors but good in the case of successfully treated cardiac trauma and bleeding diatheses, such as warfarin poisoning.

Constrictive Pericarditis

Conservative therapy for constrictive pericardial disease is usually unrewarding, as the disease appears to be progressive in nature. Surgical attempts to remove the pericardium are most successful if the disease is limited to the parietal pericardium. When the visceral pericardium is fibrotic, epicardial stripping is required; this is associated with a high incidence of complications (*e.g.,* myocardial hemorrhage, pulmonary thromboembolism). Medical management may accompany surgery, and should include salt and exercise restriction, diuretics, and possibly angiotensin-converting enzyme inhibition (captopril). The prognosis with surgical therapy is favorable.

ADDITIONAL READING

Berg R, Wingfield W. Pericardial effusion in the dog: A review of 42 cases. Journal of the American Animal Hospital Association 1984; 20:721.

Harpster NK. The cardiovascular system. In: Holzworth J, ed. Diseases of the cat: Medicine and surgery. Philadelphia: WB Saunders, 1987: 820.

Reed JR. Pericardial diseases. In: Fox PR, ed. Canine and feline cardiology. New York: Churchill Livingstone, 1988: 495.

Rush JE, Keene BW, Fox PR. Pericardial disease in the cat: A retrospective study of 66 cases. Journal of the American Animal Hospital Association 1990; 26:39.

Sisson D, Thomas W. Diagnostic value of pericardial fluid analysis in the dog. J Am Vet Med Assoc 1984; 184:51.

Thomas WP. Pericardial disorders. In: Ettinger SJ, ed. Textbook of veterinary internal medicine. Philadelphia: WB Saunders, 1989: 1132.

Thomas W, Reed J. Constrictive pericardial disease in the dog. J Am Vet Med Assoc 1984; 184:546.

24

VASCULAR DISEASE
John E. Rush, Clarke E. Atkins

The major purposes of the cardiovascular system are to provide tissues with enough blood to meet their needs for oxygen and nutrition and to remove metabolic waste products. While proper function of the heart is mandatory to achieve these goals, the delivery of blood to the tissues also depends on the integrity of the arteries, veins, capillaries, and lymphatics in both the systemic and pulmonary vascular circuits. These peripheral vessels can be involved primarily or secondarily in a number of disease processes. A list of diseases affecting the peripheral vessels and lymphatics of dogs and cats is found in Table 24-1.

Vascular diseases are probably more important in veterinary patients than is commonly realized. Arterial embolism has been recognized as a complication of feline cardiomyopathy for many years and remains one of its most severe complications. With increased awareness and diagnostic capabilities, some vascular diseases (such as systemic arterial hypertension and pulmonary thromboembolism), overlooked in the past, are being diagnosed with increasing frequency. This chapter will focus on the most frequently encountered vascular diseases in dogs and cats.

SYSTEMIC ARTERIAL HYPERTENSION

Systemic arterial hypertension can be defined as an elevation in either the systolic or diastolic arterial blood pressure above the accepted normal range. Arterial hypertension can be divided into two major categories, primary and secondary hypertension. Primary (or essential) hypertension is idiopathic in origin, while secondary hypertension is defined as hypertension secondary to a recognized disorder, such as renal or adrenal disease. The exact incidence and significance of systemic hypertension in veterinary patients remains poorly defined. Some studies estimate that systemic arterial hypertension is present in 50% to 93% of dogs with renal failure. The lack of a uniform, noninvasive, accurate, and reproducible method for measuring arterial blood pressure in dogs and cats has apparently contributed to the relative failure to diagnose hypertension in companion animals. Clinical improvement in treated hypertensive pets suggests that early diagnosis and treatment is advisable.

Causes

Primary or essential hypertension, the most common cause of systemic hypertension in human beings, is infrequently diagnosed in companion animals. Secondary causes of hypertension are more commonly recognized (Table 24-2). Systemic arterial hypertension has been frequently diagnosed in dogs and cats with renal failure, and the incidence is particularly high in animals with glomerular disease (80%). Secondary hypertension has also been associated with several endocrine disorders.

Table 24–1 *Vascular Diseases in Dogs and Cats*

DISEASES OF SYSTEMIC ARTERIES

Systemic arterial hypertension
  Primary or essential hypertension
  Secondary hypertension
Arterial thrombosis
Arterial embolism
Arteritis, vasculitis, or polyarteritis nodosa
Atherosclerosis
Arteriosclerosis
Arterial calcification
Arteriovenous shunts
  Congenital
  Acquired
Arterial aneurysm

DISEASES OF PULMONARY ARTERIES

Pulmonary arterial hypertension
Pulmonary thromboembolism
Heartworm disease

DISEASES OF SYSTEMIC VEINS

Phlebitis
Thrombophlebitis
Varicosities

DISEASES OF LYMPHATICS

Lymphangiectasia
Lymphangitis
Primary lymphedema
Lymphatic obstruction

Table 24–2 *Causes of Systemic Arterial Hypertension*

PRIMARY

Essential hypertension

SECONDARY

Renal disease
  Glomerulonephritis
  Renal parenchymal disease
  Renovascular disease (renal artery stenosis)
Endocrine disease
  Hyperadrenocorticism
  Pheochromocytoma
  Hyperthyroidism or hypothyroidism
  Hyperaldosteronism
  Diabetes mellitus
Polycythemia
Neurogenic disease (increased intracranial pressure)

Pathophysiology

Systemic arterial hypertension has been referred to as the "silent killer." It can remain clinically inapparent for long periods of time, allowing progression of pathologic changes in organs susceptible to its effects. If unsuspected, hypertension may not be recognized as the cause of clinically evident disease such as retinal detachment, renal failure, or left ventricular hypertrophy.

The pathophysiologic alterations that cause secondary hypertension are slightly different for each disease process. In renal disease, a number of compensatory changes are invoked in response to the decreased renal blood flow, recognized by the juxtaglomerular apparatus. These compensatory mechanisms include activation of the renin–angiotensin–aldosterone system and increased sympathetic stimulation; both mechanisms contribute to hypertension. Hypertension in animals with hyperadrenocorticism or primary hyperaldosteronism results when mineralocorticoids cause renal tubular retention of sodium and water, leading to hypertension. Pheochromocytomas secrete catecholamines, either continuously or intermittently; the resultant sympathetic stimulation elevates arterial blood pressure.

Regardless of the underlying cause, the importance of systemic arterial hypertension is measured by the damage inflicted on arteries and target organs throughout the body (Fig. 24-1). In hypertensive patients, intimal proliferation of collagen and elastin is apparent histologically, and muscular hypertrophy is present in the arterioles. These changes (arteriosclerosis) result in decreased luminal diameter and blood flow. Arteriolar changes appear to be most important in the kidney, where hypertension may be self-perpetuating. Glomerular capillary changes observed in dogs with hypertension include necrosis, glomerulosclerosis, fibrinoid lesions, hyalinization, and capillary occlusion. These abnormalities promote further tubular degeneration and may lead to progressive renal failure. Similar changes in small arterioles in the brain, eyes, and other tissues can result in weakness of arteriolar walls, aneurysm formation, and vessel rupture. If vessel rupture occurs in the central nervous system, intracranial hemorrhage (stroke) occurs, manifested as a central nervous system disorder of

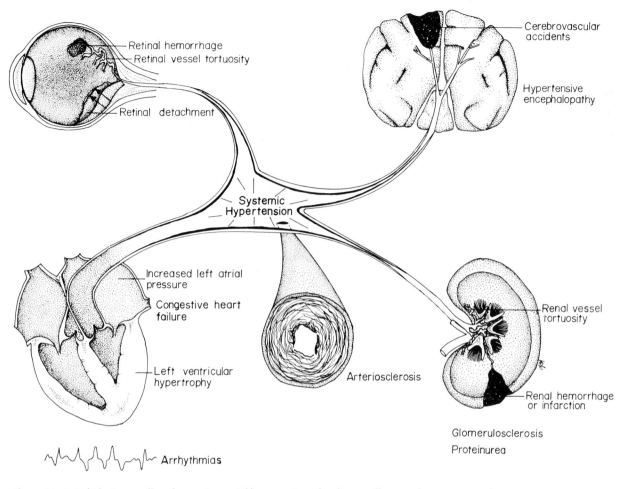

Figure 24–1 *Pathologic sequellae of systemic arterial hypertension. This diagram illustrates the important pathologic changes resulting from systemic hypertension in the heart, eyes, brain, kidney, and arterioles. Left ventricular hypertrophy is a common manifestation, while cardiac arrhythmias and increased left atrial pressure leading to congestive heart failure may occur in some animals. Retinal hemorrhages or retinal detachment may be the initial indication of hypertension. The intimal proliferation of collagen and elastin and the muscular hypertrophy of the arterioles (arteriosclerosis) are a response to hypertension and contribute to arteriolar tortuosity, which is most commonly observed in the renal and retinal blood vessels. Systemic hypertension can also lead to weakened arteriolar walls, aneurysm formation, and vessel rupture, clinically observed as cerebrovascular accidents (stroke) or renal hemorrhage and infarction. Hypertensive encephalopathy is observed in patients with malignant hypertension. Increased renal perfusion pressure can lead to glomerulosclerosis and proteinuria, and long-standing hypertension can contribute to progressive renal failure.*

rapid onset (Fig. 24-2; see Fig. 24-1). Arteriolar changes in the retinal vessels may cause retinal hemorrhage, and the elevated arterial pressure may lead to retinal detachment (Fig. 24-3; see Fig. 24-1).

Although both systolic and diastolic hypertension places an added demand on the heart, increases in the arterial diastolic pressure are of greater concern, as it is this pressure that the heart must overcome in ejecting blood into the aorta. This increases cardiac work, causes left ventricular concentric hypertrophy, and decreases cardiovascular reserves (Fig. 24-4; see Fig. 24-1). Chronic arterial hypertension may culminate in fatal cardiac arrhythmias or myocardial failure, leading to congestive heart failure.

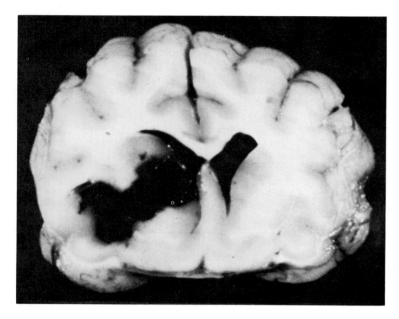

Figure 24–2 *Transverse section through the brain of a cat with long-standing hypertension. The cat died after an acute onset of neurologic signs. A large hemorrhagic infarct is present in the left cerebrum at necropsy. (Courtesy of Dr. William L. Castleman, University of Wisconsin.)*

Clinical Signs

Hypertensive animals may manifest clinical signs resulting from hypertension or the underlying disease. Presenting complaints of the former include acute blindness, ocular hemorrhage, epistaxis, congestive heart failure, renal failure, and neurologic dysfunction. Ocular changes include altered retinal arterioles (usually increased tortuosity of the vessels), swelling of the optic nerve papilla, retinal hemorrhages, and retinal detachment (see Fig. 24-3). Central nervous system abnormalities, which can include seizures, are usually of acute onset and reflect the site of vessel rupture. Auscultation of the heart may reveal a cardiac murmur or gallop, and palpation of the precordium will reveal a prominent left apical beat. The arterial pulse quality is variably hyperdynamic. Abdominal palpation may document abnormal renal size or shape in animals with secondary renal hypertension.

Diagnostic Approach

To diagnose arterial hypertension, one must be familiar with the clinical signs of hypertension as well as diseases that cause secondary hypertension. Clinicians should maintain a high degree of

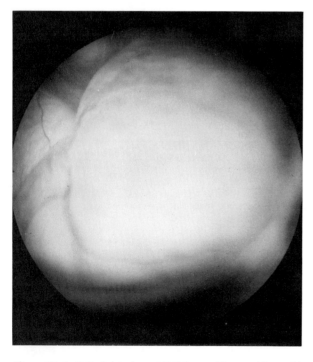

Figure 24–3 *Retinal detachment O.S. from a 12-year-old cat with hypertension. The optic disk is hidden by the detached retina, which is billowing out toward the lens. (Courtesy of Dr. Alan Bachrach, Tufts University.)*

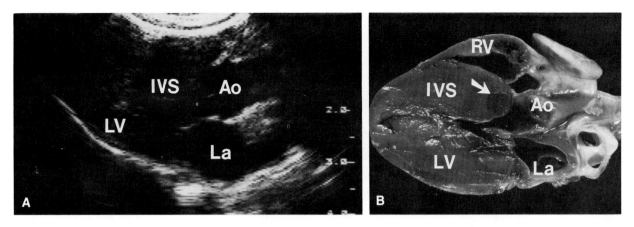

Figure 24–4 Left ventricular hypertrophy resulting from hypertension in two cats. (A) The two-dimensional echocardiogram, right intercostal long axis view of the heart demonstrates marked hypertrophy of the left ventricular wall (LV) and interventricular septum (IVS). The left atrium (La) is minimally enlarged. (Ao = aorta) (B) Pathology specimen from a cat with renal failure, hypertension, and secondary left ventricular hypertrophy. Marked hypertrophy is present in the left ventricular free wall (LV) and interventricular septum (IVS). An area of necrosis is present in the interventricular septum (arrow). (Ao = aorta; La = left atrium; RV = right ventricle) (Pathology specimen courtesy of Dr. James Cooley, University of Wisconsin.)

suspicion in patients with retinal vascular changes, hemorrhages, or detachment; unexplained left ventricular hypertrophy (hypertrophic cardiomyopathy); progressive renal failure; and neurologic disease of acute onset. Arterial blood pressure should ideally be measured in all animals with any of the diseases listed in Table 24-2.

Systemic arterial hypertension is diagnosed by documentation of reproducible, sustained elevations in systolic and/or diastolic arterial blood pressure. Measurements can be obtained using either direct or indirect methods. Serial measurements of blood pressure are required to effectively judge therapeutic response. Noninvasive, indirect measurement is preferred for evaluation of therapeutic response of systemic hypertension.

Direct blood pressure measurement is more accurate, but it requires arterial puncture, which may be painful and require tranquilization. Access to the femoral artery is obtained with a small gauge (23- to 25-gauge) needle attached to pressure recording equipment with stiff polyethylene tubing. Response to stress, fear, or excitement, associated with direct blood pressure measurement, may result in artifactual blood pressure elevations. Direct blood pressure measurement should be performed in all cases in which hypertension is suspected and the diagnosis is in question after indirect blood pressure measurement.

Indirect arterial blood pressure measurements can be obtained in companion animals using either oscillometric or Doppler techniques (Fig. 24-5). An inflatable cuff is used to occlude arterial blood flow. With gradual release, the cuff pressure obtained at the time blood flow recommences (first sound obtained with Doppler-sensed flow) is recorded as the systolic pressure. Diastolic pressure is recorded when the sounds are lost; this pressure may be difficult to determine in some animals using the Doppler technique, as the sounds may persist, with only muffling of the sounds noted at the diastolic pressure. The size of the cuff and its placement are critical to accurate blood pressure measurement, and care in selection and placement of the cuff is necessary to obtain consistent and reproducible results.

Studies to determine normal values for arterial blood pressure measurement in animals have used a variety of techniques, methods of restraint, and methods of sedation. Each practice may want to establish normal values for arterial blood pressure based on its technique, equipment, and presence or absence or sedation. Proposed normal values for canine and feline blood pressure are

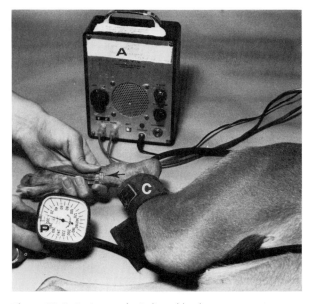

Figure 24–5 *Equipment for indirect blood pressure measurement using the Doppler technique. The transducer (black arrow) is positioned over the artery, and the amplifier (A) is adjusted until flow is detected. The pressure cuff (C) is inflated to occlude arterial blood flow. Cuff pressure is slowly released and the systolic pressure is recorded from the pressure gauge (P) when blood flow recommences.*

Table 24–3 *Normal Arterial Blood Pressures in Dogs and Cats*

	Direct	Indirect
CANINE		
Systolic	Less than 180 mmHg	Less than 160 mmHg
Diastolic	Less than 95 mmHg	Less than 95 mmHg
FELINE		
Systolic	Less than 200 mmHg	Less than 190 mmHg
Diastolic	Less than 145 mmHg	Less than 145 mmHg

listed in Table 24-3. When arterial hypertension is diagnosed, the cause of the hypertensive state should be carefully sought.

Management

The aim of antihypertensive therapy is to decrease the morbidity and mortality associated with chronic hypertension. Initial therapy for systemic arterial hypertension should be directed at the underlying disease process. If this is reversible, then chronic antihypertensive drug therapy may be avoided.

Low sodium diets (Hill's Prescription Diet h/d, k/d) are a part of all therapeutic strategies. However, sodium restriction alone will rarely return blood pressure to normal. Low sodium diets (0.1%–0.3% of the diet) used in combination with drug therapy are the most effective method of treatment. Drugs used to treat arterial hypertension include diuretics, β-blocking agents, vasodilators, angiotensin-converting enzyme inhibitors, and calcium channel blockers. Single drug therapy is often ineffective, and additional drugs are added until a successful drug regimen is found.

Although thiazide diuretics are frequently used for management of hypertension in humans, they are relatively ineffective in patients with renal failure. Since renal failure is one of the most common causes of hypertension in veterinary patients, loop diuretics like furosemide, which are effective in the face of renal failure, are usually employed.

Sympatholytic therapy (β- and/or α-blockade) has historically been the second line of antihypertensive therapy after diuretics. Sympatholytic agents reduce blood pressure by reducing cardiac output, renin secretion, and sympathetic influence on vessels. The most commonly used β-blocker is propranolol, although selective β_1-blockers like atenolol may be preferred. Selective β_1-blockade preserves the normal vasodilatory action of β_2-vascular receptors. α-Adrenergic blockers cause vasodilation by interfering with the α_1-induced vasoconstriction. Prazosin is an α-adrenergic receptor antagonist that causes vasodilation, usually without the side-effect of reflex tachycardia.

The use of captopril and enalapril, angiotensin-converting enzyme inhibitors, is based on the assumption that the renin–angiotensin–aldosterone system has been activated in the development and maintenance of the hypertensive state. Some researchers have advocated the early use of angiotensin-converting enzyme inhibitors in animals with hypertension secondary to renal failure. The intrarenal actions of these drugs in such patients may slow the progression of renal dysfunction.

Direct-acting arterial vasodilators such as hydralazine can be helpful in refractory cases. However, they may cause reflex tachycardia, increased renin release, and increased fluid retention. For these reasons, hydralazine is often used in combination with a diuretic and a β-blocker. Sodium nitroprusside, useful in hypertensive emergencies such as retinal detachments, intracranial hemorrhage, or acute heart failure, must be administered by continuous infusion. It is used only until other therapies can be initiated.

The ideal sequence of drugs for control of hypertension in companion animals is not well established and may vary for each underlying disease. For asymptomatic hypertension, we prefer to start with a low sodium diet and a diuretic while initiating additional therapies directed at the underlying disease. If these are ineffective, either a β-blocker or captopril is added. A more aggressive approach is indicated in animals with clinical signs such as retinal detachment, stroke, or heart failure. These animals are initially managed with either vasodilators (*e.g.*, hydralazine, captopril) or adrenergic blocking drugs (*e.g.*, prazosin), in addition to diuretics and sodium-restricted diets.

Patient Monitoring

Arterial blood pressure should initially be reevaluated weekly or bimonthly. Additional drugs are added or dosages adjusted until the blood pressure is consistently maintained in the normal range. When this is achieved, repeat blood pressure determinations can be obtained once every few months. In order to successfully manage hypertension, it is important to intermittently monitor end organs with potential for damage. Periodic determinations of blood urea nitrogen or creatinine concentrations, in addition to ocular examination and cardiac evaluation, are indicated. Serial thoracic radiographs, electrocardiograms, and echocardiograms are also indicated in animals with cardiovascular manifestations.

SYSTEMIC ARTERIAL EMBOLISM

A thrombus is defined as an intravascular deposit of fibrin and formed blood elements (cells). Embolisms occur when an entire or partial thrombus (or any other foreign material) breaks free from the site of origin, lodging downstream. Clinical signs, determined by the presence or absence of functioning collateral circulation, result when the tissue distal to the site of embolism is deprived of its blood supply. Arterial thromboembolic disease, common in cats, is infrequently recognized in dogs. The aortic trifurcation is the most common site of embolization in the cat (90%), while other reported sites include the front limbs, kidneys, brain, and gastrointestinal tract.

Causes

Myocardial diseases are the most common cause of arterial thromboembolism in cats. All forms of cardiomyopathy in cats have been associated with thromboembolic events. The incidence of thromboembolism in cats presented for necropsy with various myocardial diseases has been reported as high as 48% for cats with hypertrophic cardiomyopathy, 25% for dilated cardiomyopathy, and 29% for restrictive cardiomyopathy. Other causes of arterial thromboembolism in cats, such as bacterial endocarditis and neoplasia, are rare. A small number of cats have been reported with thromboembolism and no identifiable underlying disease.

Systemic arterial embolization is uncommon in the dog but has been reported with bacterial endocarditis, aberrant location of adult heartworms, hypercoagulable states such as the nephrotic syndrome, neoplasia (especially bone infarcts), and vascular foreign bodies. Dogs with myocardial disease do not appear to be significantly predisposed to arterial thromboembolism.

Pathophysiology

The three pathologic conditions thought to contribute to thrombus formation are local vessel or endocardial injury, altered blood flow (*e.g.*, circulatory stasis), and altered blood coagulability. Many believe that for thrombus formation to occur, one or more of these abnormalities must be present. Local vessel or tissue injury exposes reactive surfaces, inducing platelet adhesion and fibrin deposition and leading to thrombus formation. Injury to the endocardial surface of the atria or ventricles is often present in feline myocardial diseases; circulatory stasis in dilated atria also contributes to thrombus formation. Feline platelets are reported to contain more serotonin and to be more reactive than those of other species. Cats are also reported to have a larger platelet volume relative to body size. These factors may predispose the cat to thromboembolic events. Altered coagulability is common to many other diseases known to be associated with arterial thromboembolism. Some neoplastic and myeloproliferative disorders may cause thrombocytosis, which can promote thrombus formation. Disseminated intravascular coagulation is typically manifested as a microvascular thrombotic disease. Animals with bacterial endocarditis shed thrombi from infective valves, producing embolism of distant arteries.

When arterial embolism occurs, the development of clinical signs depends on the tissue affected and the degree of collateral circulation. It is clear that the pathogenesis of arterial thromboembolism involves more than simple mechanical obstruction to blood flow. In the case of distal aortic thromboembolism in cats, studies have demonstrated that obstruction of the distal aorta by surgical ligation causes no clinical signs, as collateral circulation is adequate. However, when a thrombus lodges in the distal aorta, vasoactive substances such as serotonin and prostaglandins, released from platelets, cause constriction of collateral vessels.

Clinical Signs

Thromboembolism results in an acute loss of function in the affected tissues. Cats with thromboembolism of the distal aorta have signs of posterior weakness and pain, with absence or weakness of femoral pulses in one or both hind limbs. The affected limbs are cold to the touch, the nailbeds are cyanotic, the nails do not bleed if clipped short, and the gastrocnemius and semitendinosus muscles may be firm and contracted. Loss of limb sensation and hyporeflexia are observed as ischemic neuropathy develops. Clinical signs in animals with unilateral embolism may progress to involve both rear legs. Thrombi may also lodge in the front limbs, renal arteries, gastrointestinal arteries, or arteries in the central nervous system. Bilateral renal artery thrombosis results in acute anuric renal failure. Disseminated intravascular coagulation has been reported in cats with aortic thromboembolism.

The most common underlying disease process in cats with thromboembolism is cardiomyopathy (see Chapter 21). Findings on physical examination that indicate cardiomyopathy as the underlying disease include cardiac murmurs or gallops, abnormal femoral pulses, and jugular venous distention. The stress and pain of thromboembolism, combined with the underlying cardiac disease, frequently precipitates congestive heart failure with cardiac gallop, arrhythmia, tachypnea or dyspnea, tachycardia, pulmonary crackles, or diminished lung sounds due to pleural effusion.

Dogs with arterial thromboembolism may also manifest signs related to the underlying disease process. For example, dogs with bacterial endocarditis (see Chapter 22) typically exhibit cardiac murmur, tachycardia, arrhythmias, fever, joint pain or distention, or evidence of urinary tract infection. Dogs with nephrotic syndrome (see Chapter 45) may have peripheral edema formation, and careful examination may help identify neoplasia in those animals for which this is the cause of thromboembolism.

Diagnostic Approach

The diagnosis of distal aortic or front limb thromboembolism can usually be established by the characteristic physical examination findings. Establishing a diagnosis of thromboembolism of arteries supplying the kidneys, gastrointestinal tract, or central nervous system is more difficult and may require angiography. Nonselective angiocardiography can be used to confirm distal aortic thromboembolism when the diagnosis is in question (see Nonselective Angiocardiography in Chapter 80; Fig. 24-6). If available, Doppler ultrasonography of peripheral vessels can be used to establish the presence or absence of blood flow.

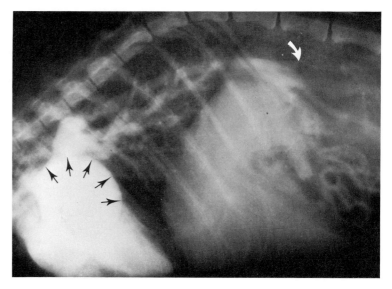

Figure 24–6 *Nonselective angiogram of a cat with cardiomyopathy and aortic thromboembolism. The column of contrast dye in the aorta ends abruptly at the site of embolism near the renal arteries (white arrow). Marked left atrial enlargement (black arrows) and pulmonary vein tortuosity are compatible with pulmonary venous hypertension and long-standing left heart failure. (Courtesy of Dr. Lawrence J. Kleine, Tufts University.)*

Laboratory abnormalities observed in animals with thromboembolism include a stress leukogram and elevated serum alanine and aspartate aminotransferase, creatine kinase, and blood glucose levels. Hyperkalemia and metabolic acidosis may result upon reperfusion of affected tissue when potassium and lactic acid are released from ischemic tissue. Azotemia may result from renal artery embolism or diminished cardiac output. Diagnostic tests should also be directed to determine the underlying disease process. In cats, an electrocardiogram, thoracic radiographs, and echocardiography or nonselective angiocardiography (see these topics in Chapter 80) are useful in establishing the presence of cardiac disease. Dogs should be evaluated for bacterial endocarditis (see Chapter 22), glomerular diseases (see Chapter 45), and neoplasia. Laboratory tests indicated in dogs with arterial thromboembolism include a complete blood count, serum biochemistry profile, heartworm test, and urinalysis. Thoracic radiography, electrocardiography, echocardiography, and blood cultures are indicated in dogs with suspected bacterial endocarditis.

Specific studies may be useful in diagnosing disorders of coagulation (see Chapter 16). Indications of hypercoagulability include shortening of the activated partial thromboplastin time, prothrombin time, and thrombin time; increased plasma fibrin degradation product concentrations; and reductions in platelets, fibrinogen, antithrombin III, and protein C.

Management

Thromboembolism can be managed medically or by surgical embolectomy. Medical therapy consists of vasodilatory drugs, anticoagulants aimed at preventing thrombus enlargement or recurrence, and thrombolytic drugs. In addition to specific therapy for thromboembolism, therapy should be directed at the underlying disease process. Propranolol should be withheld from the therapeutic regimen of cats with active thromboembolism because this nonspecific β-blocker will reverse or prevent β-adrenergic vasodilation. Additional agents, such as furosemide, potassium-poor fluid administration, or discriminative use of sodium bicarbonate may be used to control congestive heart failure, hyperkalemia, or metabolic acidosis, respectively.

Acepromazine and hydralazine are vasodilators that have been used to relieve vasospasm and promote blood flow in collateral vessels. In addition to α-blockade, acepromazine may benefit anxious cats by its tranquilizing effects. An initial dose of 0.1 mg/kg is administered intravenously, intramuscularly, or subcutaneously, and additional doses are given to achieve and maintain the desired effects of sedation.

Aspirin is commonly used to interfere with platelet function and thereby retard or prevent thrombus development. By inhibiting thromboxane A_2 synthesis and therefore platelet aggregation, aspirin is theoretically useful in preventing thrombus formation or growth, both chronically and in the setting of acute thromboembolism. While aspirin is widely used for thromboembolism, its efficacy in the prevention of reoccurrence is questionable. Serotonin antagonists, such as cyproheptadine, may be useful, given the pathogenesis of feline thromboembolism. Experimentally, cyproheptadine was shown to be useful in diminishing clinical signs when administered prior to the onset of thromboembolism (see Appendices I and II). The utility in clinical settings has not been reported.

Heparin and warfarin are anticoagulant drugs that may be useful in the management of animals with thromboembolism for slowing thrombus growth. Heparin binds to and enhances the activity of antithrombin III, which neutralizes activated clotting factors, preventing formation of thrombin and thereby interfering with coagulation. Heparin must be administered parenterally; it is most often used in animals with acute thromboembolism. The initial dose is 200 IU/kg IV, followed by 50 to 200 IU/kg subcutaneously every 6 to 8 hours. The dosage is adjusted to maintain an increase in activated partial thromboplastin time of 1.5 times the baseline level. Warfarin interferes with the hepatic metabolism of vitamin K, which is essential in the formation of clotting factors II, VII, IX, and X. A recommended initial dose is 0.05 to 0.1 mg/kg orally, or approximately 0.25 mg/day for the cat. Evaluation of the prothrombin time is required every third day, and the dose is titrated to maintain it at 1.5 to 2 times the baseline value. Some authors suggest that the use of this drug represents the most effective therapy for prevention of recurrent arterial thromboembolism. Disadvantages include a significant risk for bleeding and the added expense of frequent reevaluation.

Streptokinase, urokinase, and tissue plasminogen activator (serine proteinase) are drugs that promote thrombolysis. These drugs have been used experimentally and in some clinical trials. The fact that these drugs have not gained widespread use in veterinary patients can probably be attributed to their expense, complications associated with their use, and unresolved questions about resolution of clinical signs after thrombolysis. Of these drugs, tissue plasminogen activator shows the most promise. Tissue plasminogen activator is an enzyme that binds to fibrin within a thrombus and converts the entrapped plasminogen to plasmin, initiating local fibrinolysis and thrombus dissolution (see Appendices I and II).

Surgical embolectomy by incision or catheterization has been used in cats with aortic thromboembolism. The results of surgical embolectomy have generally been poor. Most cats have severe underlying heart disease, some have congestive heart failure or cardiac arrhythmias, and most are poor anesthetic risks. Cats surviving the procedure may not regain function of the rear legs sooner or to a greater degree than those managed medically. Cats with renal artery thromboembolism may represent an exception and should probably undergo surgical embolectomy.

Additional beneficial supportive care for thromboembolism includes maintenance of body temperature and physical therapy. Affected cats (especially those with dilated cardiomyopathy) may become hypothermic, and the affected tissues are invariably cool. Such animals should be heated to maintain normal body temperature and promote collateral circulation, but care must be taken to avoid overheating affected limbs. Following thromboembolism, the normal thermoregulatory mechanisms are lost and excessive heating can cause thermal necrosis. Physical therapy may also be useful to facilitate return of limb function, once blood flow is reestablished. Table 24-4 outlines both a conservative approach and a more aggressive approach to the management of arterial thromboembolism.

Patient Monitoring

When therapy is successful, motor function may begin to return as early as 48 hours after its institution, with most cats showing improvement within 10 to 14 days. Good return of motor func-

Table 24–4 *Therapeutic Approach to Systemic Arterial Embolism*

CONSERVATIVE APPROACH

Treat congestive heart failure
Treat metabolic acidosis and hyperkalemia when necessary
  Sodium bicarbonate (1 to 2 mEq/kg IV slowly) and 0.45% sodium chloride with 2.5%
    dextrose (usually one half of calculated maintenance requirements)
Aspirin—25 mg/kg every 2 to 3 days PO
Acetylpromazine—0.1 to 0.4 mg/kg subcutaneously, repeat three times daily or as needed to
  maintain sedation
Maintain body temperature and local heat
Physical therapy

MORE AGGRESSIVE APPROACH

Treat congestive heart failure
Treat metabolic acidosis and hyperkalemia when necessary
  Sodium bicarbonate (1–2 mEq/kg IV slowly) and 0.45% sodium chloride with 2.5% dextrose
    (usually one half of calculated maintenance requirements)
Aspirin—25 mg/kg every 2 to 3 days PO
Heparin—200 IU/kg IV followed by 50 to 200 IU/kg for 6 to 8 hours to maintain activated
  partial thromboplastin time at 1.5 to 2 times baseline value
Vasodilation
  Acepromazine—0.1 to 0.4 mg/kg subcutaneously, repeat three times daily or as needed to
    maintain sedation
  Hydralazine—0.5 mg/kg twice daily PO
Maintain body temperature and local heat
Physical therapy

*IF UNRESPONSIVE OR IF RENAL THROMBOSIS IS SUSPECTED
(OLIGURIC RENAL FAILURE)*

Thrombolytics
  Tissue plasminogen activator
  Streptokinase
  Urokinase
Surgical therapy—surgical embolectomy or balloon catheter embolectomy

tion may be achieved by 4 to 6 weeks. Residual hock flexion, rear limb weakness, or conscious proprioceptive deficits are potential persistent sequelae. The prognosis for feline aortic thromboembolism is guarded to poor. Some animals never regain rear limb function, and irreversible ischemic changes may result in gangrene that requires limb amputation or euthansia. Some cats die or are euthanized for severe and unresponsive congestive heart failure. Cats with hypertrophic cardiomyopathy may have a better chance for survival and more time to regain limb function than those with dilated cardiomyopathy. Cats that do regain function may undergo repeated episodes (75% recurrence) of thromboembolism. Aspirin or warfarin administration is continued indefinately in cats with restrictive or hypertrophic cardiomyopathy, and until left atrial size is normal in cats with taurine-responsive dilated cardiomyopathy. Recurrent throm-boembolism remains one of the most serious problems encountered in the management of cats with cardiomyopathy.

PULMONARY ARTERIAL EMBOLISM

Pulmonary arterial embolism results when venous thrombi, foreign bodies, air, fat, or tumor cells are carried by the venous system through the heart and lodge in the pulmonary arteries. The most common cause of pulmonary arterial embolism in dogs is heartworm disease (see Chapter 25).

Air emboli can result from intravenous infusions, pneumoperitoneum, retroperitoneal air injection, and other diagnostic or therapeutic techniques that involve air insufflation. The lethal dose is reported to be between 5 and 15 ml/kg of air, depending on the age, condition, and position of the patient and the rapidity of air entry. Pulmonary fat emboli may result from trauma (especially long bone fractures), fat tissue contusion, or fatty metamorphosis of the liver. Typically, the most dramatic clinical signs are similar to those of adult respiratory distress syndrome, occurring 24 to 40 hours after trauma. Tumor emboli gain access to the venous circulation from either the site of the primary neoplasm or from a metastatic focus. While these neoplastic cells may grow and eventually result in metastatic disease, such emboli are rarely large enough to result in clinical signs of pulmonary embolism. Vascular foreign bodies that lodge in the pulmonary circulation predispose to infection, vascular damage, or thrombosis and should be surgically removed.

Pulmonary Thromboembolism

The second most common cause of pulmonary arterial embolism in the dog is pulmonary thromboembolism. Pulmonary thromboembolism occurs when thrombi, which develop in large veins, break loose from their site of origin and lodge in the pulmonary arteries (Fig. 24-7). Under most circumstances, the body's fibrinolytic system is capable of dissolving small thrombi. Large thrombi that acutely block a large proportion of the pulmonary vasculature cause clinical signs of arterial hypoxemia, pulmonary infarction, or cor pulmonale.

Causes

The incidence and significance of pulmonary arterial thromboembolism in veterinary patients is not well defined. Many canine diseases have recently been recognized to be complicated by pulmonary thromboembolism; however, this syndrome is rarely recognized in the cat. The majority of associated human deaths occur in patients that were not appropriately treated, usually when the diagnosis was not established. The mortality rate is less than 10% when treatment is appropriate. These data suggest that the diagnosis should be pursued and aggressive treatment initiated in affected animals. The most commonly recognized causes of pulmonary thromboembolism in the dog are presented in Table 24-5.

Pathophysiology

The same factors that are postulated to contribute to the formation of arterial thrombi (altered coagulability, vessel wall damage, and abnormal blood flow) are important in the development of

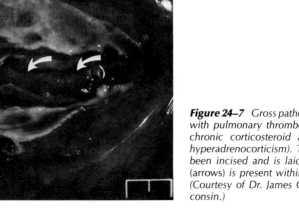

Figure 24–7 *Gross pathology specimen from a dog with pulmonary thromboembolism resulting from chronic corticosteroid administration (iatrogenic hyperadrenocorticism). The pulmonary artery has been incised and is laid open. A large thrombus (arrows) is present within the lumen of the artery. (Courtesy of Dr. James Cooley, University of Wisconsin.)*

Table 24–5 Causes of Pulmonary Arterial Embolism

Heartworm disease (embolism of worms or thrombus)
Pulmonary thromboembolism
    Hyperadrenocorticism
    Protein-losing nephropathy
        Amyloidosis
        Glomerulonephritis
    Immune-mediated hemolytic anemia
    Neoplasia
    Septic processes
    Pancreatitis
    Surgical procedures
    Congestive heart failure
    Total parenteral nutrition (long-term, large central catheter)
Air embolism
Fat embolism
Neoplastic embolism
Vascular foreign body embolism

venous thrombi. A thrombus is composed of fibrin, platelets, and other blood cells, which form in the large central veins. These thrombi can break loose from their site of attachment and be carried to the pulmonary arterial circulation. Resulting pulmonary arterial embolism prevents blood flow and oxygen exchange (ventilation–perfusion mismatching) in the affected areas of the lung. Local hypoxia and vasoactive substances, originating from platelets incorporated in the thrombus, cause pulmonary artery vasoconstriction, leading to pulmonary hypertension. If blood flow has been reduced by blockage of a large cross-sectional area of the pulmonary arteries, systemic arterial oxygen desaturation results. If pulmonary hypertension is severe, right ventricular strain (cor pulmonale) and eventual failure may occur. Finally, pulmonary infarction, an uncommon sequela, may cause intra-alveolar bleeding and chest pain.

The development of pulmonary thromboembolism in dogs with hyperadrenocorticism has been postulated to result from a "hypercoagulable state" associated with cortisol excess, hyperlipidemia, and hypercholesterolemia. Protein-losing nephropathies such as amyloidosis and glomerulonephritis lead to a hypercoagulable state early in the disease process, as large amounts antithrombin III are lost through the damaged glomerulus. Antithrombin III normally functions to prevent intravascular coagulation by neutralizing activated clotting factors. The development of pulmonary thromboembolism in dogs with immune-mediated hemolytic anemia has recently been recognized; the underlying causes are unknown.

Clinical Signs

A variety of clinical signs have been reported with pulmonary thromboembolism, including hemoptysis, acute unexplained dyspnea, cor pulmonale and right heart failure, weakness, syncope, cyanosis, and hypotension. The clinical spectrum depends on the degree of occlusion of the pulmonary arterial circulation and the presence or absence of pulmonary infarction. A large percentage of the pulmonary circulation must be occluded (probably at least 50%) for cor pulmonale to occur. Signs of cor pulmonale include dyspnea (usually with clear lung sounds), signs of right ventricular failure, or evidence of decreased cardiac output such as tachycardia, hypotension, or syncope. Hemoptysis associated with pulmonary thromboembolism is most frequently observed when pulmonary infarction has occurred. In dogs without cor pulmonale or pulmonary infarction, acute, unexplained dyspnea may be the only clinical evidence of pulmonary thromboembolism.

If an early diagnosis of deep venous thrombosis can be established, prompt treatment could prevent the development of fatal pulmonary thromboembolism. Signs of deep venous thrombosis include edema and swelling of the tissues drained by the affected vessel and palpation of a firm, thick vein. However, these classical signs are not present in all cases.

Diagnostic Approach

Initial diagnostic tests in animals with clinical signs compatible with pulmonary thromboembolism should include thoracic radiographs, electrocardiography, and arterial blood gas determination. Coagulation studies to substantiate altered coagulation might include a platelet count, prothrombin time, activated partial thromboplastin time, and fibrin degradation products. Further tests to confirm the diagnosis include pulmonary angiography or ventilation–perfusion radionuclide imaging.

Pulmonary thromboembolism should be a prime differential diagnosis in animals with moderate to severe dyspnea and minimal radiographic abnormalities, especially when upper airway diseases can be ruled out. In animals with radiographic evidence of pulmonary thromboembolism, one or more of the following abnormalities may be identified (Fig. 24-8). Uneven vascular diameter may be observed when arteries to one side of the lung are occluded. Increased diameter of the proximal pulmonary arteries, an elevated hemidiaphragm, and small pleural effusions have also been reported in dogs. Atelectasis and/or alveolar pulmonary infiltrates may indicate pulmonary infarction or hemorrhage. Dogs with cor pulmonale usually have right ventricular enlargement and may have evidence of right ventricular failure.

The electrocardiogram may demonstrate sinus tachycardia, and a right ventricular enlargement pattern may be noted if cor pulmonale is present. Cor pulmonale is suggested by the echocardiographic findings of right ventricular hypertrophy, paradoxical septal motion, and diminished left ventricular internal dimension. In addition, a thrombus may be visualized in the right atrium. The central venous pressure is typically elevated (see Central Venous Pressure in Chapter 80).

Arterial blood gases provide supportive evidence for pulmonary thromboembolism (see Chapter 71). The most common abnormalities are arterial hypoxemia (low PO_2) and hypocapnia (decreased PCO_2). Exceptions are seen in animals with mild pulmonary embolism that causes pulmonary infarction or hemorrhage. These animals, probably tachypneic from pleuritic pain, demonstrate hypocapnia, respiratory alkalosis, and normal arterial PO_2.

Ventilation–perfusion radionuclide imaging can be very useful in establishing the diagnosis of pulmonary embolism, although this mode is not yet widely available. The ventilation scan will demonstrate good ventilation to all lung fields; however, the abnormal perfusion scan should demonstrate large segmental defects in perfusion to affected lung lobes. Unfortunately, the findings on the ventilation–perfusion scan may be inconclusive, especially in animals with multiple small to medium-sized emboli.

Although invasive, pulmonary angiography is the diagnostic "gold standard" and should be performed if other tests are inconclusive. The di-

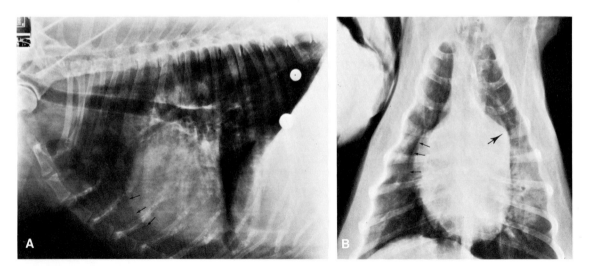

Figure 24–8 *Radiographic findings in a dog with pulmonary thromboembolism. Mild right ventricular enlargement (small arrows) is present on both the lateral (A) and the ventrodorsal (B) view. There is a bulge in the region of the main pulmonary artery segment (large arrow) on the ventrodorsal view. The remainder of the pulmonary vasculature is diminished on both views. The marked alveolar infiltrate in the left lung field on the ventrodorsal view was due to pulmonary infarction.*

agnostic angiographic finding of pulmonary embolism is the presence of an intraluminal filling defect (Fig. 24-9). Other angiographic findings that are compatible with pulmonary thromboembolism are truncation of pulmonary arteries or a lack of contrast material flowing to specific regions of the lung.

Pulmonary thromboembolism is rarely diagnosed as an isolated problem in veterinary patients. A search for the underlying predisposing disease should be part of the initial diagnostic plan. Useful tests include a complete blood count, serum biochemistry profile, heartworm test, and urinalysis. Additional tests that may be indicated in individual patients include serum amylase and lipase activities, Coomb's test, blood cultures, and ACTH stimulation or low-dose dexamethasone suppression testing.

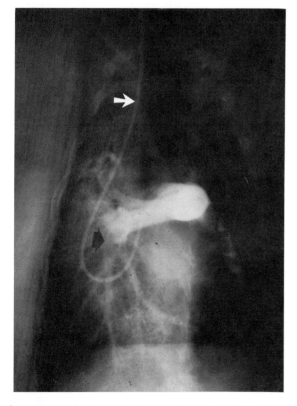

Figure 24–9 *Selective ventrodorsal pulmonary arteriogram from a dog with pulmonary thromboembolism. The catheter* (white arrow) *courses down the cranial vena cava, through the right atrium and ventricle, into the pulmonary artery. An intraluminal filling defect* (black arrow) *is present at the site of thromboembolism within the pulmonary artery supplying the right caudal lung lobe. (Courtesy of Dr. Lawrence J. Kleine, Tufts University.)*

Management

Management of pulmonary thromboembolism and deep venous thrombosis is divided into prophylactic and definitive therapies. Prophylactic therapy is based on the assumption that the body's fibrinolytic system can dissolve existent thrombi. Dissolution of the thrombus usually results in resolution of the pathophysiologic changes and clinical signs in 7 to 14 days. Prophylactic therapy is aimed at prevention of further thrombus formation or growth and resulting embolization. Heparin and warfarin are the drugs most frequently used. Heparin, which is used initially, is followed by chronic warfarin therapy for 3 to 6 months or until the predisposing cause has been resolved. Aspirin alone is probably inadequate to prevent recurrence of pulmonary thromboembolism.

The ideal care and management for naturally occurring pulmonary thromboembolism in dogs has not been well defined. We are currently using both heparin and warfarin. Heparin is started at 200 IU/kg intravenously, followed by a continuous infusion of 15 to 20 IU/kg/hour. At 4 hours, an activated partial thromboplastin time is obtained and the heparin dose is adjusted to maintain its prolongation at 1.5 to 2 times the baseline value. Simultaneously, warfarin therapy is initiated (0.5–5 mg per dog per day orally) and the dose is titrated to maintain the prothrombin time at 1.25 to 2 times the baseline. Heparin therapy, either intravenously or subcutaneously, is continued for 5 to 7 days to allow for warfarin to become fully effective.

Definitive therapy for pulmonary thromboembolism is aimed at dissolving or removing the existent thrombi. Surgical embolectomy and exogenously administered fibrinolytic agents are examples of definitive therapy. Pulmonary embolectomy requires open-heart surgery and cardiopulmonary bypass techniques, and carries a 30% to 50% mortality rate in humans. Fibrinolytic therapy with either urokinase or streptokinase has not been shown to improve survival in humans, and is associated with increased bleeding complications. Tissue plasminogen activator is a newly available fibrinolytic agent that may prove to be very useful in the management of pulmonary thromboembolism. Definitive therapy with surgery or fibrinolytic drugs is rarely used in veterinary patients.

Patient Monitoring

The disease that has led to pulmonary thromboembolism should, when possible, be aggressively treated to prevent further, potentially lethal episodes of embolism. After initiation of warfarin, prothrombin time should be measured weekly and the dosage should be adjusted to maintain the prothrombin time at 1.25 to 2 times the baseline. Once an appropriate dose is achieved, monthly reevaluations are probably adequate. Therapy should be continued for 3 to 6 months, or if the inciting cause cannot be removed, for life. Hemorrhage is the most worrisome complication.

MISCELLANEOUS VASCULAR DISEASES

Arteriovenous Malformations

An arteriovenous (A-V) fistula is a connection between an artery and vein with no interposing capillary bed. Central A-V fistulas, such as ventricular septal defect and patent ductus arteriosus, are discussed in Chapter 19. Peripheral A-V fistulas may be congenital or acquired. Congenital A-V fistulas can be located in the extremities, head, or abdomen. Those within the abdomen most frequently involve the hepatic or renal vessels. The majority of acquired A-V fistulas are located in the extremities and result from past trauma.

Arteriovenous malformations cause abnormalities of blood flow in both the heart and the peripheral blood vessels. Arterial blood, flowing directly into low pressure veins, causes increased venous pressures, with resulting venous dilation and tortuosity. The direction of blood flow in some veins distal to the fistula may reverse if the venous valves become incompetent. Blood pressure in arteries distal to the shunt is reduced, potentially resulting in inadequate tissue perfu-

sion. Blood flow through an A-V fistula provides stimulus for angiogenesis and the development of collateral circulation. After growth of new blood vessels, the volume of blood flowing through a large fistula may actually exceed the flow through the systemic circuit. The heart must eccentrically hypertrophy to increase cardiac output in response to this increased blood flow. Large A-V fistulas may ultimately lead to congestive heart failure.

Clinical signs vary with the site and size of the fistula, as well as the degree of local and central hemodynamic disturbance. Small A-V fistulas may result in few signs other than a swelling on the limb. Larger fistulas may cause pain, lameness, ischemia, edema, and ulceration of the digits. Typical findings include a soft, easily compressible swelling that is warm to the touch. Superficial veins may be distended and observed to pulsate, while palpation of a bounding or water-hammer arterial pulse is typical. A thrill, with or without an audible bruit (a musical sound heard during auscultation), may be palpable over the fistula. Large fistulas may result in abnormal blood flow to the distal limb such that the limb is cold, edematous, ulcerated, or ischemic and gangrenous. Compression of the fistula will result in loss of the machinerylike bruit and slowing of the heart rate (Branham's sign).

Animals with central or intra-abdominal A-V fistulas are typically presented for evaluation of ascites that results from portal hypertension (see Chapter 11). Those with large congenital fistulas may have stunted growth or evidence of congestive heart failure. A machinerylike bruit may be auscultated over the abdomen in some cases.

Diagnostic testing should include thoracic radiographs and selective angiography. Thoracic radiographs may demonstrate cardiomegaly, pulmonary overcirculation, or evidence of congestive heart failure in patients with very large fistulas. Selective angiography of the fistula is indicated to outline its anatomy prior to surgery. Both venous and arterial studies may be useful to help the surgeon preserve normal arterial and venous systems.

Surgery is the therapy of choice for A-V fistulas; however, very small, peripheral A-V fistulas can be treated initially with bandages or pressure wraps. Successful surgical therapy depends on ligation and excision of the abnormal blood vessels; normal circulation to the distal limb must be preserved to prevent ischemic necrosis. Acquired A-V malformations usually have fewer arteries supplying the fistula than those that are congenital and therefore are usually more amenable to surgical excision. Intra-abdominal fistulas, however, frequently have many anastomotic blood vessels, which makes surgical therapy difficult or impossible.

The prognosis for small, acquired A-V fistulas is good to guarded. While surgical therapy may be curative, regrowth of fistulae has been reported. Limb amputation is an option in animals with large or recurrent A-V fistulas. Animals with large, intra-abdominal A-V fistulas that are not amenable to surgical ligation or excision have a guarded to poor prognosis.

Vasculitis

Vasculitis most commonly involves arteries. It has been postulated that most vasculitides are caused by or associated with deposition of immune complexes in the arterial wall. Once immune complexes are deposited, complement is activated and complement components act as chemotactic factors for polymorphonuclear leukocytes. These white blood cells release lysosomal enzymes that cause further damage to the vessel wall. Some vasculitides are characterized by granulomatous reactions. These are likely the result of abnormalities in cell-mediated immunity.

Polyarteritis nodosa is the "classic" vasculitis reported in humans. This disease results in inflammation and necrotizing vasculitis of the small and medium-sized arteries. The lesions are often segmental; the characteristic histopathologic finding is the microaneurysm. Companion animals with vasculitis may have clinical and pathologic features in common with polyarteritis nodosa. Diseases that have been reported to cause vasculitis in dogs and cats include systemic lupus erythematosus, feline infectious peritonitis, and Rocky Mountain spotted fever *(Rickettsia rickettsii)*. Idiopathic (likely immune-mediated) vasculitis and immune-mediated drug reactions have also been implicated as causes of vasculitis.

Clinical signs reported in animals with vasculitis include signs of systemic illness such as fever, lethargy, and weight loss; swelling or edema (especially of the face and neck); petechial hemorrhages; and oral ulceration. Vasculitis is a multiple-system disease, and clinical signs may reflect dysfunction of many organ systems. Lymphadenopathy, polyarthritis, polymyositis, and hepatosplenomegaly have all been reported in dogs with vasculitis.

In addition to a complete blood count, serum biochemistry profile, and urinalysis, diagnostic testing in animals that manifest clinical signs compatible with vasculitis should include antinuclear antibody and rheumatoid factor titers, Rocky Mountain spotted fever titer, and feline infectious peritonitis virus titer. Biopsy of affected tissues such as skin, muscle, synovium, liver, or kidney is used to establish a definitive diagnosis.

Immunosuppressive therapy is indicated in animals with vasculitis that is not associated with systemic infection. Immunosuppressive doses of prednisone or prednisolone are used initially (2–4 mg/kg/day). Additional immunosuppressive drugs such as cyclophosphamide or azathiaprine can be employed if the disease is unresponsive to corticosteroids. Based on case reports, the prognosis for immune-mediated vasculitis in dogs appears to be good to fair. Dogs with Rocky Mountain spotted fever should receive tetracycline; appropriate therapy is usually curative. The prognosis for cats with vasculitis associated with feline infectious peritonitis virus is poor.

Atherosclerosis

Atherosclerosis, an extremely common disease in humans, is rare in dogs and unreported in the cat. Deposition of lipid and cholesterol within the intima of large and medium-sized arteries leads to smooth muscle and connective tissue proliferation within the vessel wall. The resultant luminal plaque has the potential to compromise blood flow in affected vessels. Atherosclerosis has been reported as a naturally occurring disease in dogs; however, it is suspected that hypothyroidism, hypercholesterolemia, or hyperlipidemia are prerequisites for its development. Clinical signs are nonspecific, but may include lethargy, anorexia, weakness, and dyspnea. Vomiting and collapse have been reported from affected animals, and neurologic deficits may result from vascular compromise in the brain. Electrocardiographic evidence of myocardial infarction, evidenced by ST segment elevation, ventricular arrhythmia, or conduction abnormalities, has been reported in some dogs proven to have atherosclerosis at necropsy. Thyroid function testing should be performed in dogs suspected to have atherosclerosis.

ADDITIONAL READING

Allen DG, Johnstone IB, Crane S. The effects of aspirin and propanolol, alone and in combination on hemostatic parameters in the normal cat. American Journal of Veterinary Research 1985; 46:660.

Burns MG. Pulmonary thromboembolism. In: Kirk RW, ed. Current veterinary therapy VIII. Philadelphia: WB Saunders, 1983: 257.

Cowgill LD, Kallet AJ. Systemic hypertension. In: Kirk RW, ed. Current veterinary therapy IX. Philadelphia: WB Saunders, 1986: 360.

Crawford MA, Foil CS. Vasculitis: Clinical syndromes in small animals. Compendium of Continuing Education 1989; 11:400.

Feldman BF. Thrombosis: Diagnosis and treatment. In: Kirk RW, ed. Current veterinary therapy IX. Philadelphia: WB Saunders, 1986: 505.

Flanders JA. Feline aortic thromboembolism. Compendium of Continuing Education 1986; 8:473.

Hosgood G. Arterioverous fistulas: Pathophysiology, diagnosis and treatment. Compendium of Continuing Education 1989; 11:625.

Kittleson MD, Olivier NB. Measurement of systemic arterial blood pressure. Vet Clin North Am [Small Anim Pract] 1983; 13:321.

Pion PD. Feline aortic thromboembolism and the potential utility of thrombolytic therapy with tissue plasminogen activator. Vet Clin North Am [Small Anim Pract] 1988; 18:79.

Pion PD, Kittleson MD. Therapy for feline aortic thromboembolism. In: Kirk RW, Bonagura JD, eds. Current veterinary therapy X. Philadelphia: WB Saunders, 1989: 295.

Suter PF. Peripheral vascular disease. In: Ettinger SJ, ed. Textbook of veterinary internal medicine. Philadelphia: WB Saunders, 1989: 1185.

Weiser MG, Spangler WL, Gribble DH. Blood pressure measurement in the dog. J Am Vet Med Assoc 1977; 171:364.

Wessale JL, Smith LA, Reid M et al. Indirect auscultatory systolic and diastolic pressures in the anesthetized dog. American Journal of Veterinary Research 1985; 46:2129.

25

HEARTWORM DISEASE

Clarke E. Atkins

Heartworm infection, caused by *Dirofilaria immitis*, is widely distributed, being recognized in northern and southern temperate zones as well as in the tropics and subtropics. In the United States, although the distribution favors the Southeast and the Mississippi river valley, infections have been recognized in most states (Fig. 25-1). In some endemic areas in the United States, infection rates approach 45%, and in some hyperendemic tropical regions, virtually all dogs are infected. In Canada, heartworm infection (HWI) is most prevalent in southwestern Ontario, around Montreal and Winnepeg.

When severe or prolonged, HWI may result in the pathologic process termed *heartworm disease* (HWD), which can have diverse and severe consequences. Heartworm disease may be manifested as a chronic disorder of the heart and lungs or, in the case of heartworm caval syndrome (CS), may have an acute and fulminant multisystemic presentation. Although the dog is the natural host, cats too can become infected. Because the consequences, treatment, and prognoses differ between the two species, canine and feline HWD will be discussed separately.

To effectively deal with HWI, the veterinary practitioner must have a thorough grasp of the parasite's life cycle, as this has important ramifications in the diagnosis, prevention, and treatment of HWI. In addition, an understanding of the pathophysiology of both chronic HWD and CS is important in the prognostication and successful treatment of these disorders. Diagnosis and therapy are complicated by the potential confusion with the innocuous parasite *Dipetalonema reconditum*, the number and variety of available diagnostic tests and their variable sensitivity and specificity, and the fact that therapy involves prevention of infection as well as eradication of adult worms and microfilariae.

CAUSES

Infection with the filarid parasite *D. immitis* produces HWD when worm burden and duration of infection is sufficient. This parasite is now known to be transmitted by more than 60 species of mosquitoes. The complex life cycle of *D. immitis* is depicted in Figure 25-2. Adult heartworms (L_5) reside in the pulmonary arteries and, to a lesser extent, the right ventricle. After mating, microfilarie (L_1) are produced by mature female L_5 and released into the circulation. These L_1 are ingested by feeding female mosquitoes and undergo two moults over an 8- to 17-day period. The resultant third-stage larva (L_3) is infective and is transmitted by the feeding mosquito to the origi-

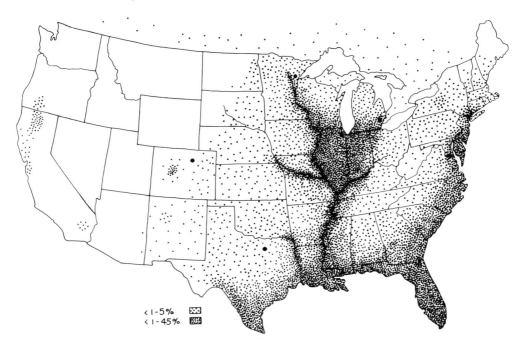

Figure 25–1. Incidence of heartworm disease infection in the United States as of 1986. (Published with permission of American Heartworm Society, Proceedings of the heartworm symposium, 1986.)

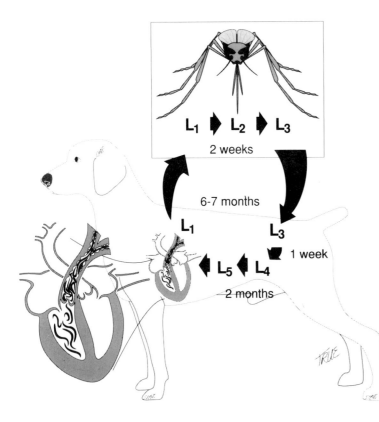

Figure 25–2. Life cycle of Dirofilaria immitis. Microfilariae (L₁) are released from gravid adult females (L₅) in the heart and pulmonary arteries of the infected dog. These L₁ are taken into feeding mosquitoes where they undergo two moults to become infective larvae (L₃) over 14- to 17-day period. Subsequent feeding on appropriate hosts results in infection or reinfection when L₃ are injected. The L₃ to L₄ moult occurs 1 to 12 days after infection with a moult to adulthood approximately 2 months after infection. These L₅ first appear 70 days after infection, completing their migration from the subcutaneous tissue to the pulmonary arteries by 4 months after infection. Microfilariae, useful in the diagnosis of heartworm infection, are found in peripheral blood 6 to 7 months after infection.

nal or another host. Another moult occurs in the subcutaneous, adipose, and skeletal muscular tissues shortly after infection (1–12 days), with a final moult to L_5 2 months (50–68 days) after infection. This immature adult soon enters the vascular system, migrating to the heart and lungs, where final maturation and mating occur. Under optimum conditions, the life cycle is 184 to 210 days, with the host becoming microfilaremic 6 to 7 months after infection. Microfilariae show both seasonal and diurnal periodicity, with greatest numbers appearing in the peripheral blood during the summer and evening hours. Adult heartworms are known to live up to 5 years and L_1 up to 30 months in the dog.

CHRONIC CANINE HEARTWORM DISEASE

Pathophysiology

In a sense, the name "heartworm" is a misnomer because dirofilariae reside in the pulmonary arterial system for the most part, and the primary insult to the health of the host is a manifestation of damage to the pulmonary arteries. The severity of the lesions and, hence, clinical ramifications are related to the relative number of worms (ranging from 1 to more than 250), the duration of infection, and the host–parasite interaction.

Immature and mature L_5 reside primarily in the pulmonary vascular tree, migrating into the right heart and great veins in heavy infections. Obstruction of pulmonary vessels by living worms is of little clinical significance. The major effect on the pulmonary arteries is produced by worm-induced (probably through immune-mediated mechanisms and trauma) villous myointimal proliferation and by arterial obstruction with and vascular reaction to "dead worm" thromboemboli.

Pulmonary vascular lesions begin to develop within days of worm arrival, with endothelial damage and sloughing as well as leukocyte and platelet activation and migration. The immigration of these cells and the release of trophic factors results in smooth muscle cell proliferation and migration, with collagen accumulation and even-

tual fibrosis. Within 4 weeks of the arrival of adult worms in the pulmonary vasculature, villous proliferative lesions are present. These eventually encroach upon and even occlude vascular lumina.

Worms that die naturally or are killed elicit an even more severe reaction, inciting pulmonary arterial thrombosis, granulomatous inflammation, and rugous villous inflammation, particularly severe in caudal lung lobes. Diseased pulmonary arteries are thrombosed, thickened, dilated, tortuous, noncompliant, and biologically incompetent, thereby resisting further vascular recruitment during increased demand. Hence, exercise capacity is diminished. The result is pulmonary hypertension, which is exacerbated with exercise or other states of increased cardiac output. The right heart, an efficient volume pump, does not withstand pressure overload. As a consequence, right heart compensation (dilatation and hypertrophy) and ultimately decompensation (right heart failure) may result in severe cases. In addition, right heart dilatation can produce secondary tricuspid insufficiency, thereby complicating cardiac dysfunction. Pulmonary infarction is uncommon because of the extensive collateral circulation provided the lung and because of the gradual onset of vascular occlusion.

Spontaneous or postadulticide thromboembolization with dead worms may precipitate or worsen clinical signs, producing right heart failure or, in rare instances, pulmonary infarction. Worm fragments worsen vascular damage and enhance coagulation, further compromising pulmonary blood flow. Consolidation of affected lung lobes may result, contributing to hypoxic vasoconstriction, which further aggravates pulmonary hypertension and diminishes pulmonary blood flow.

Pulmonary parenchymal lesions also develop by mechanisms other than post-thromboembolic consolidation. Allergic pneumonitis, a pulmonary infiltrate with eosinophils, is most often reported in true occult HWD, when immune-mediated destruction of L_1 in the pulmonary microcirculation produces amicrofilaremia. Calvert (Additional Reading) reports an incidence of 14% in 93 consecutive cases of occult HWD. This syndrome results when antibody-coated L_1, entrapped in the pulmonary circulation, incite an eosinophilic inflammatory reaction. A more sinister, but uncommon, form of parenchymal lung disease, termed *pulmonary eosinophilic granulomatosis*, has been associated with HWD. The exact cause and pathogenesis are unknown, but it is felt to be similar to HWD-related allergic pneumonitis. It is postulated that L_1 trapped in the lungs are surrounded by neutrophils and eosinophils, eventually forming granulomas and inciting bronchial lymphadenopathy. Because of the increased permeability of the diseased pulmonary vasculature and the associated increase in hydrostatic pressure, perivascular edema may develop. Although this may be evident radiographically as increased interstitial and alveolar density, it is seemingly of minimal clinical significance and does not indicate left heart failure.

Antigen–antibody complexes, formed in response to heartworm antigens, commonly produce glomerulonephritis in heartworm-infected dogs. These lesions result in proteinuria (albuminuria) and are associated with renal failure in a small percentage of cases (see Chapter 45).

Heartworms also induce disease by aberrant migration. This uncommon phenomenon has been associated with neuromuscular and ocular manifestations, as worms have been described in tissues such as muscle, brain, spinal cord, and the anterior chamber of the eye. In addition, arterial thrombosis with L_5 has been observed when worms migrate aberrantly to the aortic bifurcation. Adult heartworms may also migrate in a retrograde manner to the right heart and venae cavae, producing CS, a devastating process described below.

Clinical Signs

The clinical signs of chronic HWD depend on the severity and duration of infection, reflecting the effects of the parasite on the lungs and, secondarily, the heart. Historical findings variably include weight loss, diminished exercise tolerance, lethargy, poor body condition, cough, dyspnea, syncope, and abdominal distention. Physical examination may reveal evidence of weight loss, a split S_2 (13% of cases), heart murmur (13%), and cardiac gallop (20%). If right heart

failure is present, jugular venous distention and pulsation typically accompany hepatosplenomegaly and ascites. Cardiac arrhythmias and conduction disturbances are uncommon in chronic HWD (less than 10% of cases).

With pulmonary parenchymal manifestations of HWD, cough and pulmonary crackles are often audible. With granulomatosis, muffled lung sounds, dyspnea, and cyanosis are also reported. When massive pulmonary thromboembolization occurs, the additional signs of fever and hemoptysis may be noted. However, the majority of heartworm-infected dogs have no clinical signs at the time of diagnosis.

Diagnostic Approach

Ideally, the diagnosis is made by routine check prior to the onset of symptoms of HWD. Dogs in areas in which heartworms are endemic should undergo a yearly heartworm test. The diagnosis of HWI is made by direct or indirect identification of the parasite. This is accomplished most commonly by the microscopic identification of L_1 on a direct blood smear or above the buffy coat in a microhematocrit tube, with the modified Knott test, or after millipore filtration of blood. The accuracy of these tests, typically used for routine screening and for the diagnosis of suspected HWD, is improved by multiple testing. The modified Knott test and millipore filtration are more sensitive because they concentrate L_1, improving chances of diagnosis. The direct smear technique allows examination of larval motion, helping in the distinction of *D. immitis* from *D. reconditum* (Table 25-1). This distinction is important because the presence of the latter parasite does not require expensive and potentially toxic arsenical therapy. None of these tests can rule out HWI conclusively because of the prevalence of amicrofilaremic infections and the fact that in dogs with low numbers of L_1, false-negative results may occur. The number of circulating L_1 does not correlate well with the number of L_5 and, therefore, cannot be used to determine the severity of infection. In amicrofilaremic HWI the clinician is forced to make a diagnosis based on a combination of clinical, clinicopathologic, immunologic, and radiographic findings.

Table 25–1 *Differentiation of Microfilariae of* Dirofilaria immitis *From Those of* Dipetalonema reconditum

	Number in Blood	*Motion*	*Shape*	*Length (Knott Test)*
Dirofilaria immitis	Usually numerous	Stationary	Straight body Tapered head Straight tail	308 μ (295 to 325 μ)
Dipetalonema reconditum	Usually few	Progressive	Curved body Blunt head Curved or button-hooked tail	263 μ (250 to 288 μ)

Because many (approximately 25%) HWIs are amicrofilaremic, the utility of the tests described above in confirming suspected cases of HWD may be limited. The indirect fluorescent antibody test (IFA) is used to detect antimicrofilarial antibodies, and has particular usefulness in the diagnosis of true occult HWI (those instances in which L_1 are absent because of immune-mediated destruction). This test is specific and quite sensitive in the diagnosis of true occult HWI. Enzyme-linked immunoabsorbent assays (ELISA), which can detect either heartworm antibody or antigen, have also been developed. At this time, those tests that detect filarial antigen appear to be most specific. These "in-house" tests have rapidly gained popularity because of their accuracy (both in sensitivity and specificity) and their ease of performance. The ELISA tests have recently been shown to be useful in that serum antigen concentrations correlated to numbers of L_5. Neither type of immunodiagnostic test has been troubled by crossreaction with *D. reconditum*. Both the IFA (1 year) and ELISA (6 months) will remain positive for a period of time after successful adulticidal therapy.

Immunodiagnostic tests are currently not recommended for routine screening, with the possible exception of use in highly endemic regions. However, this is a rapidly developing research area, in which the marketing of new and refined products and changes in recommendations will likely continue. Grieve (Additional Reading) has emphasized that the test chosen should meet the needs of the practitioner, the geographic region, and the local incidence of HWI. With these considerations, the ideal test will not be the same for every practitioner.

Although not effective for screening for HWI, thoracic radiography offers an excellent method for detecting HWD, for determining its severity, and for evaluating pulmonary parenchymal changes (Table 25-2). Radiographic abnormalities, which develop relatively early in the disease course, are present in approximately 85% of cases. According to a study of 200 heartworm-infected dogs by Losonsky and associates (Additional Reading), radiographic features (Fig. 25-3) include right ventricular enlargement (60% of cases), increased prominence of the main pulmonary artery segment (70%), increased size and density of the pulmonary arteries (50%), as well as pulmonary artery tortuosity and "pruning" (50%). If heart failure is present, enlargement of the caudal vena cava, liver, and spleen, as well as pleural effusion or ascites may be evident. Thrall and Calvert (Additional Reading) suggested that pleural effusion is uncommon in heart failure due to HWD, and showed that marked enlargement of the cranial lobar pulmonary artery was a more sensitive predictor of HWD-associated heart failure than enlargement of the caudal vena cava.

Ventrodorsal thoracic radiographs are preferable for cardiac silhouette evaluation and ease, and for minimizing patient stress. However, the dorsoventral projection is superior for the evaluation of the caudal lobar pulmonary vessels, which are considered abnormal if they are larger than the diameter of the ninth rib where the rib and artery intersect. The anterior cranial pulmonary artery is best evaluated in the lateral projection, and should normally not be larger than its accompanying vein or the proximal one third of the fourth rib.

The pulmonary parenchyma can also be evaluated radiographically. In allergic pneumonitis the findings include a mixed interstitial and al-

Table 25–2 *Minimum Data Base for Chronic Heartworm Disease*

Test	Typical Abnormal Results	
	Dog	Cat
Complete blood count	Nonregenerative anemia, eosinophilia, basophilia, neutrophilia	Similar to results in dog, but less consistent
Urinalysis	Proteinuria	Inconsistent proteinuria
Blood urea nitrogen and serum creatinine	Inconsistently increased	Inconsistently increased
Serum alanine aminotransferase and alkaline phosphatase	Often increased	Inconsistently increased
Serum total protein	Variably decreased	Variably increased
Serum bilirubin concentration	Variably increased	Usually normal
BSP retention*	Usually normal; if increased, further liver evaluation may be warranted	Little information available
Thoracic radiographs	Right ventricular enlargement; pulmonary artery enlargement, tortuosity, and pruning; pulmonary interstitial and alveolar densities	Subtle changes: pulmonary artery enlargement, interstitial infiltrates
Electrocardiogram†	Right ventricular and atrial enlargement pattern, arrhythmias	Usually normal
Echocardiogram†	Right ventricular and septal hypertrophy, right ventricular dilatation. Paradoxical septal motion, small left ventricular luminal dimension, heartworms may rarely be visualized in pulmonary arteries or right ventricle	Little information available

The minimum data base is useful to detect concurrent disease, to evaluate specific organ dysfunction that may impact therapy, to identify heartworm-related manifestations such as pneumonitis or granulomatosis, and to serve as a baseline from which to gauge future abnormalities.

* BSP retention need only be measured if severe liver disease is suspected. Calvert and Rawlings (1988, Additional Reading) have observed that 30-minute BSP retention less than 15% is not associated with increased risk of therapeutic complications.

† Electrocardiograms and echocardiograms need only be obtained if there is indication of cardiac arrhythmia, heart failure, or caval syndrome.

veolar density, which is typically most severe in the caudal lung lobes (Fig. 25-4). In eosinophilic nodular pulmonary granulomatosis the inflammatory process is characterized by interstitial nodular densities, bronchial lymphadenopathy, and, occasionally, pleural effusion. With pulmonary thromboembolism, the radiographic findings reflect the increased hydrostatic pressure and increased pulmonary vascular permeability of HWD, which result in fluid accumulation (interstitial density and air bronchograms), particularly in the caudal lung lobes. Inflammation and consolidation may accompany massive embolization or pulmonary infarction.

Electrocardiography is useful in detecting arrhythmias, but is generally insensitive in detection of cardiac chamber enlargement in HWD when compared to radiography. If radiography does not suggest HWD, it is unlikely that the electrocardiogram will. The finding of a right ventricular enlargement pattern (Fig. 25-5) is supportive evidence for HWD. Lombard and Ackerman (Additional Reading) demonstrated that electrocardiographic abnormalites were present in 38% and 62% respectively of dogs with moderate and severe echocardiographic changes of HWD. Calvert and Rawlings (1988, Additional Reading) showed that the most consistent electrocardiographic parameters associated with HWD were an S wave deeper than 0.8 mV in lead V_5, mean electrical axis greater than 103°, and three electrocardiographic parameters of right heart enlargement. The latter electrocardiographic finding (greater than or equal to three enlarge-

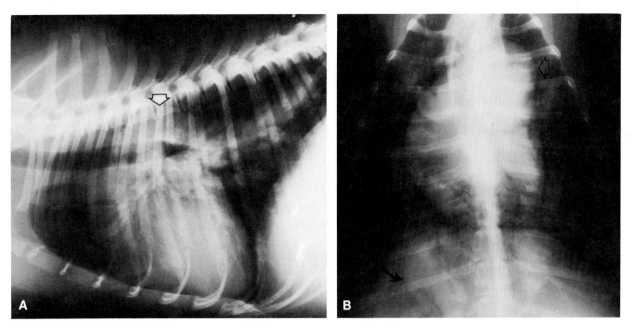

Figure 25–3. (A) Lateral and (B) ventrodorsal thoracic radiographs from a dog with heartworm disease and caval syndrome. Notice the signs of chronic heartworm disease, including right ventricular enlargement, main pulmonary artery enlargement (clear arrow), and pulmonary artery enlargement and tortuousity (dark arrow). (Published with permission: Atkins CE. Caval syndrome in the dog. Seminars in Veterinary Medicine and Surgery, 1988; 2:64.)

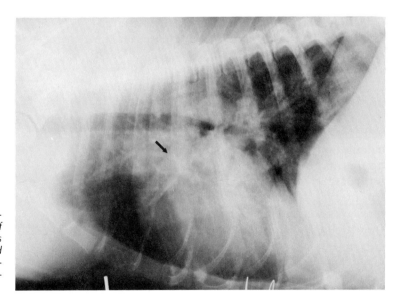

Figure 25–4. A lateral thoracic radiograph demonstrating diffuse interstitial and alveolar densities of eosinophilic pneumonitis. Parenchymal disease is most severe in the caudal lobes. Note the enlarged main and cranial (arrow) pulmonary arteries. (Photograph courtesy of Dr. Kathy Spaulding, North Carolina State University.)

ment parameters) is considered to be the most accurate. P-pulmonale is unusual in HWD, and heart failure is rare in instances in which both radiographs and the electrocardiogram fail to suggest severe right ventricular enlargement. Og-

burn and associates (Additional Reading) reported arrhythmias to be rare in HWI and HWD unless CS was present. In their study, between 2% and 4% of dogs with chronic HWD had sinus tachycardia or conduction disturbances. Calvert and

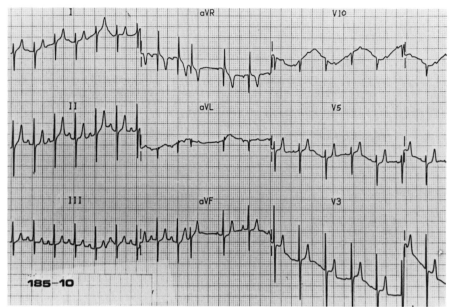

Figure 25–5. *A nine-lead ECG from a dog with heartworm disease and caval syndrome, demonstrating features of right ventricular enlargement. Note the right axis deviation, deep S waves in Leads I, II, III, aVF, V5, and V3, and positive T waves in V10. (Published with permission: Atkins CE. Caval syndrome in the dog. Seminars in Veterinary Medicine and Surgery, 1988; 2:64.*

Rawlings (1988, Additional Reading) found that only 6% of 276 dogs with HWI had cardiac rhythm disturbances.

Echocardiography is relatively sensitive in the detection of HWD-induced right heart enlargement, and is characterized by increases in the right ventricular end-diastolic dimension and septal and right ventricular free-wall thickness (Fig. 25-6). Lombard (Additional Reading) reported abnormal (paradoxical) septal motion in four of 10 dogs with HWD. The ratio of left : right ventricular internal dimensions is another useful calculation, being reduced from a normal value of approximately 3.5 to a mean value of 0.7 in dogs with HWD. Two-dimensional echocardiography can at times demonstrate worms in the pulmonary artery. Although Badertscher and associates (Additional Reading) has shown that heartworms can be similarly demonstrated in the right ventricle, this method is insensitive except in dogs with CS or worm thrombi, as the worms infrequently inhabit this location.

Hematologic and chemical abnormalities are not sufficient to make a diagnosis of HWD. They are frequently useful in providing supportive evidence and for evaluating concurrent disease that may or may not be related to HWD.

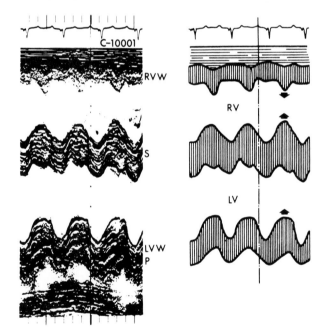

Figure 25–6. *M-mode echocardiogram and schematic demonstrating right ventricular wall and septal thickening, right ventricular luminal enlargement, and paradoxical septal motion (arrows). (Published with permission: Lombard CW. Compendium of Continuing Education. 1983; 5:971.*
RV = right ventricle; LV = left ventricle; RVW and LVW = right and left ventricular walls, respectively; S = septum; and P = pericardium.

Calvert and Rawlings (1988, Additional Reading) report that the dog with HWD in Georgia is typically found to have a low-grade, nonregenerative anemia (10% of mildly to moderately affected dogs and up to 60% of severely affected dogs), neutrophilia (20%–80% of cases), eosinophilia (85% of cases), and basophilia (60% of cases). Thrombocytopenia, which may be noted in chronic HWD, CS, and disseminated intravascular coagulation (DIC), is most common 1 to 2 weeks after adulticidal therapy. In severe cases, especially if heart failure is present, liver enzyme activities may be increased (10% of cases), and, occasionally, hyperbilirubinemia is noted. Azotemia, seen in only 5% of cases, may be prerenal in origin if dehydration or heart failure are present, or may be secondary to glomerulonephritis. If glomerular disease is severe, hypoproteinemia (hypoalbuminemia) can complicate the clinical picture. The urinalysis may rarely reveal isosthenuria; this is accompanied by the more commonly detected albuminuria (10%–30% of cases). The most pronounced clinicopathologic findings are associated with the most severe clinical findings.

The evaluation of tracheobronchial cytology is at times useful, particularly in the coughing dog with eosinophilic pneumonitis, occult HWD, and minimal radiographic evidence of HWD (see Transtracheal Wash in Chapter 80). Microscopic examination reveals evidence of an eosinophilic infiltrate. In microfilaremic dogs, L_1 may occasionally be detected in this manner. Abdominal fluid analysis in cases of congestive heart failure typically reveals a modified transudate (see Abdominal Paracentesis and Lavage in Chapter 80). Dogs with HWD and right heart failure have central venous pressure (Chapter 80) that ranges from 12 to greater than 20 cm H_2O. Ascites develops at lower central venous pressures if hypoalbuminemia is present (see Chapter 11).

Management

The medical management of HWI is complicated by the complex parasite life cycle; the marked variability in clinical manifestations and severity of HWD; the need to prevent HWI, to remove L_5, and to render the patient free of L_1; and the relative toxicity of adulticidal therapy. For these reasons, the prevention and treatment of HWI will remain a challenging endeavor to the practicing veterinarian.

Prophylaxis

Prevention of infection (Table 25-3) is the obvious aim of the veterinary clinician. Prophylactic failure results from ignorance on the part of owners as to the presence or potential severity of HWI, lack of owner compliance, or inadequate instruction of owners on preventive measures by the attending veterinarian. Amicrofilaremic dogs with HWI should be placed on preventive therapy at the time of diagnosis if the potential for further infection exists (summer months or warm climates).

Diethylcarbamazine (DEC; Filarabits, Caracide) has long enjoyed popularity as the preventive of choice. This product is safe and effective, but must be given daily (6.6 mg/kg orally), making owner compliance difficult to achieve in some instances. Diethylcarbamazine is thought to kill

Table 25–3 *Recommended Treatment and Preventive Protocols for Dogs With Canine Heartworm Infection*

PREVENTION

Diethylcarbamazine* (6.6 mg/kg PO daily) or
Ivermectin (2.5 to 5 µg/kg PO monthly)

ADULTICIDAL THERAPY

Aspirin (0.5 mg/kg twice daily to 5 mg/kg once daily) 1 to 3 weeks before and 4 to 6 weeks after adulticidal therapy in cases with heartworm disease
Thiacetarsamide sodium (2.2 mg/kg twice daily) intravenously for 2 days

MICROFILARICIDAL THERAPY†

Dithiazanine (8.8 mg/kg daily PO for 7 to 10 days) or
Ivermectin** (10% solution of ivermectin in propylene glycol, 2 ml/kg PO) or
Levamisole (11 mg/kg daily PO for 1 to 2 weeks)

* *Diethylcarbamazine should not be administered to microfilaremic dogs.*
† *Microfilaricidal therapy should be begun 4 to 6 weeks after adulticidal therapy.*
** *Ivermectin should not be used as a microfilaricide in collies.*

L₃ and early, tissue-migrating fourth-stage larvae (L₄). Unfortunately, this drug has only a small temporal "window" of therapeutic efficacy, thus explaining the need for frequent administration. Diethylcarbamazine should be administered daily from the onset of mosquito season continuously until 1 to 2 months after a killing frost. In some geographic regions the persistence of mosquitoes dictates year-round prophylaxis.

Diethylcarbamazine must only be administered to dogs free of microfilaremia, thus dictating a yearly heartworm test prior to reinstitution of preventive therapy. Inadvertent administration of DEC to microfilaremic dogs produces an adverse, possibly immune-mediated reaction approximately 25% of the time. Signs associated with this adverse drug reaction usually occur within 1 hour of medication and include depression, ptyalism, vomiting, diarrhea, weak pulses, pale mucous membranes, prolonged capillary refill time, and bradycardia. Subsequently, the dogs become recumbent, dyspneic, and tachycardic, and 9% of reactors succumb. Restated, more than 2% of microfilaremic dogs to which DEC is administered will die due an adverse drug reaction.

Not infrequently, owners inadvertently miss one or more doses of DEC. If 1 day of therapy is omitted, no problem exists and drug administration should continue. In the event that a more prolonged lapse in DEC treatment occurs, reinstitution of medication should be advised, with the realization that infection may have occurred. If a dog is found to be microfilaremic when on preventive medication, DEC prophylaxis should be continued; if inadvertently stopped, reinstitution may result in the described adverse reaction.

Ivermectin (Heartguard), a broad-spectrum anthelmintic, is effective given only once monthly because it kills L₄, thus providing a therapeutic "window" of several weeks' duration. Although it is recommended that ivermectin not be administered to dogs with HWI, the incidence and severity of reactions to this drug are far less than to DEC at the prophylactic dosage; microfilaremic dogs may, however, exhibit transient diarrhea. Ivermectin (2.5–5 μg/kg orally) is administered monthly from the onset of the mosquito season through to 1 month after the season ends. Yearly heartworm tests are advised. Although a relatively new drug, initial experience suggests that ivermectin is safe and that, at the recommended prophylactic dosage, the adverse drug reactions (*e.g.*, salivation, central nervous system dysfunction, and death) seen with the microfilaricidal dose of ivermectin in collies are absent.

Adulticidal Therapy

In most cases of HWD it is imperative to rid the patient of the offending parasite (see Table 25-2). Thiacetarsemide sodium (Caparsolate), the only drug approved for this purpose, is administered intravenously twice daily (2.2 mg/kg at no less than 8- and no more than 16-hour intervals) for 2 days (4 doses). Adult worms begin to die during the first week after treatment; this process is completed within 3 weeks. Although clinical improvement is usually achieved, the drug has been shown to effectively kill only 46% to 96% of heartworms, with immature adult and female worms being most resistant. More importantly, less than 50% of experimentally infected dogs are cleared with one course of therapy. Experience suggests that better results are obtained in the clinical situation. Persistent infection, usually detected by recurrent microfilaremia or persistent serologic evidence of HWI, requires subsequent treatment. New evidence indicates that thiacetarsemide also kills developing larvae near the time of the L₄ to L₅ moult.

Thiacetarsemide, an arsenical, is, unfortunately, toxic, with the potential to produce skin sloughing, hepatorenal dysfunction, and pulmonary embolization with dead worms. Evaluation of a pretreatment minimum data base (see Table 25-2) allows the clinician to detect underlying disorders that may complicate or dictate delaying adulticidal therapy. Because arsenicals are hepatotoxic and nephrotoxic, special attention should be paid to liver enzyme tests, blood urea nitrogen, serum creatinine, and the results of urinalysis. Certain laboratory or clinical findings may dictate that adulticidal therapy be avoided, postponed, or interrupted (Table 25-4). Because no pretreatment laboratory work predicts which dogs will suffer an adverse drug reaction, it is imperative that patients be examined before each

Table 25–4 *Indications for Omitting, Delaying, or Aborting Adulticidal Therapy*

OMIT ADULTICIDAL THERAPY

Concurrent terminal disease

DELAY ADULTICIDAL THERAPY

Severe pulmonary artery disease
Right heart failure
Allergic pneumonitis or granulomatosis
Caval syndrome
Severe renal or hepatic disease

ABORT ADULTICIDAL THERAPY

Anorexia
Icterus
Gross bilirubinuria after first or second injection
Renal failure

---

injection, with evaluation of mental status, mucous membrane color, body temperature, and appetite. In addition, a urine sample is examined for gross bilirubinuria. When discontinuation of therapy is necessary, retreatment, using the complete regime, is performed once signs have resolved (3–4 weeks).

Drug reactions to adulticidal therapy have been reported in 15% of 276 treated cases, resulting in discontinuance of treatment in only 6%. Vomiting, anorexia, and icterus were the side-effects most often encountered. Subsequent treatment was completed in most dogs (eight of 10) in which initial treatment was discontinued. Early (after the first or second dose) adverse reactions to arsenical therapy include depression, anorexia, vomiting, diarrhea, icterus, and bilirubinuria. Renal dysfunction is an unusual complication of adulticidal therapy. Reversible, acute, oliguric renal failure after two doses of thiacetarsemide sodium, which was associated with isosthenuria, azotemia, pyuria, hematuria, and urinary casts, has been described by Leib and associates (Additional Reading). Liver enzyme activities invariably rise during therapy. Elevated enzyme elevation, in the absence of evidence of severe liver disease, is not an indication to avoid beginning or to discontinue arsenical therapy.

Later complications include dead worm pulmonary embolization and skin sloughing. Embolization is most frequent in dogs with severe pulmonary artery changes; it occurs 1 to 2 weeks (or longer) after therapy. Because embolization is often precipitated by exercise, cage confinement or strict exercise restriction should be employed for 4 to 6 weeks after adulticidal therapy. Aspirin therapy has also been advocated to reduce the frequency of postadulticidal pulmonary embolization. The recommended dosage is 5 mg/kg once daily; recent work by Rackear and associates (Additional Reading) has suggested 0.5 mg/kg twice daily as the preferred dosage. Skin sloughing can be prevented by careful avoidance of subcutaneous injection of thiacetarsemide. If possible, using the same vein for two subsequent injections should be avoided. A butterfly catheter is used and saline is injected before and after drug administration to ensure proper needle placement and to rinse the drug from the line. If thiacetarsemide is inadvertently administered subcutaneously, normal saline injected at the site may minimize the reaction. Calvert and Rawlings (1988, Additional Reading) recommend dimethyl sulfoxide applied topically for treatment or prevention of signs after drug extravasation.

Ishihara and associates have recently described a method of mechanical worm removal using flexible alligator forceps. This method was 90% effective in worm removal in 36 dogs with mild to severe HWD. Only two of the nine severely affected dogs died of heart and renal failure, more than 90 days postoperatively, suggesting that in skilled hands, the technique is safe. Advantages to this technique include its high efficacy, diminished potential for arsenical toxicity (subsequent adulticidal therapy would be administered to a then asymptomatic dog), and reduced risk of thromboembolic complication. Disadvantages include the need for a light plane of anesthesia, a degree of operator skill, fluoroscopy, and subsequent arsenical administration.

Microfilaricidal Therapy

Although live microfilaria are minimally harmful to the host, they should be eliminated for several reasons. First and foremost, the dog will remain infectious to itself and other dogs for the life-expectancy of the L_1. In addition, the diagnosis of future infections is confused by persistent L_1.

Lastly, DEC cannot safely be administered to a microfilaremic dog. Microfilaricidal therapy should follow (by 4–6 weeks), not precede adulticidal therapy and should continue until the dog is amicrofilaremic (see Table 25-2). Recurrent microfilaremia suggests persistence of adult infection.

Dithiazanine (Diazan) is the only microfilaricide approved for use in the dog. This drug has the disadvantages of inconsistent availability, adverse reactions, and a tendency to discolor feces and vomitus. Drug reactions include anorexia, vomiting, and diarrhea; drug reactions are dose-related. Dithiazanine (8.8 mg/kg/day orally) is administered daily for 7 to 10 days. A modified Knott or millipore filter test is performed at that time to evaluate therapeutic success. If microfilaremia persists, treatment is continued at the same or a higher dosage. Adverse reactions can be minimized by using the lower dosage, by splitting the dose, by administering with food, or by concurrent administration of antiemetic drugs. Frequently, client dissatisfaction or drug reactions dictate the use of an alternative product.

Ivermectin is an unapproved, but commonly used and effective, microfilaricide. Ivermectin, marketed for injectable use in cattle, is diluted to a 10% solution (1 ml in 9 ml) with propylene glycol and administered orally at 2 ml/kg. A repeat heartworm test 4 weeks later dictates whether a second dose is necessary. Subsequent positive tests imply persistent adult infection. Ivermectin is quite effective, killing microfilaria in 4 to 24 hours. More than 70% of treated dogs are free of L_1 in 10 days or less, and only 4% of dogs require more than one dose.

Adverse reactions, including a shocklike syndrome or a 1- to 2-day bout of depression, anorexia, and vomiting, have been observed, each in less than 5% of treated dogs. The former more severe reaction likely has a similar pathogenesis to that seen with DEC in microfilaremic dogs, and is said to respond promptly to parenteral steroid and intravenous fluid administration. Because of the potential for drug reactions, treated dogs should be hospitalized and closely observed for the day.

Collies treated with microfilaricidal doses (0.05 mg/kg) may suffer an idiosyncratic reaction to ivermectin similar to, but more severe than, that seen in beagles given very high doses (2.5–40 mg/kg orally). Signs include salivation, tremors, confusion, ataxia, convulsions, coma, and, occasionally, death. For this reason, ivermectin should not be administered at the microfilaricidal dose to collies and related breeds.

Levamisole has adulticidal and microfilaricidal potential. The former effect is inconsistent, resulting in an average kill rate of approximately 50%; thus, although it may sterilize adult females, it is not advocated for use as an adulticide. On the other hand, though not approved, levamisole is a potent microfilaricide. Unfortunately, levamisole has a narrow therapeutic index, with lethargy, vomiting, apprehension, stiffness, trembling, and, rarely, convulsions having been noted with its use. Methods similar to those indicated for dithiazanine may be successful in preventing vomiting. The drug is administered daily (11 mg/kg/day orally) for 1 week, and, if microfilaremia persists, treatment is continued for an additional 5 to 7 days. Continued microfilaremia dictates choosing an alternative drug.

Fenthion, an organophosphate, although unapproved as a microfilaricide, has been used for this purpose. A 14% or 20% solution is administered topically weekly at a dose of 15 mg/kg. If L_1 persist after two to three treatments, an alternative drug is chosen. Signs of intoxication are those of organophosphate poisoning, and include ptyalism, gastrointestinal signs, and, potentially, convulsions and death.

Special Considerations

There are frequently manifestations and complications to HWD that require therapeutic efforts above and beyond ridding the patient of adult heartworms and L_1. In addition, the use of certain drugs in the management of HWD deserves separate discussion.

Allergic pneumonitis, which is reported to affect 14% of dogs with HWD, is a relatively early development in the disease course. Corticosteroid therapy (prednisone or prednisolone at 1–2 mg/kg/day orally) results in rapid attenuation of clinical signs with radiographic clearing in less than a week. At this point corticosteroid therapy is discontinued, as it is known to reduce the efficacy of thiacetarsemide, and adulticidal therapy is initiated immediately. Microfilaricides are generally not indicated, as infections are typically occult.

A more serious manifestation, pulmonary eosinophilic granulomatosis, responds less favorably. Treatment with prednisone at twice the dosage for allergic pneumonitis (2 mg/kg twice daily) is reported to induce partial or complete remission in 1 to 2 weeks. The prognosis remains guarded, as recurrence within several weeks is common. Prednisone may be combined with cyclophosphamide or azathioprine in an effort to heighten the immunosuppressive effect. The latter combination appears to be the most effective. Adulticidal therapy should be delayed until remission is attained. The pulmonary edema associated with increased vascular permeability and pulmonary hypertension is usually clinically silent and does not require specific treatment.

Embolism with dead worms may occur spontaneously or after adulticide administration. Fatalities result from intractable heart failure, exsanguination, or DIC, or may be unexplained and sudden. Medical management of thromboembolic lung disease is largely symptomatic, and includes cage confinement, aspirin (0.5 mg/kg twice daily to 5 mg/kg once daily), prednisone (1–2 mg/kg/day), and, in some instances, antibiotics, bronchodilators (*e.g.*, aminophylline), and fluid therapy. Although speculative at this time, vasodilators (*e.g.*, hydralazine, captopril, or enalapril) may have some future utility in the therapy of pulmonary embolism associated with HWD.

Right heart failure results from increased right ventricular afterload secondary to pulmonary artery disease and/or thromboembolic complications. Signs are worsened in the face of hypoproteinemia. In a study of 74 dogs with severe pulmonary artery disease, 58% were in heart failure (Calvert and Rawlings, 1988, Additional Reading). The survival rate was similar in dogs with or without heart failure, and was improved in both groups (by 60%) when cage rest and aspirin administration were employed. Digoxin is not recommended because it has not been shown to increase the survival rate and because toxicity and pulmonary vasoconstriction are associated with its use. However, digoxin may be beneficial in the setting of supraventricular tachycardia or refractory heart failure. Abdominal paracentesis or thoracentesis is performed only if marked discomfort is apparent (see Chapter 80 for a description of these techniques). The arterial vasodilator hydralazine has been shown by Lombard (Additional Reading) to improve cardiac output in a small number of dogs with HWD and heart failure. In my laboratory we demonstrated reduction in pulmonary artery pressure and vascular resistance, right ventricular work, and aortic pressure without changing cardiac output or heart rate in dogs with moderate HWD but without heart failure by using this drug. These data suggest that hydralazine may have utility in this setting, but that further studies are necessary to define its role, if any. Likewise, the mixed vasodilators captopril and enalapril may be of use in cases of refractory ascites for its effects on the renin–angiotensin–aldosterone system. Adulticidal therapy is delayed until clinical improvement is noted. Aspirin, through its ability to ameliorate pulmonary vascular lesions; off-loading agents (furosemide, low salt diet); and exercise restriction all reduce afterload or cardiac work, allowing improvement in cardiac function. After clinical improvement (2–4 weeks), adulticidal therapy is administered. Such therapy is generally avoided if heart failure is refractory. Antiarrhythmic therapy is seldom necessary.

Work done by Rawlings and associates (Additional Reading) has demonstrated that aspirin, through its antiprostaglandin-induced reduction in platelet function, has multiple beneficial effects in the dog with HWD. Because platelet adhesiveness and the release of platelet-derived growth factor are diminished, myointimal proliferation is slowed and reversed, even in the presence of persistent infection. As a result, dogs treated with aspirin have improved pulmonary blood flow and reduced arterial dilatation. In addition, aspirin has anti-inflammatory and analgesic effects and has been associated with an improved survival rate in dogs with HWD and heart failure when accompanied by cage rest.

Aspirin is indicated in HWD to improve pulmonary blood flow, reduce inflammation, improve the survival rate in congestive heart failure and severe pulmonary artery disease, treat DIC, and reduce the severity of thromboembolic manifestations. It has been advised that aspirin be reserved for severe HWD because of its propensity to produce gastrointestinal hemorrhage. Aspirin is administered daily (0.5 mg/kg twice daily to 5 mg/kg once daily) beginning 1 to 3 weeks prior to and continuing for 4 to 6 weeks after adulticide administration. With protracted aspirin therapy, packed-cell volume and total serum protein should be monitored periodically. Aspirin is avoided or discontinued in the face of gastrointestinal bleeding (melena or falling packed-cell volume), persistent vomiting, thrombocytopenia (less than 50,000 platelets per mm^3), and hemoptysis.

The anti-inflammatory and immunosuppressive effects inherent to corticosteroids are useful for treatment of some aspects of HWD. Prednisolone, the steroid most often advocated, reduces pulmonary arteritis, but actually worsens the proliferative vascular lesions of HWD, diminishes pulmonary arterial flow, reduces the effectiveness of thiacetarsemide, and may enhance fluid retention in heart failure. For these reasons, it has limited application other than in pulmonary parenchymal disease (*e.g.,* eosinophilic pneumonitis, pulmonary granulomatosis, pulmonary thromboembolism), in which case it has a markedly beneficial effect. In the treatment of eosinophilic pneumonitis, prednisolone is administered until signs resolve (3–5 days) at 1 to 2 mg/kg/day. Prednisolone may be used alone, but is more effective when administered with cyclophosphamide or azathioprine in the treatment of pulmonary granulomatosis. This treatment is continued for an indefinite period or until remission is achieved.

Patient Monitoring

The prognosis for asymptomatic HWI is generally good and, although the prognosis for severe HWD is guarded, a large percentage of such cases can be successfully managed. Once the initial crisis is past and adulticidal therapy has been successful, resolution of underlying manifestations of chronic HWD begins. The prognosis is poorest with severe DIC, CS, massive pulmonary embolism, eosinophilic granulomatosis, severe pulmonary artery disease, and heart failure.

After adulticidal therapy, intimal lesions regress rapidly. Improvement in the main pulmonary artery is noted as early as 4 weeks after treatment, with all pulmonary arteries having undergone marked resolution within 1 year. Radiographic and arteriographic lesions of HWD begin to resolve within 3 to 4 weeks; pulmonary hypertension is reduced within months and may be normal within 6 months of adulticidal therapy. Pulmonary parenchymal changes are often worsened during the 6 months following adulticidal therapy and then begin to lessen in severity, with marked resolution within the following 2 to 3 months. Corticosteroid therapy may be successfully employed to treat clinically significant parenchymal disease. Persistence of such lesions is suggestive of continued infection. Irreversible renal disease is uncommon with glomerular lesions resolving within months of successful adulticidal therapy. Signs of heart failure are also reversible with symptomatic therapy, cage rest, or successful clearing of infection.

HEARTWORM CAVAL SYNDROME

Heartworm CS is a severe variant or complication of HWD, characterized by a high mortality rate. The frequency of occurrence of CS varies with geography and the prevalence of dirofilariasis, as well as the diligence with which prophylactic measures are applied. Two studies in the United States have shown that 16% to 20% of dogs with HWD develop CS. Large, sporting breeds are known to be predisposed to HWD, although this predilection has not been documented for CS.

Pathophysiology

Caval syndrome is associated with heavy infestation of *D. immitis,* usually in young to middle-aged (mean 5, range 1.5–10 years) male dogs, and is most commonly diagnosed in the spring and early summer. Most studies have shown a marked sex predilection, with 75% to 90% of dogs with CS being male. This may be due to a protective factor native to the bitch or a facilitating factor in the male, and not merely to differences in exposure to infection, as is suggested for HWD. Caval syndrome is characterized by a worm burden with total numbers greater than 60, with 55% to 84% residing in the anterior and posterior venae cavae and the right atrium (Fig. 25-7). The exact reason that some heartworm-infected dogs develop this syndrome is unclear. However, a recent study has shown that the development of CS involves more than the severity of the worm burden, or even the number of worms per kg body weight. Dogs that develop CS have greater pulmonary artery pressures than those with chronic HWD and similar worm burdens.

Studies performed in my laboratory indicate that retrograde migration of adult heartworms to the venae cavae and right atrium, from 5 to 17 months after infection, produces partial inflow obstruction to the right heart and, by interfering with the valve apparatus, tricuspid insufficiency (with resultant systolic murmur, jugular pulse, and central venous pressure increase). Affected dogs also exhibit preexistent pulmonary hypertension caused by chronic HWI, which markedly worsens the adverse hemodynamic effects of tricuspid regurgitation. These combined effects substantially reduce left ventricular preload and,

hence, cardiac output. Cardiac arrhythmias may further compromise cardiac function (Fig. 25-8).

This constellation of events precipitates a sudden onset of clinical signs, including hemolytic anemia caused by trauma to red blood cells as they pass through a sieve of heartworms occupying the right atrium and venae cavae, as well as through fibrin strands in capillaries if DIC has developed. The effect of this traumatic insult to the erythron is magnified by increased red blood cell fragility due to alterations in serum-free and esterified cholesterol concentrations and lecithin acyltransferase activity. Hemoglobinemia, hemoglobinuria, and hepatic and renal dysfunction are also observed in many dogs. The cause of hepatorenal dysfunction is not clear, but it probably results from the combined effects of passive congestion, diminished perfusion, and the deleterious effects of the products of hemolysis. Hepatic lesions include hepatomegaly, cavernomatous venous dilatation and thrombosis, and centrolobular necrosis and fibrosis. Tubular necrosis with regeneration, tubular heme casts, and hemosiderosis has been described in the kidneys of affected dogs. Intravascular hemolysis, metabolic acidosis, and diminished hepatic function with impaired removal of circulating procoagulants contribute to the development of DIC. Anorexia, depression, and dyspnea (due to anxiety, anemia, reduced cardiac output, and, in some

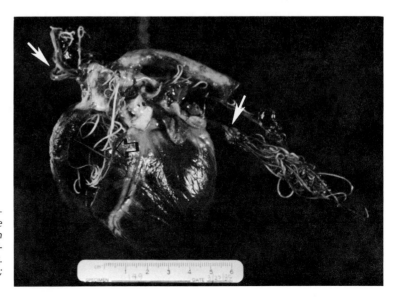

Figure 25–7. *The heart of a dog with caval syndrome. Notice the large number of worms in the venae cavae (white arrows) and the small number in the right ventricle (clear arrow). (Published with permission: Atkins CE. Caval syndrome in the dog. Seminars in Veterinary Medicine and Surgery, 1988; 2:64.)*

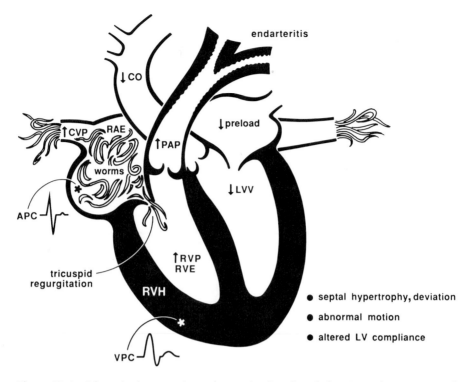

Figure 25–8. *Schematic demonstrating pathogenesis of cardiac dysfunction in heartworm caval syndrome. Caval syndrome complicates chronic heartworm disease when retrograde worm migration from the pulmonary arteries occurs, with the majority of worms relocating in the venae cavae and right atrium. Tricuspid valvular function is altered producing regurgitation; this is superimposed on preexistent pulmonary hypertension. Forward and backward heart failure result from this combination, with a decrease in tissue perfusion due to reduced left ventricular blood volume (preload). Septal deviation and abnormal motion may also contribute to diminished left ventricular preload and hence output. Right ventricular inflow obstruction and cardiac dysrhythmias probably contribute minimally to cardiac dysfunction in most cases. (Published with permission: Atkins CE. American Heartworm Society, Proceedings of the Heartworm Symposium, 1989.)*
CO = cardiac output; PAP = pulmonary artery pressure; CVP = central venous pressure; RAE = right atrial enlargement; APC and VPC = atrial and ventricular premature complexes, respectively; RVH = right ventricular hypertrophy; RVP = right ventricular pressure; RVE = right ventricular enlargement; LVV = left ventricular volume; and arrows = increased or decreased.

cases, pulmonary arterial thrombosis) also are frequently observed in dogs with CS. Without treatment, death usually ensues within 24 to 72 hours due to cardiogenic shock complicated by anemia, metabolic acidosis, and DIC.

Clinical Signs

A sudden onset of anorexia, depression, weakness, and, occasionally, coughing are accompanied in most dogs by dyspnea and hemoglobinuria. The presence of hemoglobinuria has been considered pathognomonic for this syndrome. Physical examination reveals mucous membrane pallor, prolonged capillary refill time, weak pulses, jugular distention and pulsation, hepatosplenomegaly, and dyspnea. Thoracic auscultation may disclose adventitious lung sounds, a systolic heart murmur of tricuspid insufficiency (87% of cases), a loud, split S_2 (67%), and cardiac gallop (20%). Other reported findings include ascites (29%), jaundice (19%), and hemoptysis (6%). Body temperature varies from subnormal to mildly elevated.

Diagnostic Approach

Hemoglobinemia and microfilaremia are present in 85% of dogs suffering from CS. Moderate (mean packed-cell volume 28%, or 0.28 L/L), regenerative anemia, characterized by the presence of reticulocytes, nucleated red blood cells, and increased mean corpuscular volume, is seen in the majority of cases. The normochromic, macrocytic anemia of CS has been associated with the presence of target cells, schistocytes, spur cells, and spherocytes. Leukocytosis (mean white blood cell count approximately 20,000 cells per mm^3, or 20 $\times$ 10^9/L) with neutrophilia, eosinophilia, and left shift has been described. Dogs affected with DIC are characterized by the presence of thrombocytopenia and hypofibrinogenemia, as well as prolonged one-stage prothrombin time, partial thromboplastin time, and activated clotting time, and high fibrin degradation product concentrations.

The serum biochemistry profile reveals increases in aspartate aminotransferase, alkaline phosphatase, alanine aminotransferase, and lactic dehydrogenase activities. A twofold to fourfold increase in blood urea nitrogen, unaccompanied by serum creatinine abnormality, has been described. Total and direct serum bilirubin concentrations are usually moderately high, and BSP retention is prolonged. Mild hyperglycemia (mean value 129 mg/dl, or 7.2 mmol/L), mild hypoalbuminemia, high alpha and gamma globulin concentration, and a low albumin : globulin ratio (mean value approximately 0.5) have also been described in dogs with CS. Urinalysis reveals high bilirubin and protein concentrations in 50% of cases and, more frequently, hemoglobinuria.

Central venous pressure (CVP) is high in 80% to 90% of cases (mean 11.4 cm H$_2$O). Electrocardiographic abnormalities (see Fig. 25-5) include sinus tachycardia in 33% of cases and atrial and ventricular premature complexes in 28% and 6%, respectively. The mean electrical axis tends to rotate rightward (mean + 129°), with an S$_1$, S$_2$, S$_3$ pattern evident in 38% of cases. The S wave depth in V$_5$ (CV6LU) is the most reliable indicator of right ventricular enlargement (greater than 0.8 mV in 56% of cases).

Thoracic radiography reveals signs of severe HWD with cardiomegaly, main pulmonary arterial enlargement, increased pulmonary vascularity, and pulmonary artery tortuosity, recognized in descending order of frequency (see Fig. 25-3). Massive worm inhabitation of the right atrium with movement into the right ventricle during diastole is evident echocardiographically. This finding on M-mode and two-dimensional echocardiograms is nearly pathognomonic for CS in the appropriate clinical setting (Fig. 25-9). The right ventricular lumen is enlarged and the left is diminished in size, suggesting pulmonary hypertension accompanied by reduced left ventricular loading. Paradoxical septal motion, caused by high right ventricular volume and pressure, is commonly observed. There is no echocardiographic evidence of left ventricular dysfunction. Cardiac catheterization documents pulmonary, right atrial, and right ventricular hypertension and reduced cardiac output.

Management

Caval syndrome is complex, characterized by hemolytic anemia, biochemical aberrations, diminished cardiac output and tissue perfusion, hepatic and renal dysfunction, hypoalbuminemia, hemoglobinemia and hemoglobinuria, metabolic acidosis, and the potential for pulmonary embolism and DIC. It follows then, that treatment also is complex, requiring careful monitoring in the more severe cases. Prognosis is poor unless the cause of the crisis—the right atrial and caval heartworms—is removed. Even with this treatment, the mortality rate ranges from 14% to 42%.

It is desirable to establish the degree of involvement of various organ systems. The data base should include thoracic radiographs, packed-cell volume, total serum protein, activated clotting time, alanine aminotransferase activity, blood urea nitrogen concentration, serum alkaline phosphatase activity, complete blood count, urinalysis, and CVP for determining the severity of cardiac dysfunction and monitoring fluid therapy. Ideally, prothrombin time, partial thromboplastin time, fibrin degradation products,

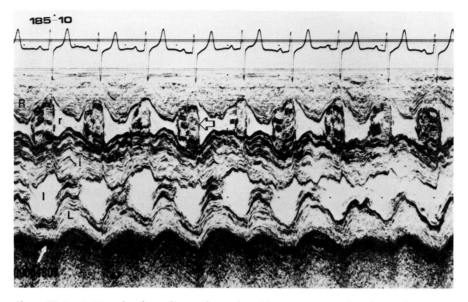

Figure 25–9. *An M-mode echocardiogram from a dog with recent onset caval syndrome, demonstrating thickening of the right ventricular (R) and intraventricular (i) septal walls, right ventricular dilation (r), and a small left ventricle (l). The echogenic mass (clear arrow) in the right ventricle represents heartworms in the atrium and atrioventricular valve area, which "fall" into the ventricle only during diastole. Paradoxical septal motion also is evident. (Published with permission: Atkins CE. Caval syndrome in the dog. Seminars in Veterinary Medicine and Surgery, 1988; 2:64.)*
L = left venticular posterior wall and white arrow designates the pericardium.

platelet count, and arterial (or venous) blood gases (see Chapter 71) should be evaluated as well. Substantial delays in worm embolectomy while awaiting laboratory results are inadvisable, however.

Fluid therapy is needed to improve cardiac output and tissue perfusion, to prevent or help reverse DIC, to prevent hemoglobin nephropathy, and to help correct metabolic acidosis. Overexuberant fluid therapy, however, may worsen or precipitate signs of congestive heart failure. In my clinic, a left jugular catheter is placed and intravenous fluid therapy is instituted with 5% dextrose in water. The catheter should not enter the anterior vena cava because it will interfere with worm embolectomy. A cephalic catheter may be substituted for the somewhat inconvenient jugular catheter, but this does not allow monitoring of CVP (see Central Venous Pressure in Chapter 80). The intravenous infusion rate for fluids is dependent on the animal's condition. A useful guideline is to infuse as rapidly as possible without raising the CVP or without raising it

above 10 cm H_2O, if it was normal or near normal at the outset. Initial therapy should be aggressive (40–80 ml/kg/hour for the first hour) if shock is accompanied by a normal CVP (less than 5 cm H_2O), and should be curtailed to approximately 1 to 2 ml/kg/hour if CVP is 10 to 20 cm of water. Whole blood transfusion is not indicated in most cases because anemia usually is not severe, and transfused coagulation factors may worsen DIC. Sodium bicarbonate is not indicated unless metabolic acidosis is severe (pH 7.15–7.2). Broad-spectrum antibiotics and aspirin (0.5 mg/kg twice daily to 5 mg/kg once daily) should be administered. Because cardiac contractility is not impaired, digitalis is not indicated. Except in rare instances when cardiac arrhythmias contribute significantly to the hemodynamic compromise or appear to be life-threatening, specific antiarrhythmic therapy is unnecessary.

Treatment for heartworm-associated DIC has been described by Calvert and Rawlings (1988, Additional Reading). Cage rest and supportive care are adequate in most cases. The platelet count should be monitored closely, and if platelets fall below 50,000 per mm³, aspirin should be discontinued and vincristine administered. Heparin may be administered subcutaneously (200 units/kg three times daily) for chronic or low-grade DIC; these authors recommend 500 units/kg three times daily for acute or end-stage DIC. The mortality rate for acute or end-stage DIC is very high.

The technique for surgical removal of caval and atrial heartworms was developed by Jackson and associates (Additional Reading). This procedure should be undertaken as early in the course of therapy as is practical. Often, sedation is unnecessary and the procedure can be accomplished with only local anesthesia. The dog is restrained in left lateral recumbency after surgical clipping and preparation of the cervical region. The jugular vein is surgically isolated distally. A ligature is placed loosely around the cranial aspect of the vein until it is incised, after which the ligature is tied. Twenty- to 40-cm alligator forceps, preferably of small diameter, are held loosely between the thumb and forefinger and guided gently down the vein. The jugular vein can be temporarily occluded with umbilical tape. If difficulty is encountered in passage of the forceps, gentle manipulation of the dog by assistants to further extend the neck will assist in passage of the forceps past the thoracic inlet, while medial direction of the forceps may be necessary at the base of the heart. Once the forceps have been placed, the jaws are opened, the forceps are advanced slightly, the jaws are closed, and the worms are removed. One to four worms usually are removed with each pass. This process is repeated until 5 to 6 successive attempts are unsuccessful. An effort should be made to remove 35 to 50 worms.

Ishihara and associates (Additional Reading) have recently described successful worm retrieval in CS using flexible alligator forceps. Following worm removal, the jugular vein is ligated proximally and subcutaneous and skin sutures are placed routinely.

After worm removal, a decline (40%) in CVP is expected. This is associated with a reduction in the intensity of the cardiac murmur and jugular pulsations, rapid clearing of hemoglobinemia and hemoglobinuria, and normalization of serum enzymatic aberrations. There is immediate and gradual improvement in cardiac function over the following 24 hours. Pretreatment clinical findings of hypothermia, ascites, and CVP greater than 20 cm H₂O carry a poor prognosis. It is important to realize that removal of worms does nothing to reduce right ventricular afterload (pulmonary vascular resistance), and, hence, fluid therapy must be monitored carefully before and after surgery to avoid precipitation of right heart failure. Cage rest should be enforced for a period of time suitable for each individual case.

Patient Monitoring

As stated above, the prognosis for CS is guarded to poor, degenerating to grave when complicated by severe DIC. Worm embolectomy through a jugular venotomy is frequently successful in stabilizing the animal, allowing adulticidal therapy to be instituted in 2 weeks to destroy the remaining heartworms. Careful scrutiny of blood urea nitrogen concentration and serum liver enzyme activities should precede the latter treatment. Aspirin therapy is continued for 3 to 4 weeks after adulticidal therapy. Substantial improvement in anemia should not be expected before 2 to 4 weeks after worm embolectomy. Microfilaricides are administered, as needed, 6 weeks after completion of adulticidal therapy.

FELINE HEARTWORM DISEASE

The parasite *D. immitis* naturally affects members of the family Canidae, but may infect other mammals as well. The domestic cat, an atypical host, can be parasitized by *D. immitis* and develop HWD. The clinical manifestations of the disease are different in this species, and the cat is afflicted approximately 20% as frequently as the dog. However, the incidence or awareness of feline HWD appear to be increasing. Similar to dogs, the male cat is at higher risk for HWI than is the female.

Pathophysiology

Experimental infection of the cat is more difficult than that of the dog, with less than 25% of L_3 reaching adulthood. This resistance is also reflected in natural infections, in which feline heartworm burdens are usually less than 10 (typically only 2–4 worms). Other indications of the cat's inherent resistance to this parasite are a shortened period of worm patency, common amicrofilaremia or low L_1 counts, and shortened L_5 life span (less than 2 years). Aberrant worm migration appears to be a greater problem in cats than in dogs.

The pulmonary arterial response to L_5 is similar to, but more severe than, that of the dog. Dillon (Additional Reading) demonstrated pulmonary enlargement within 1 week of transplantation of adults, suggesting an intense host–parasite interaction. This severe myointimal response produces pulmonary hypertension. Because the feline pulmonary artery tree is smaller than that of the dog and has less collateral circulation, embolism, even with small numbers of worms, produces disastrous results, with infarction and often death. Although uncommon, cor pulmonale and right heart failure can be associated with chronic feline HWD; these are manifested by ascites and pleural effusion (hydrothorax or chylothorax).

Clinical Signs

Even cats with severe HWD may be asymptomatic. When present, clinical manifestations are either acute or chronic (Table 25-5). Acute or peracute presentation is usually due to worm embolism, and clinical signs variably include salivation, tachycardia, shock, dyspnea, hemoptysis, vomiting and diarrhea, syncope, dementia, ataxia, circling, head tilt, blindness, seizures, and death. Postmortem examination reveals pulmonary infarction with congestion and edema. More commonly, the onset of signs is less acute (chronic form). Historical findings in chronic feline HWD include anorexia, weight loss, lethargy, exercise intolerance, signs of right heart failure, cough,

Table 25–5 *Signs Referable to Heartworm Disease in Cats*

ACUTE AND PERACUTE	CHRONIC
Dyspnea	Cough
Syncope or collapse	Dyspnea
Hemoptysis	Exercise intolerance
Tachycardia	Lethargy
Shock	Anorexia
Vomiting or diarrhea	Weight loss
Ptyalism	Vomiting
Blindness	Right heart failure
Convulsions	Death
Other neurologic dysfunction	
Sudden death	

dyspnea, and vomiting. Physical examination in these cases is often unrewarding, although a murmur, gallop, dyspnea, or diminished or adventitious lung sounds may be audible. If heart failure is present, jugular venous distention and ascites are detected.

Diagnostic Approach

Historical and physical findings are vague and nonspecific, so a high index of suspicion is necessary. Coughing cats should be suspected of having HWD; suspicion should increase if cough is accompanied by a murmur or gallop, eosinophilia, dyspnea, or vomiting.

Dillon (Additional Reading) reports that one third of all heartworm-infected cats have a nonregenerative anemia. In addition, nucleated red blood cells, leukocytosis, eosinophilia, and basophilia may be observed. Eosinophilia tends to be inconsistent (present in one third of cases) and transitory. The serum biochemistry profile and urinalysis are typically unrewarding, with hyperglobulinemia, prerenal azotemia, and proteinuria reported as inconsistent findings. More than 80% of heartworm-infected cats are amicrofilaremic. The immunofluorescent antibody test for antimicrofilarial antibodies is positive in less than one half of cases; the antigen ELISA test appears to be more sensitive. In either instance, false-negative results occur.

Because the differential diagnoses for cough in

the cat with eosinophilia include feline bronchial asthma and parasitic pneumonitis, lower respiratory cytologic evaluation, using tracheobronchial washing, is frequently performed in these cats. Cats with HWD demonstrate findings similar to those of bronchial asthma and parasitic respiratory infections (inconsistent eosinophilic inflammation), but differ from the latter in that parasite eggs or larvae are not found unless the diseases coexist.

Electrocardiographic parameters are normal in most cats with HWD, although a right ventricular enlargement pattern may be noted in some cases. Echocardiographic evaluation might demonstrate a prominent right ventricle and pulmonary outflow tract, and adult heartworms could potentially be imaged in either of these locations. Technical difficulties in the cat and the likelihood of small worm burdens limit the usefulness of this modality in the diagnosis of feline HWD.

Thoracic radiography provides the best screening test for feline HWD; however, radiographic findings differ from those of the dog with HWD. In addition, findings are subtle, making careful examination of both projections imperative. Dillon (Additional Reading) reports that right ventricular and pulmonary artery segment enlargement are not classic features of feline HWD, as they are in the canine counterpart. However, enlarged pulmonary arteries with ill-defined margins may be seen in the caudal lobes (Fig. 25-10). Nonselective angiocardiography (see Chapter 80) has been shown to be useful for demonstrating worms, as well as embolized, enlarged, tortuous, and blunted pulmonary arteries (Fig. 25-11). Pulmonary parenchymal changes typically involve the caudal lung lobes and include focal or, less commonly, diffuse interstitial infiltrates, perivascular density, and atelectasis. If heart failure is present (rare), ascites and hydrothorax may be demonstrable.

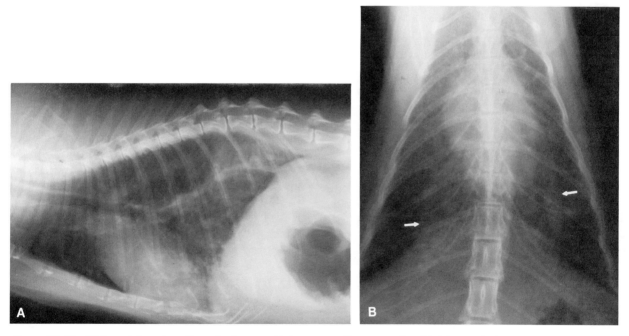

Figure 25–10. (A) Lateral thoracic radiograph of a cat with heartworm disease reveals mild right ventricular enlargement and pulmonary infiltrate, particularly severe in the caudal lobes. Evidence of aerophagia is compatible with dyspnea. (B) Ventrodorsal radiograph from a different cat demonstrating mild right ventricular enlargement and enlarged, blunted caudal pulmonary arteries (arrows), partially obscured by pulmonary infiltrate. (Photographs courtesy of Dr. Kathy Spaulding, North Carolina State University.)

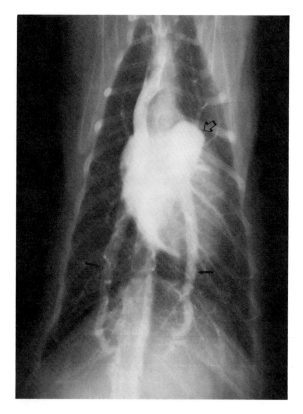

Figure 25–11. *Nonselective angiocardiogram obtained from cat with heartworm disease. Note the enlarged main pulmonary artery (open arrow) and the enlarged, tortuous, and blunted caudal pulmonary arteries (arrows.) Careful scrutiny reveals linear radiolucencies in the right caudal pulmonary artery. (Photograph courtesy of Dr. Kathy Spaulding, North Carolina State University.)*

Management

Although it has not been scientifically evaluated, thiacetarsemide sodium (2.2 mg/kg IV twice daily for 2 days) is considered to be effective for treatment of feline HWD. Adulticidal therapy is, however, of greater risk to cats than to dogs. Thromboembolic complications predominate, occurring 1 to 2 weeks after therapy. Affected cats may exhibit dyspnea and hemoptysis or may die acutely. High-dose intravenous corticosteroid therapy, intravenous fluids, oxygen, and bronchodilators have all been advocated for the treatment of thromboembolic complications. Less frequently, treated cats develop signs of vomiting and diarrhea, necessitating interruption of arsenical treatment, with reinstitution in 2 to 4 weeks. An idiosyncratic reaction to thiacetarsemide,

manifested by fulminant pulmonary edema and death, has also been reported. Other complications, such as skin sloughs, are similar to those described for the dog. Because of the frequency and severity of feline reactions to thiacetarsemide and because of the relatively short L_5 life span, adulticidal therapy is not advocated for asymptomatic cats with HWI.

Since most cats are amicrofilaremic, microfilaricidal drugs are infrequently necessary; dithiazanine (6–10 mg/kg orally for 7 days) and levamisole (10 mg/kg orally for 7 days) have been used successfully, however. Preventive medications are likewise not currently advocated for use in the cat. Treatment of pulmonary parenchymal disease and heart failure is similar to that in the dog. Eosinophilic pneumonitis is treated for 3 to 5 days with corticosteroids (prednisolone 2–4 mg/kg orally three times daily) and then discontinued when adulticidal therapy is administered. After this, prednisolone can be reinstituted if needed.

Patient Monitoring

Because of the peracute nature and high mortality associated with feline thromboembolic complications, it is advised that cats be hospitalized for 2 weeks following adulticidal therapy for observation and confinement. Signs of HWD are reversible and gradually subside after therapy. In particular, allergic pneumonitis responds quickly and dramatically to corticosteroid therapy. If treated successfully, the clinical and radiographic signs of pulmonary embolization resolve rapidly (1–2 days). Cats surviving the initial period of acute and peracute manifestations of HWD generally do well.

ADDITIONAL READING

Atkins CE. Caval syndrome in the dog. Seminars in Veterinary Medicine and Surgery 1987; 2:64.
Atkins CE, Keene BW, McGuirk SM. Investigation of caval syndrome in dogs experimentally infected with *Dirofilaria immitis*. Journal of the American College of Veterinary Internal Medicine 1988; 2:36.
Atkins CE, Keene BW, McGuirk SM. Pathophysiology of cardiac dysfunction in an experimental model of

heartworm caval syndrome in the dog: An echocardiographic study. Am J Vet Res 1988; 49:403.

Badertscher RR, Losonsky JM, Allan JP, Kneller SK. Two-dimensional echocardiography for diagnosis of dirofilariasis in nine dogs. J Am Vet Med Assoc 1988; 193:843.

Calvert CA. Feline heartworm disease. In: Fox PR, ed. Canine and feline cardiology. New York: Churchill Livingstone, 1988: 551.

Calvert CA, Rawlings CA. Canine heartworm disease. In: Fox PR, ed. Canine and feline cardiology. New York: Churchill Livingstone, 1988: 519.

Calvert CA, Rawlings CA. Therapy of canine heartworm disease. In: Kirk RW, ed. Current veterinary therapy IX. Philadelphia: WB Saunders, 1986: 406.

Dillon R. Feline heartworm disease. In: Kirk RW, ed. Current veterinary therapy IX. Philadelphia: WB Saunders, 1986: 420.

Grieve RB. Advances in the immunologic diagnosis of dirofilaria immitis infection. Seminars in Veterinary Medicine and Surgery 1987; 2:4.

Hoskins JD, Hagstad HV, Hribernik TN. Effect of thiacetarsemide sodium in Louisiana dogs with natural occurring canine heartworm disease. In: Otto GF, ed. Proceedings of the heartworm symposium '83. Bonner Springs, Kansas: Veterinary Medical Publishing Co, 1983: 134.

Ishihara K, Kitagwa H, Sisaki Y. Efficacy of heartworm removal in dogs with dirofilarial hemoglobinuria using flexible alligator forceps. Japanese Journal of Veterinary Science 1988; 50:739.

Ishihara K, Sisaki Y, Kitagwa H. Development of a flexible alligator forceps: A new instrument for removal of heartworms in the pulmonary arteries of dogs. Japanese Journal of Veterinary Science 1986; 48:989.

Jackson RF, Seymour WG, Growney PJ, Otto GF. Surgical treatment of the caval syndrome of canine heartworm disease. J Am Vet Med Assoc 1977; 171:1065.

Knight DH. Pathophysiology of dirofilariasis. Proceedings of the American College of Veterinary Internal Medicine 1979; 41.

Leib MS, Allen TA, Husted PW. Acute renal failure associated with thiacetarsemide sodium treatment for adult heartworms in a dog. Journal of the American Animal Hospital Association 1984; 20:973.

Lombard CW. Pulmonary vasodilation in heartworm dogs with cor pulmonale. Proceedings of the heartworm symposium '86. Bonner Springs, Kansas: Veterinary Medical Publishing Co, 1986: 110.

Lombard CW, Ackerman N. Right heart enlargement in heartworm infected dogs. A radiographic, electrocardiographic, and echocardiographic correlation. Veterinary Radiology 1984; 25:210.

Lombard CW, Buergelt CD. Echocardiographic and clinical findings in dogs with heartworm-induced cor pulmonale. Compendium of Continuing Education 1983; 5:971.

Lord PF, Schaer M, Tilley L. Pulmonary infiltrates with eosinophilia in the dog. Journal of the American Veterinary Radiology Society 1975; 16:4.

Losonsky JM, Thrall DE, Lewis RE. Thoracic radiographic abnormalities in 200 dogs with spontaneous heartworm infestation. Veterinary Radiology 1983; 24:120.

Ogburn PN, Jackson RF, Seymour G et al. Electrocardiographic and phonocardiographic alterations in canine heartworm disease. In: Otto GF, ed. Proceedings of the heartworm symposium '77. Bonner Springs, Kansas: Veterinary Medical Publishing Co, 1977: 67.

Rackear D, Feldman B, Farver T et al. The effect of three different dosages of acetylsalicylic acid on canine platelet aggregation. Journal of the American Animal Hospital Association 1988; 24:23.

Rawlings CA. Heartworm disease in dogs and cats. Philadelphia: WB Saunders, 1986.

Slocombe JOD, McMillan I. Heartworm in dogs in Canada in 1988. Canadian Veterinary Journal 1989; 30:504.

Takehashi N, Matsui A, Sasai H et al. Feline caval syndrome: A case report. Journal of the American Animal Hospital Association 1988; 24:645.

Thrall DE, Calvert CA. Radiographic evaluation of canine heartworm disease coexisting with right heart failure. Veterinary Radiology 1983; 24:124.

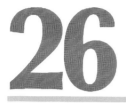

26

ANESTHESIA FOR THE CARDIAC PATIENT

Diane E. Mason, Clarke E. Atkins

This chapter is meant to serve as a guide to veterinarians faced with anesthetizing a small animal patient that has heart disease. It will discuss the approach to the patient and what must be known about the patient to choose appropriately from among many different anesthetic drugs (see Appendices I and II).

"Generic" heart disease does not exist. Anatomic, organic, and metabolic abnormalities can compromise the heart's function by varying pathophysiologic mechanisms. Anesthetic protocols used in small animals can be as diverse as the cardiac diseases themselves; therefore, there is not just one safe formula for anesthesia. Heart disease can vary from the animal with asymptomatic, subclinical disease noted as an incidental finding on the physical examination to the severely compromised animal in heart failure. Many animals that are asymptomatic are in a well-compensated stage of disease, and almost any anesthetic protocol can be administered safely. For the animal in heart failure, no matter what the underlying disease mechanism, anesthesia of any type carries great risk, and therapeutic stabilization to minimize the signs of failure is an absolute necessity before any anesthetic drugs are given. Outlined in this chapter is basic information needed for anesthetizing patients with heart disease. Cardiac disorders commonly encountered in veterinary medicine are grouped according to pathophysiologic mechanism, and anesthetic recommendations for these groups are given.

PREANESTHETIC CONSIDERATIONS

The safest approach to anesthesia in the animal with heart disease is to first make a diagnosis. Anesthesia of an animal with a murmur carries much greater uncertainty if the nature of the cardiac problem is unknown. On the other hand, if the cause of the murmur is diagnosed and the pathophysiology of this condition as well as its degree of progression and compensation is recognized, it is easier to make a decision about what anesthetic drugs to choose or avoid. It is also easier to anticipate problems the dog or cat may encounter when anesthetized. This anticipation allows the veterinarian to monitor for signs of trouble and to intervene when necessary.

History and Physical Examination

The starting point in approaching the patient is an adequate history. Is the owner aware of the presence of cardiac disease in the animal? When

365

was this problem originally diagnosed? How has the disease progressed since that time? Is the animal currently on medication for this condition? How has the animal responded to medication? Does the animal have exercise intolerance, cough, syncopal episodes, or dyspnea? A complete history gives a good indication as to the degree of compromise and relative risk for anesthesia. The risk of a planned procedure and related anesthesia should be carefully explained to the owner so that an informed decision can be made.

Physical examination and recognition of general clinical problems are addressed in detail elsewhere in this book. Two points need to be emphasized when evaluating the patient with suspected heart disease. First, the animal should be examined carefully for signs typically associated with cardiovascular dysfunction, including pallor and cyanosis (see Chapter 2), poor peripheral pulses, weakness (see Chapter 5), edema (see Chapter 10), ascites (see Chapter 11), and cough (see Chapter 13). Second, the importance of auscultation cannot be overemphasized. The stethoscope is the instrument with which most cardiovascular disease in small animal patients is first recognized. Murmurs (see Chapter 17), arrhythmias (see Chapter 18), lung sounds consistent with pulmonary edema (see Chapter 31), and

muffled heart sounds (see Chapter 17) are all significant findings in the physical examination that might go undetected without the use of a stethoscope.

Minimum Data Base

The minimum data base necessary to diagnose and assess cardiac disease in the small animal is listed in Table 26-1. This list represents only the minimum data necessary to adequately evaluate the patient's cardiovascular status. More detailed descriptions of diagnostic approaches are provided in Chapters 17 through 25 and in Chapter 80.

Hematocrit and total serum protein should be determined prior to anesthetizing any patient. These parameters are simple to obtain and relatively easy to interpret, and provide useful information. Hematocrit and total serum protein together can indicate the patient's level of hydration and the status of the erythron. Any animal undergoing anesthesia should be adequately, but not overly, hydrated. Adequate hydration helps the animal maintain an effective circulating blood volume in the face of diminished cardiac output and loss of vascular tone, which often accompany anesthesia. Adequate hydration is espe-

Table 26-1 *Minimum Data Base for the Small Animal Cardiac Patient Presented for Anesthesia*

Laboratory Test	Clinical Signficance
Hematocrit	Hydration status, anemia, oxygen-carrying capacity, blood viscosity
Total serum protein	Hydration status, risk for pulmonary edema
Serum electrolytes	Predisposition for arrhythmias
Serum urea nitrogen	Prerenal or primary renal azotemia
Thoracic radiography	Cardiac size and contour, evaluation of thoracic structures, response to therapy (e.g., pulmonary edema)
Electocardiography	Recognition and diagnosis of arrhythmias, response to therapy (e.g., antiarrhythmics), cardiac chamber enlargement
Hepatic enzymes	Liver disease and associated complications, altered drug metabolism
Urinalysis	Renal-concentrating ability, differentiation of primary from prerenal azotemia, evidence of tubular pathology
Microfilaria test	Heartworm disease and associated pulmonary, vascular, and renal complications

cially important in the individual with heart disease. These animals often have limited cardiovascular reserve and have difficulty compensating for the hemodynamic changes caused by anesthetic drugs.

The ultimate purpose of the cardiopulmonary system is to provide oxygen and nutrients to the tissues, while removing the by-products of metabolism. Tissue oxygenation results when the oxygen, carried by hemoglobin in the blood, is delivered to the tissues. Anemia can adversely affect tissue oxygenation because low hemoglobin concentration lessens the blood's ability to carry oxygen. This is particularly detrimental in a patient with heart failure because the blood's oxygen content is diminished in an animal that has impaired ability for delivery of blood to the tissues. For the patient about to undergo anesthesia, an excessively low hematocrit (less than 20%, or 0.20 L/L) is undesirable, and correction of this condition by blood transfusion should be considered prior to anesthesia (see Chapter 16).

If the oxygen-carrying capacity of the blood were the only important issue, one might assume that polycythemia (increased hematocrit) would be a beneficial state in the cardiac patient about to undergo anesthesia. Polycythemia increases oxygen-carrying capacity because the blood contains more hemoglobin. Unfortunately, polycythemia usually results from a long-standing inability of the animal to oxygenate its tissues. In cardiac patients, this is often indicative of right-to-left shunt lesions (*e.g.*, reversed patent ductus arteriosus), in which the body has attempted to compensate for this tissue hypoxia by increasing red blood cell numbers. The increased number of red blood cells causes an increase in blood viscosity, sludging of blood in peripheral capillary beds, and poor delivery of oxygen to the tissues. For the patient about to undergo anesthesia, an excessively high hematocrit (greater than 55%, or 0.55 L/L) is undesirable, and correction through fluid therapy prior to anesthesia should be considered. Occasionally, phlebotomy in conjunction with fluid therapy may be necessary if the hematocrit is greater than 65% (or 0.65 L/L) in an animal with no signs of dehydration (see Chapter 74).

Hypoproteinemia can be a special problem in the small animal with heart disease. In a normal animal several mechanisms safeguard the lung against the development of pulmonary edema (see Chapter 31). These include a large capacity to increase lymphatic flow, negative interstitial hydrostatic pressure, and the tendency for plasma protein to stay within the capillaries while interstitial proteins undergo washout through the lymphatics as fluid filters across the capillary endothelium. Although hypoproteinemia (total protein less than 4 g/dl [40 g/L] or albumin less than 2 g/dl [20 g/L]) in the dog with normal cardiovascular function rarely results in pulmonary edema, a hypoproteinemic state can potentiate the formation of edema in the dog with heart disease. Animals with left heart disease often have elevated left atrial pressure, which may lead to increased capillary hydrostatic pressure in the pulmonary circulation. Chronic increase in left atrial pressure and in fluid filtration across the capillary endothelium often means that lymphatic capacity has increased to its maximum extent. Therefore, the buffering capacity normally offered by the lymphatics has already been utilized. The animal is now highly dependent on its colloid oncotic pressure (mainly plasma albumin concentration) to oppose further fluid filtration across the capillary endothelium. Hypoproteinemia, therefore, can potentiate pulmonary edema in these patients. For the patient with cardiac disease it is important to know the concentration of plasma protein before anesthesia, and to monitor changes in plasma proteins in response to fluid therapy during and after a procedure. Prior to anesthesia, plasma transfusion (10–20 ml/kg IV) or colloid-containing fluids may be considered to counteract hypoproteinemia, and during or after anesthesia excessive administration of intravenous fluids should be avoided.

Before making an anesthetic plan, the patient should be examined for evidence of renal dysfunction. An elevated serum urea nitrogen with normal urinalysis may indicate compromised peripheral perfusion in the animal with heart disease (prerenal azotemia). If there is evidence of prerenal azotemia, cautious intravenous fluid therapy is used to reestablish adequate circulating blood volume and renal perfusion prior to anesthesia. If fluid therapy alone results in no improvement, or if the animal is in congestive heart failure, measures should be taken to improve cardiac function before administering any anesthetic drugs (see Chapter 20). If the patient has evidence for primary renal disease (*e.g.*, polyuria, polydipsia, dilute urine, elevated serum urea nitrogen and creatinine) in addition to its cardiovascular condition, this should be considered when choosing specific drugs for anesthesia. Drugs whose effect is terminated by renal elimination are likely to have a prolonged effect in these patients (*e.g.*, ketamine in the cat). More importantly, patients with renal disease can suffer acute exacerbation of their condition if improperly managed during anesthesia. Renal perfusion is highly dependent on adequate mean arterial blood pressure (greater than 60 mmHg); therefore, hypotension should be avoided. To ensure adequate renal perfusion throughout the anesthetic period, choose less hypotensive anesthetic drugs (see Tables 26-4 and 26-5), administer judicious intravenous fluid therapy, and consider dopamine hydrochloride infusion and diuretics such as furosemide and mannitol if hydration status is normal. It is essential to monitor cardiovascular parameters in these patients. Fluid overload can easily occur with aggressive intravenous fluid therapy and osmotic diuretics. An animal with subclinical heart disease could become decompensated when anesthesia and fluid overload combine to diminish cardiac function and exacerbate congestive signs.

Because heart disease often affects geriatric patients, it is prudent to evaluate serum electrolyte concentrations and identify hepatic disease if present. Serum sodium and potassium abnormalities are not common unless patients are anorexic, have concurrent disease, or are being intensively diuresed (see Chapter 72). Potassium concentrations are of particular concern because both hyperkalemia and hypokalemia predispose to arrhythmias, which may complicate the anesthetic or postoperative period. Liver disease may or may not be related to passive hepatic congestion, and should be identified so that anesthetic agents metabolized by the liver may be avoided (see Chapter 40). Elevations of serum alkaline phosphatase and alanine aminotransferase activities suggest liver disease, and liver dysfunction is

indicated by increased serum bile acids, bromsulphalein (BSP) retention, hypoglycemia, low blood urea nitrogen, and hypoproteinemia. Modest elevations in serum alkaline phosphatase and alanine aminotransferase activities are common in elderly dogs without substantial hepatic disease, and these enzymes, as well as BSP retention, are further elevated in the presence of cardiac failure.

Arterial or venous blood gases provide information on the metabolic and ventilatory status of the animal with cardiac disease and give additional evidence of the compromise caused by that patient's heart disease. Heart disease associated with low cardiac output often results in metabolic acidosis (base deficit greater than -4) due to diminished tissue perfusion, and measures should be taken (*e.g.*, fluid therapy, positive inotropes) to improve cardiac output in these patients prior to anesthesia. Hypoxemia (Pao_2 less than 65 mmHg) with or without hypercarbia ($Paco_2$ greater than 50 mmHg) can be present with congestive heart failure due to pulmonary edema. Medical therapy to diminish congestive signs (*e.g.*, diuretics, vasodilators, inotropes) is indicated prior to anesthesia, and special attention to adequate ventilation and oxygenation during the anesthetic period is recommended.

Animals with suspected disease of the cardiovascular system should be tested for heartworm infection prior to anesthesia. Heartworm disease can cause changes in the pulmonary vasculature, leading to right heart dysfunction, thromboembolic disease, and renal disease, as well as other complications (see Chapter 25). Any of these may affect that animal's ability to tolerate anesthesia.

One cannot fully assess an animal's cardiac disease without high-quality chest radiographs. Chest radiographs (see Thoracic Radiography in Chapter 80) are necessary to evaluate the heart size and changes in its contours, and may provide a diagnosis of the animal's disease. In addition, thoracic radiography allows one to evaluate the pleural cavity, esophagus, pulmonary parenchyma, and pulmonary vasculature and airways. Pulmonary edema is manifested as increased interstitial density, often in the hilar region of the lungs, while biventricular or right heart failure produces pleural effusion. These conditions should be treated prior to anesthesia to optimize ventilation and pulmonary gas exchange. Any animal who has experienced trauma should be examined for pneumothorax, fractured ribs, and pleural fluid. Removing pleural fluid or air can significantly improve an animal's tolerance of anesthesia. High peak inspiratory pressures (greater than 30 cm H_2O) should be avoided when assisting an anesthetized patient that has rib fractures or pulmonary contusions with positive pressure ventilation. Megaesophagus may be present in young animals (see Chapter 35). If present, precautions should be taken to prevent aspiration by using a rapid induction technique and immediate intubation with a cuffed endotracheal tube to protect the airway. In addition to thoracic radiography, cardiac disease is often better diagnosed or evaluated with the aid of special techniques such as angiocardiography or echocardiography (see Nonselective Angiocardiography and Echocardiography in Chapter 80) when available.

Electrocardiography has a place in the preanesthetic data base for several reasons. An electrocardiogram is necessary to diagnose arrhythmias common with certain cardiac disorders (see Chapters 18 and 80). Atrial fibrillation in large-breed dogs with dilated cardiomyopathy, ventricular arrhythmias following trauma, and sinus tachycardia in hyperthyroid cats are examples of rhythm disturbances that should be controlled prior to anesthesia to lessen risk. An electrocardiogram can be the sentinel for detrimental electrolyte imbalances such as hyperkalemia that are even more dangerous when anesthetic drugs are administered (see Chapter 72).

ANESTHETIC PLANNING BASED ON PATHOPHYSIOLOGY

The heart diseases most commonly encountered by the practicing veterinarian can be grouped into five categories based on pathophysiologic mechanism (Table 26-2). Each of these mechanisms interferes with the function of the heart in some manner. The goal in anesthetizing an animal with heart disease is to avoid exacerbating the underlying condition and, whenever possible,

Table 26–2 *Cardiac Disorders Classified According to Pathophysiology*

VOLUME OVERLOAD

Mitral regurgitation
Patent ductus arteriosus
Ventricular septal defect
Atrial septal defect

PRESSURE OVERLOAD

Pulmonic stenosis
Aortic stenosis
Canine heartworm disease

MYOCARDIAL DYSFUNCTION

Cardiomyopathy of giant-breed dogs
Boxer cardiomyopathy
Cardiomyopathy of Doberman pinschers
Feline dilated cardiomyopathy

IMPAIRED CARDIAC FILLING

Cardiac tamponade
Constrictive pericarditis
Pericardial diaphragmatic hernia
Hypertrophic cardiomyopathy

SERIOUS RHYTHM DISTURBANCES

Traumatic myocarditis
Gastric dilatation–volvulus
Feline hyperthyroidism

to help maintain the beneficial compensatory responses. Suggestions for specific conditions are outlined below.

Disorders Characterized by Volume Overload

Mitral Regurgitation

Every small animal veterinarian encounters older dogs with mitral regurgitation (MR) (see Chapter 20). This acquired valvular defect results in volume overload to the left heart. In patients with MR there is a decrease in effective forward flow into the systemic circulation because a portion of the left ventricular stroke volume regurgitates into the left atrium. Since left ventricular ejection can follow two pathways (the regurgitant and the aortic pathways), the fraction of blood that goes each way depends on the impedance that each path offers. Aortic impedance is related to the systemic vascular resistance (SVR); drugs that alter arterial impedance (arterial vasodilators) can have profound effects on forward and regurgitant flow.

In patients with MR the aim is to decrease the regurgitant fraction with drugs that reduce afterload but at the same time preserve contractility and avoid arrhythmias, so that pulmonary congestion is not exacerbated.

Xylazine is absolutely contraindicated in the dog with MR. It increases afterload, causes profound bradycardia, and diminishes contractility. Acepromazine, a potent α-adrenergic blocking drug, can reduce afterload in the patient with MR, and can be used safely for tranquilization in many of these dogs. A dose of 0.05 to 0.1 mg/kg should not be exceeded. Narcotics are safe as premedicants for MR, although they enhance vagal tone and the resulting bradycardia can aggravate the congestive signs of MR by reducing cardiac output. Anticholinergic drugs such as atropine can help prevent the vagal-induced bradycardia seen after narcotic administration. Adequate sedation prior to anesthesia minimizes the stress on the dog and allows for a reduced dose of induction agent for endotracheal intubation. Inhalant anesthetics decrease SVR, which can be helpful, but also decrease contractility and thereby stroke volume. Isoflurane is a better inhalant anesthetic than halothane in this case because it produces a greater decrease in SVR without the marked decrease in contractility that accompanies halothane at equipotent doses.

Medical therapy of chronic MR decreases volume load on the heart through diuretics, vasodilators, and a low sodium diet (see Chapter 20). When choosing intravenous fluids for use during anesthesia in the MR case, 0.9% sodium chloride should be avoided because it contains a relatively high sodium concentration (154 mEq/L). Alternatives include lactated Ringers solution (130 mEq/L sodium), 0.45% sodium chloride with 2.5% dextrose (77 mEq/L sodium) or 5% dextrose in water (0 mEq/L sodium). Large fluid loads (greater than 10 ml/kg/hour) should be avoided in animals with MR, and only the minimal amount of fluid necessary to maintain mean blood pressure (greater than 60 mmHg) and renal perfusion, while not increasing central venous pressure (see Chapter 80) or producing pulmonary edema should be used.

Congenital Left-to-Right Shunts

Both patent ductus arteriosus (PDA) and ventricular septal defect (VSD) represent congenital lesions characterized by pulmonary overcirculation that, with time, can lead to congestive heart failure from volume overload to the left (PDA, VSD) or right (rarely VSD) ventricle (see Chapter 19). These disorders are characteristically left-to-right shunts. A portion of the left ventricular output is shunted to the pulmonary artery (PDA) or right ventricle (VSD), resulting in pulmonary overcirculation and excessive venous return to the left heart. It is important to realize that the direction of flow through a shunt is not fixed, and can change with alterations in hemodynamic conditions. The amount of shunted blood is dependent on the size of the defect and the pressure difference between the two sides. We assume that anesthetic agents do not significantly alter the size of the congenital defect; however, the pressure difference between the two sides can be changed by anesthetic practices.

Many young animals with VSD or PDA are good candidates for anesthesia if congestive signs from their disease are mild. If the animal has signs of heart failure, medical therapy to control these signs is recommended prior to anesthesia (see Chapter 19). Many animals show radiographic evidence of pulmonary congestion and early pulmonary edema. These animals often benefit from diuretic therapy before anesthesia.

Again, xylazine should be avoided, as it markedly depresses contractility, causes bradycardia, and elevates SVR acutely, each enhancing the likelihood of congestive heart failure. Balanced anesthetic techniques are best in animals with left-to-right shunt lesions because they allow for lower drug doses. Benzodiazepines and narcotics are good premedicant choices. Low doses of thiobarbiturates can be used for induction, unless the animal already is in heart failure. Either halothane or isoflurane is acceptable as an inhalation agent, although isoflurane is preferred because it depresses contractility to a lesser extent.

The radiographic appearance of pulmonary

hypertension may indicate impending or existent right-to-left or bidirectional shunting, and includes an enlarged right heart and main pulmonary artery segment and enlarged pulmonary arteries that are blunted or tortuous in the periphery of the lung. If radiographic evidence of significant pulmonary hypertension exists, an attempt should be made to prevent a shift in the direction of the shunt (to right-to-left). This can be done by avoiding further elevation in pulmonary vascular resistance by preventing struggling or coughing at induction with use of good sedation prior to the induction of anesthesia. Rather than attempt intubation in an animal that is too light at induction, an induction agent should be administered to ensure a smooth intubation. High airway pressures (greater than 30 cm H₂O) should be avoided if assisting the animal's ventilation intraoperatively, as this will raise pulmonary vascular resistance as well. Marked decreases in SVR (hypotension) should also be avoided because if systemic blood pressure falls below the pulmonary artery pressure, a shift in the direction of the shunt can occur.

When choosing drugs for sedation, induction, or maintenance of anesthesia, avoid those agents most likely to produce hypotension (see Tables 26-4 and 26-5). A note of caution for all animals with shunt lesions is to avoid accidental injection of air bubbles into the circulation through veins or venous catheters. Normally, small air bubbles introduced into the venous system embolize in the pulmonary circulation and are of little consequence. However, arterial embolization of the air might result if a right-to-left or bidirectional shunt occurred at some point in the cardiac cycle. Air embolization to the brain, coronary arteries, or other major organs could be fatal.

Disorders Characterized by Pressure Overload

Aortic and pulmonic stenosis are congenital defects that cause pressure overload on the left or right ventricle, respectively (see Chapter 19). Pressure overload on the right ventricle also occurs with pulmonary hypertension, associated with canine heartworm disease. The compensatory response to pressure overload is an increase in muscle mass (concentric hypertrophy) in the affected ventricle. This ventricular hypertrophy is often not matched by an appropriate increase in myocardial perfusion, so myocardial oxygen consumption is a concern with these lesions.

Valvular Pulmonic Stenosis

In the dog, pulmonic stenosis is usually caused by valvular dysplasia. With simple valvular stenosis, blood flow is related to the size of the valvular orifice and the pressure gradient generated across it. Anesthetic drugs can cause myocardial depression and reduce the heart's ability to generate a pressure gradient across the stenosis. To maintain adequate pulmonary flow, the animal requires good cardiac contractility. While assuring good contractility, however, care should be taken to avoid inadvertently causing tachycardia. Rapid heart rates are detrimental in animals with valvular pulmonic stenosis because an increased heart rate elevates myocardial oxygen demand. Tachycardia also reduces diastolic filling time, diminishing stroke volume, and may result in hypotension and diminished coronary perfusion pressure. Consequently, in the tachycardic animal, while oxygen demand in the myocardium is high, oxygen delivery is being compromised and myocardial ischemia can result.

Myocardial depressants should be avoided so that contractility is maintained. Tachycardia, hypovolemia, and arrhythmias must also be avoided in order to maximize ventricular filling. Maintain good ventilation and oxygenation, since animals with valvular pulmonic stenosis are susceptible to myocardial ischemia from hypoxic episodes, as well as from tachycardia. Regulate SVR to maintain normotension and adequate coronary perfusion pressure.

To avoid tachycardia, minimize excitement and struggling prior to induction. This can be accomplished by the use of narcotic premedicants. Narcotics provide excellent sedation; they increase the vagal influence on the heart and slow the heart rate. Narcotics do not diminish the contractility of the myocardium significantly. Fluid therapy can be used to maintain adequate vascular volume and cardiac preload.

Subvalvular Aortic or Pulmonic Stenosis

The usual site of the obstruction in dogs with aortic stenosis is subvalvular. In addition, many dogs with pulmonic stenosis will develop a muscular infundibular hypertrophy secondary to their valvular stenosis, which creates a functional subvalvular obstruction. In both of these cases, excessive myocardial contractility can increase the degree of muscular obstruction in the ventricular outflow tract. With subvalvular aortic stenosis and with pulmonic stenosis complicated by marked muscular infundibular hypertrophy the compromise due to the obstruction can be decreased by avoiding tachycardia and hypovolemia, as above. In contrast to the uncomplicated valvular pulmonic stenosis, in which the aim is to maintain good contractility, these animals may benefit from a slightly diminished ventricular contractile state.

Excessive sympathetic tone can be avoided by preventing pain, stress, or excitement in the patient. Sedation prior to anesthesia will help, but once again, care should be taken to avoid agents that might cause hypotension. The negative inotropic and chronotropic effects of halothane may help to reduce the degree of muscular outflow obstruction. β-Blockade (*e.g.*, propanolol, atenolol, metoprolol) may be useful to decrease myocardial oxygen consumption, tachycardia, and ventricular or supraventricular arrhythmias (see Appendices I and II).

Narcotics are excellent premedicants for these patients because they alleviate pain and have an excellent calming effect. An intramuscular combination of midazolam (0.2 mg/kg) and either oxymorphone (0.05–0.1 mg/kg) or butorphanol (0.2–0.4 mg/kg) usually provides adequate and safe sedation in both the dog and cat. Narcotics can also be used for anesthetic induction. With adequate sedation from narcotics, a low-dose thiobarbiturate is a safe induction agent as well. Intravenous ketamine or diazepam and ketamine should be avoided in these animals. Ketamine stimulates the sympathetic nervous system, raises circulating levels of catecholamines, and can have both positive inotropic and chronotropic effects on the heart, therefore increasing the degree of subvalvular obstruction. The negative inotropic effects of halothane may be beneficial in these patients; however, if preoperative arrhythmias are significant, the less arrhythmogenic drug isoflurane is a better choice. β-Blockers can be used if tachyarrhythmias are significant, or if heart rates are elevated and the risk of myocardial ischemia is great. β-Blockers should always be used cautiously in combination with cardiac depressant drugs, such as halothane, as the negative inotropic effects are additive and an individual's sensitivity to the these drugs is difficult to predict.

Disorders Characterized by Myocardial Dysfunction

Dilated (Congestive) Cardiomyopathy

Idiopathic dilated cardiomyopathy of giant-breed dogs, dilated cardiomyopathy of cats, boxer cardiomyopathy, and cardiomyopathy of Doberman pinscher dogs are frequently encountered conditions in veterinary medicine (see Chapter 21). They have in common a poorly understood etiology and a pathophysiology of progressive loss of contractile function in the myocardium. The ejection fraction is low, resulting in a diminished stroke volume. Cardiac output is poor, pulmonary congestion is common, and signs of right heart failure may complicate the animal's clinical condition. Animals may have marked vasoconstriction in an attempt to maintain adequate blood pressure, manifested by cold extremities, pale mucous membranes, and weak peripheral pulses. Atrial fibrillation, tachyarrhythmias, or ventricular ectopic beats are common findings on the electrocardiogram.

Cardiomyopathic patients should be considered a very poor risk for anesthesia. Fortunately, the instances in which these animals require general anesthesia are rare. One should carefully consider the benefit to be gained from the procedure requiring anesthesia. Prior to anesthesia, medical therapy should be used to improve the clinical signs of heart failure. Diuretics, vasodilators, antiarrhythmic agents, cage rest, and inotropic drugs can be used to decrease congestion and edema and improve cardiac output (see Chapters 18 and 21). Fluid therapy is useful in hypotensive or dehydrated animals. An animal's ability to respond to a positive inotrope may be a good indicator of its ability to tolerate the risk of anesthesia.

The anesthetic aim is to avoid further myocardial depression. Generally speaking, low doses of easily eliminated drugs are the safest approach. The liberal use of inotropes (*e.g.*, dopamine, dobutamine) is encouraged during anesthesia to sustain adequate contractility. Arryhthmias should be avoided, as they may interfere with adequate ventricular filling and therefore diminish cardiac output, or may lead to terminal arrhythmias.

Cardiomyopathic animals have cardiovascular compromise and are slow-moving and depressed. They usually need very little premedication. Intravenous diazepam or midazolam is often sufficient. The cardiovascular effects of these benzodiazepines are minimal; they also reduce the dose of induction agents required and lower the minimum alveolar concentration of inhalation agents. Intravenous induction techniques should be limited to etomidate, diazepam and ketamine or narcotics. Ketamine may also be useful for short procedures, such as nonselective angiocardiography, in cats with dilated cardiomyopathy (see Chapter 80). Mask induction with isoflurane can be considered in a very quiet animal. Dopamine or dobutamine infusions (1–10 µg/kg/min) often help to improve the contractile state of the heart during anesthesia.

Disorders Characterized by Impaired Cardiac Filling

Cardiac tamponade, constrictive pericarditis, and hypertrophic cardiomyopathy are diseases in which impaired ventricular filling results in diastolic dysfunction (see Chapters 21 and 23). Despite a common pathophysiology, these disorders present slightly differing anesthetic challenges.

Cardiac Tamponade

If pericardial effusion is mild it causes little compromise of cardiac function and offers little risk for anesthesia (see Chapter 23). However, as effusion increases in the pericardial space the intracardiac pressures begin to elevate, resulting in cardiac tamponade. With tamponade there is equalization of diastolic pressures throughout the heart, and ventricular filling during diastole is limited. The subsequent decrease in stroke volume results in decreased cardiac output. With a fixed left ventricular stroke volume, cardiac output is completely dependent on heart rate. The animal's compensatory mechanisms for this disease are fluid retention and tachycardia to maintain cardiac output, and vasoconstriction to maintain arterial blood pressure. The typical result is right heart failure.

The anesthetic aims are to maintain the compensatory mechanisms of a rapid heart rate, adequate intravascular volume, and adequate vascular tone.

Pericardiocentesis is strongly encouraged prior to anesthesia (see Chapter 80). This procedure, along with cage rest, with or without diuresis often renders these patients virtually asymptomatic and minimally at risk for anesthesia. Diazepam and ketamine is a good combination for intravenous induction in both cats and dogs with tamponade. Myocardial depressants, vasodilators, and barbiturates should be avoided. Excessive positive pressure (greater than 30 cm H_2O) should be avoided if ventilating these animals during anesthesia, as this further impairs venous return and diminishes cardiac filling.

Constrictive Pericarditis

Constrictive pericarditis is similar in pathophysiology and symptomatology to cardiac tamponade, although impairment of diastolic filling occurs only in late diastole. Cardiac output can be normal when heart rate remains elevated, since systolic function is well maintained. Little fluid can be removed from the pericardial sac of these patients, so preanesthetic pericardiocentesis is not useful.

The aims are similar to those for tamponade, that is, maintaining the heart rate and intravascular volume to optimize early diastolic ventricular filling and cardiac output, and promoting normotension.

Vasodilators such as acepromazine should be used only when adequate volume expansion from intravenous fluids is possible. Narcotics are safe if the bradycardic response is prevented with anticholinergics. Thiobarbiturate inductions cause significant myocardial depression and are generally avoided. The combination of diazepam and ketamine is the induction agent of choice.

Hypertrophic Cardiomyopathy

Hypertrophic cardiomyopathy is another disorder of diastolic dysfunction. The thickened ventricular walls have impaired diastolic relaxation. Ventricular filling is slow and incomplete in the early phase of diastole, when rapid ventricular filling usually takes place. Consequently, these animals depend on adequate intravascular volume (preload) and atrial systole for optimizing their ventricular volume. Heart failure, arrhythmias, and heart rate should be controlled or optimized prior to anesthesia.

Arrhythmias and hypovolemia should be avoided. Some myocardial depression is tolerated in these hypercontractile hearts. To maintain blood pressure, supply adequate fluid volume.

Narcotics are an excellent choice in hypertrophic cardiomyopathy. The associated increase in vagal tone is well tolerated and often beneficial. In contrast to the pericardial diseases, ketamine should not be used for induction in animals with hypertrophic cardiomyopathy because it increases heart rate, elevates myocardial oxygen demand, and shortens diastolic filling time. β-Blockers may be needed in these animals to reduce heart rate and allow the necessary ventricular filling time, and to prevent arrhythmias.

Disorders Characterized by Serious Rhythm Disturbances

There are a number of situations in veterinary medicine in which a primary noncardiac disease can have profound effects on cardiac function through secondary metabolic or organic changes that occur in the myocardium. These changes are often manifested by increased incidence of cardiac arrhythmias. Either because of the presence of or potential for arrhythmias, these patients present a unique challenge in anesthetic manage-ment. Following are three examples of diseases that fit into this category and that are frequently encountered by the small animal practitioner.

Traumatic Myocarditis

Cardiac arrhythmias following trauma are a well-recognized clinical entity in canine patients. These arrhythmias may arise after blunt chest trauma, and are sometimes attributed to myocardial contusions. In addition, cardiac arrhythmias can arise without evidence of direct thoracic trauma in patients with head trauma, spinal cord trauma, or pelvic limb fractures. The suggested etiology for the arrhythmias in these cases is myocardial ischemia secondary to severe shock, or sympathetic overstimulation. The most common arrhythmias observed following trauma are premature ventricular contractions or ventricular tachycardia. The onset of these rhythm disturbances can occur from 1 to 48 hours after the traumatic incident.

When possible, these animals should be stabilized before surgery, and surgery should be delayed until arrhythmias are well controlled or resolved. When anesthesia is necessary, the less arrhythmogenic anesthetic agents are preferred; arrythmias should be treated as needed (see Chapter 18).

Fluid therapy and preoperative antiarrhythmic agents are recommended. Lidocaine at 1 to 2 mg/kg can be given and repeated several times; however, a total dose of 8 mg/kg should not be exceeded, or central nervous system toxicity (seizures) may arise. After initial bolus treatment, a continous lidocaine infusion at 50 to 80 µg/kg/min can be used to maintain serum lidocaine levels in an adequate antiarrhythmic range. Lidocaine infusions sometimes are necessary for several days. Procainamide or quinidine are also used in animals that are refractory to lidocaine therapy or for whom intravenous infusion is not practical (see Chapter 18).

After stabilization, the following considerations can be used for choosing anesthetic drugs. Acepromazine is antiarrhythmic; it decreases the heart's susceptibility to catecholamine-induced rhythm disturbances and can be an effective premedicant for the traumatized animal. However, it should not be used in an acute situation when volume depletion due to shock or blood loss may be present, as it is safe only in the well-stabilized animal that has the cardiovascular reserve necessary to handle the resultant vasodilatation. Narcotics are good premedicants following trauma because many of these animals are suffering pain and the superior analgesia of narcotics is the most humane way to facilitate their handling. The best induction agent is a combination of lidocaine and thiamylal. This combination allows a reduced dose of the depressant drug thiamylal, and lidocaine elevates blood levels to provide antiarrhythmic effect. Isoflurane is a better inhalant choice than is halothane when arrhythmias are present or anticipated. If anesthesia is necessary for a procedure involving the rear limbs, epidural anesthesia combined with heavy narcotic sedation is an option. In animals with significant thoracic trauma, endotracheal intubation and oxygen supplementation are advised. Nitrous oxide should never be used in these animals because of the likelihood of exacerbating a pneumothorax.

Gastric Dilatation–Volvulus

While the animal with traumatic myocarditis can often be managed medically and the anesthetic episode delayed until arrhythmias are resolved, the dog presented with gastric dilatation–volvulus often requires immediate life-saving surgery (see Chapter 36). The need to undergo anesthesia exists in an animal that has significant cardiopulmonary compromise as a consequence of its gastric disturbance. Inadequate circulating blood volume, impaired oxygen delivery to tissues, and acid-base and electrolyte abnormalities exist as complicating factors. These problems can often be rectified by initial aggressive treatment with intravenous fluids and gastric decompression.

Dogs with gastric dilatation–volvulus are very susceptible to the development of arrhythmias. The predominant arrhythmias encountered are premature ventricular contractions and ventricular tachycardia. Histopathologically, areas of myocardial necrosis have been identified in dogs with gastric dilatation–volvulus that are consistent with myocardial ischemia. Manage-

ment of ventricular arrhythmias in these dogs is similar to that of the dog with traumatic myocarditis (Chapter 18). Bolus administration of lidocaine followed by a continuous lidocaine infusion is the measure to take in the acute situation preoperatively when ventricular arrhythmias are noted.

It is necessary to volume expand these animals with a balanced electrolyte solution intravenously (60–90 ml/kg/hour) immediately upon admission and to attempt gastric decompression. Ventricular arrhythmias should be treated if present, and electrolyte imbalances identified and corrected. Anesthetic drugs that have minimal cardiovascular effects—not arrhythmogenic agents—should be selected.

Premedication is often not necessary in the debilitated animal. Intravenous diazepam or midazolam can be used with little untoward effect. In an animal with documented ventricular arrhythmias, induction with lidocaine and thiamylal is safe and will often temporarily abolish ventricular arrhythmias. If ventricular arrhythmias are not yet present the above technique can still be used. An alternative induction regimen is intravenous fentanyl-droperidol. This works well in dogs that remain in sinus tachycardia despite adequate intravenous fluid administration prior to anesthesia. Mask inductions are not recommended because of the likelihood of regurgitation and pulmonary aspiration injury. Isoflurane is the inhalant anesthetic of choice for animals with gastric dilatation–volvulus because the animal will experience decreased incidence of myocardial depression and arrhythmogenesis when compared with halothane or methoxyflurane. Nitrous oxide should be avoided in cases of gastric dilatation–volvulus to prevent further expansion of the gas-filled stomach. If an animal does not tolerate anesthesia well, it may be beneficial to decrease the amount of inhalation agent being given and supplement with intravenous narcotics such as fentanyl (1 ug/kg) or oxymorphone (0.05 mg/kg).

Hyperthyroidism

Feline hyperthyroidism has become a well-recognized clinical entity in small animal practice, and surgical thyroidectomy is an effective form of treatment for this disorder (see Chapter 61). Gastrointestinal, behavioral, urinary, and integumentary complaints are common from owners of hyperthyroid cats.

Thyroid hormone also has profound influence on the cardiovascular system; thus, anesthetizing the hyperthyroid cat for thyroidectomy poses a unique challenge for the small animal practitioner. The cardiovascular effects of excess thyroid hormone are a result of both its direct effects on the myocardium and its indirect effects of sympathoadrenal stimulation. Cats with hyperthyroidism often have sinus tachycardia, atrial or ventricular arrhythmias, and cardiomegaly that resembles hypertrophic cardiomyopathy. The cardiac change of hyperthyroidism is usually a reversible disease once the animal becomes euthyroid. If a cat is showing signs of cardiac failure, therapy to alleviate the signs of heart failure is indicated.

Initially, these animals are at high risk for anesthetic complications. Medical management of their hyperthyroid state is absolutely necessary prior to anesthesia. Adequate treatment for a period of 2 to 3 weeks can change a thyrotoxic cat to a euthyroid cat and markedly diminish the risk of an anesthetic episode. Preferred medical therapy consists of the oral antithyroid drug methimazole. Cats with significant cardiac involvement respond well to propanolol, atenolol, or metoprolol administration during this time period. These β-adrenergic blocking drugs help control the tachycardia, arrhythmias, and hypercontractile state of the myocardium. When heart failure is present, thoracentesis along with furosemide, rest, and a low sodium diet may be indicated (see Thoracentesis and Insertion of Chest Tubes in Chapter 80). If myocardial failure is proven echocardiographically, digoxin should be administered and β-blockade avoided.

If antithyroid therapy renders the cat euthyroid, the risks of anesthesia are reduced and many anesthetic drugs can be tolerated if the cat has not had significant cardiac involvement. Otherwise, the safest approach to anesthesia is to adequately sedate the cat to avoid excitement and sympathetic nervous system stimulation, choose less arrhythmogenic anesthetic drugs, and monitor the animal closely and be prepared to treat arrhythmias that may arise.

Premedicants with antiarrhythmic properties are highly recommended. An excellent combination is acepromazine (0.1 mg/kg) and oxymorphone (0.1 mg/kg). Acepromazine decreases the likelihood of catecholamine-induced arrhythmias, and in combination with the narcotic provides an excellent calming restraint for these often hyperexcitable cats. Thiobarbiturates are the induction agent of choice for the hyperthyroid animal. These drugs have a similar chemical structure to the antithyroid drugs and possess antithyroid activity themselves. Isoflurane is the inhalation agent of choice because it causes the least sensitization of the myocardium to catecholamine-induced arrhythmias. If tachycardia or ventricular arrhythmias appear intraoperatively, 0.1 mg propanolol can be administered intravenously to control arrhythmias.

Table 26-3 summarizes the desired hemodynamic effects one should strive for with each of the diseases mentioned above. When uncertain of the diagnosis of the patient's heart condition, the best approach is to avoid extremes. When an increased heart rate is recommended during anesthesia for a particular condition, this should be interpreted as a moderate increase (heart rate of 120–140 beats per minute in the dog) rather than a call to induce extreme tachycardia (heart rate greater than 180 beats per minute). Extremes of heart rate, vascular tone, and contractility are not well-tolerated even by animals with normal cardiovascular function, and can be disastrous in those with compromised cardiovascular function, with or without preexistent heart failure. Anesthetic recommendations for patients presented in shock are discussed in Chapter 4.

Tables 26-4 to 26-7 have been prepared as a guide for choosing appropriate anesthetic drugs for the cardiac patient. The major cardiovascular effects of drugs commonly used for premedication, induction, and inhalation anesthesia are indicated. The dosage ranges recommended are deliberately conservative. The dosages apply either to the dog or the cat unless indicated for one species only. The more compromised an animal, the less anesthetic drug it is able to tolerate. With particularly compromised animals choose the

Table 26–3 Desired Hemodynamic Changes for Selected Cardiac Conditions

Disease	Preload	PVR	SVR	HR	Contractility
Mitral regurgitation	+	N/−	−	N/+	N/+
Patent ductus arteriosus	+	N/−	N/−	N/+	N
Ventricular septal defect	+	N/−	N/−	N/+	N
Pulmonic stenosis (valvular)	+	−	N	−	N/+
Pulmonic stenosis (infundibular)	+	−	N	−	−
Aortic stenosis (subvalvular)	+	N	N	−	−
Pericardial disease	+	N	N/+	+	N
Hypertrophic cardiomyopathy	+	N	N/+	N/−	−
Dilated cardiomyopathy	+	N	N/−	N	+ +

N = maintain within normal range; + = animal typically benefits from an increase in these parameters;
− = animal typically benefits from a decrease in these parameters; PVR = pulmonary vascular resistance;
SVR = systemic vascular resistance; HR = heart rate

Table 26–4 Comparison of Premedications Used in Small Animal Practice

Drug	Intramuscular Dosage (mg/kg)	Cardiovascular Effects				
		HR	BP	CO	MVO$_2$	Rhythm
Acepromazine	0.05 to 0.1	+	−	+	+	Antiarryhythmic
Butorphanol	0.2 to 0.4	−	NC	NC/−	NC	+ Vagal tone
Diazepam	0.1 to 0.2 (IM or IV)	NC	NC	NC	NC	NC
Droperidol with fentanyl*	0.05 to 0.1 (ml/kg) (dog only)	−	NC	NC/−	NC	+ Vagal tone
Ketamine	5 to 8 (cat only)	+	+	+	+	Sinus tachyarrhythmia
Merperidine	2 to 4	−	−	NC/−	NC	+ Vagal tone
Midazolam	0.1 to 0.2 (IM or IV)	NC	NC	NC	NC	NC
Morphine	0.2 to 0.5 (dog only)	−	NC/−	NC/−	NC	+ Vagal tone
Oxymorphone	0.05 to 0.1	−	NC	NC/−	NC	+ Vagal tone
Tiletamine and zolazepam	3 to 5	+	+	+	+	Sinus tachyarrhythmia
Xylazine	0.5 to 1	−	+/−	−	−	Arrhythmogenic

* Innovar-Vet contains 20 mg/ml of droperidol and 0.4 mg/ml of fentanyl.
NC = no change; + = increase in this parameter from the resting state; − = decrease in this parameter from the
resting state; HR = heart rate; BP = blood pressure; CO = cardic output; MVO$_2$ = myocardial oxygen consumption

lowest dose possible to achieve the desired effect or consider drug combinations, such as narcotics and tranquilizers, to minimize negative side-effects while optimizing the clinical effect.

PATIENT MONITORING DURING ANESTHESIA

If a problem arises with a patient while it is under anesthesia, the problem must first be recognized in order for appropriate measures to be taken to correct the situation. Hemodynamic monitoring involves the use of observational skills and noninvasive and invasive techniques. The methods chosen depend to a great extent on the equipment available, one's comfort with use of the equipment, and the degree of reliability one places in the technique.

Much information can be obtained about the anesthetized animal without investing a large amount of money in monitoring equipment. Heart rate, pulse strength, pulse regularity, mucous membrane color, capillary refill time, bleeding at the surgical site, and respiratory rate and rhythm are among the parameters that can be

Table 26–5 *Comparison of Intravenous Induction Agents Used in Small Animal Practice*

Drug	Intravenous Dosage (mg/kg)	Cardiovascular Effects				
		HR	BP	CO	MVO$_2$	RHYTHM
Diazepam and ketamine*	0.05 to 0.1 (ml/kg)	+	+	+	+	Sinus tachyarrhythmia
Droperidol with fentanyl	0.03 to 0.05 (ml/kg) (dog only)	NC	NC	NC/−	NC	+ Vagal tone
Etomidate	1 to 2	NC	NC	NC	NC	NC
Thiamylal	6 to 12	+	−	−	+	Arrhythmogenic
Thiamylal and lidocaine	3 to 6 and 3 to 6 (dog only)	NC	−	−	NC	Antiarrhythmic
Thiopental	8 to 15	+	−	−	+	Arrhythmogenic
Tiletamine and zolazepam	1 to 3	+	+	+	+	Sinus tachyarrhythmia

* A 50:50 mixture of diazepam and ketamine contains 2.5 mg/ml of diazepam and 50 mg/ml of ketamine.
NC = no change; + = increase in this parameter from the resting state; − = decrease in this parameter from the resting state; HR = heart rate; BP = blood pressure; CO = cardic output; MVO$_2$ = myocardial oxygen consumption

Table 26–6 *Comparison of Inhalation Agents Used in Small Animal Practice*

Drug	MAC		Cardiovascular Effects				
	Dog	Cat	HR	Inotropy	CO	SVR	Arrhythmia
Halothane	0.87	0.82	−	−	−	−	+ + +
Isoflurane	1.3	1.6	+	NC/−	NC/−	−	NC
Methoxyflurane	0.23	0.23	NC/−	−	−	−	+ +
Nitrous oxide	200	255	NC	NC/−	NC/−	NC	NC

NC = no change; + = increase in this parameter from the resting state; − = decrease in this parameter from the resting state; MAC = minimum alveolar concentration; HR = heart rate; CO = cardic output; SVR = systemic vascular resistance

followed by observational techniques alone. Changes in these variables should be watched closely. Frequent checking is advised because trends are usually apparent before a crisis arises and because the cardiac patient is less stable than the normal dog or cat when hemodynamic alterations due to anesthesia or surgery are occurring.

Noninvasive monitoring techniques can be as simple as a stethoscope or as complex as a pulse oximeter. The stethoscope provides information on heart rate and rhythm and gives a crude measure of contractility, as the intensity of heart sounds changes. Intraoperative electrocardiographic monitoring is strongly encouraged. The Doppler ultrasound apparatus is an excellent monitoring tool, providing not only an audible pulse sound for following rate and rhythm changes, but also providing systolic blood pressure readings so that trends can be quantified and the response to intervention can be evaluated.

Maintaining adequate blood pressure to ensure tissue perfusion is the goal any time an animal is anesthetized. The palpable pulse feels strong when there is a large difference between the systolic and diastolic blood pressures. The pulse strength may feel adequate when the mean blood pressure is less than 60 mmHg and tissue perfusion is compromised. Urine output, as measured from a urinary catheter, can be a good indication of the adequacy of blood pressure over time, but does not reflect acute change. If mean blood pressue is greater than 60 mmHg, the normal rate of urine production should be 1 to 2 ml/kg/hour.

Invasive monitoring techniques take more time to institute and often involve the use of more complex equipment; however, the information obtained is usually quantitative and more accurate than that obtained through observational or noninvasive techniqes. The most accurate way to

Table 26-7 *Anesthetic Agents Considered Safest for Cardiac Patients*

PREMEDICATION

Butorphanol
Diazepam
Droperidol with fentanyl citrate
Midazolam hydrochloride
Morphine sulfate
Oxymorphone

INDUCTION

Diazepam and ketamine
Etomidate
Droperidol with fentanyl
Isoflurane

MAINTENANCE

Isoflurane

monitor systemic blood pressure is by placement of a catheter directly into the dorsal pedal or femoral artery of the dog or cat. With an arterial catheter in place, blood pressure can be accurately measured using an aneroid manometer or a pressure transducer and recording system. An excellent review of monitoring methods and equipment has recently been written by Haskins (Additional Reading).

The technique of central venous pressure monitoring is discussed in Chapter 80. Monitoring of central venous pressure is one of the best ways to evaluate the rate of fluid administration during anesthesia. For cardiac patients, such as those with volume overload disease, it is advisable to monitor central venous pressure when the danger of fluid overload is high yet the concern for maximizing preload is significant.

FLUID THERAPY IN THE ANESTHETIZED CARDIAC PATIENT

Bonagura (Additional Reading) has set forth the following goals for fluid therapy in cardiac patients: optimizing venous pressures, enhancing free water excretion, and inhibiting sodium retention. Patients with cardiac disease but normal or near normal function can withstand standard fluid therapy regimens recommended by anes-thesiologists (10 ml/kg/hour). However, with left heart failure, such regimens may precipitate pulmonary edema.

Complications may be minimized by controlling the signs of failure prior to anesthesia, using salt-deficient fluids (0.45% sodium chloride with 2.5% dextrose, or 5% dextrose in water, with potassium supplementation as indicated by the clinical situation), using the minimal volumes necessary to replace surgical losses and maintain blood pressure and tissue perfusion, and carefully monitoring the patient. The dilemma is to provide adequate fluid support (preload) to maintain cardiac output without precipitating the signs of congestion. Central venous pressure, while not an accurate indicator of pulmonary venous pressure, is useful as an indicator of right heart filling pressure and fluid overload. Ideally, the central venous pressure should be maintained at 8 to 11 cm H_2O, with increases or decreases counteracted by decreases or increases in fluid infusion rate, respectively.

For asymptomatic patients with little risk of low output or congestive heart failure, balanced electrolyte solutions at 10 ml/kg/hour are acceptable. Patients with volume overload defects or heart disease that requires medical therapy to maintain adequate function should be administered balanced electrolyte solutions at 5 ml/kg/hour, with blood pressure and central venous pressure dictating the necessary changes in fluid rate. For more severely affected patients, we recommend the saline-poor fluids mentioned above, administered at 2 ml/kg/hour. Potassium chloride supplementation to these fluids may be necessary at 30 mEq/L. Infusion rates are determined after careful scrutiny of the patient's needs based on underlying disease, degree of compensation, blood loss, pulmonary auscultation, central venous pressure, and systemic arterial blood pressure. Fluid administration rates will vary between individual patients and within individuals during a procedure.

ADDITIONAL READING

Bonagura JD. Fluid and electrolyte management of the cardiac patient. Vet Clin North Am [Small Anim Pract] 1982; 12:501.

Haskins SC. Monitoring the anesthetized patient. In: Short CE, ed. Principles and practice of veterinary anesthesia. Baltimore: Williams & Wilkins, 1987: 455.

Ingwersen W, Allen DG, Dyson DH, Black WD et al. Cardiopulmonary effects of a ketamin-acepromazine combination in hypovolemic cats. Canadian Journal of Veterinary Research 1988; 52:423.

Ingwersen W, Allen DG, Dyson DH, Black WD et al. Cardiopulmonary effects of a halothane-oxygen combination in hypovolemic cats. Canadian Journal of Veterinary Research 1988; 52:428.

Mason DE, Hubbell JAE. Anesthesia and the heart. In: Fox PR, ed. Canine and feline cardiology. New York: Churchill Livingstone, 1988: 591.

McDonnell W. Anesthesia for cardiovascular surgery. In: Slatter DH, ed. Textbook of small animal surgery, vol 2. Philadelphia: WB Saunders, 1985: 2634.

Moise NS, Short CE. Cardiac anesthesia. In: Short CE, ed. Principles and practice of veterinary anesthesia. Baltimore: Williams & Wilkins, 1987: 183.

Paddleford RR. Anesthetic considerations in patients with preexisting problems or conditions. In: Paddleford RR, ed. Manual of small animal anesthesia. New York: Churchill Livingstone, 1988: 253.

Seeler DC, Dodman NH, Norman W, Court M. Recommended techniques in small animal anaesthesia: IV. Anaesthesia and cardiac disease. Br Vet J 1988; 144:108.

THE
RESPIRATORY
SYSTEM

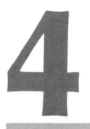

4

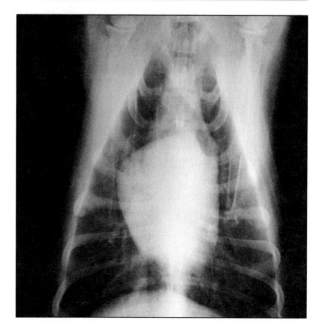

27

NASAL DISCHARGE
Ned F. Kuehn, Philip Roudebush

Nasal discharge is a common problem encountered in dogs and cats. Chronic nasal discharge is an important clinical sign that, with few exceptions, localizes a disorder to the nasal cavity or frontal sinuses. Sneezing is a clinical sign that is often associated with nasal discharge; however, intranasal diseases that cause extensive destruction of the turbinates are often not associated with sneezing despite copious nasal discharge.

Characterization of the discharge often helps the clinician choose an appropriate diagnostic approach to these patients. Nasal discharges may be categorized according to volume (copious, scant), frequency (continuous, intermittent), location (unilateral, bilateral), and appearance (serous, purulent, mucoid, mucopurulent, bloody). Serous discharges are clear and typically acellular; mucoid discharges, which are also clear and acellular, have a high protein content. Purulent nasal discharges are opaque, viscous, and pale yellow or light green, and contain abundant neutrophils and bacteria. Mucopurulent discharges are composed of both mucus and pus (mucopus) and have abundant neutrophils; the presence of bacteria is, however, variable. Depending on the underlying etiology, any of the above discharges may be blood-tinged. Finally, bloody nasal discharge (epistaxis) is indicative of active hemorrhage and primarily contains red blood cells.

CAUSES

The routine causes for the various types of nasal discharge are given in Table 27-1. The causes of purulent nasal discharges and epistaxis can be divided into intranasal and extranasal categories. Intranasal causes are those diseases confined to the nasal cavity or paranasal sinuses, whereas extranasal causes are systemic diseases associated with nasal discharge.

PATHOPHYSIOLOGY

The kind of nasal discharge is largely dependent on the type and duration of the underlying lesion. The first physical sign of upper respiratory disease is often a serous nasal discharge. These discharges are produced in response to nonspecific irritation of the nasal mucosa and therefore are generally of little diagnostic value. Serous nasal discharges are usually licked away by the animal and are often not recognized by the owner. Blood-tinged serous discharges are more likely to be recognized by the client. Blood-tinged serous discharges are often intermittent, and are typically associated with discrete intranasal lesions. Forceful or paroxysmal bouts of sneezing, however, may also result in a blood-tinged serous discharge.

Table 27–1 Causes of Nasal Discharge

SEROUS NASAL DISCHARGE

Active viral upper respiratory infection
    Feline herpesvirus (rhinotracheitis)
    Feline calcivirus
    Canine distemper
    Canine adenovirus (Types 1 and 2)
    Canine parainfluenza
    Canine reovirus or herpesvirus (rare)
Feline chlamydiosis
Intranasal parasites
    Linguatula serrata (dogs)
    Pneumonyssus caninum (dogs)
    Syngamus ierei (cats)
Oronasal fistula (canine tooth)
Rhinosporidiosis (dogs, rare)

PURULENT NASAL DISCHARGE

INTRANASAL CAUSES

Secondary bacterial infection (dogs and cats)
Mycotic rhinitis
    Aspergillosis
    Blastomycosis
    Cryptococcosis
    Penicilliosis
Foreign body rhinitis
Traumatic rhinitis or sinusitis
Cleft palate
Oronasal fistula
Neoplasia
    Adenocarcinoma
    Fibrosarcoma
    Others
Nasopharyngeal polyps (cats)
Benign nasal polyps (dogs)

EXTRANASAL CAUSES

Bacterial bronchopneumonia
Megaesophagus with aspiration pneumonia
    Congenital megaesophagus
    Acquired megaesophagus
Achalasia with nasal reflux of food
Acquired esophageal stricture

MUCOID TO MUCOPURULENT NASAL DISCHARGE

Mycotic rhinitis
    Aspergillosis
    Blastomycosis
    Cryptococcosis
    Penicilliosis
Neoplasia
    Adenocarcinoma (most common)
    Others

HEMORRHAGIC NASAL DISCHARGE (EPISTAXIS)

INTRANASAL CAUSES

Acute nasal trauma
Oronasal fistula (rare)

EXTRANASAL CAUSES

Inherited factor deficiencies
    von Willebrand's disease (common in dogs)
    Factor VIII deficiency (classic hemophilia)
    Other inherited factor deficiencies
Acquired factor deficiencies
    Vitamin K antagonists (e.g., warfarin, indandiones)
    Liver failure
Disseminated intravascular coagulation
Immune-mediated thrombocytopenia
Infectious thrombocytopenia
    Canine ehrlichiosis
    Rocky Mountain spotted fever
Hyperviscosity syndromes
Systemic hypertension (rare)

Change from a serous to purulent discharge indicates that the mucociliary clearance mechanism of the nose is no longer able to oppose bacterial colonization. For example, viruses that attack the upper respiratory system disrupt the mucociliary apparatus and permit bacterial adherence to sinonasal epithelial cells. These viruses may additionally suppress the immune response and reduce macrophage function, facilitating bacterial invasion. Other chronic intranasal lesions, such as tumors or mycotic infections, may also disturb the mucociliary clearance mechanism of the nose and permit bacterial invasion.

Bacterial infections of the nose are rarely a primary condition; they usually are secondary to some primary lesion.

Mucoid nasal discharges are a result of exuberant production of mucus by goblet cells. This type of discharge is produced in response to chronic diseases. Mucoid discharges are seen most often in older dogs and cats with intranasal carcinoma. Mucopurulent discharges indicate both chronicity and secondary infection. The presence of blood in a mucopurulent discharge suggests tissue destruction, although bleeding may occur as a result of episodes of explosive sneezing.

Epistaxis, or hemorrhagic nasal discharge, is more prevalent in dogs than in cats. The presence of epistaxis is often more suggestive of an underlying coagulation defect than of a primary intranasal lesion (see Chapter 16). Nevertheless, tumors, foreign bodies, mycosis, and trauma also commonly cause epistaxis and should be considered if a coagulation profile is normal.

CLINICAL SIGNS

The presence of nasal discharge, other than perhaps a serous discharge, is often quite apparent to the owner and veterinarian. Nasal discharge or sneezing are prominent localizing signs to disorders of the upper respiratory tract (nasal cavity and paranasal sinuses). Nasal discharge, however, may also be related to systemic disease and may be the only outward manifestation of a much more serious underlying disorder. For example, a purulent discharge may occur secondary to bronchopneumonia, and epistaxis may be the result of a coagulopathy.

Diagnostic Approach

The definitive diagnosis of diseases involving the nasal cavity and paranasal sinuses is often difficult. The anatomy and physiology of the upper respiratory tract in dogs and cats is complex and can vary considerably between breeds. Furthermore, the nasal passages in dogs and cats are often difficult to visualize and interpret radiographically. Chronic nasal discharge often poses a particularly difficult diagnostic and therapeutic challenge. When possible, it is advisable to do a complete evaluation of a patient with nasal discharge early in the course of disease rather than treat symptomatically.

The signalment may eliminate certain causes of nasal discharge from initial consideration. Most causes of nasal discharge in dogs are the same in cats; however, cats do have several unique diseases (feline infectious upper respiratory disease complex and nasopharyngeal polyps). Animals older than 6 to 8 years of age have a higher incidence of intranasal tumors, benign nasal polyps, dental disease, and mycotic

diseases. On the other hand, congenital diseases or nasopharyngeal polyps (cats) are more likely in animals younger than 6 months of age. Epistaxis may occur with von Willebrand's disease, a common bleeding disorder reported in at least 30 breeds of dogs. Chronic bilateral mucopurulent nasal discharge is often seen in young puppies or kittens with cleft palate. Finally, a purulent nasal discharge may be seen secondary to esophageal hypomotility and megaesophagus, which is frequently associated with Siamese and Siamese-related cat breeds, German shepherds, Irish setters, and several other dog breeds (see Chapter 36).

The patient history may reveal important information concerning the cause of nasal discharge. A consistently unilateral discharge strongly supports the diagnosis of intranasal disease. An acute unilateral discharge associated temporally with pawing at the face and sneezing is suggestive of a foreign body. Chronic nasal discharges that are initially unilateral and later become bilateral and sanguineous are highly suggestive of intranasal neoplasia or mycotic rhinitis.

The type of discharge is important in establishing an initial list of differentials. Serous discharges result from the initial response of the nasal mucosa to nonspecific irritation. A serous discharge that later becomes purulent would suggest secondary bacterial rhinitis as a complication of a wide variety of intranasal or systemic diseases. Mucoid discharges characteristically are seen in older animals with intranasal neoplasia. Intermittently blood-tinged nasal discharges indicate active tissue destruction or severe sneezing.

The clinical response to an adequate course of antibiotic therapy may give some clues as to the underlying cause of the nasal discharge. Purulent nasal discharges that are responsive to antibiotics only during their course of administration indicate the presence of a bacterial infection secondary to some primary intranasal disease. Purulent or mucopurulent discharges that are unresponsive to antibiotics tend to be associated with mycotic rhinitis. In older animals, mucoid discharges that are unresponsive to antibiotics often are associated with intranasal tumors. Many animals with either intranasal tumors or fungal rhinitis have secondary bacterial rhinitis. A temporary response to antibiotics may occur, but this response should not prevent the search for the primary underlying disease.

A thorough general physical examination, with attention paid to evidence of systemic disease, should be followed by careful examination of the oral, nasal, and ocular regions. Gross distortions of facial symmetry often indicate neoplasia (Fig. 27-1) and, rarely, trauma. Pain on palpation of the nose and depigmentation or ulceration of the rhinarium and external nares occurs frequently with mycotic rhinitis.

Most animals seen for evaluation of nasal discharge should receive a thorough oral evaluation. Because root abscesses of the upper canines and incisors (and, less commonly, the carnassial teeth) may cause unilateral nasal discharge, a probe should be passed into the gingival sulcus. If the probe passes easily into the deep periodontal structures, a tooth root abscess or oronasal fistula should be suspected. Most dogs will tolerate this procedure awake; however, if not, it should be performed under heavy sedation or general anesthesia.

Special attention should be given to ophthalmic examination in any patient with nasal discharge. The presence of unilateral epiphora may indicate obstruction of the nasolacrimal duct. Exophthalmus and increased intraocular pressure should direct attention to the possibility of a retrobulbar mass. Finally, the retina should be evaluated for lesions indicating the presence of systemic infection. The finding of retinitis on a fundic examination may suggest systemic infection, especially cryptococcosis in cats.

Quite often the history and physical examination do not contribute a significant amount of information helpful in establishing a diagnosis. Most patients with nasal discharge require further diagnostic procedures, which might include a complete blood count, platelet count, serum biochemistry profile, urinalysis, coagulation profile, radiographs of the nose and paranasal sinuses, rhinoscopy, biopsy, culture and sensitivity, and serology (Table 27-2). Although the majority of these procedures require general anesthesia, this may be warranted to achieve the goal of establishing a definitive diagnosis to facilitate proper management of the patient.

A complete blood count, serum biochemistry profile, and urinalysis should be done when systemic disease is suspected. A complete blood count, platelet count, and coagulation profile (activated partial thromboplastin time, one-stage prothrombin time, activated clotting time, fibrin degradation products, fibrinogen) is indicated for a patient with epistaxis unrelated to trauma. Young dogs with epistaxis may require additional tests to determine specific clotting factor deficiencies (see Chapter 16).

Radiographs of the nasal cavity and paranasal

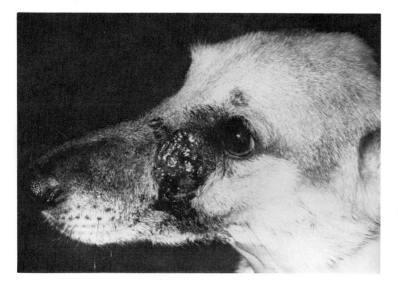

Figure 27–1 *Photograph of the face of an 11-year-old female mixed-breed dog showing a mass rostral to the left eye. The mass was an adenocarcinoma originating from the nasal cavity. The dog had had a chronic unilateral (right-side) mucopurulent nasal discharge for approximately 1 year. Unfortunately, no diagnostic procedures were performed prior to the emergence of this mass to find a cause for the chronic nasal discharge. Periodic treatment with oral antibiotics only partially decreased the volume of nasal discharge.*

Table 27–2 *Laboratory Assessment of Nasal Discharge*

Test	What to Check for
Complete blood count	Neutrophilia (pneumonia, abscess)
	Eosinophilia (allergic rhinitis)
	Thrombocytopenia
Coagulation profile	Coagulation abnormality
Skull radiographs	Loss of symmetry
	Bone destruction (fungal rhinitis, neoplasia)
	Masses
	Foreign bodies
Rhinoscopy	Fungal plaques
	Masses
	Turbinate destruction
Pharyngoscopy	Polyps
	Foreign bodies
	Masses
Cytology	
Nasal discharge	Neutrophils
	Eosinophils
	Fungal elements
Masses	Fungal elements
	Tumor cells
Culture	Bacteria (pure growth)
	Fungi
Biopsy	Histologic interpretation

sinuses are often required for diagnosing a patient with nasal discharge. It is essential that animals be anesthetized (heavy sedation is not sufficient) for any radiographic study of the nasal cavity. This is because critical positioning of the skull is imperative for correct interpretation of the films. When reading nasal films, it is important to look for symmetry and compare one side of the rhinarium and sinuses with the other. Well-positioned nasal radiographs also help direct where biopsies or surgical approach to the nose should be made. See Ticer in the Additional Reading section for descriptions on patient positioning for nasal films.

Nasal radiographs usually refine the list of differentials, although they occasionally may be diagnostic. In many instances, a final diagnosis is dependent on the cytologic and histologic appearance of tissue specimens. Radiographic studies allow one to distinguish destructive lesions, radiodense foreign bodies, traumatic injuries, and osteomyelitis. Destructive lesions indicate either fungal or neoplastic disease. Osteomyelitis of the bone surrounding tooth roots indicates an apical abcess. Inflammatory (hyperplastic) rhinitis is nondestructive and radiographically characterized by increased density in the nasal cavity due to excessive secretions and hyperplasia of the mucous membranes. Copious discharges also cause an overall increased water density to the nasal cavity and may obscure subtle primary lesions. The radiographic appearance of the nose may be normal with early infections, intranasal parasites, or radiolucent foreign bodies. Also, no demonstrable radiographic changes may be evident in animals with apical tooth root abscesses if osteomyelitis is not present.

Following radiographic studies of the skull, a comprehensive visual examination of the oral cavity should be performed with the animal remaining under anesthesia. At this time it is also prudent to reevaluate symmetry of the face. A complete examination of the oral cavity should include evaluation of symmetry of the hard and soft palate and examination of the pharynx and nasopharynx. A dental mirror aids in visualization of the nasopharynx. The oral cavity should be inspected for the presence of oronasal fistulas. To complete the examination, a probe should be passed in the medial gingival sulcus of the upper canines and incisors to search for tooth root abscesses.

Endoscopic examination of the nasal cavity should only be done after obtaining radiographs of the skull. This is because hemorrhage created during rhinoscopy may obscure subtle radiographic lesions. Rhinoscopic procedures occasionally have to be aborted because excessive nasal discharge or hemorrhage can totally obscure visualization of intranasal structures. Suctioning of the nasal passages prior to rhinoscopy sometimes aids in clearing accumulated material.

The most economical instrument to view the nasal cavity is an otoscope speculum; however, one is limited to visualization of the rostral rhinarium only. Negative findings with this instrument may mislead the clinician, since neoplastic and fungal diseases are typically found in the caudal half of the nasal cavity. Both rhinoscopy and nasopharyngoscopy can easily be performed using a flexible fiberoptic bronchoscope. Although direct visualization and biopsy of the caudal nasal cavity is possible, this technique is limited to larger dogs because of the size of the instrument. We prefer to use a needle arthroscope or cystoscope. These instruments allow direct evaluation and biopsy of structures deep in the nasal cavity and can be used in cats and small dogs.

In many instances, the histologic or cytologic appearance of tissue specimens is essential for a final diagnosis. Tissue biopsies may be obtained directly using an endoscope or blindly using a piece of rigid polyethylene tubing (see Nasal Biopsy in Chapter 80). The blind approach is useful when excessive secretions or hemorrhage obscure direct visualization of the desired lesion. It also harvests tissue samples when proper endoscopic equipment is not available. A portion of the collected tissue specimens should be examined cytologically for neoplastic changes or the presence of fungal elements. A sample of tissue should also be submitted for fungal culture whenever mycotic rhinitis is a possibility. Finally, larger pieces of tissue should be sent for histopathologic evaluation.

Fluid and debris collected during a nasal flush may also be submitted for cytologic evaluation and bacterial and fungal culture. Tissue removed either directly or blindly from the suspected lesion yields diagnostic information superior to that obtained from a nasal flush.

The interpretation of culture results from tissue recovered form the nose often causes considerable confusion. The nose normally is home to a wide variety of microorganisms, which are present as mixed bacterial and fungal populations. The vast majority (if not all) of cases of bacterial rhinitis are secondary to some underlying cause. Fungal cultures tend to be more rewarding than bacterial cultures. A positive fungal culture in a symptomatic animal usually is significant. Caution is required in the interpretation of positive fungal cultures, however. For example, *Aspergillus* sp and *Penicillium* sp are present in 30% to 40% of normal dogs and dogs with nasal tumors. On the other hand, failure to isolate a fungal organism from an animal with mycotic rhinitis may be the result of poor sampling technique, bacterial overgrowth, or poor culture technique.

The interpretation of fungal serology (see Chapter 79) may be equally as confusing. A positive test indicates that the patient's concentration of serum antibody is consistent with, but not diagnostic for, infection. False-negative tests are rare with the agar gel immunodiffusion assay for aspergillosis or penicilliosis, but positive test results will occur in animals with nasal neoplasia and concurrent fungal infection. It is recommended that confirmation be made of positive serologic tests in those patients with supporting clinical signs. This is accomplished by identification of the organism by culture, cytology, or biopsy, and by definitively ruling out any underlying (predisposing) disease, such as neoplasia.

Other Diagnostic Procedures

Surgical exploration of the nose is occasionally required when other attempts to discover a diagnosis fail. Exploratory rhinotomy affords good visualization of the nasal cavity and the opportunity to remove in toto the causative factor. Postoperative complications may result (subcutaneous emphysema, epistaxis, chronic nasal discharge), so careful planning and good communication with the client is required.

Computed tomography affords a detailed view of the nasal cavity with higher resolution and sensitivity than that possible with routine diagnostic imaging techniques. We believe that animals with nasal neoplasia should have a computed tomographic scan of the nasal cavity so that the full extent of disease is known prior to surgical debulking and radiation therapy.

MANAGEMENT

Acute Causes of Nasal Discharge

Acute Inflammatory Disease

Acute inflammatory rhinitis usually causes a serous nasal discharge and is often the result of viral upper respiratory infections. In cats, feline herpesvirus and feline calicivirus are most important. Canine distemper virus, canine adenoviruses (types 1 and 2), and canine parainfluenza virus are the most common causes of acute inflammatory rhinitis in dogs. Primary bacterial infection is an extremely rare cause of acute inflammatory rhinitis. Secondary bacterial rhinitis, characterized clinically by a purulent nasal discharge, commonly follows primary viral upper respiratory infections.

Treatment is largely symptomatic. Antibiotics are recommended for the treatment of secondary bacterial rhinitis. Occasionally animals will develop chronic rhinitis following an episode of acute rhinitis. This is a particularly bothersome sequela in many cats following infection with the feline upper respiratory disease complex (see Feline Chronic Viral Upper Respiratory Disease, below).

Epistaxis

Epistaxis commonly results from trauma, intranasal foreign bodies, and bleeding disorders. Erosive disorders, such as intranasal tumors or mycotic rhinitis, typically present with the history of intermittent epistaxis or blood-tinged discharges.

Foreign Bodies

Intranasal foreign bodies (grass awns, foxtails, porcupine quills) are a common problem in dogs, but are rarely seen in cats. The well-developed sense of smell of dogs in conjunction with their inherent curiosity results in foreign bodies being inhaled or lodged in the nasal cavity. Occasionally, sadistic individuals may place foreign objects (*e.g.*, crayons, pencils) or fire missiles into the nose of animals. Pawing at the face and sneezing are the usual clinical signs associated with intranasal foreign bodies. Epistaxis may also be seen. Epistaxis is often due to sneezing or may be a direct result of vascular damage by the foreign body.

Radiographs of the nose can help localize radiodense objects. The majority of foreign bodies, however, are radiolucent and not visible on radiographs. Rhinoscopy is generally required to visualize and remove the foreign body. Vigorous nasal flushing may also be attempted to dislodge a foreign object.

Chronic nasal discharge may result if removal of the offending object is not entirely successful. Surgical exploration and curettage of the nasal cavity may be needed.

Trauma

Acute hemorrhagic nasal discharge most often follows nasal trauma due to blunt injuries (automobile accidents or collision with fixed objects) or penetrating injuries (bullets, impalement by a stick, dog fights). Following such injuries, the skull and oral cavity should be examined carefully for displacement fractures or malalignment of facial bones. Animals with evidence of concurrent skull trauma should be observed closely for the development of abnormal neurologic signs.

Animals with epistaxis following traumatic nasal injuries should receive cage rest and close observation. Narcotic analgesics may be required to calm nervous or excitable patients unwilling to lie still. The head of the animal should be kept low to prevent aspiration of blood. The formation of blood clots in the nasal passages can result in varying degrees of upper airway obstruction. Animals exhibiting anxiety because of profound upper airway obstruction may also benefit from the administration of narcotic analgesics. The use of external ice packs to slow hemorrhage is discouraged because they often add to patient distress. Packing of the external nares to stop blood loss is also discouraged. This procedure merely diverts blood to the internal nares. Blood loss will continue, although it will not be evident externally.

Patients with severe nasal hemorrhage require crystalloid fluid replacement therapy and, occasionally, whole blood transfusions. Epinephrine 1 : 100,000 or cocaine 4% may be dripped into the nose. These drugs cause vasoconstriction and often help control hemorrhage. Cocaine has the added advantage of local anesthetic properties, which may help control local pain. Occasionally, general anesthesia is required to pack the entire nose (internal and external nares) in order to stop hemorrhage. The packing material should remain in place for at least 24 hours before attempting removal. Surgical exploration of the nose to stop uncontrollable hemorrhage is rarely required. Damaged turbinates and bone fragments should be removed.

The potential long-term sequella following traumatic injuries to the nose include bacterial or mycotic osteomyelitis, sequestra formation, sinusitis, and frontal mucocele formation. Any animal presented with chronic nasal discharge and a history of prior nasal trauma should be carefully evaluated for these complications.

Chronic Causes of Nasal Discharge

Allergic Rhinitis

Allergic rhinitis is probably an unusual (or overlooked) disorder in dogs and cats. Typically, allergic rhinitis is a type I hypersensitivity reaction to inhaled allergens by sensitized individuals. Examination of tissues or secretions from these patients will reveal large numbers of eosinophils and few neutrophils. The nasal discharge is usually serous to mucoid. Clinical signs are generally seasonal unless exposure to the inciting agent is year-round (*e.g.*, house dusts or molds). Prolonged exposure to the inciting agent may result in chronic nasal discharge, epithelial hyperplasia, and submucosal lymphocytic and plasmacytic infiltration.

Treatment ideally would be avoidance of the offending allergen; however, this is rarely possible. Prednisolone, at an oral dose of 0.25 to 0.5 mg/kg once daily, every other day, or every third day, may be effective during the allergy season. Antihistamines may also be beneficial in reducing the amount of nasal discharge (see Appendices I and II). Animals with lymphoplasmacytic rhinitis require more aggressive therapy (see Lymphoplasmacytic Rhinitis, below).

Bacterial Rhinitis

As a rule, bacterial infections of the nose are secondary to some primary lesion. Primary bacterial rhinitis is very rare and is considered unlikely when two or more bacteria are isolated concurrently or a single species is isolated in low numbers from the nose.

A common mistake in the treatment of a purulent discharge is to overlook the possibility of a primary lesion and to direct therapy solely at the bacteria recovered from the discharge. Antibiotics typically will only resolve a purulent discharge as long as the patient is receiving the drug. In most instances, the discharge will recur 2 to 3 days after discontinuing therapy. Treatment should be directed mainly at the primary condition. While initiating correction of the underlying problem, however, treatment should also be directed at the secondary bacterial infection. This is because chronic bacterial infection of the upper respiratory tract may be a principal event in the pathogenesis of bacterial pulmonary infections.

Chronic Inflammatory Rhinitis (Sinusitis)

Chronic inflammatory rhinosinusitis is a diagnostic and therapeutic challenge. Nasal discharge is often of many months to years duration in these animals. Often the discharge is unilateral initially and later becomes bilateral. At the time of presentation, the discharge has often changed character from serous or mucoid to purulent and sanguineous. Tonsillitis or pharyngitis may be present secondary to chronic postnasal drainage. Many of these animals have histories of transient responsiveness to antibiotics, with signs that relapse after discontinuation of therapy.

Often no precipitating cause or unusual circumstance that might be associated with the development of clinical signs is found. Nonetheless, owners should be questioned thoroughly regarding past events that may give a clue to the underlying cause of the chronic discharge. In all patients it is strongly advised that a complete evaluation be done relatively early in the course of disease. A thorough evaluation of the nasal cavity is recommended prior to administration of a wide range of symptomatic treatments because certain intranasal disorders, such as mycotic or neoplastic disease, are much easier to manage early in the course of disease. Some animals with chronic nasal discharge require several complete evaluations before an underlying cause is found. Owners must be made aware of the difficulty in finding the underlying cause in some animals so that they do not become overly hopeful that a quick cure will be found early in the course of disease.

The diagnostic approach to patients with chronic inflammatory rhinitis is the same as that outlined earlier for nasal discharge in general. High-quality radiographs of the nose and paranasal sinuses are extremely important in the workup of these patients. Turbinate destruction is not seen until the disease is advanced, and is most commonly associated with fungal disease or neoplasia. Radiographic evidence of turbinate destruction, erosion of the vomer bone, and increased density of the sinuses is characteristic of intranasal tumors rather than fungal disease. Malalignment of facial bones or excessive new bone formation may be sequellae of a traumatic injury. The upper dental arcade should be carefully examined for evidence of osteomyelitis secondary to an apical abcess. Unfortunately, often all that may be found is a nonspecific increased density of the nasal cavities due to excessive secretions and hyperplasia of the nasal mucosa. We recommend that nasal radiographs and rhinoscopy be repeated 3 months later if the initial studies are nondiagnostic and the nasal discharge is not resolved. If the problem persists after the second attempt to obtain a diagnosis noninvasively, an exploratory rhinotomy should be considered.

The management of chronic nasal discharge when no underlying cause can be found is difficult. Broad-spectrum antibiotics, such as tetracycline, chloramphenicol, or trimethoprim-sulfa, are given for a minimum of 4 to 6 weeks. Topical antibiotics have no advantage over oral preparations. Nasal decongestants may afford some relief to patients with copious discharges. α-Adrenergics, such as phenylephrine, cause arteriolar constriction of mucosal vessels and reduce congestion and edema by reducing arteriolar blood flow. Oral decongestants, such as phenylpropanolamine, may also reduce nasal discharge. Rebound congestion is seen after prolonged use of these drugs, but may be minimized by using them for only 3 to 4 days at a time.

Corticosteroids should probably be used only when the cause of the chronic nasal discharge has an allergic basis. Long-term use can predispose to mycotic rhinitis or allow existing mycotic rhinitis to disseminate. In cats, corticosteroids may cause shedding of virus in carrier cats with chronic viral upper respiratory disease (see below).

An aggressive therapeutic nasal flush with 10 to 20 ml of povidone–iodine solution (Betadine) diluted 1 : 10 with isotonic saline may benefit some patients. This should be done with the animal under anesthesia and only after all diagnostic procedures have been completed. The discharge may return, however, several months following treatment.

Surgical exploration of the nasal cavity is warranted when intranasal disease is not amenable to medical management. It may also be used as a diagnostic procedure when repeated attempts at defining an underlying cause by noninvasive means have failed.

Feline Chronic Viral Upper Respiratory Disease

Feline chronic upper respiratory disease is clinically characterized by signs associated with chronic rhinosinusitis, and probably results from persistent viral infection. This disease is usually diagnosed after excluding other causes of chronic rhinosinusitis in cats. Also, chronic upper respiratory disease may be the only external evidence of immunosuppression secondary to feline leukemia virus or feline immunodeficiency virus infection. Up to 80% of cats with acute upper respiratory tract disease become carriers of the causative viruses. Any number of these cats can subsequently go on to show chronic to intermittent respiratory signs. Some cats may have intermittent severe attacks of rhinosinusitis, whereas other cats may have spontaneous remission of signs after many months of illness.

One of the common upper respiratory viruses in cats, feline herpesvirus, has an affinity for sites of osteogenesis. In some severely affected cats this virus may cause necrosis and bone destruction of nasal turbinates. This may be one explanation for the chronic rhinosinusitis observed in some cats that have recovered from the acute phase of upper respiratory disease. Also, despite elimination of the viral infection, clinical signs may persist because of mucosal damage and development of a secondary bacterial infection.

Treatment is largely symptomatic. Broad-spectrum antibiotics, such as ampicillin or trimethoprim-sulfa are indicated because secondary bacterial rhinosinusitis is a common complicating factor in these cats. Chloramphenicol or tylosin are sometimes preferred because of their extended spectrum of activity against chlamydiae and *Mycoplasma* organisms. Antibiotics should be continued for at least 4 to 6 weeks. A response to antibiotic therapy should be seen within 3 to 5 days of starting treatment.

Decongestants are beneficial in reducing the amount of nasal discharge. Because a reduction in the amount of nasal discharge often improves the sense of smell, some cats with chronic rhinosinusitis and partial anorexia may have an improved appetite when given nasal decongestants. One drop of 0.25% phenylephrine hydrochloride (Neo-Synephrine) or similar preparations is given intranasally every 4 to 6 hours. By altering nostrils every 3 days, the effects of rebound congestion may be avoided. Phenylpropanolamine is an oral decongestant that is also useful in reducing the amount of nasal discharge in some cats (see Appendices I and II).

Humidification of the air increases moisture content of the secretions and facilitates their movement out of the nasal passages. An affected cat may be kept in the bathroom while a hot shower is running. Effective therapy requires a minimum of 15- to 30-minute treatments 3 to 4 times daily. An alternative is instilling a drop of normal saline in each nostril 4 to 6 times daily to decrease the viscosity and increase the outward movement of nasal secretions.

Corticosteroids should be avoided unless absolutely needed. These drugs may mask underlying neoplasia or exacerbate fungal disease if a thorough workup is not done prior to treatment. In addition to reducing the cat's ability to fight infective processes, virus carriers may start shedding virus particles during corticosteroid therapy. The short-term use of corticosteroids, however, may be beneficial to reduce inflammation.

The most important aspect in the management of these cats is good nursing care. They need to be kept in a warm, draft-free environment. Cleaning of the face several times daily often seemingly makes these cats feel better. Forced feeding or heating of the food to increase its odor is often required in severely affected cats.

Lymphoplasmacytic Rhinitis

Lymphoplasmacytic rhinitis is an uncommon cause of chronic nasal disease in dogs. Clinical signs are similar to those with chronic infectious rhinitis and nasal neoplasia. This disease is characterized by a prominent infiltration of the nasal mucosa and submucosa by lymphocytes and plasma cells. The disease appears to represent an immune-mediated process. Lymphoplasmacytic rhinitis differs from type I hypersensitivity allergic rhinitis in that infiltration of the nasal mucosa with eosinophils is not seen. It may represent a chronic form of allergic rhinitis (see Allergic Rhinitis, above).

Antibiotics typically fail to cause resolution of clinical signs. Corticosteroids appear to be the treatment of choice. A good response is generally seen to prednisolone at an oral dose of 2 mg/kg once daily for 2 weeks. Once a response is seen, the dosage of prednisolone should be gradually tapered to the lowest amount required to maintain remission of clinical signs. Therapy is generally continued for 6 weeks, although occasionally dogs require treatment for a full year. Because aspergillosis may occasionally be associated with a lymphoplasmacytic infiltrate of the nasal mucosa, one must be certain that underlying fungal disease is not present when initiating long-term corticosteroid therapy.

Mycotic Rhinitis

Aspergillosis and penicilliosis are the most common causes of mycotic rhinitis in dogs. Cryptococcosis is the most common cause in cats. The exact pathogenesis of infection with *Aspergillus* sp or *Penicillium* sp is not completely understood in the dog. In humans, immunocompromised patients are most often affected. Most dogs with infection appear otherwise healthy. Infection in the dog may be secondary to damage to the turbinates, which allows these opportunistic fungi to invade bone. In some dogs, underlying factors such as foreign bodies or neoplasia have been associated with mycotic rhinitis. In cats, a deficiency in the immune system is a prerequisite to infection with *Cryptococcus neoformans*. Consequently, most cats with nasal cryptococcosis are feline leukemia virus or feline immunodeficiency virus positive. Cell-mediated immunity is diminished in cats infected with feline leukemia virus.

The destructive rhinitis associated with nasal aspergillosis and penicilliosis occurs in younger dogs than that typically associated with intranasal tumors. Tumor may easily be differentiated from mycotic rhinitis on the basis of clinical signs if facial deformity or exophthalmus is present. Diagnosis is based on clinical signs supported by tissue or culture identification of fungal elements. Nasal radiographs will reveal destruction of turbinates with advanced mycotic rhinitis (Fig. 27-2). Fungal plaques may be directly visualized by rhinoscopy. Tissue from sites of active disease should be submitted for culture and histopathology. In cats with nasal cryptococcosis, cytologic evaluation of impression smears or aspirates from the site of disease will often reveal characteristic fungal elements. Serologic testing may support a diagnosis of mycotic rhinitis, although positive test results should always be confirmed with unequivocal identification of fungal elements in tissue samples.

Medical treatment of nasal aspergillosis and penicilliosis should be attempted first unless life-threatening complications requiring surgical intervention are deemed likely. One approach to therapy begins with a therapeutic nasal flush using 10 to 20 ml of povidone–iodine solution

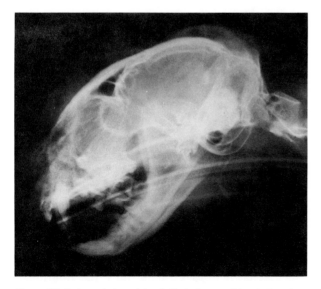

Figure 27–2 *Lateral view of the skull of a 3-year-old male American shorthair cat with severe disfigurement of the rostral nasal region. Notice the marked soft-tissue swelling, bone destruction, and osteolysis. These radiographic changes are compatible with either fungal or neoplastic processes. The final diagnosis was nasal cryptococcosis.*

diluted 1 : 10 with saline. This is followed with the oral administration of thiabendazole at an oral dose of 20 mg/kg, divided, given twice daily for 6 weeks. Anorexia, vomiting, and diarrhea are common side-effects of thiabendazole. Even though thiabendazole is currently the treatment of choice, its overall success in complete cure of patients with nasal aspergillosis and penicilliosis is not particularly encouraging. Alternative systemic medications include amphotericin B, nystatin, flucytosine, sodium iodide, and ketoconazole; however, their efficacy in the treatment of nasal aspergillosis or penicilliosis is not known at this time. Enilconazole, an imidazole similar to ketoconazole, appears very promising for the treatment of nasal aspergillosis; nevertheless, this drug is not currently available. In severe cases, surgical curettage of the nasal cavity and paranasal sinuses is recommended to remove the unhealthy tissue. Drains are then placed into the frontal sinuses to allow for daily flushing of the nasal cavities with either diluted povidone–iodine solution or a suspension of thiabendazole at 20 mg/kg. In general, the prognosis for cure for patients with nasal aspergillosis or penicilliosis is fair to poor with treatment.

In cats, amphotericin B or flucytosine, alone or in combination, is used for the treatment of nasal cryptococcosis. It is recommended, however, that flucytosine not be used as the sole agent because resistance rapidly develops to this drug. Amphotericin B is given at an intravenous dose of 0.5 mg/kg daily or 1 mg/kg every other day for a total cumulative dosage of 7.5 to 8.5 mg/kg. Nephrotoxicity and hypokalemia are potential side-effects of this drug; therefore, it is advisable to monitor serum urea nitrogen, creatinine, and potassium regularly during the course of treatment. The oral dose for flucytosine is 75 mg/kg twice daily, for a total of 6 weeks. The dosage of amphotericin B can be reduced by 50% if flucytosine is given simultaneously. This may reduce the occurrence of nephrotoxicity associated with amphotericin B therapy. Ketoconazole alone or in combination with flucytosine may also be tried for the treatment of cryptococcosis. This drug is given at an oral dose of 10 mg/kg, twice daily for a minimum of 4 to 6 months. The dosage for ketoconazole is doubled when meningitis is present.

The prognosis for cure for cats with nasal cryptococcosis treated with amphotericin B or ketoconazole combined with flucytosine is fair to good. The prognosis and success rate for cats treated with ketoconazole alone is not clear at this time.

Nasopharyngeal Polyps

Nasopharyngeal polyps are uncommon growths of uncertain etiology that arise from the middle ear in cats. They are seen most often in cats between 6 months and 5 years of age. The polyps enter the nasopharynx by way of the eustachian tube. Treatment is accomplished by surgical removal of the entire polyp and its base.

Neoplasia

Of all domestic animals, dogs, followed by cats, have the highest incidence of tumors of the nose and paranasal sinuses. Some authors indicate that dolichocephalic breeds of dogs have a higher risk than brachycephalic breeds; however, this is not universally agreed on. Most intranasal tumors are malignant. Metastasis occurs in 10% of the cases and is generally seen in the late stages of disease. Typical sites for metastasis are the regional lymph nodes, lung, and brain (through direct extension through the cribiform plate).

The clinical signs associated with nasal tumors mimic those seen with chronic rhinitis and mycotic rhinitis. Radiographic differentiation of neoplastic disease from mycotic rhinitis can be difficult (Fig. 27-3; see Fig. 27-2). Definitive diagnosis requires cytologic or histologic evaluation. Treatment is best approached with a combination of surgical debulking followed by radiation therapy. Prior to surgical debulking, a computed tomographic scan is strongly recommended to evaluate the total extent of disease in the nasal cavity and to determine whether extension into the cranial vault has occurred. Unless the disease is caught early and is amenable to total surgical excision, cures are unusual. The overall prognosis is poor if untreated, with usual survival times of 36 months from the time of diagnosis. The longest median survival times (8–13 months) are in those patients undergoing cytoreductive therapy fol-

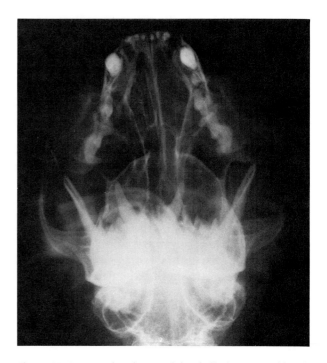

Figure 27–3 *Ventrodorsal view of the skull of a 4-year-old male Manx cat presented with the chief complaint of a chronic unilateral nasal discharge from the left nostril for 9 months. The volume of discharge was reported to decrease with antibiotic therapy. Notice the increased water density and the loss of fine bony detail within the left nasal cavity as compared to the right side. The final diagnosis was primary nasal lymphosarcoma.*

lowed by soft deep radiation (cesium or orthovoltage) treatment.

PATIENT MONITORING

The need for patient follow-up is largely dependent on the cause of the nasal discharge. In those cases in which the underlying cause can be corrected, a rapid resolution of the problem should follow. Patients with chronic nasal discharge and those in which an underlying cause for the problem cannot be found should be evaluated occasionally for changes in the nature or character of the discharge or for clinical signs that might give a clue to the underlying cause. Periodically repeating laboratory work and nasal radiographs, cytologies, and biopsies is also encouraged in patients with chronic nasal discharges of undetermined etiology.

ADDITIONAL READING

Adams WM, Withrow SJ, Walshaw R et al. Radiotherapy of malignant nasal tumors in 67 dogs. J Am Vet Med Assoc 1987; 191:311.

Barsanti JA. Cryptococcosis. In: Greene CG, ed. Clinical microbiology and infectious diseases of the dog and cat. Philadelphia: WB Saunders, 1984: 700.

Barsanti JA. Opportunistic fungal infections. In: Greene CG, ed. Clinical microbiology and infectious diseases of the dog and cat. Philadelphia: WB Saunders, 1984: 728.

Beck ER, Withrow SJ. Tumors of the canine nasal cavity. Vet Clin North Am [Small Anim Pract] 1985; 15:521.

Bradley RL. Selected oral, pharyngeal, and upper respiratory conditions in the cat: Oral tumors, nasopharyngeal and middle ear polyps, and chronic rhinitis and sinusitis. Vet Clin North Am [Small Anim Pract] 1984; 14:1173.

Burgener DC, Slocombe RF, Zerbe CA. Lymphoplasmacytic rhinitis in five dogs. Journal of the American Animal Hospital Association 1987; 23:565.

Ford RB. Sneezing and nasal discharge. In: Ford RB, ed. Clinical signs and diagnosis in small animal practice. New York: Churchill Livingstone, 1988: 189.

Harvey CE. Nasal aspergillosis and penicilliosis in dogs: Results of treatment with thiabendazole. J Am Vet Med Assoc 1984; 184:48.

Harvey CE, O'Brian JA. Nasal aspergillosis–penicilliosis. In: Kirk RW, ed. Current veterinary therapy VIII. Philadelphia: WB Saunders, 1983: 236.

Hawkins EC. Chronic viral upper respiratory disease in cats: Differential diagnosis and management. Compendium of Continuing Education 1988; 10:1003.

Norris AM, Laing EJ. Diseases of the nose and sinuses. Vet Clin North Am [Small Anim Pract] 1985; 15:865.

Parker NR, Binnington AG. Nasopharngeal polyps in cats: Three case reports and a review of the literature. Journal of the American Animal Hospital Association 1985; 21:473.

Rudd RG, Richardson DC. A diagnostic and therapeutic approach to nasal disease in dogs. Compendium of Continuing Education 1985; 7:103.

Ticer JW. Radiographic techniques in small animal practice. Philadelphia: WB Saunders, 1975.

Withrow SJ, Susaneck SJ, Macy DW et al. Aspiration and punch biopsy techniques for nasal tumors. Journal of the American Animal Hospital Association 1985; 21:551.

CHRONIC BRONCHITIS
Ned F. Kuehn, Philip Roudebush

Chronic bronchitis is essentially an incurable disease of insidious onset, usually seen in middle-aged or older small breeds of dogs. Pathologic changes compatible with chronic bronchitis may be seen in some cats with chronic feline asthma (see Chapter 30). This chapter will discuss chronic bronchitis in the dog only.

Chronic bronchitis is characterized clinically by a chronic, persistent cough, and pathologically by chronic inflammation of pulmonary airways as well as mucus hypersecretion. The cough is usually productive, with gagging and the production of sputum.

Chronic bronchitis in humans is defined as a condition identified with chronic or recurrent excessive mucus secretion in the bronchial tree, occurring on most days for at least 3 months of the year during at least 2 years. The diagnosis is made in the absence of other specific pulmonary diseases (*e.g.*, cancer, pneumonia, tuberculosis).

Because of their shorter lifespan, the definition is modified somewhat for dogs. Chronic bronchitis in dogs is defined as a condition of chronic or recurrent excessive mucus production in the bronchial tree for at least 2 consecutive months in the preceding year, and manifested clinically by chronic coughing. As in humans, the cause of the chronic hypersecretion of bronchial mucus is not attributable to other lung disease. Therefore, the diagnosis of chronic bronchitis requires fulfill-

ment of three major criteria: chronic cough, evidence of excessive mucus or mucopus (mucopurulent matter) hypersecretion, and exclusion of other chronic respiratory diseases (*e.g.*, pulmonary neoplasia, parasitism, fungal pneumonia).

CAUSES

The causes for chronic bronchitis in the dog are poorly understood. The major difficulty in determining the cause of chronic bronchitis is that the disease is detectable only in its advanced stages. This is largely because chronic bronchitis has an insidious onset and lengthy pathogenesis, and because the diagnosis is largely based on a descriptive clinical definition.

The three etiologic factors in humans that are considered most important for the hypersecretion of mucus in the bronchial tree are smoking, atmospheric pollution, and infection. Table 28-1 lists several possible causes for chronic bronchitis in dogs.

PATHOPHYSIOLOGY

Chronic bronchitis is characterized pathologically by excessive viscid mucus or mucopus in the tracheobronchial tree. The viscid mucus con-

397

Table 28–1 *Possible Causes for Chronic Bronchitis in Dogs*

Passive smoking (chronic exposure to smoke in poorly ventilated, confined spaces)
Atmospheric Pollution (chronic exposure to sulfur dioxide [SO_2], a common atmospheric pollutant, causes mucus hypersecretion, bronchial mucus gland hypertrophy, bronchiectasis, and emphysema in dogs.)
    Exposure to air pollution increases the incidence of infections in humans.
Respiratory tract infections
    In humans, childhood lower respiratory tract infections increase the incidence of chronic cough in adults.
     Possible infectious agents in dogs:
        Canine distemper virus
        Adenovirus (Types 1 and 2)
        Herpesvirus
        Bordetella bronchoseptica
        Parasites
           Filaroides milksi
           Filaroides herthi
           Crenosoma vulpis
           Capillaria aerophilia
Genetic factors
    Alpha$_1$-antitrypsin deficiency
Bronchiectasis
Allergic (hypersensitivity) lung diseases

tains a large number of neutrophils and macrophages admixed with varying amounts of cellular debris and edematous fluid. Smaller bronchi are often occluded by thick mucus plugs. The bronchial mucosa is usually hyperemic, thickened, and edematous. Polypoid proliferations often project from the mucosa into the bronchial lumen. Patchy pneumonia is a complicating factor in about one quarter of affected dogs. Emphysema is a much less important lesion in the dog than in humans, and is primarily confined to the edges of the lung lobes.

Fibrosis, edema, and cellular infiltration of the lamina propria by lymphocytes, plasma cells, macrophages, and neutrophils is seen histopathologically. A significant proportion of the tracheobronchial wall is occupied by mucus glands. There is an increase in both size and number (hypertrophy) of mucus glands, in addition to an overall increase (hyperplasia) in epithelial goblet cells. Focal ulceration, loss of cilia, and squamous metaplasia of the bronchial epithelium is also found.

Extremely severe cases may show medial hypertrophy of the small pulmonary arteries and muscularization of the pulmonary arterioles. These changes are associated with right ventricular hypertrophy secondary to chronic hypoxic pulmonary hypertension.

It is generally accepted that the development of chronic bronchitis is the result of a vicious cycle of airway damage and patient response. The airways are protected in healthy dogs by a set of pulmonary defense mechanisms, including normal ciliary action, normal quantity and quality of mucus, efficient collateral ventilation, and an efficient cough mechanism. Persistent infection or chronic inhalation of airborne irritants can result in sustained injury to the bronchial epithelium. This will stimulate metaplastic transformation of the ciliary epithelium, hyperplasia and hypertrophy of mucus-secreting glands and cells, and hyperemia and cellular infiltration of the bronchial mucosa. Chronic saccular dilatation and destruction of the walls of bronchi and bronchioles (bronchiectasis) may result from long-standing airway inflammation. Once bronchiectatic airway changes occur, they are irreversible. Furthermore, because all of these changes impede normal defense mechanisms, bacterial colonization of the airways frequently results.

Toy breeds of dogs often develop weakness of the cartilaginous rings of the trachea and major bronchi. This results in tracheobronchial collapse during expiration and during coughing (see Chapter 14). Collapse of the major airways impedes expiratory airflow and efficient clearance of mucus from the bronchial tree, factors that repeatedly exacerbate the clinical condition of patients with chronic bronchitis.

Chronic insult to the bronchial epithelium not only contributes to decreased efficiency of normal pulmonary defense mechanisms, but also promotes the development of functional obstruction to intrapulmonary gas flow. Airway diameter is reduced in chronic bronchitis by any combination of the following mechanisms:

Edema and cellular infiltration of airway walls
Copious quantities of tenacious intraluminal mucus
Localized endobronchial narrowing associated with fibrosis of the lamina propria and polypoid proliferations of the mucosa
Spasticity of bronchial smooth muscles, causing reactive airway narrowing (may not be as significant in dogs as compared to humans)
Collapse of larger bronchi associated with weaken-

ing of the bronchial walls subsequent to chronic inflammatory activity
Plugging of smaller airways by tenacious mucus
Obliteration of bronchioles as a result of inflammatory activity

Emphysema develops following flooding of the alveoli with mucus.

The most common functional sequella in chronic bronchitis is the development of chronic airflow obstruction, which is generally referred to as *chronic obstructive pulmonary disease* (COPD). Chronic obstructive pulmonary disease is an insidious condition characterized by minimally reversible airflow obstruction, and cannot be explained by any specific or infiltrative lung disease. The minimal reversibility of COPD differentiates it from asthma (see Chapter 30), which is a disease of significant reversibility of airflow obstruction. The small peripheral airways are the predominant sites of irreversible airflow obstruction. The persistent airway inflammation associated with chronic bronchitis is responsible for the development of refractory airflow obstruction.

The small airways normally contribute only a small percentage of total airway resistance, because the tremendous number of small airways dramatically increases the total cross-sectional area for gas flow. Disease of the small airways, therefore, must be diffuse and extensive before airway resistance is enhanced sufficiently to bring about clinical signs. Dogs normally have extensive interconnections between alveoli and adjacent respiratory bronchioles. Collateral ventilation through these channels allows alveoli primarily served by obstructed bronchioles to continue to be ventilated. One can therefore appreciate that small airway disease in the dog must be remarkably extensive before clinical signs are observed.

In humans, the diagnosis of COPD relies on quantitative documentation of airflow obstruction by pulmonary function testing. Enhanced airway resistance and a decline in maximum expiratory airflow rate are characteristic findings for COPD. Because pulmonary function testing is not widely available in veterinary medicine, the diagnosis of COPD is usually determined on the basis of clinical and radiographic findings. Extensive obstruction of small airways primarily manifests clinically as expiratory dyspnea (see Chapter 14). Gas trapping in COPD occurs with premature closure of the small airways during expiration. In advanced cases, gas trapping may occur during quiet breathing, resulting in a barrel-chested appearance of some patients with COPD. Hyperinflation of the lung fields is seen radiographically.

Patients with advanced chronic bronchitis and COPD develop maldistribution of ventilation in relation to blood flow through the lung. This ventilation–perfusion inequality results because ventilation is universally reduced within the lung in relationship to blood flow. Chronic hypoxemia stimulates erythropoiesis, and mild to moderate erythrocytosis (secondary polycythemia) results. The overall increase in airway resistance associated with advanced chronic bronchitis increases the work of breathing and intensifies the hypoxemic state. Vasoconstriction of the pulmonary arteries occurs in response to hypoxemia. This pulmonary hypoxic vasoconstrictor response causes an increase in pulmonary vascular resistance and pulmonary artery pressure. Chronic pulmonary hypertension may lead to right ventricular failure (cor pulmonale).

CLINICAL SIGNS

Chronic bronchitis is most frequently seen in middle-aged (5 years) and older smaller breeds of dogs (*e.g.*, terriers, poodles, cocker spaniels). The clinical signs usually seen in patients with chronic bronchitis include:

Persistent, intractable, productive cough with gagging and production of sputum (coughed up sputum may be swallowed and thus difficult to document)
Unproductive, resonant, harsh, hacking cough during the day and productive cough during the evening or early morning hours
Paroxysmal cough precipitated by exercise or excitement
Obesity
Cyanosis, collapse, exhaustion, and exercise intolerance
Pronounced sinus arrhythmia
Expiratory dyspnea
Varying periods of remission followed by exacerbation of coughing (exacerbations may be in association with changes in weather—particularly cold weather)

Systemic signs of illness that may be seen during severe exacerbations or episodes of bronchopneumonia

DIAGNOSTIC APPROACH

The clinical diagnosis of chronic bronchitis requires fulfillment of three major criteria:

1. Chronic cough on most days for at least 2 consecutive months during the preceding year
2. Evidence of excessive mucus or mucopus hypersecretion
3. Exclusion of other chronic respiratory diseases

The first two criteria may easily be established with a thorough and accurate history. The third criteria is established only after an exhaustive examination for other causes of chronic cough and dyspnea. The most important differential diagnoses that must be ruled out are cardiac diseases (mostly chronic mitral regurgitation), chronic pneumonia, pulmonary neoplasia, foreign body bronchitis, dirofilariasis, pulmonary parasites, and fungal pneumonia.

The physical examination may not contribute significantly to the patient evaluation or may reveal evidence of systemic illness (*e.g.*, pneumonia). Diligent auscultation of the chest is important, since cardiac diseases (*e.g.*, chronic mitral regurgitation, cor pulmonale) or pulmonary diseases (*e.g.*, tracheal collapse, pneumonia) are often present as coexisting problems or secondary complications in patients with chronic bronchitis. Lung sounds may be normal or abnormal, depending on the degree of airway involvement. Paninspiratory crackles and expiratory wheezes are the most commonly heard adventitious (abnormal) breath sounds auscultated in patients with chronic bronchitis. In those dogs with coexisting collapse of the intrathoracic trachea, an end-expiratory snap (click) may be heard during coughing or forced expiratory efforts. Nevertheless, it must be stressed that many dogs with COPD have normal auscultatory findings.

Dogs with severe obstructive lung disease also may show evidence of hyperinflation (barrel-chested appearance), pronounced expiratory effort, and a prolonged expiratory phase of respiration.

Laboratory assessment of patients with chronic bronchitis is summarized in Table 28-2. A complete blood count, serum biochemistry profile, and urinalysis are indicated if systemic disease is suspected. In dogs with only respiratory abnormalities, a complete blood count can be valuable, although it is often normal. An increased white blood cell count may indicate the presence of bronchopneumonia, or eosinophilia may suggest an allergic or parasitic pneumonitis. Blood gases may be indicated in some patients with severe obstructive lung disease. An increased $PaCO_2$ due to hypoventilation is a grave finding that denotes the onset of ventilatory failure associated with increased work in breathing. All dogs with chronic cough from heartworm-endemic areas should have a Knott test (or similar test) performed to rule out dirofilariasis (see Chapter 25). A fecal examination should also be performed to rule out lung parasites (see Chapter 33).

Good-quality thoracic radiographs are essential to rule out other causes of chronic cough or disclose complicating conditions (*e.g.*, pneumonia, bronchiectasis, cardiac disease). Thoracic radiographs from dogs with nonobstructive chronic bronchitis will usually show bronchial wall thickening or generalized increased airway-

Table 28–2 *Laboratory Assessment of Chronic Bronchitis*

Test	What to check for
Complete blood count	Neutrophilia Eosinophilia
Knott's test	Microfilaria
Fecal analyses	Parasitic ova and larvae
Arterial blood gas	Decreased PaO_2 Increased $PaCO_2$
Thoracic radiographs	Bronchial or bronchointerstitial lung pattern Bronchiectasis Bronchopneumonia Hyperlucency and enlargement of lung fields Cardiomegaly
Transtracheal wash	Degenerative neutrophils Bacteria (intracellular) Eosinophils

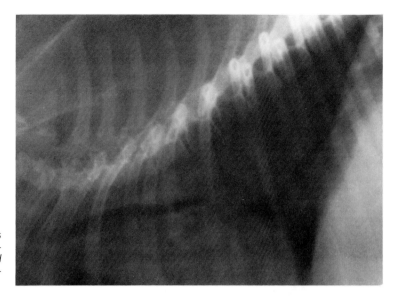

Figure 28–1 *Lateral thoracic radiograph shows close-up view of the dorsal lung fields from a 12-year-old female pug with chronic bronchitis and tracheal collapse. Notice the diffuse bronchointerstitial markings.*

oriented interstitial density (Fig. 28-1). Some dogs, however, may have normal-appearing lung fields. Bronchial wall thickening is recognized by "donut" shadows and "tram lines," which arise from end-on or longitudinal projections of thickened bronchial walls, respectively. Dogs with obstructive chronic bronchitis (chronic bronchitis and COPD) have radiographic evidence of pulmonary hyperinflation in addition to bronchial wall thickening and generalized increased airway-oriented interstitial density. Pulmonary hyperinflation is recognized by hyperlucency and enlargement of the lung fields and by caudal displacement and flattening of the diaphragm. Bronchopneumonia and bronchiectasis commonly arise as complications of chronic bronchitis. Superimposed bronchopneumonia is recognized radiographically by patchy alveolar infiltrates. Bronchiectasis is identified by saccular dilation of bronchi.

Transtracheal washing should be done in all dogs suspected of having chronic bronchitis, in order to collect material for cytology and microbiology (see Transtracheal Wash in Chapter 80). It is definitely indicated in any dog with chronic bronchitis and exacerbation of clinical signs. Cytologies typically reveal excess mucus with either normal bronchial epithelial cells or increased numbers of macrophages, goblet cells, neutrophils, lymphocytes, and hyperplastic epithe-lial cells. Purulent material characterized by increased neutrophils with engulfed bacteria indicates an associated bronchial infection or bronchopneumonia. The presence of large numbers of eosinophils suggests an allergic or parasitic etiology for the cough.

Culture of the fluid obtained during transtracheal washing is indicated to rule out secondary bacterial infections. It is essential that the material be obtained from the lower airways and not the pharynx in order for the culture results to be meaningful. The most common isolate is *Bordetella bronchiseptica*, although streptococci, *Pasturella, Escherichia coli, Pseudomonas,* and *Klebsiella* organisms have all been routinely isolated.

Bronchoscopy may be a useful procedure in helping to establish a clinical diagnosis of chronic bronchitis (see Tracheobronchoscopy in Chapter 80). Bronchocosopy is also valuable in obtaining representative samples from the deeper airways for cytology and culture. Routinely seen in the airways of chronic bronchitics during bronchoscopy is diffuse airway inflammation associated with hypersecretion and thick tenacious mucus, found in strands or small plaquelike accumulations. Mucus plugs may occasionally be visualized in small airways (Fig. 28-2). The airways typically appear roughened and hyperemic. Occasionally, polypoid or nodular proliferations are seen projecting into the bronchial lumen.

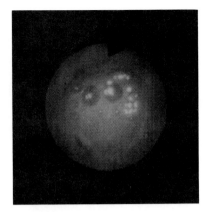

Figure 28–2 *Bronchoscopic view of a small airway containing a plug of mucopurulent material in a dog with chronic bronchitis.*

MANAGEMENT

The structural alterations in airway anatomy associated with chronic bronchitis are not readily reversible (if at all). The development of bronchiectasis, tracheobronchial collapse, and emphysema are permanent, irreversible changes that complicate the management of these patients. Because chronic bronchitis is essentially incurable, client education is very important. There should be an understanding by the client of the natural history of the problem and the goals of therapy.

Therapy is employed on the basis of an assessment of the nature and severity of each individual animal's problem(s). Basically, management of patients with chronic bronchitis is divided into five major categories:

1. Avoidance of exacerbating factors
2. Relief of airway obstruction
3. Control of cough
4. Control of infection
5. Oxygen therapy

Any one patient may or may not require therapy from all five categories.

Factors initiating chronic bronchitis are rarely identified. If exposure to the offending agent continues, cure is rarely achieved and control is simply more difficult. In the unusual situation in which cessation of exposure to the initiating factor(s) can be attained, there is a reduction in airway inflammatory changes and return of the airway anatomy toward normal. It is recommended that dogs with chronic bronchitis avoid exposure to inhaled irritants and reduce exposure to passive smoking. Events promoting stress or excitement should also be avoided to reduce the episodes of paroxysmal bouts of coughing. Exacerbation of clinical signs is most commonly seen during winter months, so during colder weather it is recommended that the owner maintain these animals in a warm, draft-free environment.

Relief of airway obstruction is generally accomplished by patient-specific combinations of four types of therapy:

1. Treatments that promote removal of accumulated airway secretions
2. Weight control
3. Bronchodilator medications
4. Anti-inflammatory medications

Methods should be attempted to facilitate removal of accumulated airway secretions in patients with chronic bronchitis. The continued accumulation of thick, tenacious airway secretions establishes an environment suited to microbial invasion. The inhalation of humidified air is beneficial in that it moistens the thick, tenacious bronchial secretions and thereby facilitates their movement from the airways. Aerosol therapy for hospitalized patients may be accomplished by placing a portable nebulizer in an enclosed cage with the animal. A more expensive alternative is the use of an oxygen cage with humidification and temperature controls. The animal should be allowed to inhale a bland aerosol (0.9% saline) for at least 15 to 30 minutes three to four times daily in order for therapy to be effective. Therapy may be accomplished at home by compelling the dog to breath aerosolized vapors from a portable nebulizer. Effective therapy at home requires a minimum of 15- to 30-minute treatments three to four times daily.

Light exercise after aerosol therapy assists in dislodging bronchial mucus and helps open small airways by promoting increased lung volumes associated with a standing posture. Chest physical therapy is also beneficial following aerosol therapy to aid in dislodging bronchial mucus.

Chest percussion (coupage) is achieved by using a cupped hand to generate vibrations on the patient's thoracic wall. This should be done three to four times daily for 5 to 10 minutes per session. The success of treatment is judged by the induction of a bout of productive coughing following therapy.

Expectorants may also be tried to promote removal of bronchial secretions. Theoretically, these drugs enhance the secretion of less viscous bronchial mucus. Their efficacy in attaining this goal, however, is questionable. Medications containing a combination of cough suppressants and expectorants should not be used. An intact cough reflex is desirable to expel bronchial secretions. Without question, the best agent to promote removal or prevent formation of thick mucus is water (maintenance of normal hydration and aerosol therapy).

Many dogs with chronic bronchitis are overweight. The excessive accumulation of intrathoracic and intra-abdominal fat imposes a restrictive defect on the respiratory system and thereby decreases lung volume. A low resting lung volume predisposes the animal to small airway closure, which decreases the efficiency of normal pulmonary defense mechanisms and reduces pulmonary ventilation. Weight reduction will improve ventilation, promote increased exercise capability, and reduce stress on the cardiovascular system. In some cases, a significant improvement in clinical signs is seen with weight loss alone (see Chapter 7).

Bronchodilators (Table 28-3) are widely prescribed in humans to relieve spasm of bronchial smooth muscle associated with chronic bronchitis. Their use in dogs with chronic bronchitis is based on the assumption that bronchoconstriction is present and is a significant component of airway obstruction. Inhalant selective β_2-agonists, such as salbutamol, are widely used in the therapy of COPD in humans. Because inhalant medications are difficult to administer to dogs, oral bronchodilator drugs are more popular in veterinary medicine. The xanthine derivatives, such as theophylline and aminophylline, are most commonly used in the management of canine chronic bronchitis. Antimuscarinics, such as atropine, may also cause bronchodilation; how-

Table 28–3 *Suggested Oral Medications for the Management of Chronic Bronchitis in Dogs*

BRONCHODILATORS

THEOPHYLLINE DERIVATIVES
Aminophylline, regular release: 10 to 11 mg/kg every 6 hours
  Various trade names
Aminophylline, sustained release: 20 mg/kg every 12 hours
  Theo-Dur (Key)
  Slo-Bid (Rorer)
  Theobid (Glaxo)
Oxtriphylline 12 to 13 mg/kg every 6 to 8 hours
  Choledyl (Parke-Davis)

ADRENERGIC DRUGS
Metaproterenol: 0.5 mg/kg every 6 hours
  Alupent (Boehringer Ingelheim)
  Metaprel (Dorsey)
Terbutaline: 2.5 to 5 mg every 8 hours
  Brethine (Geigy)
  Bricanyl Tablets (Lakeside)
Isoproterenol compound elixir: 0.44 ml/kg every 6 to 12 hours
  Isuprel Compound Elixir (Winthrop-Breon)

ANTITUSSIVES

Butorphanol: 0.5 to 1 mg/kg every 6 to 12 hours
  Torbutrol (Bristol)
Hydrocodone bitartrate: 0.25 mg/kg every 6 to 12 hours
  Hycodan (Du Pont)
Codeine: 1 to 2 mg/kg every 6 to 12 hours
  Various trade names
Dextromethorphan: 1 to 2 mg/kg every 6 to 12 hours
  Various trade names

ever, their use is undesirable because these drugs increase the viscosity of airway secretions, which may obstruct airways.

It is difficult to confirm the presence and reversibility of bronchoconstriction in dogs with chronic bronchitis because pulmonary function tests are not widely used in these animals. Furthermore, several experimental studies have demonstrated a lack of airway hyperreactivity in the dog. Therefore, as opposed to humans, spasm of bronchial smooth muscle may not be a significant feature of chronic bronchitis in dogs. Despite this possible limitation, probably all dogs with chronic bronchitis should be given the benefit of trial therapy with bronchodilators. Efficacy of therapy should be judged in terms of clinical improvement.

Anti-inflammatory drugs appear to benefit some patients, presumably by alleviating chronic airflow restriction brought about by airway inflammation and bronchoconstriction. These drugs are especially valuable if moderate to large numbers of eosinophils are found in secretions collected from the respiratory tract. The finding of eosinophils may suggest an underlying allergic cause for the chronic bronchitis (see Chapter 30). Corticosteroids are the most commonly used anti-inflammatory drugs for chronic bronchitis in dogs; however, they should not be given to patients with secondary bronchopulmonary infections. A 10- to 14-day trial using oral prednisolone at a dosage of 1 to 2 mg/kg once daily or every other day is initially recommended. If improvement is observed, a longer course of glucocorticoid therapy may be considered. The dosage of prednisolone should be reduced to the absolute minimum required to maintain improvement of clinical signs. Prolonged alternate-day therapy is beneficial in some patients. If the administration of prednisolone does not bring about significant improvement, the drug should be discontinued because of the numerous potential adverse side-effects associated with chronic glucocorticoid therapy (see Appendix II).

Cough is an important pulmonary defense mechanism (see Chapter 13). Effective removal of airway secretions is of great importance in patients with chronic bronchitis. These patients, however, frequently have paroxysmal bouts of nonproductive coughing. Antitussives (see Table 28-3) may be used to break the cough cycle. The use of antitussives should be restricted to periods of cough exacerbation, because continual use causes further retention of bronchial mucus. Moreover, it is important not to indiscriminately suppress coughing, especially in the face of bronchial infection. A cause for an acute exacerbation of cough should be found, if possible, before recommending cough suppressants.

Secondary bacterial bronchial infection or bronchopneumonia is a common cause for exacerbation of clinical signs (see Chapter 29). Prompt, effective treatment of any bacterial bronchial infection is essential in dogs with chronic bronchitis in order to prevent further perpetuation of airway damage and the development of bronchopneumonia. The use of antibiotics should be based only on demonstrated evidence of bronchial infection. Because of the unpredictable nature of organisms involved (and their anti-

microbial sensitivities), broad-spectrum antibiotics, such as trimethoprim-sulfa or the fluoroquinolones (*e.g.*, norfloxacin and enrofloxacin), should be used until culture results are known.

Oxygen therapy is used in veterinary medicine only as temporary support for a patient while correcting the underlying problem. During oxygen therapy, the inhaled air should be humidified to help liquify tenacious bronchial secretions and prevent drying of the airways. Periodic suctioning of airways or chest physical therapy (coupage) should be attempted to remove accumulated secretions. Animals receiving oxygen therapy and suffering from severe obstructive disease should be monitored frequently for hypoventilation because their hypoxic drive stimulus for respiration may be removed by the inhalation of oxygen-rich air.

PATIENT MONITORING

Chronic bronchitis is essentially incurable. The prognosis is improved when the airway inflammation can be effectively controlled and exposure to environmental respiratory irritants reduced. Periods of exacerbation, nevertheless, often characterize the chronic, progressive clinical course of disease in these patients. Fortunately, most dogs are affected only by a recurrent cough. All dogs with chronic bronchitis should have periodic examinations to evaluate the effectiveness of any current therapy and to ensure that secondary bronchopulmonary infections are not present.

The major complications associated with chronic bronchitis are the development of bronchopneumonia, bronchiectasis, and, in severely affected dogs, cor pulmonale. Bronchopulmonary infections should be treated promptly and effectively. The irreversible airway changes associated with bronchiectasis cause severe impairment of mucociliary clearance, which allows for mucus accumulation in the airways and predisposes to recurrent bronchopulmonary infections. Dogs with bronchiectasis, therefore, should be inspected more frequently (every 3 to 6 months) for the development of bronchopneumonia. Cor pulmonale (right heart failure) is a serious consequence of chronically increased pulmonary vascular resistance. This is a direct complication of advanced chronic bronchitis and indicates a grave prognosis for the patient.

ADDITIONAL READING

Amis TC. Chronic bronchitis in dogs. In: Kirk RW, ed. Current veterinary therapy IX. Philadelphia: WB Saunders, 1986: 235.

Bonagura JD, Hamlin RL, Gaber CE. Chronic respiratory disease in the dog. In: Kirk RW, Bonagura JD, eds. Current veterinary therapy X. Philadelphia: WB Saunders, 1989: 361.

Haschek WM. Response of the lung to injury. In: Kirk RW, ed. Current veterinary therapy IX. Philadelphia: WB Saunders, 1986: 235.

Moise NS, Wiedenkeller D, Yeager AE et al. Clinical, radiographic and bronchial cytologic features of cats with bronchial disease: 65 cases (1980–1986). J Am Vet Med Assoc 1989; 194:1467.

Papich MG. Bronchodilator therapy. In: Kirk RW, ed. Current veterinary therapy IX. Philadelphia: WB Saunders, 1986: 278.

Prueter JC, Sherding RG. Canine chronic bronchitis. Vet Clin North Am 1985; 15:1085.

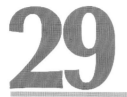

PNEUMONIA

Philip Roudebush, Ned F. Kuehn

Infections caused by bacteria, fungi, and viruses are an important cause of respiratory tract disease. Improvements in immunoprophylaxis by use of newer vaccines have significantly decreased the incidence of viral respiratory infections. However, bacterial and mycotic pneumonia are potentially life-threatening infections which are still common and should be approached in a thorough, systematic fashion.

The normal canine tracheobronchial tree and lung are not continuously sterile. One study using guarded culture swabs of the lower trachea isolated seven different bacteria from 37% of clinically healthy dogs. Another study confirmed that 47% of tracheal samples from healthy dogs contained bacteria, while aerobic bacteria were isolated from 37% of lung samples. All lung samples were sterile in only 2 of 19 dogs. Most of the bacteria cultured from the trachea and lungs (78%–80%) were identical to those found in the pharynx of those same dogs (Tables 29-1 and 29-2).

These data support the concept that oropharyngeal bacteria are frequently aspirated and may be present for an unknown interval in the normal tracheobronchial tree and lung. This bacterial population has the potential to cause clinical respiratory infection and clouds interpretation of airway and lung cultures.

BACTERIAL PNEUMONIA

Causes

Bacteria enter the lower respiratory tract primarily by the inhalation/aspiration and hematogenous routes. Whether or not a respiratory infection will develop depends on the complex interplay of many factors: size, inoculation, and virulence of the organism on the one hand vs. resistance of the host on the other. Clinical conditions that predispose the animal to bacterial pneumonia include: preexisting viral, mycoplasma, or fungal respiratory infections; regurgitation, dysphagia, and vomiting; reduced levels of consciousness (stupor, coma); severe metabolic disorders (*e.g.*, diabetes mellitus, uremia, hyperadrenocorticism); thoracic trauma or surgery; immunosuppressive therapy (*e.g.*, anticancer chemotherapeutic agents, glucocorticoids); and functional or anatomic disorders (*e.g.*, tracheal hypoplasia, primary ciliary dyskinesia). Intravenous catheter-associated bacteremia is probably the most common cause of hematogenous pneumonia, especially in patients with severe underlying disease.

Bacterial pneumonia is more common in the dog than in the cat. *Bordetella bronchiseptica* appears to be the principal primary bacterial patho-

Table 29–1 Results of Bacterial Isolation From Tonsil and Pharynx Swabs of Clinically Healthy Dogs*

Streptococcus (α- and nonhemolytic)
Staphylococcus (coagulase negative)
Neisseria species
Escherichia coli and *Enterobacter* species
Pasteurella multocida
Bacillus species
Streptococcus (β-hemolytic)
Alcaligenes species
Klebsiella pneumoniae
Proteus species
Pseudomonas species
Corynebacterium species
Staphylococcus (coagulase positive)
Clostridium species
Bacteroides species
Propionibacterium species
Peptostreptococcus species
Fusobacterium species

* Bacteria are listed in approximate order of frequency of isolation.

Table 29–2 Results of Bacterial Isolation From Tracheal Swabs and Lung of Clinically Normal Dogs

Staphylococcus (coagulase positive and negative)
Streptococcus (α- and nonhemolytic)
Pasteurella multocida
Klebsiella pneumoniae
Enterobacter aerogenes
Acinetobacter species
Moraxella species
Corynebacterium species

gen of canine pneumonia, although one report suggests that *Streptococcus zooepidemicus* may also be a primary pathogen. Most isolates in dogs with pneumonia are thought to be opportunist invaders, the most common of which are staphylococci, streptococci, *Escherichia coli, Pasteurella multocida* and *Klebsiella pneumoniae* (Table 29-3). A single pathogen is isolated in the majority of cases, but mixed infections are common (Table 29-4). Gram negative isolates predominate in both single and mixed infections.

Bacterial pathogens in feline pneumonia are poorly documented. *Bordetella bronchiseptica* and *Pasteurella* species are reported most frequently.

Clinical Signs

Historical findings and clinical signs of canine bacterial pneumonia include cough, fever, dyspnea, serous or mucopurulent nasal discharge, anorexia, depression, weight loss, and dehydration. Auscultation usually reveals abnormal breath sounds, including increased intensity or bronchial breath sounds, crackles, and wheezes.

Diagnostic Approach

The diagnosis of bacterial pneumonia is confirmed by hematologic findings, thoracic radiographs, and microbiologic and cytologic examination of material from the tracheobronchial tree or lung. A neutrophilic leukocytosis with a left shift is frequently found on a complete blood count. Arterial blood-gas values correlate well with the degree of physiologic disruption in patients with bacterial pneumonia and are a sensitive monitor of the patient's progress during treatment. Thoracic radiographs reveal an alveolar pattern characterized by increased pulmonary density in which margins are indistinct (unless they are lobar borders) and in which air bronchograms may be seen. A patchy or lobar alveolar pattern will be present in a cranial ventral lung lobe distribution.

The definitive method of establishing a diagnosis of bacterial pneumonia is to obtain aspirations, washings, or brushings for microbiologic and cytologic examinations. Multiple procedures that bypass the oropharynx have been recommended to obtain these specimens. Blood cultures can also be helpful in identifying the etiologic agent causing bacterial pneumonia.

Because animals are unable to expectorate sputum, a transtracheal washing and aspiration is a safe, simple, and clinically valuable method for obtaining tracheobronchial material for culture and cytologic examination (see Transtracheal Wash in Chapter 80). The technique is well tolerated by most dogs and cats and requires only minimal restraint of the unanesthetized patient.

Table 29–3 Most Common Isolates From the Lower Respiratory Tracts of Dogs with Suspected Bacterial Pneumonia

Isolate	Percentage of Dogs
Bordetella bronchiseptica	7 to 22
Escherichia coli	17 to 29
Klebsiella species	10 to 15
Pasteurella species	7 to 34
Pseudomonas species	6 to 34
Staphylococcus species	9 to 20
Streptococcus species	15 to 27
Others	17 to 35

Table 29–4 Number of Bacterial Isolates Per Positive Sample From Dogs with Lower Respiratory Tract Infections

Number	Percentage of Dogs
1	58 to 60
2	22 to 23
3	11 to 16
≥4	2 to 7

Preparation of material for cytologic evaluation can be done by several methods. Visible strands of exudate may be teased onto a glass slide, smeared, and stained. Small quantities of material can be centrifuged and smears made of the sediment. New methylene blue wet mounts and Wright's, Giemsa, or Gram's stains of air-dried smears can be used for identification of cellular elements and bacteria. Cytologic evaluation of tracheobronchial secretions is usually consistent with a purulent exudate. Bacteria are often not demonstrable, and their absence in cytologic specimens from transtracheal aspirations does not rule out bacterial pneumonia. An aliquot of aspirated material can be cultured directly for aerobic and anaerobic bacteria. Anaerobic culture is indicated only when aspiration pneumonia or a pulmonary abscess is suspected. Secretions that coat the distal end of the catheter can be cultured if the amount of aspirated material is minimal.

Tracheobronchoscopy is valuable for obtaining brush catheter specimens for cytologic and microbiologic examination but requires that the patient be maintained under general anesthesia (see Tracheobronchoscopy in Chapter 80). Anesthesia is of particular concern in the patients with bacterial pneumonia who may be poor anesthetic risks.

The advantages of tracheobronchoscopy are numerous when compared with other diagnostic techniques. Endoscopy allows the direct visualization of the tracheobronchial tree and the lesions associated with bacterial pneumonia. This evaluation allows a better assessment of the patient's clinical status and prognosis. The cytologic preparations obtained by mucosal brushings through the endoscope are superior to those obtained from transtracheal washing and aspiration.

Because of passage through the oropharynx, bacterial cultures obtained via bronchoscopes have been considered unreliable in the past. Sterile, open-end brush-in-catheter systems passed through the endoscope are frequently contaminated by the same organisms identified by nasopharyngeal cultures. A commercially available catheter (Microbiology Specimen Brush, Microvasive Inc.), which enhances the ability to obtain reliable cultures of lower airway secretions through a bronchoscope, has recently been developed. This system consists of a sterile brush contained within a telescoping double catheter occluded by a distal polyethylene glycol plug. The plugged telescoping double-catheter system is passed through the instrumentation channel of the bronchoscope, and the brush is extended into secretions to be cultured. The brush is retracted into the inner catheter, and the entire brush-in-telescope double-catheter system is removed from the endoscope. The brush is advanced out of the catheter, where the wire is transected with sterile scissors and the brush is placed in trypticase soy broth. The only disadvantage is the moderate price for a catheter system that can be used only once.

Transthoracic fine needle aspiration can be used to procure material for microbial culture and cytologic examination directly from the lung. Fine needle aspiration is best performed after routine diagnostic procedures such as transtracheal washing have proven negative. The technique, contraindications, and complications have been well described in the section Lung Biopsy in Chapter 80.

A recent study of diagnostic procedures in a canine model of streptococcal pneumonia found that transthoracic fine needle lung aspiration had the highest sensitivity and specificity for bacterial recovery when compared with transtracheal washing, flexible fiberoptic bronchoscopy, transbronchial lung biopsy, or blind catheter brushing. Sensitivity was enhanced when culturing was performed immediately following the procedure rather than sending the samples to the microbiology laboratory. Complications of percutaneous fine needle aspiration are common and potentially serious. Pneumothorax is the primary complication with a 20% to 30% incidence rate reported in one study.

Blood cultures have been recommended in human beings with bacterial pneumonia to help isolate the infectious agent. Documented bacteremia is also thought to be a poor prognostic finding. No studies in animals exist that document the value of blood cultures in establishing a prognosis or isolating the bacterial agent in cases of pneumonia. One study did confirm that 50% of dogs with experimentally induced streptococcal pneumonia were blood culture positive within 48 hours of onset of clinical signs.

Management

Oral or parenteral antibacterials are the principal therapy for lower airway bacterial infections. It is unrealistic to expect any single antibacterial to be routinely effective against the wide variety of organisms causing bacterial pneumonia. The most important criterion for selection of an antibacterial is identification of the bacterial organism. Substantially more patients recover if their antibacterial therapy is administered according to culture and in vitro susceptibility testing than if it is empirically administered.

Initially, choices of antibacterials can be based on the shape of bacteria noted on airways or lung cytologic preparations. Cocci are usually staphylococci or streptococci, while rods are usually members of the family Enterobacteriaceae. The members of this family are the most unpredictable with respect to antibacterial agents. A reasonable choice of antibacterial in gram positive cocci infections is ampicillin/amoxicillin, cephalosporins, chloramphenicol, quinolones, gentamicin, or trimethoprim-sulfonamide. Gram negative rod infections are best treated with amikacin, chloramphenicol, gentamicin, quinolones or trimethoprim-sulfonamide. Chloramphenicol, gentamicin, kanamycin and tetracycline are most effective against *Bordetella bronchiseptica*. Anaerobic infections should be treated with ampicillin/amoxicillin, cephalosporins, clindamycin, penicillin, tetracycline or trimethoprim-sulfonamide. Levels of antibacterials in airway secretions after oral or parenteral administration are much lower than serum levels. Therefore, systemic antibacterials should be administered in high doses for several weeks so that maximum concentrations are reached in lung tissue and airway secretions.

Maintenance of normal systemic hydration is an important therapeutic objective in patients with bacterial pneumonia. Dehydration hinders mucociliary clearance and secretion mobilization because normal respiratory secretions are greater than 90% water. Parenteral fluid therapy should be initiated if needed to repair existing fluid deficits and provide for maintenance fluid requirements (see Table 72-5).

The goal of aerosol therapy is to mobilize secretions by adding water to the mucociliary blanket. A nebulizer that produces particles between 0.5 and 3.0 microns must be used to ensure that water is deposited in the lower airways. The animal is placed in an enclosed chamber and a bland aerosol (normal saline) is nebulized into the chamber. The animal should be treated at least three or four times daily for 30 to 45 minutes per treatment. Pretreatment with bronchodilators is recommended. Water vaporizers or humidifiers are inadequate for this type of therapy.

Nebulization with bland aerosols has subjectively resulted in more rapid resolution of cases of canine bronchopneumonia when used in conjunction with physiotherapy and systemic antimicrobials. Physiotherapy should always be used immediately after aerosolization to enhance secretion clearance. Physiotherapy includes mild forced exercise, increasing cough frequency by chest wall coupage or tracheal manipulation and postural drainage. Aerosol administration of aminoglycosides substantially reduces the number of bacteria in airways of dogs with experimental infection with *Bordetella bronchiseptica*. Routine intratracheal or aerosol administration of antibacterials is not recommended.

Animals with severe tachypnea, dyspnea, or marked hypoxemia (PaO_2 less than 60 mmHg) require oxygen therapy. The early period of highest mortality with bacterial pneumonia corresponds to the greatest hypoxemia. The oxygen should be humidified to prevent drying of respiratory membranes. Oxygen can be administered by oxygen cage, mechanical ventilator, intratracheal cannula, or nasal catheter. Drugs such as antitussives and antihistamines that inhibit mucokinesis and exudate removal from the respiratory tract should be used cautiously.

PULMONARY ABSCESS

Causes

A pulmonary abscess is a necrotic area of lung parenchyma containing purulent material usually produced by pyogenic infections. Pulmonary abscesses are uncommon in dogs and cats. Most arise from aspiration of oropharyngeal or gastric contents and are termed primary lung abscess. Secondary lung abscess results from a primary underlying process such as a bronchial obstruction, septic or heartworm disease thromboemboli, parasites (paragonimiasis), foreign body, bullous emphysema, tuberculosis cavities, or neoplasia. Obligate anaerobic bacteria are identified more frequently than aerobes, but mixed infections are common. *Mycoplasma* species were recovered from a pulmonary abscess in one cat.

Clinical Signs, Diagnostic Approach, and Management

The clinical signs with pulmonary abscess depend on the etiology but closely resemble those of chronic bacterial pneumonia. Clinical findings include weight loss, chronic fever, cough, and hemoptysis. Hematologic findings include leukocytosis with a left shift, anemia, and rarely hypoproteinemia. An abscess will usually appear on a thoracic radiograph as an ill-defined pulmonary nodule or mass, with or without cavitation. Abscesses are often indistinguishable from granulomas, traumatic bullae, tumors, or pneumatocysts. Cytologic examination of brushings or aspirations is consistent with a septic or nonseptic purulent exudate.

Lung abscesses are usually treated without drainage, using long-term antibacterial therapy. Choice of antibacterials should be based on culture and susceptibility findings. Clindamycin appears to be the antibiotic of choice in treatment of human anaerobic lung abscess.

MYCOTIC PNEUMONIA

Fungi are complex organisms which are distributed widely in nature. The organisms which cause systemic or deep mycotic infections are endemic in large areas of North America. Mycotic pneumonias are common problems seen in small companion animals because of the wide environmental distribution of fungi and their use of airborne spores for reproduction.

Pathophysiology, Clinical Signs, and Diagnostic Approach

Cryptococcus neoformans is a saprophytic encapsulated yeast-like fungus with worldwide distribution. It grows best in soil enriched with pigeon or other avian excreta. Infection is thought to occur by inhalation of airborne organisms, although basidiospores of the sexual (mold) stage may also be involved. The airborne organisms vary in size, with most apparently impacting on the upper respiratory passages. The organisms can be small enough to reach the alveoli during inhalation.

The upper respiratory tract (nasal passages, sinuses), central nervous system, eye, skin, and lymph nodes are the most common sites of infection in the cat. Pulmonary lesions are reported in one fourth to one half of feline cases. Clinical signs of upper respiratory cryptococcosis include sneezing, snuffling, nasal discharge, and swellings over the nasal region. Coughing can occur due to pneumonia or aspiration of postnasal drainage from sites of upper respiratory infection.

The lesions of cryptococcosis vary from gelatinous masses to granulomas. The pulmonary lesions appear as multiple white granulomas, although lobar consolidation can occur. Cryptococcal pneumonia may represent direct infection of the lung from environmental sources or merely an extension of the infection from primary sites in the upper airways. One cat was described with tracheal but no pulmonary lesions.

Diagnosis is usually based on identification of the organism from cytologic preparations or biopsies of nasal masses, nasal exudate, cerebrospinal fluid, enlarged lymph nodes, or cutaneous masses. Cryptococcal pneumonia is rarely identified ante-mortem, but organisms were obtained by both transtracheal washing and fine needle lung aspiration in one cat with radiographic evidence of lobar consolidation.

Cryptococcus organisms are opportunistic fungi that usually cause disease in immunosuppressed cats. Feline leukemia virus infection, malignancy, chronic glucocorticoid administration, and malnutrition are commonly associated with cryptococcal infections in cats.

Central nervous system and ocular signs are most commonly reported in canine cryptococcosis. Dry cough was reported in 2 of 22 (9%) dogs, and hilar lymphadenopathy and nodular densities were reported on thoracic radiographs of one dog (Fig. 29-1). Most dogs with cryptococcal lung lesions are not diagnosed ante-mortem, but approximately 50% of reported cases had respiratory lesions.

Histoplasma capsulatum is a saprophytic dimorphic fungus which causes the most prevalent systemic mycotic infection in animals and humans. Distribution of this organism is worldwide, but it is highly endemic in the central Mississippi river valley and its major tributaries the Ohio, lower Missouri, and Tennessee river basins. Smaller foci of infection in North America include the Atlantic seaboard of Maryland, Virginia, and North Carolina, as well as the St. Lawrence river valley.

H capsulatum thrives best in moist red-yellow podzolic soil, especially that enriched by decaying wood, chicken, pigeon, starling, or bat excreta. The excreta is thought to enhance rapid growth and give rise to large numbers of infective spores. Localization of the disease in the region of rich alluvial river basins has been ascribed to periodic flooding which disseminates these infective spores.

H capsulatum shows thermal dimorphism, which means it routinely grows as a mold in soil at ambient temperatures and as a yeast in tissues at 30° to 37°C. The mycelial form produces branching septate hyphae and two types of spores: small spherical microconidia (microaleuriospore) and large thick-walled macroconidia (macroaleuriospore, chlamydospore). The yeast phase appears in tissue as a well-defined achromatic double-refractile capsule. The capsule surrounds a mass of irregularly scattered chromatin, and the organism divides by simple fission and budding.

The respiratory tract is invariably the route of infection with inhalation of windblown or soilborne spores. Contact with highly infected soil probably enhances the chance of developing infection. Infection may result from direct mucosal invasion of the oral pharynx or gastrointestinal tract and may explain the enterocolonic form of canine histoplasmosis. Spores reach the alveoli where they are phagocytized by alveolar macrophages. Within the alveolar macrophage the yeast phase develops and reproduces. The rapidly growing *Histoplasma* organisms may kill the cell with the organisms being released into the surrounding tissue.

Free organisms or infected macrophages enter the interstitium of the lung, with vascular spread toward the periphery and lymphatic spread toward the tracheobronchial lymph nodes. The organisms may multiply in the alveolus leading to a focal inflammatory response. Histoplasmosis elicits a granulomatous response, with infiltration of plasma cells, lymphocytes, and macrophages.

At this point, the course of infection is determined by the cell-mediated immune response of the host. This basic pathophysiologic scheme is shared by histoplasmosis, blastomycosis, and coccidioidomycosis in all mammals. A self-limited acute pulmonary infection often occurs in which the organism will initially reproduce but is later eliminated by the cell-mediated immune response. Transient fever and cough will signal the acute pneumonia, but these clinical signs are often indistinguishable from those of viral or bacterial tracheobronchitis. The animal may initially recover from the acute pneumonia, but the organisms remain quiescent in the lung. Endogenous reactivation of this infective focus may occur at a later time.

With an inadequate host response during the acute pneumonia the organisms continue to proliferate, and massive reticuloendothelial cell infiltration results in interstitial and alveolar flooding. Progressive pulmonary infection will ensue, with or without extrapulmonary involvement. Progressive pulmonary infection will be recognized as chronic cough, wheezing, tachypnea, dyspnea, anorexia, weight loss, fever, and occasionally death.

The second major pathophysiologic pathway encompasses the animal who does not initially exhibit clinical signs of acute pneumonia. In one group of animals, multiplication of the organism is restricted by cell-mediated immunity, and the organisms are destroyed before clinical signs develop. This subclinical form of the infection is very common in histoplasmosis. A smaller group of animals will have an insidious onset of chronic pulmonary and/or extrapulmonary infection. This form is most common of histoplasmosis which is clinically recognized. Chronic pulmonary histoplasmosis results in a granulomatous interstitial pneumonia and enlargement of the tracheobronchial lymph nodes (hilar lymphadenopathy) (see Figs. 29-1 and 29-2). The hilar lymphadenopathy can become severe enough to compress the lobar bronchi.

Dissemination to extrapulmonary sites is characterized by diffuse involvement of the reticuloendothelial system with granulomatous inflammation. Organs most commonly involved in disseminated histoplasmosis include the bone marrow, spleen, liver, and lymph nodes. Clinical signs will depend on the site involved and may coincide with respiratory signs.

Diagnosis of histoplasmosis is based on geographical location, clinical signs, thoracic radiographs, serology, and demonstration of the organism cytologically or histopathologically. Histoplasmosis is most common in young (less

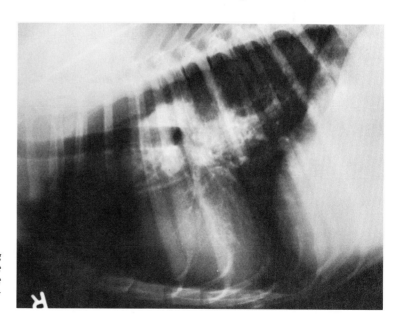

Figure 29–1 Lateral thoracic radiograph of a dog with mycotic pneumonia. The increased soft tissue density at the base of the heart surrounding the tracheal bifurcation is due to tracheobronchial (hilar) lymphadomegaly.

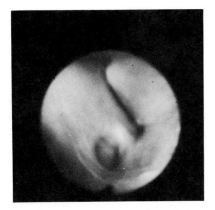

Figure 29–2 *View of the right caudal lobar bronchi through an endoscope. Note the external compression of the bronchus by hilar lymphadomegaly when compared to the normal bronchus.*

than 4 years of age) dogs of sporting or hound breeds. Clinical signs include acute or chronic cough, tachypnea, dyspnea, exercise intolerance, anorexia, fever, and weight loss. Extrapulmonary dissemination results in peripheral lymphadenopathy, splenomegaly, hepatomegaly, icterus, diarrhea, or anemia. Neutrophilic leukocytosis and mild nonregenerative anemia are common laboratory findings.

Thoracic radiographs will usually parallel the pathophysiologic changes previously described (Table 29-5). Initial changes include a linear to finely nodular interstitial pattern which corresponds with multiplication of the organism,

edema, and inflammation in the lung interstitium (Fig. 29-3). Alveolar patterns occur less commonly when progressive pulmonary infection leads to alveolar flooding. Hilar lymphadenopathy represents inflammation and enlargement of the tracheobronchial lymph nodes. Calcification of pulmonary interstitial granulomas and tracheobronchial lymph nodes represents the radiographic appearance of inactive lesions. These inactive lesions may be seen on thoracic radiographs of animals with no prior history of respiratory infection.

Serologic tests measure an animal's antibody titer rather than detect whether the organisms is actually present. Serologic tests are subject to false positive (past exposure, antigenic crossover) and false negative (anergy, early infection) reactions. Serologic methods available for histoplasmosis include the complement fixation test (CFT), with mycelial and yeast-phase suspensions, and agar-gel immunodiffusion (see Chapter 79). Accuracy of the CFT is compromised by cross reactivity with blastomycosis and the presence of anticomplementary factors in canine serum. Titers of 1 : 8 are suspicious, and titers of 1 : 16 or greater are considered positive in animals with appropriate clinical signs. Agar-gel immunodiffusion offers a promising alternative, but extensive data is unavailable for this technique in histoplasmosis.

The most rapid method of diagnosis is demon-

Table 29–5 *Pathogenesis of Thoracic Lesions and Radiographic Patterns in Mycotic Pneumonias*

Radiographic Pattern	Pathogeneis
Miliary to nodular interstitial pattern	Free organisms or macrophages containing organisms enter lung interstitium inciting pyogranulomatous inflammation and edema. Dissemination in lung is vascular toward pleural surface and lymphatic towards hilum. Smaller foci of inflammation and nodules coalesce as the disease progresses.
Bronchial pattern	Direct extension from initial focus of infection causes peribronchial inflammation and edema.
Alveolar pattern	Primary focus of inflammation in alveoli spreads with accumulation of exudate in larger areas of alveoli and airways.
Hilar lymphadenopathy	Spread of organisms and inflammation centripetally through the lymphatics to tracheobronchial lymph nodes. Enlarged lymph nodes, perilymphatic connective tissue fibrosis, extracapsular infection, and impaired lymphatic drainage result.

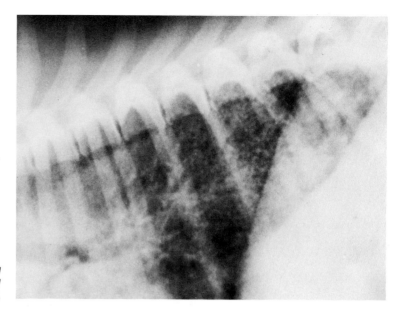

Figure 29–3 *Lateral thoracic radiograph centered over the caudal lung fields. A nodular interstitial pattern typical of mycotic pneumonia is visualized.*

strating the organism in cytological specimens. Pulmonary infection is confirmed by finding the characteristic organism in sputum, transtracheal washings, bronchoscopic brushings, pleural fluid, or fine needle lung aspirates. Infection is often confined to the lung interstitium, a fact which makes isolation of the organism difficult. In disseminated cases, the organism can be demonstrated in peripheral blood smears, buffy coat blood smears, bone marrow aspirates, lymph node aspirates, hepatic aspirates, splenic aspirates, and rectal scrapings. The organism will be found intracellularly in monocytes, macrophages, or histiocytes (Fig. 29-4*A*).

Blastomyces dermatitidis is a saprophytic dimorphic fungus which causes systemic infections in both animals and humans. The exact ecologic niche of this organism is unknown, but human and canine cases have a definite geographic distribution in North America. The endemic areas include the Mississippi, Ohio, and Tennessee river basins and the central Atlantic states. Much of the endemic area for histoplasmosis and blastomycosis overlap.

Isolation of the fungus from the environment has proven exceedingly difficult, making the ecology of the organism elusive. Current information points toward the soil as the source of the organism, but failure to culture blastomyces suggests

its ecologic niche is very restricted compared to that of *Histoplasma* organisms. Studies have shown a close correlation between canine cases and exposure to wooded areas, suggesting a focal environmental source. Dogs have become infected after contacting soil experimentally seeded with the organism.

B dermatitidis shows thermal dimorphism with a mycelial phase at ambient temperatures and a yeast phase in tissues. The mycelial form produces branching septate hyphae and chlamydospores. The yeast phase appears in tissue as a capsule with a thick double-contoured cell wall. The organism reproduces in tissue by simple fission and budding (Fig. 29-4*B*). Filamentous forms of blastomycetes have been found in man, experimentally infected mice, and the dog. The filamentous form is rare and represents true hyphae or pseudohyphae formation in tissue.

The spectrum of illness that can result from blastomycosis is extremely variable and ranges from a self-limited pulmonary infection to a rapidly progressive fatal disease. The respiratory tract is considered the portal of entry. Intratracheal inoculation of dogs with spores and exposure to seeded soil has produced pulmonary infection. The pathogenesis of pulmonary lesions and dissemination is similar to that described for histoplasmosis previously. Blastomycosis will in-

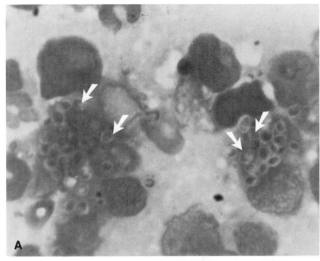

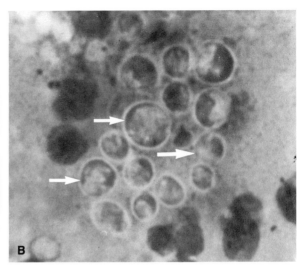

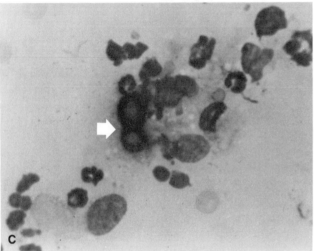

Figure 29–4 (A) Cytologic preparation of bone marrow from a dog with histoplasmosis. Note the characteristic intracellular organisms (arrows). (B) Cytologic preparation of a lymph node from a dog with blastomycosis. Note the characteristic broad-base budding organism (arrows). (C) Cytologic preparation of thoracic fluid from a dog with coccidioidomycosis. Note the characteristic endospores from a ruptured spherule (arrow).

cite a pyogranulomatous inflammation with a more intense polymorphonuclear cell response than histoplasmosis. A lower incidence of tracheobronchial lymphadenopathy occurs with blastomycosis when compared to both histoplasmosis and coccidioidomycosis. This results in less respiratory distress due to lobar bronchial constriction although dyspnea still occurs in severe pneumonia. Disseminated blastomycosis may involve any organ in the body, but skin, bone, eyes, lymph nodes, and the male genital tract are favored sites.

Canine blastomycosis is diagnosed by clinical signs in animals from endemic areas, thoracic radiographs, serology, and demonstration of the organism cytologically or histopathologically. Blastomycosis is seen most frequently in young, large-breed, male dogs. Clinical signs of thoracic involvement include cough, dyspnea, tachypnea, exercise intolerance, fever, anorexia, weight loss, and regurgitation. Extrapulmonary dissemination results in peripheral lymphadenopathy, blindness, prostatitis, testicular swelling, lameness, and painful subcutaneous swellings with fistulas or ulceration. The most consistent laboratory findings are a neutrophilic leukocytosis and nonregenerative anemia.

Thoracic radiography usually shows diffuse miliary to nodular interstitial patterns (see Fig. 29-3). Bronchial, alveolar, cavitary, pleural, and mixed patterns also occur and confuse the radiographic picture of blastomycosis. The nodular interstitial lesions may coalesce, and patchy areas of consolidation result. As mentioned earlier, the incidence of hilar lymphadenopathy is somewhat less than the other systemic mycoses.

Serologic methods available for blastomycosis include CFT, agar-gel immunodiffusion, counter immunoelectrophoresis, and antiglobulin hemagglutination test (see Chapter 79). The complement fixation test was used extensively in the past but anticomplementary factor in canine serum and cross reactivity with histoplasmosis decrease the accuracy of this test. A CFT titer of 1 : 8 or greater is presumptive evidence for infection, while a titer of 1 : 32 or greater indicates active infection. False positive and false negative CFT titers are common. Agar-gel immunodiffusion is presently considered more reliable than the CFT. The sensitivity and specificity are reported to be greater than 90%. In the same study, 10 of 13 dogs seroconverted to negative within 6 months of initiating therapy, although some clinically recovered animals remained positive for long periods of time.

Definitive diagnosis depends on identification of the organism by culture, biopsy, or cytology. Examination of cytologic specimens offers the least expensive and most rapid diagnostic technique. Pulmonary infection is confirmed by finding the characteristic budding cells with thick refractile walls in sputum, transtracheal washing, bronchoscopic brushings, pleural fluid, or fine needle lung aspirates (see Fig. 29-4*B*). In extrapulmonary dissemination, large numbers of organisms occur in aspirates of lymph nodes, testicles, and subcutaneous nodules. Impression smears of draining lymph nodes and ulcerated skin lesions are also rewarding. Recovery of the organism is less frequent in ocular paracentesis, urine sediment, prostatic washes, and bone aspirates.

Coccidioides immitis is a saprophytic dimorphic fungus which has the narrowest geographical distribution of all systemic mycoses. Coccidioidomycosis is a New World disease not found outside the western hemisphere. The endemic area includes central and southern California, Arizona, southern Nevada, southern Utah, southern New Mexico, southwest Texas, and bordering regions of northern Mexico. This endemic area is coterminous with the lower Sonoran life zone. This region has a hot, semiarid climate with short intense rainy seasons falling on sandy alkaline soil.

As a dimorphic fungus, *C immitis* proliferates in the mycelial phase in surface soil and forms abundant arthrospores (arthroconidia). These arthrospores are easily detached and readily distributed by wind, rodents, and other wild animals. The arthrospores swell into spherules for the yeast or tissue phase. The cytoplasm of spherules undergoes cleavage to produce endospores. After endosporulation the spherules burst to release hundreds of endospores. This process is unlike the other pathogenic fungi in which the tissue phase reproduces by budding.

After inhalation of infective arthrospores, clinical disease is determined by pathophysiologic mechanisms described for histoplasmosis and blastomycosis. The immunopathologic response by the host will determine the extent and severity of the lesions. The clinical spectrum will range from asymptomatic infection to fatal extrapulmonary dissemination. Coccidioidomycosis stimulates a pyogranulomatous response. Based on pathologic observations, it is thought that released endospores stimulate intense polymorphonuclear leukocyte infiltration, while intact spherules stimulate macrophages, lymphocytes, giant cells, and caseation. Macrophages ingesting arthroconidia and endospores may be unable to kill them unless cell-mediated release of lymphokines stimulates phagolysosomal fusion. In progressive pulmonary infection, the endospores disseminate throughout the lung interstitium and tracheobronchial lymph nodes through lymphohematoginous drainage. Disseminated coccidioidomycosis usually involves the skin, lymph nodes, male genital tract, bones, joints, and abdominal organs.

Coccidioidomycosis is diagnosed in dogs from endemic areas by clinical findings, thoracic radiographs, serology, and demonstration of the organism (Fig. 29-4*C*). The disease is seen most often in young, large-breed male dogs. Clinical signs of pulmonary infection include cough, dyspnea, wheezing, fever, anorexia, weight loss, and dysphagia. Extrapulmonary dissemination results in peripheral lymphadenopathy or abscessation, subcutaneous abscesses with sinus formation or ulceration, lameness, and testicular swelling. Common laboratory findings include mild to moderate neutrophilic leukocytosis, mild nonregenerative anemia, and hyperglobulinemia.

Thoracic radiographs show diffuse interstitial or mixed patterns, pleural thickening, and hilar lymphadenopathy. These radiographic changes mirror the pathophysiologic processes occurring in the dog. A summary of the radiographic appearance of mycotic pneumonia appears in Table 29-5.

Serology may help to establish a presumptive diagnosis of coccidioidomycosis (see Chapter 79). Precipitin and complement fixation tests are available, although canine anticomplementary factor makes the CFT more difficult to interpret. The precipitin test detects IgM antibodies within 3 to 6 weeks postinfection, while the CFT titer detects IgG antibodies 8 to 10 weeks postinfection. With a CFT, a titer of 1 : 4 is negative, titers of 1 : 8 are suspicious, and titers greater than 1 : 16 are positive.

Fungal culture, histopathology of affected tissue, or cytology are necessary for a definitive diagnosis. Cytologic examination of sputum, transtracheal washings, bronchial brushings, pleural fluid, or fine needle lung aspirates will often reveal the characteristic endosporulated spherule (Fig. 29-4C). However, nodular interstitial diseases, such as the systemic mycoses, may give false negative results on airway or aspirate cytology. Lymph node aspirates and impression smears of exudate from draining skin lesions are often rewarding.

Management

The development of antimycotic agents has proceeded much more slowly than that of antibacterials. Antibiotics affect physiologic processes critical only to bacteria and thus inhibit bacteria while not harming the patient. Bacteria are prokaryotic (the state of having no true nucleus), while fungi are eukaryotic (the state of having a nucleus) like mammals, which means fungi have evolved complex metabolic processes. This eukaryotic similarity between mammals and fungi has made development of nontoxic antimycotic agents difficult.

The structural integrity and permeability of all cell membranes are largely determined by lipids. Cholesterol is the sterol found almost exclusively in mammalian plasma membranes, while ergosterol is the main sterol in yeast and fungal cells. Phospholipids are components of all biological membranes. The two major drugs available for therapy of the systemic mycoses, amphotericin B and ketoconazole, both affect cell membrane sterols (Table 29-6).

Amphotericin B is a polyene antibiotic with a broad spectrum of antifungal activity; in decreasing order of susceptibility are blastomycetes and *Histoplasma, Cryptococcus,* and *Coccidioides* organisms. Aspergilli are usually resistant. Differences in susceptibility of various fungi to polyene antibiotics are attributed to varying sterol contents of cell membranes.

Crystalline amphotericin B is insoluble in water and is poorly absorbed across the gastrointestinal mucosa or skin. It is the most toxic antimicrobial drug in common use today. Nephrotoxicity represents the most serious limitation to its effective use. Amphotericin B causes marked decreases in intrarenal blood flow due to

Table 29–6 *Summary of Suggested Treatment Protocols for Mycotic Pneumonias*

AMPHOTERICIN B

0.15 to 0.50 mg/kg IV, 3 times weekly as slow IV bolus to a total dose of 8 to 12 mg/kg.
Give 1.0 mg/kg IV, 2 to 3 times weekly for severe infections.

KETOCONAZOLE

10 to 30 mg/kg/day divided 2 to 3 times daily with meals. Histoplasmosis and blastomycosis, minimum 2 months of therapy.
Coccidioidomycosis, 6 to 8 months.

AMPHOTERICIN B AND KETOCONAZOLE

Start with amphotericin B: 0.15 to 0.50 mg/kg IV, 3 times weekly to total dose of 4 mg/kg. Then follow with ketoconazole 10 mg/kg/day for minimum 2 months. (A longer treatment period is needed for coccidioidomycosis.)

arteriole vasoconstriction, subsequent decreases in glomerular filtration rate, and impaired distal tubular function. Other adverse effects include fever, anorexia, non-regenerative anemia, phlebitis, and vomiting. Amphotericin B also causes perivascular irritation if extravasated.

Dosage schedules for amphotericin B have been empirically established based on limits of nephrotoxicity, convenience, and clinical experience. The total dosage of amphotericin B that will constantly provide a cure is not precisely known for a given patient or for a given fungal infection; nor is the tolerable daily dosage of amphotericin B predictable for each patient. However, certain guidelines are available for daily doses and length of therapy.

A frequently used regimen is to give 0.15 to 0.50 mg/kg intravenously as a daily dose until a total accumulated dosage of 9 to 12 mg/kg is achieved. These doses are given on alternate days or three times weekly. In critically ill patients, an accelerated schedule of 1 mg/kg should be used. A syringe and butterfly catheter for infusion of 20 to 40 ml of amphotericin B over 5 to 10 minutes is preferred. Mild to moderate pulmonary infections will usually respond to lower accumulated doses than disseminated infections. Higher total doses and longer treatment schedules are needed for osteomyelitis and coccidioidomycosis. In human beings, a total dose of 20 mg/kg is adequate to prevent relapses of blastomycosis. The only comparable veterinary study showed a 65% cure rate in 23 dogs with blastomycosis given a total dose of 8 to 9 mg/kg.

The decision of when to discontinue therapy can be difficult. The length of therapy will vary with the organism, extent of infection, and clinical response. Treatment with amphotericin B is stopped when there is clinical improvement, failure to identify the organism cytologically, stabilization, or improvement in radiographic findings and a decrease in serologic titers (generally 8–24 weeks).

Pretreatment monitoring of blood urea nitrogen and/or creatinine will usually prevent serious renal disease. Criteria for interrupting therapy vary but values of 50 to 60 mg/dl (18–21 nmol/L) blood urea nitrogen (BUN) and 3.0 mg/dl (265 μmol/L) creatinine are frequently cited. Renal function almost always improves after brief cessation of therapy, and treatment can be reinstituted once serum levels of BUN or creatinine fall below these values. During treatment a flow sheet can be used to record the daily dosage, total accumulated dosage, BUN, and creatinine values.

Ketoconazole is a synthetic imidazole derivative with antifungal properties which has recently become available for clinical use. Ketoconazole inhibits ergosterol biosynthesis which coincides with accumulation of 14 α-methylsterols. Ketoconazole also causes a shift of unsaturated to saturated moeties of triglycerides, phospholipids, and sterol esters. These changes enhance cell membrane disturbances, decrease the activity of membrane-bound enzymes, and inhibit growth. Mammalian cells utilize dietary cholesterol in cell membranes, while fungal cells must synthesize their own sterols, especially ergosterol. This process accounts for the selective toxicity of ketoconazole. For some fungal organisms, ketoconazole may act as a pharmacologic suppressant with fungistatic rather than fungicidal activity. This difference emphasizes the role of the patients immune response in helping eliminate the infection.

Ketoconazole is effective in vitro against *Histoplasma* and *Coccidioides* organisms and blastomyces, but is less effective against *Cryptococcus* organisms and aspergilli. Only limited efficacy data is available for use of ketoconazole in human and animal patients with systemic mycotic infections. Reported clinical efficacy in animals includes successful treatment of canine blastomycosis, canine coccidioidomycosis, feline histoplasmosis, and feline cryptococcosis. The role of ketoconazole in therapy of fungal pneumonia is encouraging and further clinical investigation is awaited.

Unlike amphotericin B, ketoconazole is water soluble and well absorbed from the gastrointestinal tract. Absorption is improved in an acid environment, and higher, more consistent plasma levels are achieved in people when ketoconazole is taken with a meal. Safe oral administration over a prolonged period of time is the attractive feature of ketoconazole. Toxic side effects are fewer and less severe than those associated with amphotericin B. Adverse effects include anorexia, vomiting, hepatomegaly, increased serum alanine aminotransferase, increased serum alkaline phosphatase, lightening or graying of the hair coat color, embryotoxicity, and teratogenesis. The hepatic changes appear to be reversible, and serum enzyme levels will fall after discontinuation of the drug. Serum enzyme levels of alanine aminotransferase and alkaline phosphatase should be monitored monthly during therapy.

The oral dose of ketoconazole in dogs is 10 to 30 mg/kg/day divided 2 to 3 times daily with a meal. Use of 10 mg/kg/day for 60 to 62 days in 11 dogs with blastomycosis resulted in elimination of the organism in 36% of the animals. Use of 30 mg/kg/day in two other dogs with blastomycosis apparently eliminated the organism in both animals. A treatment schedule of amphotericin B (total dose of 4 mg/kg) followed by ketoconazole (10 mg/kg/day for 60 days) resulted in the cure of 11 of 18 dogs with blastomycosis (61%). The efficacy of low-dose amphotericin B plus ketoconazole was similar to the efficacy of using amphotericin B alone at higher total doses. Treatment of pulmonary coccidioidomycosis requires the lower end of the ketoconazole dosage for a minimum of 6 to 8 months, while disseminated infection requires 8 to 12 months of therapy. The current recommendations are to continue ketoconazole for 60 days in canine histoplasmosis and blastomycosis before reevaluating the patient. A feline dose is reported as 50 mg or 15 to 20 mg/kg given twice daily on alternate days.

Clinical responses to ketoconazole appear to be slower than with amphotericin B. This response reflects the interference of cell membrane synthesis rather than the direct attachment and damage to cell membranes. Patients with severe infections should receive amphotericin B alone or amphotericin B followed by ketoconazole. Relapses are common in both animals and man with the use of ketoconazole. This fact may reflect the fungistatic nature of the drug and the failure of the patient to mount a sufficient immune response.

Patient Monitoring

Prognosis is poor to guarded in patients with severe pneumonia, evidence of pleural effusion, skeletal lesions, and major organ failure. The decision to end therapy is based on clinical improvement, resolution of radiographic lesions, and failure to isolate the infecting organisms.

VIRAL PNEUMONIA

Primary viral pneumonia is uncommon in dogs and cats but often initiates respiratory disease that is complicated by bacterial rhinitis, tracheobronchitis, or bronchopneumonia. The viral agents capable of causing respiratory lesions will be briefly discussed (Table 29-7).

Causes, Pathogenesis, and Clinical Signs

Canine viral respiratory infections are most often described as part of the canine infectious tracheobronchitis complex. These viruses cause pharyngitis, tonsillitis, tracheitis, bronchitis, and/or interstitial pneumonia. Severe complicated cases have bacterial bronchopneumonia as a sequela.

Until 1962, canine distemper virus (morbilli virus) was thought to be the only viral cause of infectious respiratory disease in dogs. Canine distemper virus causes interstitial pneumonia and in combination with pathogenic bacteria it con-

Table 29–7 *Viruses That Cause Respiratory Infections in Dogs and Cats*

VIRUS

CANINE
Canine adenovirus type 1
Canine adenovirus type 2
Herpesvirus
Morbillivirus (Canine distemper virus)
Parainfluenza virus
Reovirus

FELINE
Calicivirus
Herpesvirus
Reovirus

tributes to a bronchopneumonia. Canine distemper virus causes a multisystemic infection of which pneumonia is a part of the disease complex.

Canine parainfluenza virus was first isolated in 1967 from dogs with respiratory disease and is the most frequently isolated viral agent from dogs with infectious tracheobronchitis. The virus replicates in nasal mucosa and bronchial epithelium causing rhinitis, bronchitis, tracheitis, and bronchiolitis. After experimental aerosol exposure, clinical signs include fever, serous to mucoid nasal discharge, and nonproductive cough. Clinical signs are more severe with concurrent infection with *Bordetella bronchiseptica* or *Mycoplasma*.

Canine adenovirus type 2 was isolated in 1962 as the first viral agent other than canine distemper virus associated with respiratory disease. After experimental aerosol exposure, clinical signs include anorexia, nasal discharge, and coughing. Lesions in these dogs include rhinitis, tonsillitis, pharyngitis, and bronchitis. In mixed infections with *B bronchiseptica* or mycoplasmas severe necrotizing tracheobronchitis, bronchiolitis, and interstitial pneumonia is found. Experimental intratracheal administration of canine adenovirus type 2 plus *B bronchiseptica*, *Pasteurella* species, or *Pseudomonas* species produces a distemper-like syndrome of mucopurulent nasal discharge, ocular discharge, and bronchopneumonia.

Herpesviruses plays major roles in respiratory infections of other species and have been isolated from dogs with respiratory disease. Herpesvirus is capable of initiating tracheobronchitis, but its overall contribution to the infectious canine tracheobronchitis complex is considered minor. Experimental aerosol exposure in dogs produces transient serous nasal discharge but no pneumonia.

Canine reoviruses are isolated rarely from dogs with respiratory infections. They produce mild pathological lesions and no clinical signs when gnotobiotic dogs are experimentally infected.

Three viruses are of importance in causing respiratory disease in cats, but only calicivirus causes pneumonia. Feline reovirus infections cause very mild clinical signs including serous ocular discharge and photophobia. Herpesviruses have a temperature dependent predilection for the upper respiratory tract and conjunctiva. Clinical signs in cats with herpesvirus infections include fever, anorexia, salivation, coughing, paroxysmal sneezing, and mucopurulent nasal and ocular discharge.

Feline calicivirus has affinity for lung and oral mucosa. Clinical signs include fever, serous ocular discharge, anorexia, salivation, oral ulcers, and dyspnea. Several pathogenic strains of calicivirus exist, and infection with virulent strains can cause fatal pneumonia, especially in young cats. Pathogenesis of the pneumonia is well documented. Calicivirus infects alveolar macrophages and pneumocytes in peripheral air exchange units. The virus stimulates these cells to produce neutrophil chemotactic factor which results in a neutrophilic exudative pneumonia.

Management

Principles of treatment for viral pneumonia are similar to those outlined under bacterial pneumonia.

ADDITIONAL READING

Green CE. Clinical microbiology and infectious diseases of the dog and cat, ed 2. Philadelphia: WB Saunders, 1990, 114.

Moser KM, Maurer J, Jassy L et al. Sensitivity, specificity and risk of diagnostic procedures in a canine model of Streptococcus pneumoniae pneumonia. Am Rev Respir Dis 1982; 125:436.

30

ALLERGIC LUNG DISEASE

Ned F. Kuehn, Philip Roudebush

The respiratory tract is in constant contact with the external environment and is therefore a major site of antigenic challenge. Diverse nonimmunologic and immunologic respiratory defense mechanisms are present to fend off potentially deleterious agents that are inhaled or aspirated. The host immune response, however, may on occasion have a detrimental function that results in tissue injury and clinical disease. These detrimental immunologic reactions are called *allergies* or *hypersensitivity reactions.*

Allergic lung disease is a result of one or several different types of hypersensitivity reactions whose consequences are detrimental to the host. We are only beginning to understand allergic lung disease in the dog and cat. Nevertheless, several lung diseases of allergic (or suspected allergic) etiology are documented or suspected in these species. These diseases include pulmonary infiltrates with eosinophilia (PIE), heartworm pneumonitis, allergic bronchopulmonary aspergillosis, parasitic pulmonary hypersensitivities, pulmonary nodular eosinophilic granulomatosis, extrinsic allergic alveolitis, and allergic or eosinophilic bronchitis (asthma).

CAUSES

The suspected causes of the allergic lung diseases are listed in Table 30-1. The classification scheme presented here is modified from that used in human medicine and is roughly based on the primary anatomic site of allergic disease and the immunologic mechanism(s) involved. Unfortunately, in many cases an etiology can not be found. The term PIE should not be used to designate disease in which a definitive etiology can be established.

PATHOPHYSIOLOGY

Allergic (hypersensitivity) reactions represent an excessive immunologic response to a substance that is usually innocuous in most individuals. Hypersensitivity reactions are classified on the basis of the different immunologic mechanisms by which they initiate tissue injury (Table 30-2). Immediate (Type I) hypersensitivities are probably the most common immune reactions causing allergic lung disease. Immune-complex (Type III)

423

Table 30–1 *Classification and Suggested Causes of Allergic Lung Disease in Dogs and Cats*

HYPERSENSITIVITY PNEUMONITIS (EXTRINSIC ALLERGIC ALVEOLITIS)
Molds
Actinomycetes
Other antigenic proteins

ASTHMA OR ALLERGIC (EOSINOPHILIC) BRONCHITIS
Pollen
Dusts
Atmospheric pollutants
Molds
Other inhaled aeroallergens

EOSINOPHILIC PNEUMONIAS (PULMONARY INFILTRATES WITH EOSINOPHILIA)
SIMPLE PULMONARY EOSINOPHILIA (LÖFFLERS'S SYNDROME)
Migrating parasites
   Ascarids
   Ancylostoma
Pulmonary mycosis
Viruses
Bacteria
Drugs
Unknown causes

PROLONGED PULMONARY EOSINOPHILIA WITHOUT ASTHMA
Pulmonary parasites
Pulmonary mycosis
Viruses
Bacteria
External inhaled aeroallergens
Unknown causes

TROPICAL PULMONARY EOSINOPHILIA
Filarial parasites (dirofilariasis)

PULMONARY NODULAR EOSINOPHILIC GRANULOMATOSIS
Filarial parasites (dirofilariasis)
Unknown causes

PULMONARY EOSINOPHILIA WITH ASTHMA
Pulmonary aspergillosis

DRUG-INDUCED PULMONARY HYPERSENSITIVITIES
Drugs incriminated in humans
   Carbamazepine
   Chlorpropamide
   Imipramine
   Mephenesin carbamate
   Para-amino salicylate
   Penicillin
   Sulfa drugs
   Tetracyclines

PULMONARY EOSINOPHILIA WITH POLYARTERITIS NODOSA
Unknown causes

PULMONARY INFILTRATES WITH EOSINOPHILA OF UNKNOWN ETIOLOGY

and Delayed (Type IV) hypersensitivity reactions are probably involved in certain allergic lung diseases; however, the mechanisms by which sensitization occurs to elicit these reactions are poorly understood. Cytotoxic (Type II) hypersensitivity reactions appear to be rarely involved in pulmonary disease. Type I allergic reactions play a major role in most pulmonary hypersensitivities. In sensitized individuals, immediate hypersensitivity reactions occur when a specific foreign antigen binds to IgE on the surface of mast cells causing degranulation and release of various factors that mediate the inflammatory response and provoke an infiltration of eosinophils. Eosinophils help regulate and dampen the Type I hypersensitivity reaction by inhibiting mast cell degranulation, facilitating degradation of mast cell mediators of inflammation, and phagocytosis of mast cell granules and IgE complexes. Eosinophils also release major basic protein, which normally neutralizes heparin released from mast cells. Major basic protein, however, may have a detrimental effect on the lung by damaging respiratory epithelial cells. Necrosis and sloughing of respiratory epithelial cells can impair the mucociliary apparatus and disrupt an important nonimmunologic defense mechanism of the pulmonary system. In situations of intense antigenic stimulation, eosinophilic lung injury can be extensive.

Pulmonary Infiltrates With Eosinophilia

Pulmonary infiltrates with eosinophilia (PIE) describes a group of allergic lung diseases characterized by the presence of both pulmonary associated and peripheral eosinophilia. Unfortunately, this combination is found in most allergic lung diseases. In the broadest sense, PIE is a generic designation of numerous allergic lung diseases of unrelated causes involving a spectrum of pulmonary hypersensitivity reactions, ranging from mild to severe, transient to chronic, and self-limiting to fatal.

Eosinophilic infiltrates may be limited to airways or the alveoli or may be present to varying degrees in both structures. Thoracic radiographs typically show combined alveolar and interstitial

Table 30–2 *Types of Hypersensitivity (Allergic) Reactions in Allergic Lung Disease*

TYPE I: IMMEDIATE (ANAPHYLACTIC) HYPERSENSITIVITY REACTIONS

Initiated by interaction of antigen with IgE antibody bound to surface of mast cells in sensitized individuals.

Antigen-antibody interaction causes degranulation of mast cells and rapid release of vasoactive and immunoregulatory substances.

TYPE II: CYTOTOXIC HYPERSENSITIVITY REACTIONS

Initiated by binding of IgG or IgM antibody to antigenic components on cell or tissue surfaces. Binding of antibody to the cells causes activation of the complement cascade, resulting in cell lysis and then cell phagocytosis by macrophages and neutrophils.

TYPE III: IMMUNE-COMPLEX HYPERSENSITIVITY REACTIONS

Initiated by deposition of circulating antigen-antibody complexes in various tissues or blood vessels.

Binding of and activation of complement to these immune complexes attracts neutrophils, which release various proteolytic and lysosomal enzymes that destroy surrounding host tissues.

TYPE IV: CELL-MEDIATED (DELAYED) HYPERSENSITIVITY REACTIONS

Initiated by interaction of sensitized T lymphocytes with immune complexes or specific antigens.

Response of these T lymphocytes is either direct cytotoxicity or release of lymphokines, which recruit inflammatory cells that secondarily cause tissue damage.

---

patterns. A bronchial pattern may also be present. Peripheral eosinophilia is a variable finding and may be absent (for example, because of prior corticosteroid administration), or its presence may be due to unrelated causes (*e.g.*, skin disease, gastrointestinal parasitism).

Because PIE is caused by diverse factors (see Table 30-1), the use of this term should probably be restricted to those cases in which an underlying cause is not found. We urge that the term PIE not be used to describe allergic lung diseases in which a definitive etiology can be established.

Simple Pulmonary Eosinophilia (Löffler's Syndrome)

Simple pulmonary eosinophilia (Löffler's syndrome) is a mild eosinophilic pneumonitis most often associated with migrating parasites and fungal infections. The accumulation of eosinophils in the lungs of patients with parasitic diseases may either be due to endogenous substances secreted by some parasites or to release of eosinophilic chemotactic factors during inflam-matory reactions. Immediate (Type I) and delayed (Type IV) hypersensitivity reactions may be mounted by the host toward invading helminths. The pulmonary migration of intestinal parasites (*Toxocara* species, *Strongyloides stercoralis*, *Ancylostoma* species) through the lung is generally associated with mild and transient or subclinical signs. Treatment is rarely required.

Pulmonary Eosinophilia Without Asthma

Pulmonary eosinophilia without asthma is a severe hypersensitivity pneumonitis associated most often with nonfilarial parasites and less commonly with fungal or chronic bacterial infections in dogs and cats. Type I and Type IV hypersensitivity reactions are probably involved. Infection of the respiratory tract by primary pulmonary parasites (*Capillaria aerophilia*, *Filaroides osleri*, *F. herthi*, *F. milksi*, *Crenosoma vulpis*, *Paragonimus* species, *Aelurostrongylus abstrusus*) typically elicits an intense chronic eosinophilic pneumonitis or bronchitis or both. Moderate to severe clinical signs are often present in these patients.

Pulmonary Eosinophilia With Asthma (Allergic Bronchopulmonary Aspergillosis)

Pulmonary eosinophilia with asthma is an uncommon cause of allergic asthma in dogs. Also called *allergic bronchopulmonary aspergillosis* (ABPA), this disease is caused by multiple (Type I and Type III) immunologic reactions against *Aspergillus fumigatus*. This organism colonizes the mucus secretions of the bronchopulmonary tree without invading tissue; however, the release of antigen materials during its colonization is responsible for sensitization of the host. Thoracic radiographs usually show ill-defined pulmonary infiltrates, which may transiently disappear to reappear at a different location. Occasionally atelectasis and pneumonia may occur. Bronchiectasis involving proximal airways and pulmonary fibrosis may develop in chronic cases.

Tropical Pulmonary Eosinophilia (Heartworm Pneumonitis)

Tropical pulmonary eosinophilia, caused by a Type I hypersensitivity reaction to filarial parasites, is a common cause of allergic lung disease in dogs and cats. Approximately 10% to 15% of all dogs with immune-mediated occult heartworm infection develop eosinophilic (allergic) pneumonitis. Microfilarial antigen is normally present in excess in heartworm disease. Therefore, all of the antimicrofilarial antibody produced by the host is consumed and microfilaremia persists. Immune-mediated occult heartworm disease, on the other hand, generally develops in a state of antimicrofilarial antibody excess. In this situation, all of the filarial antigen is complexed; therefore, microfilaria become entrapped in the pulmonary circulation and do not enter the systemic circulation.

Thoracic radiographs from dogs or cats with heartworm pneumonitis typically show diffuse linear interstitial infiltrates with concomitant diffuse alveolar lung disease. The alveolar infiltrate often is most prominent in the caudal lung lobes. Occasionally the pneumonitis may be so severe that the pulmonary infiltrates observed on thoracic radiographs may be mistaken for pulmonary edema or pulmonary blastomycosis. In many cases, little to no radiographic evidence of vascular or cardiac changes indicative of heartworm is present, a fact that often complicates the diagnosis of this disease.

Pulmonary Nodular Eosinophilic Granulomatosis

Pulmonary nodular eosinophilic granulomatosis (PNEG) is a rare, severe PIE-like syndrome occurring in dogs and is most often associated with heartworm. Types I, III, and IV (and perhaps Type II) hypersensitivity reactions to microfilaria may be involved. The hypersensitivity reactions to microfilaria are typically characterized by granulocytic inflammation with large numbers of eosinophils and small granulomas consisting of eosinophils and mononuclear cells. In PNEG, however, the granulomatous reaction becomes unusually severe and progressive during the course of the disease. Associated pathology may include eosinophilic granulomatous lymphadenitis, tracheitis, tonsillitis, splenitis, enteritis, gastritis, eosinophilic pericholangitis, and, occasionally, eosinophilic infiltration of liver and kidney. The granulomatous inflammation found in other organs suggests that soluble antigens or immune complexes may also be important, as are the adult or microfilarial antigens in the lung that trigger the pulmonary inflammation.

Thoracic radiographs from dogs with PNEG usually show mixed alveolar and interstitial infiltrates plus variably sized multiple pulmonary nodules scattered throughout the lung fields. Hilar and mediastinal lymphadenopathy and pleural effusion may also be present, though these findings are inconsistent.

Drug-Induced Pulmonary Hypersensitivities

Drug-induced pulmonary hypersensitivities are poorly documented in dogs and cats, either because they are rare or because they are largely unrecognized. Immediate (Type I) hypersensitivity is the suspected mechanism for the majority of these allergic reactions. The clinical signs may either be transient and mild, responding to drug withdrawal alone, or prolonged and severe, requiring glucocorticoid and supportive care.

Asthma or Allergic (Eosinophilic) Bronchitis

Asthma or *allergic (eosinophilic) bronchitis* is a reversible obstructive airway disease caused by an immediate (Type I) hypersensitivity in response to a wide variety of inciting agents (see Table 30-1). The airway response in asthma is different from that in chronic bronchitis (see Chapter 28) because asthma is a condition characterized by reversible airway obstruction and occurs only when an inciting agent stimulates the tracheobronchial tree.

The hypersensitivity reaction in asthma differs from other Type I pulmonary hypersensitivities in that the reaction principally involves the airways and not the parenchymal tissue. Mast cell degranulation causes the release of various factors, which provoke an eosinophilic infiltration and cause bronchial smooth muscle contraction, mucus gland hypersecretion, increased capillary permeability, and granulocyte chemotaxis. The outcome is airway obstruction due to bronchoconstriction, mucus plugging, edema, and the accumulation of cellular debris. The degree of physical airway obstruction is often particularly profound in cats, because bronchial mucus glands are more abundant in cats than other species.

Bronchoconstriction in asthma may also result from neurogenic imbalance of the cholinergic, β2-adrenergic, and adrenergic systems that innervate the airways. Any factor that blocks the β2-adrenergic or stimulates the adrenergic or cholinergic systems will cause bronchoconstriction. Neurogenic bronchoconstriction may be set off by infections, exercise, excitement, or air pollutants. The neurogenic bronchoconstriction elicited by these factors may also exacerbate the bronchoconstriction and bronchial obstruction resulting from hypersensitivity reactions.

Feline asthma is an acute respiratory disease characterized by a sudden onset of severe dyspnea. This disease is often accompanied by peripheral eosinophilia, and chronic recurrent episodes of coughing are not uncommon. Eosinophils, neutrophils, lymphocytes, and plasma cells are typically found within the lumen and walls of primary bronchi. The use of the term "asthma" to describe this bronchopulmonary disease of unknown etiology in cats is controversial. Although an allergic etiology is suspected, the exact cause(s) and pathophysiologic process responsible for this disease have not been elucidated. Interestingly, the pathologic changes in the lungs of some of these cats are more consistent with a diagnosis of chronic bronchitis.

Hypersensitivity Pneumonitis (Extrinsic Allergic Alveolitis)

Hypersensitivity pneumonitis (extrinsic allergic alveolitis) is a diffuse inflammatory disease of the distal portions of the lungs in reaction to inhaled organic allergens by sensitized individuals. Immune-complex (Type III) and cell-mediated (Type IV) hypersensitivity reactions appear to be involved primarily in the pathogenesis of hypersensitivity pneumonitis. Terminal airways and alveolar and interstitial tissues rather than the large airways are primarily affected.

In humans, repeated inhalation of certain actinomycetes and fungus-laden organic dust or foreign animal and plant proteins can cause this type of allergic reaction. The extent of the role inhaled allergens play in pulmonary hypersensitivities in dogs and cats is not clear at this time. However, inhaled allergens may be responsible for many of the suspected pulmonary hypersensitivities that defy etiologic diagnosis.

The pneumonitis in this allergic lung disease is characterized by a prominent mononuclear (macrophage lymphocyte) infiltrate associated with neutrophils. Normally, the accumulation of neutrophils and macrophages and their subsequent release of various inflammatory mediators in response to foreign substances are protective functions designed to eliminate the offending antigenic substances and promote repair of damaged tissues. Chronic antigen exposure or persistence of nondegradable antigen, however, will result in the continuous release of inflammatory mediators, which exert their potent biologic effects on surrounding tissues by producing substantial tissue destruction.

Acute hypersensitivity pneumonitis is characterized by fever, dry cough, and dyspnea 4 to 6 hours after exposure of a sensitized patient to antigen. Clinical signs generally last only 12 hours, providing no additional exposure occurs. Chronic hypersensitivity pneumonitis results from repeated or continuous exposure to the inciting antigen(s). Granuloma formation, interstitial and pulmonary fibrosis, and chronic respiratory failure are the sequela.

CLINICAL SIGNS

Clinical signs rarely suggest allergic lung disease, unless exposure to a specific antigen or air pollutant is known to provoke an attack. The clinical signs observed, however, help localize the patient's problem to a disorder of the cardiorespiratory system. The spectrum of clinical signs depend largely on the severity of the pulmonary hypersensitivity reaction. Expected clinical findings in patients with allergic lung disease include one or more of the following: exercise intolerance, coughing (acute or chronic, paroxysmal or continuous, productive or nonproductive), dyspnea (primarily expiratory), tachypnea, wheezing, gagging, hemoptysis, open-mouthed breathing, cyanosis, frantic behavior, and debilitation or emaciation.

The patient's history may give some clue to an underlying cause for the respiratory difficulty. Precipitating factors, such as exposure to a specific antigen or seasonal predisposition, suggest an allergic etiology. Clients owning dogs or cats from areas endemic for certain pulmonary parasites should be questioned about exposure of their pets to intermediate hosts or environments favored by the parasites (see Chapter 33). Owners of dogs from heartworm endemic areas should also be questioned concerning their animal's heartworm status and whether their dog actually receives a regular heartworm preventative (see Chapter 25).

Physical examination findings are generally not specific for allergic lung disease. Some animals may have a slight increase in body temperature due to increased respiratory effort. Auscultation of the lung fields may reveal inspiratory crackles or expiratory wheezes or both. A split second (S_2) heart sound may be due to heartworm, as well as other causes of pulmonary hypertension. The finding of a "silent chest" (near to total absence of lung sounds) often correlates with a high degree of airway obstruction and should be considered an ominous sign. This finding occurs most often in association with severe cases of asthma (particularly in cats).

DIAGNOSTIC APPROACH

The aggressiveness with which one approaches the diagnostic workup of a patient with suspected pulmonary disease depends on the degree of respiratory distress. Patients with mild or moderate respiratory distress can handle most diagnostic procedures without additional compromise of their respiratory reserve. Patients with severe respiratory distress should be stabilized before attempting diagnostic procedures. An attempt should be made in every case of suspected allergic disease to define an underlying cause. The laboratory assessment of allergic lung diseases is summarized in Table 30-3.

Thoracic radiographs are essential to the documentation and assessment of pulmonary disease. Unfortunately, many of the pulmonary hypersensitivities have no definitive radiographic find-

Table 30–3 *Laboratory Assessment of Allergic Lung Disease*

Test	What to Check For
Complete blood count	Eosinophilia, basophilia
Fecal analysis	Parasitic ova or larvae
Knott's test	Microfilaria
Chest radiographs	Interstitial or alveolar infiltrates, bronchial changes
Transtracheal wash	
Cytology	Eosinophils
Culture	Bacterial infection

ings. Findings common to many of the allergic lung diseases are irregular patchy alveolar infiltrates and increased bronchial markings.

Radiographic patterns associated with parasitic pulmonary diseases often include increased linear or nodular interstitial markings or large solid to cavitary pulmonary densities. An associated pneumothorax or pneumonia may rarely be present with parasitic pulmonary diseases. Heartworm typically causes characteristic changes in the cardiac silhouette and pulmonary vasculature, which are easily recognized radiographically (see Chapter 25). The massive alveolar infiltrates occurring with heartworm pneumonitis may, however, obscure the cardiac and pulmonary vascular shadows. Also, many of the cases with heartworm pneumonitis have few of the changes characteristic of heartworm, a fact that makes this diagnosis difficult at times (Fig. 30-1).

Typical radiographic findings in patients with allergic bronchitis (asthma) are often nonspecific and include increased bronchial markings with patchy alveolar infiltrates (Fig. 30-2). Cases associated with severe airway obstruction may show radiographic evidence of aerophagia and air-trapping (increased pulmonary radiolucency, flattening of the diaphragm, forward expansion of the rib cage). Radiographic lesions usually subside following acute exacerbation; however, a chronic bronchitic component may be evident in patients with recurrent attacks (increased bronchial markings, bronchiectasis, right middle lobe collapse).

A complete blood count may yield useful information. Allergic lung diseases may be accompanied by eosinophilia and basophilia; however, this finding is inconstant. Nonpulmonary hypersensitivities, such as intestinal parasitism and various skin diseases, may also have an associated eosinophilia. A mild leukocytosis may be found in patients with allergic lung disease, although a moderate to marked leukocytosis should alert the clinician to the possibility of pneumonia. Occasionally a mild anemia is also present, presumably due to the anemia of chronic inflammatory disease.

Fecal analysis for parasitic ova should be done in all suspected cases of allergic lung disease. The

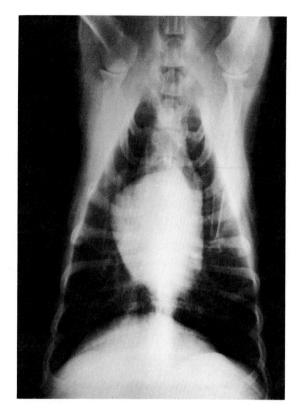

Figure 30–1 *Ventrodorsal thoracic radiograph of a 7-year-old female Irish setter with peripheral eosinophilia and pulmonary infiltrates of eosinophils secondary to occult heartworm. Notice the moderate bronchointerstitial changes throughout the lung fields. The cardiovascular changes are minimal in this particular patient with heartworm pneumonitis.*

Baermann technique is required to detect larval stages in feces. All dogs from heartworm endemic areas should have a microfilaria test performed. Serologic testing for heartworm should be done in cases where the microfilaria test is negative but clinical signs, hematologic tests, and radiographs are consistent with heartworm. Cats suspected of having dirofilariasis should be tested by both an enzyme-linked immunosorbent assay test and indirect fluorescent antibody test specific for feline heartworm.

A transtracheal wash (see Transtracheal Wash in Chapter 80) should be performed if the history, clinical signs, radiographs, fecal analyses, and hematologic and serologic tests do not establish the specific cause of the pulmonary disease. The fluid recovered from the wash should be submit-

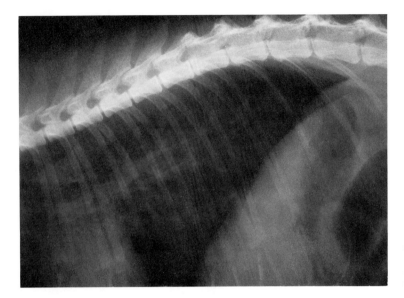

Figure 30–2 *Lateral thoracic radiograph of a 10-year-old female American shorthair cat with asthma. Notice the prominant bronchial pattern. The lung fields are hyperinflated and hyperlucent because of air-trapping by obstructed bronchioles during expiration.*

ted for culture and cytologic analysis. The finding of large numbers of eosinophils supports a diagnosis of allergic bronchitis (asthma) or eosinophilic pneumonitis. Rarely, chronic bacterial or fungal infections may produce an eosinophilic response, and culturing of a portion of the wash fluid is highly recommended. Cytologic examination may also reveal parasitic larva or ova overlooked on fecal analyses.

A spectrum of cytologic changes are seen in feline asthma. Large numbers of nontoxic neutrophils often represent the predominate cell type in many cases of feline asthma. Some cases may have a preponderance of eosinophils, while other cases may have a mixture of eosinophils and neutrophils. Culture is recommended to rule out bacterial infection if degenerative neutrophils are present.

Skin testing may be tried if no cause for suspected allergic lung disease is found and a seasonal or environmental influence is evident from the history. However, one must be careful in interpreting the results because the allergens identified by intradermal skin testing may not be the ones causing the pulmonary hypersensitivity. A difference in mast cell distribution between the lungs and skin could be one explanation for this discrepancy.

Lung biopsy should be performed in those cases in which a definitive diagnosis has not been established by noninvasive means (see Lung Biopsy in Chapter 80). In human medicine, lung biopsy is an accepted procedure for establishing a diagnosis and prognosis in patients with a wide variety of chronic interstitial lung diseases.

MANAGEMENT

The major goal in the management of allergic lung disease is correction or treatment of the underlying problem. A careful search for known causes of pulmonary hypersensitivities (*e.g.,* parasites, heartworms, infections, aeroallergens, drugs) should be attempted for every patient. In cases where environmental allergens are suspected, some, but not all, animals respond favorably to a change in environment or to removal of allergy-inducing objects. Most of the primary pulmonary parasites are effectively eliminated with levamisole, albendazole, fenbendazole, or thiabendazole (see Chapter 33). Suspected drug-induced pulmonary hypersensitivities are treated successfully often by mere withdrawal of the drug only.

In many cases, the severity of the hypersensitivity reaction is such that glucocorticoids are required to reduce the inflammatory activity prior to successful management of the underlying condition. Prednisolone is usually effective at a daily dose of 1 to 2 mg/kg orally tapered over 10 to 14 days. Chronic low dose glucocorticoid therapy (0.5 mg/kg/day) may be required in situations where exposure to an environmental allergen (*e.g.*, plant pollen, mold, dust) can not be eliminated or where the underlying cause of the pulmonary hypersensitivity remains undetermined. To minimize the numerous potential side effects of chronic glucocorticoid therapy, alternate day or every third day therapy is recommended whenever possible. Bronchodilators may be indicated if bronchoconstriction is suspected or only a partial response to steroids is observed.

The management of cats with feline asthma may be particularly challenging (Table 30-4). Cats without cyanosis but having mild to moderate respiratory distress generally respond favorably to cage rest and glucocorticoids. Bronchodilators may be needed if only a partial response to glucocorticoids is found. Cats with severe respiratory distress or cyanosis require immediate respiratory support. Supplemental oxygen is essential. Glucocorticoids and bronchodilators are also required to treat these patients. A dramatic response to oxygen and glucocorticoids in cats with compatible historical and clinical findings may be used to add support to a diagnosis of feline asthma. Management of recently stabilized acute asthmatics or cats presented for paroxysms of cough due to feline asthma require daily administration of glucocorticoids. Prednisolone or triamcinolone are usually effective. These medications should be gradually tapered over a period of several weeks. Antibiotics should be given if tracheobronchial cytology reveals septic inflammation. Broad spectrum antibiotics such as ampicillin are suggested initially. The initial antibiotic of choice should be reevaluated based on findings from culture and sensitivity results. Antibiotic therapy should be continued for a minimum of 34 weeks. Cats experiencing recurrent attacks frequently require chronic glucocorticoid therapy. Alternate day or every third or forth day therapy is advisable to prevent potential complications of long-term glucocorticoid therapy. Cats with chronic bronchial disease often become increasingly refractory to glucocorticoids and may benefit from bronchodilator therapy. A sustained release formulation of theophylline (Theo-Dur)

given at a dosage of 50 to 100 mg orally once daily is often effective. Avoidance of offending agents (*e.g.*, aerosols, smoke, or dusts) may improve clinical signs or reduce the frequency of attacks in feline asthma.

PATIENT MONITORING

In many cases of allergic lung disease, an underlying cause is not found. Periodic exacerbation of clinical signs or recurrent attacks should be anticipated in these patients. Further episodes often

Table 30–4 *Suggested Medications for the Medical Management of Feline Asthma*

MILD TO MODERATE RESPIRATORY DISTRESS

Corticosteroids
 Dexamethasone: 0.2 to 2.2 mg/kg/day, IV or IM
Bronchodilators
 Aminophylline: 4.5 to 5.0 mg/kg/day, PO, IM, or slowly IV

SEVERE RESPIRATORY DISTRESS OR CYANOSIS

Supplemental oxygen therapy
Corticosteroids
 Dexamethasone: 0.2 to 2.2 mg/kg/day, IV or IM
Bronchodilators
 Aminophylline: 4.5 to 5.0 mg/kg/day, PO, IM, or slowly IV
 Epinephrine: 0.5 to 0.75 ml of 1 : 10,000 solution, IM or SC
  Side effects: tachycardia, arrhythmogenic
 Isoproterenol: 0.1 to 0.2 ml of 1 : 5000 solution, IM or SC
  Side effects: tachycardia, arrhythmogenic
 Atropine: 0.05 mg/kg IM or SC
  Comments:
   acute management only (do not use long term); useful for resistant bronchospasm; give prior to airway manipulation;
  Side effects: decreases mucociliary clearance

MAINTENANCE THERAPY

Corticosteroids
 Prednisolone or prednisone:
  Initially: 1.0 to 2.0 mg/kg PO 2 to 3 times daily
  Taper: 2.5 mg PO once daily, every other day, or less frequently
 Triamcinolone:
  Initially: 0.25 to 0.5 mg/kg PO once daily
  Taper: 0.25 to 0.5 mg/kg PO once daily, every other day, or less frequently
 Methylprednisolone acetate: 10 to 20 mg per cat IM every 6 to 8 weeks (only use for cases with problems in compliance)
Bronchodilators
 Theophylline, sustained release (Theo-Dur[R]): 50 to 100 mg PO per cat per day
 Terbutaline: 1.25 mg PO every 12 hours

require additional medical care. This fact particularly should be communicated to owners of cats with feline asthma.

Those animals requiring chronic glucocorticoid therapy should be monitored periodically to ensure that the dose of medication is not higher than actually needed to control clinical signs. Clients of animals requiring chronic glucocorticoid therapy should be warned of the adverse long-term side effects of these medications (see Appendix).

In those cases where the underlying cause is identified and corrected, the long-term prognosis is excellent.

ADDITIONAL READING

Bauer TG. Pulmonary hypersensitivity disorders. In: Kirk RW, ed. Current veterinary therapy X. Philadelphia: WB Saunders, 1989: 369.

Calvert CA, Mahaffey MB, Lappin MR, Farrell RL. Pulmonary and disseminated eosinophilic granulomatosis in dogs. Journal of the American Animal Hospital Association 1988; 24:311.

Felsburg PJ. Respiratory immunology. In: Kirk RW, ed. Current veterinary therapy IX. Philadelphia: WB Saunders, 1986: 228.

Halliwell REW, Gorman NT. Hypersensitivity lung disease. In: Halliwell REW, Gorman NT, eds. Veterinary clinical immunology. Philadelphia: WB Saunders, 1989: 359.

Moise NS, Spaulding GL. Feline bronchial asthma: pathogenesis, pathophysiology, diagnostics, and therapeutic considerations. Compendium of Continuing Education 1981; 3:1091.

Moses BL, Spaulding GL. Chronic bronchial disease of the cat. In: Spaulding GL, ed. Symposium on respiratory diseases. Vet Clin North Amer 1985; 15:929.

Noone KE. Pulmonary hypersensitivities. In: Kirk RW, ed. Current veterinary therapy IX. Philadelphia: WB Saunders, 1986: 285.

Papich MG. Bronchodilator therapy. In: Kirk RW, ed. Current veterinary therapy IX. Philadelphia: WB Saunders, 1986: 278.

Pechman RD. Newer knowledge of feline bronchopulmonary disease. In: August JR, Loar AS, eds. Symposium on advances in feline medicine I. Vet Clin North Amer 1984; 14:1007.

Suter PF. Lower airway and pulmonary parenchymal diseases. In: Suter PF, ed. Thoracic radiography: a text atlas of thoracic diseases of the dog and cat. Wettswil, Switzerland: PF Suter 1984: 517.

31

PULMONARY EDEMA

Ned F. Kuehn, Philip Roudebush

Pulmonary edema is a condition characterized by the abnormal, diffuse, extravascular accumulation of fluid within the peribronchial, interstitial, or alveolar areas of the lung. Edema fluid originates most often from endogenous sources; however, in some diseases, or in a near drowning, for example, aspirated exogenous fluids have a significant contribution to the total volume of accumulated edema fluid. Pulmonary edema is an important complication in a spectrum of cardiac and pulmonary diseases and may be life-threatening. Respiratory failure is manifested by an inability to oxygenate arterial blood, often despite the ability to ventilate sufficiently to excrete carbon dioxide. Successful treatment of patients with pulmonary edema often depends on discovery of the underlying cause of fluid formation.

CAUSES

A pathophysiologic classification of known and suspected causes of pulmonary edema is given in Table 31-1. It is convenient to group the various causes of pulmonary edema into categories based on the primary pathophysiologic mechanism responsible for fluid formation. In certain circumstances, however, multiple factors may be involved in the fluid formation, and in certain causes of pulmonary edema the mechanisms for fluid formation are not clearly understood. The most common cause for pulmonary edema in dogs and cats is left heart failure.

PATHOPHYSIOLOGY

In health, fluid movement between the capillaries, lymphatics, and interstitial and alveolar tissues is a dynamic process. The lungs are normally a site of constant liquid filtration and removal, at a rate similar to that found in most other organs. Pulmonary edema results only when the rate of fluid filtration in the lungs exceeds the rate of its removal.

The capillary endothelium ordinarily is highly permeable to water and small molecules and ions, but relatively impermeable to large proteins. On the other hand, the alveolar epithelium usually is considerably less permeable than the capillary endothelium to the passage of small molecules and proteins. The alveolar epithelium does allow passage of water, but even small molecules typically are prevented from crossing into the alveolar space. The capillary endothelium, therefore, is the major site of filtration of liquid in the lungs.

The factors determining the rate of fluid filtra-

Table 31–1 *Causes of Pulmonary Edema Based on Pathophysiologic Mechanisms*

INCREASED CAPILLARY HYDROSTATIC PRESSURE

Cardiogenic:
  Myocardial failure
    Dilated cardiomyopathy
  Chronic pressure or volume overload
    Mitral regurgitation
    Congenital heart disease
      Patent ductus arteriosus
      Subaortic stenosis
    Obstruction to left ventricular filling
      Hypertrophic cardiomyopathy
      Left atrial thrombus
      Left atrial neoplasm
  Arrhythmias
Overinfusion of blood or fluids
Pulmonary venous diseases
  Pulmonary veno-occlusive disease
  Pulmonary venous stenosis
    Mediastinal masses

INCREASED CAPILLARY PERMEABILITY

Infectious pulmonary disease
  Bacterial or viral pneumonia
Toxic damage
  Inhaled toxins
    Smoke inhalation
    Oxygen toxicity
  Aspiration syndromes
    Gastric contents
    Near drowning and drowning
    Hypertonic substances
  Circulating exogenous toxins
    Snake venom
    Paraquat
    Endotoxins
    ANTU (rodenticide)
  Circulating endogenous toxins
    Uremia
    Vasoactive substances
      Histamine
      Kinins
      Prostaglandins
    Shock lung (vasoactive substances?)
Pulmonary contusion
Disseminated intravascular coagulation
  Post-infectious immune-complex disease
  Heatstroke
Immunologic reactions
  Idiosyncratic drug reactions
  Allergic alveolitis
Adult respiratory distress syndrome (ARDS)

LYMPHATIC INSUFFICIENCY

Neoplastic infiltration
  Lymphangitis carcinomatosis
  Lymphoma
Fibrosing lymphangitis
Tracheobronchial lymphadenopathy

DECREASED COLLOID OSMOTIC PRESSURE

Hypoalbuminenia
  Protein-losing nephropathies
  Protein-losing enteropathies
  Protein-losing skin diseases
  Chronic liver failure
  Nutritional disorders
Over infusion of crystalloid fluids

INCREASED NEGATIVE INTERSTITIAL PRESSURE

Re-expansion pulmonary edema

UNKNOWN MECHANISMS

Neurogenic pulmonary edema
Pulmonary embolism
Pulmonary parenchymal disease
Postanesthetic
Cardioversion
High-altitude pulmonary edema

tion across the pulmonary capillary endothelium (and across the capillary endothelium in most other tissues) are defined by Starling's equation: $Qi = K[(Pc - Pi) - \sigma d(\pi c - \pi i)]$; where, Qi is the net flow out of the capillary into the interstitium; K is the filtration coefficient (an expression of the leakiness of the membrane); Pc and Pi are the hydrostatic pressures in the capillary and interstitial space, respectively; πc and πi are the colloid osmotic pressures in the capillary and interstitial space, respectively; and, σd is the reflection coefficient (a measure of the effectiveness of the membrane in preventing or reflecting the passage of protein as compared to that of water across the membrane). Careful examination of Starling's equation reveals that the volume of fluid leaving the capillary and flowing into the interstitium is: 1) directly related to the leakiness (permeability) of the capillary membrane; and, 2) directly related to the differences in osmotic and hydrostatic forces across the capillary membrane. The permeability of the capillary endothelium normally remains constant in health. Therefore, the regular movement of fluid across the capillary endothelium and into the interstitial space is brought about by differences in hydrostatic and osmotic forces across the capillary membrane.

The hydrostatic and osmotic pressures within the capillary are usually greater than the hydrostatic and osmotic pressures found in the interstitial spaces.

In general, hydrostatic forces tend to move fluid from within the capillaries to the interstitial space, while colloid osmotic forces tend to keep fluid within the capillary lumen. The overall net difference between the hydrostatic and osmotic pressures is such that a slight continuous flow of fluid goes out of the capillary lumen and into the interstitial space. The fluid that leaves the capillaries moves within the interstitial space along the alveolar walls and then trails to the perivascular and peribronchial interstitium, which contain the lymphatics. The lymphatic vessels then collect the interstitial fluid, an act that causes a continuous slow lymph flow and prevents the accumulation of fluid within the pulmonary parenchyma. Pulmonary edema develops when one or more of the intravascular or extravascular forces governing filtration (hydrostatic

and osmotic pressures) changes by a critical amount, the permeability of the capillary endothelium is enhanced, lymphatic drainage is impaired, or some combination of these factors is altered significantly (Fig. 31-1).

Only a very small amount of fluid can be accommodated within the interstitial space nearby the alveolar wall. In contrast to this, a substantial volume of fluid can accumulate in the interstitial spaces surrounding the airways and vessels. During the early stages of pulmonary edema, the accumulation of free fluid in the interstitial spaces surrounding the airways and vessels forms a band around the bronchioles and veins. This peribronchovascular fluid accumulation can be recognized on thoracic radiographs as increased interstitial densities, perivascular smudging, and peribronchial cuffing. With advancing pulmonary edema, peribronchial fluid accumulation continues to increase. The intensifying ring of fluid surrounding bronchioles may lead to narrowing and premature closure of the airways during expiration (expiratory dyspnea and end-inspiratory crackles). Clinically this problem is accentuated in older and recumbent animals.

Alveolar flooding occurs only after the peribronchovascular interstitial spaces are filled with fluid and when the rate of fluid filtration continues to exceed that of lymphatic removal. As alveoli become progressively filled with fluid, total pulmonary gas exchange gradually deteriorates. The pulmonary capillaries encircling flooded alveoli become a pure venous-arterial shunt because no ventilation can occur within these flooded units. Dyspnea, tachypnea, and hypoxemia are seen clinically. Thoracic radiographs will reveal an alveolar pattern characterized by air bronchograms.

Blood-gas determinations may be useful to gauge the severity of alveolar flooding and the need for supplemental oxygen therapy. In dogs, however, the magnitude of arterial hypoxia occasionally correlates poorly with the severity of edema. This event probably occurs because dogs normally have an extensive collateral airway network. Therefore, regional ventilatory changes associated with pulmonary edema are less likely to result in ventilation-perfusion mismatching sufficient to cause severe hypoxia.

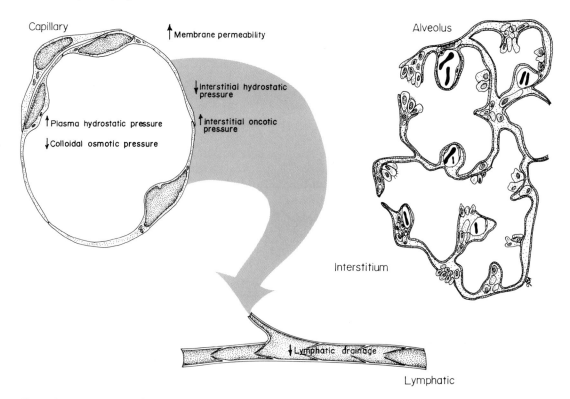

Figure 31–1 *Factors contributing to the formation of pulmonary edema.*

The presence of foam in the airways represents the last stage in the sequence of pathophysiologic events associated with pulmonary edema. The development of foam indicates that air and liquid have intermixed, the site of which is probably the small airways. The exceptionally low surface tension of surfactant stabilizes the tiny bubbles. Blood tinged foam may be present in some forms of pulmonary edema, particularly those of cardiac origin. These pink frothy secretions are produced by the mixture of small quantities of blood that oozes from ruptured blood vessels, presumably the result of increased hydrostatic pressure. Blood tinged foam does not develop because of alterations in the permeability of the alveolar capillary membrane sufficient to permit passage of particles as large as red blood cells.

Lung compliance, or the ease with which the lung can be expanded, is severely impaired in pulmonary edema. As lung compliance decreases (lung stiffness increases) the patient increases work and energy expenditure to support ade-

quate ventilation. Fluid in alveoli causes an increase in surface tension, which also contributes to decreased lung compliance. Chronic interstitial edema induces reactive tissue changes and lung fibrosis, which furthermore decrease pulmonary compliance. Compliance changes and hypoxemia cause tachypnea, dyspnea, and apprehension. With increased stiffness to the lungs, breathing becomes more shallow and rapid. Hyperventilation (and coughing) may likewise develop from stimulation of specialized pulmonary juxtacapillary receptors (J receptors) by interstitial edema.

An important underlying difference exists between pulmonary and nonpulmonary tissues. Nonpulmonary tissues (except the brain) have a relatively large interstitial space, which can store relatively large quantities of fluid without causing life-threatening derangement of function. In the lung, the interstitial space has a limited storage capacity. When the rate of fluid accumulation in the interstitial space exceeds lymphatic drainage, excess fluid will move into the airspaces and interfere with gas exchange. The anatomic classification of pulmonary edema as either interstitial edema or alveolar edema is often clinically relevant. Interstitial pulmonary edema occurs earlier clinically and is recognized radiographically by increased interstitial densities, perivascular smudging, and peribronchial cuffing.

A brief discussion of the pathophysiological processes responsible for the formation of fluid based on the various categories of pulmonary edema given in Table 31-1 follows.

Increased Capillary Hydrostatic Pressure

This condition is the most common cause of pulmonary edema in dogs and cats and frequently complicates heart failure. In cardiogenic pulmonary edema, left atrial pressure rises, causing an increase in pulmonary venous and capillary pressures. The development of alveolar edema in these conditions is dependent on the rate of increase of venous pressure. For example, in dogs with chronic mitral regurgitation, venous pressures gradually rise over a period of time, and remarkably high venous pressures are tolerated without clinical evidence of alveolar edema. Alveolar flooding is prevented because the caliber or number (or both) of pulmonary lymphatics increases to accommodate higher lymph flow, even despite the presence of marked interstitial edema. On the other hand, dogs with acute mitral regurgitation resulting, for example, from sudden rupture of chordae tendineae may rapidly develop alveolar edema. Alveolar flooding occurs rapidly in this situation because this sudden (but smaller) rise in venous pressure does not allow sufficient time for pulmonary lymphatics to adjust to higher lymph flow rates.

Increased Permeability

Various clinical syndromes result in damage to the alveolar capillary membrane and are often referred to as *adult respiratory distress syndrome* (ARDS). Direct physical or chemical damage to either the alveolar epithelial or pulmonary capillary endothelial cells may increase permeability of these structures and lead to pulmonary edema. An increase in pulmonary microvascular permeability causes leakage of virtually pure plasma into the interstitium and raises the interstitial osmotic pressure to equal that of plasma. Therefore, the normal protective effect of the transmural osmotic pressure difference is lost. Samples of fluid obtained from the lower respiratory tract in patients with permeability edema are identical to those of plasma. This finding is in distinct contrast to cardiogenic pulmonary edema, in which the protein concentration of fluid from the lower respiratory tract is lower than that in blood.

Lymphatic Insufficiency

Normal lymphatic drainage may be slowed because of obliteration or distortion of the lymphatics or lymph nodes. Pulmonary edema may occur at a lower rate of enhanced filtration (or even in the absence of an increase in filtration) because the normal capacity of the lymphatics to accommodate fluid is compromised by disease.

Decreased Colloid Osmotic Pressure

A decrease in colloid osmotic pressure is rarely responsible for the formation of pulmonary edema alone. A decrease in colloid osmotic pressure typically will exaggerate the volume of edema, which occurs when some other precipitating factor is present (*e.g.*, left heart failure). A decrease in serum protein concentration causes a decline in the transmural protein osmotic pressure difference and results in increased filtration (assuming hydrostatic forces and permeability are unchanged). Pulmonary edema does not normally develop under these circumstances because the removal of fluid by the lymphatics increases to keep pace with the augmented rate of fluid formation. One major consequence of a reduced transmural protein osmotic gradient is that pulmonary edema may occur at a lower level of increased hydrostatic pressure difference than that expected when serum protein concentrations are normal. For example, milder forms of left heart failure may be associated with pulmonary edema earlier in the course of disease in patients with hypoproteinemia than would be expected in patients with normal plasma protein concentrations.

Decreased Interstitial Pressure

Decreased interstitial pressure would be expected to promote pulmonary edema by increasing the hydrostatic pressure difference across the capillary wall. The rapid removal of fluid or air from patients with large unilateral pleural effusions or pneumothorax may cause the development of pulmonary edema on the side of the lung that is rapidly expanded. It is proposed that the formation of pulmonary edema in these instances may be related to mechanical forces acting on the interstitial space, which serve to create a large negative (decreased) interstitial pressure as the lung is expanded. Evidence also exists of altered (increased) capillary permeability in these patients.

CLINICAL SIGNS

The scope of associated historical and physical examination findings depends to some extent on the cause of the pulmonary edema and its severity. Historical information and clinical signs often support a diagnosis of cardiac or pulmonary disease but are infrequently specific for pulmonary edema. The clinical signs most often observed include the following: dyspnea, rapid and shallow breathing, exertional dyspnea (possibly the only sign with mild edema), orthopnea, cough (dogs mainly, cats rarely), paroxysmal dyspnea during recumbency, Cheyne-Stokes respiration (few short breaths followed by a period of apnea followed again by a few short breaths), open mouth breathing (sign of severe respiratory distress in the cat), cyanosis, and expectoration of foamy liquid (indicates fulminant edema). As pulmonary fluid accumulation intensifies, dogs, unlike cats, are generally reluctant to lie down. Af-

fected dogs tend to stand or sit with their elbows abducted. Cats, however, often crouch in a sternal position with elbows abducted.

Auscultatory findings vary as well as the clinical signs. Abnormal respiratory sounds, regardless of their intensity, are not specific for pulmonary edema and only allude to the presence of lung disease. With early interstitial edema, no audible abnormalities may be found. As smaller airways become compressed from peribronchial edema, inspiratory crackles may be heard as these previously closed airways pop open. As edema worsens, both inspiratory and expiratory crackles and wheezes may be heard.

Additional historical and physical examination abnormalities may suggest a possible cause for the pulmonary edema. The presence of a heart murmur, gallop rhythm, or arrhythmia during auscultation may suggest a cardiac cause for the edema. A frayed electrical cord and burns in the mouth of a dog or cat might suggest electrocution.

DIAGNOSTIC APPROACH

When the historical and clinical findings suggest the possibility of pulmonary edema, thoracic radiographs should be obtained for confirmation and assessment of its severity (Fig. 31-2). Evaluation of the cardiac silhouette is especially important, as congestive heart failure is the most common cause of pulmonary edema in dogs and cats (see Chapter 20). In severely compromised patients, emergency therapy may be required to stabilize the patient before thoracic radiographs can be obtained safely.

Following initial stabilization of the patient, other ancillary diagnostic procedures are often required to determine the underlying cause for the edema (Table 31-2). Unless the history and physical examination findings suggest otherwise, it is recommended to first rule out cardiogenic causes for the edema, since they are most common. Cardiac auscultation, thoracic radiography, electrocardiography, and, if necessary, echocardiography will ordinarily disclose evidence supporting primary heart disease.

A complete blood count, serum biochemistry

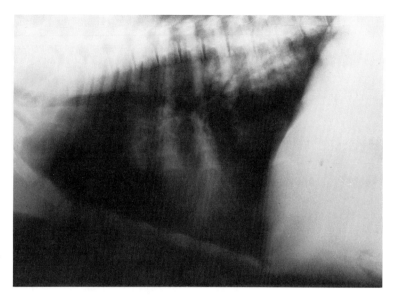

Figure 31-2 *Lateral thoracic radiograph of a 2-month-old male Great Dane with mild neurogenic pulmonary edema as a result of status epilepticus. Notice the diffuse interstitial pattern throughout the lung fields. Recovery was uneventful, and specific therapy was not required to manage the pulmonary edema.*

panel, and urinalysis are generally indicated. These tests may disclose underlying disorders (*e.g.*, hypoproteinemia, renal failure), which might exacerbate an otherwise clinically stable primary cardiac disease, or disclose non-cardiac

Table 31-2 *Laboratory Assessment of Pulmonary Edema*

Test	What to Check For
Complete blood count	Neutrophilia
	Neutropenia
	Toxic neutrophils
	Anemia
	Thrombocytopenia
Serum biochemistry	Hypoproteinemia
	Hypoalbuminemia
	Azotemia
Urinalysis	Proteinuria
Thoracic radiographs	Increased interstitial markings
	Peribronchial cuffing
	Perivascular cuffing
	Air bronchograms
	Cardiomegaly
	Left atrial masses
	Heartworm disease
Electrocardiogram	Heart rate and rhythm
	Chamber enlargement
Echocardiogram	Chamber enlargement
	Myocardial contractility
	Valvular abnormalities
	Intracardiac mass(es)

edematogenic diseases such as uremia or endotoxemia. Blood-gas determinations may be necessary to gauge the need for or effectiveness of supplemental oxygen therapy.

If the primary disease responsible for the edema formation is still not disclosed, sophisticated diagnostic procedures are often required. Selective pulmonary vascular catheterization for measurement of pulmonary artery and pulmonary artery wedge pressures may disclose the presence of pulmonary hypertension (which may be contributory to the development of pulmonary edema) or pulmonary venous hypertension, respectively. Several direct and indirect methods are available to assess alterations in vascular permeability. Availability of equipment and clinicians trained for these procedures, however, is limited.

MANAGEMENT

Therapeutic measures beneficial for the management of dogs or cats with pulmonary edema are outlined in Table 31-3. The basic therapeutic objectives are: 1) restoration of arterial oxygenation; 2) mobilization of the edema fluid; 3) correction of acid-base imbalances; and 4) successful treatment of the underlying cause of the pulmo-

(text continues on page 442)

Table 31–3 *Therapeutic Measures Helpful for Treatment of Pulmonary Edema*

GENERAL MEASURES USEFUL IN MOST FORMS OF PULMONARY EDEMA

Avoid unnecessary stress on the animal
Provide cage rest
Measures to improve oxygen exchange
  Provide supplemental oxygen
    Avoid >50% O_2 concentration for >24 hrs
  Intubate and provide mechanical ventilation, if critical
    Positive end-expiratory pressure ventilation
    Continuous positive airway pressure ventilation
  If frothing evident
    Airway suction
    Nebulization with 20% to 50% ethanol
  Bronchodilation
    Aminophylline (dogs and cats)
      PO, slowly IV: 5 to 10 mg/kg every 6 to 8 hrs as needed
Reduce anxiety
  Morphine (avoid in neurogenic edema)
    Dogs
      IV: 0.05 to 0.1 mg/kg every 2 to 3 min until relief evident
      SC, IM: 0.2 to 0.5 mg/kg every 4 to 6 hrs as needed
    Cats
      IM: 0.1 mg/kg every 4 to 6 hrs as needed
      SC: 0.1 mg/kg every 4 to 6 hrs as needed
  Acetylpromazine (dogs and cats)
    SC, IM: 0.05 to 0.25 mg/kg every 4 to 8 hrs as needed
  Diazepam
    Dogs
      IV: 5 to 10 mg every 2 to 6 hours as needed
    Cats
      IV: 2 to 5 mg every 2 to 6 hrs as needed
  Pentobarbitol (dogs and cats)
    IM, IV: 6 to 10 mg/kg every 6 to 12 hrs as needed
Decrease lung liquid accumulation
  Loop diuretics
    Furosemide (IV, IM, SC)
      Dogs: 2 to 8 mg/kg; may repeat every 1 to 12 hrs
      Cats: 1 to 2 mg/kg; may repeat every 8 to 12 hrs
Correct or improve acid-base derangement
Guard against congestion or atelectasis in dependent lobes
  Alternate patient position if animal recumbent

THERAPY PRIMARILY AGAINST INCREASED CAPILLARY HYDROSTATIC PRESSURE

Cardiogenic edema
  Increase myocardial contractility
    Dopamine
      IV: 2 to 8 μg/kg/min constant rate infusion
    Dobutamine
      IV: 2 to 10 μg/kg/min constant rate infusion
    Milrinone (dogs and cats)
      PO: 0.5 to 1.0 mg/kg every 8 to 12 hrs
    Digitalis (rapid IV digitalization not suggested)
      Dogs: PO: 0.22 mg/m^2 every 12 hrs
      Cats: PO: 0.008 mg/kg every 12 hrs

(continued)

Table 31–3 (continued)

Decrease afterload
  Morphine (see above)
  Hydralazine (dogs)
    PO: 0.5 to 3 mg/kg every 12 hrs
  Sodium nitroprusside (dogs and cats)
    IV: 5 to 20 μg/kg/min constant rate infusion
Decrease preload
  Morphine (see above)
  Loop diuretics (see above)
  Nitroglycerin (administer topically on hairless area)
    Dogs: 1/4 to 3/4 inch 2% ointment every 8 hours
    Cats: 1/8 to 1/4 inch 2% ointment every 8 hours
  Isosorbide dinitrate (dogs and cats)
    PO: 0.5 to 2.0 mg/kg every 8 hrs
  Phlebotomy (dogs and cats)
    6 to 10 ml/kg once
Control or abolish arrhythmias
  Antiarrhythmics (drug indicated by type of arrhythmia)
Non-cardiogenic edema
  Blood or fluid overload
    Stop blood or fluid administration
    Diuretics (see above)
    Phlebotomy (see above)
  Pulmonary venous diseases
    Surgical or medical intervention as situation dictates

THERAPY PRIMARILY AGAINST INCREASED CAPILLARY PERMEABILITY

Hypovolemia
Anti-inflammatory drugs
  Methylprednisolone (dogs and cats)
    IV: 10 to 30 mg/kg
  Prednisolone (dogs and cats)
    IV: 1 to 2 mg/kg
Free radical scavengers (see text)
  Superoxide dismutase (DMSO)
    IV: 2 mg/kg dose, interval unknown
  Orgotein
    SC: 5 mg total dose every 24 hrs
Prostaglandin synthesis inhibitors (see text)
  Indomethocin (dogs)
    IV: 10 mg/kg follow with 5 mg/kg/hr
  Flunixin meglumine (dogs)
    IV, IM: 0.25 to 1.0 mg/kg once daily
Increase plasma oncotic pressure
  Albumin
  High-molecular-weight dextran
Suppression of intravascular coagulation
  Heparin?
  Low-molecular-weight dextran?

nary edema. A responsible approach to treatment requires the succession of rapid decisions based on clinical findings. Acute fulminating pulmonary edema demands prompt attention directed at the life-threatening signs. In subacute or chronic pulmonary edema, identification of the primary cause should be attempted first, and then therapy specifically directed at the underlying problem should be initiated.

The general measures outlined in Table 31-3 are applicable to most forms of pulmonary edema. Mild pulmonary edema may require no more than cage rest. In more severe forms of edema, the degree of therapeutic intervention is dictated by the patient's clinical condition. If a cause for the edema is not immediately discernible, further diagnostic tests are deferred until the patient is stabilized.

Animals with moderate to severe pulmonary edema should be maintained in an oxygen-enriched environment. Oxygen can be provided by means of a face mask, nasal catheter, or oxygen cage. The administration of elevated levels of oxygen (40%–60%) at the start of therapy is useful because it increases the driving force for diffusion of oxygen into the alveolar capillaries. High oxygen concentrations (greater than 70%), however, can injure lung tissue. Animals with severe pulmonary edema benefit from endotracheal or tracheostomy tube placement and mechanical ventilation with either positive end-expiratory pressure or continuous positive airway pressure. Suctioning of airways is necessary if frothing is present. Bronchodilators, such as aminophylline, may facilitate oxygen delivery to the alveoli.

Sedation of patients with moderate to severe pulmonary edema is generally necessary. Morphine is the sedative of choice. Morphine exerts three direct beneficial effects in the treatment of pulmonary edema: relief of anxiety, depression of respiratory centers, and venodilation. Relief of anxiety reduces energy expenditure and also improves ventilation in patients with violent breathing patterns. Depression of respiratory centers is beneficial because it will change the character of the respirations from rapid, violent movements to slow, deep respirations. The venodilatory effects of morphine increase the volume of blood sequestered in capacitance vessels. This pooling will divert blood volume from the pulmonary to the systemic veins and decrease pulmonary capillary pressure. Cats become hyperexcited at high dosages of morphine; therefore, this drug should be used cautiously in cats. Low dosages of phenothiazines are also effective in cats. Morphine will increase intracranial pressure and is contraindicated in dogs or cats suspected of having neurogenic pulmonary edema. Diazepam may be a useful sedative in this situation.

Potent loop diuretics, such as furosemide, are particularly effective in mobilizing edema fluid from the lung. Intensive diuresis (to the point of hypovolemia) may improve pulmonary mechanics and gas exchange in patients with pulmonary edema due to altered membrane permeability (*e.g.*, adult respiratory distress syndrome). The overzealous use of these drugs, nevertheless, may dramatically reduce cardiac output and cause shock (see Chapter 4).

Measures directed toward normalization of acid-base derangements may be needed (see Chapter 71). Respiratory alkalosis is usually not of sufficient magnitude to require specific treatment other than measures designed to relieve the pulmonary edema. Metabolic acidosis principally occurs because of the combination of severe reduction in cardiac output and functional impairment of the liver. Treatment with sodium bicarbonate and measures designed to relieve the pulmonary edema are required when severe metabolic acidosis is present.

Measures Directed Primarily Against Increased Capillary Pressure

The most common cause of increased pulmonary capillary pressure in the dog and cat is left heart failure. General measures directed at control of the pulmonary edema and specific therapy directed at the cause of the heart failure is indicated (see Table 31-3). Specific therapy is contingent on the determination of the cause of the heart failure. The clinician is directed to the appropriate chapters in the section on problems of the cardiovascular system (see Chapter 20).

Measures Directed Primarily Against Increased Capillary Or Alveolar Membrane Permeability

Relatively few therapies are available at this time with demonstrable clinical efficacy for the management of increased alveolar capillary membrane permeability. Pulmonary edema due to increased membrane permeability is generally more difficult to treat than that due to cardiogenic factors. Often the site and extent of injury is not established. In cases of pulmonary edema due to septicemia, specific therapy is directed primarily against the infectious agent. Glucocorticoids may have beneficial anti-inflammatory properties in the management of septic shock (see Chapter 4). Corticosteroids have also been advocated for the treatment of smoke inhalation, electric shock, anaphylaxis, snake bites, and ARDS. With pulmonary edema related to altered clotting mechanisms (*e.g.*, disseminated intravascular coagulation), correction of the underlying problem, if possible, is essential (see Chapter 16). The clinical use of free radical scavengers (*e.g.*, DMSO, orgotein) and prostaglandin synthesis inhibitors is limited at this time. On empirical grounds, flunixin meglumine appears beneficial in the management of septic shock (see Chapter 4).

PATIENT MONITORING

Continuous monitoring of patients with moderate to severe pulmonary edema is essential. Once the patient is stabilized, a thorough search is made to find and correct the underlying cause. Long-term patient management is dependent on the cause of the edema.

ADDITIONAL READING

Bauer TG, Thomas WP. Pulmonary edema. In: Kirk RW, ed. Current veterinary therapy VIII. Philadelphia: WB Saunders, 1983: 252.

Crowe DT. Traumatic pulmonary contusions, hematomas, pseudocysts, and acute respiratory distress syndrome: an update. Part I. Compendium of Continuing Education 1983; 5:396.

Davis LE. Management of acute pulmonary edema. J Am Vet Med Assoc 1979; 175:97.

Fitzpatrick RF, Crowe DT. Nasal oxygen administration in dogs and cats: experimental and clinical investigations. Journal of the American Animal Hospital Association 1986; 22:293.

Harpster N. Pulmonary edema. In: Kirk RW, Bonagura JD, eds. Current veterinary therapy X. Philadelphia: WB Saunders, 1989: 385.

Morgan RV. Respiratory emergencies. Part I. Compendium of Continuing Education 1983; 5:228.

Olivier NB. Pulmonary edema. In: Symposium on respiratory diseases. Vet Clin North Am 1985; 191:1011.

Pascoe PJ. Short-term ventilatory support. In: Kirk RW, ed. Current veterinary therapy IX. Philadelphia: WB Saunders, 1986: 269.

Suter PF, Ettinger SJ. Pulmonary edema. In: Ettinger SJ, ed. Textbook of veterinary internal medicine: diseases of the dog and cat, 2nd ed. Philadelphia: WB Saunders, 1983: 797.

Tams TR. Aspiration pneumonia and complications of inhalation of smoke and toxic gases. In: Symposium on respiratory diseases. Vet Clin North Amer 1985; 191:971.

Tams TR, Sherding RG. Smoke inhalation injury. Compendium of Continuing Education 1981; 3:986.

32

PLEURAL EFFUSION
Ned F. Kuehn, Philip Roudebush

Pleural effusion is the presence of increased amounts of fluid of any kind within the pleural space. The detection of pleural effusion does not represent a definitive diagnosis, since a diverse group of diseases may have pleural effusion as part of their syndrome. Pleural effusions cause an increase in pleural volume at the expense of lung volume, resulting in varying degrees of respiratory distress or difficulty. Pleural effusions are principally classified by the type of effusion present (transudative, exudative, hemorrhagic, pyogranulomatous, neoplastic, chylous, pseudochylous). Pleural effusions may be further classified based on the pathophysiologic mechanisms underlying their formation.

Several terms are used to describe pleural effusions. *Hydrothorax* is a term used in the broad sense to include any pleural effusion with a low fibrin and cell count (transudates or modified transudates). *Pyothorax* or *empyema* pertains to effusions characterized by purulent fluid with high fibrin and neutrophil counts. *Hemothorax* denotes the accumulation of blood in the pleural space. *Chylothorax* refers to the accumulation of lymph (chyle) in the pleural space; whereas, *pseudochylothorax* denotes chyloid or chyloform effusions that appear grossly similar to chyle. In general, therapy for any type of pleural effusions is directed at the underlying disease responsible for fluid formation.

CAUSES

The general causes for pleural effusions, based on the clinicopathologic properties of the pleural fluid itself, are listed in Table 32-1. Depending on chronicity, several of the causes for pleural effusions may exhibit more than one fluid type.

PATHOPHYSIOLOGY

Normally, the pleural space is only a potential space containing a very small amount of fluid, which serves as a lubricant for the lung during respiration. The pleural space is surrounded by two serosal surfaces: the visceral pleura, which covers the surface of the lungs, and the parietal pleura, which covers the thoracic walls, the mediastinum, and the diaphragm. The movement of fluid through the pleural space is a dynamic process whereby fluid principally moves through capillaries of the parietal pleura and into the pleural space and then is absorbed by capillaries of the visceral pleura and thoracic lymphatics. The passage of fluid through the pleural membranes is in accordance with Starling's forces (see Chapter 31). That is, fluid movement is dependent on the hydrostatic, colloid osmotic, and intrapleural pressures.

Fluid movement into the pleural space is more

445

Table 32–1 *Causes of Pleural Effusions Based On Clinicopathologic Properties of the Effusion*

PURE TRANSUDATES

Hypoalbuminemia
  Protein-losing enteropathy
  Protein-losing nephropathy
  End-stage liver disease
Early congestive heart failure
  Right herat failure
  Biventricular heart failure

MODIFIED TRANSUDATES (OBSTRUCTIVE EFFUSIONS)

Congestive heart failure
  Primary right heart failure
    Pericardial tamponade
    Constrictive pericarditis
    Tricuspid insufficiency
    Myocardial failure
  Biventricular heart failure
Atelectasis
Diaphragmatic hernias
Lung lobe torsion
Intrathoracic neoplasia
  Right atrial tumors
  Heart base tumors
  Mediastinal tumors
  Pleural tumors
Pulmonary embolism
Idiopathic

EXUDATES (INFLAMMATORY EFFUSIONS)

Septic exudates
  Bite wounds
  Iatrogenic (post-surgical, post-thoracentesis)
  Pneumonia (parapneumonic effusion)
  Hematogenous spread
  Mediastinitis
  Ruptured esophagus
  Penetrating thoracic wound
  Foreign bodies
    plant awns or foxtails
  Peritonitis
Nonseptic exudates
  Pyogranulomatous effusions
    Feline infectious peritonitis
    Actinomycosis
    Nocardiosis
  Immune-mediated pleuritis
    Systemic lupus erythematosis (SLE)
  Idiopathic
    Occult infections
    Hypersensitivity reaction
  Acute pancreatitis

HEMORRHAGIC

Trauma
  Fractured ribs
  Pulmonary contusion
  Injury to chest wall, diaphragm, mediastinum
  Iatrogenic (surgery)
Diaphragmatic hernia
  Ruptured spleen
  Ruptured liver
Coagulopathies
  Hemophilia
  Dicoumarol toxicosis
  Disseminated intravascular coagulation
  Thrombocytopenia
Neoplasia
  Hemangiosarcoma
  Other
Dirofilariasis
Aortic aneurysm
  Spirocerca lupi
Pulmonary infarction
Lung lobe torsion

NEOPLASTIC

Mediastinal lymphosarcoma
Mesothelioma
Thymoma
Primary lung tumor
Carcinomatous effusions
Other

CHYLOUS

Thoracic lymphangiectasia
  Congenital
  Acquired
    Lymphangitis
    Neoplasia
  Lymphatic hypertension
    Venous thrombi
    Heart failure
    Pericardial disease
    Dirofilariasis
    Lung lobe torsion
    Neoplasia
Traumatic
  Post-surgical
  Coughing
  Diaphragmatic hernia

PSEUDOCHYLOUS

Chronic heart failure
  Cardiomyopathies (cats)
Neoplasia (cats)
Low-grade infections (cats)
Any chronic pleural effusion

complex than that in other areas of the body because two separate capillary networks, those of the parietal and visceral pleura, govern fluid movement within the pleural space. The capillaries of the parietal pleura are supplied by way of the intercostal arteries, which have hydrostatic pressures similar to those of the systemic circulation. On the other hand, the capillaries of the visceral pleura are served by the lower pressure pulmonary circulation. The pressure in the pleural space is subatmospheric. The net pressure of Starling's forces across the pleural space favors movement of fluid from the parietal pleura across the pleural space and reabsorption of fluid through the visceral pleura. The visceral pleura also is a more vascular structure than the parietal pleura, lending it a larger capillary surface area. Thus, the reabsorptive capacity of the visceral pleura exceeds the transudative capacity of the parietal pleura. The majority of fluid moved across the pleural space is reabsorbed by the venous end of the capillaries, whereas the lymphatics only return 10% to 20% of the fluid to the circulation.

Normally the capillary endothelium is only slightly permeable to large molecules; therefore, just a small amount of protein (albumin) leaks into the pleural space. The lymphatic vessels provide the only means for this protein to leave the parietal space. If protein were allowed to accumulate, the intrapleural colloid osmotic pressure would increase and favor fluid movement into the pleural space from both the parietal and visceral pleura. In addition to the reabsorption of proteins, the lymphatics also provide the only means for red blood cells and other particulate matter to return to the circulation. Lymphatic reabsorption in animals occurs primarily in the lower mediastinal pleura and along the caudal margins of the thorax.

Pleural fluid accumulates when the dynamic equilibrium of pleural fluid production and reabsorption is disrupted by disease conditions (Fig. 32-1). Alterations in this dynamic equilibrium include increases in hydrostatic pressure, decreases in colloid osmotic pressure, increases in capillary permeability, and obstruction of lymphatics. When alterations in any one or more of these conditions occur, pleural fluid continues

to accumulate until another equilibrium is established.

Pleural effusions are best characterized by the clinicopathologic properties of the pleural fluid itself. The physiochemical and general cytologic features of these fluids make it possible to classify these effusions into one of seven patterns (Table 32-2). The pathophysiologic derangements responsible for the formation of these patterns are discussed.

Pure Transudates

Pure transudates result secondarily to diseases that bring about extreme hypoalbuminemia (serum albumin less than 1.0 mg/dl or 10 g/L). Severe hypoalbuminemia causes a decreased colloid osmotic pressure, which allows fluid to move out of both the parietal and visceral pleura into the pleural space. This increased movement of fluid into the pleural space overloads the lymphatics and results in sequestration of a low protein transudate in the pleural space.

Modified Transudates (Obstructive Effusions)

Modified transudates, also called obstructive effusions, frequently result from increased hydrostatic pressure in blood vessels or from lymphatics draining the pleural cavity. Obstruction, constriction, or congestion of lymph or blood vessels will increase venous or lymphatic hydrostatic pressures or both. Right or biventricular heart failure is the most common cause of modified transudates. Systemic venous hypertension results from increased right atrial or right ventricular pressures. Left heart failure alone does not result in pleural effusion. Compression of pleural lymphatics and veins by masses, such as infiltrative tumors, can also produce increased hydrostatic pressure.

Modified transudates are poorly cellular initially; however, they eventually become modified by a secondary inflammatory response that increases cellularity. Similarly, long standing pure

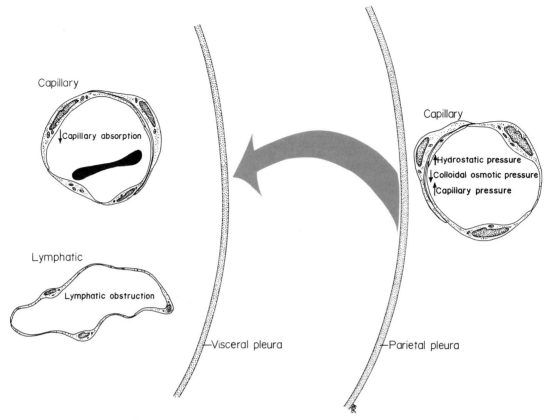

Figure 32–1 *Factors contributing to the formation of pleural effusion.*

transudates may also become modified by the same mechanism.

Exudates (Inflammatory Effusions)

Septic and nonseptic exudates evolve when inflammation of the capillary walls allows protein, cells, and fluid to leak into the pleural space. A subsequent increase in intrapleural colloid osmotic pressure facilitates the movement of fluid into the pleural space from capillaries in both the visceral and parietal pleura. Inflammation of the pleura also produces increased regional blood flow resulting in capillary hypertension. With the loss of favorable oncotic and hydrostatic gradients, fluid removal must be maintained by regional lymphatics. The effectiveness of lymphatic flow, however, is compromised by fibrosis or in-

traluminal obstruction with cellular, infectious, or inflammatory debris.

Septic effusions are caused by a wide variety of infectious agents. The bacteria Bacteroides sp and Fusobacterium sp (both anaerobes) and *Pasteurella multocida* are probably the most frequent causes of pyothorax in the cat. In the dog, Actinomyces sp and *Nocardia* species are the most common isolates. Other bacteria isolated from septic pleural effusions in the dog and cat include streptococci, staphylococci, *Escherichia coli, Klebsiella* species, *Proteus* sp, *Enterobacter* species, and corynebacteria. Additional organisms occasionally isolated include *Cryptococcus* species, *Toxoplasma* species, Aspergillus sp, and *Coccidioides immitis.* Differentiation between actinomyces and *Nocardia* species should be attempted because treatment for these two organisms is dissimilar.

Table 32-2 *Physiochemical and Cytologic Features of Pleural Effusions*

	Pure Transudates	Modified Transudates	Exudates		Hemorrhagic Effusions	Neoplastic Effusions	Chylous Effusions	Pseudochylous Effusions
			Nonseptic	Septic				
COLOR	Colorless-pale amber	Yellow-pink	Yellow-pink	Yellow	Red	Yellow-red	White-pink	White-pink
TRANSPARENCY	Clear	Clear-cloudy	Clear-cloudy	Cloudy-flocculent	Opaque	Opaque	Opaque	Clear-opaque
PROTEIN (g/dl)	<2.5 (<25 g/L)	>2.5 (>25 g/L)	>3.0 (>30 g/L)	>3.0 (>30 g/L)	>3.0 (>30 g/L)	>2.5 (>25 g/L)	>2.5 (>25 g/L)	>2.5 (>25 g/L)
SPECIFIC GRAVITY	<1.020	1.020–1.030	>1.025	>1.025	>1.025	>1.020	>1.020	>1.020
RED BLOOD CELLS	None–rare	Variable	Moderate	Moderate-high	Acute: high chronic: moderate	Variable	Variable	Variable
NUCLEATED CELLS/µl	<1000 (<1 × 10^9/L)	>1000 (>1 × 10^9/L)	>2000 (>2 × 10^9/L)	>5000 (>5 × 10^9/L)	>1000 (>1 × 10^9/L)	>1000 (>1 × 10^9/L)	>2000 (>2 × 10^9/L)	>1000 (>1 × 10^9/L)
NEUTROPHILS	Rare	Variable nondegenerative	Moderate nondegenerative	Moderate-high nondegenerative-degenerative	Variable nondegenerative	Variable nondegenerative	Acute: low chronic: moderate nondegenerative	Variable nondegenerative
LYMPHOCYTES	Rare	Variable	Variable	Variable	Variable	Variable	Acute: high chronic: low	Variable
MACROPHAGES	Occasional	Variable	Increased Ingested debris	Increased Ingested debris	Chronic: moderate increase Erythrophagocytosis	Moderate increase erythrophagocytosis	Present	Present
MESOTHELIAL	Occasional	Occasional	Rare	Rare	Chronic: present	Present	Occasional	Occasional
OTHER						Neoplastic cells		
BACTERIA	Absent	Absent	Absent	Present intra- and extracellular	Absent	Absent	Absent	Absent
LIPID	Absent	Absent	Absent	Absent	Absent	Absent High cholesterol	Triglycerides-high Cholesterol-low Sudan III-positive Ether-clears	Triglycerides-low Cholesterol-high Sudan III-negative Ether-no clearing

Pyogranulomatous effusions are nonseptic inflammatory exudates characteristic of feline infectious peritonitis and sometimes Actinomyces and *Nocardia* species in the dog. The coronavirus causing feline infectious peritonitis elicits an immune-complex vasculitis, which affects all serosal surfaces. This immune-complex vasculitis is accompanied by a secondary pyogranulomatous serositis. The resulting pyogranulomatous pleuritis provokes subsequent exudation of thick, viscous, protein-rich straw-colored fluid into the pleural space. Occasionally, these effusions become secondarily infected with bacteria and complicate the primary disease process by causing an active septic pleuritis.

Hemorrhage

Hemorrhagic effusions result from hemorrhage into the pleural space caused by trauma, vessel erosion, or coagulopathies. The packed-cell volume, cell counts, total protein, and myeloid : erythroid ratio are similar in these effusions to that of peripheral blood. Fluid samples obtained from patients with acute hemorrhage (within 45 minutes) may clot. Platelets may also be present. Chronic hemorrhagic effusions undergo mechanical defibrination as a result of agitation by thoracic viscera and will not clot after aspiration. Chronic hemorrhagic effusions typically are devoid of platelets and usually contain macrophages with phagocytized red blood cells (erythrophagocytosis).

Neoplastic

Thoracic neoplasia can cause an exudative (inflammatory), transudative (obstructive), pseudochylous, or hemorrhagic effusion. The cytologic presence of neoplastic cells identifies this type of effusion. The absence of tumor cells, however, does not rule out neoplasia as the primary cause of any type of effusion. In fact, in the majority of neoplastic effusions, tumor cells are never detected by cytologic analysis.

Chyle

Chylous effusions arise from obstruction or disruption of chyle flow in the thoracic duct with subsequent accumulation in the pleural space. Chyle consists of lymph and droplets of triglycerides (chylomicrons) in a stable emulsion. Chyle is formed when dietary fat absorbed through the intestinal lacteals mixes with lymph. The thoracic duct is the main pathway for transport of lymph, chylomicrons, and newly formed lymphocytes to the peripheral blood. The bulk of plasma proteins that leave the circulation at the capillary level are also returned to the vascular compartment as lymph by way of the thoracic duct.

The major cause of chylothorax in animals is thoracic lymphangiectasia, which is characterized by abnormal dilation of the thoracic duct and collateral lymphatics. Thoracic lymphangiectasia may be a result of several disease process: 1) congenital, due to an abnormality of the lymphatic system; 2) acquired, due to involvement of the lymphatic ducts by inflammatory process or neoplasia; or, 3) a result of increased lymphatic pressure, as in heart failure or other diseases causing obstruction of thoracic duct flow into the cranial vena cava. Trauma may cause rupture of the thoracic duct and result in accumulation of chyle within the pleural space. In some situations, an underlying disease process cannot be proved.

Animals with chylothorax often have serious metabolic sequela (in addition to the adverse cardiorespiratory consequences of the pleural effusion itself). The sequestration of chyle within the pleural space results in a steady loss of proteins, fats, fat-soluble vitamins, water, and electrolytes. These losses invariably lead to severe metabolic deficits and weight loss. This problem is accentuated when repeated aspirations of the chest occur, thereby permanently removing these essential metabolites from the system. A marked loss of circulating lymphocytes also occurs, which may seriously compromise the patients immune function. Lymphopenia is a common hematologic finding in animals with chylothorax.

Chyle is generally relatively inert; however, it may cause a secondary nonseptic pleuritis in some cats and dogs. This pleural reaction will elicit pleural fibrosis and secondary complications, such as severe atelectasis and alveolar fibrosis. Pulmonary dysfunction in patients with pleural fibrosis is often severely compromised. Chyle is bacteriostatic due to its high fatty acid content. Therefore, pyothorax is an unusual complication of patients with chylothorax.

Pseudochylous Effusions

Pseudochylous effusions are also high in lipid content and look grossly similar to chylous effusions; however, their mode of formation and physiochemical characteristics are markedly different. Pseudochylous effusions are associated with any chronic pleural effusion, especially chronic heart failure and intrathoracic neoplasia. Pseudochylous effusions do not result from the seepage of chyle into the pleural space. Rather, lecithin and cholesterol, which are thought to be breakdown products of cells undergoing fatty degeneration, account for the high lipid content of these effusions. The suspected source of these lipids are malignant or exfoliated pleural membrane cells.

Pseudochylous effusions may be differentiated from chylous effusions on the physiochemical properties of the fluids. Pleural fluid triglyceride concentrations are higher and the pleural cholesterol : triglyceride ratios are lower in chylous effusions than in nonchylous effusions in both dogs and cats. Pleural cholesterol : triglyceride ratios less than 1 are supportive of a chylous effusion. Pseudochylous effusions have a high cholesterol concentration, typically twice that of the serum cholesterol. The chylomicrons in chylous effusions stain with Sudan III, but globules in pseudochylous effusions will not stain with Sudan III. Pseudochylous effusions do not clear with ether, as they do with chylous effusions.

CLINICAL SIGNS

Clinical signs exhibited by animals with pleural effusion vary depending on the volume of fluid, the rate of its accumulation, the underlying disease process, and the presence of concurrent cardiopulmonary disease. Most animals have one or more of the following signs on clinical presentation: dyspnea, rapid and shallow breathing, restrictive breathing pattern (increased inspiratory component with an accentuated abdominal component), barrel chested appearance, standing or sitting position with abducted elbows and extended neck, orthopnea, coughing, open mouth breathing (sign of severe respiratory distress in the cat), and cyanosis.

Physical examination findings largely depend on the primary disease process. Upon auscultation, animals with pleural effusion will generally be found to have muffled heart sounds and muffled to silent lung sounds. The attenuation of heart and lung sounds is particularly noticeable ventrally. Percussion of the chest reveals dullness or flatness. A fluid line may be percussed in larger patients.

Some animals with pleural effusion may only present with signs referable to the respiratory system. Others may also have evidence of multisystemic disease with nonspecific signs such as anorexia, fever, depression, weight loss, pale mucous membranes, ascites, lymphadenopathy, chorioretinitis, and anterior uveitis. Occasionally, clinical findings are helpful in identifying the underlying etiology. For example, the presence of pulse deficits, arrhythmias, or heart murmurs may indicate that the effusion is due to heart failure; or, the presence of ventral edema may suggest the cause for the effusion to be secondary to hypoproteinemia.

DIAGNOSTIC APPROACH

The approach taken to the initial workup of a patient suspected of having pleural effusion depends on the degree of respiratory embarrassment the patient is suffering. Severely affected animals may require immediate needle thoracentesis or chest tube placement to stabilize respiratory function (see Thoracentesis and Insertion of Chest Tubes in Chapter 80).

Thoracic radiographs should be obtained in all patients suspected of having pleural effusion to assess the amount and location of the fluid. Most of the pleural effusions in dogs and cats are bilateral because the mediastinum in these species is not entirely impermeable to the crossing of fluid from one side of the chest to the other. Exudative effusions (*e.g.*, pyothorax), however, may be unilateral because reaction of the parietal pleura to inflammatory activity may close any partial mediastinal communication between each side of the chest. The radiographic signs indicative of pleural effusion include one or more of the following: interlobar fissure lines, rounding of lung margins at the costophrenic angles, retraction of lung borders from the thoracic wall, scalloping of lung margins dorsal to sternum, partial to total obliteration of the cardiac silhouette, and widening of the cranioventral and caudoventral mediastinum (Fig. 32-2).

Thoracic radiographs are also useful to document associated pulmonary, mediastinal, and cardiac pathology. Suspected mass lesions or cardiac disease may further be evaluated by ultrasound prior to removal of the pleural fluid. Radiographs should also be obtained following removal of the pleural fluid to obtain better images of the

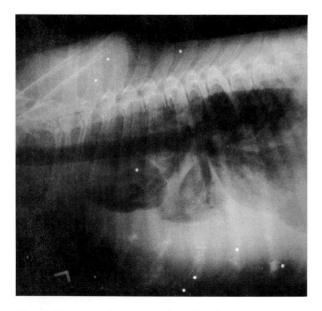

Figure 32–2 *Lateral thoracic radiograph of a 9-year-old female Labrador retriever with a malignant pleural effusion (undifferentiated carcinoma). Notice the scalloping of lung margins dorsal to the sternum and the partial obliteration of the cardiac silhouette due to the effusion.*

lung fields for assessment of pulmonary parenchymal disease (*e.g.*, pneumonia) and of the heart and other intrathoracic structures for documentation of associated pathology (*e.g.*, cardiomyopathy, mediastinal lymphoma).

To a large degree, the diagnostic approach to a patient with pleural effusion is determined by the type of effusion present. Thoracentesis allows for aseptic collection of pleural fluid for physiochemical and cytologic analysis and culturing (see Thoracentesis and Insertion of Chest Tubes in Chapter 80). Approximately 5 ml of fluid should be placed in a tube with anticoagulant (EDTA) for cell counts. Another 5 to 10 ml of fluid is stored without anticoagulant for physiochemical determinations. Fluid should also be obtained for aerobic and anaerobic cultures and for determination of sensitivities to different antimicrobials. A Gram's stain of the fluid can be made for rapid assessment of the presence of microorganisms. The classification of pleural fluids is based on physical, chemical, cytologic, and bacteriologic characteristics (see Table 32-2). The differentiation of chylous and pseudochylous effusions is given in the section above.

Laboratory evaluation, including a complete blood count, serum chemistry profile, urinalysis, microfilaria check, and fecal analysis, is indicated in all animals with pleural effusion because of the many diseases that can cause the condition (Table 32-3). These tests may be particularly important when a cause for the effusion is not readily found.

A complete cardiac evaluation, including thoracic radiographs and an electrocardiogram, should be performed when the clinical signs and fluid analysis are suggestive of heart disease. Removal of fluid from the chest is desirable prior to radiography in order to facilitate visualization of the entire cardiac silhouette. An electrocardiogram should also be obtained following removal of fluid from the chest because the fluid contained within the chest cavity may damp cardiac electrical activity and result in low voltage (small) complexes in all ECG leads, thereby making interpretation of the ECG difficult. Echocardiography may be required to thoroughly evaluate cardiac function. Echocardiography or angiocardiography or both may be required to delineate intra- or

Table 32–3 *Laboratory Assessment of Pleural Effusions*

Test	What to Check for
Complete blood count	Neutrophilia Lymphopenia Neoplastic lymphocytes
Serum biochemistry	Hypoproteinemia Hypoalbuminemia
Urinalysis	Proteinuria
Fecal analyses	Parasitic ova or larvae
Knott's test	Microfilaria
Chest radiographs	Extent of pleural effusion Evidence of concurrent pulmonary disease Chest masses Cardiac size
Electrocardiogram	Rate and rhythm Arrhythmias Chamber enlargement
Echocardiogram	Chamber enlargement Valvular abnormalities Myocardial contractility Intracardiac mass(es) Pericardial effusion
Pleural fluid analysis	Color Protein content Specific gravity Cellularity Differential cell count Lipid content Microorganisms

extra-cardiac defects and masses such as congenital cardiac defects and right atrial tumors or pericardial effusions and heart base tumors, respectively (see Echocardiography and Nonselective Angiocardiography in Chapter 80).

In some situations an underlying cause for the effusion cannot be found. In these situations, an exploratory thoracotomy may be considered.

MANAGEMENT

Management of patients with pleural effusion is largely dependent on identification of an underlying etiology. Patients with severe respiratory distress require immediate removal of the fluid either by needle thoracentesis or placement of a chest tube (see Thoracentesis and Insertion of Chest Tubes in Chapter 80). Results from the fluid

analysis and cultures, laboratory tests, and thoracic radiographs generally indicate a cause for the effusion. The management of selected causes follows.

Hypoalbuminemia

Hypoalbuminemia is the cause for the majority of pure transudates. Hypoalbuminemia results from either decreased production (chronic liver failure or malabsorption/maldigestion syndromes) or increased loss (protein losing enteropathies or protein losing nephropathies). Occasionally both decreased production and increased loss of protein may be involved. Prompt investigation into and correction of the underlying cause for protein loss is essential to the management of these patients. For management of these problems, the clinician is referred to those chapters specifically dealing with these diseases. In situations where abatement of the underlying disease is not possible (*e.g.*, end stage cirrhosis), the prognosis is grave.

Congestive Heart Failure

Congestive heart failure is a particularly common cause of massive pleural effusion in the cat, but somewhat less common in the dog. Pleural effusion usually results from biventricular heart failure. The type of effusion associated with heart failure is generally a modified transudate; although, with long standing effusions (especially in cats with cardiomyopathy) the effusions can become pseudochylous. Therapy is directed at improving cardiac function. The reader is directed to Chapters 20 and 21 for information on management of pleural effusion and heart disease.

Modified Transudates From Causes Other Than Heart Failure

The majority of effusions due to modified transudates from causes other than heart failure are initiated by an obstructive lesion causing increased venous or lymphatic hydrostatic pressure or both. Identification of an underlying etiology can occasionally be difficult, although a thorough workup should be made to rule out pericardial tamponade, diaphragmatic hernia, lung lobe torsion, or neoplasia. Exploratory surgery may be required when an underlying cause is not demonstrable.

Correction of the underlying condition is required for resolution of these effusions. When the effusion is secondary to tumors unresponsive to attempts at medical and surgical management, pleurodesis (see Chronic Pleural Effusions, below) can be attempted to obliterate the pleural space and reduce the formation of fluid.

Pyothorax (Empyema)

The cause of pyothorax frequently cannot be determined, despite a thorough search for evidence of penetrating chest, neck, or mediastinal wounds or esophageal perforation. In patients with severe respiratory distress, the majority of fluid should be removed by needle thoracentesis to stabilize cardiopulmonary function. Continuous drainage of the thorax through a chest tube is preferred for the initial management of these patients. Patients will not do well clinically until effective drainage is accomplished. Continuous drainage facilitates a more complete removal and resolution of the pyothorax. Once the patient is stable, a chest tube is placed at the level of the seventh or eighth intercostal space. Dual chest tube placement is required occasionally when persistent loculation or a complete mediastinum prevents adequate evacuation of both hemithoraces. Cytologic examination of the pleural fluid should be done frequently to evaluate the efficacy of therapy. Gram's stains are performed every 24 to 48 hours throughout the period of drainage. Chest evacuation is discontinued when: 1) thoracic radiographs show complete clearing of the chest for 48 hours; 2) the Gram's stain is negative; and, 3) there is production of less than 30 ml or 15 ml of nonpurulent fluid for 24 hours in dogs or cats, respectively.

Intermittent pleural lavage is less than ideal, but may be attempted if continuous water seal drainage is not possible. Continuous pleural lavage permits more complete evacuation and rapid resolution of the pyothorax. The patient's chest is lavaged twice to four times daily. Prior to each lavage, the chest should be evacuated of all fluid possible. Slides of this fluid may be made for cytologic evaluation and Gram's stains. Ten ml/kg of body weight of warm sterile saline is instilled into the chest over 5 to 10 minutes. The saline is left in the chest for 45 to 60 minutes, during which time the animal is gently rolled several times. The lavage fluid is then evacuated from the chest. Approximately 25% of the instilled volume of saline will be reabsorbed during this process.

Antibiotic therapy is used with, not in lieu of, continuous or intermittent drainage of the chest. The initial choice of antibiotic should be made on examination of a Gram stained smear of the fluid. In most cases, therapy should be instituted with relatively high doses of parenteral ampicillin (22–33 mg/kg every 6 hours, IV). Instillation of antibiotics into the pleural space is not recommended because adequate levels of antibiotic in the thoracic space can be attained with either oral or parenteral therapy. When improvement is noted, the patient may be switched to oral ampicillin (22–33 mg/kg every 6–8 hours). The initial choice of antibiotic may occasionally need to be modified based on results from culture sensitivities or poor response to therapy. Serial cultures may be needed when a patient continues to produce a septic effusion despite antibiotic therapy or when a change in organism morphology is noted on Gram's stains. In most cases, treatment is continued for a minimum of 6 weeks.

Penicillin is the drug of choice for anaerobic infections. However, 15% of feline and a lesser percentage of canine empyemic infections are associated with *Bacteroides fragilis*, an organism that typically is not sensitive to penicillin in vitro. Therefore, if *B fragilis* is isolated, chemotherapy using either chloramphenicol or clindamycin is suggested. Hospital-acquired (nosocomial) infections often have sensitivity patterns that are less predictable. Treatment with a combination of antibiotics, such as ampicillin and gentamicin, is recommended until culture results are known.

Surgical exploration of the chest cavity for a possible foreign body should be contemplated in cases having recurrence of the problem or those nonresponsive to conservative therapy.

Pyogranulomatous Effusions

These effusions are most characteristic of feline infectious peritonitis and occasionally actinomycosis and nocardiosis in the dog. Diagnosis of feline infectious peritonitis is aided by analysis of the fluid, presence of systemic signs, and titers. Because the basic lesion of feline infectious peritonitis is a consequence of an immune-mediated vasculitis, cytotoxic therapy using immunosuppressive doses of prednisolone combined with cyclophosphamide may offer some relief. However, because of the poor prognosis, attempts at therapy generally fail.

Hemothorax

Identification of hemothorax should prompt the clinician to initiate an immediate investigation as to its cause. Patients with pleural space hemorrhage resulting from trauma should also be evaluated for pneumothorax. Chest tube drainage may be required if blood or air or both cannot be removed at a rate sufficient to keep up with its accumulation. Depending on the rate of blood accumulation, intermittent or continuous pleural evacuation may be necessary. Bleeding from ruptured pulmonary vessels tends to be self-limiting as the compression from the accumulated effusion collapses the lung and stops active bleeding.

Nontraumatic hemothorax often is the result of acquired or congenital coagulopathies or neoplasia. A complete coagulation profile should be obtained, including platelet count, activated clotting time, prothrombin time, partial thromboplastin time, fibrinogen, and fibrin degradation products (see Chapter 16). Specific factor analyses may be required for a definitive diagnosis when congenital coagulopathies are suspected. Therapy will largely depend on the cause of the coagulation defect. Blood transfusion or vitamin K therapy may be needed. If a diagnosis of disseminated intravascular coagulation is made, identification and correction of the under-lying disease, if possible, is necessary. When coagulopathies are identified, thoracentesis should be limited only to patients exhibiting signs of cardiopulmonary compromise because the procedure may contribute to further bleeding.

Tumors cause hemorrhagic effusions by erosion of blood vessels, rupture of the tumor mass, or by initiation of hemorrhagic diathesis (*e.g.*, disseminated intravascular coagulation). Treatment options are dependent on the anatomic location and type of tumor involved.

Neoplastic Effusions

Depending on the neoplastic process, the resulting effusion may be a modified transudate or an inflammatory, pseudochylous, or hemorrhagic effusion. A tissue or cytologic diagnosis or both is required. Treatment is directed at therapy appropriate for the tumor type. Pleurodesis may be attempted when tumor related pleural effusion cannot be controlled by medical or surgical means (see Chronic Pleural Effusions, in this chapter).

Chylous Effusions

Determination of the cause for chylothorax can be difficult, but an attempt should be made to define the underlying defect. In patients with a history of trauma, a rent in the wall of the thoracic duct should be suspected. Thoracic neoplasia is a potential cause of chylothorax, which should be considered in older animals. Typically, no definable inciting cause can be discovered by noninvasive methods. Lymphangiography has shown that many of these idiopathic cases are due to thoracic lymphangiectasia.

The results of conservative, nonsurgical management of chylous effusions are generally poor, with only about 25% of patients showing a satisfactory response. Multiple needle thoracocentesis or intermittent chest tube drainage with a low-fat diet (Hill's Prescription Diet r/d), parenterally administered fat and water soluble vitamins, and exercise restriction may be tried initially. This approach may obviate the need for duct repair following traumatic injuries. If, however, this approach fails to remedy the situation within 3 to 4 weeks, surgery is indicated.

Thoracic duct ligation is the preferred approach to treatment of most causes of chylous effusion. Although this approach to management may be considered aggressive, the expense of maintaining satisfactory long-term conservative management, the problems encountered in the proper care of chest tubes for long periods of time, and the unpredictable outcome of conservative treatment justifies early surgical intervention. The clinician is recommended to read articles on surgical techniques (Harpster; Birchard, Additional Reading).

Lung lobe torsion is an uncommon cause, but well known complication, of chylothorax. Surgical removal of the affected lobe (most often the right middle lobe) and simultaneous thoracic duct ligation should be carried out.

Intrathoracic infection is a rare complication of chylothorax. However, nonsterile needle thoracocentesis or contamination of chest tubes may establish an infection. Treatment for this complication is outlined above in the section on pyothorax.

Chronic Pleural Effusions

Patients are occasionally encountered with a recurrent pleural effusion and no demonstrable underlying cause. These idiopathic effusions typically are low grade inflammatory with variable mixtures of inflammatory cell types. Some of these contain a large percentage of eosinophils. Conservative treatment can include diuretics, antibiotics, corticosteroids, and intermittent drainage of the chest. If conservative management fails, pleurodesis can be tried.

Pleurodesis may be used to stop chronic effusions and provide some relief of respiratory compromise. An irritant is entered into the pleural space to cause an acute inflammatory reaction of the pleural membranes and subsequent development of diffuse adhesions between the visceral and parietal pleura. The most common indication for pleurodesis is chronic pleural effusion secondary to malignancy. Pleurodesis can be used to treat chylothorax; however, the results are mostly inconsistent. Still, animals with persistent chylous effusion following ligation of the thoracic duct may respond favorably to pleurodesis.

Prior to infusion of the sclerosing agent, the pleural space should be thoroughly evacuated using a chest tube. Bilateral chest tubes should be placed in the patient to facilitate complete evacuation of the pleural space. The sclerosing agent of choice for dogs is tetracycline solution (Panmycin). A single intrapleural dose of 35 mg/kg of tetracycline is diluted in 30 to 75 ml of sterile isotonic saline. Five to fifteen ml of 1% lidocaine is added to the tetracycline-water mixture to help prevent pleural pain. One half of the tetracycline-lidocaine mixture is instilled into the pleural space through one thoracic tube and the other half of the mixture is given through the second tube in the opposite side of the chest. This procedure is followed by administering air (25–100 ml, depending on size of the dog) through each chest tube to ensure contact of the tetracycline mixture with the pleural surfaces. The animal is gently rolled several times to distribute the solution. The pleural space is drained 2 hours later. Continuous suction drainage of the chest is maintained for 12 to 36 hours after pleurodesis (or until the effusion stops) to enhance contact between the visceral and parietal pleura. The chest tube is removed when the drainage from the chest is less than 2 to 4 ml/kg/day. Satisfactory results are not usually obtained by repeated thoracocentesis with a needle.

Guidelines for pleurodesis in cats are not established at this time. Although high dose tetracycline will cause renal toxicity in dogs, this single intrapleural dose should be safe in dogs with normal renal function. Nonetheless, careful monitoring of renal function is advisable.

PATIENT MONITORING

The frequency of checks on patient progress is largely dependent on the ability of the clinician to define and treat the underlying cause of the effusion. Successful correction of the underlying problem usually affords the patient a good prognosis.

ADDITIONAL READING

Bauer T. Pyothorax. In: Kirk RW, ed. Current veterinary therapy IX. Philadelphia: WB Saunders, 1986: 292.

Berg J. Chylothorax in the dog and cat. Compendium of Continuing Education 1982; 4:986.

Birchard SJ, Fossum TW, Gallagher L. Pleurodesis. In: Kirk RW, ed. Current veterinary therapy X. Philadelphia: WB Saunders, 1989: 405.

Birchard SJ, Gallagher L. Use of pleurodesis in treating selected pleural diseases. Compendium of Continuing Education 1988; 10:826.

Birchard SJ, Smeak DD, Fossum TW. Results of thoracic duct ligation in dogs with chylothorax. J Am Vet Med Assoc 1988; 193:68.

Forrester SD, Troy GC, Fossum TW. Pleural effusions: pathophysiology and diagnostic considerations. Compendium of Continuing Education 1988; 10:121.

Fossum TW, Birchard SJ. Chylothorax in 34 dogs. J Am Vet Med Assoc 1986; 188:1315.

Fossum TW, Birchard SJ. Chylothorax. In: Kirk RW, ed. Current veterinary therapy X. Philadelphia: WB Saunders, 1989: 393.

Fossum TW, Jacobs RM, Birchard SJ. Evaluation of cholesterol and triglyceride concentrations in differentiating chylous and nonchylous pleural effusions in dogs and cats. J Am Vet Med Assoc 1986; 188:49.

Harpster NK. Chylothorax. In: Kirk RW, ed. Current veterinary therapy IX. Philadelphia: WB Saunders, 1986: 295.

Jonas LD. Feline pyothorax: a retrospective study of twenty cases. Journal of the American Animal Hospital Association 1983; 19:865.

Noone KE. Pleural effusions and diseases of the pleura. In: Spaulding GL, ed. Symposium on respiratory diseases. Vet Clin North Am 1985; 15:1069.

Willauer CC, Breznock EM. Pleurovenous shunting technique for treatment of chylothorax in three dogs. J Am Vet Med Assoc 1987; 191:1106

33

RESPIRATORY PARASITES

Philip Roudebush, Ned F. Kuehn

The dog and cat are often infected by parasites that reproduce in the nasal cavity, trachea, bronchi, and pulmonary parenchyma. These parasitic infections must be differentiated from parasites whose larval forms only migrate through the respiratory system and parasites that migrate aberrantly into the respiratory system.

A wide variety of clinical signs and pathologic lesions develop from primary parasitic infection of the respiratory tract. The severity of clinical manifestations is quite variable, ranging from asymptomatic to fatal infections. This broad range of clinical syndromes depends largely on the number of organisms that infect the respiratory tract, the site of predilection within the respiratory system by a particular parasite, and the nature of the host's response to the presence of the parasite.

CAUSES

Four respiratory parasites are of clinical and practical importance in the dog and cat (Table 33-1). Other primary parasitic infections of the respiratory system occur, but are uncommon and

sporadic in nature (Table 33-2). Individual clinical entities are best discussed in terms of the causative organism. An understanding of the biology of each parasite is necessary to develop a rational approach to diagnosis, treatment, and control of each organism.

PATHOPHYSIOLOGY, CLINICAL SIGNS, AND DIAGNOSTIC APPROACH

Filaroides (Oslerus) osleri

The dog is host to three species of metastrongylid lungworms belonging to the genus *Filaroides*. *Filaroides osleri* is a slender worm (up to 1 cm in length) that causes the formation of eosinophilic granulomatous nodules in the distal trachea and principal bronchi.

Unlike other metastrongylids, which require molluscan intermediate hosts to develop into the infective third-stage larvae (L$_3$), *Filaroides* organisms are directly infective as first-stage larvae (L$_1$). Females are ovoviviparous, depositing larvae encapsulated by a single shell membrane into

Table 33–1 _Common Respiratory Parasites_

CANINE

Filaroides (Oslerus) osleri
Capillaria aerophila
Paragonimus kellicotti

FELINE

Aelurostrongylus abstrussus
Capillaria aerophila
Paragonimus kellicotti

Table 33–2 _Respiratory Parasites of Lesser Concern_

Filaroides milksi
Filaroides hirthi
Crenosoma vulpis
Pneumonyssus caninum
Linguatula serrata
Spirocerca lupi
Toxoplasma gondii

the respiratory passage. The L₁ isolated from tracheal scrapings, adult worm dissection, and freshly passed canine feces are directly and immediately infective when ingested by a dog. Regurgitant feeding at weaning has been shown to be the likely mode of transmission in wild canines. After ingestion, the parasite is thought to penetrate the intestinal mucosa and migrate to the distal trachea and principal bronchi, where submucosal eosinophilic granulomas or nodules are formed.

Clinical cases occur in young dogs 6 months to 3 years of age, and mimic infectious tracheobronchitis. The dog is usually admitted with the chief complaint of a chronic paroxysmal nonproductive to slightly productive cough of several months' duration. In the early stages of infection there are no systemic signs, with the dog exhibiting a good appetite and normal exercise tolerance. Dyspnea, bouts of wheezing, anorexia, and weight loss become progressively worse as the granulomas further occlude the primary bronchi. The clinical signs are often exacerbated during exercise or when the dog becomes excited. The coughing and wheezing are unresponsive to all forms of symptomatic therapy, including antibiotics, antihistamines, and antitussives. Physical examination is often normal in early cases, while inspiratory dyspnea and auscultation of crackles and wheezes are prevalent in advanced cases.

Diagnosis of _F. osleri_ infections is accomplished with the aid of a complete blood count, thoracic radiographs, transtracheal washing, fecal examination, and tracheobronchoscopy. The complete blood count may be normal, but frequently exhibits a mild to moderate eosinophilia. Thoracic radiographs also may be normal,

while some cases reveal nonspecific signs of peribronchial infiltration, pleural thickening, and increased linear interstitial markings. The actual tracheobronchial nodules are very difficult to visualize without the aid of positive contrast bronchography. Bacterial bronchopneumonia and pneumothorax have been reported as secondary complications and may be detected on radiographs.

Fecal examination should include zinc sulfate flotation, a direct saline smear of fresh feces, or the Baermann technique to look for larvae. If larvae are found in fresh feces that are not contaminated with soil or extraneous organic material, then one need only distinguish between lungworm larvae of metastrongylids _(Filaroides, Aelurostrongylus, Crenosoma)_ and the rhabdid larvae of _Strongyloides stercoralis_. If the feces are stale, then hookworm larvae may have developed and hatched. In fecal specimens contaminated with soil or extraneous organic material, freeliving nematodes and their larvae may also confuse the issue by their presence. Larvae of _F. osleri_ average 230 μ in length and have a characteristically kinked tail. Larval numbers are often small, and multiple negative fecal examinations may occur.

Transtracheal washing and aspiration is a valuable technique in the diagnosis of all respiratory parasitic infections (see Transtracheal Wash in Chapter 80). Cytologic examination of the material obtained by transtracheal washing will reveal characteristic embryonated eggs of _F. osleri_ (Fig. 33-1). A final method of diagnosis and evaluation of _F. osleri_ infection is tracheobronchoscopy (see Tracheobronchoscopy in Chapter 80). This procedure involves using a rigid or flexible bronchoscope to visually evaluate the trachea and principal bronchi. Examination will reveal

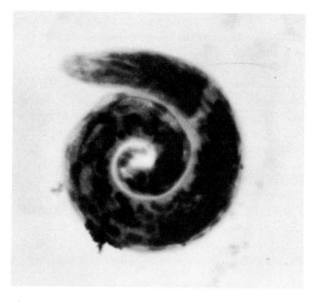

Figure 33–1. *Embryonated ovum characteristic of* Filaroides osleri *obtained via transtracheal washing and aspiration from a young dog with chronic coughing and wheezing.*

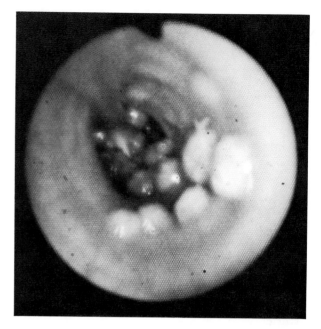

Figure 33–2. *Nodular lesions characteristic of* Filaroides osleri *noted during bronchoscopy at the tracheal bifurcation and extending into the primary bronchi of a dog with chronic cough.*

numerous 1- to 10-mm nodules protruding into the distal tracheal lumen and occluding the principal bronchi (Fig. 33-2). Endoscopy serves as both a diagnostic tool and a method to evaluate the severity of the lesions. Along with clinical response, periodic endoscopic examination during therapy serves as a means to assess improvement.

Filaroides milksi

This is a natural parasite of wildlife, with the dog serving as a rare accidental host. *Filaroides milksi* differs from *F. osleri* by its smaller size and its location in the parenchyma of the lungs.

The life cycle of *F. milksi* is probably similar to *F. osleri*. It is not known whether the L_1 are directly infective, or whether terrestrial mollusks, principally slugs, serve as intermediate hosts.

Adult parasites are found throughout the lung, principally in the bronchioles and alveoli. Inflammation and granulomatous reaction surround both live and dead parasites, primarily in subpleural regions. Clinical signs include dyspnea and cough. Thoracic radiographs may reveal an interstitial pattern.

Filaroides hirthi

This is the smallest of the three *Filaroides* species that infect dogs. It also has a direct life cycle in which L_1 are the infective stage. Autoinfection (reinfection of the host with L_1 before larvae leave the host) may increase the potential for serious infection. Adult *F. hirthi* infect bronchioles and alveoli, similar to *F. milksi*.

Natural infections were originally reported only from beagle breeding colonies. The infection described in beagles was characterized by small numbers of worms, focal granulomatous reactions, no clinical signs, and an inability to recover larvae from the feces. Zinc sulfate flotation was subsequently found to be much more efficient than the Baermann technique in concentrating the larvae in feces from these beagles.

Infection of *F. hirthi* in five individual pet dogs has recently been reported. Large numbers of adult lungworms caused diffuse suppurative and granulomatous lesions. These dogs demonstrated clinical signs of dyspnea, coughing, cyanosis, and respiratory distress. Three dogs suffered fatal infections, while two were treated successfully.

Thoracic radiographs revealed mixed interstitial, nodular, bronchial, or alveolar patterns. Larvae were successfully recovered from feces by direct smears and sodium nitrate flotation.

Control of *F. hirthi* in breeding colonies includes treating bitches before whelping and separating pups from older, infected dogs. Good hygiene is essential in infected dogs, and pups can be hand-raised or foster-raised on uninfected bitches.

Aelurostrongylus abstrussus

The domestic cat is the only known definitive host for this parasite, which has worldwide distribution. The adult worms reside in the respiratory bronchiole, alveolar ducts, and alveoli, and occasionally in the smaller branches of the pulmonary arteries. Eggs are laid by the adults in the alveoli, alveolar ducts, and interstitial spaces. The eggs embryonate to L_1, which ascend the respiratory tree and are coughed up, swallowed, and deposited in the feces. The L_1 can survive for several weeks to months in moist soil, but require a molluscan intermediate host, such as snails or slugs, for further development. The cat is infected by ingesting the snail or slug containing the infective L_3. The natural mode of infection is probably through predation of paratenic or transport hosts. A transport host (*e.g.,* amphibians, birds, reptiles, rodents) may eat the infected mollusks, and the L_3 merely reencysts in their tissues and undergoes no further development. The L_3 are thus found unchanged and alive in tissues of the transport hosts to serve as a source of infection to the feline predator. When ingested, the L_3 penetrates the gastrointestinal mucosa and follows a blood migration to the lungs.

The clinical signs and lesions of aelurostrongylosis in the cat depend to a great extent on the number of parasites involved and the response of the individual cat to the adult parasites, eggs, and larvae. The parasites, eggs, and larvae can stimulate an intense granulomatous inflammatory response consisting of mononuclear cells and eosinophils, which may develop as nodules throughout the lungs, especially in the subpleural region. No signs of pulmonary hypertension or associated right ventricular changes were documented with experimental infection. Many affected cats show little or no clinical disease due to infection.

Typical clinical signs of aelurostrongylosis include a chronic, harsh nonproductive cough, dyspnea, tachypnea, anorexia, fever, and lethargy. These signs may be quite progressive and severe. The most dangerous period is 6 to 13 weeks after infection, when great numbers of eggs and larvae are deposited in the pulmonary parenchyma. Auscultation during clinical disease will reveal diffuse low-pitch crackles and wheezes.

Aelurostrongylosis may be diagnosed on the basis of history, physical examination, hematology, thoracic radiographs, transtracheal washing, and fecal examination. The most commonly infected cat is one that is an outdoor predator with the previously described signs. Leukocytosis and eosinophilia are the most common hematologic findings.

The radiographic findings in experimental aelurostrongylosis have been well described. The earliest radiographic sign of lung disease in the infected cat is a mixed bronchial and patchy alveolar pattern. During the most severe stages of experimental disease, an alveolar pattern was predominant. As the alveolar pattern subsequently resolved, the nodular interstitial and peribronchial pattern became more obvious. Pleural effusion has been reported in one cat. Thus it can be seen that aelurostrongylosis can cause the entire gamut of radiographic pulmonary patterns in the cat.

Identification of the characteristic notched, S-shaped tail of L_1 is the most accurate and practical method of diagnosis. The L_1 can easily be identified in exudate obtained by transtracheal washing or tracheobronchoscopy. The L_1 can also be identified in direct smears and flotation of fresh feces. Fecal examination and transtracheal washings will not reveal early infections when adults are not yet mature, nor late infections when worms are no longer laying eggs.

Capillaria aerophila

The "fox lungworm" is a slender (15–40 mm in length) parasite that infects the nasal cavity, trachea, and bronchi of wild carnivores and sometimes the domestic dog and cat. *C. aerophila* is not a metastrongylid, but is a member of the Tricurid, and thus is closely related to whipworms.

The adult parasites inhabit the nasal or tracheobronchial mucosa. Eggs are laid on the mucosal surface and are coughed up, swallowed, and passed as an intact ovum in the feces. The eggs are very resistant to environmental conditions, and require 5 to 7 weeks to mature. Infection occurs by ingestion of the infective egg (direct life cycle) or may involve earthworms as facultative intermediate hosts. The eggs hatch, and larvae penetrate the gastrointestinal mucosa on a migration to the lungs through the blood.

Capillariasis may be an asymptomatic and self-limiting infection. Clinical disease usually occurs in young dogs and cats. A kitten as young as 10 weeks of age has been reported to be infected with clinical signs. Most dogs and cats exhibit a chronic mild to moderate, nonproductive cough and occasional periods of dyspnea, respiratory distress, anorexia, and weight loss. In both dogs and cats the cough is usually very intermittent, with periods of acute exacerbation. Physical examination may vary from normal to occasional crackles on auscultation. A cough is easily elicited upon tracheal palpation, due to the tracheitis and bronchitis.

Diagnosis of capillariasis involves a clinical history, physical examination, hematology, thoracic radiographs, transtracheal washing, cytology of nasal exudate or brushings, endoscopy, and fecal examination. Mild leukocytosis, eosinophilia, or basophilia are consistent hematologic findings. Thoracic radiographs usually reveal a mild to diffuse peribronchial and interstitial pattern without evidence of vascular enlargement or alveolar involvement. Demonstration of the characteristic oval, pale yellow unembryonated eggs (35 × 60 μ) with bipolar plugs in fecal flotation, tracheobronchial washing, or nasal discharge is the best method of diagnosis (Fig. 33-3). Endoscopy will reveal an increased amount of serous to mucoid exudate and inflamed mucosa.

Paragonimus kellicotti

Paragonimus kellicotti is a digenetic fluke that forms fibrous cysts in the lungs of many different wild carnivores and domestic dogs and cats. The

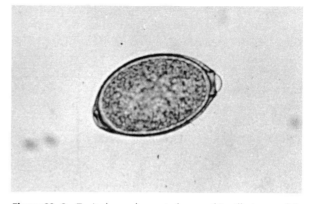

Figure 33–3. *Typical unembryonated ovum of* Capillaria aerophila *with bipolar plugs. These ova are found in transtracheal washings and on routine fecal flotation. They must be distinguished from whipworm ova.*

parasite is widely distributed in the United States and portions of Canada, and as far as can be ascertained is the only species of *Paragonimus* in North America. The distribution of *P. kellicotti* is regulated by the distribution of its intermediate hosts.

The life cycle of this trematode involves two intermediate hosts. Eggs passed in the feces of carnivores develop into miracidia, which infect the first intermediate host, small aquatic snails. The miracidia multiply asexually in the snail and produce mature cercariae. These cercariae leave the snail and penetrate the second intermediate host, the crayfish, and become metacercariae in the crayfish heart. Dogs, and cats become infected by ingesting crayfish with metacercariae.

Young flukes encyst in the intestines and migrate through the peritoneal cavity, diaphragm, and pleural cavity, where they penetrate the pulmonary parenchyma. Here they form cystic cavities in the parenchyma, which establish communication with bronchioles. Eggs are produced, which enter these bronchioles to be coughed up and swallowed. The prepatent period is 34 to 56 days. The risk of natural infection in dogs and cats that are predators may be quite high when one considers that in a local watershed near Columbus, Ohio, 42% to 80% of crayfish were documented to be infected with *P. kellicotti* metacercariae.

Clinical signs again vary with the number of parasites infecting the host and the host's reaction to the presence of adults and ova. Experimentally inoculated cats have been clinically normal despite radiographic evidence of lesions. This may also occur in natural infection. Typical clinical signs of pulmonary paragonimiasis include a chronic productive cough, respiratory distress, acute dyspnea associated with spontaneous pneumothorax, hemoptysis, excessive salivation, and systemic signs such as anorexia, lethargy, and weight loss. The pathologic features of pulmonary paragonimiasis that produce clinical signs consist of parasitic cysts or cavities and an intense eosinophilic inflammatory response to both the adult and ova. Pneumothorax occurs frequently, and is associated with communication of a parasitic cyst with the pleural space.

Diagnosis of pulmonary paragonimiasis is based on environmental history, physical examination, hematologic studies, radiographic findings, fecal examination, and transtracheal washing. The environmental history usually relates to an animal that is an active predator with access to streams or lakes. Physical examination often reveals an unthrifty animal that is easily induced to cough, with or without hemoptysis. Auscultation will vary with the severity of the infection. Mild neutrophilic leukocytosis with a left shift and eosinophilia are the usual hematologic findings.

The radiographic features of pulmonary paragonimiasis in the dog and cat have been well documented. The lesions are most often detected in the caudal lung lobes; this probably reflects the migratory pathway of the fluke. Ill-defined interstitial nodular densities and distinct multiloculated, air-filled pneumatocysts are the most consistent radiographic findings in the lungs of infected animals. Radiographically, the interstitial nodular densities are more common in cats, while pneumatocyst formation is the rule in dogs. Once the pneumatocyst forms around an adult fluke there is little change in the radiographic appearance of the lesions, even over a period of several months. Pneumatocysts may be confused on radiographs with bronchial cysts, pulmonary abscesses, or cavitational neoplasms. Pneumothorax with pulmonary atelectasis is also a radiographic finding.

Diagnosis is best confirmed by the presence of the characteristic *P. kellicotti* eggs, which have a single operculum, measure 50 × 100 μ, and are gold–brown in color (Fig. 33-4). The eggs are easily demonstrated on fecal examination or transtracheal washing. The sedimentation technique of fecal examination is more sensitive in detection of *Paragonimus* ova at low counts than is sodium nitrate flotation. However, at peak egg production there is no apparent difference in diagnostic efficacy between sedimentation and flotation techniques.

Linguatula serrata

The tongueworm is an internal parasite of the respiratory tract of vertebrates. The taxonomic position of this parasite is a pentastomid; adults are helminthlike, while preadult stages are arthropodlike. Animals become infected by eating viscera of sheep, cattle, rabbits, or rodents. Adults are tongue-shaped, and attach to the caudal nasal mucosa of the dog, fox, and wolf. Clinical signs in the dog include sneezing, coughing, rubbing at the nose, serosanginous mucoid nasal discharge,

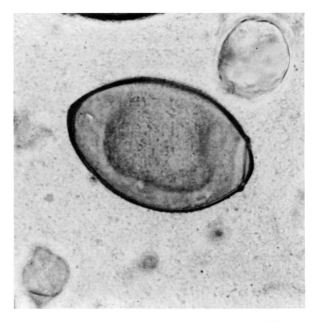

Figure 33–4. *Single opercular ovum of* Paragonimus kellicotti. *These ova are found in a transtracheal washing, fecal sediment, or fecal flotation.*

and continued swallowing attempts. Diagnosis is confirmed by finding characteristic eggs in feces or nasal secretions. Eggs appear yellowish, with hooks surrounded by a thin, transparent bladderlike envelope. Surgical removal of the adult is the only therapy that is described.

Crenosoma vulpis

Crenosoma vulpis is a small helminth that infects the trachea, bronchi, and bronchioles of dogs, wolves, foxes, raccoons, badgers, and black bears. Animals are infected by ingesting infected land snails or slugs. Pathogenesis of lesions and clinical signs closely parallel capillariasis. Diagnosis of crenosomiasis is confirmed by finding characteristic larvae in fresh feces by direct smear, flotation, or the Baermann technique.

Pneumonyssus caninum

Pneumonyssus caninum is a small mite that inhabits the nasal passages and sinuses of dogs. The effects of mite infection are generally not serious. Infection is often asymptomatic, although sneezing, rubbing at the nose, head shaking, and inflamed mucosa are reported. The mode of transmission is unknown, but is probably direct contact. Diagnosis is based on finding the mites crawling from the external nares. No specific therapy has been investigated, but anecdotal reports suggest that environmental pest strips impregnated with organophosphates may be effective.

MANAGEMENT AND PATIENT MONITORING

Treatment of asymptomatic individuals with respiratory parasite infection, especially capillariasis, may not be necessary. Periodic examination of feces and careful observation for signs of clinical disease may suffice in these patients.

Severely affected dogs and cats require supportive treatment for the dehydration and emaciation that often accompany the chronically ill indi-

vidual. Little or no success has been reported from the use of diethylcarbamazine citrate, phenothiazine, tetrachlorethylene, stibophen, cyanacethydrazide, lithium antimony thioanalate, antimony biscatechol disulfonate, sodium iodide, emetine hydrochloride, dihydrostreptomycin, sulfonamides, dichlorvos, dithiazanine iodide, methyridine, intratracheal injection of phenol or phenothiazine, or surgical removal of parasites. The most successful reported mode of therapy for the respiratory parasites is use of the drugs levamisole, thiabendazole, albendazole, fenbendazole, ivermectin, and praziquantel.

Levamisole is effective against filaroidiasis, capillariasis, aelurostrongylosis, and probably crenosomiasis. Adverse side-effects are frequent, especially in cats, and include vomiting, salivation, diarrhea, and restless behavior. Reported oral levamisole doses are 7 to 20 mg/kg daily for 7 to 14 days. Treatment for 20 to 30 days or longer is probably needed for infection with *F. osleri*.

Thiabendazole is effective against *F. osleri*, but has not been used routinely for other respiratory parasites. For *F. osleri*, thiabendazole is used at dosages of 30 to 70 mg/kg twice daily in food for 10 to 30 days. Thiabendazole must be introduced gradually because high initial doses are poorly tolerated and may be associated with severe emesis. Therapy with thiabendazole and levamisole should continue until remission of all clinical signs or until there is a decrease in the quantity and size of the nodular *F. osleri* lesions as viewed by tracheobronchoscopy.

Albendazole and fenbendazole are benzimidazole anthelmintics that are effective for treatment of filaroidiasis, aelurostrongylosis, and paragonimiasis. Efficacy against capillariasis and crenosomiasis probably also exists. Albendazole is not currently available on the veterinary market, but fenbendazole is safe in the dog and cat and readily available. Oral dosages for both drugs is 25 to 50 mg/kg twice daily for 5 to 14 days. Treatment should continue until at least 2 days of negative fecal examinations have been observed. Benzimidazoles kill helminths and cause temporary suppression of egg production by female worms that survive treatment. Results of fecal examination for eggs or larvae may be negative for several weeks after treatment. Fecal examinations should be repeated in 6 to 8 weeks to further evaluate benzimidazole therapy. Pneumothorax from the migration of irritated or dying flukes and anaphylactic reactions are the only reported complications of therapy.

Ivermectin has known efficacy against lungworm infections of cattle, horses, sheep, and swine. It is the newest anthelmintic recommended for treatment of small animal respiratory parasites. Efficacy in selected case reports appears to be good against nematodes, but efficacy against trematodes is not documented. Dosages are 200 to 400 μg/kg subcutaneously or orally. Treatment should be given weekly until fecal examinations remain negative or clinical signs resolve.

Praziquantel is approved for use in dogs and cats with cestodiasis, and has recently been used for treatment of paragonimiasis in humans and dogs. The dosage reported to be successful in one dog (25 mg/kg orally three times daily for 2 consecutive days) is several times higher than that given for elimination of cestodes. Oral administration of praziquantel for treatment of paragonimiasis is suggested because relatively large volumes of the injectable formulation are required.

ADDITIONAL READING

Barsanti JA, Prestwood AK. Parasitic diseases of the respiratory tract. In: Kirk RW, ed. Current veterinary therapy VIII. Philadelphia: WB Saunders, 1983: 241.

Georgi JR. Parasites of the respiratory tract. Vet Clin North Am 1987; 17:1421.

THE
DIGESTIVE
SYSTEM

5

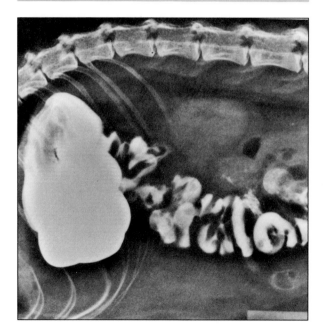

34

DYSPHAGIA, DROOLING, AND HALITOSIS

Michael D. Willard

Oral disorders may cause halitosis, drooling, anorexia, or dysphagia. Commonly seen in clinical practice, these problems are often treated symptomatically because of difficulty in properly examining the patient's mouth or lack of familiarity with the area.

CAUSES

Dysphagia (the inability to prehend or swallow food normally) may be due to pain, mass lesions, trauma, or neuromuscular dysfunction (Table 34-1).

Pain is usually due to trauma or inflammation, and may be so intense that the patient refuses to swallow. The most common causes of oral pain are foreign objects, fractures, osteomyelitis, gingivitis, periodontitis, stomatitis, glossitis, or retrobulbar inflammation (Table 34-2). Depending on their location, tumors occasionally cause sufficient pain to produce dysphagia.

Oral inflammation is usually secondary to underlying systemic disease or continued disruption of the oral mucosa. Mechanical disruption is typically caused by foreign objects, tumors, granulomas, or dental abnormalities (e.g., tartar-promoting periodontitis or rubbing against the buccal mucosa). However, periodontitis usually produces halitosis instead of dysphagia. Immune-mediated oral disease (pemphigus vulgaris or systemic lupus erythematosus) may cause continual epithelial disruptions, allowing bacterial proliferation.

Masses must be large or strategically placed to produce dysphagia. Most localized oral growths are malignant. The most common oral canine malignancies are malignant melanomas, squamous carcinomas, and fibrosarcomas. Acanthomatous epulis is a relatively benign although locally invasive tumor. Squamous carcinomas are the most common oral feline neoplasia and often produce dysphagia due to lingual involvement. Eosinophilic and histoplasmocytic granulomas also occur on the tongue. Marked tonsillar enlargement often causes dyspnea and may also cause gagging. Finally, sialoceles in the pharynx or under the tongue (ranulas) may produce similar results.

Trauma typically causes transient pain unless there is a fracture or secondary infection. Occasionally, the mouth is so deformed that the pa-

469

Table 34–1 Causes of Dysphagia in Dogs and Cats

ORAL PAIN

See Table 34-2

ORAL MASS

Tumor
  Melanoma (dogs)
  Squamous cell carcinoma
  Fibrosarcoma (dogs)
  Epulis
Granuloma
  Eosinophilic granuloma

TRAUMA

Fractured bones
  Mandible
  Maxilla
  Hard palate
  Hyoid apparatus
Fractured teeth
Cranial nerve damage

NEUROMUSCULAR DISEASE

Oral (prehensile) dysphagia
  Cranial nerve deficits (cranial nerve V damage causing
    "dropped" lower jaw)
  Acute or chronic masseter or temporal myositis (dogs)
Pharyngeal dysphagia
  Acquired neuromuscular disease
    Myasthenia gravis
    Rabies
    Idiopathic
  Congenital neuromuscular disease
Cricopharyngeal dysphagia (dogs)
  Achalasia
  Incoordination

MISCELLANEOUS

Pharyngeal foreign object
Temporomandibular joint abnormalities

Table 34–2 Causes of Oral Pain in Dogs and Cats

INFLAMMATION

Gingivitis or periodontitis
Stomatitis, glossitis, or pharyngitis
  Idiopathic
  Pemphigus vulgaris
  Systemic lupus erythematosus
  Contact dermatitis (allergic or irritant)
  Upper respiratory viral infection (cats)
  Bacterial infection
  Trauma or foreign objects
  Feline leukemia virus or feline immunodeficiency virus-
    associated stomatitis (cats)
  Lymphocytic–plasmacytic gingivitis
  Histoplasmosis
  Uremia
  Heavy metal intoxication (especially thallium)
  Drug eruption (any drug)
  Chemical (caustics such as lye)
  Traumatic (plant awns such as burdock)
Osteomyelitis
  Tooth root abscess
Acute temporal or masseter myositis
Retrobulbar abscess

FOREIGN OBJECTS

Bones
Needles
Sticks

TRAUMA

Fractured mandible or maxilla
  Automobile-associated trauma
  Fights with other animals (especially dogs)
  "High-rise" syndrome (especially cats)
Fractured teeth

MISCELLANEOUS

Neoplasia

---

tient cannot eat. Mandibular and maxillary fractures are examples; they may occur secondary to automobile-associated trauma or falling from great heights. Cats especially, may have compressive cranial fractures with separation of the left and right maxillary or nasal bones.

Neuromuscular disease is a more complex and potentially more subtle cause of dysphagia. Complete inability of the cranial or oropharyngeal muscles to prehend, chew, or swallow food is rare but obvious. Partial neurologic deficits may be difficult to recognize.

Drooling may be due to ptyalism or pseudoptyalism. Ptyalism is excessive production of saliva; it is principally caused by nausea, oral pain, and hepatic encephalopathy (Table 34-3). Pseudoptyalism is due to an inability to swallow and is typically secondary to dysphagia.

Halitosis is usually due to bacterial proliferation, with production of odiferous metabolites (Table 34-4). Occasionally, the smell may be a reflection of the diet (*e.g.*, manure).

PATHOPHYSIOLOGY

Pain, trauma, and masses may produce dysphagia; however, their location determines the symptomatology. The best example is a retrobulbar abscess. Whenever the mouth is opened, the verti-

Table 34–3 *Causes of Pseudoptyalism and Ptyalism in Dogs and Cats*

INABILITY TO SWALLOW (PSEUDOPTYALISM)

Rabies
Oral pain of any cause
Dysphagia due to any cause

OVERPRODUCTION OF SALIVA (PTYALISM)

Chemical or toxin
  Organophosphate drugs or chemicals
Bitter-tasting drugs
  Ophthalmic atropine which the animal tastes when it licks the nares (the drug travels to the nares through the nasolacrimal duct)
Salivary gland overproduction (rare)
Behavioral cause (Pavlovian reaction)

NAUSEA (PTYALISM)

Nausea due to any cause

MISCELLANEOUS

Hepatic encephalopathy (especially cats)
Facial nerve paralysis

Table 34–4 *Causes of Halitosis in Dogs and Cats*

BACTERIAL METABOLISM

Tartar
Retained food
  Between teeth or their roots
  Impaction of food into tonsillar fossulae
  Into cavities or defects in the oral cavity
Damaged oral tissue
  Stomatitis or glossitis due to any cause
  Tumors
  Granulomas

MISCELLANEOUS

Eating of foul-smelling material, such as manure

cal ramus of the mandible exerts pressure in this region. If there is inflammatory disease, then opening the mouth can cause severe pain, despite otherwise minimal discomfort.

Neuromuscular disorders also cause dysphagia. These disorders are easier to comprehend if one considers that swallowing normally consists of three main phases: the prehensile or oral phase, the pharyngeal phase, and the cricopharyngeal phase.

The oral or prehensile phase consists of those actions necessary to bite into the food and keep it within the mouth while chewing. The masticatory and facial muscles are used extensively. Cranial nerve deficits affecting these muscles prevent the animal from taking a normal bite or chewing effectively. These deficits may be due to primary central nervous system disease (*e.g.*, tumor) or traumatized cranial nerves.

Muscular disorders may also cause oral phase dysphagia. Swollen, inflamed, painful muscles make the patient unwilling to use these muscles to open the mouth, while fibrotic, scarred muscles (*e.g.*, chronic masseter myositis) prevent the patient from opening its mouth. Occasionally, temporomandibular joint problems may also prevent normal opening or closing of the mouth.

The pharyngeal phase consists of moving food to the base of the tongue, forming a bolus, and propelling it into the esophagus. Cranial nerve deficits are the primary reasons for weakness or uncoordination of these muscles. Such deficits may be permanent or transitory. Pharyngeal dysfunctions sometimes cause more difficulty when the patient swallows liquids versus solids because the former cannot be controlled by the dysfunctioning muscles as well as the latter.

Neurologic disorders causing pharyngeal dysphagia often concurrently affect the proximal esophagus, producing dilatation just caudal to the cricopharyngeal muscle. Severe aspiration is possible if anything (*e.g.*, cricopharyngeous myotomy) prevents the cricopharyngeous muscle from remaining closed and keeping such material in the esophagus.

Rabies is an ascending viral infection of nerves. Although the presentation may be quite variable, it may produce a lower motor neuron paralysis of the pharyngeal muscles and mandible or cause painful pharyngeal spasms when the animal attempts to drink. This can result in dysphagia plus drooling copious amounts of saliva.

Cricopharyngeal disorders principally consist of achalasia (inability of the cricopharyngeal muscle to relax). This produces an obstruction when the base of the tongue tries to propel a bolus of food into the esophagus. In some cases there seems to be incoordination between the pharyngeal and cricopharyngeal phases so that cricopharyngeal relaxation does not occur at the proper time. Although cricopharyngeal disorders are usually congenital, they may rarely be acquired. The cause of congenital achalasia is uncertain; acquired disease may be due to cranial nerve dysfunctions.

Gingivitis is inflammation of the gingiva surrounding the teeth. Periodontitis is gingivitis that has progressed into the periodontium. As tartar accumulates, the bacterial flora in the tartar changes and produces enzymes, which damage the free gingival margin and cause gingival proliferation or recession. In either case, further bacterial proliferation results in gingival destruction. Increased tartar increases the likelihood and severity of the inflammation; however, some animals with minimal tartar have severe gingivitis whereas others with excessive tartar accumulations have no gingivitis. Cats may have excessive gingival inflammation in response to minimal tartar. Although not described in dogs and cats, oral disease due to immunoglobulin A deficiency may exist.

Because the mouth has a profuse normal flora, immunosuppression can produce stomatitis. Collies with cyclic neutropenia and cats with feline leukemia virus-associated neutropenia may have severe oral ulceration that persists until the peripheral neutrophil count increases. Likewise, Feline immunodeficiency virus (FIV)-associated gingivitis ostensibly occurs due to immunosuppression. Hypoproteinemia may be responsible for oral ulcers that resolve once proteins are replenished.

Halitosis is due to bacterial degradation of food or tissue; thus, food must be retained in the mouth or tissue must be damaged in order for bacterial colonization to occur. The normal, constant turnover of oral mucosa helps prevent bacterial colonization, and oral tissue destruction allowing bacterial proliferation is uncommon unless there is abnormal tissue (*e.g.*, tumor) or continual trauma. However, tartar is a common cause of halitosis because tartar is partially composed of bacteria. This means that as the tartar accumulates, bacterial populations increase.

CLINICAL SIGNS

In most instances of oral disease, several clinical signs occur simultaneously (Table 34-5).

An acute onset of clinical signs suggests

Table 34–5 *Clinical Signs of Oral Disease in Dogs and Cats*

Dysphagia
  Anorexia
  Coughing during eating or drinking
  Food dropping from the mouth
  Inability to eat
  Regurgitation
  Repeated attempts or difficulty in swallowing
Drooling
  Dried saliva on legs or chin
  Saliva dripping from mouth
Pain
  "Head shy"
  Refuses oral examination or cries out when examination is attempted
Halitosis
Aspiration pneumonia
  Cough
  Fever
Weight loss
Severe atrophy of cranial muscles

trauma, a foreign object, or ingestion of a noxious substance, while a gradual onset may be due to almost anything. Dysphagia may be detected when the owner sees abnormal efforts or failed attempts at chewing and swallowing, such as food falling from the mouth, repeated attempts to swallow, stretching out the head and neck when swallowing, and coughing associated with eating or drinking. Signs may be worse when liquids are consumed. Patients may refuse to eat because of pain, discomfort, or aspiration experienced when trying to eat or drink. Oropharyngeal disorders can also cause regurgitation, which occurs minutes to hours after eating. Cough and fever may be the major signs if severe aspiration pneumonia is present. Some patients lose weight due to malnutrition secondary to refusal or inability to eat. In short-haired dogs, the clients may notice severe atrophy of the cranial muscles, while dogs with rabies may evidence behavioral change ("furious" rabies or "dumb" rabies) or other vague central nervous system signs.

Other signs attending dysphagic disorders may initially be more dramatic to the owners. Halitosis is often the first sign that clients note, especially in pets with tartar, periodontitis, and tumors.

Drooling may be obvious or may be noted by finding dried saliva around the mouth or on the front legs. Oral pain may not be reported, but clients may state that the pet is "head shy." Occasionally, the pet may paw at the mouth, rub its muzzle on the ground, or whine. In areas where rabies is possible or in pets that may have been exposed to rabies, a careful history should ascertain the vaccination status of the dysphagic pet and whether there has been any behavioral change.

Halitosis is readily identified, although occasional clients must be informed that their pet's breath smells normal. Pathological odor is usually so foul that there is no doubt that it is a problem.

DIAGNOSTIC APPROACH

First one must identify which problems are present. The history should be used to search for obvious causes (*e.g.,* electrical cord burns, ingestion of caustic agents).

If one is unsure whether dysphagia is present, the pet should be observed while eating. Sometimes the owners may have to describe the act if the animal will not eat at the veterinary clinic. Sometimes the pet must be fed several times before dysphagia is obvious. Some patients with oropharyngeal disorders will have food impacted in the tonsillar fossulae, and regurgitation may occur hours after eating; however, this is uncommon.

Once dysphagia is identified, the history should search for an acute onset consistent with rabies, trauma (*e.g.,* automobile-associated, dog fight, snake bite, or electric cord shock), noxious chemicals (*e.g.,* strong alkali), abscess, or foreign objects (Fig. 34-1). One should be sure that the onset was acute and that it is not a case of the owner suddenly noticing a chronic problem. Chronic or slowly progressive dysphagia may be due to almost anything.

If rabies seems possible, the owners should be advised, the patient isolated, and the proper authorities notified. One may confine the patient and, if it dies within 7 to 10 days, send the brain for histologic or fluorescent antibody examination. Alternatively, immunofluorescence of skin biopsies, including the base of the maxillary sensory vibrissae, seems to be a reliable means of antemortem diagnosis if it is not done too early in the course of the disease. Occasionally, patients

with rabies may have atypical presentations and may not die within the expected 2 weeks. Therefore, any patient with unexplained central nervous system signs should be approached with the thought that rabies is possible. Fortunately, canine and feline rabies is relatively uncommon in many areas, and other causes of dysphagia will usually be found. However, the veterinarian should take precautions to guard against exposure while examining the patient (gloves and careful sanitation) and should not attempt to examine a vicious animal without chemical restraint, regardless of prophylactic rabies immunizations that the pet or the veterinarian have had.

If swollen, painful temporal or masseter muscles are found, a muscle biopsy is indicated. If the temporal and masseter muscles are severely atrophied, one must consider chronic myositis, although some patients with temporal and masseter muscle atrophy are not diseased. Chronic myositis may cause scarring that prevents the mouth from opening, even when the animal is anesthetized. Insertional electromyelographic activity may appear normal if the muscles have been replaced by fibrous connective tissue. A muscle biopsy is indicated to confirm the diagnosis and eliminate other causes of myopathy (*e.g.,* toxoplasmosis). Serology (antibodies to 2 M muscle fibers) to separate masseter myositis from polymyositis is available (Shelton, Additional Reading).

Next, the dysphagic patient should have a careful oral and cranial examination. Compliant patients without evidence of pain, a foreign object, or a mass may have a neuromuscular disorder. Patients with oral pain and those resisting oral examination are likely to have a significant oral lesion. If necessary, chemical restraint (*e.g.,* a thiobarbiturate) should be used to allow thorough oral examination. All gingival and lingual surfaces, as well as the pharynx and hard and soft palates, must be closely examined so as to confidently eliminate oral masses, foreign objects, and areas of inflammation. A laryngoscope is useful. Teeth should be inspected for fractures, neck lesions (in cats), and looseness. Often, oral foreign objects are wedged between the teeth, especially the carnassial teeth (upper fourth premolars), or lodged in the posterior pharynx.

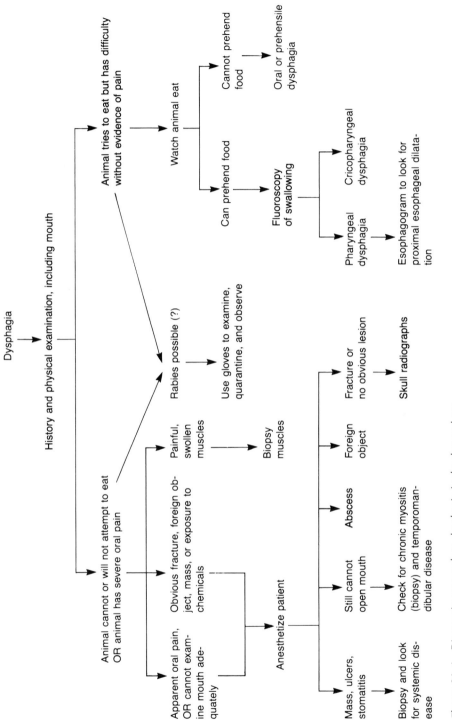

Figure 34–1. *Diagnostic approach to dysphagia in the dog and cat.*

Distribution of oral lesions may be informative. Stomatitis due to trauma from tartar or broken teeth will be closely associated with the responsible teeth. Mucocutaneous ulceration suggests an immune-mediated disease; however, some of these diseases do not have lesions limited to these sites. Papillomatosis may cause multiple smooth or cauliflowerlike growths on the oral mucosa or tongue. Fibromatous and ossifying epulides may be single, but often present as multiple pedunculated growths around the teeth.

Masses must be biopsied unless the diagnostician is absolutely certain of the diagnosis, papillomatosis and some fibrous epulides being the only reasonable examples of such lesions. If a mass is found that may be a sialocele, needle aspiration is advised before an incisional biopsy. Cytologic examination of fine needle aspirates or scrapings may be diagnostic for melanomas (if they are melanotic) and squamous carcinomas. However, fibrosarcomas do not exfoliate well. Furthermore, amelanotic melanomas can be epithelioid or resemble connective tissue tumors (fibrosarcomas). Aspiration of submandibular lymph nodes (even when normal-sized) and thoracic radiographs are indicated regardless of the type of malignancy, as all forms can eventually metastasize.

A mass cannot be assumed to be or not be neoplastic based on size and how localized it is.

Eosinophilic granulomas can become sizable and resemble carcinomas (Fig. 34-2). Although more common in cats, they occur in Siberian husky dogs and rarely in other breeds. Laceration and granulation of the frenulum of the tongue secondary to a linear foreign body may resemble a carcinoma. Some malignancies do not form discrete masses, but diffusely infiltrate the dental arcade, resembling severe periodontitis (Fig. 34-3). Single or multiple masses due to calcinosis circumscripta may occur on the tongue of dogs, especially the larger breeds. Lymphocytic–plasmacytic gingivitis of cats can be proliferative and resemble a diffuse neoplasia.

Any area of inflammation that cannot clearly be attributed to a foreign object or tartar should be biopsied. These biopsies must be relatively deep so that the underlying disease process is not obscured by superficial inflammation from the normal bacterial flora. The biopsy site may be cauterized with silver nitrate to stop the hemorrhage. Buccal mucosa that comes into contact with the carnassial teeth may be severely inflamed. These teeth usually have the worst tartar accumulations; however, relatively mild tartar accumulations can produce severe inflammation. After biopsying the tissue, it is reasonable to clean the teeth. Unexplained stomatitis or glossitis is an indication for a complete blood count, serum biochemistry profile, and urinalysis (Table 34-6).

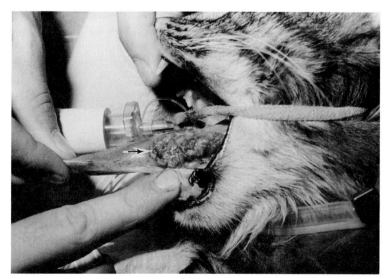

Figure 34–2. *A large, ulcerated mass (arrow) at the base of the tongue of a cat. It looks like a carcinoma but is an eosinophilic granuloma.*

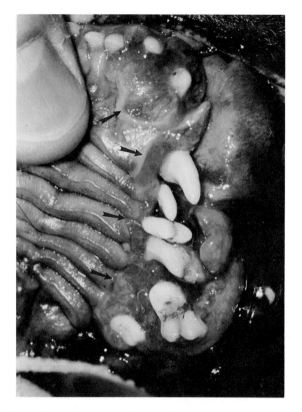

Figure 34–3. *There is a diffuse swelling around the teeth in the upper arcade (arrows) of this Pekingese dog that resembles an inflammatory lesion but is an advanced amelanotic melanoma.*

Uremia commonly causes ulcerative stomatitis or necrotic glossitis. Hypoproteinemia, diabetes mellitus, hyperadrenocorticism, and heavy-metal intoxication may also be responsible. If these tests are not helpful, then oral biopsies should be done. Culture of oral lesions is usually of minimal value due to contamination from the profuse normal flora. If immune-mediated disease is suspected, very recent lesions (bullae) should be biopsied and submitted for histopathology and immunofluorescence. ANA titers may also be helpful. Cats with persistent stomatitis or gingivitis should be tested for feline leukemia virus and FIV infections.

Glossitis affecting the anterior lingual margin plus stomatitis of the hard palate can occur in cats that clean chemicals (disinfectants) off their hair coats or dogs that ingest caustic substances (*e.g.*, lye). Electrical cord burns of the tongue often have concomitant burns on both sides of the mouth, often at the commissure of the lips. Ulcerative glossitis or stomatitis, epiphora, and nasal discharge suggest feline upper respiratory viral infection (calicivirus or herpesvirus). Diffuse glossitis not clearly associated with stomatitis or trauma from teeth suggests foreign objects (*e.g.*, burrs). Necrosis of the anterior portion of the tongue suggests uremia or an electrical cord burn. Occasionally, hair is found growing on the tongue. This is usually asymptomatic unless accompanied by severe inflammation.

Patients that experience pain when they open their mouths but in which no apparent cause is found at oral examination should also have their eyes examined and their pharynx and temporomandibular joints radiographed for foreign objects. Concurrent unilateral ocular disease suggests a retrobulbar problem.

Skull radiographs should include lateral, dorsoventral, open-mouth, or oblique views. The temporomandibular joints should also be evaluated. Adequate radiographs cannot be obtained without anesthesia. Many foreign objects are obvious (*e.g.*, needle lodged in the pharynx), while radiolucent ones may be suggested by soft-tissue swelling or emphysema. Diffuse, non-neoplastic bony proliferation of the caudal mandible or tympanic bullae (craniomandibular osteopathy) occurs in West Highland white, Scottish, and cairn terriers, and occasionally in other breeds.

Marked pain upon opening the mouth without any obvious cause may be due to a retrobulbar abscess. This may not cause other physical or radiographic changes. The presence of unilateral ocular disease (conjunctivitis, chemosis, uveitis) may suggest retrobulbar abscess; however, these signs may be absent. Such disease must sometimes be diagnosed by ruling out other causes in a patient with a suggestive physical examination.

Dysphagic animals without oral pain, a mass, a foreign object, or bony destruction and with normal muscles of mastication need dynamic studies of the mouth and pharynx using barium contrast to distinguish pharyngeal from cricopharyngeal dysfunction. This distinction is critical because surgery is necessary for cricopharyngeal disorders but usually contraindicated in pharyngeal disease. Almost all patients with cricopharyngeal dysfunction present as a congen-

Table 34–6 Laboratory Assessment of Dysphagia, Drooling, and Halitosis

Test	What to Check For
Complete blood count	Inflammation (aspiration pneumonia, oral infection extending into the deeper oral tissues)
	Neutropenia (oral ulceration in cats due to feline leukemia virus, cyclic neutropenia in collies)
	Lymphopenia, eosinopenia (hyperadrenocorticism)
Serum biochemistry profile	Hypoalbuminemia (may cause ulcers)
	Uremia (oral ulcers, lingual necrosis)
	Hypercholesterolemia (hyperadrenocorticism)
	Increased serum alkaline phosphatase (hyperadrenocorticism)
	Hyperglycemia (diabetes mellitus)
Urinalysis	Isosthenuria (renal disease causing uremia)
	Glucosuria (diabetes mellitus)
Radiographs	Fractures
	Osteomyelitis
	Foreign objects
	Temporomandibular joint problems
ANA, LE cell preparation	Systemic lupus erythematosus
Antibodies to 2M muscle fibers	Masticatory myositis

ital defect, while pharyngeal disorders usually present as an acquired disease. However, exceptions occur with both syndromes, and contrast procedures utilizing static images are seldom adequate for differentiation. Fluoroscopy is adequate, but cinefluorography is better. Unfortunately, these radiographic studies are seldom available outside of referral practices and academic institutions. One should also determine if the proximal esophagus retains material, which generally contraindicates cricopharyngeal myotomy.

Drooling that cannot be attributed to oral pain or dysphagia may be due to nausea or hepatic encephalopathy. Some animals develop such aversions to certain drugs (e.g., cephalothin) that even the odor of the drug causes nausea and salivation.

Halitosis in nondysphagic patients necessitates a thorough oral examination. Excessive tartar accumulation, gingival proliferation, and gingival recession are usually obvious. Because the odor is dependent on the types and not just numbers of bacteria, small amounts of tartar may be responsible. It is often reasonable to remove the tartar, treat the periodontitis, and see what happens to the halitosis.

MANAGEMENT

Oral foreign objects, lacerations, and fractures should be corrected, and secondary infections treated. Nasogastric, pharyngostomy, or gastrostomy tubes are useful for animals that are unable to eat or those with severe oral lesions (see descriptions of these techniques in Chapter 80).

Inflammatory Diseases

It is always preferable to treat an underlying cause of stomatitis (e.g., pemphigus vulgaris, systemic lupus erythematosus, fungal infection, or uremia) or to at least identify an underlying cause that will eventually resolve if the patient can be supported long enough with symptomatic therapy (e.g., feline calicivirus, feline herpesvirus, ingestion of a caustic agent, or drug eruption).

Idiopathic stomatitis, by definition, can only be treated symptomatically. Antibiotics with a broad spectrum, including anaerobic bacteria, are needed (e.g., amoxicillin, chloramphenicol, and clindamycin). Metronidazole is also effective against anaerobic bacteria. Flushing a lesion with saline, dilute chlorhexidine solutions (0.2%), or dilute povidone–iodine solutions to remove debris and kill bacteria is useful if the animal does not drink the solution. Hydrogen peroxide is occasionally useful as a cleansing rinse, but it is seldom tolerated by pets. Cleaning the teeth may be helpful even when there is relatively little tartar present. Extraction of teeth adjacent to severely affected areas is often beneficial. Feline leukemia virus- and FIV-associated stomatitis must often be treated in the same manner, although glucocorticoids (*e.g.*, prednisolone 1.1–2.2 mg/kg once daily, orally or intramuscularly) may help alleviate the stomatitis in neutropenic, feline leukemia virus-positive cats.

Glossitis is treated similarly to idiopathic stomatitis. However, granulomatous glossitis due to foreign bodies (*e.g.*, "burr tongue") requires cutting off the superficial proliferative tissue. Lingual necrosis must be treated symptomatically; subsequent dysphagia may necessitate various diets (liquid that can be sucked into the mouth or food made into balls that the patient can learn to "toss" into the back of the mouth).

Retrobulbar abscesses are drained by incising the gingiva immediately behind the last upper molar and directly under the eye. Mosquito hemostats are inserted dorsally until they enter the retrobulbar region and then are pulled out with the jaws opened. After establishing drainage, systemic antibiotics (*e.g.*, amoxicillin, cefazolin, enrofloxacin) are utilized.

Tumors

Malignant melanomas metastasize early and are not responsive to surgery, chemotherapy, or radiation therapy. Aggressive surgery (partial maxillectomies and hemimandibulectomies) with adjunctive radiation may be curative or palliative for gingival squamous carcinomas and fibrosarcomas. Acanthomatous epulis is readily treatable with surgery or radiation therapy. Tonsillar and lingual squamous carcinomas are usually untreatable. Fibromatous and ossifying epulides do not require resection unless they are causing mechanical problems with chewing, in which case localized resection is sufficient. Oral papillomatosis usually regresses spontaneously in 1 to 2 months. Other malignancies must be considered, especially those that metastasize early or are disseminating in nature (*e.g.*, lymphosarcoma). However, osteosarcomas of flat bones do not metastasize as readily as those of the long bones, and surgery may be more useful.

Eosinophilic granulomas may superficially resemble tumors, but usually respond to high-dose corticosteroid therapy (*e.g.*, prednisolone 2.2 mg/kg/day orally or intramuscularly) and rarely require surgery. Megestrol acetate may also be used, but cats must be monitored carefully for drug-associated diabetes mellitus and female reproductive disorders (see Appendix II). Feline lymphocytic–plasmacytic gingivitis may be helped by removing teeth in the more severely affected areas; resecting proliferative tissue and corticosteroids may also be tried. Many cats with severe lymphocytic–plasmacytic gingivitis respond best to multiple tooth extractions. Calcinosis circumscripta may be resected or left alone. Salivary mucoceles should not only be drained, but the responsible salivary glands should be removed to prevent recurrence.

Tooth Problems

Fractured teeth, tooth root abscesses, and severe stomatitis due to chronic trauma from teeth (especially the carnassial teeth) often necessitate extractions. Feline tooth neck lesions require filling of the lesions or extraction of the affected teeth. Some cats with proliferative gingival lesions respond best if the teeth are removed.

The most useful therapy for preventing problems is cleaning the teeth. It is important that the tooth crown be scaled (an ultrasonic scaler is useful), the subgingival area cleaned with curettes, the root planed, and the crown polished to prevent rapid recurrence of the tartar. Simply removing large flakes of tartar with hemostats or dental hoes is easy but ineffective, as the subgingival area is untouched and tartar recurs rapidly. Prophylactic antibiotics are begun 1 hour before and repeated until 24 hours after the procedure. If tartar and periodontitis are severe, antibiotic therapy should commence 2 to 3 days before the procedure. The choice of antibiotics is the same as for idiopathic stomatitis. Gingival hyperplasia producing periodontal pockets greater than or equal to 5 mm should be resected to remove the deep sulcus that allows bacterial proliferation and predisposes to periodontitis.

Once the teeth are cleaned, it is advantageous to have the clients brush them with veterinary dentifrices (products for humans have detergents that foam and are objectionable to pets) or rinse the mouth with 0.2% chlorhexidine for 1 minute daily.

Neuromuscular Disorders

Muscular disease causing swelling or atrophy must be carefully defined before therapy is initiated. Nonseptic cranial myositis of dogs usually responds to anti-inflammatory therapy; prednisolone (2.2 mg/kg/day) with or without azathioprine (2 mg/kg/day) usually provides some benefit within 7 to 10 days, although occasional patients require 20 to 30 days of therapy. Once the patient can open the mouth normally, the glucocorticoid dose is slowly reduced to an alternate-day dosage and the azathioprine is switched to an alternate-day dosage. If the drugs are withdrawn too quickly the disease often recurs and may be difficult to put back into remission.

Oral dysphagia due to neuromuscular disease can be resolved only if the underlying disease is treatable. Trauma (*e.g.*, bruising or stretching of a nerve) may cause temporary dysfunction, resolving spontaneously. Apparently delayed maturation of nerves, causing pharyngeal dysfunction, may eventually resolve much like congenital esophageal weakness if the patient does not die of aspiration pneumonia first.

True cricopharyngeal dysfunction (both achalasia and asynchrony) is often amenable to cricopharyngeal myotomy. If a scar occurs at the myotomy site, the cicatrix may produce obstruction. Pharyngeal dysfunction with concurrent proximal esophageal dilatation must not be treated with such a myotomy lest subsequent aspiration kill the patient. Age of onset helps differentiate the two, but is not foolproof. Pharyngeal dysfunction must be treated by seeking to identify the underlying neuropathies or myopathies

and resolving them. Pharyngostomy tube feeding may be done while awaiting resolution of the cause.

Craniomandibular osteopathy may sometimes be helped by glucocorticoid therapy or surgical removal of excess periosteal bone. However, the bony proliferation may recur and prevent the patient from eating. Bony proliferation usually stops once the patient matures.

PATIENT MONITORING
Neoplasia

Failure to treat malignant neoplasms early and aggressively is usually fatal. Melanomas and lingual or tonsillar squamous cell carcinomas have a very poor prognosis regardless of therapy. Early treatment of gingival squamous cell carcinomas and rostral fibrosarcomas may be curative. After resecting oral malignancies, examination every 6 to 12 weeks is recommended to detect recurrence as quickly as possible. Acanthomatous epulis is curable. Although uncommon, neoplasia secondary to radiotherapy has occurred and should be considered, especially if high doses of radiation are used.

Idiopathic stomatitis is usually controlled with symptomatic therapy. Failure to control signs results in weight loss due to anorexia or euthanasia due to the client's intolerance of the halitosis. These patients, as well as those with stomatitis due to foreign objects, eosinophilic granuloma, and systemic diseases should be reexamined every 1 to 4 weeks until resolved.

Chronic atrophic myositis and acute myositis can usually be controlled with medical therapy. The patient must be monitored carefully, as drug therapy is gradually withdrawn lest the disease recur. If the tongue has been burned chemically or electrically, it should be observed weekly until it becomes obvious which portions will survive and which will slough.

Dental Disease

After a dental cleaning, the mouth should be examined every 6 to 8 months. If severe tartar and periodontitis are not resolved, the patient will usually have an eventual loss of teeth plus an increased chance of other infections. Many patients with severe gingivitis do not seem to feel well.

Neuromuscular Disorders

Failure to control neuromuscular dysphagia often results in fatal aspiration pneumonia or emaciation. Congenital cricopharyngeal achalasia has a good prognosis with surgery, while some acquired pharyngeal dysfunctions will respond to medical therapy.

ADDITIONAL READING

Burrows CF, Miller WH, Harvey CE. Oral medicine in veterinary dentistry. In: Harvey CE, ed. Veterinary dentistry. Philadelphia: WB Saunders, 1985: 34.

Dillon AR. The oral cavity. In: Jones BD, ed. Canine and feline gastroenterology. Philadelphia: WB Saunders, 1986: 1.

McKeever PJ. Stomatitis. In: Kirk RW, ed. Current veterinary therapy IX. Philadelphia: WB Saunders, 1986: 846.

Norris AM, Withrow SJ, Dubielzig RR. Oropharyngeal neoplasms. In: Harvey CE, ed. Veterinary dentistry. Philadelphia: WB Saunders, 1985: 123.

Shelton GD, Cardinet GH. Canine masticatory muscle disorders. In Kirk RW, ed. Current veterinary therapy X. Philadelphia: WB Saunders, 1989: 816.

35

REGURGITATION

Michael D. Willard

Most clinicians will see several vomiting or regurgitating patients weekly. However, despite being common problems for the primary care veterinarian as well as the referral specialist, vomiting and regurgitation are often confused.

CAUSES

The major causes of regurgitation are given in Table 35-1.

PATHOPHYSIOLOGY

Vomiting is a centrally mediated reflex resulting in expulsion of gastric or intestinal contents, whereas regurgitation causes loss of food, water, or saliva from the esophagus or pharynx.

For regurgitation to occur, material must be retained in the esophagus or pharynx due to mechanical obstruction of the lumen or muscular weakness. The retained material must next move orad so that a gag reflex occurs and the material reenters the oral cavity, where it is either spit out or reswallowed.

Mechanical Esophageal Obstruction

Mechanical esophageal obstruction may be congenital or acquired. The former is usually due to an extramural vascular ring anomaly (e.g., persistent right fourth aortic arch), but may be caused by agenesis of an esophageal segment.

Acquired obstructions are intraluminal, intramural, or extraesophageal. Acquired intraluminal and intramural obstructions are usually due to foreign objects, scarring following esophagitis, or neoplasia. The stomach will rarely intussuscept into a grossly enlarged esophagus. Extraesophageal obstructions are usually due to neoplastic mediastinal or cervical masses. True achalasia (failure to open) of the lower esophageal sphincter rarely occurs, and is a poorly characterized neuromuscular dysfunction.

Esophageal diverticula not caused by vascular ring obstructions are rare in dogs and cats. Pulsion diverticula are the result of a rent in the esophageal musculature, with subsequent pushing of luminal contents through the weakened area. Traction diverticula (which are not well documented in dogs or cats) are due to adhesions between the esophagus and other structures. As

Table 35–1 *Causes of Esophageal Regurgitation in Dogs and Cats*

OBSTRUCTION

Congenital
  Vascular ring anomaly (especially persistent right aortic arch)
  Esophageal deviation (often asymptomatic; especially bulldogs and Shar Peis)
  Agenesis (partial or complete)
Acquired
  Ingestion of foreign object (especially dogs)
  Cicatrix
  Extraluminal mass
    Mediastinal tumor (lymphosarcoma)
    Thyroid tumor (carcinoma; especially dogs)
  Primary esophageal tumor
    Carcinoma
    Fibrosarcoma due to *Spirocerca lupi* (especially dogs)
  Achalasia of the lower esophageal sphincter (especially dogs)
  Gastroesophageal intussusception (especially dogs)
  Esophageal diverticula

WEAKNESS

Congenital
  Idiopathic esophageal weakness
Acquired
  Myopathy
  Neuropathy
  Myasthenia gravis (localized to the esophagus or generalized; especially dogs)
  Esophagitis
    Gastroesophageal reflux
    Hiatal hernia (especially Shar Peis)
    Ingestion of foreign object
    Ingestion of caustic agents (alkali)
    Secondary to persistent vomiting (especially due to gastrinoma)
  Metastatic neoplasia
    Thyroid carcinoma (especially dogs)
    Respiratory tract carcinoma
  Infection with *Spirocerca lupi* (especially dogs)
  Hypothyroidism (dogs)
  Systemic lupus erythematosus
  Dysautonomia (Key–Gaskell syndrome in cats)
  Heavy metal intoxication (thallium, lead)
  Hypoadrenocorticism
  Dermatomyositis (collies)
  Chagas' disease (trypanosomiasis)

the adhesion contracts, that side of the esophagus is pulled away and an outpouching is formed.

Esophageal Weakness

The esophagus is a tube of muscle, striated in dogs and smooth plus striated in cats. Esophageal weakness may be caused by anything that produces lower motor neuron dysfunction of these muscles.

Congenital canine esophageal weakness has been attributed to delayed maturation of nerves or areas of the central nervous system. Acquired esophageal weakness may be due to muscular disease (myopathies), destruction of acetylcholine receptors (*e.g.*, myasthenia), altered resting membrane potentials (*e.g.*, hyperkalemia), lack of efferent innervation (*e.g.*, destruction of the vagus nerve, polyneuropathy, or primary central nervous system disease) or lack of the afferent innervation necessary for bolus-dependent reinforcement of esophageal waves (esophagitis).

Secondary Effects

Regurgitating animals principally lose ingested food or water; saliva is the main endogenous secretion lost. Dehydration and electrolyte abnormalities are uncommon, the principal secondary effect of regurgitation being aspiration pneumonia. Aspiration may occur secondary to vomiting, but regurgitating patients are at increased risk, possibly from concurrent incoordination of laryngeal and pharyngeal muscles.

CLINICAL SIGNS

While ejection of material from the mouth is the principal complaint, a patient may have life-threatening regurgitation despite failure of the client to notice it (Table 35-2). Some animals swallow the material after it enters the mouth or quickly re-eat what was ejected from the mouth. In such cases, the only evidence of regurgitation may be a spot of dried mucus on the floor or carpet. Vomiting is usually not this subtle, and animals rarely re-eat vomited material.

Regurgitation may never be suspected by the client, the only sign being respiratory disease due to aspiration tracheitis or pneumonia. Aspiration disease principally causes a cough, which may range from acute to chronic and from mildly productive to productive, with dyspnea or mucopurulent nasal discharge. An esophageal foreign object may compress the airways, producing

Table 35-2 *Clinical Signs Suggesting Regurgitation*

Ejection of food or phlegm from the mouth (especially if it is tubular in shape; however, this shape is uncommon)
Spots of mucus, water, or food on floor or carpet
Chronic cough
Fever or depression
Difficulty swallowing
Weight loss
Anorexia
Flaccid dilatation in neck, especially one that moves with respirations (uncommon)
Mass near thoracic inlet (uncommon)
Swollen, painful distal extremities (due to thoracic mass and hypertrophic osteopathy uncommon)

acute dyspnea and choking. Occasionally, the esophagus becomes so dilated that it prevents normal lung expansion, resulting in dyspnea. The cervical esophagus can become so dilated with air that the negative pressure changes in the thorax are reflected by a bellowslike activity, seen as a mass in the neck getting alternatively bigger and smaller in phase with respiration. Finally, large foreign objects may lodge at the thoracic inlet and produce a mass effect there.

Marked weight loss occasionally occurs from malnourishment. Likewise, patients may be anorectic due to severe aspiration pneumonia, pain associated with eating (due to a foreign object or severe esophagitis), or systemic disease (*e.g.*, neo-

plasia or myopathy) that is responsible for the esophageal dysfunction. Esophageal foreign objects may perforate, resulting in septic pleuritis or mediastinitis, which causes depression or fever. Sometimes patients refuse to eat in order to avoid esophageal pain. Rarely, esophageal disease secondary to infection with *Spirocerca lupi* or neoplasia causes hypertrophic osteopathy with lameness from swollen, firm, warm, painful distal extremities. Rare individuals with esophageal diverticula may regurgitate or demonstrate anorexia, fever, or pain. Finally, some animals have severe esophageal lesions that are asymptomatic and found fortuitously on thoracic radiographs taken for other reasons.

DIAGNOSTIC APPROACH

Material is ejected from the mouth due to regurgitation, vomiting, or expectoration. When a patient is presented because of "vomiting," the first step is to distinguish these three possibilities by examining the history (Table 35-3). Expectoration is seen as coughing or ejection of phlegm. Although the history usually permits accurate differentiation between regurgitation and vomiting, it can occasionally be misleading. The vigorous retching typically associated with vomiting is not present in all vomiting patients; also,

Table 35-3 *Differentiation of Vomiting and Regurgitation by History*

	Regurgitation	Vomiting
PRODROMAL SALIVATION	−	+
PRODROMAL ANTICIPATION	−	+
RETCHING	− (although patient may gag)	+
MATERIAL		
Tubular shape	Rare, but suggestive when found	−
Bile	−	+/−
Fresh blood	+/−	+/−
Digested blood	−	+/−
Digested food*		
Amount	Any amount	Any amount
Time relative to eating	Any time	Any time

* This is hard to determine and is often misleading.
+ = is present; − = is not present

clients may empathize with the patient and describe the relatively mild abdominal press due to the gag reflex as prodromal retching. Finally, some patients that sound like they are regurgitating are actually vomiting.

If the history is confusing or unavailable or does not fit with the clinician's impression of the patient, a plain chest radiograph, possibly followed by a barium contrast esophagogram, is probably the quickest way of determining whether esophageal disease is present. If there is no evidence of esophageal disease on such a study, then the patient is usually vomiting, although some esophageal diseases (*e.g.*, sliding hiatal hernias, gastroesophageal reflux, mild esophageal motor dysfunction, and esophagitis) may be difficult to detect by this procedure.

Once the clinician has decided that regurgitation is occurring, the next concerns are deciding, first, whether it is due to esophageal or pharyngeal disease and, second, whether it is due to obstruction or weakness. The first question is best answered by the history and by watching the patient eat (Fig. 35-1). Dysphagia suggests pharyngeal or cricopharyngeal dysfunction (see Chapter 34); pharyngeal dysphagia may have concurrent proximal esophageal dilatation. If the regurgitating patient is not dysphagic, then the esophagus is usually the site of the problem. The history should be reexamined to see if there was an acute onset, as might occur with a foreign object or in esophagitis following anesthesia.

Radiographs are indicated next to decide if there is obstruction or weakness. Plain films (including the cervical and thoracic areas) should always precede contrast films to search for evidence of esophageal disease such as aerophagia (which can also be seen in normal dogs that are excited), increased esophageal density, and, especially foreign objects or pleural fluid or air. Foreign objects may be obvious from the history and physical examination, but most foreign objects are bones, particularly from poultry and pigs. This presents a potential source of diagnostic confusion. Patients that have overeaten often have abdominal or gastric discomfort and vomit due to an acute gastritis, which spontaneously resolves. However, the acutely regurgitating patient probably has an esophageal foreign object. Good-quality plain thoracic radiographs are often diagnos-

tic, but they must be carefully scrutinized, as poultry bones are less dense than most canine or feline bones and are easily overlooked (Fig. 35-2).

If even slight pleural effusion or pneumothorax is noted, pleurocentesis and culture should be done because of the possibility of esophageal perforation. Perforation due to an esophageal foreign object may occur 1 to 10 days after ingestion, depending on the object and the amount of pressure and mucosal ischemia present. Esophaeal perforation may be difficult to detect. If pleural or mediastinal air or fluid is noted, then one has good reason to suspect perforation. However, the absence of these findings does not eliminate perforation. A radiographic contrast study may or may not detect perforation. Whenever an esophageal foreign object is removed endoscopically, the chest should be radiographed after the procedure to ensure that pneumothorax (a sign of occult perforation) is not present.

Finding a foreign object that seems unlikely to cause obstruction (dog food or hair ball) indicates looking for a partial esophageal obstruction (mild vascular ring anomalies, scars, or neoplasia) by contrast radiographs or endoscopy.

Most primary esophageal cancers are asymptomatic until they are large enough to be seen on plain chest radiographs, usually as a tissue density in the caudal lung fields (Fig. 35-3). Any density in this area should evoke suspicions of esophageal disease, even in asymptomatic patients. Esophageal diverticula must also be considered. Finally, it is important to note that failure to find obvious esophageal disease on plain radiographs in no way eliminates esophageal disease.

Contrast esophagograms are indicated to confirm the presence of esophageal disease, to look for esophageal perforation in selected cases, and to define known esophageal dysfunction. Even patients with obvious megaesophagus may have additional problems (*e.g.*, neoplasia, foreign object, achalasia) that need to be addressed. Some patients with apparent esophageal disease on plain radiographs (such as that due to aerophagia) will be found to have a normal esophagus with contrast radiographs. Even an undefined thoracic density should be evaluated with a contrast esophagogram. Barium sulfate is preferred over iodine contrast agents unless esophageal perforation is suspected (and even then some may

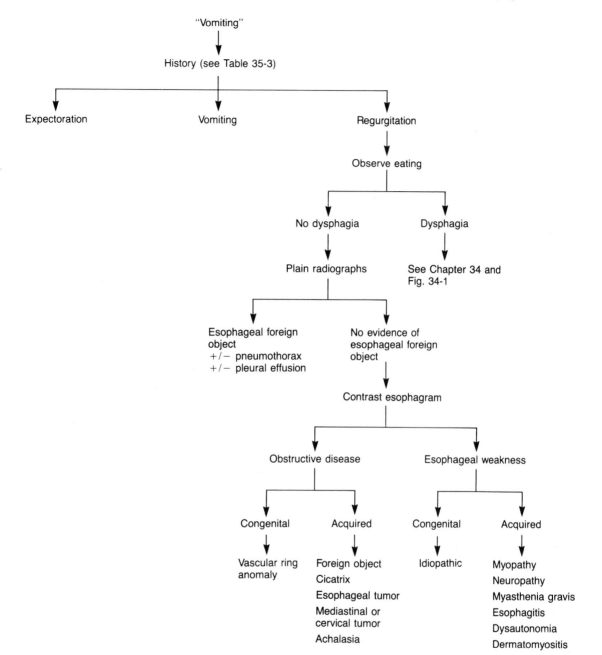

Figure 35–1. *Diagnostic approach to regurgitation in the dog and cat.*

argue that barium provides such an improved contrast study that it should be used). To differentiate esophageal weakness from obstruction, liquid or paste preparations are usually better than barium mixed with food. However, some cases of partial obstruction (*e.g.,* achalasia) and a few pa-

tients with esophageal weakness are better defined with barium mixed with food. If regurgitation is suspected and the liquid or paste barium preparations are unrevealing, then barium mixed with food should be used.

Esophageal obstruction is denoted by the dye

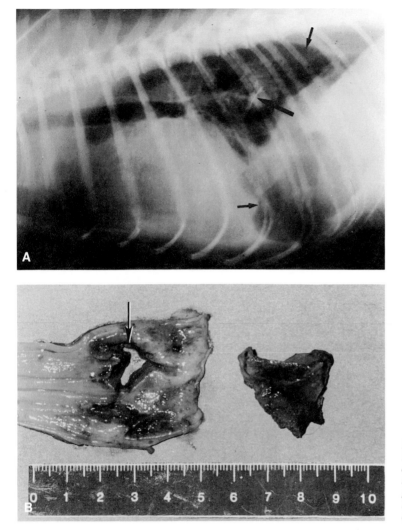

Figure 35–2. *(A) Plain thoracic radiograph showing pleural effusion (short arrows) plus a small radiodense shadow in the region of the esophagus (long arrow). (B) The esophagus from the dog radiographed in A. Note the perforation (arrow) caused by the bone, which was only in the esophagus for 4 days.*

column coming to an abrupt stop or having a filling defect, while esophageal weakness is suggested by generalized distention of the esophageal lumen without evidence of obstruction (Fig. 35-4). Esophageal weakness must be distinguished from the distention typically seen proximal to obstructive lesions (Fig. 35-5) and the effects of drugs such as ketamine or xylazine. Occasionally, generalized weakness can produce focal distentions resembling vascular ring anomalies (Fig. 35-6). Focal accumulations of contrast media especially near the diaphragm may suggest diverticula. Other changes on the esophagogram indicating esophageal disease include gastroesopha-

geal reflux, roughened esophageal mucosa, or displacement of the esophagus from its normal position (O'Brien, Additional Reading). However, the absence of marked changes on the esophagogram does not eliminate the possibility of esophagitis.

If obstruction is present, the next question is whether it is intraluminal, intramural, or extraesophageal. This determines whether the patient will be approached endoscopically or with thoracotomy. Acquired intraluminal obstructions usually produce filling defects (Fig. 35-7) or an abrupt cessation to the barium column; they are usually due to foreign objects or neoplasia. Intra-

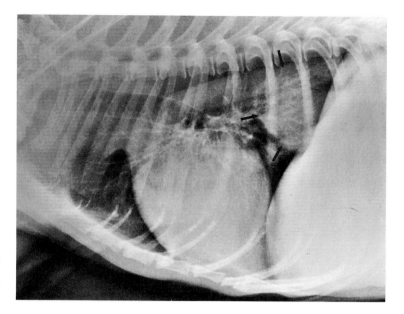

Figure 35–3. *Plain thoracic radiograph showing a previously unsuspected soft-tissue mass in the diaphragmatic lung field (arrows) that was subsequently determined to be an esophageal carcinoma.*

mural obstructions may have a similar radiographic appearance or extensive areas of constriction. These are usually due to scar formation, but occasionally are caused by neoplasia. Congenital extraesophageal obstruction due to a vascular ring anomaly produces an abrupt cessation to the contrast, but its location (just cranial to the base of the heart) and the history will usually suggest the diagnosis (see Fig. 35-5). Acquired extraesophageal obstructions due to masses (carcinoma or lymphosarcoma) usually produce less discrete obstruction, plus there may be an obvious soft-tissue density (Fig. 35-8). Deviation of the esophagus, especially near the thoracic inlet, may suggest obstruction. Usually due to breed predisposition, such deviations rarely cause clinical signs and one should not be hasty in pronouncing them to be the cause of the regurgitation.

If an obstruction cannot be defined by contrast radiographs, then esophagoscopy is indicated

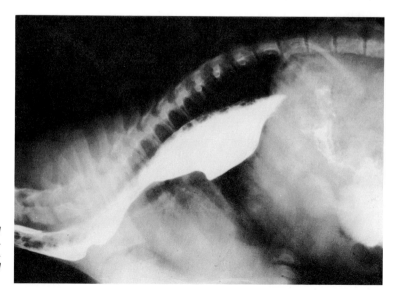

Figure 35–4. *Contrast esophagogram (lateral view) of a 3-month-old collie demonstrating retention of barium throughout the length of the esophagus. This is most compatible with generalized esophageal weakness.*

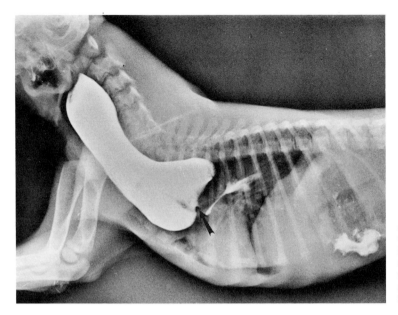

Figure 35–5. Contrast esophagogram (lateral view) of a 6-week-old dog with a persistent right fourth aortic arch causing extramural obstruction. Note the abrupt cessation of the dilated esophagus (arrow) cranial to the heart and the lack of significant retention of barium caudal to the point of obstruction.

(Figs. 35-9 to 35-11). Esophagoscopy detects and defines foreign objects as well as cicatrices and proliferative lesions. A cicatrix is seen as a scar with little or no proliferation, while most esophageal cancers are obviously proliferative. These can usually be diagnosed by endoscopic biopsy. Fibrosarcomas tend to be smooth-surfaced with a necrotic pungent odor. Carcinomas are usually cauliflowerlike and bleed readily.

Achalasia of the canine lower esophageal sphincter rarely occurs as an acquired disorder, and is difficult to discern by static image contrast esophagograms. This disorder is best diagnosed fluoroscopically by finding adequate esophageal waves that have difficulty propelling a bolus through the otherwise apparently normal lower esophageal sphincter. If fluoroscopy is unavailable, one can feed a barium meal, hold the patient vertically for 5 to 10 minutes, and re-radiograph the patient. If little or no barium passes into the stomach and the lower esophageal sphincter is endoscopically normal, achalasia should be considered.

Finally, a large filling defect in the lower esophagus (which can sometimes extend up past the heart) and failure of barium to pass into the stom-

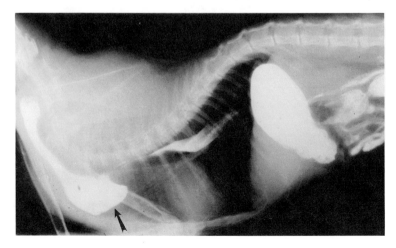

Figure 35–6. Contrast esophagogram (lateral view) of a young cat with generalized esophageal weakness that was diagnosed fluoroscopically (lack of esophageal motility) and at necropsy (lack of constriction around the esophagus). Note the accumulation of barium near the thoracic inlet (arrow), which mimics the diverticulum expected with a vascular ring anomaly.

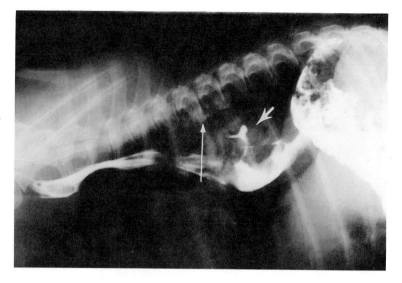

Figure 35–7. *Contrast esophagogram demonstrating a filling defect due to an intraluminal neoplasia (short arrow). Note the unusual spondylosis suggestive of* Spirocerca lupi *(long arrow).*

ach might be due to a gastroesophageal intussusception. This is uncommon, but the lack of a normal gastric shadow coupled with the above findings is suggestive. Gastroesophageal intussusception seems to be more common in younger patients.

The diagnostic approach to so-called *megaesophagus* depends on the patient's age. Young animals with apparent congenital weakness should be treated conservatively. Pets with apparent acquired esophageal weakness generally have a primary neuromuscular disease or esopha-

gitis. Esophagitis may be undetectable radiographically or it may produce obvious roughening of the mucosa. Therefore, even though esophagitis is less common than primary neuromuscular disease, esophagoscopy may be useful in patients with acquired esophageal weakness. Esophagitis usually causes roughening of the mucosa, hyperemia, or bleeding, which may be difficult to discern with contrast radiographs. Some breeds (chow chow) normally have pigmented esophageal mucosa. Biopsies may be definitive if the gross appearance is questionable, but an oral

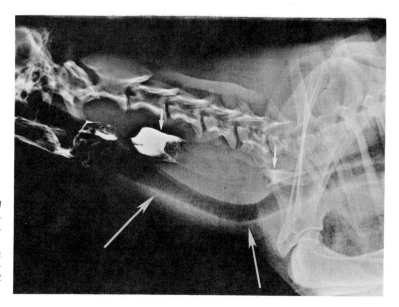

Figure 35–8. *Contrast esophagogram of an old Doberman pinscher with a thyroid carcinoma compressing the cervical esophagus and causing a diffuse extraesophageal obstruction of the esophagus. Note the soft-tissue swelling displacing the trachea ventrally (long arrows), with barium in the esophagus on both sides of the swelling (short arrows) but especially cranial to the swelling.*

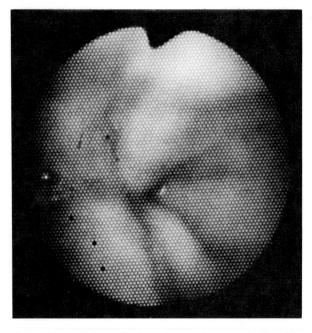

Figure 35–9. *Endoscopic view of an esophagus at the site of an extraesophageal obstruction. Despite insufflating the esophagus, it is not distended and the mucosa has a "gathered" appearance, suggesting that something outside the esophagus is constricting it.*

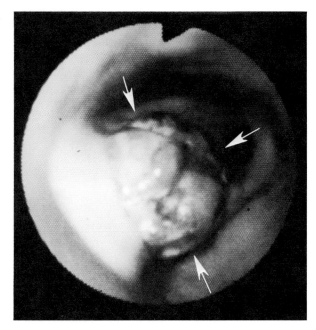

Figure 35–11. *Endoscopic view of an esophagus with an intraluminal obstruction due to a fibrosarcoma secondary to Spirocerca lupi. The esophagus is insufflated but there is a large mass within the lumen (arrows), which is the tumor.*

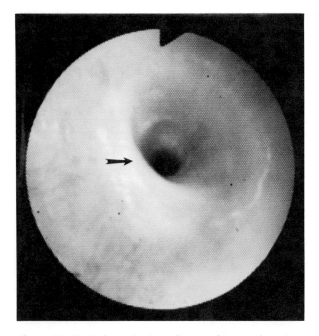

Figure 35–10. *Endoscopic view of an esophagus with an intramural stricture due to a cicatrix. Despite insufflating the esophagus, the distal portion remains constricted. In contrast to Figure 35–9, there is an obvious scar (arrow).*

biopsy capsule (Quinton multipurpose biopsy instrument) must be used, as biopsies through flexible endoscopes are often inadequate.

If acquired esophageal weakness is not due to esophagitis, an underlying cause (see Table 35-1) should be sought (Table 35-4), even though one is uncommonly found. Antibody titers to acetylcholine receptors, ANA titers, LE cell preparations and serum T3 and T4 concentrations are indicated, even if there are no other signs of systemic disease. Electromyography and selected muscle or nerve biopsies are sometimes helpful, as is searching for heavy-metal intoxication (*e.g.*, lead and thallium), hypoadrenocorticism, or Chagas' disease.

If esophagitis is present, one must consider whether it is due to a prior foreign body, spontaneous or anesthetic-associated gastroesophageal reflux, hiatal hernia, an early esophageal neoplasia, ingestion of a caustic substance, or vomiting of acidic gastric contents. Recent general anesthesia is suggestive of gastroesophageal reflux. A focal area of esophagitis may mean there was a

Table 35–4 Laboratory Assessment of Regurgitation

Test	What to Check For
Complete blood count	Inflammation (aspiration pneumonia) Nucleated red blood cells (lead intoxication)
Serum biochemistry	Hyperkalemia (hypoadrenocorticism) Hypercholesterolemia (hypothyroidism)
Chest radiographs	Esophageal dilatation Esophageal foreign object Spondylosis of thoracic vertebrae (spirocercosis) Mediastinal mass Pleural fluid or air (perforation) Mass (esophageal tumor) Pulmonary infiltrate or air bronchograms (aspiration pneumonia)
Titer to acetylcholine receptors	Myasthenia gravis
ANA, LE cell preparation	Systemic lupus erythematosus
Serum T4 concentration	Hypothyroidism
Serum creatinine phosphokinase or electromyelography	Myopathy or neuropathy
Serum gastrin concentration	Increased values (gastrinoma, uremia, gastric outflow obstruction)

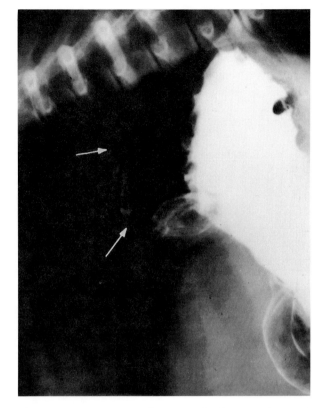

Figure 35–12. Contrast esophagogram of a Shar Pei with a hiatal hernia. Note the stomach extending cranial to the diaphragm (arrows). (Courtesy of Dr. Ross Stickle, Michigan State University.)

foreign object that spontaneously passed into the stomach or was regurgitated. Oral and lingual ulcers may be from ingestion of a caustic agent. Gastrinomas (tumors producing excessive gastrin and gastric hyperacidity) cause vomiting, duodenal dysfunction, diarrhea, and esophagitis secondary to the copious amounts of acidic gastric contents being vomited. These patients are typically older. Fasting serum gastrin concentrations are usually increased, although the serum gastrin response to secretin or calcium occasionally has to be determined.

Hiatal hernias may be seen radiographically as collections of contrast media in a stomach protruding through the diaphragm (Fig. 35-12). Because some of these hernias can slide from the thorax to the abdomen and back again, exposing the radiographs while applying constant abdominal pressure may promote herniation of the stomach into the thorax, allowing diagnosis. Occasionally, endoscopy may reveal hernias and

similar abnormalities that would otherwise go undefined. Hiatal hernias may be more common than reported and should be sought in patients with regurgitation or esophagitis due to unknown cause, especially in Shar Pei dogs.

Some esophageal motility defects do not markedly dilate the esophagus. In some patients with strong histories of regurgitation and normal esophagograms, repeated esophagograms (use both liquid barium and barium mixed with food) that include fluoroscopy of the entire esophagus (especially the area immediately caudal to the cricopharyngeal muscle) may be needed. Finally, fluoroscopy may allow the detection of reflux of contrast into the pharynx (Fig. 35-13). This appears to be uncommon, but may be important prognostically, as these patients seem to have severe problems with aspiration pneumonia.

Small filling defects may occasionally be found on esophagograms. *Spirocerca lupi* should be con-

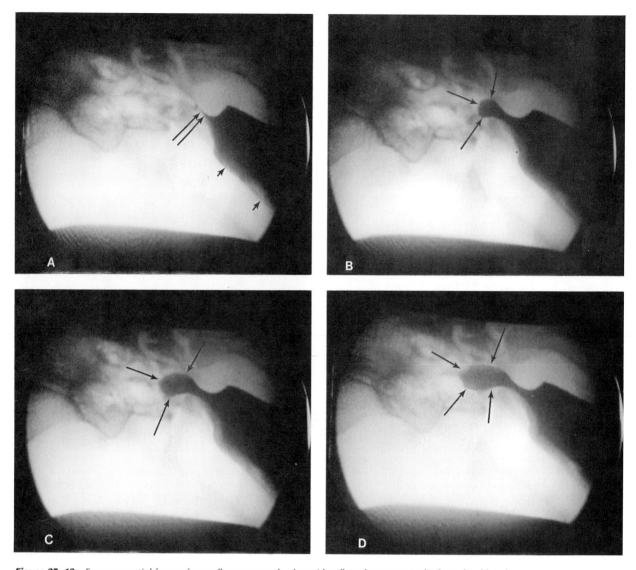

Figure 35–13. *Four sequential frames from a fluoroscopy of a dog with reflux of contrast media from the dilated esophagus (short arrows) into the oropharynx. In A, the cricopharyngeal region is denoted (double arrows). In B, C, and D, progressive movement of contrast into the oropharynx is seen (long arrows).*

sidered, and fecal sedimentation examination may detect the small, delicate ova. Often, these patients have an unusual spondylosis on the ventral aspect of the thoracic vertebrae that does not initially bridge from one vertebrae to another (see Fig. 35-7). Endoscopically, one may see small nodules or slightly raised ulcerated lesions. Rarely, a red worm will be seen protruding from the lesion.

Thyroid neoplasms occasionally grow into the esophagus, disrupting normal function and caus-

ing poor motility. Other neoplasms (*e.g.*, respiratory tract carcinomas) may rarely do likewise.

Esophageal diverticula are rare in dogs and cats. When present they are typically pulsion types; they typically cause a focal collection of contrast and are near the diaphragm.

Finally, the diagnostician must be aware of breed predispositions. Bulldogs and Shar Pei dogs commonly have mild to marked esophageal deviations between the thoracic inlet and the base of the heart (Fig. 35-14). These deviations rarely cause symptoms, but one must be aware of them lest the regurgitation be inappropriately attributed to them.

MANAGEMENT

For regurgitating patients resolution of the underlying disease is desired; however, if that is not possible or will not be effective quickly enough to prevent aspiration, symptomatic therapy is necessary. Symptomatic therapy consists of rehydration, treatment of aspiration pneumonia, or dietary manipulation so that food is less likely to be retained in the esophagus. The latter consists of feeding and watering the patient from an elevated platform so that it has to stand in a near vertical position on its hind legs to eat, making the patient remain standing for 5 to 10 minutes following feeding, changing the character of the food (some patients respond better to gruel, while others with a remnant of esophageal motility tolerate dry food better), feeding multiple small feedings per day (if dry food is used, free choice feeding is preferred), and, occasionally, bypassing the esophagus (gastrostomy or enterostomy feeding or total parenteral nutrition) for a time.

Esophageal obstructions should not be treated with conservative dietary management except as an adjunct to surgery; they must be removed. Congenital vascular ring anomalies must be re-sected by a thoracotomy before the esophagus is irrevocably distended. Even mild or partial obstructions should be removed lest a foreign object someday cause acute obstruction or perforation. Care must be taken during surgery not to damage the vagus nerve and produce esophageal weakness and dilatation.

Removal of nonperforating foreign objects should first be attempted with endoscopy. Foreign objects should be withdrawn through the mouth. Excessive force can damage the esophagus. With rigid endoscopy one uses retrieval forceps to pull the object into the rigid scope, protecting the esophageal mucosa from further damage. Flexible scopes permit removal of foreign objects that are further from the mouth (as in larger dogs). However, it is often difficult to pull the object through the cricopharyngeal sphincter with flexible endoscopes. If necessary, one can pass a rigid endoscope through this area and then pass the flexible scope through it. The foreign object is pulled into the rigid scope as far as possible and then the scopes and object are removed as one unit. Rarely, the object may be pushed into the stomach with an endoscope, but great care must be taken to ensure that a sharp point does not perforate the esophagus or that the object is not pushed through a devitalized section of the esophagus, again possibly perforating it. After removing the object, the chest should be radio-

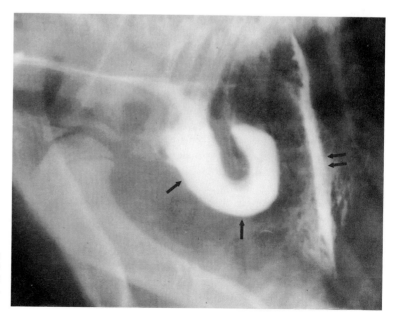

Figure 35–14. *Lateral contrast esophagogram of a Shar Pei showing a marked esophageal deviation (arrows). The linear streak of contrast material to the right (double arrows) is an artifact. (Courtesy of Dr. Russ Stickle, Michigan State University.)*

graphed to check for pneumothorax, a sign of probable perforation. Objects that cannot be removed by endoscopy indicate thoracotomy. If the esophagus may have been perforated, endoscopy is contraindicated as it may produce a tension pneumothorax or further contaminate the chest.

After removing an esophageal foreign object, therapy depends on the severity of the esophagitis. Ulceration or erosion requires antibiotic therapy that will also be effective against anaerobes (*e.g.*, amoxicillin, ampicillin, or cephalothin). Severe ulceration may necessitate a gastrostomy tube (see Surgical Tube Gastrostomy and Percutaneous Tube Gastrostomy in Chapter 80) or corticosteroid therapy to prevent cicatrix formation (prednisolone 1 mg/kg once daily, intramuscularly). Obstruction due to cicatrix following esophagitis is treated by bougienage, or preferably by balloon dilatation. The latter produces less trauma than bougienage.

Most esophageal malignancies are inoperable because they are asymptomatic until advanced. Extraesophageal obstructions (*e.g.*, mediastinal lymphosarcoma or thyroid carcinoma) are often inoperable, but may respond to chemotherapy or radiotherapy. Surgically correctable lesions are occasionally found.

Esophageal diverticula should be removed even if they are asymptomatic. Such structures provide fertile ground for foreign objects to obstruct or perforate the esophagus.

Lower esophageal achalasia, which rarely occurs, necessitates esophagomyotomy. However, the myotomy must not be too aggressive or gastroesophageal reflux and esophagitis that is as bad or worse than the original disease may result. Nifedipine, a calcium channel blocking agent has been used in humans and suggested in dogs (0.25–0.5 mg/kg sublingually, 20–30 minutes before meals) to relax smooth muscle and decrease lower esophageal sphincter pressure (Chandra et al, Additional Reading).

Congenital esophageal weakness is generally idiopathic. Symptomatic therapy is designed to prevent further esophageal dilatation and aspiration until the esophageal innervation matures and the patient is able to maintain itself. Metoclopramide has not been useful.

Acquired esophageal weakness is an indication to treat the underlying problem, which, unfortunately, is often undefined. Symptomatic therapy is the only option if the cause is unknown. Metoclopramide has not been useful in stimulating esophageal motility in these patients.

If the underlying cause is found, it is sometimes possible to resolve the esophageal weakness. Localized myasthenia is sometimes treatable. Some patients with myasthenia, hypothyroidism, and acquired esophageal weakness respond dramatically to thyroid supplementation, as seen by resolution of esophageal weakness and disappearance of the antibodies to acetylcholine receptors. Other patients with localized myasthenia may respond to acetylcholinesterase inhibitors such as pyridostigmine bromide (dogs: 2 mg/kg orally as needed). However, one must be careful not to create problems by overdosing the acetylcholinesterase inhibitor. Some cases of myasthenia gravis respond to immunosuppressive doses of glucocorticoids alone.

Esophagitis is usually treatable. Regardless of whether it is due to gastroesophageal reflux, persistent vomiting of acidic gastric contents, ingestion of caustics, or foreign objects, it requires an antibiotic with or without corticosteroid therapy, the latter to prevent cicatrix formation. There is often gastroesophageal reflux (either as a cause or an effect of the esophagitis); therefore, histamine (H_2) antagonists (*e.g.*, cimetidine 5–10 mg/kg orally three to four times daily, or ranitidine 2.2–4.4 mg/kg orally twice daily) and metoclopramide hydrochloride are used to decrease gastric acidity, keep the stomach empty, and increase lower esophageal sphincter tone. Sucralfate (dogs: $1/4$–1 g orally two–four times daily; cats: $1/4$ g orally twice daily) may help resolve and prevent esophageal ulceration. Gastrostomy tubes (see Surgical Tube Gastrostomy and Percutaneous Tube Gastrostomy in Chapter 80) are used in patients with severe disease to prevent contamination by food of inflamed esophageal mucosa and aspiration. Pharyngostomy tubes should be avoided, as they may perpetuate esophagitis and produce gastroesophageal reflux.

The presence of a hiatal hernia does not necessitate surgical correction, as many produce minimal clinical signs. If a hiatal hernia is symptomatic it usually requires surgical correction, although rare hiatal hernias will apparently resolve spontaneously as the patient matures.

Esophageal weakness associated with *Spirocerca lupi* is difficult to control. The parasites may seemingly be killed by anthelmintics (Fox et al, Additional Reading), but the esophageal disease may persist or worsen.

PATIENT MONITORING

Failure to control or resolve regurgitation due to any reason often causes fatal aspiration pneumonia or weight loss. All regurgitating patients should be closely observed for signs of aspiration.

The prognosis of young animals with congenital megaesophagus partly depends on their conditions when first seen. Emaciation, severe regurgitation, and severe pneumonia are poor prognostic indicators. In one study, only 3 of 18 dogs with congenital esophageal weakness were alive after 3 months (Boudrieau and Rogers, Additional Reading). However, a significant number of animals that are regurgitating may be managed successfully despite persistence of the esophageal disease (Fig. 35-15). If irreversible dilatation has occurred the prognosis is grave (Fig. 35-16).

The prognosis of acquired esophageal weakness due to an identifiable cause depends on the prognosis of the underlying cause as well as the severity of aspiration disease at the time of diagnosis. Acquired esophageal weakness of unknown cause has a guarded prognosis, as many of these patents die from aspiration pneumonia. In one study, 16 of 32 dogs with acquired esophageal disease were alive after 3 months (Boudrieau and Rogers, Additional Reading). Patients with iatrogenic or spontaneous incompetence of the cricopharyngeal muscle are at particular risk for aspiration. Even if they are not being fed, they tend to regurgitate and aspirate saliva.

Failure to remove esophageal foreign objects usually results in eventual perforation and death due to septic mediastinitis or pleuritis. Occasionally, the object will pass spontaneously, but it can still produce esophageal stricture if not treated properly. If a foreign object has been removed or if there has been esophagitis for any reason, then the patient should be watched; persistent regurgitation should prompt repeat radiographic or endoscopic examination. Most cases of esophagitis, including gastroesophageal reflux that is not due to structural defects (severe hiatal hernia), can be resolved by medical therapy. Surgery is needed for severe hiatal hernias and is often successful. Cicatrix is typically cured by balloon dilatation, but repeated dilatation and prolonged medical treatment may be needed. Animals that have had esophageal surgery should be watched for stricture formation. Partial esophageal strictures and diverticula that are not removed may be responsible for sudden obstruction or perforation due to an otherwise innocuous for-

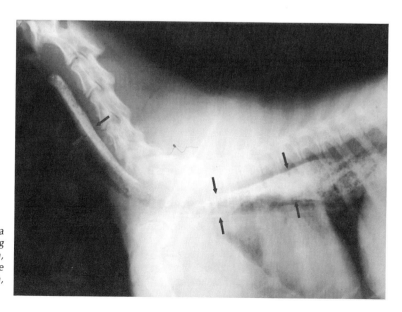

Figure 35–15. *Lateral contrast esophagogram of a dog with congenital esophageal weakness. The dog was managed successfully by dietary manipulation, and no further regurgitation was seen despite the persistence of the esophageal disease (see retention, arrows).*

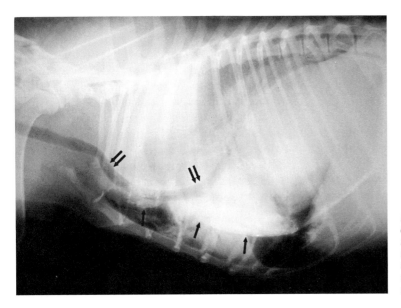

Figure 35–16. *Lateral contrast esophagogram of a dog with uncontrolled congenital esophageal weakness of 3 years' duration. The esophagus (arrows) fills most of the chest and is causing dyspnea. The trachea (double arrows) is markedly depressed due to the weight of the esophagus. Therapy cannot reverse or compensate for dilatation this severe.*

eign object. Delay in correcting vascular ring anomalies may or may not lead to irreversible dilatation of the esophagus and persistence of vomiting after surgical relief of the obstruction.

The prognosis of extraesophageal lesions causing esophageal obstruction depends on the lesion. Many are due to malignancies that carry a poor prognosis. Esophageal malignancies and gastroesophageal intussusception have a very poor prognosis due to the typically advanced nature of the lesion at diagnosis.

ADDITIONAL READING

Boudrieau RJ, Rogers WA. Megaesophagus in the dog: A review of 50 cases. Journal of the American Animal Hospital Association 1985; 21:33.

Chandra NC, McLeod CG, Hess JL. Nifedipine: A temporizing therapeutic option for the treatment of megaesophagus in adult dogs. Journal of the American Animal Hospital Association 1989; 25:175.

Ellison GW, Lewis DD, Phillips L, Tarvin GB. Esophageal hiatal hernia in small animals: Literature review and a modified surgical technique. Journal of the American Animal Hospital Association 1987; 23:391.

Fingeroth JM, Fossum TW. Late-onset regurgitation associated with persistent right aortic arch in two dogs. J Am Vet Med Assoc 1987; 191:981.

Fox SM, Burns J, Hawkins J. Spirocercosis in dogs. Compendium of Continuing Education 1988; 10:807.

Harvey CE, O'Brien JA, Durie VR. Megaesophagus in the dog. J Am Vet Med Assoc 1974; 165:433.

Hoffer RE. Surgical diseases. In: Slatter DH, ed. Textbook of small animal surgery. Philadelphia: WB Saunders, 1985: 654.

Lantz BC, Cantwell HD, VanVleet JF et al: Pharyngostomy tube induced esophagitis in the dog: An experimental study. Journal of the American Animal Hospital Association 1983; 19:207.

O'Brien TR. Radiographic diagnosis of abdominal disorders in the dog and cat. Covell Park Vet Co, Davis CA, 1981: 141.

Pearson H, Darke PGC, Gibbs C et al. Reflux esophagitis and stricture formation after anesthesia. Journal of Small Animal Practice 1978; 19:507.

Ridgway FL, Suter PF. Clinical and radiographic signs in primary and metastatic esophageal neoplasms of the dog. J Am Vet Med Assoc 1979; 174:700.

Roudebush P, Jones BD, Vaughan RW. Medical aspects of esophageal disease. In: Jones BD, ed. Canine and feline gastroenterology. Philadelphia: WB Saunders, 1986: 54.

Shelton GD, Willard MD, Cardinet GH, Lindstrom J. Acquired myasthenia gravis: Selective involvement of esophageal, pharyngeal and facial muscles. Journal of Veterinary Internal Medicine 1990, in press.

Woods CB, Rawlings C, Barber D et al: Esophageal deviations in four English bulldogs. J Am Vet Med Assoc 1978; 172:934.

Zimmer JF. Canine esophageal foreign bodies: Endoscopic, surgical and medical management. Journal of the American Animal Hospital Association 1984; 20:669.

36

VOMITING
Michael D. Willard

CAUSES

Vomiting is a common clinical problem. The major causes of acute and chronic vomiting are given in Tables 36-1 and 36-2, respectively, and the major causes of hematemesis are given in Table 36-3. These lists are not complete, as there are myriad potential etiologies. For example, almost any oral medication may produce vomiting in an intolerant patient.

PATHOPHYSIOLOGY

Vomiting refers to a centrally mediated reflex causing expulsion of gastric or intestinal contents; regurgitation is not centrally mediated and results in the loss of food, water, or saliva from the esophagus or pharynx.

Vomiting requires stimulation of the medullary vomiting center. This is usually due to input from the chemoreceptor trigger zone or abdominal vagal afferents. The chemoreceptor trigger zone responds to blood-borne substances (*e.g.*, drugs or uremic toxins), while vagal stimulation may arise from alimentary tract inflammation (gastritis or enteritis), stretching of the bowel (distention due to obstruction), or irritation of the liver, pancreas, kidneys, spleen, or peritoneum. Input from the vestibular apparatus (*e.g.*, motion sickness) or central nervous system inflammation

or pressure (*e.g.*, encephalitis) may also be responsible for vomiting. Whenever the medullary vomiting center is stimulated, prodromal salivation, gastroparesis, reversed duodenal peristalsis, contraction of abdominal muscles, which increases intra-abdominal pressure (causing retching), and ejection of gastric or intestinal contents from the mouth may occur.

Regardless of cause, vomiting causes loss of endogenous gastric or intestinal secretions. Dehydration is common in vomiting patients. Effects on electrolyte and acid-base balance depend on which portions of the alimentary tract are involved. Gastric vomiting (especially due to gastric outflow obstruction) classically produces hypokalemic, hypochloremic, metabolic alkalosis with paradoxical aciduria due to the loss of secretions rich in potassium, chloride, and hydrogen ions. However, concurrent dehydration may decrease tissue perfusion, causing lactic acidosis. If there is substantial loss of duodenal secretions, then bicarbonate loss may cause acidemia despite relatively mild dehydration. Therefore, one cannot accurately predict a vomiting patient's acid-base status even in those with known gastric vomiting, much less when the cause of the vomiting is uncertain.

Whenever the alimentary tract is obstructed, the clinical signs will be influenced by the position of the obstruction. The further aborad the obstruction, the less severe the vomiting, dehy-

Table 36–1 *Causes of Acute Vomiting in Dogs and Cats*

VESTIBULAR APPARATUS INPUT

Motion sickness

DIET OR DRUGS

Food intolerance
Food poisoning
Foreign objects
  Obstructing foreign object
  Linear foreign object (especially cats)
  Intussusception (especially dogs)
Chemical
  Iatrogenic
    Digitalis
    Cyclophosphamide
    Erythromycin
    Various other medications
  Intoxication
    Pesticides
    Herbicides
    Ethylene glycol

INFLAMMATION

Canine or feline parvoviral enteritis
Canine distemper
Pancreatitis (especially dogs)
Postoperative irritation
Peritonitis
  Uroabdomen
  Septic peritonitis due to intestinal leakage

OBSTRUCTION

Gastric dilatation–volvulus (patient does not usually vomit, but does retch; dogs, especially large or giant breeds)
Gastric or intestinal foreign object (including linear foreign objects)
Intussusception
Intestinal torsion or volvulus (especially dogs)
Intestinal incarceration

dration, and electrolyte or acid-base abnormalities tend to be. Conversely, compensation is less likely and electrolyte or acid-base aberrations are more severe with more orad obstructions.

Of the many causes of vomiting or nausea, there are five whose pathophysiology should be considered separately: gastric dilatation–volvulus, linear foreign body, intestinal intussusception, strangulated intestinal obstruction (intestinal incarceration), and gastroduodenal ulceration.

Gastric dilatation–volvulus (GDV) occurs when the stomach becomes progressively dilated. Although overeating can produce gastric dilatation (especially in young dogs), gaseous distention is the primary problem in mature patients.

The source of the gas is uncertain. As the stomach becomes progressively distended, the patient becomes unable to pass contents out the pylorus, eructate, or vomit. At that point, the gastric dilatation has become self-sustaining. As the stomach enlarges, it puts pressure on the large veins in the abdomen, preventing adequate blood return from the posterior vena cava and the hepatic portal vein. This venous obstruction produces splanchnic congestion and hypovolemic shock. The stomach wall may eventually become necrotic due to impaired perfusion secondary to the pressure as well as the long axis twisting (volvulus) of the stomach. As the stomach twists, the spleen is often malpositioned, leading to obstruction of splenic vessels with consequent engorgement. The severe shock and splanchnic congestion promote disseminated intravascular coagulation, and may allow sepsis to develop. The cause

Table 36–2 *Causes of Chronic Vomiting in Dogs and Cats*

GASTROINTESTINAL OBSTRUCTION

Foreign object
Tumor or granuloma
Benign pyloric stenosis (especially dogs)
Gastric antral mucosal hypertrophy (especially dogs)
Chronic, partial gastric volvulus (dogs, especially large or giant breeds)
Idiopathic gastric hypomotility (rare)
Pseudo-obstruction (rare)

ABDOMINAL INFLAMMATION

Chronic gastritis or enteritis
Gastrointestinal ulceration or erosion
Colitis
Pancreatitis (especially dogs)
Peritonitis
  Septic peritonitis
  Uroabdomen
  Bilious ascites
Splenic torsion

OTHER DISEASES

Diabetic ketoacidosis
Hypercalcemia
Uremia
Hypoadrenocorticism (especially dogs)
Hepatic insufficiency or disease
Cholecystitis
Feline heartworm disease
Feline hyperthyroidism
Central nervous system disease
Behavioral disorders
Pyometra

Table 36–3 *Causes of Hematemesis in Dogs and Cats*

COAGULOPATHY (ESPECIALLY WHEN THERE IS CONCURRENT INTERRUPTION OF THE GASTRIC MUCOSA)

Vitamin K antagonists (warfarin, pindone, brodifacoum)
Disseminated intravascular coagulation
Drug-induced (aspirin, other nonsteroidal anti-inflammatory drugs)

GASTROINTESTINAL BLEEDING

Ulceration or erosion
  Tumor
  Inflammatory bowel disease
  Infiltrative disease (fungal)
  Foreign object
  Stress (hypoperfusion due to hypovolemic or septic shock)
  Hyperacidity
    Gastrinoma
    Mast cell tumor
  Renal failure
  Hypoadrenocorticism
  Hepatic failure
  Drug-induced (aspirin, indomethacin, naproxen, indomethacin, flunixin meglumine, other nonsteroidal anti-inflammatory drugs, possibly corticosteroids—especially dexamethasone)
  Caustic ingestion (lye)
  Bile reflux
Gall bladder pathology (emptying blood into the duodenum)

EXTRAGASTROINTESTINAL BLEEDING THAT IS SWALLOWED AND THEN VOMITED

Esophageal
  Esophagitis
  Tumor
  Laceration
Oral
  Tumor
  Laceration
Respiratory
  Lung lobe torsion
  Tumor
  Posterior nares

---

for GDV is uncertain, but breed conformation, gastric motility patterns and engorgement with food or water and subsequent vigorous exercise have been suggested.

Linear foreign bodies (such as a string) may behave differently than other foreign objects. If one end of a linear object attaches to a point in the alimentary tract, becoming fixed (usually at the base of the tongue or at the pylorus), the rest may trail down into the intestines. The intestines try to move the latter portion in an aborad fashion like they would other objects. However, because the object is fixed at one end, the intestines cannot move it; rather, the intestines gather around the object as they repeatedly try to propel it. The

result is that the peristaltic activity of the intestines eventually causes the object to saw through the tissue and contaminate the peritoneal cavity, often in multiple areas.

Intussusception is the prolapsing or telescoping of one part of the intestine into the lumen of an immediately adjacent loop. Such a prolapse usually occurs when one portion of the intestine is hypermotile; however, if there is a mass lesion in the intestine (*e.g.,* tumor, granuloma, or scar), it may serve as a fixation point that is "pushed" into the adjacent intestinal lumen. In dogs and cats, the most common type is that in which the ileum prolapses into the colon (ileocolic intussusception), probably because it is relatively easy for the smaller ileum to enter the larger colon. However, intussusceptions may occur elsewhere (*e.g.,* enteroenteric, cecocolic, gastroesophageal). An intussusception may produce luminal obstruction, mucosal congestion, or infarction, depending on the length of the intussusception and the size of the intestinal loops involved. Therefore, some intussusceptions cause severe, acute signs, whereas others have relatively few signs despite a chronic course. When congestion occurs, it decreases intestinal mucosal viability, with subsequent absorption of bacteria and their toxins. Eventually, there can be rupture of the affected area and peritoneal contamination.

Strangulated intestinal obstruction (also called *incarceration*) occurs when an intestinal loop is trapped in a tissue rent (an abdominal wall hernia or tear in the mesentery). The entrapped intestinal loop receives arterial blood flow, but the venous return is obstructed, causing venous congestion of the affected loop. Occlusion of the lumen at each end of the strangulation produces a closed loop in which fluid accumulates secondary to the venous congestion. Subsequent bacterial proliferation in this loop and devitalization of the mucosa allows bacteria and their toxins to be absorbed, so that there is not only hypovolemic but also septic shock (see Chapter 4).

Gastrointestinal ulceration may be caused by mechanical or physiologic mechanisms. Foreign objects and tumors are the most common mechanical causes of mucosal disruption, although ingestion of caustics may occasionally be responsible. The major physiologic mechanisms are poor mucosal perfusion, hyperacidity, and excessive bile acids entering the stomach. Any of these may be responsible by themselves or they may augment one another. Increasing back diffusion of acid (hydrogen ion concentration) into the gastric mucosa is probably the final common pathway by which these latter three mechanisms promote gastric ulceration. Certain drugs (*e.g.,* nonsteroidal anti-inflammatory agents) promote this back diffusion and its detrimental effects.

CLINICAL SIGNS

Ejection of fluid or food from the mouth is due to regurgitation, vomiting, or expectoration. Many but not all vomiting patients are anorectic (Table 36-4). The severity of the disease causing the vomiting cannot be correlated with weight loss or the frequency or severity of vomiting. In fact, diseases that typically cause vomiting (*e.g.,* gastric foreign object or uremia) may not do so in a particular patient. There may be prodromal signs (salivation, excessive swallowing, pacing, or restlessness) without actual vomiting. Pacing and restlessness are ostensibly due to the animal knowing that something is amiss and feeling uncomfortable. Because dogs with GDV are unable to vomit, one typically only sees signs of nausea (pacing, drooling, retching, or discomfort).

Occasionally, vomiting pets will have obvious abdominal pain. Such pain may be noted when the animal assumes a "praying" position (called the *position of relief*), whines, or cries out or bites when the abdomen is handled (*e.g.,* when the animal is picked up). However, many dogs and cats with painful abdomens will not display such obvious signs.

Table 36–4 *Clinical Signs That May Accompany Vomiting*

Abdominal pain
Anorexia
Depression
Drooling
Ejection of water, phlegm, food, bile or blood from the mouth
Gagging, retching
Pacing
"Praying position"

Pets with acute abdomens (acute abdominal disease, typically causing shock, pain, or sepsis) usually manifest obvious depression due to discomfort or shock. From the client's perspective, shock may be denoted by weakness, pale mucous membranes, and nonresponsiveness. Septic shock may produce dark or muddy-colored mucous membranes (see Chapters 2 and 4).

Hematemesis can be obvious (red blood) or subtle. Coffee-groundlike particles in the vomitus strongly suggest digested blood. The clinician should specifically query every client with a vomiting pet regarding the appearance of the vomitus.

DIAGNOSTIC APPROACH

When a patient is presented because of "vomiting," the first step is to differentiate vomiting, regurgitation, and expectoration. The history usually allows separation (see Table 35-3), but the diagnostician can be misled by the client. Vigorous retching is not present in all vomiting patients, plus prodromal retching due to vomiting can be confused with the relatively mild abdominal press due to the gag reflex in regurgitating patients. Finally, some patients with histories suggestive of passive regurgitation are actually vomiting.

If the history does not clearly distinguish between vomiting and regurgitation or does not seem consistent with laboratory findings or the clinician's impression of the patient, plain and barium contrast radiographs are probably the quickest way of determining whether esophageal disease is present. If there is no evidence of esophageal disease on such a study (*e.g.,* esophageal dilatation, barium retention, vascular ring anomaly, foreign body), then the patient is usually vomiting, although some esophageal diseases (*e.g.,* sliding hiatal hernias, gastroesophageal reflux, and mild esophagitis) can be difficult to define by this procedure.

Once vomiting is confirmed, the next questions are: Is it acute or chronic? Does the patient have an acute abdomen? and Is blood present in the vomitus? We will consider acute abdomen and other acute disorders first.

Acute Disorders

Many acute disorders producing nonbloody vomiting are self-limiting (*e.g.*, motion sickness, dietary indiscretion, parasites, and bacterial or viral gastritis or enteritis). However, the syndrome of acute abdomen must be identified early and treated aggressively. *Acute abdomen* refers to acute disease, usually producing shock or sepsis, that originates from the abdomen. The abdomen is identified as the likely source of problems by finding abdominal pain, distention, a mass, or fluid. The most common causes of acute abdomen are gastric or intestinal obstruction or a foreign body; peritonitis due to gastric or intestinal perforation or devitalization; ischemia due to a foreign object, torsion, intussusception, or volvulus; and abdominal bleeding due to trauma, tumor, or ulceration.

History and physical examination are used to determine if the problem is acute or if an acute abdomen is likely (Fig. 36-1). The history should determine how rapidly progressive the disease is, while the physical examination reveals whether shock is present. Abdominal palpation is used to detect masses, distended bowel loops, and evidence of pain. Masses surrounded by the costal arch can be difficult to palpate, but raising the cranial end of the animal may cause them to fall into more caudal portions of the abdomen, making them easier to palpate. One must be careful that a "mass" is not a kidney hanging low in the abdomen, or a colonic fecal mass. The latter can often be deformed if palpated carefully.

Abdominal pain can be difficult to detect. Relatively few animals cry out when palpated; instead, they arch their back, try to move away, shift their back legs from side to side, or tense their abdominal muscles to guard the abdomen. When a painful abdomen seems to be present, one must also consider whether palpating techniques are at fault. Rough palpation may be resented by animals without abdominal disease.

Gastric dilatation–volvulus must be identified early; it is a true emergency. It is typically seen in large-breed dogs with deep chests, but is not limited to these. Nonproductive retching is noticed first. The cranial abdomen will become progressively larger and tympanic due to gaseous distention. Obvious findings on physical examination are adequate for diagnosis. If the clinician is unsure of the diagnosis, plain abdominal radiographs should be done. Simple aerophagia must be distinguished from true dilatation. The latter causes rounding of the stomach shadow. Compartmentalization, or *double bubble* (Fig. 36-2), is diagnostic of gastric volvulus. Usually with an acute problem requiring immediate therapy, occasional dogs will have chronic, partial gastric volvulus causing intermittent vomiting, nausea, or abdominal pain and predisposing to later acute GDV.

Linear foreign bodies occur in dogs, but are more common in cats. The base of the tongue should always be examined thoroughly in vomiting cats (if necessary use chemical restraint) to look for objects such as string wrapped around it. Failure to find string fixed there does not eliminate a linear foreign object, which can fix elsewhere (*e.g.*, pylorus). Abdominal palpation may reveal bunched intestines that are painful when palpated. Bunched intestines with small gas bubbles on radiographs are suggestive of a linear foreign body (Fig. 36-3*A*). Barium contrast radiographs may reveal intestinal pleating (Fig. 36-3*B*). However, contrast radiographs should not be done if it seems likely that the foreign object has caused perforation (*e.g.*, abdominal effusion, fever, or other signs of peritonitis), lest barium make the peritonitis worse. Endoscopy often reveals a portion of the foreign object at the pylorus. If such an object is seen, one must not try to pull the object out (or must at least be extremely careful) lest the object perforate devitalized intestines.

Intussusceptions classically produce vomiting, abdominal pain, and scant, bloody diarrhea. Usually ileocolic in nature, they can produce a thickened bowel loop (sometimes described as a "sausage"); however, they are not always turgid and can be difficult to find during abdominal palpation. Short ileocolic intussusceptions are sometimes only palpated high in the cranial abdomen. Plain radiographs are rarely diagnostic. If one suspects this disorder but cannot document it, barium contrast radiographs (especially a barium enema) may be definitive (Fig. 36-4). Flexible colonoscopy may also be useful in finding an il-

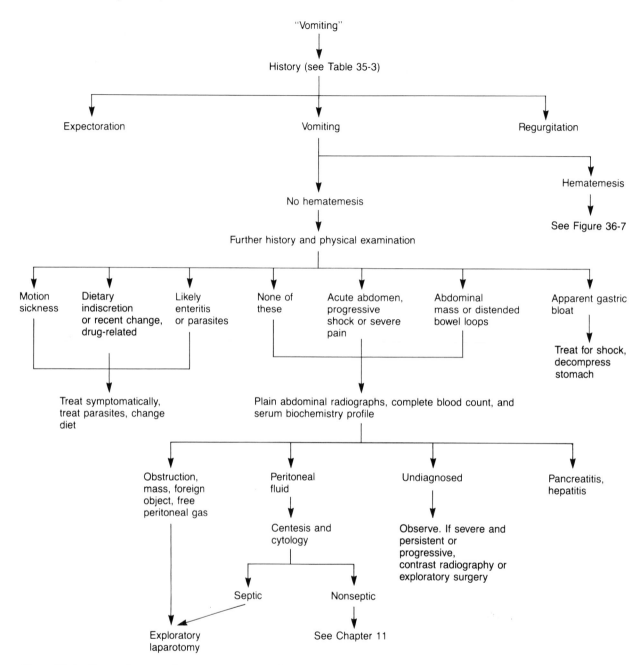

Figure 36–1. *Diagnostic approach to acute vomiting in the dog and cat.*

eocolic intussusception. Some ileocolic intussceptions will protrude from the anus and mimic an anal prolapse. Occasionally, chronic intussusceptions may occur and produce diarrhea with or without blood as the major clinical sign. Hypoproteinemia with or without iron-deficiency anemia due to gastrointestinal blood loss is common in chronic intussusception. This syndrome usually occurs in relatively young dogs (typically less than 6–8 months old).

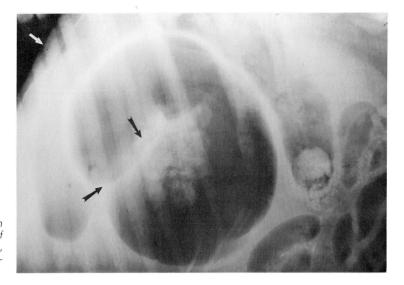

Figure 36–2. *Plain lateral abdominal radiograph of a dog showing gastric distention and a "shelf" of tissue causing compartmentalization (black arrows), which is diagnostic of gastric volvulus. The diaphragm is denoted by a white arrow.*

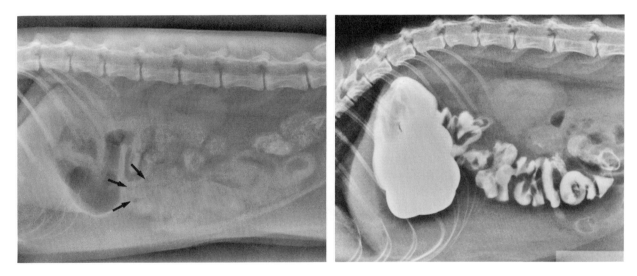

Figure 36–3. *(A) Lateral abdominal radiograph of a cat with a linear foreign body causing bunching of the intestines with small, intraluminal gas bubbles (arrows). (B) Contrast abdominal radiograph showing the pleating of the intestines typical for linear foreign bodies.*

Strangulated intestinal obstructions typically present with an acute history of a painful abdomen and rapidly progressive hypovolemic or septic shock (see Chapter 4). These obstructions typically occur after trauma (*e.g.*, automobile-associated or surgical) produces a hernia. Abdominal palpation typically reveals a distended, painful intestinal loop. Plain radiographs should document a dilated segment of small intestine (Fig. 36-5).

Any object, mass or ulcer may perforate and cause peritonitis. These patients may be depressed to the point of no longer evidencing abdominal pain.

If the patient seems excessively ill, if the disease is prolonged or progressive, or if the clinician believes that the patient may have a serious problem, plain or contrast radiographs, a complete blood count, and a serum biochemistry profile are the next steps. Plain abdominal radiographs

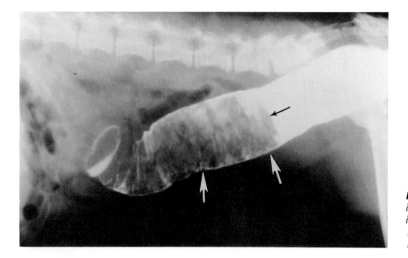

Figure 36–4. *Barium contrast enema demonstrating a filling defect characteristic of an ileocolic intussusception (arrows). (Reprinted with permission, Bailey MQ, Greenfield CL. What's your diagnosis. J. Am Vet Med Assoc 1987; 191:115.)*

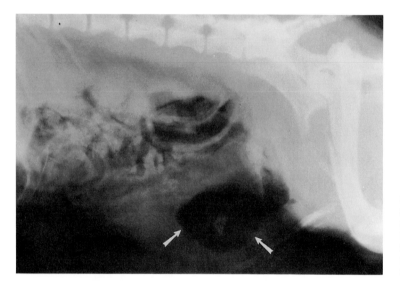

Figure 36–5. *Lateral plain radiograph of a dog's abdomen. Note the distended bowel loop, which is outside the normal confines of the abdomen (arrows). This is due to a segment of intestine that has slipped through a hernia where the prepubic tendon was avulsed from the pelvis after automobile-associated trauma.*

may reveal intestinal obstruction (Fig. 36-6), masses, or abdominal fluid that was not detected by abdominal palpation. If abdominal fluid is present, it should be sampled and analyzed as soon as possible (see Abdominal Paracentesis and Lavage in Chapter 80). If alimentary tract obstruction, a foreign object, or a mass is likely, then the patient should be supported as needed with fluid, electrolyte, or acid-base therapy, and a diagnostic laparotomy done as soon as the patient can tolerate surgery. Likewise, patients with acute abdomen that are deteriorating but do not have an obvious diagnosis should have an exploratory laparotomy.

Acutely vomiting patients that do not have an acute abdomen and are not becoming progressively worse may be pursued more conservatively. Many of these animals are young and likely have an infectious enteritis (*e.g.*, parvovirus), dietary intolerance, or parasites. The history should be examined for evidence of contagion or exposure to toxins. Fecal examinations are indicated, as is switching to a bland diet (*e.g.*, chicken plus rice or cottage cheese plus rice). These patients should all be treated as though they were infectious, and proper disinfection and sanitation procedures should be followed. If parvoviral disease seems likely in a dog, the feces

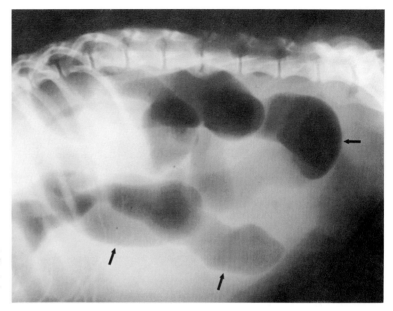

Figure 36–6. *Lateral plain radiograph of a dog's abdomen. Note the generalized, air-filled, dilated small intestinal loops (arrows), suggesting obstruction. The lack of serosal contrast in this patient is due to loss of fat.*

may be assayed for viral antigen and a complete blood count may be requested to look for neutropenia.

Hematemesis

With hematemesis one must consider coagulopathy, blood being swallowed and then vomited (*e.g.*, bleeding oral lesion or blood coughed up from the lungs), and bleeding alimentary tract lesions (Fig. 36-7). Hematemesis is more common in dogs than in cats. A careful description of the act helps eliminate oral bleeding (blood dripping from the mouth that is not associated with vomiting) and nasal and respiratory bleeding (blood being coughed up or sneezed). Next, iatrogenic causes (*e.g.*, nonsteroidal anti-inflammatory drugs) and causes of severe stress (*e.g.*, severe hypotension due to trauma, anesthesia or surgery, or generalized sepsis) should be sought. Coagulopathy should be ruled out by history (exposure to rodenticides), physical examination (bleeding elsewhere in the body), or appropriate screening procedures (platelet estimate, activated clotting time, and bleeding time) (see Chapter 16). Next, a physical examination is performed to look for abdominal masses and cutaneous mast cell tumors. The latter can look like almost anything (they

often mimic lipomas); therefore, every mass should be aspirated. Fortunately, mast cell tumors are generally easy to diagnose cytologically. Next, clinical pathology data should eliminate renal and hepatic failure, especially if the hematemesis is chronic.

If none of these causes of hematemesis is found in a patient with acute disease, then simple, acute gastritis of unknown etiology and hemorrhagic gastroenteritis must be considered. Acute gastritis is usually idiopathic or due to dietary indiscretion, and tends to be self-limiting. There are no diagnostic laboratory or radiographic findings. Hemorrhagic gastroenteritis causes hematemesis and/or hematochezia characterized by polycythemia (packed-cell volume greater than 60%), often with normal plasma total solids. Clinically, hemorrhagic gastroenteritis may resemble canine parvoviral disease; it tends to be more serious than acute gastritis.

Hematemesis that is not clearly due to respiratory tract disease, coagulopathy, drug therapy, renal failure, hepatic failure, shock, acute gastritis, or hemorrhagic gastroenteritis usually indicates gastroduodenoscopy, especially if it is chronic. A contrast gastrogram may be performed to look for ulcers, foreign objects, or tumors (Fig. 36-8); however, endoscopy is more sensitive for finding ulcers and erosions, allows bi-

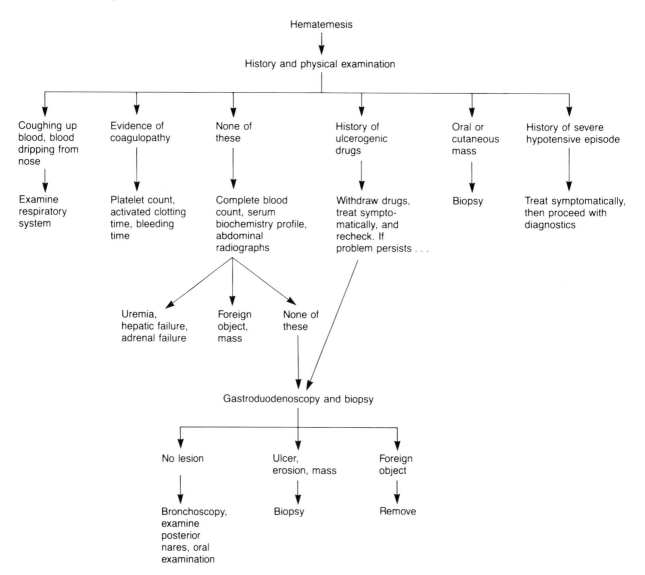

Figure 36–7. *Diagnostic approach to hematemesis.*

opsy of lesions, and differentiates the patient with one or two potentially resectable gastric lesions from one with diffuse, inoperable disease. Foreign objects may be removed endoscopically. The stomach must be examined carefully, employing adequate distention so that the entire mucosal surface can be inspected. If the stomach is not properly distended, large ulcers can remain hidden in the rugal folds. The duodenum and esophagus should be examined as well.

The margin of ulcers or erosions should be bi-

opsied to look for neoplasia and inflammatory diseases. Most ulcerating carcinomas and lymphosarcomas are easily diagnosed by endoscopic biopsy. However, scirrhous tumors may not allow endoscopic diagnosis despite causing large ulcers. It is uncommon that one can identify the initial cause of inflammatory ulcers, although *Campylobacter pyloridis* (also called Helicobacter pylori) might be found. Phycomycosis produces large ulcerations, but the organism will almost never be identified in endoscopic biopsies. In pa-

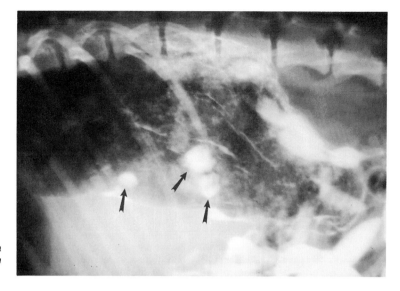

Figure 36–8. Contrast abdominal radiographs of a dog demonstrating circular areas retaining barium (arrows). These areas suggest ulcers.

tients with duodenal ulcers and suggestive histories (*e.g.,* older dogs with vomiting or diarrhea unresponsive to most therapies, except possibly histamine [H₂] antagonists), serum gastrin concentrations may diagnose or eliminate gastrinomas.

If the site of bleeding is not obvious during endoscopy, gastric and duodenal mucosal biopsies are indicated, as nonulcerating inflammatory bowel disease can be responsible. If the cause of bleeding is still uncertain, one may perform endoscopy of the respiratory tract (including the posterior nares and bronchi) (see Tracheobronchoscopy in Chapter 80), evaluate the gallbladder with ultrasonography, and test adrenal gland function with a ACTH stimulation test (see Chapter 60). If these are also unrevealing, one may have to wait until the hematemesis recurs and then reevaluate.

Chronic Nonbloody Vomiting

There are three main categories causing this problem: alimentary tract obstruction, alimentary or abdominal inflammation, and diseases best diagnosed by clinical pathology testing (Fig. 36-9). There are other possibilities (*e.g.,* central nervous system disease such as limbic epilepsy), but they are less common. Diagnostics may take

the form of tests or may include therapeutic trials. The latter often involves dietary change (*e.g.,* hypoallergenic diet). Such a diet should be used for at least 1 to 2 weeks before its efficacy is evaluated.

A thorough history and physical examination should search for obvious causes (*e.g.,* abdominal masses). Next, blood and urine should be analyzed for evidence of renal, adrenal, or hepatic failure, hypercalcemia, acute pancreatitis, diabetic ketoacidosis, feline hyperthyroidism, and feline heartworm disease (Table 36-5). Some of these diseases resemble each other and require careful consideration of the serum biochemistry profile (Table 36-6). If hepatic or adrenal failure are suspected, adrenal function testing (ACTH stimulation) and hepatic function testing (preprandial and postprandial serum bile acids; see Chapter 40) may be done. Increased serum amylase or lipase are suggestive of pancreatitis; however, these values may be normal despite severe pancreatitis (see Chapter 39). While peripheral white blood cell counts are usually increased in acute pancreatitis, they are often normal in patients with gastritis or enteritis and in some with peritonitis.

Plain radiographs should be examined for evidence of intestinal obstruction (*e.g.,* distended bowel loops), foreign objects, abdominal mass or organomegaly (mass or displacement of intes-

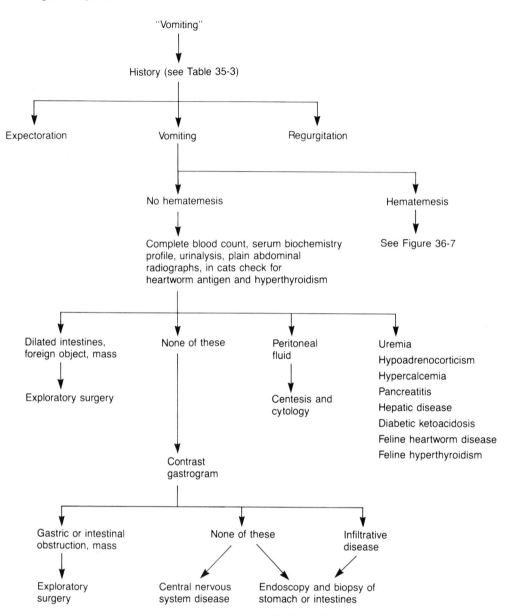

Figure 36–9. *Diagnostic approach to chronic vomiting in the dog and cat.*

tines), and abdominal fluid (decreased serosal detail). If a foreign object is found, vomiting can usually be ascribed to it; however, some animals with gastric foreign objects (*e.g.*, balls, rocks, plastic toys) not causing obstruction can be asymptomatic for weeks to months. Before seeking to remove an object, always radiograph the patient again just before the procedure, as some objects will spontaneously pass, and bones, espe-

cially cancellous ones, may be destroyed by the stomach in 12 hours.

Free abdominal fluid indicates abdominocentesis or diagnostic peritoneal lavage (see Abdominal Paracentesis and Lavage in Chapter 80). Spontaneous septic peritonitis always indicates exploratory surgery, as alimentary tract leakage is the most common cause. Nonseptic peritonitis necessitates considering uroabdomen, bilious ab-

Table 36–5 *Laboratory Assessment of Vomiting*

Test	What to Check For
Complete blood count	Neutropenia (parvovirus, septic shock) Anemia (blood loss due to hematemesis) Neutrophilia (infection, especially peritonitis or pancreatitis)
Serum biochemistry profile	Azotemia (prerenal azotemia, uremia) Hyperglycemia (diabetes mellitus) Hypoglycemia (especially young animals, also due to hepatic disease) Hypercalcemia (especially due to malignancy) Increased serum alanine aminotransferase (hepatic disease) Increased serum alkaline phosphatase (hepatic or pancreatic disease) Hypoalbuminemia (hepatic or intestinal disease) Hyperkalemia (renal or adrenal failure) Hypokalemia (losses due to vomiting) Hypochloremia (losses due to gastric vomiting) Increased total carbon dioxide (gastric vomiting) Decreased total carbon dioxide (lactic acidosis) Hyperamylasemia or hyperlipasemia (prerenal azotemia, renal azotemia, acute pancreatitis) Hyperlipidemia (pancreatitis)
Urinalysis	Low specific gravity (renal insufficiency) Glucosuria (diabetes mellitus, acute renal tubular damage) Ketonuria (diabetic ketoacidosis) Bacteriuria (upper urinary tract infection causing renal failure)
Abdominal radiographs	Gaseous distention of stomach or intestine (obstruction) Fluid distention of stomach or intestine (obstruction) Mass Foreign object Lack of serosal contrast (fluid, loss of fat) Displacement of organ or intestine (mass, splenic torsion) Organomegaly
ACTH stimulation test	Deficient response (hypoadrenocorticism)
Serum bile acids	Increased values (hepatic insufficiency)
Serum gastrin concentration	Increased values (renal failure, gastric outflow obstruction, gastrinoma)
Serum T4	Increased values (feline hyperthyroidism)
ELISA for heartworms	Positive values (feline heartworm disease)
Feline leukemia virus test	Positive values (various diseases) Negative values (most abdominal lymphosarcomas are negative)
ELISA for parvovirus	Canine parvovirus disease

domen, pancreatitis, and parasitic or fungal peritonitis, as well as feline infectious peritonitis.

If plain radiographs and clinical pathology data are not diagnostic, then contrast radiographs of the stomach and intestines or gastroduodenoscopy are the next steps.

Contrast radiographs may reveal radiolucent foreign objects (filling defects), gastric outflow obstruction (failure of the contrast to adequately leave the stomach), complete or partial intestinal obstruction (narrowing of a segment of intestine), or mucosal infiltration (roughened, cobblestone surface). All of these are indications for either surgical exploration or gastroduodenoscopy plus biopsy. Contrast gastrograms must be done correctly. Food should be withheld for 12 to 24 hours and fecal matter eliminated through enemas. Barium sulfate is preferred over iodine solutions

Table 36-6 *Differentiation of Selected Causes of Vomiting*

	Blood Urea Nitrogen and Creatinine	Urine Specific Gravity	Serum Calcium	Serum Sodium to Potassium Ratio	Serum Amylase and Lipase
UREMIA	↑	Isosthenuric	N, ↑	N	<2 × N
HYPERCALCEMIA	N, ↑	Isosthenuric Hyposthenuric	↑	N	<2 × N
HYPOADRENOCORTICISM	N, ↑	Concentrated Isosthenuric	N, ↑	↓	<2 × N
PANCREATITIS	N, ↑	Concentrated	N, ↓	N	should be >2 × N but may be less

N = normal; ↑ = increased; ↓ = decreased

because the former is not excessively diluted with secretions, as is the latter. Enough barium sulfate must be administered to distend the stomach (10-12 ml/kg for small dogs and cats and 5-7 ml/kg for large dogs, as per O'Brien [Additional Reading]). Radiographs should be taken immediately in dorsoventral, ventrodorsal, right lateral, and left lateral projections to allow thorough evaluation of the stomach. Dorsoventral and right lateral projections can be retaken in 15 minutes, 60 to 90 minutes, and at 3 to 4 hours if needed. Gastric outflow obstruction is denoted by finding that barium has not begun to exit the stomach within 30 minutes or that there is substantial barium remaining in the stomach longer than 3 to 4 hours after administration. Filling defects, abnormal rugal patterns, or roughened mucosal surfaces may also be found (Fig. 36-10). Likewise, intestinal obstructions and mucosal infiltrative diseases may be noted during such contrast radiographs. For more discussion on contrast gastrograms and contrast intestinal radiographs, see O'Brien in the Additional Reading list.

Gastric outflow obstruction may be due to benign muscular hypertrophy (called *pyloric stenosis*), benign gastric antral mucosal hypertrophy, a foreign object, tumor, phycomycosis, inflammatory infiltrates, or gastric volvulus. Filling defects may be due to foreign objects, tumors, granulomas, or food material. Abnormal rugal patterns and roughened mucosal surfaces may also be due to infiltrative inflammatory or neoplastic disease.

Pyloric stenosis is defined at surgery by finding the pylorus thickened due to muscular hypertrophy, with no evidence of infiltrative disease. Gastric antral mucosal hypertrophy is due to redundant mucosa blocking the gastric antrum. It may grossly resemble neoplasia, although hypertrophy is limited to the mucosa without infiltrating the muscularis. Mucosal hypertrophy usually has a softer texture than neoplasia. However, one should not guess, but biopsy.

Gastric adenocarcinoma and lymphosarcoma are the most common malignancies of the canine and feline stomachs, respectively. Adenocarcinomas may be principally infiltrative and ulcerative, or they may be more proliferative. Proliferative masses may sometimes be detected on plain radiographs (Fig. 36-11), while infiltrative masses require barium contrast studies (Fig. 36-12). Both are diagnosed by biopsy or cytology. Deep biopsies should be taken that will represent the infiltrative process and not just the ulcerated, inflamed mucosa overlying the tumor. Occasionally, a carcinoma is scirrhous or is principally in the submucosa and does not erupt into the lumen. These types sometimes cannot be diagnosed endoscopically. Phycomycosis is more difficult to definitively diagnose. Principally found in the southeastern United States, it causes a dense submucosal fibrous connective tissue proliferation plus widespread mucosal necrosis. A dark line sharply demarcating the affected mucosa (possibly a line of infarction) is suggestive of this disorder. The fibrous connective tissue pre-

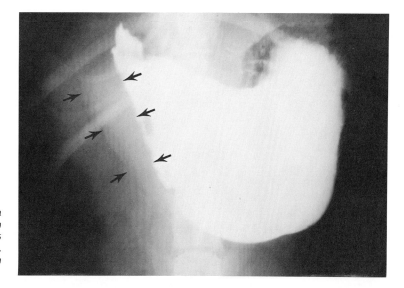

Figure 36–10. *Contrast abdominal radiograph of a dog with gastric phycomycosis. This film was taken 30 minutes after administering barium. There is complete retention of the barium in the stomach, and the wall of the antrum is thickened and rough (arrows).*

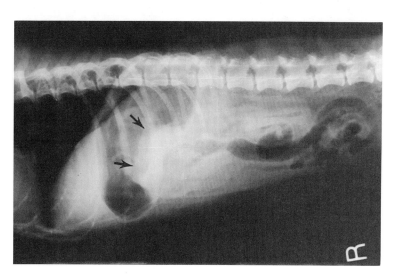

Figure 36–11. *Plain abdominal radiograph of a dog with a gastric adenocarcinoma. Note the intraluminal soft-tissue density (arrows).*

vents normal peristalsis and emptying (see Fig. 36-10). The organism is in the dense fibrous connective tissue and is often difficult to find, even with special stains of large biopsy samples.

Occasionally, contrast radiographs reveal little or no gastric emptying despite lack of outflow obstruction. Idiopathic gastric hypomotility is diagnosed in these patients if they have no evidence of obstruction, abdominal inflammation, or systemic disease. One must ascertain that failure to empty is not from recent surgery, occult inflammation, or atony secondary to drugs (*e.g.*, ketamine hydrochloride, xylazine, or parasympatholytics that may have been used thera-

peutically or for restraint). Gastric and intestinal biopsies are normal.

Intestinal obstruction that is not evident on plain abdominal radiographs can be diagnosed by contrast radiographs. Tumors, foreign objects, cicatrices, and extramural compression are possible and will have to be approached endoscopically or surgically for a definitive diagnosis.

Infiltrative mucosal disease is not always evident on contrast gastric or intestinal radiographs. However, when present (see Fig. 37-5), it clearly indicates mucosal biopsy.

If an infiltrative pattern is found on contrast radiographs, or if the cause of the vomiting is still

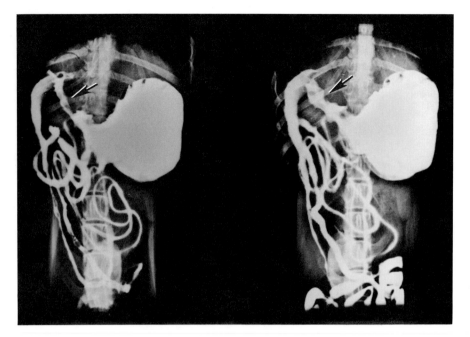

Figure 36–12. *Sequential contrast abdominal radiographs of a dog with a gastric adenocarcinoma. Note that the antrum is irregular and does not expand (arrows).*

unknown after contrast radiographs, then alimentary tract biopsy using gastroduodenoscopy or exploratory laparotomy is necessary. Multiple mucosal biopsies should be taken of the stomach and duodenum regardless of their appearance. Some patients with significant mucosal disease may have one or more normal biopsies. It is important that the intestines (especially the duodenum) also be biopsied.

Dogs and cats may have severe chronic gastritis despite relatively mild or infrequent vomiting. The clinical signs do not necessarily reflect the severity of the inflammatory infiltrate. Inflammatory infiltrates may be composed of lymphocytes, eosinophils, neutrophils, macrophages, or histiocytes.

Cats, in particular, may have inflammatory bowel disease (lymphocytic–plasmacytic enteritis), causing vomiting (which is often intermittent) with or without diarrhea. There may be no laboratory evidence of this disease except on the biopsies. While some of these cats have obvious mucosal abnormalities, many have grossly normal-appearing mucosa. Many nondiarrheic dogs vomit due to duodenitis. Lymphocytic–plasmacytic and eosinophilic duodenitis are more likely, although occasional patients will have a purulent or necrotic duodenitis of unknown cause. Cytology is often diagnostic, but histopathology is needed to identify lymphocytic–plasmacytic disease.

If the cause of the chronic vomiting is still undiagnosed after the above workup, then central nervous system disease, including tumors, encephalitis, limbic epilepsy, and behavior disorders, must be considered. Electroencephalography, cerebrospinal fluid analysis (see Chapter 80), or computed tomography may be useful.

MANAGEMENT

Acute Disorders

Treatment depends on the suspected cause. Whenever acute GDV is diagnosed, immediate therapy for shock with concurrent removal of gastric contents is indicated. The former usually involves bilateral cephalic vein catheters, aggressive intravenous fluid therapy, and corticosteroids. Hypertonic 7% saline solution may be more useful in treating the shock than isotonic solutions (see Chapter 4). Orogastric intubation is followed by gastric lavage. If one cannot intubate the stomach, then a temporary gastrostomy is performed, as per Walshaw and Johnston (Additional Reading). If there is gastric volvulus, surgery is needed to reposition the stomach and a gastropexy is advisable. If dilatation alone was present, surgery is optional. Care must be taken during the postoperative period to treat potentially severe cardiac arrhythmias (see Chapter 18). Hypokalemia can make resolution of these cardiac arrhythmias more difficult, and potassium chloride may be supplemented in the intravenous fluids (see Chapter 72).

Obstructions (especially strangulated), foreign objects, masses, and perforations causing acute abdomen must be removed as soon as the patient is stable. Symptomatic therapy involves correction of electrolyte, fluid, and acid-base aberrations. Laboratory determinations are necessary, as one cannot accurately predict changes. If sepsis seems likely, broad-spectrum antibiotics that are also effective against anaerobic bacteria (*e.g.*, ampicillin plus amikacin) are indicated.

Intussusceptions may be manually reduced or resected if tissue viability is questionable or if recurrence seems likely. One should search for underlying causes of irritation that may have predisposed the patient to the intussusception.

Linear foreign objects should be removed. Some will pass through the alimentary tract without problems if the point of fixation is cut or if they never became fixed. If surgery is not done immediately, then the patient should be carefully monitored for the next 24 to 36 hours. If there is any doubt that these objects will pass through the alimentary tract safely, they should be removed. When removing them, one should not pull them out through one incision unless they come readily, but make as many enterotomies as necessary. Excessive force often causes a devitalized ruptured intestinal loop to perforate and contaminate the abdomen.

Symptomatic Therapy

Treatment of acute vomiting not complicated by shock or excessive abdominal pain is principally symptomatic. Fluid, electrolyte, or acid-base therapy is used as needed (see Chapters 71 and 72). The vomiting will often stop if one simply withholds oral feeding and waits for 24 to 36 hours. However, if the patient is very uncomfortable or if there is excessive loss of fluids and electrolytes, then pharmacologic control of vomiting is indicated (Table 36-7).

Central-acting dopamine antagonist drugs such as acepromazine, chlorpromazine, prochlorperazine, and metoclopramide hydrochloride effectively inhibit the chemoreceptor trigger zone. Additionally, promazine derivatives directly affect the medullary vomiting center. Metoclopramide also stimulates gastric motility and emptying. Narcotics (*e.g.*, fentanyl) are effective antiemetics, although they may produce vomiting before they penetrate and block the medullary vomiting center. Trimethobenzamide may be effective in some patients, but is not as consistent as the promazine derivatives. Parasympatholytics (*e.g.*, atropine or aminopentamide) are often used, but are less effective than the promazine derivatives or metoclopramide. Orally administered, locally acting antiemetics (Kaopectate or bismuth subsalicylate) are seldom effective in severely vomiting patients and should only be used in patients with mild signs.

Persistent vomiting may also necessitate parenteral or enteral nutrition if patients are in sustained negative nitrogen balance (see Chapter 8).

Specific Therapy

Chronic, nonbloody vomiting necessitates removal of the underlying cause. This may mean surgery to remove or bypass obstructions and foreign objects. Foreign objects may often be removed endoscopically. Pyloric stenosis is amen-

Table 36–7 *Selected Antiemetic Drugs*

Acetylpromazine: 0.1 mg/kg PO two to three times daily
Chlorpromazine: 0.4 mg/kg PO or IM two to three times daily
Prochlorperazine: 0.06 to 0.1 mg/kg IM two to four times daily
Metoclopramide: 0.25 to 0.5 mg/kg PO or subcutaneously two to three times daily *or* 1 mg/kg IV infused over 24 hours
Trimethobenzamide: 3 mg/kg IM two to three times daily

able to pyloroplasty or pyloromyotomy. Gastric antral mucosal hypertrophy is resolved by resection of redundant mucosa. Gastric malignancy is almost never cured by surgery, probably because clinical signs are often delayed until the lesion is advanced, but gastroduodenostomy is sometimes palliative for obstruction due to gastric cancer. Phycomycosis is rarely amendable to surgery, as it tends to be extensive and spreads to adjacent organs and structures. Idiopathic gastric hypomotility may respond to metoclopramide hydrochloride (0.25–0.5 mg/kg orally) given 30 minutes before meals, three times daily. Intestinal obstruction due to foreign objects or scars is often cured by surgery. If the obstruction is neoplastic, surgical success depends on the tumor. Lymphosarcoma is typically disseminated, whereas carcinomas may be resectable. Idiopathic intestinal hypomotility (pseudoobstruction) may cause obstruction that responds poorly to medical therapy (metoclopramide), although cisapride (canine and feline dosages not currently available) will probably be more effective than metoclopramide for intestinal lesions.

Chronic gastritis is usually treated with metoclopramide, histamine (H₂) antagonists (cimetidine, ranitidine, or famotidine), dietary change, or, in the case of lymphocytic gastritis, prednisolone. Lymphocytic–plasmacytic enteritis (especially duodenitis) may require anti-inflammatory or immunomodulatory drugs such as prednisolone, azathioprine, or metronidazole. Canine eosinophilic gastroenteritis often responds to a strict elimination diet (mutton plus rice); feline eosinophilic disease typically responds poorly to therapy. Purulent and necrotic duodenitis often fails to respond to therapy, although antibiotics and steroids may be tried.

Nonalimentary tract diseases causing vomiting must be treated as needed. Uremia, a relatively common cause of chronic vomiting, usually produces hypergastrinemia and gastric hyperacidity. Therefore, histamine (H₂) antagonists are often helpful. The antiemetic metoclopramide is excreted through the kidneys, thus care must be exercised when this drug is used in uremic patients. Treatment of feline heartworm disease is discussed in Chapter 25. Therapy of pancreatitis and hepatic disease are discussed in Chapters 39 and 40, respectively.

Limbic epilepsy may be treated with routine anticonvulsants (phenobarbital) (see Chapter 53). Other central nervous system diseases must be treated based on individual case requirements.

Gastrointestinal ulcers may be treated by removal of the ulcer, specific therapy of the underlying cause, or symptomatic therapy.

Resection of the ulcer is indicated if there is excessive blood loss that is not amendable to medical management and there are limited, potentially resectable lesions.

Ideally, the underlying cause should always be treated. However, such causes are often occult, and even when they are treated the ulcers may initially persist, necessitating symptomatic therapy. All foreign objects, no matter how soft or small, should be removed. Even if they rarely cause the ulcer, they can inhibit healing. Hydration and splanchnic perfusion must be maintained to allow mucosal healing. Parenteral nutrition may be considered in patients with intractable vomiting, ulceration, and malnutrition.

Decreasing gastric acidity may help resolve ulcers, even when they are not caused by hyperacidity. This may be done by not stimulating acid secretion (nothing orally), by neutralizing acid that is present (orally administered antacids such as aluminum hydroxide with or without magnesium hydroxide), and by blocking gastric gland stimulation (histamine (H₂) antagonists such as cimetidine or ranitidine). These latter two drugs prevent histamine from stimulating the parietal cell. Ranitidine (2.2–4.4 mg/kg twice daily, orally or intramuscularly) is more potent than cimetidine (5–10 mg/kg three–four times daily, orally or intravenously) and may succeed when the latter fails. Famotidine and nizatidine are newer histamine (H₂) antagonists that may eventually be used in dogs and cats because they are more potent and have longer effective half-lives. Omeprazole (0.5–1.5 mg/kg once daily orally in dogs) has recently become available and is probably the most effective drug available for blocking gastric acid secretion (see Appendix II). Oral antacids may be used, but they usually must be given at least four to six times per day to consistently keep gastric pH levels greater than 5. Furthermore, oral antacids containing calcium and magnesium often stimulate gastric acid secretion, so that as soon as the buffering capacity is exceeded, hyperacidity occurs.

The ulcer may also be protected medically. Although Kaopectate and barium sulfate have been used for this purpose, these are not very effective. Sucralfate is a sucrose–aluminum hydroxide complex that adheres tightly to the exposed ulcerated tissue. Given orally at 0.25 to 1 g twice to three times daily, it prevents acid from reaching the ulcer base, neutralizes pepsin, adsorbs bile acids, and stimulates prostaglandin synthesis. Although this drug supposedly works best in an acid environment, it seems to be effective at higher *p*Hs. Sucralfate decreases the bioavailability of orally administered cimetidine (and possibly other drugs). These drugs should be given 2 hours apart if the cimetidine is administered orally. There is minimal absorption of sucralfate, and the only common side-effect is constipation; however, it adsorbs other drugs that are simultaneously given orally.

Metoclopramide stimulates gastric emptying, helping to prevent gastroduodenal reflux and the associated exposure of the gastric mucosa to bile acids.

Not yet evaluated in veterinary medicine, misoprostol is a prostaglandin analog that is supposed to protect the gastric mucosa. Likewise, pirenzepine hydrochloride is a selective anticholinergic that is an effective antacid. Finally, omeprazole blocks the parietal cell proton pump and is probably the most effective antacid available.

PATIENT MONITORING

Failure to detect alimentary tract obstruction, foreign objects, intussusception, or GDV usually leads to death from septic peritonitis or hypovolemic shock. Resolving these problems before sepsis or irreversible shock occurs is usually curative. Gastric malignancies and phycomycosis have a poor prognosis despite treatment. Nonseptic peritonitis (uroabdomen, bilious abdomen) has a reasonably good prognosis if treated appropriately. Failure to identify the systemic causes of vomiting (*e.g.*, uremia, hypoadrenocorticism, hypercalcemia) leads to worsening of the disease and may cause death.

Most patients with acute gastritis recover. Hemorrhagic gastroenteritis is usually curable if treatment is begun early enough. If symptomatic therapy is utilized for patients with acute, nonbloody vomiting, one should watch the electrolyte, acid-base, and fluid status.

Most nonmalignant ulcers can be cured with medical therapy, although surgical resection is needed in patients that are hemorrhaging badly. Failure to resolve ulcers may lead to severe gastrointestinal bleeding with anemia or shock, or to perforation and septic peritonitis. Patients with hematemesis should have their hematocrit monitored and, if the signs resolve, the clients should check for melena in case alimentary tract bleeding continues without further vomiting.

Most patients with inflammatory bowel disease and chronic gastritis can be managed medically, although purulent duodenitis seemingly has a poor prognosis.

If the alimentary tract is opened for any reason, one should watch the patient for signs of leakage and subsequent peritonitis. Such complications usually occur 3 to 5 days after surgery. Any signs of vomiting or abdominal pain should alert the clinician to this possibility. Patients with inflammatory bowel disease do not require rechecking unless potentially myelosuppressive therapy (*e.g.*, azathioprine in cats) is being used, in which case weekly complete blood counts may be done for the first 4 to 6 weeks. Then periodic reevaluations may be done.

Patients with pancreatitis need special consideration as discussed in Chapter 39.

ADDITIONAL READING

Happe RP, Van Der Gaag I, Lamers CRHW et al. Zollinger–Ellison syndrome in three dogs. Vet Pathol 1980; 17:177.

Lantz GC. The pathophysiology of acute mechanical small bowel obstruction. Compendium of Continuing Education 1981; 3:910.

Muir WW, Lipowitz AJ. Cardiac dysrhythmias associated with gastric dilatation–volvulus in the dog. J Am Vet Med Assoc 1978; 172:683.

Murray J, Robinson PB, McKeating FJ et al. Peptic ulceration in the dog. Vet Rec 1972; 91:441.

O'Brien TR. Radiographic diagnosis of abdominal disorders in the dog and cat. Covell Park Vet Co, Davis CA, 1981:204.

Stanton ME, Bright RM. Gastroduodenal ulceration in dogs. Journal of the American College of Veterinary Internal Medicine 1989; 3:238.

Tams TR. Chronic feline inflammatory bowel disorders. Compendium of Continuing Education 1986; 8:371.

Todorff FJ. Gastric dilatation–volvulus. Compendium of Continuing Education 1979; 1:142.

Twedt DG, Grauer GF. Fluid therapy for gastrointestinal, pancreatic and hepatic disorders. Vet Clin North Am 1982; 12:463.

Walshaw R, Johnston DE. Treatment of gastric dilatation–volvulus by gastric decompression and patient stabilization before major surgery. Journal of the American Animal Hospital Association 1976; 12:162.

Weaver AD. Canine intestinal intussusception. Vet Rec 1977; 100:524.

Willard MD. Some newer approaches to the treatment of vomiting. J Am Vet Med Assoc 1984; 184:590.

Wingfield WE. Acute gastric dilatation–volvulus. Vet Clin North Am 1981; 11:147.

37

DIARRHEA
Michael D. Willard

Patients with diarrhea are routinely seen in primary care as well as referral veterinary practices. The problem ranges from mild, self-limiting episodes to persistent, life-threatening syndromes.

CAUSES

The most common causes of acute canine and feline diarrhea are infections, diet, and parasites (Table 37-1). If these persist (especially the latter two) and result in inflammatory infiltrates or intestinal bacterial overgrowth, chronic diarrhea may result. The causes of chronic diarrhea are usually categorized as small intestinal (Table 37-2) or large intestinal (Table 37-3); this differentiation aids in diagnosis and treatment.

PATHOPHYSIOLOGY

Diarrhea is due to increased fecal water. Diarrhea does not denote the presence of fecal blood or mucus, although these may be seen in diarrheic feces.

Small Intestinal Diarrhea

The small intestine absorbs nutrients; therefore, small intestinal disease often produces weight loss. Diarrhea occurs when the amount of ileal fluid entering the colon is greater than the colon can absorb. This means that small intestinal disease can cause severe malabsorption and weight loss without diarrhea, or that weight loss may precede diarrhea due to small intestinal disease.

Increased fluid may enter the intestines due to excessive secretion of water into the lumen or due to increased osmotic pressure within the lumen, causing water retention. Hypermotility is rarely, if ever, the primary cause for increased fecal water. While hypersecretion and lumenal distention may produce increased peristalsis, this is usually the effect and not the cause.

Increased intestinal secretion is usually due to one of three major classes of secretagogues: bacterial enterotoxins, hormones, or detergentlike substances. Bacterial enterotoxins are a relatively common cause, but they are seldom documented in dogs and cats, probably because they are typically associated with self-limiting diseases not requiring definitive diagnosis. Prostaglandins, as mediators of inflammation, are increased in inflamed tissues, but also function with cyclic adenosine monophosphate to cause hypersecretion. Detergentlike substances, including hydroxylated fatty acids, deconjugated bile acids, and select drugs such as castor oil, probably act by increasing prostaglandin synthesis in the colonic mucosa. Detergents are probably common in patients that have malabsorptive diseases or chronic intestinal bacterial overgrowth. Regard-

Table 37–1 *Causes of Acute Diarrhea in Dogs and Cats*

DIET

Intolerance
Allergy
Poor quality diet
Food poisoning due to bacterial toxins

PARASITES

Hookworms
Roundworms
Whipworms (especially dogs)
Giardia
Others
    Coccidia (especially cats)
    Strongyloides

INFECTION

Bacterial
    Campylobacteriosis
    Salmonellosis
    Clostridial infection
Viral
    Parvovirus
    Coronavirus
    Canine distemper
    Feline leukemia virus (cats)
    Feline immunodeficiency virus (cats)

MISCELLANEOUS

Intoxication
    "Garbage eaters"
    Chemicals
    Heavy metals (thallium, arsenic)
    Drug-related (digitalis)
Hemorrhagic gastroenteritis (dogs)
Acute pancreatitis (especially dogs)

less of cause, secretion occurs from the crypt epithelium and does not presuppose damage to the absorptive villus epithelium.

Osmotic diarrhea can be iatrogenic (*e.g.,* magnesium sulfate) or spontaneous. Spontaneous osmotic diarrhea may be due to severe villus atrophy or maldigestive disorders (*e.g.,* pancreatic insufficiency or lactase deficiency) that allow carbohydrates to persist in the intestinal lumen. Lactase deficiency may be congenital or secondary to intestinal mucosal damage, which destroys this brush border enzyme and delays its replenishment by the enterocytes. However, undigested and unabsorbed nutrients will not always produce diarrhea because they may be scavenged by large intestinal bacteria.

While diarrhea is often described by placing it in one of these pathophysiologic categories, dogs and cats rarely have diarrhea readily classified as being purely one type. Many diseases probably have a combination of mechanisms. For example, an inflammatory disease may destroy villi and decrease lactase (which allows undigested carbohydrate particles to remain in the lumen) plus increase prostaglandin synthesis (which produces hypersecretion).

Viral diarrheas destroy selected enterocyte populations. Parvovirus affects rapidly dividing cells (intestinal crypt epithelium and bone marrow precursors), resulting in severe villus atrophy (due to lack of crypt cell precursors) with bleeding plus secondary infections (due to the denuded intestinal mucosa). Destruction of bone marrow precursors may produce neutropenia, which also promotes sepsis. Canine parvovirus can damage

Table 37–2 *Causes of Chronic Small Intestinal Diarrhea*

PARASITES

Giardia (especially dogs)
Hookworms
Roundworms

MALDIGESTIVE DISEASES

Exocrine pancreatic insufficiency (especially dogs)
Lactase deficiency (especially cats)

NONPROTEIN-LOSING MALABSORPTIVE DISEASES

Dietary intolerance or allergy
Inflammatory bowel disease
    Lymphocytic–plasmacytic enteritis
    Eosinophilic enteritis
    Granulomatous enteritis
Neoplasia
    Lymphosarcoma
Infection
    Histoplasmosis (especially dogs)
    Chronic intestinal bacterial overgrowth (especially dogs)
    Feline leukemia virus (cats)
    Feline immunodeficiency virus (cats)
    Campylobacteriosis
    Clostridial infection (dogs)
Villus atrophy
    Idiopathic atrophy
    Gastrinoma
    Gluten-responsive atrophy

PROTEIN-LOSING ENTEROPATHY

Intestinal lymphangiectasia or other lymphatic disorders (dogs)
Any of the disorders listed under nonprotein-losing
    malabsorptive diseases

MISCELLANEOUS

Feline hyperthyroidism

Table 37–3 *Causes of Chronic Large Bowel Diarrhea*

DIET

Intolerance
Allergy

INFECTION

Salmonellosis
Campylobacteriosis
Clostridial infection
Histoplasmosis (dogs)
Prototothecosis (rare)
Feline leukemia virus (cats)
Feline immunodeficiency virus (cats)
Infection with *Yersinia* organisms (rare)

PARASITES

Whipworms (especially dogs)
Giardia (especially dogs)
Amebiasis (rare)

INFLAMMATORY BOWEL DISEASE

Lymphocytic–plasmacytic colitis
Eosinophilic colitis
Granulomatous colitis
Histiocytic ulcerative colitis (principally boxer dogs and related breeds)
Ulcerative colitis

NEOPLASIA

Lymphosarcoma
Colonic adenocarcinoma (especially dogs)

MISCELLANEOUS

Cecocolic intussusception (rare, but mostly in dogs)

the myocardium if the patient is infected while the cells are replicating. This damage results in severe congestive cardiomyopathy, but is now unusual because most neonates have enough maternal immunity to prevent infection during the early period of life when myocardial fibers are dividing.

Coronavirus infects mature villus epithelium, which causes villus atrophy, albeit not as severe as that due to parvovirus. Furthermore, coronavirus damage tends to heal more rapidly because the crypt epithelium is intact.

Large Intestinal Diarrhea

The colon normally stores feces and absorbs water. Therefore, colonic dysfunction is usually more often associated with inappropriate elimination than with small bowel disease. Seemingly, the colon does not need to be as severely diseased as the small intestine does to produce diarrhea. This is because there is no organ that modifies the feces after they enter the colon.

Protein-Losing Enteropathy

A special category of diarrhea is protein-losing enteropathy. This is usually due to small intestinal disease, although large bowel disorders may be responsible. Such enteropathies cause protein loss in excess of what the intestine can reabsorb. Although many intestinal diseases can cause protein-losing enteropathy, intestinal lymphangiectasia is the classic example of a severe protein-losing enteropathy causing serum albumin less than or equal to 1.5 g/dl (15 g/L). The intestinal lymphatics are obstructed for uncertain reasons, and lipogranulomas can often be found along lymphatics; however, it is uncertain whether the granulomas are the cause or the effect of the disease. Lymphangiectasia can be secondary to processes that block lymphatics by cellular infiltrates (*e.g.*, severe lymphocytic–plasmacytic enteritis and lymphosarcoma); however, these diseases are not referred to as *intestinal lymphangiectasia*. The latter term is usually applied to diseases in which there is no obvious primary cause for the obstruction or lipogranulomas.

Regardless of cause, the villus lacteals swell as they collect chylomicrons. They eventually rupture into the intestinal lumen and release absorbed fat plus lymph that contains serum proteins and lymphocytes, resulting in hypoalbuminemia and often hypoglobulinemia and lymphopenia. Diarrhea, ostensibly due to hydroxylated fatty acids causing colonic secretion, is expected but not always present.

CLINICAL SIGNS

Diarrhea due to small intestinal disease tends to present differently than that due to large intestinal disease. Table 37-4 provides the major clinical signs of both types. Intermittent or repeated bouts of diarrhea (especially small intestinal) is

Table 37-4 *Clinical Signs of Large Intestinal Vs. Small Intestinal Diarrhea*

	Small Intestinal Diarrhea	*Large Intestinal Diarrhea*
Weight loss	Probable	Uncommon
Appetite	May be ravenous	Often normal
Vomiting	Possible	Possible
Frequency of defecation	Normal to slightly increased	Often very increased, with multiple attempts per bowel movement
Volume of feces	Individual defecations are normal to increased	Individual movements are normal to less, due to lack of accumulation prior to defecation
Fecal mucus	Unlikely	Likely
Hematochezia	No	Often present
Melena	Possible	No
Steatorrhea (slate-gray stools or obvious fat in stools)	Possible	No
Tenesmus or dyschezia	Uncommon unless there is secondary anal or perineal irritation	Common
Borborygmus	Possible	Unlikely

probably due to one persisting disease, as opposed to the several episodes typical of different intestinal diseases. The periodicity is probably due to the colonic compensation that occurs when the amount of ileal effluent is decreased.

The clinician must carefully consider the client's description of the frequency of defecation and volume of feces. It is easy for the client to give vague generalities that are misunderstood. It is better to identify the client's ignorance than to believe wrong data. The response to such questions as "Does your pet defecate more frequently than normal?" may be useless, as some clients assume that diarrhea presupposes increased frequency. Other clients may never have noticed how frequently their pet defecated until the diarrhea occurred. Instead, the question should be worded, "How many times per day does your pet defecate or attempt to defecate?" It is also important to determine whether the pet completely evacuates its colon the first time it defecates or if repeated attempts are necessary. If the client cannot provide an accurate description of the feces or the act of defecation, then the veterinarian should observe them. Another important consideration is whether the character of the stool or defecation

has changed during the disease. The description of the stool early in the course of the disease (before anorexia, different diets, and medications have altered it) may allow more accurate localization of the problem.

Some colonic problems produce hematochezia without diarrhea. In particular, rectal neoplasms and cecocolic intussusceptions may produce severe bleeding associated with normal or loose stools.

DIAGNOSTIC APPROACH

Acute Diarrhea

The first issue is whether the diarrhea is acute or chronic. Acute diarrhea (that which has come on suddenly and has lasted less than 5–7 days) tends to be self-limiting. In general, mild or moderately severe acute diarrhea is an indication for few tests. If a public health risk is possible (*e.g.*, salmonellosis or campylobacteriosis), if several animals are at risk (a kennel or pet store), or if the illness becomes severe, then more diagnostics are appropriate. The need for fluid, electrolyte, and acid-base therapy can often be determined by physical examination and history; however, prolonged disease or a depressed, weak animal in shock indicate clinicopathologic testing. If immediate therapy is needed, blood and urine should first be obtained for later analysis—unless the patient is literally dying before one's eyes.

Mild to moderately severe acute diarrhea is usually due to diet, parasites, bacteria, or a viral agent. The history should be searched for obvious causes (*e.g.*, recent dietary change or exposure to animals that may have been infectious). At least two to three fecal flotation and direct examinations are indicated. Food intolerance is diagnosed by eliminating other common causes (*e.g.*, parasites or infections), finding that a suspicious diet has been fed, substituting a more appropriate diet, and noting a clinical response. A history suggesting contagion or a public health risk may be an indication to look for specific etiologic agents.

Severe acute diarrhea (as noted by marked depression, severe dehydration, hematochezia, or hematemesis) is usually due to bacteria or virus (especially parvovirus), although various intoxications, heavy hookworm infestations, and hemorrhagic gastroenteritis may be responsible. Fecal analysis, a complete blood count, serum electrolytes, and blood glucose determinations are reasonable (Table 37-5).

Intestinal parasites (hookworms and roundworms) are usually relatively easy to diagnose by fecal examination. However, neonatal hookworm infestations from transmammary transmission may produce severe diarrhea and blood loss before ova are shed into the feces. These patients must be diagnosed by finding anemia plus bloody stool. Tapeworm ova are usually retained in tapeworm segments, which prevents the ova from being found on fecal examination. However, they rarely cause diarrhea. Larvae of *Strongyloides* species are found on direct fecal examination, but unless the fecal sample is fresh, one may confuse them for hookworm larvae that have hatched.

Giardia can be easy or difficult to find. Although classically producing large volumes of loose stool ("cow patty") with perhaps a little mucus, this organism can cause almost any type of diarrhea. Direct examination of fresh feces may reveal motile trophozoites. Zinc sulfate flotation utilizing centrifugation offers the best chance of diagnosing these parasites. Even then, it is may be necessary to perform three or more examinations before finding them. Sometimes giardia cysts will be damaged by flotation solutions and mistaken for coccidial oocysts. Recently, ELISA methods have been tried on feces, but the test has not been validated for the dog. Cytology of duodenal mucosa or duodenal flushes is a reasonable test for giardiasis, although it is invasive unless duodenoscopy is available. Cats are also infected by giardia.

Canine parvoviral diarrhea may be a severe, life-threatening disease; it can also produce relatively mild gastrointestinal upset (diarrhea and inappetence for 1–2 days), depending on the patient's immunity and the degree of exposure. Younger dogs and some breeds (Doberman pinscher, Rottweiler) tend to become sicker. In severely affected patients, vomiting (sometimes hematemesis) and bloody diarrhea may persist for days. Signs may progress rapidly, some patients becoming prostrate within hours. Hypovolemic and septic shock are possible (see Chapter 4). Cardiac failure due to cardiomyopathy is rare and is usually not associated with diarrhea. Feline parvoviral diarrhea (panleukopenia) is similar to canine parvoviral diarrhea.

Leukopenia is common, but is neither sensitive nor specific for canine parvoviral diarrhea. An ELISA for fecal parvoviral antigen seems to be sensitive and specific. Electron microscopic examination of feces takes longer and cannot differentiate between pathogenic canine parvovirus and nonpathogenic minute virus of canines. Samples for electron microscopic evaluation should be taken early in the course of the diarrhea, before the number of shed viral particles diminishes. Serology is not recommended. Fortunately, it is rarely necessary to definitively diagnose canine parvoviral diarrhea in order to treat it appropriately.

Hemorrhagic gastroenteritis may resemble canine parvoviral diarrhea in having an acute onset, vomiting, and bloody stools. Classically affecting small-breed dogs that have not had access to garbage, hemorrhagic gastroenteritis tends to produce hematocrits greater than 60% (0.60 L/L) and

Table 37–5 Laboratory Assessment of Diarrhea

Test	What to Check For
Complete blood count	Neutropenia (parvovirus, overwhelming sepsis) Lymphopenia (intestinal lymphangiectasia) Anemia (gastric or intestinal bleeding)
Serum biochemistry profile	Hypoalbuminemia (protein-losing enteropathy) Hypoglobulinemia (protein-losing enteropathy) Hypoglycemia (in stressed young or neonatal animals) Increased serum alanine aminotransferase (hepatic disease) Increased serum alkaline phosphatase (hepatic disease) Hypocholesterolemia (protein-losing enteropathy) Hypokalemia (losses due to diarrhea) Hypercalcemia (lymphosarcoma or other malignancy)
Fecal flotation and direct examination	Parasites or their ova
Sudan black B fat stain of feces	Positive (steatorrhea due to EPI or small bowel disease)
Iodine stain of feces for starch	Positive (amylorrhea due to EPI or small bowel disease)
Film digestion test for trypsin	Unreliable, should not be done
Abdominal radiographs	Mass or foreign object
Serum vitamin B_{12}	Decreased (EPI, bacterial overgrowth, villus atrophy)
Serum folate	Decreased (malabsorption of small bowel) Increased (bacterial overgrowth)
Trypsin-like immunoreactivity	Decreased (EPI)
BT-PABA	No absorption (EPI) Partial absorption (EPI or small intestinal disease)
Fat absorption test	Decreased (EPI or small intestinal disease)
Fat absorption test and pancreatic enzymes	Decreased (small intestinal disease)
d-Xylose absorption	Decreased (bacterial overgrowth or small intestinal disease)
Glucose tolerance test	Not recommended for intestinal disorders
Fecal culture	Salmonellosis, campylobacteriosis, or infection with *Yersinia* organisms or *Clostridium perfringens*
ELISA for fecal parvoviral antigen	Present (parvoviral diarrhea)

EPI = exocrine pancreatic insufficieny.

may have normal plasma total solids. The cause is unknown.

Canine coronavirus seldom needs to be diagnosed, as it rarely causes severe disease. However, electron microscopy of feces obtained early in the disease is the best diagnostic test.

Campylobacteriosis is a bacterial disease caused by *Campylobacter jejuni*. This organism is infectious for human beings, thus recent gastroenteritis in persons or pets in the same household is a reasonable indication to culture feces for *C. jejuni*. This bacteria is present in feces from many normal dogs and cats, especially young animals. Nonetheless, some diarrheic dogs have *C. jejuni* cultured from their feces, and improve quickly when treated with appropriate antibiotics. Specific techniques are necessary for successful culturing. The laboratory must be contacted for directions before the feces are collected. One should not attempt to culture this bacteria without specific instructions.

Salmonellae seldom cause diarrhea in dogs and cats, although they may harbor the organism. Fecal culture should be considered if the history suggests contagion.

Chronic Diarrhea

Chronic diarrhea (that which has persisted for more than 10–14 days) requires a more aggressive diagnostic approach. Symptomatic therapy is seldom needed in such patients, although nutritional support (enteral or total parenteral nutrition) may be necessary in animals with severe nutritional deficits due to the diarrhea.

Repeated fecal examinations are always appropriate, and empirical parasiticide therapy despite negative fecal analysis is reasonable if the parasite is potentially difficult to find (*e.g.*, giardia and whipworms). A complete blood count, serum biochemistry profile, and urinalysis are useful in eliminating extra-alimentary disease causing diarrhea (*e.g.*, hypoadrenocorticism, uremia) and identifying potential protein-losing enteropathies (see Table 37-5).

Next, the diarrhea should be classified as principally small or large intestinal in origin. As per Table 37-4, this should be done with the history and physical examination. If the diarrhea clearly has attributes of both, then the large intestinal disease may be the easier one to pursue initially.

Chronic Large Intestinal Diarrhea

Chronic large intestinal disease is an indication for repeated direct and flotation fecal examinations (Fig. 37-1). Rectal examination is needed because colonic neoplasia, usually occurring within 5 to 8 cm of the anus, is common. Histoplasmosis and other granulomatous diseases may also cause proctitis and rectal strictures. Careless rectal examination may suggest that the dog was uncomfortable and had a rectal spasm; however, careful palpation may reveal the "spasm" to be a band of granulation or neoplastic tissue.

Whipworms can be difficult to detect because ova are shed periodically and are dense enough to sink in some flotation solutions. Thus it is reasonable to empirically treat for whipworms despite several negative fecal examinations.

Colonoscopy and multiple biopsies are indicated next (see Colonoscopy, Mucosal Scraping, and Biopsy in Chapter 80). A flexible endoscope allows examination of the ascending colon and ileocecal area; however, rigid colonoscopy is usually adequate. Colonoscopy allows visualization and biopsy of lesions beyond the 6 to 8 cm accessible through the use of proctoscopy. Multiple mucosal biopsies should be performed regardless of the appearance of the colonic mucosa because many diseases do not always cause gross changes. These biopsies should detect inflammatory bowel diseases (lymphocytic–plasmacytic colitis, eosinophilic colitis, histiocytic ulcerative colitis, and chronic ulcerative colitis), neoplasia, histoplasmosis, and prototothecosis. If a mass lesion or an obvious proliferation is being biopsied, the tissue must be biopsied deep enough to ensure that the underlying infiltrate is sampled. A superficial biopsy may reveal inflamed colonic mucosa but not the underlying adenocarcinoma.

Intestinal histoplasmosis typically causes bloody diarrhea, fever, weight loss, hypoproteinemia, or thrombocytopenia; however, signs vary markedly between patients, some having protracted mild diarrhea without systemic involvement. Histoplasmosis may cause corrugated rectal mucosa, rectal strictures, or normal-appearing mucosa. Occasionally, it is localized to focal areas in the colon. If histoplasmosis is possible, cytology of scrapings is often diagnostic (Fig. 37-2) and is faster than histopathology. Some lesions are missed by biopsies but found by scrapings that sample larger surface areas. The mucosa is gently scraped (especially any thickened, corrugated areas) with a spatula or dull scalpel blade. The smears are air dried and stained with methylene blue, Wright's stain, Giemsa stain, or the like. Serology is rarely diagnostic.

Prototothecosis is a rare infection with algae. The colon and eyes are typically involved. Colonic biopsy should be definitive.

Lymphocytic–plasmacytic colitis can be diagnosed by histology but not cytology. This is a relatively common inflammatory bowel disease

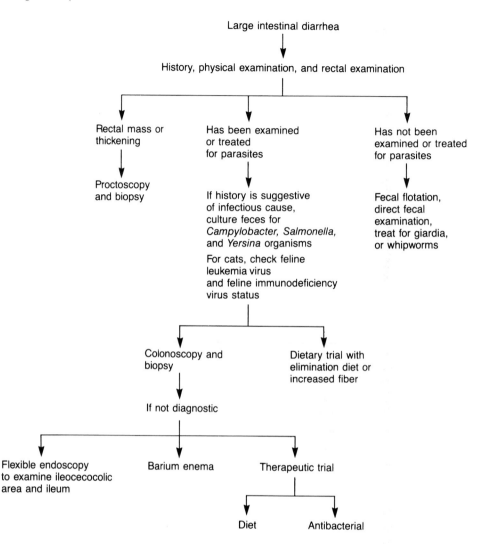

Figure 37–1. *Diagnostic approach to chronic large intestinal diarrhea.*

of cats and dogs; however, the pathologist must be familiar with intestinal pathology, as lymphocytes and plasma cells are normally found in the colonic mucosa. If mild lymphocytic–plasmacytic colitis is diagnosed, the tissue may be normal and a second opinion from a gastrointestinal pathologist might be sought.

Eosinophilic colitis may occur in any breed, but German shepherd dogs seem to be disproportionately affected. Peripheral eosinophilia is inconsistent. Cytology of colonic mucosa is suggestive if many eosinophils are seen. However, eosinophils are normally present in colonic mu-

cosa and a diagnosis of mild eosinophilic colitis should arouse suspicion regarding its accuracy. Eosinophilic colitis may be associated with similar gastric, intestinal, or respiratory infiltrates. Concurrent lymphocytic–plasmacytic infiltrates are common. Fortunately, this disease is rare in cats.

Histiocytic ulcerative colitis is principally seen in boxer dogs, although bulldogs and similar breeds are occasionally affected. Ulcers are not consistent, but if present, one should biopsy near their edge plus in nonulcerated areas.

Occasionally, one will diagnose granuloma-

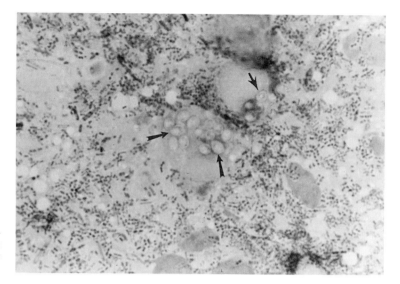

Figure 37–2. *Cytologic preparation of colonic mucosa showing numerous* Histoplasma capsulatum *organisms (arrows) within a macrophage (Wright's stain, 1000 ×).*

tous colitis, atrophic colitis, or chronic ulcerative colitis. These are not as well characterized in dogs and cats as the previous types.

Colonic adenocarcinoma is the most common canine colonic malignancy. Typically found near the rectum in older animals, hematochezia and tenesmus are common signs. These masses usually have obvious submucosal infiltration and may be circumferential or localized. Some constrict the rectal lumen with minimal proliferation, while others protrude far into the lumen. One must be sure to biopsy deep enough, as some tumors are principally in the submucosa and have inflamed mucosa overlying them. Colonic neoplasia is rare in the cat, but is often lymphosarcoma when it occurs. Colonic phycomycosis may occur near the rectum and may clinically mimic rectal adenocarcinoma.

Adenomatous polyps are principally found near the rectum. While some have a small, hard mass on the end of an obvious stalk, others have brood "heads" that obscure the underlying linear stalk. These latter lesions can be so extensive that it is difficult to discern that they are polyps. Adenomatous polyps are relatively soft and do not infiltrate underlying tissues. They should be histologically examined, as carcinoma "in situ" rarely occurs.

Granulomatous proctitis occurs infrequently. It may resemble malignancy because it is diffuse and infiltrative. Biopsy is needed to differentiate the two. Cecocolic intussusceptions differ from ileocolic intussusceptions in that the former do not obstruct and rarely produce acute abdomen or sepsis. They typically cause hematochezia with or without diarrhea. Occasionally, they may be palpated or seen on plain abdominal radiographs (a "coiled spring" in the ascending colon), but they are typically hard to diagnose.

Sometimes colonic biopsy samples are normal despite obvious large intestinal signs (e.g., mucoid stools). The cause of this is uncertain, although it has been attributed to irritable bowel syndrome or bacterial overgrowth. See under Management, below, for therapy of these patients.

If the cause of large bowel diarrhea is still undiagnosed after the approach described above, then rebiopsy of the colon should be considered. Histoplasmosis, in particular, can produce a low-grade infection that is missed despite multiple colonic biopsies.

Chronic Small Intestinal Diarrhea

Chronic small intestinal disease not due to parasitism is either maldigestive, nonprotein-losing malabsorptive, or protein-losing. Among the first tests done should be the staining of feces for undigested fats and the measurement of serum protein and albumin concentrations (Fig. 37-3). If serum albumin is less than 2 g/dl (20 g/L), then protein-losing enteropathy should be considered, as the other two conditions generally do not produce severe hypoalbuminemia. If hypoalbuminemia is not present, maldigestion is considered

next, especially (but not only) if undigested fats are found in the feces.

MALDIGESTION. Lactase deficiency is anecdotally reported in cats, especially Siamese. Intolerance to milk is documented by the occur-

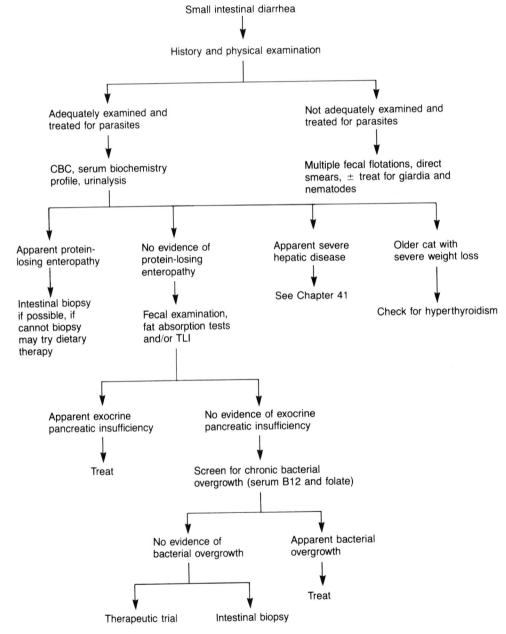

TLI = trypsin-like immunoreactivity.

Figure 37–3. *Diagnostic approach to chronic small intestinal diarrhea.*

rence of diarrhea after feeding diets containing milk products. While lactase deficiency is a concern whenever small intestinal mucosal disease may prevent normal lactase production, it is not tested for specifically.

If canine feces contain excessive undigested fats, then maldigestion due to exocrine pancreatic insufficiency, the principal cause of canine maldigestion, is likely (not all dogs with exocrine pancreatic insufficiency have identifiable fat in their feces). Undigested fats in the feces do not diagnose exocrine pancreatic insufficiency, but indicate further tests to confirm it or a trial of appropriate pancreatic enzyme therapy. Definitive diagnosis is preferable due to the cost of appropriate enzyme replacement and its life-long nature.

The best tests to confirm exocrine pancreatic insufficiency are serum trypsinlike immunoreactivity, the bentiromide test, and undigested and digested fat absorption tests. The first is the most sensitive and specific. The bentiromide (BT-PABA) test is reliable but expensive, and requires multiple blood samples or a 6-hour quantitated urine sample. The fat absorption tests are convenient and inexpensive, but are not as sensitive or specific as the other two. If serum vitamin B_{12} concentrations are determined, a lowered value suggests exocrine pancreatic insufficiency, bacterial overgrowth, or severe villus atrophy. However, normal serum vitamin B_{12} concentrations do not eliminate this disease.

If pancreatic enzyme replacement is to be used as a therapeutic trial, one should remember that failure to respond does not eliminate exocrine pancreatic insufficiency, because some patients require dietary change, antacids, or antibacterial therapy for the pancreatic enzymes to be effective. Even if the enzyme therapy seems effective, it is wise to stop it and see if the diarrhea recurs to be certain that the clinical improvement and the enzyme administration were not fortuitously associated. Many clients have spent large sums on unneeded pancreatic enzyme supplements because of supposed clinical response to supplementation. Because of the potential difficulty in diagnosing patients with exocrine pancreatic insufficiency, it is advisable to use definitive tests before initiating aggressive diagnostics for primary intestinal disease.

MALABSORPTION. Once maldigestive disease has been eliminated, the small intestine is investigated. There are two main diagnostic approaches to nonprotein-losing malabsorptive disease: therapeutic trials and intestinal biopsy. The former is a valid diagnostic test if it is carefully planned and implemented.

Because diet is a common cause of small bowel diarrhea, it is reasonable to prescribe a trial elimination diet (*e.g.,* boiled mutton and rice). Such a diet contains substances to which the patient has not been previously exposed and should not be sensitized. This is not the same as a bland diet. The elimination diet should be the sole substance fed to the patient for at least 2 and preferably 4 weeks. The better elimination diets tend to be more expensive or cumbersome than the less restrictive diets. However, if an excellent elimination diet does not work, then the owner need not try several others. If a strict elimination diet is successful, then a less expensive and more convenient diet will probably be found eventually.

Empirical antibacterial therapy is reasonable because chronic small intestinal bacterial overgrowth can cause or exacerbate other intestinal diseases. The drug should kill aerobic and anaerobic bacteria (*e.g.,* tetracycline, tylosin, and amoxicillin), and should be used for at least 2 to 3 weeks before assessing efficacy. Neomycin is not effective against anaerobic bacteria. Because bacterial overgrowth is probably secondary to underlying intestinal disease, it is not unusual for antibacterial therapy to resolve the diarrhea but for signs to recur after withdrawing the drugs.

Serum vitamin B_{12} and folate concentrations are useful in screening for chronic bacterial overgrowth and severe intestinal villus atrophy. Decreased serum B_{12} plus a normal to increased folate concentration suggests bacterial overgrowth; however, not all patients with bacterial overgrowth have these changes. Quantitated aerobic and anaerobic culture of duodenal fluid is useful but probably unavailable unless one is at an institution. Obligate pathogens are not required, only excessive numbers of bacteria (usually mixed populations). Performing D-xylose absorption tests before and after antibiotic administration may diagnose bacterial overgrowth if the absorption remarkably improves after antibiotic therapy.

Although not commonly available, analysis of expired H_2 after a carbohydrate meal is useful in looking for carbohydrate malabsorption due to any reason, as well as for bacterial overgrowth. In the latter case, one expects excessive expired hydrogen soon after ingesting a meal (before the food has the chance to reach the colon).

Plain abdominal radiographs are seldom helpful in patients with chronic small intestinal diarrhea. However, they may occasionally reveal a mass, tumor, or stagnant loop. The latter may be a partially obstructed loop of intestine or one that has a focal dilatation due to intramural disease (Fig. 37-4). Care must be taken not to mistake a loop that is transiently dilated for one that has intrinsic disease. Repeat plain radiographs should reveal persistence of the dilated loop if there is intrinsic disease. Such a dilatation allows food retention and bacterial overgrowth. Regardless of cause, a persistently dilated intestinal segment indicates surgical exploration.

Feline leukemia virus and feline immunodeficiency virus (FIV) tests are worthwhile in ill cats. Although the syndromes have not been comprehensively defined, there appear to be significant enteropathies associated with these viral infections in cats.

Contrast upper gastrointestinal radiographs and intestinal function tests are useful if one is trying to decide whether or not the small intestine is diseased. Radiographic signs of intestinal infiltration document significant disease (Fig. 37-5). Likewise, a clearly abnormal D-xylose absorption test is consistent with bacterial overgrowth or primary intestinal disease. The fat absorption test is readily available, but is more subjective in its interpretation. Failure to find abnormalities with these tests does not rule out intestinal disease. If these tests document small intestinal disease, then intestinal biopsy is indicated. However, despite failure of these tests to document an abnormality, one can still reasonably biopsy the intestines because biopsy is more sensitive and specific for diagnosing intestinal disease. It is often reasonable to skip these tests and proceed to intestinal biopsy, especially if endoscopy is available. The major value of these other tests is to convince the diagnostician of the need for biopsy in patients with particularly obscure disease.

Occasionally, culture for selected pathogens (*C. jejuni, Yersinia enterocolitica, Clostridium perfringens, Clostridium difficile*) may be helpful if the history is suggestive of contagion or if intestinal biopsy is unrevealing. *C. difficile* rarely has been associated with chronic diarrhea in dogs. Likewise, *Y. enterocolitica* has rarely been responsible for large bowel diarrhea. Successful culture and identification of causative organisms requires selective media. One may also assay for the toxin in the feces.

Intestinal biopsy is the most definitive test in

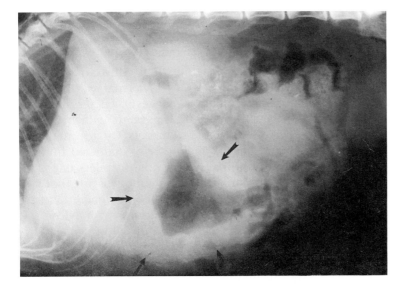

Figure 37–4. Plain radiograph of a cat with a dilated segment of small intestine (arrows). This was later found to be due to lymphosarcoma invading that segment of intestine.

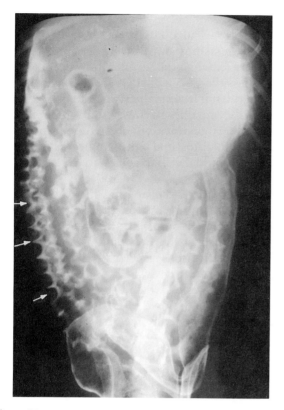

Figure 37–5. *Barium contrast radiograph showing pattern consistent with intestinal infiltrative disease. Note the scalloped appearance (arrows) of the intestinal mucosa.*

patients with malabsorption, although it generally does not diagnose bacterial overgrowth. Full-thickness biopsies of the stomach, duodenum, jejunum, ileum, and mesenteric lymph node may be performed at laparotomy. However, gastroduodenoscopy plus ileocolonoscopy usually provides diagnostic tissue samples, poses less risk to the patient, and requires less anesthetic time. If the endoscopist needs help passing through the pylorus or preanesthesia including ketamine or xylazine may be advantageous, although experience should eliminate the need for these drugs. The disadvantages of small intestinal endoscopic biopsy are that, first, the lesion may be inaccessible due to its location (in the middle of the jejunum) or the patient's size (less than 2 kg or greater than 50–60 kg) and, second, the biopsies are small and subject to distortion if mishandled. Occasionally, the shallow nature of the biopsy

samples may cause misdiagnosis. In particular, intestinal lymphosarcoma may be too deep to reach with the flexible biopsy instrument, and yet there may be a reactive lymphocytic–plasmacytic infiltrate above it, resulting in a misdiagnosis of lymphocytic–plasmacytic enteritis. If the endoscopic biopsies are not diagnostic or if the diagnosis obtained through flexible endoscopy is suspect, then exploratory laparotomy can be performed next with no detriment to the patient due to the endoscopic procedure.

Lymphocytic–plasmacytic enteritis and eosinophilic enteritis are the inflammatory bowel diseases most commonly found in dogs and cats. Lymphocytic–plasmacytic enteritis requires histopathology for diagnosis. It may be more common in German shepherd dogs, in which it can be associated with intestinal bacterial overgrowth and can occasionally produce protein loss. Lymphocytic–plasmacytic enteritis is also reasonably common in cats, in which it typically causes vomiting, but may also produce malabsorption or diarrhea.

Eosinophilic enteritis seems to be more common in German shepherds than other dogs. Peripheral eosinophilia is inconsistent. Histopathology is definitive, but mucosal cytology is sometimes diagnostic.

Severe villus atrophy may also be detected by biopsy. The lesion may have total villus collapse and may morphologically resemble sprue in humans.

Lymphosarcoma is the most common feline intestinal neoplasia, and is reasonably common in dogs. The intestines may be thickened, but can appear grossly normal. Mesenteric lymph nodes are commonly infiltrated and enlarged, but this finding is inconsistent. Feline intestinal lymphosarcoma is often unassociated with feline leukemia virus infection, and rarely has circulating neoplastic cells. Pseudohyperparathyroidism (hypercalcemia of malignancy) is uncommonly seen with this type of lymphosarcoma. Diagnosis requires identification of neoplastic lymphocytes or other evidence of malignancy.

PROTEIN-LOSING ENTEROPATHY. Protein-losing enteropathy is suggested by hypoproteinemia, especially panhypoproteinemia. However, panhypoproteinemia is inconsistent. If the disease causes excessive globulin production (as in the basenji), then intestinal globulin losses may be associated with normal globulin levels or hyperglobulinemia. Lymphopenia is common in lymphangiectasia but less common in other causes of protein-losing enteropathy. Intestinal lymphangiectasia classically produces the most severe protein-losing enteropathy, but lymphosarcoma, severe lymphocytic–plasmacytic enteritis, and intestinal histoplasmosis may also produce significant protein loss. Yorkshire terriers and soft-coated wheaten terriers seem to have a high incidence of lymphangiectasia, while basenjis are noted for intestinal lymphoproliferative disease with associated protein loss. A special consideration in young animals (less than 6–8 months of age) that have protein-losing enteropathy not due to parasitism is a chronic intussusception.

The first step in diagnosis is to eliminate renal protein losses by checking the urine protein: creatinine ratio, and hepatic insufficiency by hepatic function testing (*e.g.*, serum bile acid concentrations). Hypoalbuminemia with normal or increased globulin concentrations is more consistent with renal losses or hepatic failure; however, there are enough exceptions that one should use tests to try to definitively eliminate these causes before proceeding. With these causes eliminated, if protein-losing enteropathy is suspected, intestinal biopsy will confirm it and determine which

disease is responsible. Large intestinal biopsies are sometimes adequate in disseminated disease (*e.g.*, histoplasmosis). Full-thickness intestinal biopsy is risky when the serum albumin concentration is less than 1.5 g/dl (15 g/L). However, serosal patch-grafting lessens the risk of dehiscence. Occasionally, one may find white granulomas (Fig. 37-6) on the intestines, which are lipogranulomas suggestive of intestinal lymphangiectasia. The intestines should be biopsied if these lesions are found.

Occasionally, a therapeutic trial designed to prevent further rupture of intestinal lacteals is elected instead of biopsy. If this is done, then the trial should consist only of dietary management, as some medications used for lymphangiectasia (*e.g.*, corticosteroids) may make other diseases causing protein-losing enteropathy (*e.g.*, histoplasmosis) worse. The diet for lymphangiectasia is discussed below.

MANAGEMENT

Acute Diarrhea

Most acute diarrheas of unknown etiology may be managed by treating for parasites, switching to a bland diet (*e.g.*, chicken and rice), restoring fluid, electrolyte, and acid-base status as needed, and perhaps withholding food for 12 to 24 hours. The

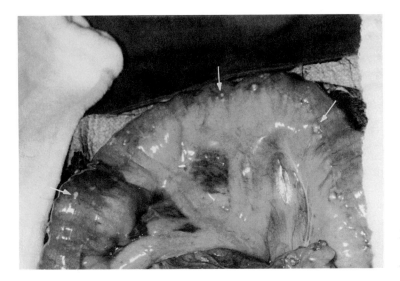

Figure 37–6. *Gross view of the intestines of a dog with hypoalbuminemia and hepatic dysfunction. The white nodules (arrows) are lipogranulomas associated with intestinal lymphangiectasias.*

value of withholding food in patients with acute diarrhea is debatable; the patient should probably be allowed to eat bland food as soon as it wants to, as long as it does not clearly make the diarrhea worse.

Fluid and electrolyte therapy may be needed (see Chapters 71 and 72). Intravenous administration is the best route in severely dehydrated patients. Fluid rates should be calculated instead of guessed (maintenance = 60 ml/kg/day and deficit [in milliliters] = weight in kilograms × estimated percent of dehydration × 1000); otherwise, it is common to give less than is needed. Once the patient is rehydrated, its body weight should be monitored daily to detect occult water losses. Potassium may have to be supplemented, and can be given intravenously (usually at 0.1–0.2 mEq/kg/hour) or orally. Serum potassium concentrations should be monitored if administration is prolonged or aggressive.

Very young pets (less than 6–12 weeks old) and very small dogs (less than 2–4 kg) that are anorectic should have glucose supplementation either orally or parenterally (5% dextrose in water, either alone or with electrolyte solutions at a maintenance rate). These animals are at risk for hypoglycemia whenever they are severely ill and anorectic.

Alternatively, oral rehydration therapy may be used. These solutions contain electrolytes and glucose. If the intestinal villus epithelium is functioning, it will absorb the glucose, which, because it is tied to sodium absorption, forces concomitant water absorption. Marked mucosal destruction, as with severe parvoviral diarrhea, may render this therapy futile, but it is often effective. The patient should be given at least one part of plain water for every two parts of rehydration solution that it drinks. Thirst should be satisfied by plain water. The solution can be given hourly, either by free choice or by a nasoesophageal or gastric tube (see Nasoesophageal Intubation in Chapter 80). One should plan to replace existing deficits over 8 to 12 hours when using these solutions. These solutions must be used as directed to avoid hyperkalemia and hypernatremia.

Patients with acute diarrheas (especially if they are young) are potentially contagious to other animals and humans; therefore one should observe strict sanitation. Hypochlorite solution (bleach diluted 1 : 32 with water) is a satisfactory disinfectant for canine parvovirus and many other pathogens.

If the patient is febrile, then systemic antibiotics (β-lactams, parenteral aminoglycosides, potentiated sulfa drugs) should be used. Oral aminoglycosides (neomycin) are useful if diarrhea is due to campylobacteriosis. Other antibiotics commonly effective for this organism are erythromycin and tetracycline. β-Lactam antibiotics are seldom effective against *C. jejuni*, which typically produces β-lactamase. Hepatic encephalopathy is another indication for oral aminoglycosides (see Chapter 40). If anaerobic bacteria are suspected, then amoxicillin, metronidazole, tetracycline, or chloramphenicol should be used. For specific pathogens, sensitivity testing is recommended.

Parasiticides commonly consist of metronidazole for giardia and broad-spectrum anthelmintics for nematodes (fenbendazole, mebendazole, or dichlorvos). For younger animals with acute diarrhea, pyrantel pamoate is useful for hookworms and roundworms. *Strongyloides* are treated with thiabendazole or a 5-day regime of fenbendazole. Tapeworms are rarely pathogenic, although they are offensive to clients. They can be effectively treated with praziquantel.

Antidiarrheal drugs (Table 37–6) are indicated in patients that have excessive loss of fluids and electrolytes. The most effective are the antiprostaglandins (bismuth subsalicylate) and the opiates (diphenoxylate, loperamide, or paregoric). Bismuth causes the feces to become black (mimicking melena). The salicylate is absorbed, warranting caution in cats. Opiates must be used cautiously in animals weighing less than 10 kg; also, they may allow bacterial proliferation due to intestinal stasis.

Table 37–6 *Selected Antidiarrheal Drugs for Use in Dogs*

Bismuth subsalicylate: 1 to 2 ml/kg PO, two to three times daily for 1 to 2 days
Diphenoxylate: 0.05 to 0.1 mg/kg PO, two to three times daily
Loperamide: 0.08 mg/kg PO, three to four times daily
Codeine: 0.2 to 0.5 mg/kg PO two to four times daily

Adsorbents are usually of dubious value. Kaopectate (1–2 ml/kg orally one to four times daily) improves the stool consistency, but that is probably due to adding particulate matter to the feces, which improves their consistency until the disease spontaneously resolves. Similarly, dietary fiber supplementation sometimes improves stool consistency. Cholestyramine resin (1/4–1/2 g twice daily with food or in water) has been useful in selected human disorders, and has been tried in dogs. It binds to bile acids and possibly other toxins in the intestinal lumen.

Anti-inflammatories, especially flunixin meglumine (0.3 mg/kg IM), have been used in canine parvoviral diarrhea. The rationale has been that decreasing the intestinal inflammation is beneficial to the patient. Although there are no studies to prove that this treatment is beneficial for the intestines, severe parvoviral diarrhea often has secondary bacteremia, and flunixin meglumine is useful in endotoxic shock. However, this drug is ulcerogenic, especially if used repeatedly or with corticosteroids.

Chronic Diarrhea

Pancreatic enzyme supplementation must be done carefully to procure a response from dogs with exocrine pancreatic insufficiency. Powdered enzymes mixed with food are usually effective, even when the same product in tablet form is not. A relatively low fat diet may also aid therapy. Because the enzymes are sensitive to low pH, concurrent use of histamine (H_2) antagonists (cimetidine 5–10 mg/kg orally three–four times daily) may prevent enzyme inactivation. Bacterial overgrowth occurs frequently in patients with exocrine pancreatic insufficiency, and appropriate antibacterial therapy may make previously ineffective enzyme therapy successful.

Elimination diets for inflammatory bowel disease are often useful for canine and feline lymphocytic–plasmacytic disease of the small and large intestines as well as canine eosinophilic infiltrative disease. Boiled mutton (1/4 lb), boiled rice (1 cup), vegetable oil (1 teaspoon), and dicalcium phosphate (1.5 teaspoon) is an excellent elimination diet (Lewis, Additional Reading). Cats do not seem to like mutton, and one may substitute rabbit. Cottage cheese and boiled rice is often useful. Commercial products are also available. Various commercial diets that are not particularly restrictive may often be successful in cats with lymphocytic–plasmacytic enteritis (e.g., Hill's Feline c/d, Purina's Tender Vittles, and Iams Kitten Food.

Rare dogs with severe villus atrophy seem to respond favorably to gluten-free diets.

Diets for protein-losing enteropathy due to intestinal lymphangiectasia often consist of an extremely low fat diet plus a medium-chain triglyceride oil (1–2 ml/kg/day in food). The absence of long-chain fatty acids prevents chylomicron formation from rupturing the lacteals, while the water-soluble medium-chain fatty acids bypass the lacteals and enter the portal circulation. However, the medium-chain triglycerides have a disagreeable taste and initially must be added sparingly to the diet lest the patient refuse to eat. Cooking the food may improve its palatability.

Dietary therapy includes restrictive diets and, in the case of colitis, addition of fiber. The latter may be beneficial in feline lymphocytic–plasmacytic colitis and perhaps canine irritable bowel syndrome. Insoluble fiber seems to be the most useful type in colonic disease. Coarse wheat bran (1–2 tablespoons per can of food) or processed cellulose (1 teaspoon of Metamucil per can of food) may be used. One should probably allow at least 2 to 3 weeks to see results. Currently, it is controversial how beneficial fiber is for inflammatory colonic disease compared to elimination diets, especially in dogs.

Antibiotic therapy for chronic intestinal bacterial overgrowth usually consists of tetracycline, tylosin, or amoxicillin. It may be necessary to treat the patient for 2 to 3 weeks before response is seen. Furthermore, because bacterial overgrowth is apparently secondary to other diseases, the treatment may have to be prolonged lest overgrowth reoccur. Supposedly, *C. perfringen-* or *C. difficile*-induced diarrhea is resolved with drugs active against anaerobes (metronidazole).

Inflammatory bowel disease is usually treated

with diet or drugs. Other ancillary therapy may include cleaning and applying soothing ointments to an inflamed anus as well as enforcing rest to avoid stimulating colonic evacuation.

Canine and feline lymphocytic–plasmacytic colitis and enteritis may be responsive to elimination diets. In German shepherd dogs, lymphocytic–plasmacytic enteritis may be associated with bacterial overgrowth, which should be treated simultaneously.

Severe cases of inflammatory bowel disease that do not respond to diet alone may require anti-inflammatory therapy. If anti-inflammatory therapy is needed, prednisolone is often administered orally at 2.2 to 4.4 mg/kg/day. Cats may also require anti-inflammatory therapy, but tend to have fewer side-effects from corticosteroids. Azathioprine may be used in both species to augment the effects of the prednisolone, but the feline dose (0.3 mg/kg orally every other day) is much less than the canine dose. Concurrent metronidazole has also been used for its supposed effects on the immune system.

Protein-losing enteropathy will occasionally require anti-inflammatory therapy (prednisolone 1.1–2.2 mg/kg/day) in addition to dietary management. Patients with many lipogranulomas may especially benefit from the steroid therapy.

Canine eosinophilic enteritis and colitis usually responds to strict elimination diets, even when it does not respond to steroid therapy. Corticosteroid therapy may be effective, but is seldom needed. However, feline eosinophilic infiltrates may be part of a hypereosinophilic syndrome, which is poorly responsive to therapy. If glucocorticoids are used, they should initially be administered in high doses (prednisolone 2.2–4.4 mg/kg/day).

Ulcerative colonic diseases may respond to sulfasalazine (Azulfidine) (dogs: 35–50 mg/kg orally divided; cats: 15 mg/kg orally divided), which consists of a sulfa drug joined to 5-aminosalicylic acid. The bond is broken by colonic bacteria, and the salicylate is essentially "applied" directly to the diseased colonic mucosa. However, the sulfa moiety may produce keratoconjunctivitis sicca, and idiosyncratic vasculitis or arthritis may occur, especially in Doberman pinschers and rott-

weilers. Up to 2 weeks of therapy may be needed before beneficial effects are seen. 5-Aminosalicylic acid (Asacol) by itself (10 mg/kg orally twice daily) will hopefully reduce side-effects. The efficacy and dose of this drug in small animals is yet to be determined. It appears that keratoconjunctivitis sicca may still be a problem with long-term (longer than 4 months) use in dogs.

Other anti-inflammatory therapy for various colitides, particularly those that are severe and nonresponsive to other medications, may consist of retention enemas of corticosteroids or sulfasalazine. While this is a means of applying large concentrations of the drug to the affected area, inflamed tissues may absorb the drug, resulting in systemic effects (*e.g.*, iatrogenic hyperadrenocorticism). Products that are not readily defecated following the enema (foam products instead of solutions) should be used.

Intestinal histoplasmosis often responds to ketoconazole, itraconazole, or amphotericin B therapy. Therapeutic success depends on whether the disease can be controlled before other organ failure occurs. Colonic adenocarcinoma can be treated with surgical excision if the lesion is not extensive and there is no evidence of metastasis. Care must be taken to avoid causing incontinence by the surgery. Lymphosarcoma is usually treated by combination chemotherapy, although solitary masses may rarely be resected. Rectal polyps can be resolved with simple surgical excision. Granulomatous proctitis typically responds to corticosteroids with or without azathioprine. Cecocolic intussusception is resolved by removing the cecum surgically.

There seems to be a syndrome of chronic canine large-bowel mucoid diarrhea for which no reason can be found by tests or biopsies. Colonic mucosa is usually histologically normal. These patients often respond to empirical therapy with tylosin. In other instances, high fiber diets may be beneficial.

Feline leukemia virus- and FIV-associated diarrheas have no specific therapy, and at times must be treated symptomatically with diet, antibiotics, and anthelmintics. Here one must search for secondary problems and treat them aggressively.

PATIENT MONITORING

Failure to control severe fluid, electrolyte, or acid-base changes and hypoglycemia are the major causes of mortality in acute enteritis, except in parvoviral diarrhea, which may also have severe sepsis. While mild parvoviral diarrhea often resolves spontaneously, severe parvoviral diarrhea has a guarded prognosis in dogs and cats. Likewise, severe hookworm infestations of neonates must be treated quickly. Otherwise, patients with acute diarrhea need minimal monitoring after the signs are brought under control other than to ensure that the diarrhea does not recur and that it does not appear in other exposed animals. Animals in which acute diarrhea persists for more than 10 days without improvement should be approached as having chronic diarrhea.

In patients with chronic diarrhea, once the disease has been diagnosed and therapy begun, monitoring principally consists of evaluation of stools and, in the case of small intestinal disease, body weight. It is important that the clients be aware that prolonged therapy may be needed and that 2 to 3 weeks is the minimum time needed to accurately evaluate response to many therapies.

Canine and feline lymphocytic–plasmacytic colitis usually responds well to therapy, as does canine eosinophilic enteritis or colitis. Feline eosinophilic enteritis or colitis has a poor prognosis. Intestinal histoplasmosis has a good prognosis if other organ failure does not occur. Histiocytic ulcerative colitis may often be controlled, but can recur despite therapy. Lymphosarcoma may be palliated for weeks to months. The enteropathies apparently associated with feline leukemia virus and FIV seem to have a guarded to poor prognosis. Colonic adenocarcinoma is rarely cured, but may be surgically palliated if it is not too advanced when first seen. Adenomatous polyps are typically resolved by surgery, while granulomatous proctitis can usually be controlled medically.

Protein-losing enteropathy due to intestinal lymphangiectasia often responds well to dietary therapy with or without corticosteroids. Patients with protein-losing enteropathy should have their serum proteins rechecked every 5 to 7 days initially. If the disease is controlled, then the proteins should be evaluated every 3 to 6 months to check for recurrence of disease.

Repeat endoscopy and biopsy is useful in determining whether therapy for chronic diarrhea can be stopped or if it should persist. However, its cost : benefit ratio cannot be accurately judged yet.

ADDITIONAL READING

Barlough FJ. Canine giardiasis. Journal of Small Animal Practice 1979; 20:613.

Breitschwerdt EB, Halliwell WG, Foley CW et al. A hereditary diarrheic syndrome in the basenji characterized by malabsorption, protein losing enteropathy, and hypergammaglobulinemia. Journal of the American Animal Hospital Association 1980; 16:551.

Ewing GO, Gomez JA. Canine ulcerative colitis. Journal of the American Animal Hospital Association 1973; 9:395.

Ford RB. Canine histoplasmosis. Compendium of Continuing Education 1980; 2:637.

Hendrick M. A spectrum of hypereosinophilic syndromes exemplified by six cats with eosinophilic enteritis. Vet Pathol 1981; 18:188.

Hill FWG. Malabsorption syndrome in the dog. Journal of Small Animal Practice 1972; 13:575.

Jacobs RM, Weiser MG, Hall RL. Clinicopathologic features of canine parvoviral enteritis. Journal of the American Animal Hospital Association 1980; 16:809.

Lewis LD, Morris ML Jr, Hand MS. Small animal clinical nutrition III. Topeka, KS: Mark Morris Associates, 1987.

Romatowski J: Use of oral fluids in acute gastroenteritis in small animals. Modern Veterinary Practice 1985; 4:261.

Seiler RJ. Colorectal polyps of the dog. J Am Vet Med Assoc 1979; 174:72.

Tams TR. Chronic canine lymphocytic plasmacytic enteritis. Compendium of Continuing Education 1987; 9:1184.

Tams TR, Twedt DC. Canine protein-losing gastroenteropathy syndrome. Compendium of Continuing Education 1981; 3:105.

Willard MD, Sugarman B, Walker RD. Gastrointestinal zoonoses. Vet Clin North Am 1987; 17:145.

Williams DA. New tests of pancreatic and small intestinal function. Compendium of Continuing Education 1987; 9:1167.

38

CONSTIPATION, DYSCHEZIA, AND TENESMUS

Michael D. Willard

Constipation is the inability to defecate without undue difficulty and is commonly seen in private practice. Obstipation is complete inability to eliminate feces (intractable constipation). Dyschezia refers to painful or difficult evacuation of feces from the colon. Tenesmus is painful or ineffectual straining to urinate or defecate. Megacolon refers to a colon distended with feces until it is much larger than normal. These problems may be severe, or they be mild and reflect a client's undue concern.

CAUSES

There are seven main causes of constipation: inappropriate intake, drugs, refusal to defecate due to pain, refusal to defecate due to behavior or environment, obstruction of the colon or rectum, deviation of the large intestine, and weakness of the colonic musculature (Table 38-1).

Most of these also cause tenesmus or dyschezia; however, tenesmus and dyschezia are not always related to constipation. Urethral obstruc- tion in male cats produces tenesmus, which is often mistakenly attributed to constipation. Likewise, stranguria from urinary tract infection in females may be mistaken for constipation, especially if urine is not seen. Finally, colitis and proctitis typically cause tenesmus due to rectal irritation.

PATHOPHYSIOLOGY

Very low residue diets may be constipating in dehydrated patients. Excessive fiber without adequate fluid intake also produces hard feces that are difficult to evacuate. Excessive fiber may come from an inappropriate diet (*e.g.*, popcorn) or from attempted therapy (*e.g.*, excessive supplementation of processed cellulose). Occasionally, diets with reasonable amounts of fiber constipate particular patients for uncertain reasons. Ingested hair and bones are especially common causes of constipation.

Drugs uncommonly cause canine and feline constipation. Sucralfate (Carafate) can be respon-

Table 38–1 *Causes of Constipation in Dogs and Cats*

DIET	**COLONIC OBSTRUCTION**
Foreign objects	Intraluminal
Excessive fiber plus lack of water	Tumor
Indigestible substances (popcorn, bones, hair)	Foreign object
	Intramural
DRUGS	Tumor
Narcotics	Cicatrix
Sucralfate	Granuloma
Kaopectate	Extracolonic
Barium sulfate	Tumor (colonic or prostatic)
Aluminum hydroxide	Cicatrix
Anticholinergics	Granuloma
Antihistamines	Pelvic abscess
	Prostatomegaly (dogs, especially sexually intact ones that have benign prostatic hyperplasia)
REFUSAL TO DEFECATE DUE TO PAIN	Paraprostatic cyst (dogs)
Proctitis	Pelvic fracture
Inflammatory bowel disease	Enlarged sublumbar lymph nodes
Histoplasmosis	Screwtail growing into anal region (bulldogs and Boston terriers)
Idiopathic	Pseudocoprostasis
Rectal neoplasia (especially dogs)	Imperforate anus
Benign rectal stricture	
Pelvic or rear leg fracture	**COLONIC DEVIATION**
Perianal fistulas (dogs, especially German shepherds)	Perineal hernia
Anal sacculitis or abscess	
Perineal abscess (cat bite abscess)	**COLONIC NEUROMUSCULAR DISEASE**
	Electrolyte abnormality
REFUSAL TO DEFECATE DUE TO BEHAVIOR OR ENVIRONMENT	Hypokalemia
	Hypercalcemia
House-trained animals that have their routine broken	Neuromuscular disease
Cats in new or altered environments, soiled litterbox	Dysautonomia (cats)
Lack of exercise	Congenital defects (Manx cats)
Paraplegia	Spinal cord disease
	Hypothyroidism (dogs)

sible if too much is used for too long. Overdosing sucralfate is easy, as the dose must be estimated from recommendations for humans. Opiates are constipating, but because they are typically used to treat diarrhea, constipation is seldom a complaint. Excessive barium sulfate or Kaopectate in dehydrated patients may be responsible. Anticholinergics and antihistamines occasionally produce constipation.

Refusal to defecate is typically due to either pain or behavior. Pain may be from inflammation or mechanical obstruction. Foreign bodies may cause obstruction, but this is uncommon because objects that pass through the pylorus and ileocolic valve will pass through the rectum—un-less a sharp point catches at the anus. Severe spasm may result, which intensifies the pain and promotes retention of the foreign object.

Rectal inflammation causing constipation has multiple causes. Severe proctitis may be due to trauma (foreign object), bacteria, or immune-mediated mechanisms. Perirectal pain is commonly due to anal sacculitis or perianal fistulas. Some patients cannot assume a normal posture for defecating due to pain from arthritis or hindlimb fractures, while others have disease preventing normal ambulation (spinal cord disease or orthopedic problems).

Well house-trained pets or nervous animals, especially cats, may refuse to defecate unless familiar conditions are present. Other cats may refuse to defecate because the litter box is soiled or different, or because of the addition of a new pet or a new person to the household. Some dogs will not defecate if their normal routine of walks or activity is interrupted, in part because physical activity is needed to stimulate defecation.

Colonic or anal obstruction may be intraluminal, intramural, or extracolonic. Intraluminal obstruction is primarily due to rectal neoplasms and, occasionally, foreign objects. Not all neoplasms are malignant (adenomatous polyps); however, benign polyps are rarely large enough to obstruct. Obstructing foreign objects are invariably at the rectum unless there is a partial stricture in front of it. As the object tries to pass through the rectum, it usually causes pain, resulting in reflex tightening of the anus, causing more pain and obstruction, which causes rectal spasm and so on.

Intramural obstructions can occur anywhere along the colon. Colonic adenocarcinomas are usually rectal. Benign rectal strictures and granulomatous proctitis or colitis are due to uncertain causes. Cicatrix may be due to chronic colitis or other lesions.

Extracolonic obstructions are typically due to a fractured pelvis, enlarged prostate gland, paraprostatic cyst, sublumbar or pelvic lymphadenopathy, or tumors in the posterior abdomen. Occasionally, pelvic abscesses of undetermined origin may be responsible.

Colonic wall weakness is uncommonly documented, and when it occurs it is often debatable whether it is the cause of the constipation or the result of chronic colonic distention secondary to constipation. Some breeds (Manx cats) have a predisposition for pelvic neurologic deficits leading to constipation. Hypothyroidism and perhaps hypercalcemia or hypokalemia may produce colonic weakness. The idiopathic constipation and megacolon described in cats may be due at least in part to primary colonic dysfunction or behavior leading to voluntary fecal retention.

Hirschsprung's disease is often mentioned when pets with megacolon are discussed. Hirschsprung's disease is a congenital aganglionosis of the rectum preventing the rectal sphincter from relaxing, which in turn produces a functional ob-

struction. This is not well documented in dogs and cats.

CLINICAL SIGNS

Dogs and cats do not have to defecate daily to be normal. When constipation occurs, tenesmus and dyschezia are usually the major signs noticed by the client. Sometimes the client recognizes that a pet without tenesmus has not defecated for an inappropriately long time. Finally, the owner may observe excessively hard stools, which usually indicate some degree of constipation, even if the frequency of defecation is normal.

Constipated patients usually have tenesmus preceding elimination of feces and may assume a half-squatting position when attempting to defecate. Some vocalize because of pain when defecating. Obstipated patients may be depressed and anorectic, losing weight and, if perforation occurs, in acute septic shock.

Patients with colitis and proctitis typically have tenesmus persisting after defecation. They continue to strain despite there being nothing left in the colon. In this respect they resemble stranguric pets that continue to strain after all the urine has been evacuated from the urinary bladder.

DIAGNOSTIC APPROACH

When tenesmus occurs, one should first determine whether it indicates colorectal or urinary disease (Fig. 38-1 and Table 38-2).

Male cats with urethral blockage causing large, hard, inexpressible urinary bladders are often believed to be constipated. Male and female cats with nonobstructed cystitis causing a small, obviously uncomfortable urinary bladder also strain; however, they typically void at least small amounts of urine allowing recognition of the urinary problem.

After urinary tract disease is eliminated by history and physical examination, visual and digital rectal examination are indicated. Visual examination may reveal rectal prolapses, congenital imperforate anus, pseudocoprostasis, peri-

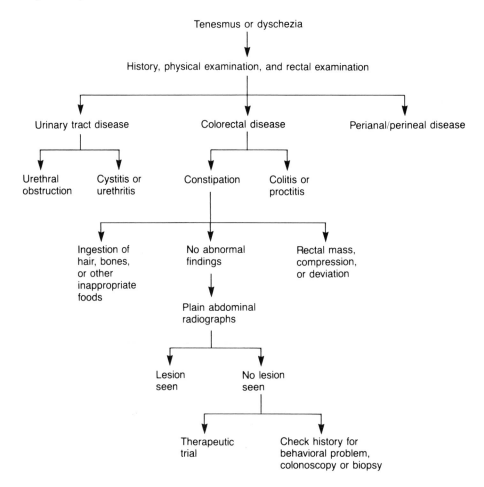

Figure 38–1. *Diagnostic approach to tenesmus or dyschezia.*

anal fistulas, small lesions on the exterior of the anus that would be missed by digital examination, and even some perineal hernias. If necessary, the patient should be chemically restrained to allow examination.

Digital rectal examination should be done on a conscious animal, anesthesia being reserved for intractable patients or those in extreme pain. The examiner should search for hard feces, soft-tissue obstruction, bony obstruction, foreign objects, deviation of the rectal canal, and inappropriate rectal or perirectal pain. In male dogs, the prostate gland should be carefully considered, as benign prostatic hyperplasia is a common cause of tenesmus (see Chapter 57). Fecal material should be retrieved and examined for foreign objects,

hair, bones, and other inappropriate substances. Special care should be taken to feel for partial rectal strictures that are not obvious during a hasty palpation. Anal sacs should be expressed and their contents examined for evidence of inflammation.

One must determine whether constipation is present. Hard, dry feces in the colon, or intestines distended with feces may be detected by digital rectal examination or abdominal palpation. If diarrhea is present, then large bowel disease is suspected and the case is approached as discussed in Chapter 37. Pseudocoprostasis occurs when hair and fecal matter has matted over the anus, thus effectively obstructing it. The perianal tissues are usually inflamed and painful.

Table 38–2 *Laboratory Assessment of Constipation*

Test	What to Check For
Serum biochemistry profile	Hypercalcemia (due to malignancy, including anal sac carcinoma) Hypokalemia (due to many causes; see Chapter 72) Hypercholesterolemia (hypothyroidism)
Abdominal radiographs	Mass (especially in or near pelvis) Pelvic fracture Megacolon
Serum T4	Decreased level (hypothyroidism)

Anal prolapses may protrude several centimeters from the anus or may be an area of eventration only occurring along a segment of the anal circumference. Rectal prolapses are especially common in young animals, in which they are secondary to rectal straining associated with diarrhea. If a rectal prolapse is evident, one should carefully palpate around the everted colonic mucosa to ascertain that it is a rectal prolapse and not a long ileocolic intussusception extending out of the anus.

Perianal fistulas classically occur in German shepherd dogs, although other breeds are afflicted. These dogs may display pain and vigorously resist lifting of the tail. Once the area is visualized, one or more draining tracts are usually obvious. Perineal hernias may result in impacted feces in a rectal diverticula, with subsequent bulging of one side of the perineum. Careful rectal examination reveals a diverticula on the side of the rectum due to lack of muscular support.

Anal sacculitis is detected by finding a painful anal sac filled with purulent secretions. There is often associated soft-tissue swelling. Occasionally, these sacs cannot be expressed due to occlusion of the duct, but a developing abscess or obvious cellulitis is present.

Constipation requires a review of the history and physical examination for obvious causes (*e.g.*, drug or dietary considerations, a Manx cat with neurologic defects, or English bulldog with a screwtail growing into the anal region). However, one should always search for colonic obstruction and rectal pain to ascertain that there is not another problem (a partial obstruction) that has been made manifest by poor diet or drug therapy.

Plain radiographs are indicated to look for undetected soft-tissue masses or pelvic fractures. Feces stopping abruptly before the rectum (Fig. 38-2) suggest obstruction, although foreign material (sand or bones) may cause similar findings. Sometimes it is helpful to repeat the radiographs after feces have been removed with enemas.

Soft-tissue masses should be biopsied regardless of size, as many are not neoplastic. Fine needle aspiration should be done on extracolonic

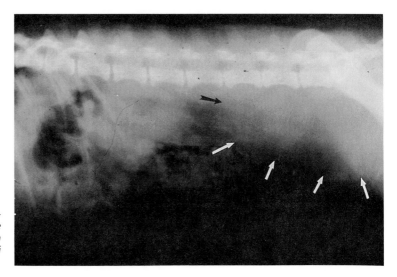

Figure 38–2. *Lateral thoracic radiograph of a constipated dog that has a megacolon due to a massive pelvic lymph node (arrows) compressing the colon ventrally. (Courtesy of Dr. Gregg Boring, Mississippi State University.)*

masses before endoscopic or incisional biopsies. Pelvic canal abscesses can be large and so hard that clinicians believe them to be a bony proliferation. Such abscesses often contain sterile, necrotic fluid. Biopsy of enlarged lymph nodes may reveal metastatic neoplasia. Sublumbar lymph nodes large enough to cause colonic obstruction should be palpable, allowing transabdominal fine needle aspiration (see Fig. 38-2).

If the cause of constipation is not found radiographically, colonoscopy and biopsy are indicated to look for inflammatory and obstructive diseases (see Colonoscopy, Mucosal Scraping, and Biopsy in Chapter 80). Barium enemas are rarely useful, but can be done if one does not have access to a colonoscope. Feces should be removed if possible. Endoscopy may reveal strictures or ulcers undetected by radiographs. Ulcerated or cauliflowerlike obstructions are usually diagnosed by endoscopic biopsy (Fig. 38-3). However, smooth-surfaced masses may represent extracolonic or submucosal proliferations. Fine needle aspirates should be done first. Next, a biopsy deep enough to reach the submucosa is needed, something which does not always happen unless a rigid endoscope is used and the operator purposefully seeks to obtain the deeper, firmer tissue. Finally, colonic biopsies should be done if lesions have not been noted.

Patients without evidence of dietary, iatrogenic, obstructive, or pain-related causes may have behavioral problems or colonic weakness. For the former, one may resolve the constipation with enemas and then see how well the patient does once it is returned to its normal environment or daily routine. For the latter, the patient's thyroid status may be determined by resting or thyroid stimulating hormone-stimulated serum T4 values. Serum calcium and potassium concentrations should be checked. If a cause cannot be determined, then the constipation is termed *idiopathic*.

MANAGEMENT

Treatment for tenesmus and constipation may be symptomatic or specific in nature. Specific therapy to correct the underlying cause is preferable, but the problem is not always obvious. One must search for underlying causes because successful symptomatic therapy may allow a previously treatable lesion to progress and eventually become untreatable.

Symptomatic Therapy

Symptomatic therapy for constipation consists principally of dietary change, laxatives, or enemas. Dietary therapy refers to providing a diet with adequate fiber. Insoluble fiber (coarse wheat bran) or soluble fiber with insoluble characteristics (psyllium hydrocolloid [Metamucil]) can increase stool bulk and moisture content. However, adequate water must be available or else the increased fiber may cause constipation. Canned pumpkin pie filling may also be used as a source of fiber; it is more often accepted by cats.

Laxatives and stool softeners are typically used (Table 38-3) because clients desire more immediate results. Laxatives should be mild if one is unsure whether the fecal mass can be expelled by

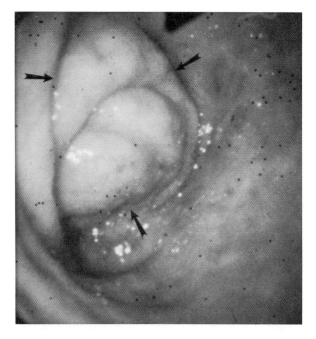

Figure 38–3. *Endoscopic view of a colon from a constipated German shepherd with a colonic obstruction (arrows) not seen radiographically. This is a granuloma due to blastomycosis.*

Table 38–3 *Selected Laxatives and Stool Softeners*

Bisacodyl: 5 mg/day (cat); 5 to 10 mg/day (dog)
Mineral oil: 5 to 20 ml once to twice daily (dog)
Docusate sodium: 50 mg/day (cat); 50 to 200 mg/day (dog)
Psyllium hydrocolloid: 1 teaspoon per can of food
Coarse wheat bran: 1 to 3 tablespoons per can of food
Lactulose: 1 ml/4.5 kg PO up to three times daily

this means, because strong laxatives or cathartics may cause pain or rupture if the patient is obstructed. Bisacodyl (Dulcolax) is a mild, irritant laxative that can also be used in conjunction with dietary fiber therapy in the conservative management of idiopathic constipation. Orally administered mineral oil is a good lubricant, but careless administration can cause aspiration pneumonia. Petrolatum (Laxatone 1–5 ml orally once daily) may be given instead, and is safer. Wetting agents such as docusate sodium (colace) have a detergent action, promoting water penetration into hard, dry feces. However, it is not advisable to use these wetting agents in conjunction with mineral oil. Osmotic laxatives such as lactulose (initially give 1 ml/4.5 kg orally three times daily, and then adjust dose to maintain desired fecal consistency) may be used chronically to increase fecal water. Be careful that severe overdosage of lactulose does not cause significant free water loss and hypernatremia. Glycerin suppositories also stimulate defecation.

Warm water enemas with or without Ivory or castile soap (do not use products with hexachlorophene) usually resolve constipation. The patient should be adequately hydrated lest the water simply be absorbed from the colon instead of softening the fecal mass. Large volumes of water are administered by gravity flow as far into the colon as possible, but rapid administration can cause vomiting. Be especially careful if a syringe is used to deliver the fluid (as in a cat) because acute colonic distention may cause pain.

For especially hard feces retention enemas may be required. As much water as can be administered without stimulating elimination is given six to eight times per day so that the feces can absorb and retain it. Even with such therapy, 2 to 4 days may be required to defecate the fecal mass.

Osmotic enemas (hypertonic phosphate preparations) should not be used unless the patient can assuredly defecate the material promptly. Otherwise, smaller dogs and cats may have colonic sequestration of fluid, causing depression, ataxia, vomiting, hypernatremia, hyperphosphatemia, hypocalcemia, and metabolic acidosis. Some patients have died from such treatment.

If the constipation is not responding to the enemas and mild laxatives, one should resist the temptation to manually break down the mass per rectum with hemostats. While this approach can be effective, it can also damage the already insulted colonic mucosa if it is done carelessly. Given time, conservative therapy should work. Metoclopramide is not useful, although cisapride (canine and feline doses not yet determined) may be helpful in stimulating colonic motility.

If megacolon exists, it may be necessary to remove the feces through a laparotomy. In animals that have had megacolon for a short time, removal of feces may allow the colon to return to normal size. However, severe, intractable constipation with irreversible colonic dilatation may necessitate colectomy and ileorectal anastomosis (Rosin, Additional Reading). The latter has been effective in some cats with intractable, idiopathic megacolon.

Symptomatic therapy may also be performed for tenesmus or dyschezia of unknown origin. If there is pain at defecation but the reason is occult despite appropriate diagnostics, empirical antibacterial therapy with drugs effective against anaerobic bacteria (*e.g.*, chloramphenicol, amoxicillin, cefazolin, metronidazole) is reasonable. If that is also unsuccessful, corticosteroid therapy (prednisolone 1.1 mg/kg orally once daily) may be considered on a trial basis.

Specific Therapy

Specific therapy for constipation varies with the cause. Controlling access of patients to bones and other undesirable food stuffs plus withdrawing constipating drugs is obvious. Long-haired animals should be groomed to remove the source of hair. Pelvic canal obstructions generally necessitate surgery. Castration may reduce benign prostatic hyperplasia. Surgery is needed for paraprostatic cysts, perineal hernias, growth of a misshapened tail into the anal area, congenital imperforate anus, abscesses in the pelvic canal, and fractured pelvic bones. Systemic diseases (*e.g.*, hypothyroidism, hypercalcemia, or hypokalemia) must also be treated as needed.

Neoplasms must be histologically defined because colonic adenocarcinoma, the most common canine rectal neoplasm, requires aggressive surgery if metastasis is not obvious. On the other hand, benign rectal strictures may be resected or the anus mechanically dilated to break down the fibrous ring. Rectal polyps are readily resected. Sublumbar lymph nodes that are enlarged often contain lymphosarcoma or carcinoma cells. Neither tumor can be cured by resection, because lymphosarcoma is disseminated and carcinoma in the node represents metastasis. Lymphosarcoma may be treated with chemotherapy, often with rewarding results.

Animals with constipation due to proctitis or colitis should have the feces removed by way of enemas, and then the inflammatory disease treated as per Chapter 37. Rectal foreign objects should be removed digitally or during proctoscopy. Fecal material causing pseudocoprostasis is first soaked and then gently removed. A topical steroid–antibiotic ointment (Panalog, Cortisporin) is usually helpful in alleviating irritation.

Anal sacculitis is usually treated medically (express the contents, infuse an antibiotic–steroid combination [Panalog] into the sac, and apply warm compresses), but treatment of anal sac abscesses varies. A ruptured abscess should be irrigated with saline or povidone–iodine and a hot pack should be applied. Systemic antibiotics (*e.g.*, amoxicillin, cefazolin) are indicated. If intact, it should be lanced if there is an obvious head or soft spot. Otherwise, hot compresses should be used until a soft spot occurs. If recurrent, the anal sacs can be excised.

Chronic, idiopathic constipation of cats that do not have a megacolon should be treated with a combination of insoluble dietary fiber, mild laxatives (bisacodyl or lubricants), and enemas as needed. There should be no reason why the cat would be reluctant or unable to use the litter box, such as failure to remove feces, new animals in the household, or moving the litter box to a new location. Recurrent megacolon may necessitate subtotal colectomy.

Rectal prolapses may be treated in several ways. The rectal mucosa is carefully replaced digitally, and a rectal examination then ensures that there is not an intussuscepted section. In mild cases, replacement of the rectum with or without the use of a topical antibiotic–steroid ointment may be all that is needed. One should always look for a cause of irritation that was probably responsible, such as infectious enteritis or intestinal parasites. In more severe or persistent cases, a purse-string suture may be placed in the rectum for 1 to 3 days so that the animal can defecate but cannot reprolapse the rectum. Retention Kaopectate or barium sulfate enemas alleviate some discomfort and decrease straining. If there is still recurrence, epidural anesthesia, colopexy, or resection of the prolapse may be considered. Colopexy is usually successful unless there is devitalized tissue requiring resection.

Perianal fistulas require surgical excision and fulguration of the tracts, plus postoperative antibiotics. Antibiotics by themselves are ineffectual. These tracts may recur after surgery and necessitate repeated operations. Care must be taken during the surgery to avoid destroying the anal sphincter. Likewise, postoperative anal stricture formation may necessitate surgery.

PATIENT MONITORING

Untreated constipation eventually produces megacolon. Megacolon is a lower intestinal obstruction, and although not an immediate problem, it can eventually cause the patient's death. If the underlying cause can be resolved, the prognosis is good. Otherwise, conservative medical management is often successful, except when there is untreatable neurologic disease of the pelvic area or idiopathic megacolon in cats. Once therapy for constipation is begun, the clients will usually be able to determine whether or not it is effective by observing the animal.

Although not reported in veterinary medicine, extended overuse of laxatives in humans has been found to result in temporary or permanent colonic damage. Consequently, clients should be cautioned against overuse of these drugs.

Benign prostatic hyperplasia responds well to castration, and paraprostatic cysts do not usually recur after surgery (see Chapter 57). Perineal hernias may recur and necessitate repeated surgery. Colonic adenocarcinomas have a very poor prognosis, as they have often spread by the time of diagnosis. Proctitis can usually be resolved, allowing normal defecation. Anal sac disease should be cured by appropriate therapy, including surgery. Cats with idiopathic constipation must be carefully monitored, especially if there are multiple cats in the household. They should be fed separately to ensure that they are receiving fiber and they should have a separate litter box to ensure that they are defecating normally. Failure to adequately control constipation may result in megacolon. Rectal prolapses should be curable. Animals with rectal prolapses should be checked twice daily for the first 2 to 4 days to guard against reprolapse. Perianal fistulas are apt to recur after surgery, and the prognosis is guarded for cure. Dogs with perianal fistulas need to be examined every 3 to 6 months for the first year after apparent resolution of the problem to ensure that there is no recurrence. Pain of occult cause often responds to antibiotics or corticosteroid therapy.

ADDITIONAL READING

Burrows CF. Constipation. In: Kirk RW, ed. Current veterinary therapy IX. Philadelphia: WB Saunders, 1986: 904.

Dimske DS. Using dietary fiber to manage constipation. In: Managing fiber-responsive disease. Veterinary Medicine Publishing Co, 1988: 25.

Greiner TP, Johnson RG, Betts CW. Diseases of the rectum and anus. In: Ettinger SJ, ed. Textbook of veterinary internal medicine, 2nd ed. Philadelphia: WB Saunders, 1983: 1493.

Rosin E, Walshaw R, Mehlhaff C et al. Subtotal colectomy for treatment of chronic constipation associated with idiopathic megacolon in cats: 38 cases (1979–1985). J Am Vet Med Assoc 1988; 193:850.

39

PANCREATITIS
Michael D. Willard

Canine pancreatitis is a relatively common recurrent disease that is often misdiagnosed because of its varied clinical presentations and the lack of sensitive, specific tests. It is rare in cats. The majority of cases in cats are documented only at surgery or necropsy.

CAUSES

There are numerous causes of experimental pancreatitis, but these will not be discussed. Traumatic pancreatitis occurs secondary to automobile-associated trauma, the high-rise syndrome, and surgery, in which it is particularly prevalent following major gastric and duodenal resection–reconstruction and prolonged procedures requiring manipulation in the region of the pancreas. Pancreatitis may rarely be associated with toxoplasmosis, feline infectious peritonitis, and infection with *Eurytrema procyonis*. Of uncertain significance in dogs and cats is drug-induced pancreatitis. Azathioprine and L-asparaginase have been implicated in pets, while furosemide and corticosteroids are possible causes in humans. Hypercalcemia may cause canine pancreatitis, although this is uncommon. Pancreatic adenocarcinoma may cause pancreatitis.

The conditions most commonly associated with canine pancreatitis typically involve lipids: excessive fat ingestion, hyperlipidemia, and obesity. Hyperlipidemia seems to be a major risk factor. Most hyperlipidemia is postprandial; true fasting hyperlipidemia (opalescent to white plasma after a 12-hour fast) is usually due to diabetic ketoacidosis, hypothyroidism, or idiopathic hyperlipidemia. The cause of the latter is uncertain, but an enzymatic abnormality is likely. Idiopathic hyperlipidemia may be found in any dog, but schnauzers have a higher than expected incidence of it and acute pancreatitis.

PATHOPHYSIOLOGY

Fat (in the diet or the blood) seems to be the most important cause of spontaneous canine pancreatitis, and appears to induce it by activation of pancreatic phospholipase or elastase. Ostensibly, the activated enzymes leak into surrounding tissues, causing destruction of pancreatic acinar tissue and subsequent nonseptic inflammation. This process can be self-perpetuating because the inflammation impairs normal pancreatic circulation, which allows the inflammation and enzyme leakage to persist or worsen. This has been referred to as "autodigestion" of the pancreas.

Pancreatic inflammation stimulates vagal afferent nerves and the medullary vomiting center. Abdominal pain or fever may occur, and the liver and transverse colon, due to their close proximity to the pancreas, can be damaged by leaking enzymes.

In mild to moderate cases with adequate pancreatic perfusion, there is usually spontaneous resolution. This milder form is called *edematous pancreatitis*. The more severe forms usually have gross pancreatic bleeding and have been called *hemorrhagic pancreatitis*. In hemorrhagic pancreatitis, extensive inflammation may cause significant abdominal fluid sequestration, which, plus the fluid losses due to vomiting and anorexia, causes severe hypovolemic shock. Serum albumin and calcium concentrations may also decrease; however, the poor perfusion is more serious, as it may worsen the pancreatitis. Severe inflammation may cause sludging of pancreatic blood flow and disseminated intravascular coagulation. Fat embolization may result in renal or other organ failure. Release of myocardial depressant factor (a small polypeptide that inhibits cardiac function) has also been described. This peptide supposedly produces a positive feedback loop, which decreases cardiac output, leading to more severe pancreatitis.

Severe acute pancreatic swelling or chronic scarring can occlude the main bile duct as it courses through the pancreas. Chronic pancreatitis may also produce granulomas and similar obstruction, thus causing icterus.

Destruction of the islets of Langerhans', with resultant diabetes mellitus or destruction of exocrine pancreatic tissue, producing exocrine pancreatic insufficiency, is an uncommon sequela. In dogs, diabetes mellitus and exocrine pancreatic insufficiency are infrequently attributable to pancreatitis. The common association of acute pancreatitis with diabetic ketoacidosis may be due to the hyperlipidemia commonly accompanying uncontrolled diabetes.

A severe complication is pancreatic abscess formation. Although the precise mechanism by which a pancreatic abscess occurs is unknown, this accumulation of necrotic tissue or fluid can produce relentless vomiting, depression, and abdominal pain. Most pancreatic abscesses are nonseptic, although septic abscesses are rarely seen.

Occasionally, fat necrosis occurs in areas remote from the pancreas (*e.g.*, the subcutaneous tissues), ostensibly due to extensive release of lipase into the circulation. This syndrome is uncommon.

CLINICAL SIGNS

Animals with pancreatitis may be asymptomatic or may have clinical disease ranging from mild to severe and peracute to chronic. Asymptomatic disease is suggested by finding patients that have severe pancreatic scarring or granuloma formation despite no history of vomiting or other signs suggesting pancreatitis.

The most common and consistent sign of acute canine pancreatitis is vomiting; it is usually coupled with anorexia. Vomiting can be postprandial or may occur on an empty stomach. Bile is commonly present in the vomitus, but hematemesis is uncommon. Noticeable abdominal pain and fever are less consistent. Icterus and acholic stools may occur if the bile duct is occluded from swelling or scarring. Azotemia and uremia may also occur. Rarely, generalized subcutaneous fat necrosis produces sterile abscesses over the body, which can be extremely painful.

Feline pancreatitis may or may not have such obvious signs. Some cats will only evidence chronic weight loss, while others will have varying degrees of vomiting. Anorexia, dehydration, jaundice, and abdominal discomfort have also been reported.

DIAGNOSTIC APPROACH

Although possible in any dog or cat, pancreatitis is most common in dogs that are obese, are fed table scraps, have access to fatty scraps (*e.g.*, trimmings or waste baskets), or have fasting hyperlipidemia. There may be a history of repeated bouts of what clients describe as a "sensitive stomach." The clients have often reached this conclusion because the pet vomits when there is a minor dietary change, or for no obvious reason. This can produce a self-perpetuating problem in which a spoiled pet will eat only certain foods from the owners' table. The tendency of the patient to vomit reinforces to the clients that the animal needs "special dietary consideration," and they persist in feeding inappropriate foods. Many of these clients do not feed commercial dog foods or they supplement them with table scraps. The diagnostician must carefully consider this aspect of the history lest the owners, who may suspect the diet to be partially responsible and consequently feel some guilt, volunteer a less than complete description of the animal's diet.

Miniature schnauzers are so commonly affected with idiopathic hyperlipidemia and pancreatitis that any vomiting miniature schnauzer should be suspected of having acute pancreatitis. Likewise, a history of prior vomiting in this breed suggests pancreatitis. Finally, all dogs with diabetic ketoacidosis or icterus not due to hemolysis should be screened for pancreatitis.

Cranial abdominal pain is common in pancreatitis, although it may be difficult to detect, especially in severely depressed patients. More stoic dogs do not readily show evidence of abdominal discomfort. If a vomiting patient has anterior abdominal pain, pancreatitis is likely, but one must also consider a perforating linear foreign body, peritonitis, acute hepatitis, necrotizing cholecystitis, and, occasionally, gastritis.

Severe pancreatitis can produce hypovolemic shock, and most patients with pancreatitis are somewhat dehydrated. However, dehydration may be difficult to detect, as many of these patients are obese, which makes skin-tenting unlikely despite extracellular volume depletion. Nausea may cause oral mucous membranes to be moist despite volume depletion. Vomiting patients should be screened for acute pancreatitis. Severe, progressive acute abdomen may necessitate surgery before all test results are received; however, one should seek to eliminate pancreatitis from the differential diagnosis before surgery.

The most common screening tests for acute pancreatitis are serum amylase and serum lipase activities. Dogs and cats with acute pancreatitis often have increased serum amylase or lipase activities. If either of these values is greater than twice normal, it suggests pancreatitis, assuming that other consistent clinicopathologic changes are present. However, these tests can be insensitive, and some patients with severe pancreatitis (even pancreatic abscesses) have normal or minimally increased values, while others with marked increases do not have significant pancreatic disease (low serum lipase concentration almost always eliminates a diagnosis of pancreatitis). Therefore, one should request both determinations plus a complete blood count, serum biochemistry profile, and urinalysis if pancreatitis is possible. Serum lipase activity may be more sensitive in the cat. The saccharogenic method of assaying serum amylase is misleading in dogs due to naturally occurring serum maltase activity. Urinary amylase excretion is a valuable diagnostic aid in humans, but has not been useful in dogs.

Serum amylase and lipase activities are typically increased less than two times normal by decreased glomerular filtration, although they may occasionally be increased more than that. This can cause diagnostic confusion, because pancreatitis can cause prerenal azotemia due to shock. The question then arises whether pancreatitis produced the increased amylase or lipase and blood urea nitrogen or creatinine values, or if something caused azotemia and secondarily increased serum amylase or lipase activities. A urinalysis should aid in differentiating these situations. Renal azotemia should prevent adequate concentration of the urine (urine specific gravity less than 1.030 in the dog or 1.035 in the cat), whereas azotemia secondary to pancreatitis is the result of poor cardiac output plus decreased renal perfusion, which should produce appropriately concentrated urine (urine specific gravity greater than 1.030 in the dog or 1.035 in the cat).

Patients with acute pancreatitis usually have a mild to dramatic neutrophilic leukocytosis with or without a left shift. In addition, many dogs with pancreatitis have increased alanine aminotransferase and serum alkaline phophatase activities due to the close proximity of the pancreas to the liver and the main bile duct. Increased serum alkaline phosphatase activity may occur regardless of whether or not the patient becomes icteric. Hypocalcemia is due to uncertain reasons; however, it is not usually of diagnostic or therapeutic

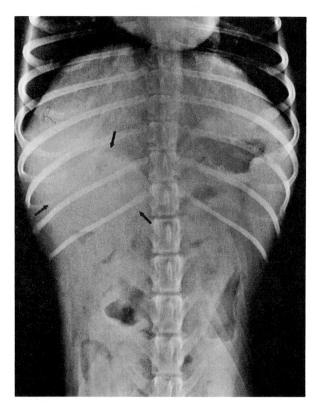

Figure 39–1. *Ventrodorsal radiograph of a schnauzer with acute pancreatitis. Note the loss of contrast within the right cranial abdominal quadrant (arrows).*

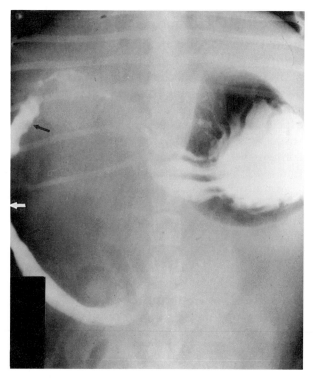

Figure 39–2. *Ventrodorsal barium contrast radiograph of a schnauzer with diabetic ketoacidosis that was vomiting profusely. Note the lateral deviation of the duodenum (arrow), suggesting a mass in the region of the pancreas.*

significance. Hyperlipidemia in a vomiting dog is suggestive of pancreatitis, but the hyperlipidemia may simply be postprandial or an incidental finding.

Plain radiographs may aid in the diagnosis of pancreatitis (Fig. 39-1). Decreased serosal contrast in the right cranial abdominal quadrant, a mass-effect displacing the duodenum, a widening of the angle between the stomach and the duodenum, or localized dilatation of the duodenum ("sentinel loop") may be seen with acute pancreatitis. Contrast radiographs may reveal duodenal changes not detected otherwise: duodenal dilatation, constriction, or displacement (Figs. 39-2 and 39-3). However, lack of radiographic changes does not make pancreatitis less likely. If ultrasonography is available, pancreatic masses may be detected.

Rarely, abdominal exudate will be caused by pancreatitis. In such cases, the amylase activity

of the fluid will supposedly be greater than that of serum. However, most patients with pancreatitis have relatively little abdominal fluid, and, if present, it will be in the region of the pancreas.

Surgery may be diagnostic in patients that do not have expected changes in serum amylase or lipase activities or abdominal radiographs. In dogs, this approach is usually only taken when there is a severe progressive acute abdomen or chronic, undiagnosed vomiting. Surgery should not be done hastily, as it is rarely therapeutic in these patients unless there is a pancreatic abscess. In fact, surgery can be counterproductive in patients with medically manageable disease. At surgery, pancreatitis can be grossly obvious (*e.g.,* edema, hemorrhage or abscess) or inapparent. Even marked pancreatitis may not have grossly evident disease. Therefore, careful biopsy may be warranted.

Not as well defined as its canine counterpart,

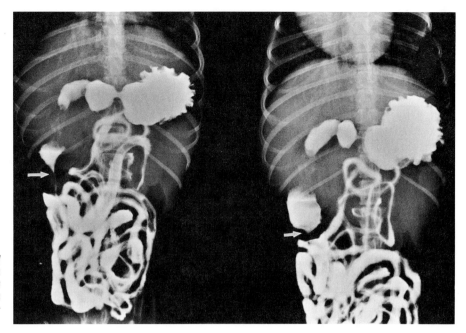

Figure 39–3. *Two ventrodorsal barium contrast radiographs of a schnauzer with chronic pancreatitis that show duodenal dilatation and a focal constriction (arrows) consistent with pancreatitis.*

feline pancreatitis seems more prone to cause chronic weight loss without vomiting and abdominal pain. Pancreatitis seems to be relatively infrequent, while pancreatic adenocarcinoma seems to be more prevalent in cats than in dogs. Therefore, exploratory surgery may be more likely to be the means of diagnosing feline pancreatitis. If a localized or diffuse pancreatic mass is found, histopathology is indicated. The size of the mass does not indicate whether it is neoplastic or inflammatory. Furthermore, both pancreatitis and pancreatic adenocarcinoma may cause multiple mesenteric lesions due to fat saponification or metastasis, respectively. Finding neoplastic cells on cytologic examination of these lesions is definitive. However, many patients with pancreatic adenocarcinoma have inflamed areas within the tumor that, if evaluated cytologically, may result in a misdiagnosis of pancreatitis.

Trypsinlike immunoreactivity (used for diagnosing exocrine pancreatic insufficiency) may be increased due to pancreatitis. Other assays for similar circulating peptides indicative of pancreatitis are being tested, but no such test is currently available.

Methemalbuminemia can be associated with pancreatitis. Most dogs with acute pancreatitis

that have been tested had increased serum methemalbumin concentrations, but the test has not been widely used and is not readily available for veterinarians.

Cats with pancreatitis should be screened for toxoplasmosis or feline infectious peritonitis. Serology (especially immunoglobulin M titers) and retinal examination are useful for the former, while analysis of effusions, retinal examination, or protein electrophoresis on serum or effusions may be helpful for the latter.

MANAGEMENT

Therapy principally consists of fluid, electrolyte, and acid-base support plus preventing oral intake until the pancreatic inflammation resolves (see Chapters 71 and 72). All oral intake should be stopped until the patient has not vomited for at least 48 to 72 hours. During that time, aggressive fluid therapy must ensure adequate pancreatic perfusion to prevent edematous disease from becoming hemorrhagic. The most common mistake is failure to adequately maintain the intravascular compartment and cardiac output. Even when one calculates maintenance and deficit fluid requirements, ongoing losses from vomiting and abdominal sequestration must be considered. It is usually better to give a little too much fluid therapy rather than too little.

Other therapies have been tried, but none have clearly been beneficial in human studies. Parasympatholytics (*e.g.*, atropine or propantheline bromide) have been used to decrease pancreatic secretions, as have glucagon and somatostatin. Antibiotics have been used prophylactically; however, septic pancreatitis appears to be rare and, when present, indicates surgery. Analgesics have been advocated, but these are rarely needed in dogs and cats (Chapter 12). Even radiation therapy has been tried. At this time, aggressive fluid therapy, preventing oral intake, antiemetics for severe vomiting, and alleviation of underlying causes are the backbone of successful therapy for canine pancreatitis.

Searching for underlying causes is appropriate, albeit rarely successful. Drug-induced canine and feline pancreatitis appears to be rare. Even though steroid administration increases serum lipase activity, this increase is usually not due to pancreatitis. Sulfa drugs and azathioprine may be responsible, and if they are being used in a patient with pancreatitis they should be withdrawn. Hypercalcemia, if present should be resolved (see Chapter 72).

Surgery is not generally indicated because pancreatitis is rarely a surgically correctable lesion. However, severe cases that progress despite appropriate therapy may be helped, especially if a pancreatic abscess can be drained. Conceivably, traumatic pancreatitis may be due to surgically correctable pancreatic duct disruption, but this is unlikely.

Occasionally, a pancreatic mass may be found during abdominal exploratory surgery. The mass should always be biopsied to determine if it is neoplastic. Resection of such a lesion should not be attempted, as the surgery may cause more morbidity and mortality than the mass. Most dogs with chronic pancreatitis causing extrahepatic obstruction will improve with conservative medical therapy. For those that remain obstructed, a cholecystojejunostomy may relieve the icterus. If this bypass procedure is performed, one should be sure that the opening between the intestine and gallbladder is large enough, so that food entering the gallbladder does not become impacted and cause an ascending infection.

Once the acute episode is controlled, the clients should be educated so as to prevent recurrence. Risk factors such as fasting hyperlipidemia, obesity, or fatty meals should be resolved by maintaining the patient on a very low fat diet (Hill's r/d or w/d). One should also look for hypothyroidism, even if the patient's clinical appearance is not suggestive. If hyperlipidemia persists despite 14 days of an appropriate low fat diet, then drug therapy (*e.g.*, gemfibrozil 150 mg orally two–three times daily for a 10-kg dog) may be used to lower serum triglyceride concentrations.

PATIENT MONITORING

Once pancreatitis has been resolved, there is little need for monitoring except to ascertain that predisposing factors (*e.g.*, hyperlipidemia or obesity) have been controlled. Failure to adequately treat acute pancreatitis may not alter the outcome if the episode is mild; however, it could result in progression to hemorrhagic pancreatitis and even death. Failure to prevent recurrence of pancreatitis may eventually lead to a severe or fatal episode of acute pancreatitis or may rarely produce exocrine pancreatic insufficiency or diabetes mellitus.

ADDITIONAL READING

Fittschen C, Bellamy JEC. Prednisone treatment alters the serum amylase and lipase activities in normal dogs without causing pancreatitis. Canadian Journal of Comparative Medicine 1984; 48:136.

Garvey MS, Zawie DA. Feline pancreatic disease. Vet Clin North Am 1984; 14:1231.

Kleine LJ, Hornbuckle WE. Acute pancreatitis: The radiographic findings in 182 dogs. Journal of the American Veterinary Radiology Society 1978; 19:102.

Matthiesen DT, Rosin E. Common bile duct obstruction secondary to chronic fibrosing pancreatitis: Treatment by use of cholecystoduodenostomy in the dog. J Am Vet Med Assoc 1986; 189:1443.

Murtaugh RJ. Acute pancreatitis: Diagnostic dilemmas. Seminars in Veterinary Medicine and Surgery 1987; 2:282.

Owens JM, Drazner FH, Gilbertson SR. Pancreatic disease in the cat. Journal of the American Animal Hospital Association 1975; 11:83.

Salisbury SK, Lantz GC, Nelson RW, Kazacos EA. Pancreatic abscess in dogs: Six cases (1978–1986). J Am Vet Med Assoc 1988; 193:1104.

Schaer M. A clinicopathologic survey of acute pancreatitis in 30 dogs and 5 cats. Journal of the American Animal Hospital Association 1979; 15:681.

40

HEPATIC DISEASE

Michael D. Willard

Hepatic disease is varied in its presentation, and thus requires increased awareness on the part of the clinician for diagnosis and treatment.

CAUSES

Hepatic disease may be due to processes centered in the liver (primary hepatic disease) or it may be secondary to problems in other organs that secondarily damage the liver. Infiltrative, infectious, metabolic, toxic, or congestive disorders (Table 40-1) typically affect the liver. Congenital portovascular anomalies (venous shunts) may cause atrophy and hepatic insufficiency.

PATHOPHYSIOLOGY

The causes of hepatic disease may be divided into three principal processes: impairment of biliary flow, hepatocyte destruction or dysfunction, and vascular anomalies. Each of these will be considered separately, and then the results of hepatic failure or insufficiency will be considered as a group. The pathophysiology of icterus will not be considered in detail here, as it is dealt with in Chapter 3.

Impairment of Biliary Flow

Obstruction of biliary structures (cholestasis) may be due to focal disease that blocks a major duct (e.g., a stone, tumor, or granuloma of the bile duct) or diffuse changes causing obstruction of bile canaliculi throughout the hepatic parenchyma (e.g., hepatocellular swelling, diffuse fibrosis, or infiltration). Increased serum alkaline phosphatase activity due to enzyme induction is one of the first clinicopathologic changes. This happens more quickly in the dog than in the cat. Next, urine bilirubin increases, and eventually the serum bilirubin concentration may increase; thus, the patient becomes jaundiced and the urine turns orange. Unless there is concurrent hepatocyte dysfunction or other underlying disease, the patient may have few other signs. Pruritus (due to bile salt deposition in the skin) rarely occurs in dogs with hepatobiliary disease.

553

Table 40–1 *Causes of Hepatic Disease*

INFILTRATIVE DISEASES

Neoplastic
   Hepatocellular carcinoma
   Bile duct carcinoma
   Disseminated disease (lymphosarcoma)
   Metastatic disease (hemangiosarcoma and others)
Inflammatory
   Cholangitis or cholangiohepatitis (especially cats)
   "Chronic active hepatitis" (dogs, especially Doberman
     pinschers)
   Lobar dissecting hepatitis
   Acute pancreatitis (especially dogs)

INFECTION

Histoplasmosis
Blastomycosis
Leptospirosis (dogs)
Infection with *Bacillus piliformis,* (Tyzzer's disease [rare])
Infectious canine hepatitis (dogs)
Feline infectious peritonitis (cats)
Infection with *Amphimerus pseudofelineus* (cats)
Septicemia

METABOLIC DISEASES

Lipidosis
   Idiopathic (cats)
   Diabetes mellitus
Copper storage disease (dogs, especially Bedlington terriers and
   West Highland White terriers)
Vacuolar hepatopathy (dogs)
   Spontaneous hyperadrenocorticism
   Iatrogenic hyperadrenocorticism
Hyperthyroidism (cats)
Intrahepatic cholestasis (dogs)
Glycogen storage disease (rare; dogs)
Urea cycle enzyme deficiencies (rare; dogs)

TOXINS

See Table 40–4

CONGESTIVE DISEASES

Right heart failure
Postcaval syndrome (especially dogs)

END-STAGE LIVER DISEASE

Cirrhosis

MISCELLANEOUS

Congenital portosystemic shunts or other congenital portal vein
   anomalies
Congenital hepatic arteriovenous fistulas
Portal vein thrombosis
Hepatic veno-occlusive disease

Hepatocyte Destruction or Dysfunction

Lack of functional hepatocytes may also produce icterus; however, other signs of hepatocellular dysfunction may be more important. Hepatocellular dysfunction may be due to hepatocyte necrosis, replacement of functional hepatocellular mass, or shunting of blood around functional hepatocytes.

Necrosis of hepatocytes is principally caused by anoxia, toxins, viral infections, or inflammation. Anoxia may be due to severe, acute anemia or passive congestion, as seen in acute right heart failure (*e.g.,* heartworm postcaval syndrome). Inflammation may be granulomatous (fungal disease such as histoplasmosis or blastomycosis), bacterial (especially in cats), or immune-mediated (suspected but seldom proved). Toxic hepatopathy may be caused by toxins (*e.g.,* heavy metal, acetaminophen, phenacetin, various petroleum derivatives), dose-dependent drug toxicity (*e.g.,* mercaptopurine or acetaminophen), or idiosyncratic, dose-independent drug toxicity (*e.g.,* halothane). The resulting hepatocellular loss may be acute, and may be responsible for severe signs. Neoplastic infiltration (lymphosarcoma) may disrupt hepatic function by crowding out hepatocytes, causing inflammation, or disrupting blood flow.

Normal hepatocellular cytosol may be replaced by proteinaceous fluid (vacuolar hepatopathy) or fat (feline hepatic lipidosis or diabetes mellitus). Vacuolar hepatopathy is principally due to glucocorticoids and is rarely responsible for clinical signs of hepatic dysfunction.

Hepatocellular fat accumulation (lipidosis), if severe, may cause hepatic failure. Fat entering the hepatocyte must be incorporated into a lipoprotein to be removed. Protein is required to make lipoproteins, and cats do not conserve protein well. Cats with excessive fat mobilization (an obese cat that becomes anorectic) or a negative nitrogen balance are at risk for hepatic lipid accumulation. Once begun, this process can become self-perpetuating: hepatocellular lipid accumulation decreases hepatic function, which causes anorexia, which causes more lipid breakdown, which causes more hepatic lipid accumulation, and so on.

Vascular Anomalies

Blood is shunted around hepatocytes by single congenital shunts or multiple acquired shunts. Congenital anomalies may produce abnormal connections between the hepatic portal vein and other large vessels, such as the azygous vein or the posterior vena cava. Usually solitary, such connections allow hepatic portal blood to preferentially flow into the larger vein with less resistance, thus bypassing the liver. If enough portal blood bypasses the liver, substances that would normally be removed or extracted from the blood will remain. In addition, the liver will atrophy. The pancreas normally empties into the portal vein, resulting in the liver being exposed to a higher concentration of insulin than the rest of the body. This increased exposure to insulin is necessary for the liver to maintain its size; therefore, shunting of portal blood around the liver causes progressive hepatic atrophy. Thus, a congenital portosystemic shunt not only prevents the liver from adequately metabolizing blood-borne substances, but also reduces its functional capacity through atrophy. The degree of hepatic atrophy and the patient's diet will determine what signs occur.

Acquired portosystemic shunting is usually due to portal hypertension secondary to hepatic cirrhosis, a condition in which extensive fibrosis occurs secondary to some prior insult. This fibrosis causes hepatic pseudolobule formation, altering normal blood flow through the hepatic sinusoids and increasing hepatic portal flow resistance. In this sense, acquired shunts are a "safety valve" that prevent splanchnic venous congestion by keeping portal venous pressures from becoming too great. However, there is also intrahepatic shunting, in which the blood that does enter the pseudolobules is shunted around many of the remaining functional hepatocytes. Ascites is more common in patients with acquired portosystemic shunts than in those with congenital shunts (see Chapter 11).

Recently, other causes of portal hypertension have been found. Veno-occlusive disease (obliteration of central veins due to fibrosis or hypertrophy) has been documented in cocker spaniel dogs. Various other congenital malformations of the portal vasculature (arterio-venous fistula) or

acquired thrombosis of the portal vein may likewise be responsible, although the cause of the latter is uncertain.

Regardless of the cause, deficient hepatic function may produce clinical signs by failure to metabolize endogenous or exogenous compounds or by inadequate synthesis of selected proteins and carbohydrates. The liver normally metabolizes toxic substances into nontoxic metabolites or excretes them. Failure to do this may cause vomiting, anorexia, weight loss, neurologic dysfunction, and various drug intoxications.

The term given to central nervous system disease secondary to hepatic failure is *hepatic encephalopathy*. It can be functional without identifiable morphologic abnormalities or may cause degenerative central nervous system changes and cerebral edema. Hepatic encephalopathy (HE) is most easily induced with anesthetics, sedatives, and narcotics that are extensively metabolized by the liver. Barbiturates may persist in the blood, resulting in very slow recoveries, while routine doses of phenothiazine derivatives may produce seizures. This problem may be worsened by the brain becoming more sensitive to the effects of these drugs.

Endogenous toxins may produce similar signs. If ammonia, aromatic amino acids, mercaptans, and skatols from the gastrointestinal tract are not removed from the portal blood, clinical signs of HE may develop. Any combination of seizures, coma, stupor, cortical blindness, ataxia, head pressing, hypermetria, or behavioral change may occur. The precise function of each substance in the pathogenesis of HE is yet unclear. It is probably multifaceted, which would explain the range of clinical signs. The signs in any given patient may vary if the diet causes greater or lesser amounts of these substances to be formed.

Hepatic failure often causes vomiting. Stimulation of the chemoreceptor trigger zone by circulating drugs or toxins is the probable cause, although hepatic inflammation may stimulate vagal afferent innervation to the medullary vomiting center. Diarrhea, possibly from maldigestion secondary to bile acid deficiency, may occur. Weight loss is common, and may be due to maldigestion, anorexia, or interruption of intermediary metabolism.

Hematuria may be due to cystic calculi. Failure of the liver to metabolize ammonia from the intestines allows blood ammonia concentrations to increase, with resultant spillage into the urine. Ammonium biurate crystals and calculi can then form (see Chapter 47).

Albumin, blood urea nitrogen, glucose, and clotting factors are synthesized in the liver; hence, hepatic failure may cause corresponding deficiencies. Hypoalbuminemia due to hepatic failure is classically associated with normal to increased serum globulins, and may be severe enough (less than 1.5 mg/dl, or 15 g/L) to produce ascites without portal hypertension (see Chapter 11). Blood urea nitrogen is important in maintaining the renal medullary concentration gradient, and lowered levels may explain why some patients with hepatic insufficiency have polyuria–polydipsia (see Chapter 9). Mild to moderate hypoglycemia can occur, producing weakness, disorientation, stupor, seizures, or coma (see Chapter 77).

The coagulation system can be affected in at least two ways. Severe hepatic failure (less than 80% of normal functional mass) may cause decreased clotting factor production. Hepatic inflammation may result in sludging of hepatic sinusoidal blood flow, resulting in disseminated intravascular coagulation. Antithrombin III, also produced in the liver, is often decreased in hepatic insufficiency, which may make disseminated intravascular coagulation more difficult to treat (see Chapter 16).

Ascites secondary to hepatic disease is typically a transudate or a modified transudate (see Chapter 11). Different hepatic diseases may cause ascites, but those producing portal hypertension are more consistently associated with ascites. Cirrhosis is a more common cause than most others, probably because it can produce hypoalbuminemia and portal hypertension simultaneously. Portal hypertension may be due to intrahepatic obstruction secondary to hepatic fibrosis and/or renal salt retention leading to overhydration. When hypertension and hypoalbuminemia occur simultaneously, ascites occurs at higher than expected serum albumin concentrations and lower than expected portal venous pressures.

CLINICAL SIGNS

The liver performs many functions, and signs may vary dramatically between patients with similar diseases (Table 40-2).

Clinical signs due to acute hepatic dysfunction may be more severe than those due to chronic hepatic disease, despite similar amounts of functional liver. This is probably because the patient with acute disease has had less time to compensate. Patients with slowly progressive hepatic disease may not show clinical signs until essentially all hepatic compensatory mechanisms are exhausted (severe cirrhosis), and even then the initial signs may be subtle (*e.g.,* polyuria–polydipsia).

Unfortunately, the most common signs of hepatic disease are nonspecific: anorexia, weight loss, or vomiting. Other reasonably common signs include polyuria–polydipsia, ascites, hepatomegaly, icterus, or HE. The latter may be particularly variable between patients. Classically peaking within hours of eating a meal (especially high protein diets and diets of low biologic value protein), some patients have constant evidence of HE, while others have intermittent signs not as-

Table 40–2 *Clinical Signs Consistent with Hepatic Disease in Dogs and Cats*

Vomiting (common)
Anorexia (common)
Weight loss (common)
Hepatomegaly (common)
Hepatic encephalopathy
    Ataxia
    Behavioral change (this is common and may mimic lethargy)
    Coma
    Cortical blindness
    Drooling (cats)
    Head pressing
    Hypermetria
    Seizures
    Slow recovery from anesthesia
    Stupor
Ascites
Diarrhea
Hematuria
Icterus
Microhepatica
Polyuria–polydipsia
Pruritus (rare)

sociated with meals. Icterus is not a sensitive sign of canine hepatic disease.

DIAGNOSTIC APPROACH

The diagnostic approach to the patient with hepatic disease consists of settling three issues. First, one must determine whether hepatic disease exists in a given patient. Second, one must determine whether that disease is clinically significant and distinguish any obvious causes. Finally, the issue of whether to biopsy and, in cases of suspected congential portosystemic shunts, whether to perform exploratory surgery or radiography must be decided (Fig. 40-1).

Determining that hepatic disease is present may occasionally be done by the history and physical examination if obvious hepatomegaly, classic HE predictably occurring after meals, or jaundice despite a near-normal hematocrit are present. More often, the history and physical examination arouse suspicion of hepatic disease, but that suspicion must be confirmed by clinical pathology laboratory testing or abdominal radiographs (Table 40-3).

The routine serum biochemistry profile tests that are most commonly examined to determine whether hepatic disease is present are the serum activities of alanine aminotransferase (ALT) and serum alkaline phosphatase (SAP). However, the diagnostic ability of these tests is limited. One must acknowledge that: there are major species differences between dogs and cats; many patients with severe hepatic disease do not have increased ALT or SAP; these tests detect hepatic disease but do not specifically identify any particular disease; these tests are not prognostic; these are not hepatic function tests; and there are other complete blood count, serum biochemistry profile and urinalysis parameters that may indicate hepatic disease even when ALT and SAP are normal.

The major differences between dogs and cats involve SAP and urine bilirubin. Canine SAP is easily induced, especially by glucocorticoids. In fact, vacuolar hepatopathy secondary to iatrogenic or spontaneous hyperadrenocorticism is a major cause of high canine SAP. Dogs commonly have significant increases in SAP (greater than four times normal) without the presence of clinically significant hepatic disease. In contrast, any increase in feline SAP suggests clinically significant hepatic disease or hyperthyroidism or diabetes mellitus. Likewise, while normal dogs commonly have small amounts of urine bilirubin, any bilirubinuria in a cat is suggestive of hemolytic or significant hepatic disease.

Increased ALT means that hepatocyte membranes have been damaged by primary, secondary, acute, or chronic hepatic disease. Alanine aminotransferase is readily released from hepatocytes; in fact, ALT activities 1½ to 2 times normal are commonly not associated with any identifiable hepatic disease and may spontaneously return to normal (Fig. 40-2). Serum ALT values greater than four times normal suggest that significant hepatic damage is present, but severe diseases with minimal inflammation (e.g., neoplastic infiltration, congenital shunting, cirrhosis) often have normal serum ALT.

Increased aspartate aminotransferase is similar to ALT, but it is also increased by muscular damage and hemolysis. Bound to hepatocellular mitochondria, aspartate aminotransferase is not released from hepatocytes as readily as is ALT.

Increased SAP due to increased enzyme production is usually caused by obstruction of bile flow or induction from various drugs or hormones (Fig. 40-3). Young dogs typically have a two- to three-fold increase, ostensibly due to widespread, rapid bone growth. Glucocorticoids usually increase canine SAP levels, hyperadrenocorticism probably being the major cause of marked increases in canine SAP. Even small amounts of steroids absorbed from ocular medications may noticeably increase canine SAP. Inflammatory diseases without hepatocellular swelling or fibrosis, as well as congenital vascular anomalies, may or may not increase SAP. Even obvious cirrhosis may not increase SAP. Acquired bone lesions almost never cause significant increases (greater than 3–4 times normal) in SAP in dogs or cats.

Cats produce less SAP and excrete it faster than dogs. They usually do not reliably increase SAP after steroid therapy. Because it is harder to increase feline SAP activity, any increase is indicative of significant hepatic disease, although hy-

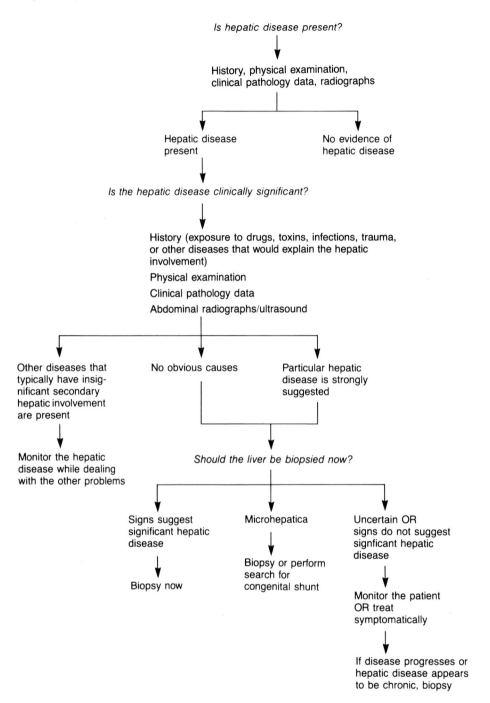

Figure 40–1. *Diagnostic approach to hepatic disease.*

Table 40-3 Laboratory Assessment of Hepatic Disease

Test	What to Check For
Complete blood count	Anemia (due to chronic disease)
	Neutrophilia (due to inflammatory disease or stress)
	Thrombocytopenia (due to disseminated intravascular coagulation)
Serum biochemistry profile	Increased alanine aminotransferase (hepatocyte damage due to any cause)
	Increased aspartate aminotransferase (hepatocyte damage due to any cause)
	Increased serum alkaline phosphatase (cholestasis or induction due to drugs)
	Increased γ-glutamyltransferase (cholestasis or induction due to drugs)
	Hyperbilirubinemia (hepatic insufficiency, cholestasis, or hemolytic anemia)
	Hypoalbuminemia (hepatic insufficiency)
	Hypoglycemia (hepatic insufficiency)
	Decreased blood urea nitrogen (hepatic insufficiency or polyuria-polydipsia)
Urinalysis	Bilirubinuria (not always significant in dogs, always significant in cats; hepatic insufficiency, cholestasis, or hemolytic anemia)
	Increased urobilinogen (hepatic insufficiency or hemolytic anemia)
	Lack of urobilinogen (complete cholestasis)
	Ammonium biurate crystals (hepatic insufficiency)
	Low specific gravity (hepatic insufficiency)
Coagulogram	Decreased antithrombin III (hepatic insufficiency)
Abdominal radiographs or ultrasound	Microhepatica (hepatic atrophy or cirrhosis)
	Hepatomegaly (hepatic infiltration or congestion)
	Asymmetry (tumor, cyst, or granuloma)
Serum bile acids	Increased (hepatic insufficiency)
BSP retention	Increased (hepatic insufficiency, poor cardiac output, or artifact)
Blood ammonia	Increased (hepatic insufficiency)

perthyroidism and diabetes mellitus may also be responsible.

γ-Glutamyltransferase is similar to SAP, but may be more specific for the liver. It is not increased by bone growth in young animals, as is SAP.

Serum bilirubin is not increased as consistently as ALT or SAP in patients with hepatic disease. Even when hyperbilirubinemia occurs, it is not diagnostic of hepatobiliary disease unless hemolysis has been eliminated.

Decreased serum albumin, urea nitrogen, or glucose is consistent with hepatic insufficiency. However, these are not consistently found, even in severe hepatic disease. Likewise, each of these may be produced by other organ dysfunction; thus, one must confirm that the liver is responsible by eliminating other causes or finding other evidence of hepatic disease.

Urinalysis findings may be helpful. Any bilirubin in feline urine is significant, while there must be an inappropriately increased amount in canine urine to be noteworthy. Increased urobilinogen is suggestive of hepatocellular or hemolytic disease. However, bright light degrades bilirubin and urobilinogen so that it cannot be measured in urine or serum if these samples are not promptly analyzed. Ammonium biurate crystals are suggestive of hepatic insufficiency, and are usually due to hyperammonemia. In dalmatian dogs, however, ammonium urate crystals may be normal.

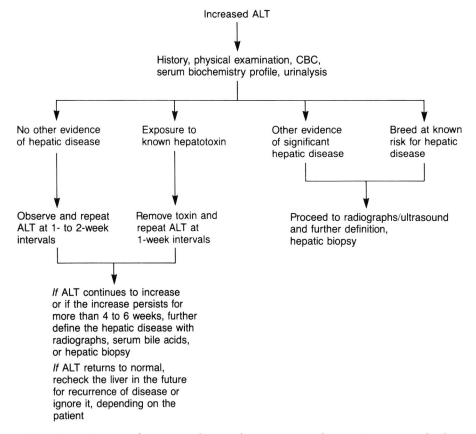

Figure 40–2. *Diagnostic approach to increased serum alanine aminotransferase (ALT) activity in the dog and cat.*

Complete blood count findings are less helpful in detecting hepatic disease than the aforementioned tests. Nonregenerative anemia associated with many leptocytes is suggestive of hepatic dysfunction, but this is neither sensitive nor specific.

If one is uncertain whether hepatic disease is present despite history, physical examination, complete blood count, serum biochemistry profile, and urinalysis, then abdominal radiographs or hepatic function tests may be performed. A patient with hypoalbuminemia or hypoglycemia despite normal ALT and SAP should be tested for hepatic insufficiency.

Preprandial and postprandial serum bile acid concentrations are relatively sensitive and specific tests for hepatic insufficiency. A preprandial bile acid that is more than five to ten times normal suggests significant hepatic dysfunction. If the patient has been chronically anorectic, the preprandial value may not reflect the severity of the hepatic dysfunction. When the patient eats, the gallbladder empties bile acids into the intestine, from which they will be absorbed when they reach the ileum. Assuming a normal intestinal transit time, such feeding ensures that bile acids have recently entered the blood and prevents prolonged anorexia from allowing the liver excessive time to remove bile acids that were absorbed from the intestine days before.

Bromsulphalein (BSP) dye retention may be used instead of serum bile acids to evaluate hepatic function, but decreased cardiac output, extravasation of the dye, lipemia, icterus, hemolysis, ascites, and hypoalbuminemia may alter results significantly. Indocyanine green clearance has been used in dogs and cats, but there is little clinical experience with it at this time.

Blood ammonia concentrations are indicative

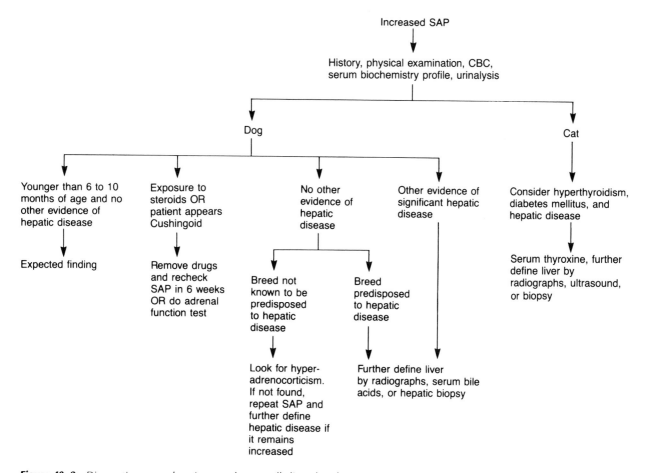

Figure 40–3. *Diagnostic approach to increased serum alkaline phosphatase (SAP) activity in the dog and cat.*

of hepatic disease when increased; however, many patients, including some currently experiencing HE, may have normal blood ammonia concentrations. Rarely, urinary tract infection with urea-splitting bacteria may increase blood ammonia, especially if there is urinary tract obstruction. The ammonia tolerance test is more sensitive in identifying hepatic dysfunction, but is technically difficult and cumbersome. Blood samples for ammonia determinations must be collected in ice-chilled tubes and quickly transported to the laboratory while on ice. Oral administration of ammonia chloride may cause vomiting or produce HE. Ammonia chloride can be given per rectum to avoid vomiting, but then it may be defecated.

Once hepatic disease has been identified, one next determines if it is clinically significant by considering the liver's size and shape, any obvious causes of hepatic disease, and the patient's clinical condition.

Radiographic changes may detect and better define hepatic disease. Although not as sensitive as hepatic function tests, they are often more readily available. Hepatomegaly, microhepatica, and asymmetry all indicate hepatic disease. Focal hepatic enlargements (Fig. 40-4) are usually due to tumors, although cysts, granulomas, and masses of fatty liver with scarring are possible. Any focal enlargement is an indication for hepatic biopsy. A fine needle aspirate should be used first in case the mass is a cyst or a hemorrhagic tumor. The size of the mass is not prognostic or diagnostic.

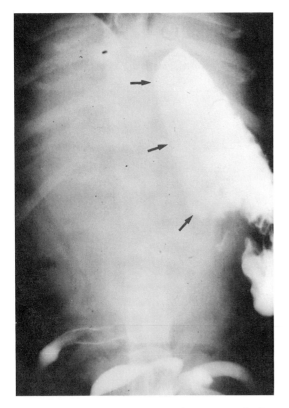

Figure 40–4. *Radiograph of a dog with a mass on the liver, as indicated by displacement of the barium-filled stomach to the left (arrows).*

If the hepatic shape is normal, the next concern is the size. Microhepatica is diagnosed by considering the angle of the gastric shadow on the lateral projection. When the stomach assumes a near-vertical position or if the ventral region of the stomach is directed cranially instead of caudally, microhepatica is usually present (Fig. 40-5). Dogs with deep chests may have a somewhat vertical stomach gas shadow and still be normal. If these criteria are not considered, microhepatica may be misdiagnosed. True microhepatica is usually due to fibrosis or scarring (cirrhosis) or atrophy (as due to congenital portovascular anomalies), and as such is important.

A normal-sized liver does not diagnose or eliminate hepatic disease.

If the liver is obviously cirrhotic (fine or coarse nodules present, blunt or rounded margins), biopsy is useful to define the causative, underlying disease. If the liver does not appear cirrhotic (normal color and texture plus thin, leaflike margins), this does not eliminate cirrhosis, but necessitates careful exploration for a portovascular shunt, arteriovenous fistula, or obstructed portal vein.

Hepatomegaly is detected on the lateral projection by finding the gastric shadow becoming more horizontal and the ventral hepatic margin extending significantly beyond the costal arch (Fig. 40-6). One also expects a more rounded he-

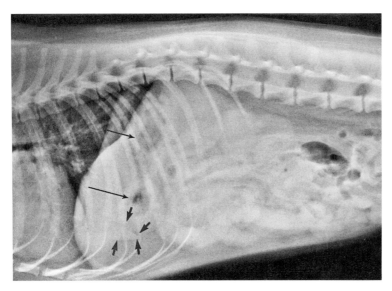

Figure 40–5. *Radiograph showing microhepatica in a dog (short arrows), as noted by the forward displacement and altered angle of the gastric air bubble (long arrows).*

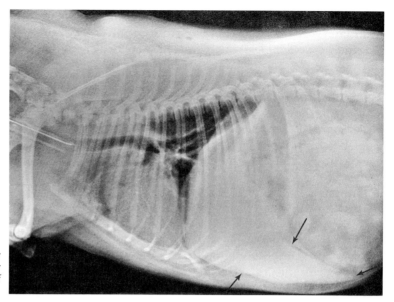

Figure 40–6. *Radiograph showing hepatomegaly in a dog, as noted by the protrusion of the liver beyond the costal arch (arrows) and the rounding of the edge of the liver.*

patic margin. Hepatomegaly means that hepatic disease is present; it may be clinically significant or insignificant.

Ultrasonographic analysis of the liver is more sensitive in finding intrahepatic masses and infiltration. If possible, this analysis should be done in conjunction with radiography.

Simultaneously, the diagnostician should search for obvious causes of hepatic disease. Anticonvulsants, endogenous or exogenous glucocorticoids, various hepatotoxins (carbon tetrachloride), and genetic predisposition (Bedlington terrier or Doberman pinscher) should be sought.

Patients with hepatic disease of uncertain cause and uncertain significance force a decision. If the patient is stable and not particularly ill, one may reasonably observe or symptomatically treat the patient and then repeat selected tests in 1 to 8 weeks to assess disease progression. Alternatively, if the patient is too ill to wait that long, if the patient appears to have severe, progressive, or chronic disease, or if the clients desire an answer now, the liver should be biopsied (see Liver Biopsy in Chapter 80).

Unless an obstruction of the biliary tree is anticipated, fine needle aspiration or laparoscopy are the preferred techniques for hepatic biopsies. A sterile otoscope or anoscope is a suitable laparoscope for most cats and many dogs. Larger animals (especially if obese) may require a regular laparoscope or surgical exploration.

If the hepatic biopsy is performed during a laparotomy, then a complete exploratory procedure should be done. Hepatic disease may be secondary to other problems (pancreatitis and inflammatory bowel disease), so one should not hesitate to biopsy the alimentary tract if it is unclear whether the hepatic disease is primary or secondary. Hepatic tissue should be submitted for histopathology, culture, or quantification of elements (copper).

If there are multiple portosystemic shunts in a young animal or in one that does not have obvious cirrhosis, then measurement of portal venous pressure should be done using a water manometer to determine if portal hypertension is present. Such hypertension strongly suggests an acquired disorder. If portal pressures are normal, then congenital, multiple shunts must be considered.

Diagnosis of Specific Hepatic Diseases

Most hepatic diseases will be diagnosed by the above approach. However, specific comments about selected diseases are in order, as some diseases are strongly suggested by select findings and diagnostic shortcuts may be appropriate.

Feline hepatic lipidosis is suggested by a history of an obese cat that became anorectic. There is minimal inflammation, but the liver enlarges and usually becomes very yellow. Cats are typically icteric, and have increased SAP but minimally increased ALT. Fine needle aspiration can provide presumptive diagnosis. Tissue samples placed in formalin often (but not always) float due to the excessive fat. Fatty liver may also be found in animals with diabetes mellitus, which rarely causes clinically significant hepatic dysfunction in dogs but may cause feline icterus.

Cholangitis–cholangiohepatitis is more common in cats. An inflammatory disease that may be caused by infectious (bacterial) or immune-mediated mechanisms, cellular infiltrates principally occur around bile ducts; they may consist of neutrophils or mononuclear cells. Increased SAP and ALT, hepatomegaly, and icterus are typical. Aspiration cytology is often not definitive. Histopathology is required, and hepatic tissue should be cultured if possible. This disease may resemble hepatic lipidosis, but classically has greater increases in ALT. This disease also occurs in dogs, ostensibly due to similar causes.

Inflammatory infiltration of the liver usually causes hepatocellular necrosis, and typically increases ALT to more than four times normal values.

Chronic active hepatitis is a name given to a collection of hepatic diseases that have mononuclear infiltrates plus piecemeal or bridging necrosis. Of uncertain cause, systemic immunologic mechanisms are suspected. Cirrhosis is a common sequela. These changes can be seen in various breeds, but are especially associated with hepatocellular copper accumulation in Doberman pinschers.

Copper-associated diseases with inflammatory infiltrates occur in Bedlington terriers, Doberman pinschers, and West Highland white terriers. The pathogenesis is different in the three breeds, but Bedlingtons and Dobermans may have similar clinical signs. Chronic inflammation produces mononuclear infiltrates, fibrosis, and cirrhosis, while concurrent acute disease causes hepatocellular necrosis and neutrophilic infiltrates. In Doberman pinschers, particularly, the disease is usually chronic; microhepatica is typical by the time the patient is clinically ill. A history of a female Doberman pinscher younger than 5 years of age with signs compatible with hepatic dysfunction (especially polyuria–polydipsia) is suggestive. Owners may have difficulty believing that a disease that "appeared so suddenly" is chronic. If the pet is stressed, acute hepatic failure may occur with little warning. These three breeds are so predisposed to this hepatic disease that any increase in ALT or SAP (including minor, "insignificant" elevations) should be viewed as indicating potentially severe problems. They may indicate the need for hepatic biopsy.

Infectious agents may cause hepatic infiltrative disease. Histoplasmosis and blastomycosis cause granulomatous infiltrates and hepatomegaly. Increases in ALT and SAP are expected. In both infections, hepatic involvement usually indicates systemic disease, with other organs being involved. Disseminated histoplasmosis commonly affects the lungs, bone marrow, colon, spleen, or lymph nodes; many patients have low-grade fevers. Serology is notoriously insensitive for histoplasmosis. Aspiration cytology of the liver or other enlarged organs is usually definitive. Blastomycosis often affects lymph nodes, eyes, skin, and lungs; fever is common. Agar gel immunodiffusion for antibodies to *Blastomyces dermatitidis* is sensitive and specific in chronic cases (see Chapter 79). Aspiration cytology of any affected organ is definitive if the organism is found.

Feline infectious peritonitis may cause hepatopathy and icterus, but often has other signs of the disease (*e.g.*, nonseptic exudate, uveitis, hyperglobulinemia), aiding diagnosis. Other infectious agents are less common (*Bacillus piliformis*, infectious canine hepatitis, *Amphimerus pseudofelineus*), and should be diagnosed by biopsy or, in the case of feline hepatic trematodes, also by fecal shedding of ova. Vacuolar hepatopathy occurs when normal hepatocellular cytosol is replaced with proteinaceous fluid or glycogen. Due to endogenous or exogenous corticosteroids, it is one of the major causes of increased canine SAP concentrations plus hepatomegaly. It can also significantly increase serum bile acid concentrations and BSP dye retention. Aspiration cytology of the liver may be suggestive, but histopathology is needed for definitive diagnosis. However, definitive diagnosis is rarely needed if the history is suggestive. It is often reasonable to remove the source of the steroids and recheck the SAP over the next 4 to 8 months. The SAP should decrease after removing the corticosteroid influence.

Glycogen storage disease of dogs is often mentioned, but seldom documented. If present, one would expect to see hypoglycemia plus hepatomegaly due to glycogen accumulation in a relatively young animal.

Acute fulminant hepatic failure is often due to hepatocellular necrosis caused by infectious agents (*e.g.*, infectious canine hepatitis) or various toxins. A history of administration of potential hepatotoxins should be sought (Table 40-4). Infectious canine hepatitis due to adenovirus is relatively rare now, but histopathology is definitive. Regardless of cause, these patients usually have major increases in ALT and SAP, hyperbilirubinemia, HE, or disseminated intravascular coagulation. Many cannot be biopsied because of fulminant disease, coagulopathy, and poor anesthetic risk, and must be treated symptomatically until biopsy is feasible.

Postcaval syndrome due to sudden obstruction

Table 40–4 *Selected Known and Suspected Hepatotoxins of Dogs and Cats*

Acetaminophen (especially cats)
Aflatoxin (rare, but when occurs is often severe)
Azathioprine (rare)
Carbon tetrachloride (rare)
Chlordane
Chloroform
Furosemide (in very large doses)
Heavy metals
Ketoconazole (uncommon)
Mebendazole (questionable, idiosyncratic)
Mercaptopurine
Methotrexate
Oxibendazole (questionable, may be idiosyncratic)
Phenobarbital (when used chronically)
Primidone (when used chronically)
Tetracycline
Thiacetarsamide

of the right atrium or posterior vena cava by heartworms can cause hemolysis and hepatic necrosis. Heart murmur, hemoglobinuria, weakness, or collapse are expected in severe cases (see Chapter 25).

Pancreatitis may obstruct the bile ducts, while leakage of enzymes may damage adjacent hepatic parenchyma, increasing SAP, bilirubin, and/or ALT. Serum amylase and lipase activities may be diagnostic in some cases, but normal amylase and lipase do not eliminate pancreatitis (see Chapter 39).

Cirrhosis can be caused by anything that destroys hepatocytes. Signs may be mild or severe. Many patients with cirrhosis have microhepatica, but some (particularly cats) may have normal-sized livers. Alanine aminotransferase and SAP are often, but not invariably, increased. Hepatic function tests should reflect insufficiency. Ascites is common, but inconsistent. Aspiration cytology is seldom helpful; histopathology is needed for diagnosis. Some cirrhotic livers have fine nodules (micronodular cirrhosis), while others have large nodules (macronodular cirrhosis), the gross appearance sometimes being deceiving. Sometimes diabetics with macronodular cirrhosis have severe crusting lesions at mucocutaneous junctions. If contrast venography is performed, tortuous vessels are expected in the region of the kidneys (Fig. 40-7).

Neoplastic infiltration may be primary or metastatic. The liver is a common site for metastasis from alimentary, pancreatic, and splenic carcinomas or sarcomas and from mast cell tumors, plus it is commonly infiltrated by lymphosarcoma. Increased SAP is expected due to compression of bile canaliculi, but many patients have normal ALT and SAP plus radiographically normal or enlarged livers. Obvious hepatic masses are principally due to hepatomas or hepatocellular carcinomas. If ultrasonography is available, it is a sensitive means of detecting neoplasia, especially hemangiosarcomas. Patients with diffuse hepatic involvement due to lymphosarcoma may often be diagnosed by fine needle hepatic aspirates (see Liver Biopsy in Chapter 80). Not all hepatic masses are neoplastic.

Congenital portosystemic shunts are most

commonly found in dogs and cats younger than 6 months of age, although they are sometimes found in patients older than 3 years. Poor weight gain, abnormal behavior (especially after eating), vomiting, polyuria–polydipsia, or ptyalism (especially in cats) is suggestive of this disorder. Animals with minor shunts or on diets that help prevent central nervous system signs may not be diagnosed for years. These patients typically have normal or insignificant increases in ALT and SAP values, and may have normal or decreased serum albumin, blood urea nitrogen, or glucose. Microhepatica is expected. These findings indicate exploratory surgery to identify and partially ligate the shunt. If the shunt cannot be found, then a mesenteric portogram is indicated. A single shunt between the portal vein and some other vein is expected (Fig. 40-8), although multiple congenital shunts are rarely seen. If microhepatica is equivocal, then pre- and especially postprandial serum bile acid concentrations will usually confirm or deny hepatic insufficiency.

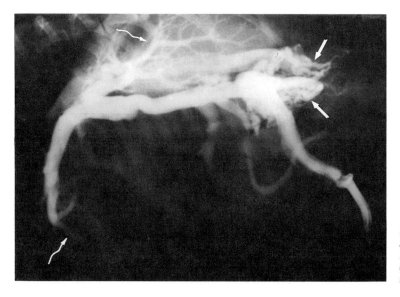

Figure 40–7. *Mesenteric portogram of a dog with acquired portosystemic shunting due to cirrhosis. Note multiple shunts in the region of the kidney (straight arrows), in addition to the arborization in the liver (curved arrows).*

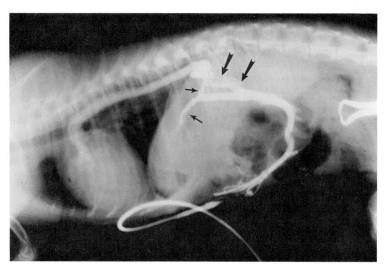

Figure 40–8. *Mesenteric portogram of a dog with a congenital portosystemic shunt. Note the large vessel connecting the hepatic portal vein to the azygous vein (large arrows), in addition to the diminished arborization in the liver (small arrows).*

MANAGEMENT

Symptomatic Therapy

If a definitive diagnosis is obtained, specific therapy may commence. Symptomatic therapy can be used in patients without a diagnosis or when specific therapy will not resolve the clinical signs quickly enough. Symptomatic therapy principally consists of fluid and electrolyte replacement, antibacterial drugs, nutritional support, treatment of coagulopathies, control of ascites, and prevention or treatment of HE. Fluids and electrolytes, especially potassium, should be replaced as needed (see Chapter 72). Systemic antibacterial therapy (*e.g.,* amoxicillin) may help, as diseased livers may be unable to remove and destroy bacteria that enter the portal blood from the intestines. Antibiotics (neomycin 20 mg/kg orally twice daily) may also help control HE.

In cats with hepatic lipidosis, supplying adequate nutrition is the specific therapy. In anorectic animals with other hepatic disease, force-feeding or using oxazepam to stimulate the appetite may be useful. B-complex vitamins are also reasonable (see Chapter 8). Nutritional therapy includes supplying glucose to hypoglycemic patients. However, nutritional therapy should by no means include indiscriminate use of nutritional aids such as lipotrophic factors, which often contain methionine, an amino acid that can produce HE in patients with severe hepatic insufficiency.

Coagulopathy must be defined before it can be symptomatically treated. If poor absorption of vitamin K is due to cholestasis, parenteral administration of vitamin K_1 should resolve signs. If clotting factors are decreased due to lack of functional hepatic parenchyma, little can be done other than to provide these factors by way of transfusions (see Chapter 16). The most problematic coagulopathy is disseminated intravascular coagulation, particularly in patients with acute hepatic necrosis. Antithrombin III, which is needed for heparin therapy to be effective, is produced in the liver; hence, fresh plasma transfusions may be needed in disseminated intravascular coagulation accompanying hepatic failure.

Ascites may be due to hypoalbuminemia or portal hypertension plus salt retention (see Chap-

ter 11). The animal rarely requires relief from the effusion unless there is dyspnea or severe discomfort. If necessary, the fluid may be removed directly by syringe and needle, although there is risk of infection plus further depletion of body proteins (see Abdominal Paracentesis and Lavage in Chapter 80). Diuretics are effective, but can cause hypokalemia or acute hypovolemia, leading to renal failure. Use of salt-restricted diets may be sufficient to control the ascites or at least allow lower doses of diuretics to be used.

Hepatic encephalopathy may present as an acute emergency or as a chronic condition. In patients with acute signs, a cause for the acute decompensation should be sought and resolved (Table 40-5). Cleansing enemas should remove all colonic fecal matter. Retention enemas with neomycin or lactulose should then be administered to inhibit further ammonia production and absorption. All oral intake should stop, and the patient must be given parenteral fluids. Alkalinizing fluids such as lactated Ringer's injection should be avoided (alkalosis increases intracellular transport of ammonia and amines), and hypokalemia should be resolved because it promotes alkalosis, reduces the conversion of ammonia to glutamine, and causes the increased production of ammonia by renal tubular cells. Glucose may be included in the fluids to avoid hypoglycemia. Systemic antibiotics that kill anaerobes (*e.g.,* amoxicillin) reduce colonic bacterial populations. If cerebral edema occurs, mannitol admin-

Table 40–5 *Causes of Acute Hepatic Encephalopathy in Dogs and Cats*

Alkalosis (due to drugs, lactated Ringer's injection)
Azotemia
Constipation
Dehydration
Diuretics (by producing hypokalemia and alkalosis)
Drugs (especially sedatives [acepromazine], narcotics [morphine sulfate, meperidine hydrochloride], anesthetic agents [thiobarbiturates], and methionine)
Gastrointestinal bleeding (by providing protein substrate)
High protein diet
Hypokalemia
Infection
Uremia (increased enterohepatic circulation of urea nitrogen with increased ammonia production)

istration is helpful. Sedatives and tranquilizers should be avoided unless they are absolutely necessary to control convulsions, in which case the lowest effective dose of diazepam or phenobarbital should be used.

Chronic HE may be controlled by using a low protein diet that contains highly digestible protein (*e.g.*, Hill's k/d, u/d), by reducing colonic bacterial populations with oral neomycin or metronidazole, by preventing ammonia absorption with lactulose, or by resolving the underlying cause (ligating a portosystemic shunt).

Specific Therapy

Specific therapy will depend on the disease that is present. Feline hepatic lipidosis is treated by supplying adequate protein and calories so that hepatocellular fat may be removed by lipoprotein synthesis. Mild cases may be treated with appetite stimulants (*e.g.*, oxazepam 0.2–0.5 mg/kg orally once to twice daily) or force feedings. More severely affected cases require a conduit allowing consistent alimentation. Nasoesophageal tubes (see Nasoesophageal Intubation in Chapter 80) sometimes work, although many cats do not tolerate them as long as is necessary. Pharyngostomy tubes may interfere with the feline larynx; therefore, gastrostomy tubes are often used (see Surgical and Percutaneous Tube Gastrostomy in Chapter 80). These allow easy feeding and are well tolerated by most cats. From 1 to 16 weeks of such feeding may be needed. A specially formulated diet, Clinicare Feline Liquid Diet, may be usd for nutritional support. There is currently no evidence that corticosteroid therapy is useful in this disease.

Feline cholangitis–cholangiohepatitis is probably caused by various disease processes. If the inflammatory infiltrate is principally neutrophilic, then aggressive antibacterial therapy is used (*e.g.*, amoxicillin or cephalothin). If the infiltrate has a large mononuclear component, then prednisolone 1.1 to 2.2 mg/kg/day may be useful. Choleretics (dehydrocholic acid 10–15 mg/kg orally three times daily for 7–10 days) have been used to stimulate watery biliary secretion, although their effectiveness in this disease is uncertain. Oxazepam may be useful in stimulating appetite.

Copper storage disease is documented in Bedlington terriers and West Highland white terriers, although the disease appears to be dissimilar in the two breeds from the standpoint of severity of clinical signs. If the disease can be identified before cirrhosis or acute failure occurs, then copper reduction therapy may be used. Most dog foods have relatively high copper concentrations, although Hill's Prescription Diet u/d is copper-restricted. Copper chelators may be used; however, currently available drugs work slower than desired and may have adverse side-effects. Penicillamine (10–15 mg/kg orally twice daily) has been used, but trientine hydrochloride (15 mg/kg orally twice daily) seems to be more effective and has fewer complications. Oral zinc acetate administration (100–200 mg twice daily) prevents intestinal copper absorption in humans, but this has not yet been well documented in dogs. Corticosteroids may stabilize hepatocyte membranes in acute episodes.

Doberman pinscher hepatic disease has been called *chronic active hepatitis* and *copper storage disease*, although its pathogenesis is not yet clear. Often not causing signs until the patient has severe cirrhosis, there may be little that can be done if all hepatic compensatory reserves have been exhausted by the time it is diagnosed. However, if a reasonable amount of functional hepatocellular tissue is left, glucocorticoids may reduce the inflammation and improve the quality and quantity of life. Corticosteroids should only be administered long enough to reduce the inflammation without causing severe vacuolar hepatopathy. One may also seek to reduce hepatic copper stores as mentioned above, or fibrosis as mentioned below.

Chronic active hepatitis in other breeds is treated symptomatically, and corticosteroids are judiciously used as needed to improve quality of life. Copper accumulation is not usually expected in other breeds, but the disease will otherwise be somewhat similar to Doberman pinscher hepatic disease.

Infectious causes of hepatopathy must be

treated depending on the agent. For example, histoplasmosis and blastomycosis require ketoconazole, itraconazole, or amphotericin B therapy.

Vacuolar hepatopathy is due to steroid therapy, stress, or hyperadrenocorticism. Resolving the underlying disease should be adequate, although it may require weeks or months before the vacuolar hepatopathy resolves. However, vacuolar hepatopathy itself is rarely of clinical significance.

Infectious canine hepatitis is rarely seen now, but requires symptomatic management for acute hepatic failure, often with disseminated intravascular coagulation.

Cirrhosis may occur following acute or chronic hepatic insults. Once it exists, there is little that can be done other than to treat symptomatically and prevent progression. Patients with cirrhosis may have years of quality life if they are well managed symptomatically. Attempts to reverse cirrhosis with colchicine have benefited some humans and perhaps some dogs (dogs: 0.03 mg/kg orally once daily or every other day). This is currently considered experimental therapy, and may have side-effects that have not yet been reported.

Congenital portosystemic shunts are best treated by complete or partial surgical ligation of the shunt. While relatively easy in patients with extrahepatic shunts, intrahepatic shunts are technically more difficult unless one has advanced surgical training. Portal pressures should be measured during the procedure to avoid splanchnic congestion, which can lead to death. After ligation, the portal pressures should not exceed 10 mmHg over preligation pressures, nor should they exceed 18 mmHg. In rare cases when there are multiple congenital shunts that cannot be ligated, the posterior vena cava may be banded to increase its pressure and force blood back into the liver. Currently, there is no surgical treatment acknowledged to benefit patients with acquired portosystemic shunts secondary to hepatic cirrhosis.

Intrahepatic cholestasis is a poorly defined syndrome of cholestasis without evidence of cholangitis or obstruction. Treatment is uncertain, but protracted fluid therapy has benefited some cases. Conceivably, dietary cholestyramine resin (dogs: 0.25–0.5 g orally with food twice daily) may be useful, because lithocholic acid (a bile acid) has been implicated as a cause in humans.

Toxic hepatopathy is treated symptomatically and by withdrawing the offending agent.

Hepatic neoplasia may be resected if it is focal (*e.g.,* hepatoma). Many hepatic neoplasms are metastatic growths, and in this case chemotherapy is the only option. Surgery with or without chemotherapy is infrequently successful, except for lymphosarcoma, in which it is often palliative (see Chapter 15).

PATIENT MONITORING

The prognosis for properly treated feline hepatic lipidosis is reasonable for cure. Likewise, many cats with cholangitis can be cured. Copper storage diseases can often be cured if a low copper diet and copper chelators are utilized before end-stage hepatic disease is present. Many Doberman pinschers with chronic active hepatitis have a poor prognosis due to the advanced nature of the disease when it is diagnosed. However, some of these patients live for months or longer with symptomatic therapy. Histoplasmosis and blastomycosis can often be cured if the patient does not die of systemic complications first. Vacuolar hepatopathy should not cause clinical signs. Acute hepatic failure due to any cause (infectious canine hepatitis or drug-induced) carries a guarded prognosis, and many of these patients die despite removing the underlying cause and initiating therapy quickly.

Patients with cirrhosis may often be palliated for weeks to years if care is taken to prevent progression of the disease and if symptomatic therapy controls signs. If colchicine is used chronically, care should be taken to monitor for side-effects reported in humans (*e.g.,* agranulocytosis; see Appendix II). Patients with cirrhosis and ascites may sometimes be managed successfully for months or years with low salt diets and intermittent diuretics (see Chapter 11). Failure to control or resolve chronic hepatic disease may lead to death due to cirrhosis (end-stage hepatic disease) or hepatic insufficiency. Congenital portosystemic shunts have a good prognosis if the shunt is surgically approachable and if intraoperative hemorrhage and postoperative pancreatitis, splanchnic congestion, and thrombus formation do not kill the patient. Most hepatic malignancies (primary and metastatic) are fatal, although rare lesions are solitary and may be successfully resected.

Monitoring may be by clinical signs or by repeated biochemical determinations. In particular, following serum enzyme activities or serum albumin or bile acid concentrations may allow one to determine if the disease is static, progressive, or resolving. Appetite is also a good means of evaluating patients with hepatic disease. This is especially true in dogs receiving potential hepatotoxins, such as ketoconazole or thiacetarsamide. As long as the patient has a good appetite, the treatments may continue; however, if appetite declines the patient should be further evaluated or therapy postponed.

ADDITIONAL READING

Bunch SE, Polak DM, Hornbuckle WE. A modified laparoscopic approach for liver biopsy in dogs. J Am Vet Med Assoc 1985; 187:1032.

Center SA, Baldwin BH, Erb HN, Tennant BC. Bile acid concentrations in the diagnosis of hepatobiliary disease in the cat. J Am Vet Med Assoc 1986; 189:891.

Center SA, Baldwin BH, Erb HN, Tennant BC. Bile acid concentrations in the diagnosis of hepatobiliary disease in the dog. J Am Vet Med Assoc 1985; 187:935.

Crawford MA, Schall WD, Jensen RK, Tasker JB. Chronic active hepatitis in 26 Doberman pinschers. J Am Vet Med Assoc 1985; 187:1343.

Dillon AR, Spano JS, Powers RD. Prednisolone-induced hematologic, biochemical and histologic changes in the dog. Journal of the American Animal Hospital Association 1980; 16:831.

Hardy RM. Chronic hepatitis. Vet Clin North Am. 1985; 15:135.

Herrtage ME, Seymour CA, White RAS et al. Inherited copper toxicosis in the Bedlington terrier. Journal of Small Animal Practice 1987; 28:1141.

Hirsch VM, Doige CE. Suppurative cholangitis in cats. J Am Vet Med Assoc 1983; 182:1223.

Johnson CA, Armstrong PJ, Hauptman JG. Congenital portosystemic shunts in dogs. J Am Vet Med Assoc 1987; 191:1478.

Maretta SM, Pask AJ, Greene, RW, Liu SK. Urinary calculi associated with portosystemic shunts in six dogs. J Am Vet Med Assoc 1981; 178:133.

Meyer DJ, Noonan NE. Liver tests in dogs receiving anticonvulsant drugs. J Am Vet Med Assoc 1978; 173:377.

Polzin DF, Stowe CJ, O'Leary TP et al. Acute hepatic necrosis associated with the administration of mebendazole. J Am Vet Med Assoc 1981; 179:1013.

Strombeck DR, Miller LM, Harrold D. Effects of corticosteroid treatment on survival time in dogs with chronic hepatitis. J Am Vet Med Assoc 1988; 93:1109.

Tams TR. Hepatic encephalopathy. Vet Clin North Am 1985; 15:177.

Thornburg LP, Show D, Dolan M et al. Hereditary copper toxicosis in West Highland White terriers. Vet Pathol 1986; 23:148.

Twedt DC. Cirrhosis: A consequence of chronic liver disease. Vet Clin North Am 1985; 15:151.

THE URINARY SYSTEM

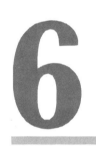

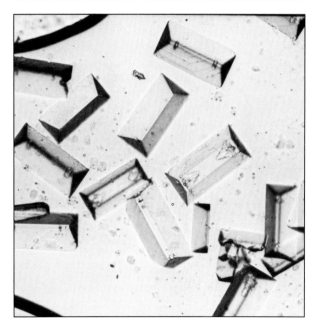

41

HEMATURIA

Cynthia A. Culham, Gregory F. Grauer

Hematuria, the abnormal presence of red blood cells in the urine, is a problem frequently encountered in clinical veterinary medicine. Hematuria may be overt (gross or macroscopic hematuria) or occult (microscopic hematuria). Occult hematuria (greater than five red blood cells per high power field) is often an incidental finding in an animal that presents with pollakiuria, stranguria, or dysuria. Hematuria is not a specific disease entity; rather, it is a clinical sign associated with an underlying disease process of the urogenital tract. Diagnostic efforts are directed toward identifying the origin of the hemorrhage within the urogenital tract as well as the cause.

PATHOPHYSIOLOGY AND CAUSES

The majority of hematuria is caused by inflammation, trauma, or neoplasia of the urogenital tract (Table 41-1); however, exceptions include hematuria caused by bleeding disorders, strenuous exercise, heat stroke, renal infarcts, and renal telangiectasia of Welsh corgi dogs. The timing of overt hematuria during voiding often provides clues as to the origin of the hemorrhage. Hematuria that occurs at the beginning of voiding suggests the hemorrhage originates from the lower urinary tract (bladder neck, urethra, vagina, vulva, penis, or prepuce). Additionally, extraurinary causes such as proestrus, metritis, pyometra, prostatic disease, or neoplasia of the genital tract may cause hematuria predominately at the beginning of voiding. Hematuria that occurs at the end of voiding usually results from hemorrhage originating from the upper urinary tract (bladder, ureters, or kidneys). In this case, the hemorrhage may be intermittent, allowing the red blood cells to settle to the cranioventral portion of the bladder and be expelled with the last of the bladder contents. When hematuria occurs throughout voiding, the origin of the hemorrhage is usually either the bladder, ureters, or kidneys. Pseudohematuria may be caused by muscle or blood pigments, drugs, and natural or artificial food colorants in urine. Examination of the urine sediment after centrifugation will allow differentiation of pseudohematuria from hematuria.

CLINICAL SIGNS

In patients with hematuria due to inflammation, trauma, or neoplasia of the lower urinary tract, pollakiuria and stranguria or dysuria are fre-

Table 41–1 *Potential Causes of Hematuria*

Urinary	Extraurinary
Inflammation	Inflammation
Bacterial infection (pyelonephritis, cystitis, urethritis)	Bacterial infection (prostatitis, metritis/ pyometra, vaginitis, balanoposthitis)
Urolithiasis (renal, ureteral, cystic, urethral)	Prostatic cyst/abscess
Feline lower urinary tract inflammation	
Drug-induced (cyclophosphamide, sulfonamides, gentamicin)	
Leptospirosis	
Parasitism (*Capillaria plica, Dioctophyma renale, Dirofilaria immitis* microfilariae)	
Glomerulopathy	
Trauma	Trauma
(kidneys, ureters, bladder, urethra)	(prostate, uterus, penis, prepuce, vagina, vulva)
Neoplasia	Neoplasia
(kidneys, ureters, bladder, urethra; primary or metastatic)	(prostate, uterus, penis, prepuce, vagina, vulva)
Miscellaneous	Miscellaneous
Amyloidosis	Proestrus
Exercise-induced	Subinvolution of placental sites
Bleeding disorders	
Heat stroke	
Renal infarcts	
Renal telangiectasia (Welsh corgi)	

quently observed clinical signs (Table 41-2). Urge incontinence and increased grooming or licking of the prepuce and vulva are additional signs of lower urinary tract disease. Owners may occasionally confuse straining to defecate due to constipation, prostatic disease, rectal disease, or anal sac disease with stranguria and dysuria. Upper urinary tract disease causing hematuria may also be associated with systemic signs including depression, lethargy, anorexia, vomiting, diarrhea, weight loss, and abdominal pain. When hemorrhage from the genital tract causes hematuria, spontaneous bleeding unassociated with voiding may also be observed. Additional signs that suggest the genital tract as the source of hemorrhage include purulent vaginal (see Chapter 56) or urethral discharge independent of voiding, behavioral changes (*e.g.,* proestrus), or straining to defecate with a stilted gait (*e.g.,* prostatic disease; see Chapter 57).

DIAGNOSTIC APPROACH

A complete history (Table 41-3) and physical examination will often help localize the source of the hematuria. Findings of depression, lethargy, and fever in association with hematuria often indicate involvement of the kidneys, prostate, or uterus. When possible, the kidneys should be palpated and assessed as to size, shape, consistency, symmetry, and pain. The urinary bladder should be palpated before and after voiding, as a full bladder may obscure intraluminal masses, uroliths, or wall thickening. Observation of voiding should also be part of the physical examination and provides the opportunity to obtain a voided urine sample. The timing of the hematuria can be confirmed and the character of the urine stream and the presence or absence of dysuria can be noted. Rectal palpation allows evaluation of the prostate in male dogs and the pelvic urethra

Table 41–2 Causes of Hematura and Potential Associated Clinical Signs

Causes	Clinical Signs
INITIAL HEMATURIA	
Trauma	
Urethra, vagina, vulva, penis, or prepuce	History of trauma, stranguria, dysuria, anuria, bleeding unassociated with voiding, normal urinalysis from cystocentesis sample, increased licking of genital region, subcutaneous accumulation of urine
Proestrus	Intermittent dripping of blood from vulva, history consistent with estrus, vaginal cytology consistent with proestrus/estrus, estrus-like behavior
Transmissible veneral tumor	Stranguria or dysuria, spontaneous bleeding, penile or vaginal mass, increased licking of genital region
Prostatitis or prostatic adenocarcinoma	Abnormal prostate on rectal palpation, stranguria or dysuria, straining to defecate, stilted gait
Uterine or vaginal lieomyosarcoma	Stranguria or dysuria, intermittent bleeding unassociated with voiding
Metritis/Pyometra	Depression, lethargy, vaginal discharge, history of recent estrus, fever, polyuria-polydipsia, leukocytosis
Vaginitis	Pollakiuria, swollen vulva, history of recent sexual activity
TOTAL OR TERMINAL HEMATURIA	
Cystitis, cystic urolithiasis, feline lower urinary tract inflammation	Pollakiuria, dysuria, urge incontinence, bladder pain, bacteriuria
Trauma	
Kidneys, ureters, bladder	History of trauma, depression, abdominal pain and/or distension, vomiting, fever, anuria
Pyelonephritis	Acute: fever, renal pain, leukocytosis, pyuria, bacteriuria, white blood cell casts, history of bacterial cystitis, azotemia Chronic: depression, anorexia, weight loss, polyuria-polydipsia, azotemia, or asymptomatic
Leptospirosis	Fever, anorexia, weight loss, vomiting, petechia, ecchymosis, diarrhea, icterus, lack of immunization
Bleeding disorder	Evidence of generalized petechia or ecchymosis
Renal infection	Occult hematuria with small infarcts, overt hematuria with large infarcts and signs of renal failure
Hematuria of Welsh corgi dogs	Intermittent occult and overt hematuria
Cyclophosphamide-induced cystitis	History of drug administration
Parasitism	Bladder: pollakiuria, stranguria, dysuria Renal: usually asymptomatic
Neoplasia	
kidney, ureter, bladder	Bladder: pollakiuria, stranguria, dysuria Kidney or ureter: kidney pain, polyuria-polydipsia, azotemia, anemia, or asymptomatic

Table 41–3 *Historical Evaluation of the Patient With Hematuria*

1. Duration of the hematuria? Is it constant, getting worse or better?
2. What is the frequency and extent of the owner's observation?
3. Is the hematuria persistent, recurrent, or a single episode?
4. History of trauma, exposure to toxicants, or current medications?
5. What is the frequency of urination? What is the volume of urine produced?
6. Is the hematuria observed throughout voiding or is it more prominent at the beginning or end of voiding?
7. Does the animal strain or have difficulty passing urine?
8. Does the animal have urinary incontinence?
9. What is the reproductive cycle status in females, and has there been recent sexual activity in males or females?
10. Is there evidence of bleeding or discharge from the vulva or penis that is unassociated with voiding?
11. Is there increased grooming or licking of the genital region?
12. Are any systemic signs present, for example, depression, anorexia, weight loss, coughing, vomiting, diarrhea, or abdominal pain?
13. Has there been a previous diagnosis? If so, what was the treatment and response to treatment?

in both sexes. The trigone region of the bladder can also be palpated through the rectum in small dogs and cats and is facilitated by concurrent abdominal palpation and pushing the bladder toward the pelvic inlet. In larger female dogs, digital vaginal palpation and the use of a vaginal speculum allow evaluation of the urethral orifice and the presence of vaginal masses, strictures, or lacerations to be ruled in or out. In male dogs, the perineal urethra should be palpated subcutaneously from the ischial arch to the os penis, and the penis should be extruded from the prepuce and examined for masses, signs of trauma, and urethral prolapse. Finally, catheterization of the urethra will allow urethral patency to be assessed.

A complete blood count and serum biochemistry profile should be evaluated in animals with hematuria that have concurrent systemic signs. An inflammatory leukocytosis is compatible with metritis/pyometra and acute bacterial pyelonephritis or prostatitis. Azotemia in association with hematuria usually indicates renal parenchymal disease or a rent in the urinary excretory pathway; however, prerenal causes of azotemia should be ruled out. If blood loss due to hematuria is severe or signs of generalized bleeding exist, a clotting profile and platelet count should be evaluated (see Chapter 16).

Comparison of urine obtained by cystocentesis (see Cystocentesis in Chapter 80) with voided urine may help differentiate lower urinary tract or genital tract disease from upper urinary tract disease. Cystocentesis avoids urine contamination with bacteria, cells, and debris from the urethra, vagina, vulva, prepuce, and uterus; however, prostatic disease (see Chapter 57) may alter urine characteristics. Abnormal urinalysis findings in urine collected by cystocentesis indicates involvement of the bladder, ureters, kidneys, or prostate. Cystocentesis, as well as catheterization or bladder expression, may result in minor hemorrhage into the urine; however, the number of red blood cells in the urine sediment is usually less than five per high power field.

Urinalysis should be performed as soon as possible following collection. Greater than 30 minutes at room temperature will allow urease-producing bacteria in urine to proliferate and increase urine *p*H. Alkaline urine may cause fragmentation and lysis red and white blood cells and casts and may change crystal composition. Additionally, hyposthenuric urine will cause lysis of red and white blood cells. Lysed red blood cells in urine may create confusion between hemoglobinuria and hematuria. Refrigeration is the easiest way to preserve the stability of a urine sample. Overnight refrigeration is acceptable for bacterial culture samples but is not ideal for chemical and cellular analysis.

Reagent strips used for the detection of blood in urine detect peroxidase-like activity of hemoglobin from lysed cells. The sensitivity of the test is approximately 0.05 to 0.3 mg hemoglobin/dl of urine (equivalent to 10,000 lysed red blood cells per ml of urine or approximately three lysed red blood cells per high power field). Myoglobinuria will also cause a positive reaction for blood on these reagent test strips.

In addition to checking the urine sediment for red blood cells, the presence of white blood cells, epithelial cells, casts, crystals, parasite ova, and bacteria should be noted. Increased numbers of white blood cells, with or without observed bacteria, suggest the possibility of infection and warrant bacterial culture of the urine (see Chapter 46). Transitional epithelial cell numbers in urine sediment may be increased with urinary tract inflammation or neoplasia; however, it is difficult to differentiate neoplastic transitional cells from hyperplastic transitional cells associated with severe inflammation. Crystals may be observed in the urine of normal dogs and cats, or they may be associated with drug treatment, bacterial infection of the urinary tract, or urolithiasis. The type of crystalluria in patients with urolithiasis often suggests the type of urolith present (see Chapter 47). Cooling of urine samples at room temperature or by refrigeration facilitates in vitro crystal formation. Casts originate in the renal tubules, and, therefore, the presence of casts in a urine sample indicates renal involvement. White blood cell casts are highly suggestive of pyelonephritis and red blood cell casts indicate hemorrhage at the level of the renal tubules. Finally, parasites associated with the urinary tract, although rare, may cause hematuria. The ova of *Dioctophyma renale* and *Capillaria plica* or microfilariae of *Dirofilaria immitis* in the urine sediment suggest parasitism as the cause of the hematuria.

Plain and contrast radiography as well as ultrasonography of the urinary tract often facilitate determining the location and cause of hematuria (Table 41-4). Lateral and ventrodorsal radiographs should be obtained prior to contrast radio-

Table 41–4 *Radiographic Procedures and Potential Findings in Patients With Hematuria*

Procedure	Indication	Potential Findings
Plain abdominal films or ultrasonography	Suspected upper urinary tract hematuria or genital tract hematuria	Radiopaque uroliths Kidney enlargement Abdominal mass(es) Bladder distension Emphysematous cystitis Enlarged uterus Enlarged prostate
Contrast urethrography	Suspected lower urinary tract hematuria or genital tract hematuria	Intraluminal filling defects Extraluminal compression Extravasation of contrast material Enlarged prostate Reflux of contrast material into prostate*
Contrast cystography or ultrasonography	Suspected bladder involvement	Radiolucent uroliths Intraluminal mass(es) Wall thickening Urachal remnant Extravasation of contrast material Enlarged prostate Reflux of contrast material into ureters*
Excretory urography	Suspected upper urinary tract hematuria	Renal parenchymal filling defects Renal pelvic dilatation or filling defects Hydronephrosis or hydroureter Ureteral obstruction Ectopic ureter(s) Extravasation of contrast material

* *May be observed in normal dogs.*

graphic procedures. Survey films of the abdomen will provide information about kidney and urinary bladder size, shape, location, and radiographic density. Patient preparation for radiographic evaluation of the urinary system should include withholding food for 24 hours and cleansing enemas given the evening before and morning of (1–3 hours prior) the evaluation. Contrast urethrography may be employed to identify the presence and location of mucosal and mural lesions, luminal filling defects, extramural compression, and urethral rupture or laceration. Abnormalities that may be identified by contrast cystography include mucosal and mural lesions, luminal filling defects, urachal remnants, vesicoureteral reflux, extraluminal mass lesions, and bladder tears. Catheter biopsy (see Catheter Biopsy of the Urethra, Bladder, and Prostate Gland in Chapter 80) of suspected lesions of the urethra or bladder may provide a histologic diagnosis. Excretory urography will provide information about the kidneys and ureters, for example: kidney and ureter number, location, size, and shape; kidney parenchymal filling defects; renal pelvic dilatation or filling defects; hydronephrosis or hydroureter; ureteral obstruction; ectopic ureters; and extravasation of contrast material.

Abdominal exploratory and biopsy may be necessary in some cases to arrive at a diagnosis (Fig. 41-1). Biopsies may be obtained from the kidneys, bladder, and prostate gland, and, if indicated, ureteral catheterization by way of cystotomy may be performed to determine if renal hematuria is unilateral or bilateral.

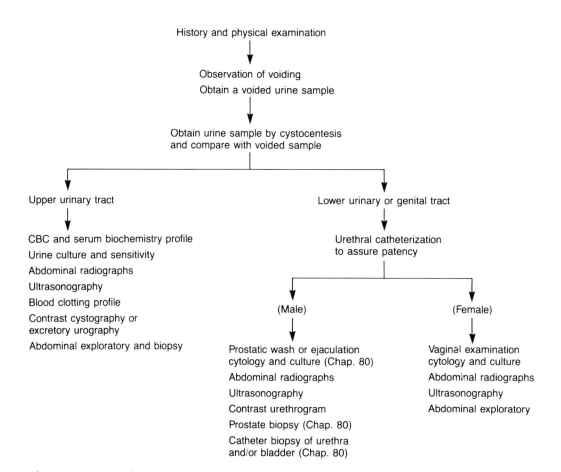

Figure 41–1. *Potential diagnostic procedures for suspected upper and lower urinary tract hemorrhage.*

MANAGEMENT AND PATIENT MONITORING

The management and follow up of the patient with hematuria depends on the underlying disease process.

ADDITIONAL READING

Crow SE. Hematuria: An algorithm for differential diagnosis. Compendium of Continuing Education 1980; 2:941.

Hitt ME. Hematuria of renal origin. Compendium of Continuing Education 1986; 8:14.

Holt PE, Lucke VM, Pearson H. Idiopathic renal hemorrhage in the dog. Journal of Small Animal Practice 1987; 28:253.

Meyer DJ, Senior DF. Hematuria and dysuria. In: Ettinger SJ, ed. Textbook of veterinary internal medicine: Diseases of the dog and cat. Philadelphia: WB Saunders, 1983: 129.

Stone EA, DeNovo RC, Rawlings CA. Massive hematuria of nontraumatic renal origin in dogs. J Am Vet Med Assoc 1983; 183:868.

Wolf AM. Hematuria and dysuria. In: Ford RB, ed. Clinical signs and diagnosis in small animal practice. New York: Churchill Livingstone, 1988: 541.

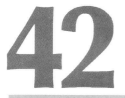

DISORDERS OF MICTURITION

Susan L. Longhofer, Gregory F. Grauer

Micturition is the normal physiologic process of passive storage and active voiding of urine. *Incontinence* may be defined as the inappropriate passage of urine and can occur as a failure of urine storage or as a disorder of urine voiding. The most commonly encountered forms of urinary incontinence are urge and hormone-responsive incontinence. While the exact incidence of either syndrome is unknown, both presentations are frequently observed in practice.

Urge incontinence in a canine or feline patient may be the first sign of lower urinary tract inflammation and is often the sign that leads owners to seek medical care for their pet. Not all forms of urinary incontinence are as easy to diagnose and treat as urge incontinence; but with an understanding of the basic physiology and the drugs currently available, many forms of urinary incontinence can be controlled.

CAUSES

The etiologies of incontinence can be divided into two major categories: neurogenic and non-neurogenic (Table 42-1). Neurogenic incontinence may be caused by any condition that creates compression, damage, or degeneration of the spinal cord, pelvic nerve, or pudendal nerve. Overdistension of the bladder for a prolonged period of time may also create a neurogenic incontinence by affecting depolarization of the bladder detrusor muscle. Non-neurogenic urinary incontinence is a broader category and includes a few forms of incontinence with either an unknown or unproven etiology. Since the neurogenic forms of incontinence usually warrant a poor prognosis it is fortunate that non-neurogenic disorders of micturition are more common.

PATHOPHYSIOLOGY

Micturition is controlled by a combination of autonomic and somatic innervation (Fig. 42-1). Parasympathetic innervation to the bladder is provided by the pelvic nerve which arises from the sacral spinal cord segments S-1 to S-3. Stimulation of the pelvic nerve results in depolarization of pacemaker fibers throughout the detrusor muscle. The subsequent spread of excitation to adjoining muscle fibers through tight junctions of smooth muscle cells leads to contraction of the detrusor muscle.

Table 42–1 *Disorders of Micturition*

Type	Causes
NEUROGENIC	
Lower Motor Neuron (LMN)	Lesion to sacral spinal cord segments S_1–S_3 (at or below 5th lumbar vertebral body)
	neoplasia
	trauma
	cauda equina syndrome
	Trauma to pelvic nerve
	Detrusor atony
	Feline dysautonomia (Key-Gaskell syndrome)
Upper Motor Neuron (UMN)	Lesion cranial to spinal cord segment S1 (above 5th lumbar vertebral body)
	intervertebral disk protrusion
	neoplasia
	trauma
	fibrocartilaginous infarct
	meningitis
	Cerebral disease
	Cerebellar disease
	Brain stem disease
Reflex dyssynergia (detrusor-urethral dyssynergia)	Spinal cord disease or peripheral neuropathy
	Idiopathic
NON-NEUROGENIC	
Hormone-responsive	Estrogen-responsive
	Testosterone-responsive
Urge incontinence	Bladder or urethral irritation
Congenital	Ectopic ureters
	Patent urachus
	Urethral fistula (rectal of vaginal)
	Pseudohermaphroditism
Outflow obstruction (paradoxical incontinence)	Urethral stricture
	Neoplasia
	Cystic or urethral calculi
	Granulomatous urethritis
	Prostatic disease
Idiopathic	Feline leukemia virus
	Inappropriate elimination (senility, excitement, behavioral)

The sacral spinal cord segments S-1 to S-3 are also the source of the somatic innervation to the external urethral sphincter by way of the pudendal nerve. The external urethral sphincter is located in the mid portion of the female urethra and in the membranous portion of the male urethra. Stimulation of the pudendal nerve causes contraction of the striated skeletal muscle of the external urethral sphincter. This contraction is under conscious control; additional somatic functions under conscious control are relaxation of the pelvic musculature and an initiation of the abdominal press which facilitate voiding.

Sympathetic innervation to the bladder through the hypogastric nerve is composed of preganglionic fibers exiting the lumbar spinal cord from the L-1 to L-4 segments and synapsing in the caudal mesenteric ganglion. B-Adrenergic fibers terminate in the detrusor muscle; stimulation results in detrusor muscle relaxation.

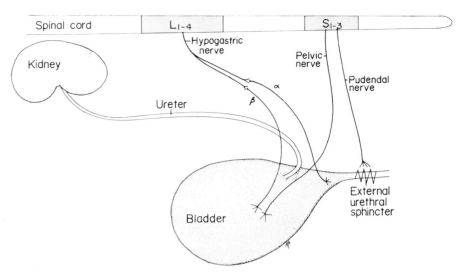

Figure 42–1. *Autonomic and somatic innervation to the bladder.*

α-Adrenergic fibers innervate the smooth muscle fibers in the trigone and urethra, resulting in contraction of these fibers to form a functional internal urethral sphincter (Fig. 42-2). α-Adrenergic receptors also have a modulating effect on the external urethral sphincter.

The normal storage phase is created by sympathetic autonomic domination which results in a relaxed detrusor muscle from β-adrenergic stimulation and urethral sphincter contraction created by α-adrenergic stimulation (Fig. 42-3). Voiding is consciously inhibited by contraction of striated urethral muscle distal to the bladder and reflexively inhibited by a spinal reflex which tightens the external urethral sphincter when a sudden increase in intra-abdominal pressure occurs (*e.g.*, barking, coughing, sneezing, or retching). Incontinence occurs if the pressure in the bladder exceeds the pressure exerted by the urethral sphincter.

Stretch receptors in the bladder sense increased mural tension, and the impulse is transmitted through spinal pathways to the thalamus and cerebral cortex. Voluntary control of micturition is mediated by the cerebral cortex, pons (main micturition center), and the cerebellum through the reticulospinal tract to the sacral nuclei. The voiding phase of micturition is characterized by parasympathetic activity (Fig. 42-4). The detrusor muscle contracts and simultaneous inhibition of the sympathetic stimulation to the

urethral sphincters occurs. When the bladder has emptied, the normal sympathetic domination resumes, and the detrusor muscle relaxes for filling. The normal residual volume of urine is less than 0.2 to 0.4 ml/kg for both the dog and cat.

CLINICAL SIGNS

The age of onset, sexual status of the animal, age at neutering, current medications, and history of trauma or previous urinary tract disorders are important anamnestic points to cover when obtaining the history of an animal with urinary incontinence (Table 42-2). The veterinarian

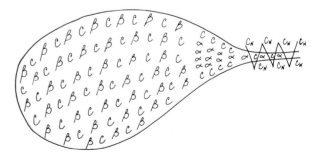

Figure 42–2. *Autonomic and somatic receptors within the bladder and external urethral sphincter. α, α-adrenergic receptors; B, β-adrenergic receptors; C, cholinergic receptors in the detrusor and urethra (muscarinic); C_N, cholinergic receptors in the external urethral sphincter (nicotinic).*

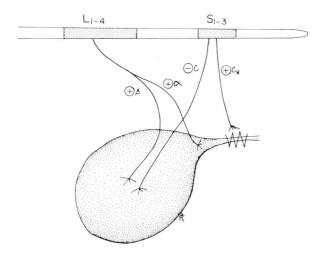

Figure 42–3. *The storage phase of micturition. β-adrenergic stimulation results in relaxation of the detrusor (+ β). α-adrenergic stimulation results in contraction of the smooth muscle fibers in the trigone, resulting in a functional internal urethral sphincter (+ α). Cholinergic (nicotinic) stimulation via the pudendal nerve results in contraction of the external urethral sphincter (+ C$_N$) During the storage phase, no pelvic nerve stimulation to the detrusor exists (− C).*

should question if the incontinence occurs when the animal sleeps; if it is a continuous or an intermittent problem; if the animal is aware that it is urinating; if the animal assumes a normal position as it attempts to void; if there are large or small amounts of urine being passed; and if the

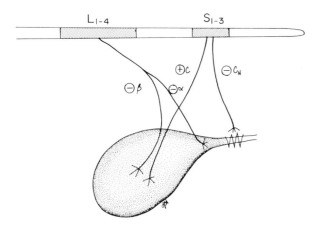

Figure 42–4. *The voiding phase of micturition. No action on the detrusor by the β-adrenergic supply (− β). Lack of stimulation by the α-adrenergic supply results in relaxation of the internal urethral sphincter (− α). Active contraction of the detrusor muscle (+ C). Lack of stimulation by way of the pudendal nerve results in relaxation of the external urethral sphincter (− C$_N$).*

animal is experiencing any difficulty passing urine.

Owners frequently mistake submissive urination, which may be a normal behavior pattern for young dogs, with urinary incontinence (see Chapter 69). Another normal behavior pattern that is misunderstood by some owners is the voiding pattern used by males to mark territory. Evaluation of the owner's description of the animal's voiding pattern may reveal a behavioral basis for the abnormal voiding, although a physical examination and a urinalysis should be performed. The physical examination should include examination of the perineum for evidence of urine scalding or staining (Table 42-3). A thorough palpation of the bladder for size and wall thickness and a rectal examination for assessment of anal tone, prostate gland, pelvic urethra, and trigone region of the bladder should be performed on all dogs. A digital vaginal examination is indicated and vaginoscopy may be used to help identify congenital defects and strictures.

A neurologic examination should include evaluation of the perineal reflex and bulbocavernosus reflex. The perineal reflex causes contraction of the anal sphincter and ventroflexion of the tail after a noxious stimulus. The perineal reflex is usually evaluated during the rectal examination; however, hemostats may be used to prod or pinch the skin in the perineal region to elicit the reflex. The bulbocavernosus reflex is elicited by gently compressing the bulb of the penis or the vulva, with the normal response being contraction of the anal sphincter. Both of the above reflexes are dependent on an intact pudendal nerve (sensory and motor) and the sacral spinal cord segments S-1 to S-3. If both reflexes are normal, the sacral reflex arc is intact.

Dogs should be walked outside so that the voiding posture and urine stream size and character can be observed. Immediately after the animal has attempted to void, the bladder should be palpated to determine residual volume. Catheterization for quantitation of residual volume is indicated if a large bladder is palpable following voiding.

A urinalysis should be performed in all cases presenting with urinary incontinence. Cystocen-

Table 42–2 *Clinical Signs Associated With Micturition Disorders*

Types	Clinical Signs
NEUROGENIC	
Lower Motor Neuron (LMN)	Dribbling of urine
	Distended bladder
	Easily expressed bladder
	History of trauma or surgery to the pelvis
Upper Motor Neuron (UMN)	Distended bladder
	Bladder is difficult to express
	History of paresis or paralysis
Reflex dyssynergia (detrusor-urethral dyssynergia)	Distended bladder
	Urine stream initiated then interrupted
	Easy to catheterize bladder
NON-NEUROGENIC	
Hormone-responsive	Middle-aged to older neutered animal
	Dribbling of urine when asleep or relaxed
	Normal voiding otherwise
Urge incontinence	Pollakiuria
	Hematuria
	Stranguria
Congenital	Young animal
	Constant dribbling of urine
	+/− normal voiding
Outflow obstruction (paradoxical incontinence)	Stranguria
	Dribbling of urine
	Distended bladder
	Difficult to express bladder
	Difficult catheterization
Idiopathic	Dribbling of urine
	Inappropriate voiding

tesis is the preferred method of collection when a urine culture is indicated; however, patients with a distended bladder should be catheterized to empty the bladder and to prevent the possibility of urine leakage from the cystocentesis site. If the

Table 42–3 *Diagnostic Plan for Urinary Incontinence*

1. Obtain history.
2. Perform physical examination, including bladder palpation and rectal examination for assessment of anal tone, prostate gland, and palpation of pelvic urethra and trigone region.
3. Perform neurologic examination, including evaluation of the perineal and bulbocavernosus reflexes.
4. Perform urinalysis.
5. Observe urination and palpate bladder after voiding is complete.
6. Define the condition as neurologic or non-neurologic.

history, physical and neurologic examinations, and urinalysis do not suggest a cause for the incontinence, further laboratory analysis or diagnostic testing may be required (Tables 42-4 and 42-5).

DIAGNOSTIC APPROACH

If neurologic lesions or deficits are detected on neurologic examination, the voiding pattern will help localize the lesion, determine the nature of an injury to the spinal cord, and help classify the injury as an upper motor neuron lesion (above the fifth lumbar vertebral body) or a lower motor neuron lesion (at or below the fifth lumbar vertebral body).

Table 42–4 *Laboratory Evaluation of Urinary Incontinence*

Test	What to Check For
Urinalysis	Evidence of urinary tract inflammation: WBCs, RBCs, crystals, bacteria, proteinuria, alkaline pH Evidence of neoplasia: neoplastic cells Evidence of parasitic disease: ova of *Capillaria* species
Urine culture	Evidence of urinary tract infection: >1,000 organisms/ml in cystocentesis samples, or >10,000 organisms/ml in catheterized samples, or >100,000 organisms/ml in voided urine samples
Serum creatinine, urea nitrogen, and potassium concentrations	Rule out postrenal obstruction

Lower Motor Neuron Injuries to the Bladder

The most characteristic sign of a lower motor neuron lesion to the bladder is a distended bladder that is easily expressed. A lower motor neuron injury affecting the bladder will create both sphincter and detrusor hyporeflexia, and, if the lesion involves spinal cord segments S-1 to S-3, both perineal and bulbocavernosus reflexes will be absent. No voluntary control of bladder function exists, but, if the bladder is not expressed, incomplete emptying will occur as the pressure within the bladder exceeds the resistance created by the nonfunctional urethral sphincters. The bladder empties incompletely because the detrusor muscle does not contract fully and cannot maintain enough pressure to keep the muscles of the urethral sphincter from collapsing. An intramural reflex develops within the detrusor muscle to aid in emptying the bladder, but it is a weak reflex and takes time to develop.

If the detrusor muscle cannot contract, or the tight junctions between smooth muscle cells are

Table 42–5 *Diagnostic Evaluation of Urinary Incontinence*

Test	What to Check for
Abdominal radiographs	Rule out radiopaque cystic calculi, evaluate size of prostate, rule out skeletal abnormalities in the vertebral column and pelvis
Ultrasound of bladder	Rule out mass lesions, urolithiasis, bladder wall thickening
Contrast cystogram and/or urethrogram	Rule out mass lesions, urolithiasis, bladder wall thickening, urachal remnants
Intravenous pyelogram	Rule out evidence of inflammatory or neoplastic disease of kidneys and ureters and ectopic ureter(s)
Myelogram or epidurogram	Rule out spinal cord neoplasia, intervertebral disc protrusion, and cauda equina syndrome
Cerebrospinal fluid analysis	Rule out infectious/inflammatory/neoplastic spinal cord disease
Electromyogram	Evaluate integrity of pudendal nerve
Cystometrogram	Localize area of increased urethral resistance and evaluate bladder tone

disrupted, the bladder is termed atonic, and a large residual volume remains after the overflow of urine occurs. Detrusor atony can occur secondary to a spinal cord lesion, or it may result as a consequence of outflow obstruction, such as that caused by mucous and struvite plugs in male cats with feline lower urinary tract inflammation (see Chapter 48). Other causes include cystic or urethral calculi, neoplasia of the trigone or the urethra, granulomatous urethritis, urethral stricture, or prostatic disease. Even when the urine outflow obstruction is relieved, bladder distention may have damaged the tight junctions so that depolarization of smooth muscle is unable to transverse the bladder, and therefore organized contraction cannot occur.

Feline dysautonomia (Key-Gaskell syndrome) is a syndrome recognized in Great Britain, although an imported cat with the disease has been reported in the United States. Characteristic signs of the disorder are mydriasis, decreased tear and saliva production, megaesophagus, constipation, bradycardia, and urine retention. The etiology of the disease is unknown, but the pathologic lesion is described as an autonomic polyganglionopathy. The bladder of an affected cat is easily expressed and detrusor activity is weak and ineffective.

Any type of injury to the pelvic nerve (trauma or surgery to the pelvic region) may create a lower motor neuron lesion to the bladder. While urethral sphincter incompetence has been observed after feline perineal urethrostomies, urinary incontinence following prostatic surgery in the dog is a much more frequent occurrence.

The diagnostic approach to lower motor neuron lesions should be aimed at determining whether the nature of the lesion is reversible. Traumatic lesions to the pelvic nerve or the sacral nerve roots are potentially reversible since peripheral nerves may regenerate. Detrusor atony is also potentially reversible if the bladder can be kept decompressed long enough to allow reestablishment of the tight junctions. Dysfunction caused by compression lesions of the sacral spinal cord may respond to decompression, but the overall prognosis is poor. A myelogram or epidurogram may reveal the extent of the lesion and guide the prognosis.

Upper Motor Neuron Lesions to the Bladder

Upper motor neuron lesions to the bladder are characterized by a large, distended bladder, especially in the dog with paresis or paralysis (see Chapter 54). No voluntary control of micturition exists, and the urethral sphincter shows reflex hyperexcitability because there is a lack of inhibition to the somatic efferents in the pudendal nerve. Expression of the bladder is difficult. If the lesion is located between spinal cord segments L-4 and S-1, even more resistance will occur because the sympathetic supply will maintain α-adrenergic tone. Reflex micturition (automatic bladder) initiated by an increase in bladder intramural pressure will usually develop 5 to 10 days after the spinal cord injury. When reflex micturition does develop, the voiding is incomplete and a large residual volume remains.

A neurologic examination will help localize the lesion to the brain or the spinal cord. Several diseases and disorders of the brain and brainstem may create upper motor neuron signs to the bladder, including cerebellar disorders, hydrocephalus, and brain tumors. Cerebrospinal fluid analysis may be useful in ruling out infectious (bacterial meningitis, toxoplasmosis, canine distemper, feline infectious peritonitis), inflammatory, or neoplastic disease (sterile meningitis, granulomatous meningoencephalitis, spinal lymphosarcoma) of the central nervous system (see Cerebrospinal Fluid Collection in Chapter 80). A myelogram will usually help determine if a spinal cord lesion (intervertebral disc protrusion or neoplasia) can be surgically approached.

Reflex Dyssynergia

Reflex dyssynergia or detrusor-urethral dyssynergia is a condition observed in male dogs. The etiology is usually difficult to determine but may include any of several neurologic lesions of the spinal cord or autonomic ganglia. The pathophysiology of reflex dyssynergia is created by active contraction of the detrusor without relaxation of the internal or external urethral sphincters.

Characteristic signs of reflex dyssynergia include normal or near normal initiation of voiding which is interrupted by contractions of the external urethral sphincter. The urine stream becomes narrowed or it may be delivered in spurts or it may be completely disrupted. The dog often strains and assumes a squatting position. Differential diagnoses that must be ruled out include urethral calculi or urethral and/or prostatic neoplasia. The bladder is usually distended and difficult to express but is easily catheterized. A neurologic examination is usually normal in these animals. A myelogram or an epidurogram may be performed to rule out compression or mass lesions of the spinal cord.

Hormone-Responsive Urinary Incontinence

Estrogens are believed to contribute to the integrity of urethral muscle tone. Middle-aged to older, spayed female dogs are prone to developing incontinence associated with sleeping and relaxation. The urine volume ranges from a "dribble" to a large volume, and dogs are not conscious of the incontinence. Intensive investigation into the sex hormone concentrations of these dogs has not been performed; however, the condition often responds to estrogen replacement therapy. Less frequently observed are male dogs that develop incontinence after castration; the condition seems to occur most commonly in dogs castrated at an older age. The condition in male dogs frequently responds to testosterone administration. Diagnosis of both disease processes is based on history, physical examination, and response to therapy.

Urge Incontinence

Urge incontinence is the inability to control voiding due to a strong urge to urinate. Inflammation of the bladder or urethra may create a sensation of bladder fullness which triggers the voiding reflex. Clinical signs of urge incontinence include stranguria, pollakiuria, and frequently hematuria. Bacterial urinary tract infection is the most common cause in the dog, and feline lower urinary tract inflammation is the most common cause in cats. A urinalysis with evidence of a urinary tract infection or inflammation (crystalluria, pyuria, or hematuria) is an adequate initial diagnostic approach for most animals with urge incontinence. If symptoms persist after the urinary tract inflammation has been successfully treated, further diagnostics, including contrast radiography, are indicated.

Infiltrative disease of the bladder (neoplasia or chronic cystitis) can produce pollakiuria and stranguria due to the lack of distensibility of the bladder. The bladder may be small and thickened on palpation, and ultrasonic examination or contrast radiography of the bladder usually demonstrates a thickened bladder wall. Infiltrative disease of the urethra (neoplasia or granulomatous urethritis) may decrease sphincter closure and create incontinence. A retrograde urethrogram is usually necessary to diagnose infiltrative disease of the urethra.

Polyuria and polydipsia can create urge incontinence by placing continual stress on the bladder wall and urethral sphincter; however, in these cases urine volume is large. A normally well-housebroken animal may start urinating in the house if frequent access to the outdoors is not provided. If increased thirst and large urine volume are described by the owners, conditions that cause polyuria and polydipsia should be ruled out (*e.g.,* diabetes mellitus, pyometra, hyperadrenocorticism, and hypercalcemia) and appropriate diagnostic tests should be performed (see Chapter 9). Iatrogenic causes, such as corticosteroid or diuretic administration, should not be overlooked.

Congenital and Anatomic Disorders

Urinary incontinence in a young animal may be associated with a variety of congenital defects of the urinary and genital systems. The most common defect is an ectopic ureter, but patent urachus, urethrorectal and urethrovaginal fistulas, female pseudohermaphroditism, and vestibulovaginal stenosis have been associated with urinary incontinence. Ectopic ureters are most commonly observed in female dogs, and breeds with the highest incidence include Siberian huskies, miniature and toy poodles, Labrador retrievers, fox terriers, West Highland white terriers, collies, and Welsh corgis. Ectopic ureters are rarely seen in cats, but the sex incidence is reversed with males having the greater incidence of occurrence.

The most common clinical sign associated with an ectopic ureter is almost constant dribbling of urine, although dogs with a unilateral ectopic ureter may void normally. Since 70% of ectopic ureters terminate in the vagina, endoscopic examination of the vagina can be used to visualize the opening of the ectopic ureter into the vagina; however, the opening is often difficult to see. An intravenous urogram is the diagnostic test of choice; alternatively, retrograde vaginourethrography may be used to characterize the defect.

Iatrogenic causes of urinary incontinence may be a result of pudendal or pelvic nerve trauma during surgery. Ureterovaginal fistula after ovariohysterectomy, uterine stump inflammation/infection, and urethral fistula after trauma or surgery have been associated with urinary incontinence. A history of trauma or recent surgery will provide a diagnostic clue in these cases, and contrast radiography will often help delineate the nature of the disorder.

Outflow Obstruction

Incontinence in an animal with urinary outflow obstruction is called paradoxical incontinence. When intravesicular pressure exceeds the pressure within the urethra, urine leaks past the outflow obstruction. Clinical signs include dribbling of urine, straining to urinate without producing urine, restlessness, and abdominal pain. The most common causes are urethral calculi and neoplasia in dogs (see Catheter Biopsy of the Urethra, Bladder, and Prostate Gland in Chapter 80) and feline lower urinary tract inflammation in cats; however urethral strictures and granulomatous urethritis can also create an obstruction to urine flow. Any type of prostatic disease may create an outflow obstruction (see Chapter 57). Older male dogs with benign prostatic hyperplasia may present with stranguria and tenesmus; however, prostatic neoplasia and prostatic abscessation are more likely causes of urinary outflow obstruction.

The very real possibility that paradoxical urinary incontinence may progress to complete urinary outflow obstruction necessitates an aggressive approach to the diagnosis and management of this condition. Diagnostics should include passage of a urinary catheter to assess urethral patency and diameter. Contrast radiography of the urethra and bladder is indicated, as well as evaluation of serum creatinine, urea nitrogen, and potassium concentrations.

Idiopathic Urinary Incontinence

In addition to the above non-neurogenic forms of urinary incontinence, there is a group of diseases that are not easily classified. Incontinence has been observed in a group of cats positive for feline leukemia virus infection. These cats were middle-aged males and females, and the pattern of urinary incontinence was similar to that of hormone-responsive urinary incontinence. Incontinence occurred primarily when the cats were asleep or resting, and normal voiding occurred otherwise. In one report, six of eleven cats had concurrent anisocoria, although neurologic examinations were otherwise normal.

Stress incontinence is a condition observed in women characterized by leakage of urine whenever intra-abdominal pressure is suddenly increased (*e.g.,* laughing, sneezing, standing, or climbing stairs). The exact condition may not occur in dogs, but a similar clinical presentation is observed in dogs that are incontinent whenever excited or frightened. Nervous dogs are especially prone to this condition, and it may also be observed in geriatric dogs. Urethral sphincter incompetence is the most likely cause, but this has not been proven.

Inappropriate urination associated with a behavioral problem is frustrating for both the owners and the veterinarians. Veterinarians can eliminate physical causes of inappropriate urination, but determining the reason for the behavior is often difficult (see Chapter 69). Incontinence may be caused by senility, decreased bladder capacity, or decreased physical control in geriatric patients. Physical problems, especially polyuric disorders and disabilities that impair mobility should be evaluated and treated. Diuretics and corticosteroids should be avoided if possible, as they will often exacerbate incontinence.

MANAGEMENT

Lower Motor Neuron Injuries to the Bladder

Patients with lower motor neuron diseases resulting from sacral spinal cord lesions or from feline dysautonomia require expression or catheterization of the bladder at least three times a day. Strict aseptic technique should be adhered to during bladder catheterization. During the initial stages, urinalysis or examination of a urine sediment should be performed weekly, and a urine culture should be initiated if any evidence of a urinary tract infection is found. Care should be taken to prevent urine scalding. Bethanechol may be administered to increase detrusor contractility if urethral patency is assured (Table 42-6). Side effects of bethanechol include salivation, vomiting, diarrhea, or colic-like signs indicating intestinal cramping. These signs are normally noticed within an hour of drug administration, and, if observed, the dosage of bethanechol should be decreased.

Management of detrusor atony requires intermittent or indwelling urinary catheterization to keep the bladder empty for a period of days to weeks. A closed urine collection system should always be employed with indwelling catheters. Urinalysis should be performed every 3 to 4 days, and a urine culture and antibiotic sensitivity obtained if there is any evidence of urinary tract inflammation. Bethanechol may be administered to increase detrusor contractility.

Upper Motor Neuron Lesions to the Bladder

Management of patients with an upper motor neuron lesion to the bladder is dependent on the presence or absence of an automatic bladder.

Prior to the development of the automatic bladder, treatment should include aseptic catheterization three times a day. Use of corticosteroids for neurologic disease may create polyuria, necessitating more frequent catheterization to prevent overdistension of the bladder. Corticosteroids will also predispose patients to urinary tract infection. During the initial stages, urinalysis or examination of urine sediment should be performed every 3 to 4 days, and a urine culture and antibiotic sensitivity should be obtained if there is evidence of urinary tract inflammation (corticosteroids will frequently mask signs of inflammation in urine; see Chapter 46). Because these animals are usually painful and reluctant to move, prevention of urine scalding is important. Use of elevated racks or absorbent bedding is indicated and petroleum jelly around the perineum or prepuce may minimize urine scalding.

After the development of an automatic bladder, the bladder should be palpated after urination to determine residual urine volume. Bladder expression two to three times a day may still be required to minimize urine stasis. Urinalysis should continue on a bimonthly schedule (at least monthly if the animal is receiving corticosteroids), and the owners should be instructed to bring in a urine sample if a change in urine color or odor is noted. Nursing care to prevent urine scalding should be continued.

Reflex Dyssynergia

Reflex dyssynergia will often respond to pharmacologic management; however, therapeutic response may require 2 to 3 weeks. Drugs that are usually incorporated include phenoxybenzamine, a somatic muscle relaxant (diazepam), and occasionally bethanechol (see Table 42-6). Intermittent urinary catheterization should be used as required to keep the bladder empty and combat detrusor atony created by overdistension.

Phenoxybenzamine has a slow onset of action, and the dosage should be increased slowly at 4-day intervals. The urinary stream is used as an indication of drug effectiveness. If the stream is weak but continuous, bethanechol may be used to increase detrusor contractility; however, bethanechol must not be used until the functional

Table 42–6 *Drugs Used in the Pharmacologic Management of Disorders of Micturition*

Drug	Action	Dosage
Aminoproprazine	Smooth muscle relaxant	2.0 mg/kg two times daily, IM (dog and cat)
Bethanechol	Parasympathomimetic increased detrusor contractility	5 to 15 mg three times daily, PO (dog) 1.25 to 5 mg three times daily, PO (cat)
Diazepam	Somatic muscle relaxant	2 to 10 mg three times daily, PO (dog) 2 to 5 mg three times daily, PO (cat)
Diethylstilbestrol	Increase urethral sphincter tone	0.1 to 1 mg once daily, PO 3 to 5 days then 0.1 to 1 mg q 7 days (dog)
Ephedrine	α-adrenergic increase urethral sphincter tone	12.5 to 50 mg three times daily, PO (dog) 2 to 4 mg/kg three times daily, PO (cat)
Oxybutynin	Direct antispasmodic effect on smooth muscle	5 mg two or three times daily, PO (dog)
Phenoxybenzamine	α-blocker decrease urethral sphincter tone	5 to 15 mg three times daily, PO (dog) 2.5 to 7.5 mg three times daily, PO (cat)
Phenylpropanolamine	α-adrenergic increase urethral sphincter tone	12.5 to 50 mg three times daily, PO (dog) 12.5 mg three times daily, PO (cat)
Propantheline bromide	Anticholinergic decrease detrusor contractility	5 to 30 mg three times daily, PO (dog) 5.0 to 7.5 mg three times daily, PO (cat)
Testosterone cypionate	Increase urethral sphincter tone	2.2 mg/kg IM, q 30 days (dog)

urethral obstruction has been relieved. If the urine stream is intermittent or narrowed, increased dosage of diazepam or phenoxybenzamine is required. Because diazepam has a very short duration of action (approximately 1–2 hours when administered orally), administering diazepam 30 minutes prior to walking the animal will sometimes aid in the management of dyssynergia. It may be several weeks before a correct combination of drugs is determined, and drug dosages may need modification over time. Periodic urinalysis are indicated to detect urinary tract inflammation at an early stage.

Hypotension is the major side effect of phenoxybenzamine administration, and the dosage should be immediately decreased if the animal shows any indication of weakness or disorientation. The dosage of phenoxybenzamine should only be increased if a favorable response is not observed after 4 days. The drug has a slow onset of action, and rapid increases in dosage should be avoided. Nausea is a side effect which can be minimized by administering the medication with a small meal. Glaucoma is a rare complication of phenoxybenzamine administration in humans.

Hormone-Responsive Urinary Incontinence

Treatment of hormone-responsive urinary incontinence includes hormone replacement and/or the use of α-adrenergic drugs (see Table 42-6). The usual induction therapy for estrogen-responsive incontinence is 0.1 to 1 mg diethylstilbestrol (DES) orally, every 24 hours for 3 to 5 days. The frequency of administration is then decreased to the lowest possible dose that will maintain continence. Some dogs can be successfully tapered to a very low maintenance dose of DES (0.1–1 mg every 7 days). Phenylpropanolamine or ephedrine (12.5–50 mg every 8 hours) may be used as an alternative drug or in addition to DES. Clients with dogs on phenylpropanolamine or ephedrine should be cautioned to observe their dog for hyperexcitability, panting, or anorexia. If these signs develop, the dosage should be decreased. While initially administered on an 8-hour schedule, in some animals, the dose of phenylpropanolamine can be decreased to a 12- or 24-hour schedule of administration. The owner's careful observation for recurrence of signs will indicate when the dose needs to be increased. Dogs with increasing resistance to DES present the greatest worry, since development of estruslike symptoms and bone marrow toxicity are possible side effects of DES administration. Endocrine alopecia is another possible side effect of DES administration. If DES-resistant dogs are not on concurrent phenylpropanolamine or ephedrine, a trial should be instituted before the DES dose exceeds recommended levels (1 mg once a day).

Testosterone-responsive urinary incontinence is best managed by parenteral testosterone since most oral testosterone undergoes rapid hepatic degradation. Depository forms injected intramuscularly may be effective for 3 to 6 weeks. Male dogs receiving testosterone should have regular rectal examinations to evaluate prostate size, especially if benign prostatic hyperplasia was the reason for castration. Testosterone-responsive incontinence will frequently respond to phenylpropanolamine or ephedrine, and these drugs can be used in male dogs with prostatic enlargement or perianal adenomas.

Urge Incontinence

Smooth muscle relaxants and anticholinergics (aminoproprazine, oxybutynin, propantheline bromide) have been used in addition to antibiotics to decrease the detrusor spasticity associated with urinary tract infections. Caution must be used to avoid the phenazopyridine dyes commonly used as urinary analgesics in human patients as they have been associated with methemoglobinemia, especially in cats.

Chronic or recurrent cystitis requires a thorough evaluation of the cause of the urinary tract infections (see Chapter 46). Antispasmodics may provide a small degree of relief; however, the underlying cause of the detrusor spasticity should be identified and corrected. Neoplastic growths within the bladder may be successfully removed, especially if they are located in the apex of the bladder. Neoplastic growths involving the trigone are more difficult to manage, although intra-operative radiation may be available at referral centers, or veterinary oncologists may be consulted to design a chemotherapy program. In cases where bladder ablation is indicated or invasive urethral neoplasia is causing outflow obstruction, transplantation of the ureters into the colon or small intestine may be attempted. Ascending pyelonephritis is a common complication of ureteral-colonic anastomosis, as are impaired renal function, gastrointestinal disturbances, diarrhea, and fecal incontinence.

Congenital and Anatomic Defects

Correction of congenital defects will depend on the nature and the extent of the defect. For example, a patent urachus and urachal diverticulum are surgically correctable as are many forms of ectopic ureters. However, urethral sphincter incompetence may occur in conjunction with an ectopic ureter, and surgical reimplantation of the ureter may not guarantee continence. Use of α-adrenergic drugs after surgery increases the percentage of successfully treated cases.

Outflow Obstruction

The size and nature of the lesion will usually determine if complete or incomplete obstruction occurs. Prevention of renal damage secondary to urinary obstruction and relief of urinary obstruction to prevent detrusor atony from overdistension are the main priorities in cases of urine outflow obstruction. The bladder should be catheterized and contrast urethrography performed. If the obstruction is created by urethral calculi, retropulsion of the urethral calculi into the bladder may be successful. If the calculi cannot be moved by retropulsion, a temporary or permanent perineal urethrostomy may be necessary.

In cases of benign prostatic hyperplasia, castration will usually result in a rapid decrease in the size of the prostate (see Chapter 57). The use of estrogens to decrease prostatic size is not recommended because of the potential for systemic side effects and squamous metaplasia of the prostate (see Appendix II). Surgical marsupialization may be necessary to manage prostatic abscessation. In some cases of prostatic neoplasia, partial or complete prostatectomy may be beneficial. Urethral neoplasia is often inoperable since clinical signs are usually not observed until the neoplasia is invasive.

PATIENT MONITORING

In general, the prognosis for neurogenic forms of urinary incontinence is poor. The long-term prognosis for most spinal cord lesions is unfavorable unless decompression of an intervertebral disc protrusion or removal of an extradural mass is successfully accomplished. Even if the lesion is decompressed, complete return of normal micturition may not occur since the central nervous system has a minimal capacity for regeneration. Damage to the pudendal nerve, pelvic nerve, or the sacral nerve roots has a more favorable prognosis since peripheral nerves have the potential to regenerate.

Long-term care of paralyzed patients is necessary in most cases. Many owners can be taught to express the animal's bladder, and many can learn to catheterize the urinary bladder. While animals kept outdoors are easiest to manage, a modified diaper may be useful for indoor pets. Some owners can not or will not deal with an incontinent animal; however, many will take the necessary steps to help their animal. Frequent urinalysis should be performed in these patients because of the high risk of urinary tract infection. Reflex dyssynergia may respond to pharmacologic management for a variable period, but occasionally the underlying disease process worsens, making pharmacologic management ineffective. Drug dosages should be re-evaluated and increased, but this approach is not always successful. Diagnostic procedures, such as a myelogram or an epidurogram, may be indicated in these refractory cases. Catheterization may be necessary for long-term management and aseptic technique must be emphasized.

Periodic urinalysis to rule out urinary tract infections is an important follow-up procedure for any disorder of micturition. The frequency of the urinalysis will depend on the nature of the disorder. The owners can be instructed to evaluate the color and odor of the urine and to bring in a urine sample immediately if they have any suspicions of an infection; however, routine monitoring is the cornerstone of prevention of severe urinary tract infections.

In contrast to a dog with neurogenic urinary incontinence, monitoring a dog with hormone-responsive urinary incontinence includes infrequent urinalysis. The prognosis for hormone-responsive urinary incontinence is usually excellent, although some dogs will require multiple drugs for management.

Dogs treated for urge incontinence secondary to a urinary tract infection should receive a follow-up urinalysis or urine culture if the animal is on corticosteroids to verify that the urinary tract infection has been eliminated. If urolithiasis (see Chapter 47) or feline lower urinary tract inflammation (see Chapter 48) is present, long-term dietary management may help prevent recurrences.

ADDITIONAL READING

Barsanti JA, Finco DR. Feline urinary incontinence. In: Kirk RW, ed. Current veterinary therapy IX. Philadelphia: WB Saunders, 1986: 1159.

Chew DJ, DiBartola SD, Fenner WR. Pharmacologic manipulation of urination. In: Kirk RW, ed. Current veterinary therapy IX. Philadelphia: WB Saunders, 1986: 1207.

Krawiec DR, Rubin SI. Urinary incontinence in geriatric dogs. Compend Contin Educ 1985; 7:557.

Moreau PM. Neurogenic disorders of micturition in the dog and cat. Compend Contin Educ 1982; 4:12.

Oliver JE, Osborne CA. Neurogenic urinary inconti- nence. In: Kirk RW, ed. Current veterinary therapy VII. Philadelphia: WB Saunders, 1980: 1122.

Osborne CA, Oliver JE, Polzin DE. Non-neurogenic urinary incontinence. In: Kirk RW, ed. Current veterinary therapy VII. Philadelphia, WB Saunders, 1980: 1128.

Rosin AH, Ross L. Diagnosis and pharmacologic management of disorders of urinary continence in the dog. Compendium of Continuing Education 1981; 3:601.

43

ACUTE RENAL FAILURE

Gregory F. Grauer

Acute renal failure (ARF) results from an abrupt decline in renal function and is characterized by impaired regulation of water and solute balance. Toxic and ischemic insults are the most common causes of acute renal dysfunction, usually resulting in damage to the epithelium of the proximal tubules. Nephrotoxicants interfere with essential tubular cell functions and cause cellular injury and death. Renal ischemia causes cellular hypoxia and substrate insufficiency, which lead to adenosine triphosphate depletion, cellular swelling, and death. Vasoconstriction occurs secondary to proximal tubular injury and further decreases glomerular filtration. Importantly, tubular lesions and dysfunction caused by toxic and ischemic insults are often reversible. The incidence of ARF in dogs and cats is unknown; however, in comparison to chronic renal insufficiency or failure, ARF is less common.

CAUSES AND PATHOPHYSIOLOGY

The kidneys are susceptible to ischemia and toxicants because of their unique anatomic and physiologic features (Table 43-1). The dispropor-

tionately large renal blood flow (approximately 20% of the cardiac output) can result in increased delivery of blood-borne toxicants to the kidney as compared to other organs. The renal cortex is especially vulnerable to toxicant exposure because it receives 90% of the renal blood flow and contains the large endothelial surface area of the glomerular capillaries. Additionally, decreased renal perfusion may result in severe renal cortical vasoconstriction and redistribution of blood flow away from the renal cortex decreasing glomerular filtration.

Within the renal cortex, the proximal tubular epithelial cells are most frequently affected by ischemia and toxicant-induced injury because of their transport functions and high metabolic rate. Hypoxia and substrate insufficiency associated with ischemia can decrease proximal tubular cell adenosine triphosphate stores, causing inactivity of the sodium/potassium pump, cell swelling, and death. In the process of reabsorbing water and electrolytes from the glomerular filtrate, proximal tubular epithelial cells may also be exposed to increasingly high concentrations of toxicants. Toxicants that are either secreted or reabsorbed by tubular epithelial cells (*e.g.*, gen-

Table 43–1 Factors That Predispose the Kidney to Ischemia and Toxicant-Induced Injury

- Kidneys receive 20% of cardiac output; the cortex receives 90% of the renal blood flow
- Large glomerular capillary endothelial surface area
- Proximal tubule cells have a high metabolic rate and are susceptible to hypoxia and nutrient deficiency
- Tubular secretion and reabsorption may concentrate toxicants within cells
- Countercurrent multiplier system may concentrate toxicants within the medulla
- Drug metabolism within kidney can create toxic metabolites

tamicin) may accumulate in high concentrations within these cells. Similarly, in the medulla, the countercurrent multiplier system may concentrate toxicants.

Finally, the kidneys also play a role in the biotransformation of many drugs and toxicants. Biotransformation usually results in the formation of metabolites that are less toxic than the parent compound; however, in some cases (*e.g.,* ethylene glycol), metabolites are more toxic.

Table 43-2 contains a partial list of potential nephrotoxicants. It should be noted that toxic insults to the kidney are often caused by therapeutic agents in addition to the more well known nephrotoxicants. In my experience, gentamicin is the most common cause of toxicant-induced ARF

Table 43–2 Common Potential Nephrotoxicants

Antimicrobials	Anesthetics
aminoglycosides	methoxyflurane
cephalosporins	Heavy metals
polymixins	lead
sulfonamides	mercury
tetracyclines	cadmium
Antifungals	chromium
amphotericin B	Organic compounds
Anthelmintics	ethylene glycol
thiacetarsamide	carbon tetrachloride
Analgesics	chloroform
acetaminophen	pesticides
ibuprofen	herbicides
phenylbutazone	solvents
Intravenous radiographic	Pigments
contrast agents	myoglobin
Chemotherapeutic agents	hemoglobin
cis-platinum	Miscellaneous
methotrexate	hypercalcemia
daunorubicin	snake venom

followed by ethylene glycol. Table 43-3 contains a partial list of ischemic causes of ARF. Prolonged anesthesia with inadequate fluid therapy in older dogs and cats is a frequent cause of renal ischemia and ARF.

Nephrotoxicants damage tubular epithelium by interacting with cell membranes or intracellular organelles. Cell membrane function may be impaired by lipid peroxidation, decreased adenosine triphosphate-mediated transport, or disruption of normal sterol-lipid interactions. Changes in cell membrane permeability impair cellular osmoregulation and result in swelling and death. Toxicants may also act as haptens and initiate immune-mediated damage subsequent to cell membrane attachment. Toxicants that accumulate within epithelial cells may interact with cellular proteins, nucleic acids, or lipids. Cellular injury and death can occur by uncoupling of the mitochondrial chain or by disrupting critical enzymatic activity.

The kidneys can maintain adequate renal perfusion pressure by autoregulation as long as mean arterial blood pressure is greater than 60 mm Hg. Maintenance of renal blood flow and perfusion pressure are necessary for both glomerular filtration and cellular delivery of oxygen and nutrients. Cellular swelling secondary to decreased sodium/potassium pump activity results in osmotic extraction of water from the extracellular space and decreased plasma water. The consequences of decreased plasma water in the renal vasculature are erythrocyte aggregation, vascular congestion, and stasis, which tend to potentiate and perpetuate the decrease in glomerular filtration, cellular oxygen, and nutrient deficiency. The

Table 43–3 Common Causes of Renal Ischemia

Dehydration	Hyperthermia
Hemorrhage	Hypothermia
Hypovolemia	Burns
Deep anesthesia	Trauma
Hypotension	Renal vessel thrombosis/
Sepsis	microthrombus formation
Analgesic administration/	Transfusion reactions
causing decreased renal	
prostaglandin formation	
and vasoconstriction	

common result of ischemic- or toxicant-induced tubular cell injury and death is nephron dysfunction and decreased glomerular filtration rate.

At the nephron level, dysfunction and reduced glomerular filtration occur in ischemic and toxicant-induced ARF due to a combination of tubular obstruction, tubular backleak, renal vasoconstriction, and decreased glomerular permeability (Fig. 43-1). Cellular debris within the tubule may inspissate and obstruct flow of filtrate through the nephron. Backleak of filtrate occurs due to loss of tubular cell integrity, allowing filtrate to escape from the tubular lumen to the interstitial space where it may be reabsorbed. Ischemic or toxicant-induced tubular damage and tubuloglomerular feedback are thought to play a role in causing renal vasoconstriction. Decreased reabsorption by damaged proximal tubule segments increases solute delivery to the distal nephron and macula densa, which results in afferent glomerular arteriolar constriction. The exact mediator of this vasoconstriction is not known, but renal prostaglandins, natriuretic factor, or the renin-angiotensin system may be involved. A decrease in the permeability of the glomerular capillary wall can also lead to a reduction of glomerular filtration. Aminoglycosides have been shown to decrease both the number and size of fenestrae in glomerular capillary endothelial cells, thereby decreasing the available surface area for ultrafiltration.

Acute renal failure has three distinct phases that are categorized as initiation, maintenance, and recovery. Ischemic episodes and nephrotoxicants that are responsible for initiating ARF may only be present for a matter of minutes or hours. During the initiation phase, therapeutic measures that reduce the renal insult can prevent development of established ARF. The maintenance phase is characterized by tubular lesions and established nephron dysfunction. Therapeutic intervention during the maintenance phase, although often life saving, usually does little to diminish existing renal lesions or improve existing dysfunction. The recovery phase is the period when renal lesions resolve and function improves. Tubular damage may be reversible if the tubular basement membrane is intact and viable epithelial cells are present. Although additional nephrons cannot be produced and irreversibly dam-

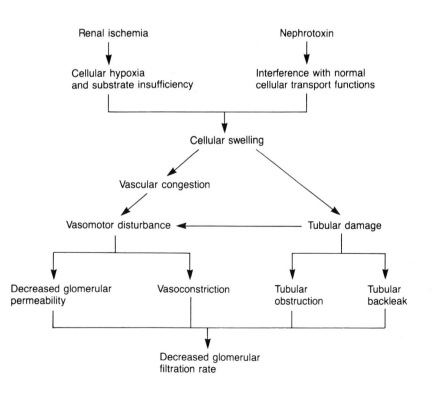

Figure 43–1. *Pathophysiology of acute renal failure.*

aged nephrons can not be repaired, functional and morphologic hypertrophy of surviving nephrons can often adequately compensate for the decrease in nephron numbers. Even if renal function recovery is incomplete, adequate function may be reestablished over a period of weeks or months.

CLINICAL SIGNS AND DIAGNOSTIC APPROACH

Clinical signs of ARF are nonspecific and include lethargy, depression, anorexia, gastroenteritis, and dehydration. Occasionally uremic breath or oral ulcers may be present. A diagnosis of renal failure is confirmed when azotemia with concurrent isosthenuria or minimally concentrated urine is documented. Often the greatest diagnostic challenge is differentiating between prerenal azotemia, ARF, and chronic renal failure (CRF).

Extraurinary disorders may cause a decrease in renal blood flow and glomerular filtration rate and cause prerenal azotemia. Examples include severe dehydration, congestive heart failure, and hypoadrenocorticism. Prerenal azotemia is initially associated with structurally normal kidneys; however, renal ischemic damage may result if the prerenal abnormality is severe or prolonged. Although treatment is initially the same for prerenal azotemia and ARF (fluid therapy and volume replacement), the prognosis is quite different. In cases of prerenal azotemia, the kidneys produce hypersthenuric urine (urine specific gravity greater than 1.030 in dogs and greater than 1.035 in cats) with a relatively low concentration of sodium and high concentration of creatinine (Table 43-4).

Acute renal failure occurs within hours or days. Unique clinical signs and laboratory findings associated with ARF include enlarged or swollen kidneys, elevated hematocrit, good body condition, an abnormal urine sediment, and relatively severe hyperkalemia and metabolic acidosis. In contrast to ARF, CRF occurs over a period of weeks, months, or years and clinical signs associated with CRF are often relatively mild for the magnitude of the azotemia. Unique signs of CRF include a history of weight loss and polydipsia-polyuria, poor body condition, nonregenerative anemia, small and irregular kidneys, and hyperparathyroidism (Table 43-5).

The hallmark of ARF due to any cause is a decrease in glomerular filtration rate. Azotemia, however, is not evident until two thirds to three fourths of the nephrons are not functioning; therefore, significant tubular lesions and decreases in glomerular filtration are often present before azotemia is detected. Urine volume may be increased, normal, or decreased, but the quality of the urine is always poor. For example, gentamicin-induced ARF is usually nonoliguric, whereas ARF induced by ethylene glycol is oliguric; however, both conditions result in urine that is isosthenuric or minimally concentrated containing high concentrations of sodium (greater than 40 mEq/L or 40 mmol/L) and relatively low concentrations of creatinine. In addition, urine may contain glucose, abnormal quantities of protein, and, depending on urine volume, casts and renal epithelial cells. Calcium oxalate crystals (most commonly monohydrate calcium

Table 43–4 *Differentiation of Prerenal Azotemia From Acute Renal Failure*

Indices	Prerenal Azotemia	Acute Renal Failure
Urine specific gravity	Hypersthenuric	Isosthenuric or minimally concentrated
Urine Na (mEq/L)	<10 to 20	>25 to 40
Urine creatinine to plasma creatinine ratio	>20:1	<10:1
Renal failure index (urine Na/urine to plasma creatinine ratio)	<1	>2

Table 43–5 *Differentiation of Acute From Chronic Renal Failure*

Acute Renal Failure	Chronic Renal Failure
History of ischemia or toxicant exposure	History of renal disease or polyuria-polydipsia
Normal or increased hematocrit	Nonregenerative anemia
Swollen kidneys	Small, irregular kidneys
Hyperkalemia	Normal or hypokalemia
Metabolic acidosis	Normal or mild metabolic acidosis
Abnormal urine sediment	Normal urine sediment
Good body flesh	Weight loss, hyperparathyroidism (osteodystrophy)
Relatively severe clinical signs for level of renal dysfunction	Relatively mild clinical signs for level of renal dysfunction

oxalate crystals) may be observed in the urine sediment in approximately 50% of dogs and cats ingesting ethylene glycol.

Histologic examination of renal biopsy specimens (see Kidney Biopsy in Chapter 80) will reveal proximal tubular cell degeneration ranging from cloudy swelling to necrosis. The interstitium may be edematous and infiltrated by polymorphonuclear leukocytes. Although these changes do not allow differentiation of toxicant-induced ARF from ARF due to ischemia, evaluation of renal histology is often helpful in establishing a prognosis. Evidence of tubular regeneration (flattened, basophilic epithelial cells with irregular nuclear size, mitotic figures, and high nuclear to cytoplasmic ratios) and generally intact tubular basement membranes are good prognostic signs. Conversely, large numbers of granular casts and extensive tubular necrosis and interstitial mineralization and fibrosis are poor prognostic signs. In addition to renal histology, the degree of functional impairment and response to therapy should be considered when formulating a prognosis.

MANAGEMENT AND PATIENT MONITORING

Since ARF is frequently iatrogenic (*e.g.*, therapeutic nephrotoxic agents or inadequate fluid therapy during anesthesia), prevention is the best therapy. Several risk factors have been identified

that predispose dogs to gentamicin-induced ARF (Table 43-6). These factors may also predispose dogs and cats to other types of toxicant-induced ARF as well as ARF induced by ischemia.

Preexisting conditions associated with decreased glomerular filtration and renal blood flow increase the risk of ARF in animals exposed to nephrotoxicants or ischemic episodes. Renal disease or renal insufficiency, advanced age, dehydration, and decreased cardiac output will decrease glomerular filtration and thereby renal excretion of nephrotoxicants. In addition, dehydration and decreased cardiac output may cause increased tubular reabsorption of nephrotoxicants. Fever, sepsis, liver disease, electrolyte abnormalities, and concurrent use of diuretics or other potential nephrotoxicants are

Table 43–6 *Acute Renal Failure: Potential Risk Factors*

Pre-existing renal disease or renal insufficiency
Advanced age
Dehydration
Decreased cardiac output
Sepsis, pyometra
Fever
Liver disease
Electrolyte abnormalities, for example, hypokalemia or hypercalcemia
Concurrent use of diuretics
Concurrent use of potentially nephrotoxic drugs, for example, aminoglycosides and intravenous radiographic contrast agents or methoxyflurane
Diabetes mellitus?

additional predisposing factors. In particular, concurrent use of furosemide and gentamicin has been associated with increased risk and severity of ARF. Furosemide probably potentiates gentamicin-induced nephrotoxicity by causing dehydration and a reduction in volume of distribution or by increasing the renal cortical concentration of gentamicin.

Acute renal failure is also common in dogs with pyometra and *Escherichia coli* endotoxin-induced urine concentrating defects. If fluid therapy is inadequate during anesthesia for ovariohysterectomy, dehydration and decreased renal perfusion may result in ARF. In humans, diabetes mellitus has also been identified as a risk factor for ARF. When anesthesia or potentially nephrotoxic drugs are indicated, recognition of these risk factors should alert the clinician to assess the risk : benefit ratio for the patient.

If renal damage is suspected, all potentially nephrotoxic drugs should be withdrawn. Induction of emesis or gastric lavage should be considered to decrease absorption of recently ingested toxicants. In addition, use of gastrointestinal adsorbents and cathartics (*e.g.,* activated charcoal and sodium sulfate, see Appendix I and II) may also be beneficial. Peritoneal dialysis (see Peritoneal and Pleural Dialysis in Chapter 80) can be used to decrease blood concentrations of dialyzable toxicants (*e.g.,* ethylene glycol and gentamicin), and diuresis initiated by intravenous administration of isotonic saline will help increase renal perfusion and excretion of toxicants. Recognition and appropriate treatment of renal injury in the initiation phase of ARF is associated with improved prognosis; therefore, patients receiving potentially nephrotoxic drugs and high risk patients undergoing anesthesia should be monitored closely.

Urine production is an excellent parameter to monitor during anesthesia. Ideally, urine production should be greater than 1 ml/kg/hr. For patients receiving potentially nephrotoxic drugs, increased urinary excretion of protein, glucose, or casts may be an early indication of renal tubular damage.

As an alternative to standard clinicopathologic tests, detection and quantitation of urine enzymes (enzymuria) has been used experimentally to recognize early nephrotoxity in the dog (Greco, Additional Reading). Most enzymes in serum are not filtered by the glomerulus because of their large molecular weight; therefore, enzymuria can be an indication of renal tubular activity, leakage, or necrosis. Several enzymes originate from specific cellular organelles and thus can serve as markers for damage to a specific site. γ-Glutamyl transpeptidase originates from the proximal tubular brush border, and N-acetyl-β-D-glucosaminidase is a lysosomal enzyme. Other enzymes (*e.g.,* lysozyme and β 2-microglobulin) are released from numerous tissues and have molecular weights that allow glomerular filtration. Once in the glomerular filtrate, these small molecular weight enzymes are extensively reabsorbed by the proximal tubule so that virtually none appears in normal urine. Decreased proximal tubular function will result in increased urinary excretion of these small molecular weight enzymes. Enzymuria precedes other manifestations of proximal tubular injury by several days; however, measurement of these enzymes in urine is normally beyond the scope of routine veterinary laboratories.

The goal of treatment of established ARF is correction of renal hemodynamic disorders and alleviation of water and solute imbalances in order to "buy time" for renal repair and regeneration. A positive response to therapy is indicated by an increase in glomerular filtration rate and urine production. Induction of diuresis facilitates management of ARF by decreasing serum urea nitrogen and potassium concentrations and by lessening the tendency for overhydration to occur. Even though glomerular filtration rate and renal blood flow may improve with diuresis, these parameters are frequently unchanged, and the increased urine production is actually a result of decreased tubular resorption of filtrate (Table 43-7). Increased urine production alone does not indicate an improvement in glomerular filtration rate.

Volume replacement (percent dehydration $\times$ body weight [kg] $\times$ 1000 = milliliters of fluid deficit) to reduce any prerenal component of the disease process is the first step of therapy in ARF (see Chapter 72). Mild volume expansion, in addition to volume replacement, has been recom-

Table 43–7 *Comparison of Glomerular Filtration Rate and Urine Production in the Normal and Nonoliguric Acute Renal Failure State*

	Normal	*Acute Renal Failure*
Glomerular filtration rate	100 L/day	20 L/day
Tubular reabsorption	99 L/day	16 L/day
Urine production	1 L/day	4 L/day

mended when replacement fluid therapy alone does not result in diuresis, since mild dehydration (less than 3%–5% of body weight) is difficult to detect clinically. Correction of fluid deficits and volume expansion, however, seldom result in improved renal function in ARF; therefore, additional therapeutic agents are often employed.

Mannitol, furosemide, and dopamine may be used in patients with ARF following volume replacement in an attempt to increase glomerular filtration rate and urine production (Table 43-8). Mannitol and furosemide are both weak renal vasodilators (probably by way of increased renal prostaglandin activity); however, both drugs are used more commonly for their diuretic effects. Low dose dopamine infusion induces renal and mesenteric vasodilatation with minimal systemic effects, and, therefore, recent interest has focused on the use of dopamine to improve glomerular filtration rate in ARF. In addition, the use of dopamine in combination with furosemide appears to enhance the diuretic action of furosemide by increasing intrarenal delivery of fur-

osemide. Caution should be used when administering mannitol since expansion of the intravascular volume may precipitate pulmonary edema in oliguric patients. Furosemide should not be used in patients that have received aminoglycosides because of the potential for prolonged antibiotic retention and enhanced nephrotoxicity. Whether or not furosemide can potentiate the toxicity of other nephrotoxicants is not known.

Hypertonic glucose is often recommended as a diuretic for dogs with ARF. No controlled comparisons exist, however, between hypertonic glucose, mannitol, and furosemide with regard to preservation of urine production or influence on duration of ARF. Mannitol might be expected to be a superior osmotic diuretic because it is an impermeable solute and is not reabsorbed by the tubular epithelium.

A list of treatment guidelines for toxicant-induced ARF is presented in Table 43-9. Identification and correction of any prerenal or postrenal abnormalities is essential. Fluid deficits should be replaced intravenously within 6 hours with 0.45% saline and 2.5% dextrose or normal saline. Maintenance and continuing loss fluid needs should be provided over a 24-hour period using 0.45% saline and 2.5% dextrose so as not to enhance hypernatremia and hyperkalemia.

Oliguria is common with ARF and was once thought to be a hallmark of the syndrome; however, nonoliguric ARF is being recognized with increasing frequency. Urine production should be quantitated so that maintenance fluid needs can

Table 43–8 *Comparison of the Effects of Mannitol, Furosemide, and Dopamine in Acute Renal Failure*

Parameter	*Mannitol*	*Furosemide*	*Dopamine (low dose)*
Renal blood flow	I	I (transient)	I
Glomerular filtration rate	?	?	I
Blood volume	I	D or NC	NC
Blood viscosity	D	I	NC
Blood pressure	I or NC	D	NC
Pulmonary edema	+	–	–
Urine volume	I	I	I
Potentiation of drug nephrotoxicity	–	+	–

I = increase, D = decrease, NC = no change, + = potential problem, – = not a potential problem, ? = questionable affect

Table 43–9 *Treatment Guidelines for Acute Renal Failure*

1. Discontinue all potentially nephrotoxic drugs.
2. Start specific antidotal therapy if applicable, for example, alcohol dehydrogenase inhibitors for ethylene glycol.
3. Identify and treat any prerenal or postrenal abnormalities.
4. Start intravenous fluid therapy:
    rehydrate patient within 6 hours
    provide maintenance and continuing loss fluid needs
5. Assess volume of urine production.
6. Correct acid-base and electrolyte abnormalities, rule out hypercalcemic nephropathy
7. Provide mild volume expansion while monitoring urine volume, body weight, plasma total solids, hematocrit, and central venous pressure
8. Administer vasodilators and/or diuretics
9. Consider peritoneal or pleural dialysis if no response to above treatment
10. Control hyperphosphatemia
11. Treat gastroenteritis and gastric hyperacidity
12. Provide caloric requirements (70–100 Kcal/kg/day)

be properly assessed. Since two thirds of maintenance fluid needs are due to fluid loss in urine, oliguric and nonoliguric patients can have large variations in their fluid needs (Table 43-10).

Measurement of urine volume also facilitates assessment of endogenous creatinine clearance, providing an estimation of glomerular filtration rate. If indwelling urinary catheters are used to measure urine volume, strict aseptic technique and closed collection systems must be employed. Uremic patients have depressed cellular immunity and phagocytic function, and infection is a leading cause of death in renal failure. Intermittent urinary bladder catheterization is usually recommended over indwelling catheterization.

During the period of rehydration, acid-base and electrolyte status should be evaluated and

Table 43–10 *Examples of Daily Maintenance Fluid Requirements*

	Normal Urine Production	Oliguric ARF	Nonoliguric ARF
Insensible loss	20 ml/kg	20 ml/kg	20 ml/kg
Urine volume	40 ml/kg	6 ml/kg	165 ml/kg
Total maintenance needs	60 ml/kg	26 ml/kg	185 ml/kg

treated. Metabolic acidosis and hyperkalemia are common in oliguric ARF. The acidosis is usually partially compensated for by a respiratory alkalosis. Bicarbonate therapy (0.3 × body weight [kg] × base deficit) should be reserved for patients whose blood *p*H is 7.15 or less (see Table 72-6). In the absence of base deficit data, bicarbonate needs may be estimated as 1 to 2 mEq/kg. Overzealous sodium bicarbonate therapy can create ionized calcium deficits and sodium excesses, which may contribute to hypervolemia in the oliguric patient.

Hyperkalemia can cause cardiac conduction abnormalities and is the most life threatening electrolyte disturbance that occurs in ARF. Diagnosis of hyperkalemia is based on serum potassium concentrations; however, bradycardia and the electrocardiographic changes of decreased P wave amplitude, increased PR interval, widened QRS complexes, and tall, spiked T waves are clinical signs frequently associated with hyperkalemia. If severe, hyperkalemia can cause atrial standstill, sinoventricular rhythms, ventricular tachycardia, fibrillation, and asystole. Hyperkalemia should be promptly treated with slow intravenous bolus administration of 1 to 2 mEq/kg of sodium bicarbonate. Insulin, dextrose, and calcium gluconate may also be used to decrease or counteract hyperkalemia (see Chapter 72).

If signs of overhydration are not present and oliguria persists after apparent rehydration, mild volume expansion (3%–5% of the patient's body weight in fluid) may be initiated. Monitoring body weight, plasma total solids, hematocrit, and central venous pressure (see Central Venous Pressure in Chapter 80) will help protect against overhydration. When fluid therapy alone fails to induce diuresis, either mannitol or dopamine and furosemide in combination are the therapeutic strategies of choice (see Tables 43-8, 43-9, and 43-11). If one regimen does not work, the other may be tried. Dopamine and furosemide therapy is probably a better choice for overhydrated patients; however, it appears that dopamine and furosemide treatment is more efficacious in ischemic ARF compared to toxicant-induced ARF and may potentiate gentamicin-induced nephrotoxicosis. Whether or not diuresis occurs, mainte-

Table 43–11 *Drugs and Dosages Used in Treatment of Acute Renal Failure*

Drug	Action	Dosage
Aluminum hydroxide (Dialume)	Enteric phosphate binder	500 mg at each feeding (pull capsule apart and mix contents into food)
Cimetidine (Tagamet)	H₂ blocker	5 to 10 mg/kg q 6 to 12 hours IV or PO
Dopamine HCL (Intropin)	Renal vasodilator	1 to 3 μg/kg/min IV (50 mg of dopamine in 500 ml of 5% dextrose results in a 100 μg/ml solution)
Furosemide (Lasix)	Loop diuretic	2 to 4 mg/kg IV
Mannitol	Osmotic diuretic	0.25 to 0.5 g/kg as a 20% or 25% solution given as a slow IV bolus
Metoclopramide (Reglan)	Antiemetic	0.2 to 0.4 mg/kg q 6 to 8 hours SC
Ranitidine	H₂ blocker	2.2 to 4.4 mg/kg q 12 hours PO
Trimethobenzamide (Tigan)	Antiemetic	3 mg/kg q 8 hours IV

nance fluid requirements should be derived from the volume of urine produced. If diuresis occurs, polyionic solutions (*e.g.*, lactated Ringer's) should be used for maintenance fluid requirements and potassium supplementation is often necessary. The latter should be determined by measuring serum potassium concentrations (Table 43-12).

Provision of daily caloric requirements is an important aspect of conservative management of renal failure. Energy requirements have a higher priority than do protein requirements, and, therefore, if caloric needs are not met, endogenous proteins will be catabolized for energy. Protein catabolism not only causes weight loss and

muscle wasting but also increases blood urea nitrogen concentrations. Protein breakdown in humans can be reduced by providing as little as 100 g of carbohydrate per day. Supplementation of essential amino acids in anephric dogs has been shown to stabilize serum urea nitrogen concentrations and increase survival time. Inappetence due to gastric hyperacidity and vomiting can usually be controlled by the use of an H₂ receptor blocker (*e.g.*, cimetidine or ranitidine), aluminum-containing antacids, and antiemetics that act at the chemoreceptor trigger zone (*e.g.*, trimethobenzamide or metoclopramide). Administration of food blended with water via a stomach tube may be tolerated by animals that are anorexic but not vomiting. Reduced protein diets (Hill's g/d or k/d) and enteric phosphate binders (aluminum hydroxide) should be used to reduce serum urea nitrogen concentrations and combat hyperphosphatemia (see Chapter 44). Sucralfate has also been used to help normalize serum phosphorus levels (see Mikiciuk, Additional Reading).

Peritoneal dialysis (see Peritoneal and Pleural Dialysis in Chapter 80) should be considered in patients with severe, persistent uremia, acidosis, or hyperkalemia. Dialysis may also be used to

Table 43–12 *Potassium Supplementation Guidelines*

Measured Serum Potassium Concentrations (mEq/L)	Amount of KCl (mEq) Added to Each Liter of Fluid Administered*
3.0 to 3.5	28
2.5 to 3.0	40
2.0 to 2.5	60
<2.0	80

* *Do not administer at a rate >0.5 mEq/kg body weight/hour.*

treat overhydration and in some cases hasten elimination of toxicants. Renal biopsy (see Kidney Biopsy in Chapter 80) should be performed if the diagnosis is in doubt, the patient does not respond to therapy within 4 to 5 days, or long-term dialysis is considered. Long-term prognosis for ARF is usually fair to good if the patient survives the period of renal dysfunction. Several weeks may be required for renal function to improve. The severity of the azotemia, histologic lesions, and the response to therapy are the most important prognostic indicators.

ADDITIONAL READING

Allen TA, Fettman MJ. Comparative aspects of non-oliguric acute renal failure. Compendium of Continuing Education 1987; 9:293.

Brown SA, Barsanti JA, Crowell WA. Gentamicin-associated acute renal failure in the dog. J Am Vet Med Assoc 1985; 186:686.

Engelhaedt JA, Brown SA. Drug-related nephropathies. Part II. Commonly used drugs. Compendium of Continuing Education 1987; 9:281.

Fox LE, Grauer GF, Dubielzig RR, Bjorling DE. Reversal of ethylene glycol-induced nephrotoxicosis in a dog. J Am Vet Med Assoc 1987; 191:1433.

Grauer GF, Thrall MAH. Ethylene glycol (antifreeze) poisoning. In: Kirk RW, ed. Current veterinary therapy IX. Philadelphia: WB Saunders, 1986: 206.

Greco DS, Turnwald GH, Adams R et al. Urinary τ-glutamyl transpeptidase activity in dogs with gentamicin-induced nephrotoxicity. Am J Vet Res 1985; 46:2332.

Mikiciuk MG, Thornhill JA. Control of parathyroid hormone in chronic renal failure. Compendium of Continuing Education 1989; 11:831.

Rubin SI. Nephrotoxicity of amphotericin B. In: Kirk RW, ed. Current veterinary therapy IX. Philadelphia: WB Saunders, 1986; 1142.

Rubin SI. Nonsteroidal antiinflammatory drugs, prostaglandins and the kidney. J Am Vet Med Assoc 1986; 188:1065

Senior DF. Acute renal failure in the dog: A case report and literature review. Journal of the American Animal Hospital Association 1983; 19:837.

Willard MD. Treatment of hyperkalemia. In: Kirk RW, ed. Current veterinary therapy IX. Philadelphia: WB Saunders, 1986; 94.

44

CHRONIC RENAL FAILURE

Gregory F. Grauer

Renal failure results when two thirds to three quarters of the nephrons of both kidneys are not functioning. Whether the underlying disease process primarily affects glomeruli, tubules, interstitial tissue, or renal vasculature, irreversible damage to any portion of the nephron renders the entire nephron nonfunctional. Healing of irreversibly damaged nephrons occurs by replacement fibrosis and a specific etiology is rarely determined. *Chronic renal failure* (CRF) occurs over a period of weeks, months, or years and is a leading cause of death in dogs and cats. Improvement of renal function is usually not possible with CRF, and, therefore, treatment is directed at reducing the clinical signs associated with the decreased renal function.

Many different and sometimes confusing terms are used to describe the deterioration of renal function (Fig. 44-1). *Renal disease* refers to the presence of renal lesions but does not imply anything about etiology, severity, or distribution of the lesions or degree of renal function. *Renal reserve* may be thought of as the percentage of nephrons that is not necessary to maintain normal renal function. Renal reserve probably varies from animal to animal but is usually greater than 50%. *Renal insufficiency* begins when renal reserve is lost. Animals with renal insufficiency appear normal but have reduced capacity to compensate for stresses such as infection or dehydration. *Azotemia* is increased concentrations of urea nitrogen and creatinine in the blood. *Renal azotemia* denotes azotemia due to renal parenchymal lesions. *Renal failure* is a state of decreased renal function that allows persistent abnormalities (*e.g.,* azotemia and inability to concentrate urine) to exist. Renal failure is a term used to indicate a level of organ function rather than a specific disease entity. *Uremia* is the presence of abnormal amounts of urine products in the blood. The uremic syndrome is a constellation of clinical signs including anemia, gastroenteritis, acidosis, pneumonitis, osteodystrophy, and encephalopathy that occur secondary to uremia.

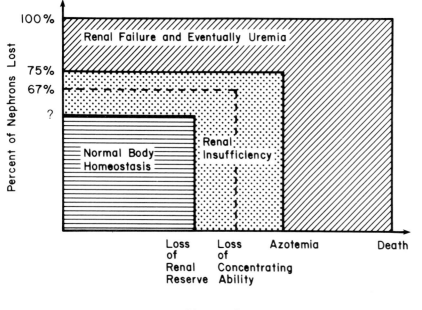

Figure 44–1. *Diagram of the stages of renal dysfunction.*

CAUSES

The cause of CRF is usually difficult to determine. Due to the interdependence of the vascular and tubular components of the nephron, the end point of irreversible glomerular or tubular damage is the same. Morphologic heterogeneity between nephrons exists in the chronically diseased kidney with the spectrum of changes ranging from severe atrophy to marked hypertrophy. The histologic changes are not process specific, and, therefore, an etiologic diagnosis is frequently not possible. Recent studies, however, indicate that primary glomerular disorders are a leading cause of CRF in the dog. Since reduction of glomerular filtration is uniformly present, CRF may be considered a single pathologic entity, although many diverse pathways can lead to this end point. Table 44-1 lists potential causes of CRF.

Progressive diseases that destroy nephrons at a slow rate allow intact nephrons to undergo compensatory hypertrophy. When renal failure finally occurs, viable nephron hypertrophy can no longer maintain adequate renal function. In animals with CRF, renal reserve is absent. Repair and regeneration of nephron damage as well as functional and anatomic hypertrophy of intact nephrons has had a chance to occur and has failed to establish adequate renal function. Renal lesions associated with CRF are usually irreversible and often progressive; therefore, improvement of renal function is usually not possible.

PATHOPHYSIOLOGY

The pathophysiology of CRF can be considered at both the organ and systemic level. At the level of the kidney, the fundamental pathology of CRF is loss of nephrons and decreased glomerular filtration. Reduced glomerular filtration results in increased plasma concentrations of substances that are normally eliminated from the body by renal excretion. A large number of substances have been shown to accumulate in the plasma in renal failure (Table 44-2). The constellation of clinical signs known as the uremic syndrome is thought to be due, at least in part, to an accumulation of these substances. Components of the uremic syndrome include sodium and water imbalance, anemia, carbohydrate intolerance, neurologic disturbances, gastrointestinal disturbances, osteo-

Table 44–1 *Potential Causes of Chronic Renal Failure*

IMMUNOLOGIC DISORDERS Systemic lupus erythematosus Glomerulonephritis Vasculitis (FIP) **NEOPLASIA** Primary Metastatic **AMYLOIDOSIS** **NEPHROTOXICANTS** (see Table 43-2) **INFLAMMATORY/INFECTIOUS** Pyelonephritis Leptospirosis Renal calculi	**HEREDITARY AND CONGENITAL DISORDERS** Renal hypoplasia/dysplasia Polycystic kidneys Familial nephropathies (Lhasa apsos, Shih Tzus, Norwegian elkhounds, Chinese Shar Pei dogs, Doberman pinschers, Samoyeds, standard poodles, soft-coated Wheaton terriers, cocker spaniels, Abyssinian cats) **RENAL ISCHEMIA** (see Table 43-3) **URINARY OUTFLOW OBSTRUCTION** **IDIOPATHIC**

dystrophy, immunologic incompetence, and metabolic acidosis. Associations between certain uremic signs and the concentration of specific compounds in plasma have been difficult to document since a number of substances tend to be retained together as renal function deteriorates. It is probable that several compounds act synergistically to produce the toxic effects associated with uremia.

In addition to excretion of metabolic wastes and maintenance of fluid and electrolyte balance, the kidneys also function as endocrine organs and catabolize several peptide hormones. Therefore, hormonal disturbances also play a role in the pathogenesis of CRF. For example, decreased production of erythropoietin and active vitamin D_3

Table 44–2 *Substances Increased in Plasma in Renal Failure*

Urea	Creatinine
Ammonia	Uric acid
Phosphate	Aromatic and aliphatic amines
Cyclic adenosine monophosphate	Amino acids
	Phenols
Indols	Middle molecules
Polyols	Guanidinium compounds
Ribonuclease	Purine and pyrimidine
Peptides	derivatives
Parathyroid hormone	Renin
Glucagon	Growth hormone
Gastrin	

contribute to the nonregenerative anemia and hypocalcemia of CRF, respectively, and decreased metabolism and excretion of parathyroid hormone and gastrin contribute to osteodystrophy and gastritis, respectively.

Part of the pathophysiology of CRF is brought about by compensatory mechanisms. The osteodystrophy of CRF occurs secondary to hyperparathyroidism, which develops in an attempt to maintain normal plasma calcium and phosphorus concentrations. Similarly, the glomerular filtration rate of intact nephrons increases in CRF in an attempt to maintain adequate renal function; however, proteinuria and glomerulosclerosis are consequences of this hyperfiltration. These observations have lead to the development of the "trade-off" hypothesis to explain the pathogenesis of CRF. Many of the components of the uremic syndrome are not easily explained by this hypothesis; therefore a combination of the above mechanisms is most likely involved.

CLINICAL SIGNS AND DIAGNOSTIC APPROACH

Clinical signs of CRF are nonspecific and include depression, lethargy, vomiting, weight loss, polydipsia-polyuria, and poor body condition. Physical examination findings may include pale mucous membranes (anemia), oral ulcers, small and irregular kidneys, and signs of osteodystrophy or "rubber jaw." In comparison to acute renal failure, clinical signs associated with CRF are often relatively mild for the magnitude of azotemia. For a more in depth discussion about differentiating acute and chronic renal failure, see Chapter 43 and Table 43-5.

The object of laboratory testing in CRF is to identify the extent of renal dysfunction and monitor response to treatment or progression of disease. It is also desirable to identify any potentially reversible component of the disease process, for example, pyelonephritis. Several laboratory determinations can be used to grossly assess the extent of renal failure. Serum urea nitrogen and creatinine concentrations are elevated as glomerular filtration decreases; however, approximately three fourths of the nephron mass must be nonfunctional before azotemia is observed. Compared to serum urea nitrogen, serum creatinine is a more reliable indicator of glomerular filtration rate, since it is less subject to extrarenal influences. Serum creatinine levels greater than 10 mg/dl (884 μmol/L) are often associated with severe CRF and may be refractory to management.

Serum inorganic phosphorus concentration is another useful index of renal function. Concentrations of serum inorganic phosphorus greater than 10 mg/dl (3.23 mmol/L) indicate moderate to severe renal failure. However, serum phosphorus should not be used by itself to evaluate renal function, since growing dogs may have some degree of hyperphosphatemia (2–3 times normal). Additionally, the degree of hyperphosphatemia does not correlate linearly with the extent of renal impairment. Urine specific gravity may also be used as a crude measure of renal function. A persistent isosthenuric specific gravity (1.008–1.012) or minimally concentrated urine specific gravity (greater than 1.012 but less than 1.030 in dogs or less than 1.035 in cats) in the face of dehydration or azotemia indicates loss of two thirds to three quarters of nephron mass.

Assessment of glomerular filtration rate is a more accurate and sensitive indicator of renal excretory function than is assessment of serum creatinine concentration. The most practical way to determine glomerular filtration rate in azotemic patients is measurement of endogenous creatinine clearance. This procedure requires 24-hour urine collection and the measurement of urine and serum creatinine. Normal values for dogs and cats are between 2.0 and 4.0 ml/min/kg of body weight. Sodium sulfanilate clearance is also a more sensitive measure of renal function than serum creatinine concentration and does not require urine collection (Maddison, Additional Reading).

MANAGEMENT

The goal of treatment of acute renal failure is to allow the patient to remain alive long enough for the viable and partially damaged nephrons to hypertrophy, repair, and compensate for the decrease in numbers. In the CRF patient, adaptive and compensatory changes have had time to occur: the presence of signs of renal failure indicates the inadequacy of these compensatory processes. Even though CRF is usually irreversible, with proper treatment, clinical signs can generally be reduced. Therapy usually must be continued for the life of the patient.

Polyuria and compensatory polydipsia occur in CRF due to a decrease in urine concentrating ability. As the number of functional nephrons decreases a compensatory increase in glomerular filtration rate occurs in each intact nephron. Thus, the quantity of fluid presented to the proximal and distal tubule is increased. In addition, a decrease in renal medullary sodium concentration gradient occurs because of the decreased number of functional nephrons and, therefore, sodium chloride pumps. Decreased medullary hypertonicity decreases the medullary osmotic pressure that drives passive reabsorption of water from the distal tubules and collecting ducts. Treatment of the polyuria is unnecessary; however, it is important that the animal with CRF always have water available for ad libitum consumption. Dehydration, as can occur with vomiting and diarrhea, may cause a rapid and severe decline in renal function. Polyuria also results in increased loss of water soluble vitamins B and C. These losses should be compensated for by dietary supplementation.

If anorexia, vomiting, or diarrhea result in dehydration, fluids should be aggressively replaced parenterally. The volume of fluid needed (in milliliters) is determined by considering the extent of dehydration (percent dehydration × body weight [kg] × 1000), the maintenance (60 ml/kg/day), and continuing loss fluid needs of the patient.

Salt should not be supplemented to patients with CRF in an attempt to maintain extracellular fluid volume and increase urine production. In fact, evidence suggests that sodium intake should be reduced in proportion with the decrease in glomerular filtration. In dogs with reduced renal mass, decreased dietary sodium intake results in decreased urinary sodium excretion without evidence of volume depletion or other adverse effects. It has been proposed that the maintenance of sodium excretion in CRF is accomplished only at the risk of one or more of the abnormalities of the uremic syndrome. Increases in sodium excretion per nephron is thought to be an adaptation to maintain sodium balance.

Hypertension is common in dogs and cats with CRF. Although the exact mechanism of the hypertension is not known, a combination of glomerular capillary and arteriolar scarring, decreased production of renal vasodilatory prostaglandins, increased responsiveness to normal pressor mechanisms, and activation of the renin-angiotensin system may be involved. Restriction of dietary salt intake is the first line of treatment. In some cases, however, β-blockers (*e.g.*, propranolol) or vasodilators (*e.g.*, hydralazine or captopril) may be necessary in addition to dietary sodium restriction to control hypertension (Tables 44-3 and 44-4 and Chapter 24).

The kidneys normally excrete hydrogen ions as phosphate salts or ammonium ions. To a point in CRF, renal acid excretion per intact nephron is increased due to increased ammonia production. In addition, respiratory compensation and bone buffering help minimize the metabolic acidosis associated with CRF. Supplementation of sodium bicarbonate is not indicated for every patient with CRF; however, dietary management (decreased dietary protein and phosphorus) may further compromise renal ammoniagenesis and acid excretion and worsen the metabolic acidosis. Oral sodium bicarbonate should be administered at an initial dosage of 8 to 12 mg/kg every 8 to 12 hours if plasma bicarbonate concentrations are less than 12 mEq/L (12 mmol/L) or blood pH is less than 7.20 (see Chapter 72 and Table 72-6). Overzealous bicarbonate supplementation may aggravate hypertension and create ionized calcium deficits. If plasma bicarbonate increases above 18 to 20 mEq/L (18−20 mmol/L), bicarbonate supplementation should be discontinued. Recent evidence suggests that increased renal ammoniagenesis may be detrimental. Increased renal tissue ammonia concentrations may have local toxic and inflammatory effects resulting in the loss of more nephrons. On the basis of these findings, sodium bicarbonate supplementation may be indicated for patients with mild metabolic acidosis; however, more information is needed before these recommendations can be made.

Restriction of dietary protein intake is the cornerstone of management of CRF and provides an internal environment that allows the animal to live more comfortably with decreased renal function. Benefits of reduced protein intake in dogs with CRF include reduced mortality and severity of clinical signs and reduced serum urea nitrogen and phosphorus concentrations. In addition, much evidence suggests that high dietary protein intake in patients with CRF causes glomerular hyperfiltration leading to glomerulosclerosis and the progression of renal lesions (Fig. 44-2). It must be noted, however, that undesirable effects associated with reduced protein intake in dogs with CRF can be found. If protein restriction is too severe, reduced renal hemodynamics, protein depletion (decreased body weight, muscle mass, and serum albumin), anemia, and acidosis will occur or be aggravated in dogs with CRF.

Ideally, dietary therapy allows all essential amino acid requirements to be met without excesses. This requirement is accomplished by feeding low quantities of high biological value protein and results in decreased need for renal clearance of urea and other nitrogenous metabolites. Nonessential amino acids can be produced by the amination of keto acids derived from carbohydrates. The ammonia for this amination comes from body and dietary protein catabolism and bacterial action on intestinal urea. Energy re-

Table 44–3 *Drugs Used in the Management of Chronic Renal Failure*

Drug	Action	Dosage
Aluminum hydroxide (Dialume)	Enteric phosphate binder	500 mg sprinkled on food and mixed in at each feeding
Captopril (Capoten)	Mixed vasodilator	0.5 to 2 mg/kg q 8 to 12 hours PO (dog) 2 mg q 8 to 12 hours PO (cat)
Chlorpromazine (Thorazine)	Antiemetic	1.1 to 4.4 mg/kg q 6 to 24 hours IM
Cimetidine (Tagamet)	H$_2$ blocker	5.0 to 10 mg/kg q 6 to 12 hours PO, SC (dog) 4.0 mg/kg q 6 hours PO, IM (cat)
Hydralazine (Apresoline)	Arterial vasodilator	0.5 to 2.0 mg/kg q 12 hours PO (dog) 2.5 mg q 12 hours PO (cat)
Metoclopramide (Reglan)	Antiemetic	0.2 to 0.4 mg/kg q 6 to 8 hours PO, SC
Nandrolone deconate (Deca Durabolin)	Anabolic steroid	1.0 to 1.5 mg/kg q week IM (dog) 0.5 to 10 mg/kg q week IM (cat)
Propranolol (Inderal)	β-blocker	0.2 to 1.0 mg/kg q 8 hours PO (dog) 2.5 to 5.0 mg q 8 to 12 hours PO (cat)
Ranitidine (Zantac)	H$_2$ blocker	2.2 to 4.4 mg/kg q 12 hours PO (dog) 2.2 mg/kg q 12 hours PO (cat)
Sodium bicarbonate	Combat metabolic acidosis	8.0 to 12.0 mg/kg q 8 to 12 hours PO
Trimethobenzamide (Tigan)	Antiemetic	3.0 mg/kg q 8 hours IM (dog)

quirements of the body have higher priority than does protein anabolism; therefore, if the available carbohydrates and fats are insufficient to meet caloric requirements, proteins will be broken down as a source of energy. Catabolism of protein for energy increases the nitrogenous waste the kidney must excrete and exacerbates the clinical signs of renal failure.

Researchers have established that minimum protein requirements for dogs and cats with CRF are higher than those of normal dogs and cats. Ideally, dogs and cats with CRF should receive protein at the rate of 2.0 to 2.2 g/kg/day and 3.3 to 3.5 g/kg/day, respectively. A good recommenda-

tion for dietary protein restriction is to feed the maximum amount of high biological value, highly digestible protein that the animal can tolerate at his or her level of renal function. The diet is restricted relative to normal pet food protein content, not relative to the animal's requirements. A favorable response to therapy is a stable body weight and serum creatinine concentration and a decreasing serum urea nitrogen concentration. Moderate dietary protein restriction should be employed early in the course of renal failure, and use of severely restricted protein diets should be reserved for patients that are refractory to moderate dietary protein restriction. Hill's ca-

Table 44–4 *Goals and Management of Chronic Renal Failure*

Goal	Management
1. Avoid dehydration	Fresh water available at all times Parenteral fluid therapy when necessary
2. Control azotemia	Dietary protein restriction
3. Control renal secondary hyperparathyrodism	Dietary phosphorus restriction Enteric phosphate binders Cimetidine
4. Control systemic hypertension	Dietary sodium restriction β-blockers and vasodilators if necessary
5. Minimize metabolic acidosis	Oral sodium bicarbonate
6. Minimize gastric irritation	Antiemetics Cimetidine
7. Avoid stress	Treat on out-patient basis Treat infections promptly Avoid corticosteroids Avoid adverse drug reactions

nine prescription diets g/d, k/d, and u/d provide 2.6 g, 2.0 g, and 1.3 g of high quality protein per kilogram of body weight respectively, and Hill's feline prescription diet k/d provides 3.3 g of high quality protein per kilogram of body weight.

Management of the hyperphosphatemia that occurs in CRF is closely related to dietary protein restriction inasmuch as protein restricted diets are also phosphorus restricted. An increase in plasma phosphorus concentration occurs in CRF as a result of decreased ability of the kidney to excrete phosphorus. Concurrently, a decrease in the active form of vitamin D decreases intestinal absorption of calcium, which, in conjunction with impaired renal reabsorption of calcium, decreases plasma ionized calcium concentrations. Hypocalcemia then stimulates parathyroid hormone secretion, which facilitates renal excretion of phosphorus and increases serum calcium concentrations by increasing renal calcium reabsorption and calcium absorption from bones and the gastrointestinal tract (Figs. 44-3 and 44-4).

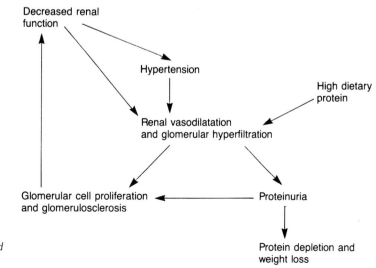

Figure 44–2. *Progression of renal disease associated with glomerular hyperfiltration.*

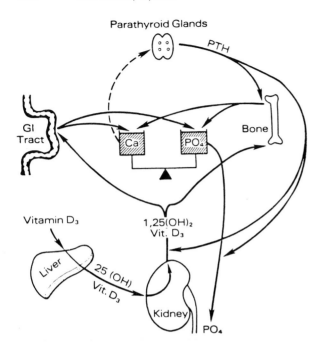

Figure 44–3. *Some of the major interactions of plasma calcium (Ca), phosphorus (PO₄), parathyroid hormone (PTH), and vitamin D and its metabolites. The dashed arrow represents inhibition of PTH release by high plasma calcium concentrations. (From Harrington AR, Zimmerman SW: Renal Pathophysiology. New York: John Wiley & Sons, 1982.)*

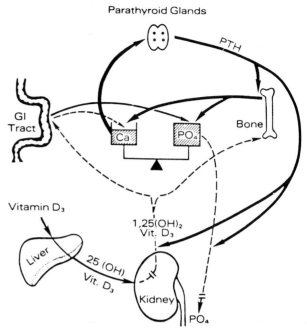

Figure 44–4. *The disturbed relationships among plasma calcium (Ca), phosphorus (PO₄), parathyroid hormone (PTH), and vitamin D and its metabolites in chronic renal failure. Heavy lines represent the overstimulation of PTH release by decreased plasma calcium concentrations and the high concentrations of PTH acting on target organs. Dashed or interrupted lines indicate pathways that are at least partially inoperative or blocked in renal failure. (From Harrington AR, Zimmerman SW: Renal Pathophysiology. New York: John Wiley & Sons, 1982.)*

The trade-offs for this hyperparathyroidism, however, are many and include osteodystrophy, neuropathy, bone marrow suppression, and soft tissue mineralization. Soft tissue mineralization may occur in the kidneys and potentially result in a progressive decline in renal function. If the product of the serum calcium and phosphorus concentrations is greater than 50 to 70 mg/dl, the patient is at risk for soft tissue mineralization.

Studies in cats with CRF have shown that normal dietary phosphorus intake is associated with microscopic renal mineralization and fibrosis and that these changes were prevented by reducing dietary phosphorus intake (renal functional abnormalities, however, were not observed in conjunction with these histologic changes). In addition to feeding a phosphorus restricted diet, administration of enteric phosphate binders such as aluminum carbonate or aluminum hydroxide will help combat hyperphosphatemia. Enteric phosphate binders are generally ineffective if dietary phosphorus intake is not restricted. Sucral-

fate has also been used to help normalize serum phosphorus concentrations (see Mikiciuk, Additional Reading).

In some cases of CRF, 1,25-dihydroxycholecalciferol (calcitriol) supplementation has been associated with increased serum calcium concentrations and decreased parathyroid hormone concentrations. Calcium or calcitriol supplementation should be used cautiously and only if hypocalcemia is documented and the product of the serum calcium and phosphorus is less than 50 to 70 mg/dl.

Vomiting and anorexia are common in dogs and cats with CRF and can often result in decreased caloric intake. Causes of vomiting and anorexia include: 1) stimulation of chemoreceptor trigger zone by uremic toxins; 2) decreased excretion of gastrin and increased gastric acid secretion (serum gastrin concentrations in dogs with renal failure may be as high as 5 times the normal concentrations); and 3) visceral irritation secondary to uremia, which stimulates the emetic center. Vomiting may be treated with trimethobenzamide or metoclopramide, which block the chemoreceptor trigger zone or chlorpromazine, which blocks the emetic center. Metoclopramide also increases gastric motility and emptying without causing gastric acid secretion. H_2 receptor blockers (cimetidine and Tanitidine) have been shown to effectively decrease gastric acid secretion and attenuate vomiting in dogs with CRF. In addition, cimetidine is thought to suppress parathyroid gland secretion, lower serum phosphorus, and improve calcium balance in uremic dogs. Oral ulcers, stomatitis, and glossitis may occur as a result of gastritis and vomiting or the effect of uremic toxins on mucosal membranes. Xylocaine Viscous (0.5–1.0 ml) orally before feeding often decreases pain associated with oral ulcerations and encourages the patient to eat.

The nonregenerative anemia observed in animals with CRF is due to a combination of decreased erythropoietin production, shortened red cell survival, gastrointestinal blood loss, and the effects of uremic toxins such as parathyroid hormone on erythropoiesis. Anabolic steroids may be of benefit to CRF patients since they promote red cell production and a positive nitrogen balance. These agents stimulate red cell precursors in the bone marrow, increase renal activation of erythropoietin, and promote protein anabolism if caloric intake is adequate. In addition, increases in red blood cell 2,3-diphosphoglycerate stimulated by anabolic steroids facilitate release of oxygen from hemoglobin to the tissues. However, several months of treatment with anabolic steroids is usually required before a response is observed, and benefits are usually minimal. Short-term studies in uremic dogs treated with anabolic steroids have failed to demonstrate any benefit with regard to body weight, serum albumin concentration, nitrogen balance, or muscle mass. In contrast, preliminary studies assessing the effects of recombinant erythropoietin treatment on anemia in dogs and cats with CRF have been quite successful; however, the cost of this treatment is high and not readily available at this time.

Impaired immune response to infectious agents occurs in the uremic animal due to an altered inflammatory response and a defect in cellular immunity. As a result the uremic animal is more susceptible to infection, and infection is a leading cause of death. Indwelling urinary catheters should be placed using aseptic technique and removed as soon as possible. Prophylactic antibiotic treatment is not recommended in conjunction with indwelling urinary catheters; urinary tract infections should be treated on the basis of culture and sensitivity results.

Caution should be taken to avoid antibiotics with known nephrotoxic effects (gentamicin). Chronic renal failure patients are good candidates for adverse drug reactions. Many drugs or drug metabolites are excreted by the kidneys and, therefore, may accumulate in patients with renal failure. Certain drugs may be nephrotoxic and further contribute to renal disease. Package inserts should be read to ascertain the route of drug excretion, potential toxicity, and how to adjust dosage in renal failure. Usually adjustment of drug dosage is not necessary if serum creatinine concentration is less than 2.5 mg/dl (221 μmol/L).

In dogs and cats with CRF, stressful situations should be avoided if at all possible. Stress is associated with release of endogenous corticosteroids that results in protein catabolism. Additionally, many CRF patients are geriatric patients that respond better to outpatient treatment than to hospitalization.

PATIENT MONITORING

Follow up examinations of CRF patients should be performed at least every 2 to 4 months. Body weight, complete blood count, serum urea nitrogen, creatinine, calcium, phosphorus, total protein, and urinalysis should be assessed at each recheck. Data flow charts facilitate monitoring the progress of these patients.

Recently, a plot of the reciprocal of the serum creatinine concentration vs. age was shown to be an indicator of the progression of CRF in dogs (Allen, Additional Reading). A linear correlation was found between the reciprocal of the serum creatinine concentration and dog age; projection of the regression line to the abscissa may predict the dog's age at the time of death attributable to renal failure. These findings indicate that nephrons may be lost at a constant rate in dogs with CRF, and changes in the slope of this line may be used to indicate the effectiveness of treatment regimes. The progression of canine CRF, however, remains in question, and use of the reciprocal serum creatinine vs. age plot needs to be validated in large numbers of dogs.

ADDITIONAL READING

Allen TA, Jaenke RS, Fettman MJ. A technique for estimating progression of chronic renal failure in the dog. J Am Vet Med Assoc 1987; 190:866.

Barsanti JA, Finco DR. Dietary management of chronic renal failure in dogs. Journal of the American Animal Hospital Association 1985; 21:371.

Bovee KC, Kronfeld DS. Reduction of renal hemodynamics in uremic dogs fed reduced protein diets. Journal of the American Animal Hospital Association 1981; 17:277.

Finco DR, Crowell WA, Barsanti JA. Effects of three diets on dogs with induced chronic renal failure. Am J Vet Res 1985; 46:646.

Krawiec DR. Renal failure in immature dogs. Journal of the American Animal Hospital Association 1987; 23:101.

Maddison JE, Pascoe PJ, Jansen BS. Clinical evaluation of sodium sulfanilate clearance for the diagnosis of renal disease in dogs. J Am Vet Med Assoc 1984; 185:961.

Mikiciuk MG, Thornhill JA. Control of parathyroid hormone in chronic renal failure. Compendium of Continuing Education 1989; 11:831.

Polzin DJ, Osborne CA, Hayden DW, Stevens JB. Effects of modified protein diets in dogs with chronic renal failure. J Am Vet Med Assoc 1983; 183:980.

Polzin DJ, Osborne CA, Leininger JR. The influence of diet on the progression of canine renal failure. Compendium of Continuing Education 1984; 6:1123.

Osborne CA, Polzin DJ, Abdullahi S et al. Role of diet in management of feline chronic polyuric renal failure: Current status. Journal of the American Animal Hospital Association 1982; 18:11.

Ross LA, Finco DR, Crowell WA. Effect of dietary phosphorus restriction on the kidneys of cats with reduced renal mass. Am J Vet Res 1982; 43:1023.

45

GLOMERULAR DISEASE AND PROTEINURIA

Gregory F. Grauer

The increased evaluation of renal biopsy specimens has greatly improved our knowledge of primary glomerular disease in veterinary medicine. Amyloidosis and glomerulonephritis are the two most common causes of glomerular disease in dogs and cats. Glomerulonephritis is usually caused by the presence of immune complexes in glomerular capillary walls and is now thought to be one of the major causes of chronic renal insufficiency and renal failure. Several studies indicate the incidence of glomerulonephritis in randomly selected dogs is as high as 50%. Amyloidosis, although less common than glomerulonephritis, is a progressive disease that also leads to chronic renal failure. Loss of plasma proteins, principally albumin, in the urine is the hallmark of glomerulonephropathy, and use of the urine protein : creatinine ratio to identify and quantitate proteinuria has greatly facilitated diagnosis of glomerular disease. Recent trials in dogs with glomerulonephritis utilizing immunosuppressive and anti-inflammatory treatment have shown much promise, whereas treatment of amyloidosis is largely unrewarding.

CAUSES AND PATHOPHYSIOLOGY

The majority of glomerular disease in dogs is mediated by immunopathogenic mechanisms. The presence of immune complexes in the glomerular capillary wall is the most important mechanism responsible for initiating glomerulonephritis. Soluble circulating immune complexes may be deposited or trapped in the glomerulus, or alternatively, immune complexes may form in situ in the glomerular capillary wall (Fig. 45-1). In situ immune complex formation occurs when circulating antibody reacts with endogenous glomerular antigens or "planted," non-glomerular antigens in the glomerular capillary wall. Recent evidence suggests in situ immune complex formation occurs in dogs with dirofilariasis. Non-glomerular antigens may localize in the glomerular capillary wall prior to antibody interaction due to electrical charge interaction or biochemical affinity.

Although antibody directed against endogenous glomerular basement membrane material has not been demonstrated in dogs and cats with

615

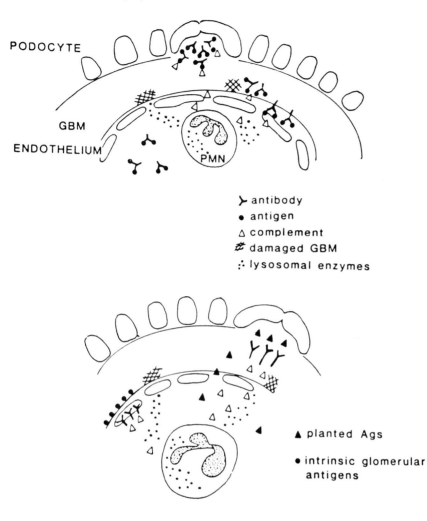

PODOCYTE

GBM

ENDOTHELIUM

PMN

⊱ antibody
● antigen
△ complement
✖ damaged GBM
∴ lysosomal enzymes

▲ planted Ags

● intrinsic glomerular antigens

Figure 45–1. *Schematic representation of the two major types of immunologically mediated glomerular injury. Circulating soluble immune complexes have become trapped in the glomerular filter and have fixed complement. Chemotactic complement components have attracted neutrophils to the area. The release of free oxygen radicals and lysosomal enzymes from the neutrophils has resulted in damage to the glomerulus (top). Damage may also result from the attachment of autoantibodies directed against fixed intrinsic glomerular antigens (bottom, left). Finally, damage may result from attachment of antibodies directed against planted nonglomerular antigens (bottom, right). (From Chew DJ, DiBartola SP. Manual of small animal nephrology and urology. Churchill Livingstone, Inc. 1986.)*

naturally-occurring glomerulonephritis, several infectious and inflammatory diseases have been associated with glomerular immune complex disease (Table 45-1). In the majority of cases, however, the antigen source or underlying disease process is not identified, and the glomerular disease is labelled as idiopathic. Identification of endogenous immunoglobulin or complement within glomerular capillary walls with immunofluorescent techniques is not difficult, but identification of exogenous antigens within glomerular tissue is rarely accomplished.

Subsequent to formation or deposition of immune complexes in the glomerular capillary wall, several factors including activation of the complement system, platelet aggregation, infiltration of polymorphonuclear leukocytes, activation of the coagulation system, and fibrin deposition contribute to glomerular damage (Fig. 45-2). Platelet activation and aggregation occur secondary to vascular endothelial damage or antigen-antibody interaction. Platelets, in turn, exacerbate glomerular damage by release of vasoactive and inflammatory substances (thromboxanes) and by facilitation of the coagulation cascade. The glomerulus responds to this injury by cellular proliferation, thickening of the glomerular basement membrane, and, eventually, hyalinization and sclerosis (Figs. 45-3 through 45-5).

Amyloidosis is characterized by extracellular deposition of nonbranching fibrillar proteins that stack into a specific β-pleated sheet conformation

Table 45–1 *Diseases That Have Been Associated With Glomerulonephritis*

Dogs	Cats
INFECTIOUS	**INFECTIOUS**
Canine adenovirus I	Feline leukemia virus
Bacterial endocarditis	Feline infectious peritonitis
Borreliosis (Lyme's disease)	Mycoplasmal polyarthritis
Brucellosis	
Dirofilariasis	
Ehrlichia organisms	
Leishmaniasis	
Pyometra	
NEOPLASIA	**NEOPLASIA**
INFLAMMATORY	**INFLAMMATORY**
Pancreatitis	Pancreatitis
Systemic lupus erythematosis	Systemic lupus erythematosis
OTHER	**OTHER**
Hyperadrenocorticism and long-term, high dose corticosteroids	Idiopathic
Idiopathic	Familial?
Familial?	Nonimmunologic-hyperfiltration
Nonimmunologic-hyperfiltration	

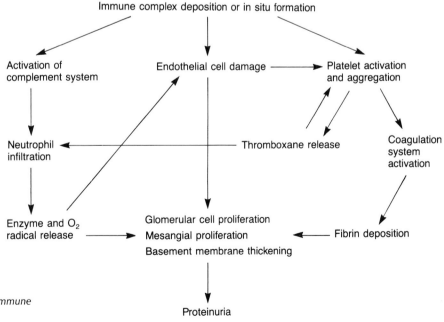

Figure 45–2. *Pathophysiology of immune complex glomerulonephritis.*

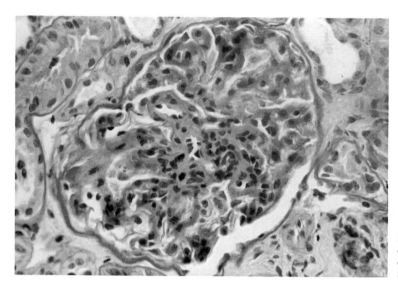

Figure 45–3. Proliferative glomerulonephritis characterized by cellular proliferation and increased mesangial matrix (PAS stain, original magnification × 400).

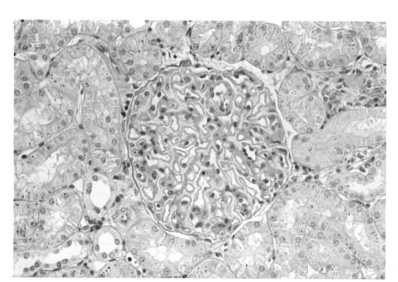

Figure 45–4. Membranous glomerulonephritis characterized by capillary basement thickening (PAS stain, original magnification × 200).

and exhibit green birefringence under polarized light when stained with Congo red. Amyloidosis in dogs and cats is the reactive systemic form in which amyloid may be deposited in several organs in addition to the kidneys. Reactive systemic amyloid deposits contain amyloid protein AA which is an amino terminal fragment of the acute phase reactant protein serum amyloid A. Serum amyloid A is produced by hepatocytes in response to tissue injury. Amyloidosis may be associated with an underlying inflammatory or neoplastic process; however, in the majority of dogs and cats

with amyloidosis, no predisposing disease can be identified. Renal amyloidosis is a familial disease in the Abyssinian cat resulting in medullary as well as glomerular amyloid deposits.

Once a glomerulus has been irreversibly damaged, the entire nephron becomes nonfunctional and is replaced by fibrous scar tissue. As more and more nephrons become involved, glomerular filtration in total decreases and sodium retention and hypertension often occur. Remaining viable nephrons compensate for the decrease in numbers with increased individual glomerular filtra-

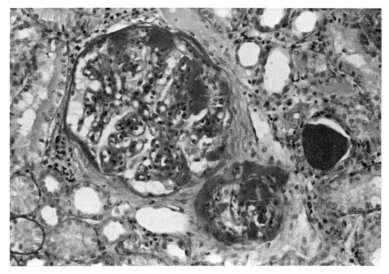

Figure 45–5. *Advanced membranoproliferative glomerulonephritis. The large glomerulus shows hypercellularity with prominent focal accumulations of mesangial matrix material and thickened glomerular capillary walls. Adhesions to Bowman's capsule and periglomerular fibrosis are also present. The smaller glomerulus is obsolescent. Notice the hyaline cast in a tubule (right) (PAS stain, original magnification × 200).*

tion rates. This hyperfiltration can cause glomerular hyalinization and sclerosis and result in progressive nephron loss independent of the above immunologic glomerular disorders.

CLINICAL SIGNS

The clinical signs associated with mild to moderate urinary protein loss are usually nonspecific, such as weight loss and lethargy; however, if protein loss is severe (serum albumin less than 1.5–1.0 g/dl or 15–10 g/L), edema and or ascites will often occur (Table 45-2). If the glomerular disease process is extensive, rendering three fourths of the nephrons nonfunctional, azotemia, polydipsia-polyuria, anorexia, nausea, and vomiting may occur. Occasionally, signs associated with an underlying infectious, inflammatory, or neoplastic disease may be the reason for presentation. Rarely, dogs may be presented with acute dyspnea due to a pulmonary thromboembolism.

Persistent proteinuria, greater than 3.5 g/day,

Table 45–2 *Clinical Signs Associated With Different Manifestations of Glomerular Disease*

Manifestations	Clinical Signs	Laboratory Findings
Mild to moderate proteinuria	Lethargy, mild weight loss, decreased muscle mass	Serum albumin <3.0 g/dl (30 g/L) but >1.5 g/dl (15 g/L)
Marked proteinuria (>3.5 g/day)	Severe muscle wasting, weight gain may occur due to edema or ascites	Serum albumin <1.5 g/dl (15 g/L) Hypercholesterolemia
Renal failure	Depression, anorexia, nausea, vomiting, weight loss, polyuria-polydipsia	Azotemia, isosthenuria or minimally concentrated urine, hyperphosphatemia
Pulmonary thromboembolism	Acute dyspnea	Hypoxia, normal or low PCO_2, fibrinogen >300 mg/dl (3 g/L) Antithrombin III <70% of normal

will often lead to clinical signs of the nephrotic syndrome. The combination of significant proteinuria, hypoalbuminemia, ascites or edema, and hypercholesterolemia is defined as the nephrotic syndrome. Classically, a combination of decreased plasma oncotic pressure and increased aldosterone activity causing sodium retention was thought to be the cause of ascites and edema. In human studies, however, aldosterone concentrations are frequently normal or low in nephrotic patients, and treatment with captopril does not prevent sodium retention. It has recently been hypothesized that intrarenal mechanisms, independent of aldosterone, contribute to sodium retention. The hypercholesterolemia associated with the nephrotic syndrome is thought to occur due to a combination of decreased catabolism of lipoproteins and increased hepatic synthesis of cholesterol-rich lipoproteins.

In addition to the above clinical signs, hypertension and hypercoagulability are frequent complications in dogs with nephrotic syndrome. Hypertension probably occurs due to a combination of sodium retention, glomerular capillary and arteriolar scarring, decreased renal production of vasodilators, increased responsiveness to normal pressor mechanisms, and activation of the renin-angiotensin system. Hypercoagulability and thromboembolism associated with the nephrotic syndrome occur secondary to several abnormalities in the clotting system. In addition to a mild thrombocytosis, a hypoalbuminemia-related platelet hypersensitivity increases platelet adhesion and aggregation proportional to the magnitude of hypoalbuminemia. Loss of antithrombin III (molecular weight 64,000) in urine also contributes to hypercoagulability. Antithrombin III inhibits serine proteases (clotting factors II, IX, X, XI, XII) and normally plays a large role in modulating thrombin and fibrin production. Finally, altered fibrinolysis and relative increases in the concentration of large molecular weight clotting factors (fibrinogen, V, VII, VIII, X) lead to an abnormal distribution of clotting factors and regulatory proteins. The pulmonary arterial system is the most common location for thromboembolism. Dogs with pulmonary thromboembolism are usually dyspneic and hypoxic with minimal radiographic abnormalities.

DIAGNOSTIC APPROACH

Persistent proteinuria with a normal urine sediment or accompanied by hyaline or granular cast formation is strongly suggestive of glomerular disease. Recently, calculation of the urine protein : creatinine ratio from random, voided canine urine samples has been shown to accurately reflect the quantity of protein excreted in the urine over a 24-hour period. This test has greatly facilitated the diagnosis of glomerulonephritis in veterinary medicine. In addition, the magnitude of proteinuria has been shown to correlate with the severity of glomerular lesions making the urine protein : creatinine ratio a useful parameter to assess response to therapy or progression of disease.

Proteinuria may be caused by pathologic or physiologic conditions (Table 45-3). Physiologic or benign proteinuria is often transient and abates when the underlying cause is corrected. Pathologic proteinuria may be caused by renal or extrarenal abnormalities. Prerenal and postrenal proteinurias can usually be identified on the basis

Table 45–3 *Classification of Proteinuria*

Type	Causes
Physiologic	Strenuous exercise
	Seizures
	Fever
	Exposure to extreme heat or cold
	Stress
Pathologic	
Nonurinary	Bence Jones proteinuria
	Hemoglobinuria/myoglobinuria
	Congestive heart failure
	Genital tract inflammation
Urinary	
Nonrenal	Urolithiasis
	Urinary tract infection
	Trauma
	Neoplasia
	Cyclophosphamide-induced
Renal	Glomerular disease
	Decreased tubular reabsorption
	Renal parenchymal inflammation or hemorrhage, for example, renal neoplasia, trauma, or pyelonephritis

of history, physical examination, and urine sediment changes. Quantitation of renal proteinuria helps evaluate the severity of renal lesions, formulate dietary therapy, and assess response to treatment or progression of disease. Proteinuria is initially detected using qualitative or semiquantitative tests such as the urine dipstick method or the sulfosalicylic acid turbidimetric test. If these tests are repeatedly positive for protein in dogs or cats without hematuria, pyuria, or urinary tract infection, urine protein excretion should be quantitated. Trichloroacetic acid Ponceau S or Coomassie blue are the most common methods used to quantitate urine protein. Collection of urine and measurement of urine protein excretion in milligrams per kilogram body weight per 24 hours has been the time honored method to quantitate proteinuria, since errors caused by variation in protein concentration due to changes in urine osmolality are minimized by 24-hour collection. Such collections, however, require the use of a metabolism cage or an indwelling urinary catheter, making the procedure cumbersome and expensive. In addition, incomplete collection of all urine produced over the 24-hour period will result in errors.

Renal proteinuria occurs mainly due to lesions involving the glomerular capillary wall. The renal tubules, however, by reabsorbing water from the glomerular filtrate, can markedly alter the protein concentration in a random urine sample. Inasmuch as creatinine is freely filtered through the glomerulus and not significantly secreted or reabsorbed by the renal tubules, the concentration of creatinine in urine is a reflection of urine osmolality. By dividing the urine protein concentration by the urine creatinine concentration, the effect of urine osmolality on the urine protein concentration is negated.

Most studies suggest that normal urine protein excretion in dogs is less than 20 mg/kg/24 hours. A regression line equation allows the urine protein : creatinine ratio when multiplied by 20 to be converted to milligrams of protein per kilogram every 24 hours. Therefore a urine protein : creatinine ratio less than 1 is considered normal in dogs. The ratio has not been fully evaluated in cats at the present time, although a value less than 0.33 may be considered normal (Hoerauf,

Additional Reading). A complete urinalysis should always be obtained prior to or along with the urine protein : creatinine ratio since dogs with hematuria or pyuria may have significant postrenal proteinuria.

There does not appear to be a relationship between urinary protein excretion and glomerular filtration rate in canine renal disease; however, the magnitude of proteinuria does appear to roughly correlate with the nature of the glomerular lesion. In two different studies, although overlap occured, urine protein excretion in dogs with glomerulonephritis was greater than in dogs with glomerular atrophy or interstitial nephritis but less than dogs with amyloidosis.

Evaluation of a renal biopsy specimen (see Kidney Biopsy in Chapter 80) is necessary for a definitive diagnosis of glomerulonephritis. Amyloidosis is a major differential diagnosis for glomerulonephritis, and histopathology is necessary to rule out renal amyloid deposition. Examination of renal histology establishes the presence, type, severity, and distribution of glomerular lesions and provides guidelines for prognostication. Glomerular hyalinization and sclerosis, extensive glomerular adhesions, fibrin deposition, epithelial crescent formation, and amyloid deposition tend to be irreversible lesions warranting a guarded to poor prognosis.

MANAGEMENT AND PATIENT MONITORING

Generation of immune complexes is dependent on the presence of antigen; therefore, the most important treatment for glomerular disease is identification and correction of underlying disease processes (Table 45-4). However, since an antigen source or underlying disease process is rarely identified or is impossible to eliminate (neoplasia), immunosuppressive drugs are often employed in the treatment of glomerulonephritis. Corticosteroids, azathioprine, cyclophosphamide, and cyclosporin A have been used clinically or experimentally to prevent immunoglobulin production by B cells or to alter the function of T helper or T suppressor cells. Unfortunately, no completed controlled clinical trials exist in veter-

Table 45–4 *Treatment Guidelines for Glomerulonephritis*

1. Identify and correct underlying disease processes
2. Immunosuppressive treatment
   a. cyclophosphamide 6.6 mg/kg PO q 24 hours for 3 days, then 2.2 mg/kg q 24 hours
   b. azathioprine 2 mg/kg PO q 24 hours (dogs only)
3. Anti-inflammatory-hypercoagulability treatment
   a. aspirin 0.5 mg/kg PO q 12 hours
4. Supportive care
   a. dietary: sodium restriction, high quality-low quantity protein (Hill's prescription diets k/d and g/d) supplemented with hard-boiled eggs to offset urine protein loss
   b. hypertension: dietary sodium restriction
      captopril 1–2 mg/kg PO q 12 hours
   c. edema/ascites: dietary sodium restriction
      furosemide 2.2 mg/kg PO as needed if necessary

inary medicine that demonstrate the efficacy of immunosuppressive drugs in the treatment of glomerulonephritis; however, early results from a study evaluating cyclosporin A treatment are encouraging.

The recent association between hyperadrenocorticism (and long-term corticosteroid therapy) and glomerulonephritis and thromboembolism in the dog, as well as the lack of consistent therapeutic response to treatment of glomerular disease with corticosteroids, indicates that corticosteroids should be used with caution in dogs with glomerulonephritis. Clinical results suggest corticosteroid treatment of glomerulonephritis may be more efficacious in cats compared to dogs. If immunosuppressive drugs are employed, proteinuria should be evaluated frequently to assess the effects of treatment. In some instances, immunosuppressive treatment may exacerbate glomerular lesions and proteinuria. Increasing evidence suggests that platelets and arachidonic acid metabolites (thromboxanes) are integrally involved in the pathogenesis of glomerulonephritis. Beneficial responses to anti-platelet therapy including aspirin, indomethacin, dipyridamole, and platelet-activating factor antagonists have been demonstrated in several studies. Dosage appears to be important when nonspecific cyclooxygenase inhibitors such as aspirin are employed. Low dose aspirin therapy can selectively inhibit platelet cyclooxygenase without preventing beneficial prostacyclin (vasodilator and platelet aggregation antagonist) formation. In several studies with mice, rats, rabbits, and dogs, thromboxane synthetase inhibitors and receptor antagonists have attenuated experimental glomerulonephritis as evidenced by decreased proteinuria, decreased glomerular cell proliferation and infiltration, decreased fibrin deposition, and preservation of glomerular filtration rate. Treatment of glomerular disease with prostaglandin analogues or dietary supplementation with marine (n-3) polyunsaturated fatty acids (as in DVM Derm Caps, Efa Vet, Efa Z Plus) to enhance prostacyclin activity has also generally attenuated glomerular disease.

Dimethyl sulfoxide (DMSO) has been shown to dissolve amyloid fibrils in vitro and in vivo in mice. It has been hypothesized that DMSO may have a similar amyloid-dissolving effect in domestic animals. The anti-inflammatory effects of DMSO may also serve to decrease production of the acute phase reactant serum amyloid A and inflammation associated with an underlying disease process. Decreased urinary protein excretion was observed in a dog with amyloidosis treated with DMSO; however, the effects of DMSO were difficult to determine since two potential underlying causes (interdigital pyoderma and a Sertoli cell tumor) were treated prior to DMSO treatment. The dosage of DMSO used in this dog was 80 mg/kg administered subcutaneously 3 times a week, and treatment was continued for more than a year without apparent adverse side effects. Other studies assessing the effects of DMSO in dogs with amyloidosis, however, have shown the treatment to be ineffective.

Colchicine is another drug that is frequently mentioned for the treatment of amyloidosis. Colchicine prevents production of serum amyloid A by hepatocytes and has been shown to have a preventative effect on amyloidosis in humans and mice when employed early in the disease process. Colchicine has not been evaluated in dogs or cats with amyloidosis. Inasmuch as glomerular amyloid deposition results in severe proteinuria with its attending side effects, and inasmuch as the disease is progressive, resulting in chronic renal failure and uremia, and no specific treatment has been proven to be effective, the prognosis for renal amyloidosis is poor.

Supportive therapy is important in the management of glomerulonephritis and amyloidosis and should be aimed at decreasing hypertension, edema, and the tendency for thromboembolism to occur. Sodium restricted diets (less than 0.3% dry matter—Hill's k/d and g/d) should be strongly recommended and vasodilators, β-blockers, and diuretics may be used as necessary (see Chapter 24). Although captopril may not prevent sodium retention in nephrotic patients, it has been shown to decrease proteinuria and intrarenal hypertension. Measurement of antithrombin III and fibrinogen concentrations may be helpful in determining which patients should be treated with anticoagulant therapy. Dogs with antithrombin III concentrations less than 70% of normal and fibrinogen concentrations greater than 300 mg/dl (3 g/L) are candidates for therapy. Anti-platelet drugs, heparin, and Coumarin have been employed for anticoagulant therapy. Inasmuch as antithrombin III deficiency is marked in some patients with protein-losing nephropathies, Coumarin should be more effective than heparin in reducing hypercoagulability. Finally, protein restricted diets (Hill's k/d and g/d) should be recommended to decrease glomerular hyperfiltration and nonimmunologic progression of glomerular disease. If proteinuria and edema are severe, hard-boiled eggs may be used to supplement reduced protein diets.

ADDITIONAL READING

Boyce JT, DiBartola SP, Chew DJ, Gasper PW. Familial renal amyloidosis in Abyssinian cats. Vet Pathol 1984; 21:33.

DiBartola SP, Chew DJ. Glomerular disease in the dog and cat. In: Kirk RW, ed. Current veterinary therapy IX. Philadelphia: WB Saunders, 1986: 1132.

DiBartola SP, Benson MD. The pathogenesis of reactive systemic amyloidosis. Journal of the College of Veterinary Internal Medicine 1989; 3:31.

Center SA, Smith CA, Wilkinson E et al. Clinicopathologic, renal immunofluorescent, and light microscopic features of glomerulonephritis in the dog: 41 cases (1975–1985). J Am Vet Med Assoc 1987; 190:81.

Center SA, Wilkinson E, Smith CA et al. 24-Hour urine protein/creatinine ratio in dogs with protein losing nephropathies. J Am Vet Med Assoc 1985; 187:820.

Grauer GF, Culham CA, Cooley AJ et al. Clinicopathologic and histologic evaluation of Dirofilaria immitis-induced nephropathy in dogs. Am J Trop Med Hyg 1987; 37:588.

Grauer GF, Culham CA, Dubielzig RR et al. Effects of a specific thromboxane synthetase inhibitor on development of experimental Dirofilaria immitis immune complex glomerulonephritis in the dog. J Vet Int Med 1988; 2:192.

Grauer GF, Thomas CB, Eicker SW. Estimation of quantitative proteinuria in the dog, using the urine protein-to-creatinine ratio from a random, voided sample. Am J Vet Res 1985; 46:2116.

Green RA, Kabel AL. Hypercoagulable state in three dogs with nephrotic syndrome: Role of acquired antithrombin III deficiency. J Am Vet Med Assoc 1982; 181:914.

Green RA, Russo EA, Greene RT et al. Hypoalbuminemia-related platelet hypersensitivity in two dogs with nephrotic syndrome. J Am Vet Med Assoc 1985; 186:485.

Hoerauf A, Reusch C, Minkus G, Hermanns W. On the significance of the urine protein/creatinine ratio for distinguishing between feline nephropathies. A diagnostic–bioptic comparative study. Proceedings of the American College of Veterinary Internal Medicine 1990; 1134.

Jaenke RS, Allen TA. Membranous nephropathy in the dog. Vet Pathol 1986; 23:718.

Jergens AE. Glomerulonephritis in dogs and cats. Compendium of Continuing Education 1987; 9:903.

MacDougall DF, Cook T, Steward AP et al. Canine chronic renal disease: Prevalence and types of glomerulonephritis in the dog. Kidney Int 1986; 29:144.

46

URINARY TRACT INFECTIONS

Gregory F. Grauer

Bacterial infection of the urinary tract occurs more frequently in dogs than cats. Approximately 15% to 40% of urinary tract inflammation in dogs is caused by urinary tract infection (UTI), whereas only 1% to 10% of urinary tract inflammation in cats is caused by infection. The majority of UTI involves bacterial inflammation of the lower urinary tract (bladder and urethra); however, ascension of bacteria to involve the ureters and kidneys is a potential sequelae of lower UTI. In comparison to bacterial UTI, mycoplasmal, chlamydial, viral, and fungal UTI are rare. Most bacterial infections of the lower urinary tract respond quickly to appropriate antibiotic treatment; however, UTI associated with defects in the host immune system (complicated UTI) often fail to respond to antibiotic therapy or relapse shortly after antibiotic withdrawal.

CAUSES

The most common bacterial pathogens associated with UTI in the dog and cat include *Escherichia coli*, staphylococci, streptococci, *Entero-*

bacter organisms, *Proteus* organisms, *Klebsiella* organisms, and *Pseudomonas*. *Escherichia coli* is by far the most common isolate from canine and feline urine (Table 46-1). Although UTI usually involves a single organism, as many as 20% may be mixed bacterial infections with two or more species. Most bacterial UTI is thought to be caused by intestinal flora that migrate up the urethra to the bladder. Although many enteric flora are anaerobes, the oxygen tension in urine probably inhibits growth of strict anaerobic bacteria; therefore, anaerobes rarely cause UTI. Bacterial virulence and the number of invading organisms are two major factors that influence establishment of UTI (Table 46-2). The ability of bacteria to adhere to the epithelial surface of the urinary tract prevents bacterial washout during voiding and allows bacterial proliferation to occur during the intervoiding period. Infection of the urinary tract usually involves bacterial colonization of the genitalia, migration along the urethra, and adherence to the uroepithelium, which is facilitated by fimbriae. Fimbriae are rigid, filamentous proteinaceous appendages found on many gram-negative bacteria. In addi-

Table 46–1 *Bacterial Isolates in Canine Urinary Tract Infections*

Isolates	Percent of Total
Escherichia coli	40
Staphylococcus aureus	15
Proteus species	12
Streptococcus species	10
Enterobacter species	10
Klebsiella species	8
Pseudomonas species	2

Table 46–2 *Factors Affecting Bacterial Virulence*

Fimbriae: allow attachment to uroepithelium
Capsular K antigens: increase invasiveness and interfere with opsonization and phagocytosis
O antigens in endotoxin: decrease smooth muscle contractility
Drug resistance:
   inherent resistance
   mutation and selection
   resistance factor transfer
Cell wall deficient bacterial variants: these bacteria can exist in hypertonic environments (urine and renal medulla) where host defense mechanisms may be compromised

tion to fimbriae, other factors that increase bacterial virulence include capsular K antigens, which interfere with opsonization and phagocytosis and O antigens in endotoxin, which decrease smooth muscle contractility. Decreased smooth muscle contractility may stop ureteral peristalsis and facilitate bacterial ascension from the lower to upper urinary tract.

Bacterial resistance to antimicrobial drugs may result from inherent resistance, mutation and selection, or transfer of resistance factors (R-factors) between organisms through DNA transfer. An entire bacterial population can acquire resistance by genetic transfer after only one dose of an antibiotic. The R-factor phenomenon has been identified in gram-negative bacteria including *E coli, Enterobacter, Klebsiella,* and *Proteus* species. R-factor resistance to multiple drugs is common, and R-factors are known to confer resistance to penicillins, cephalosporins, aminoglycosides, tetracyclines, chloramphenicol, sulfonamides, and trimethoprim.

Mycoplasmal organisms have recently been associated with UTI in dogs. Clinical signs of mycoplasmal cystitis include hematuria, pollakiuria, stranguria, incontinence, polydipsia-polyuria, and fever; however, some dogs with positive urine cultures may be asymptomatic. Whether mycoplasmas are primary urinary tract pathogens remains unclear.

PATHOPHYSIOLOGY

The status of host defense mechanisms appears to be the most important factor influencing the pathogenesis of UTI (Table 46-3). Normal voiding is the most efficient natural defense mechanism against UTI. Mechanical washout as a result of complete voiding (normal residual volume is less than 0.2–0.4 ml/kg) is responsible for removing more than 95% of bacteria that gain entrance into the urinary bladder. Washout of bacteria is enhanced by increased urine production and frequency of voiding. Disorders that decrease the frequency or volume of voided urine or that permit urine to remain in the bladder following voiding predispose animals to UTI.

Bacteria are normally present in increasing numbers from the mid to distal urethra; seldom do these organisms cause UTI in normal dogs. The high pressure zone in the mid urethra and spontaneous urethral contractions help prevent ascension of bacteria. Differences in epithelial morphology also help decrease bacterial colonization in the proximal and mid urethra. The length of the urethra and bacteriocidal prostatic secretions contribute to a decreased incidence of UTI in male dogs compared to female dogs. In both sexes, the specialized nature of the junction of the ureters with the bladder, provide valve-like protection against bacterial ascension.

Colonization of vulval and preputial luminal mucous membranes by nonpathogenic flora decreases colonization by uropathogens. Normal flora occupy most of the epithelial receptor sites, produce bacteriocins that interfere with uropathogen metabolism, and have a high affinity but low requirement for essential nutrients needed by uropathogens. Mucosal secretions help prevent adherence of uropathogens to epithelium; immunoglobulins coat pathogenic bacte-

Table 46–3 *Host Defense Mechanisms and Abnormalities That May Lead to Complicated Urinary Tract Infection*

Host Defenses	Abnormalities
Normal Micturition	
Normal urine volume	Urinary incontinence
Normal voiding frequency	Urine outflow obstruction
Small residual urine volume	Incomplete bladder emptying
Anatomic Structures	
Urethral high pressure zone	Urethral anomalies
Urethral contraction and peristalsis	Urethrosotomy surgery
Urethral length	Ectopic ureter
Vesicoureteral valve-like junction	Urachal diverticula
	Vesicoureteral reflux
	Indwelling urinary catheter
Mucosal Defense Barriers	
Antibody and mucoprotein production	Mucosal trauma
Nonpathogenic flora colonization	urolithiasis
	catheterization
	Neoplasia
	Cyclophosphamide-induced damage
Antimicrobial Properties of Urine	
Hyperosmolality	Decreased urine production
High urea concentration	Decreased frequency of voiding
Acidic pH	Glucosuria
Systemic Immunocompetence	
Cell-mediated immunity	Immunosuppressive drug therapy
Humoral-mediated immunity	Hyperadrenocorticism
	Diabetes mellitus
	Renal failure

ria, and glycosaminoglycans form a protective barrier over the epithelial surface.

Urine is frequently bacteriostatic and sometimes bacteriocidal. The antibacterial properties of urine are dependent on its composition; low pH and high concentrations of urea and weak organic acids in urine inhibit bacterial growth. In dilute urine, growth inhibition may be due to a lack of nutrients.

Uncomplicated UTI is defined as infection in which no underlying structural, neurological, or functional abnormalities can be identified. This form of disease is easiest to treat and usually undergoes rapid remission when appropriate antibiotic therapy is initiated. Complicated UTI is associated with a defect in the host's immune system; that is, interference with normal micturition, anatomic defects, damage to mucosal barriers, or alterations in urine volume or composition. Elimination of clinical and laboratory signs of complicated UTI with antibiotic treatment is usually not possible; either signs will persist or they will recur shortly after antibiotic withdrawal. Due to the relatively long urethra and antibacterial prostatic secretions, any UTI in the male dog should be considered complicated.

Interference with normal micturition often results in retention of urine, allowing multiplication of bacteria without complete washout. Distention of the bladder wall may compress intramural vessels and therefore decrease the number of white blood cells and other antimicrobial factors that may enter the bladder lumen. Damage to mucosal barriers may result in UTI depending on the extent of the lesion and concurrent introduction of uropathogens, for example, catheterization. It is interesting to note that bacterial inoculation of the urinary bladder in experimental animals usually fails to establish a UTI beyond 2 to 3 days unless the uroepithelium is first damaged by chemical or mechanical insult. Anatomic defects may allow ascending migration of bacteria (*e.g.*, indwelling urinary catheter or ectopic ureter) or may damage mucosal barriers (*e.g.*, urolithiasis, neoplasia, urachal remnant, thickened bladder wall due to chronic inflammation). Decreased urine volume is also associated with increased potential for UTI, and altered urine composition (*e.g.*, glucosuria or excretion of irritating drugs like cyclophosphamide) can enhance the environment for bacterial growth. In addition to the above local factors, systemic disorders such as renal failure, hyperadrenocorticism, prolonged steroid administration, and diabetes mellitus can result in complicated UTI.

Recurrence of clinical and laboratory signs of UTI can be classified into two groups: relapses and reinfections. Relapses are infections caused by the same species of bacteria within several weeks of cessation of treatment. Relapses may be due to use of improper antibiotic or dose, failure to eliminate predisposing causes that alter normal host defense mechanisms, or emergence of drug-resistant pathogens. Relapses in male dogs may be caused by chronic prostatic infections. Due to the blood-prostate barrier, lipid solubility and alkaline or neutral pKa appear to be necessary characteristics of antibiotics (*e.g.*, trimethoprim-sulfa, chloramphenicol, carbenicillin, erythromycin) to gain access to the prostate. Reinfections are infections caused by different pathogens. Reinfections often indicate failure to eliminate predisposing causes that alter normal host defense mechanisms. Alternatively, reinfections may be iatrogenic (*e.g.*, follow-up catheterization) or spontaneous.

CLINICAL SIGNS

Inflammation of the lower urinary tract often results in pollakiuria, urge incontinence, stranguria or dysuria, and gross or microscopic hematuria. Gross hematuria, when present, is often most pronounced at the beginning of voiding. Lower urinary tract inflammation in dogs is most commonly associated with bacterial infection; however, in cats bacterial inflammation of the

urinary tract is rare (see Chapter 48). Differentiating lower urinary infection from upper tract involvement as well as prostatitis is difficult. Acute bacterial pyelonephritis and prostatitis may manifest nonspecific systemic signs of lethargy, depression, anorexia, fever, and leukocytosis, which rarely occur with bacterial infections of the bladder and urethra; however, these signs are often not present with chronic pyelonephritis and prostatitis. Bilateral pyelonephritis may result in renal failure and subsequent azotemia and loss of urine concentrating ability. Cylindruria, especially cellular casts, indicates renal disease and, if coupled with significant bacteriuria, is suggestive of bacterial pyelonephritis.

DIAGNOSTIC APPROACH

It is important to try to identify those patients with immune system defects; therefore, a complete physical examination should be performed on all animals that present with signs of UTI. Although antibiotic treatment is the cornerstone of management, the status of host defense mechanisms is thought to be the single most important determinant in the pathogenesis of UTI. Abdominal palpation of the bladder before and after voiding may help diagnose a thickened bladder wall, mass lesion, or urolithiasis. Digital rectal examination in males and females will often allow palpation of the bladder trigone region as well as the pelvic urethra.

Laboratory confirmation of UTI usually includes urinalysis and urine culture. Urinalysis findings compatible with UTI include bacteria and increased numbers of red blood cells, white blood cells, and epithelial cells in the urine sediment (see Tables 80-11 and 80-12). Additionally, increased urinary excretion of protein and an alkaline urine *p*H are frequently observed. It should be noted, however, that sterile inflammation of the urinary tract (*e.g.*, some cases of calcium oxalate urolithiasis, neoplasia, and cyclophosphamide-induced cystitis) can also result in proteinuria, pyuria, and hematuria and that bacteria are not always observed on urine sediment examination in cases of bacterial UTI. Therefore, urine culture should be employed to confirm the presence and type of bacteria. Ideally, urine should be collected by cystocentesis (see Cystocentesis in Chapter 80) to avoid urine contamination by bacterial inhabitants of the distal urethra, prepuce, or vulva. If urine collected by catheterization, voiding, or bladder expression is cultured, it is important to quantitate the number of organisms per milliliter to differentiate infection from contamination (Table 46-4). Bacterial antibiotic sensitivity testing should be performed to guide antibiotic treatment choices and, in cases of recurrent UTI, help differentiate relapses from reinfections.

Ideally, urine specimens should be plated within 30 minutes of collection. If this is not possible, the urine sample should be refrigerated. Bacteria may double their numbers in urine every 45 minutes at room temperature, resulting in false-postive cultures. False-negative urine cultures may be obtained from urine that has been frozen or refrigerated for more than 12 to 24 hours.

Differentiation of upper from lower UTI is difficult but should be attempted in order to prevent renal damage in dogs and cats with pyelonephritis that need long-term antibiotic treatment and close monitoring (Table 46-5). The presence of cellular casts in the urine of animals with UTI is good evidence of pyelonephritis; however, the absence of casts does not rule out pyelonephritis. Fever, leukocytosis, and renal pain are compatible with but not diagnostic for pyelonephritis. Appropriate abnormal findings on an excretory urogram or a renal biopsy (see Kidney Biopsy in Chapter 80) can confirm a diagnosis of pyelonephritis; however, a lack of abnormal findings does not rule out the diagnosis. Several tests have been developed to differentiate upper and lower UTI in people (see Table 46-5); however, these tests are difficult to perform and in some

Table 46–5 Clinicopathologic Findings Associated with Upper Urinary Tract Infections

Fever, leukocytosis, renal pain
Cellular casts in urine sediment
Renal failure, i.e., azotemia and inability to concentrate urine
Excretory urogram abnormalities, i.e., renal pelvis dilatation or assymetrical filling of diverticula
Bacterial inflammation observed on renal histology
Positive bacterial culture from ureteral urine (Stamey test)
Positive bacterial culture from urine obtained after bladder washout (Fairley test)
Bacteria in urine are coated with antibody?
Increased urinary excretion of enzymes, indicating renal tubular damage or dysfunction

cases have not proven reliable in veterinary medicine.

MANAGEMENT AND PATIENT MONITORING

The goal of UTI treatment is control of pathogenic bacterial growth for a period sufficient to allow normal host defense mechanisms to prevent colonization of the urinary tract without further antibiotic administration. Although evaluation of bacterial sensitivity to antimicrobial drugs is advisable, treatment of acute onset, uncomplicated UTI is often dictated by economic and time considerations. If bacterial sensitivity results are not available, antibiotic treatment should be based on bacterial identification or the gram-staining characteristics of the bacteria involved. Clinical experience at several different veterinary teaching hospitals indicates that intelligent guesses may be made about bacterial susceptibility to antibiotics. Without benefit of bacterial sensitivity testing, the following are the drugs of choice

Table 46–4 Numbers of Bacteria/ml Considered Significant According to Method of Urine Collection in Dogs

Collection Method	Significant	Questionable	Contamination
Cystocentesis	>1,000	100 to 1,000	<100
Catheterization	>10,000	1,000 to 10,000	<1,000
Voided or expressed	>100,000	10,000 to 90,000	<10,000

for the bacteria listed: *E coli*, trimethoprim-sulfa; *Proteus* species, ampicillin; staphylococci, ampicillin; streptococci, ampicillin; *Enterobacter* species, trimethoprim-sulfa; *Klebsiella* species, cephalosporins; *Pseudomonas*, tetracycline (Table 46-6). If bacterial identification is unknown, treatment is best based on the gram-staining characteristics; that is, ampicillin for gram-positive bacteria and trimethoprim-sulfa for gram-negative bacteria.

Steps to follow for management of a UTI and a flow diagram are given in Table 46-7 and Figure 46-1. The duration of therapy of lower UTI must be individualized and should be based on the cessation of clinical signs and elimination of abnormal urine sediment as well as a negative urine culture. In general, uncomplicated lower UTI should be treated for 14 to 21 days, while recur-

Table 46–7 *Steps to Follow for Management of Urinary Tract Infections*

1. Diagnosis based on history, urine sediment, and, ideally, urine culture and sensitivity.
2. Selection of antimicrobial agent.
3. Reculturing of urine in 3 to 5 days to ascertain effectiveness of selected antimicrobial agent.
4. Examine urine sediment 3 to 4 days before discontinuing antibiotic treatment.
5. Recheck urine 10 or more days following cessation of therapy.
6. Recurrent urinary tract infections should be evaluated for underlying predisposing factors utilizing contrast radiography and/or ultrasonography.
7. Frequent reinfections may need to be treated with prophylactic doses of antibiotics after initial inflammation has been cleared up with standard dose antibiotic treatment.

rent or complicated UTI should be treated for a minimum of 4 weeks. Verification of proper selection of antibiotic therapy can be made after 3 to 5 days of therapy. Verification is accomplished by assuring that the urine is sterile. Urine sediment, however, may be still abnormal at this time.

Recurrent UTI should always be evaluated by urine culture and sensitivity. Additionally, attempts should be intensified to identify defects in the host immune system. Double contrast cystography and ultrasonography may be used to rule out anatomic abnormalities and mucosal lesions of the bladder. In male dogs, semen and prostatic wash cytology and culture (see Prostatic Massage, Urethral Brush Technique, and Ejaculation in Chapter 80) as well as ultrasound examination should be employed to rule out bacterial prostatitis. Excretory urography, ultrasonography, and renal biopsy (see Kidney Biopsy in Chapter 80) may confirm the presence of pyelonephritis; however, these parameters may be normal with chronic pyelonephritis. Finally, consideration should be given to the possibility of otherwise asymptomatic hyperadrenocorticism causing recurrent UTI, especially UTI without increased numbers of white blood cells and red blood cells in the urine.

Long-term (4–6 week) antibiotic treatment is required for recurrent UTI and careful follow-up examinations should be employed (see Table

Table 46–6 *Antimicrobial Agents to Which Greater Than 90% of the Urinary Isolates are Susceptible In Vitro at Concentrations Less Than ¼ of the Expected Urine Concentration*

Organism	Antimicrobial Agents*
Escherichia coli	Trimethoprim-sulfa
	Nitrofurantoin
	Cephalexin
	Gentamicin
Coagulase positive staphylococci	Ampicillin
	Chloramphenicol
	Trimethoprim-sulfa
	Nitrofurantoin
	Cephalexin
	Kanamycin
	Gentamicin
Proteus mirabilis	Ampicillin
	Trimethoprim-sulfa
	Cephalexin
	Gentamicin
Klebsiella pneumonia	Cephalexin
	Gentamicin
Streptococcus species	Ampicillin
	Trimethoprim-sulfa
	Gentamicin
Pseudomonas aeruginosa	Gentamicin (89%)
	Tetracycline (>80%)
Enterobacter species	Trimethoprim-sulfa (>80%)

* *Information for enrofloxacin is not available at this time.*

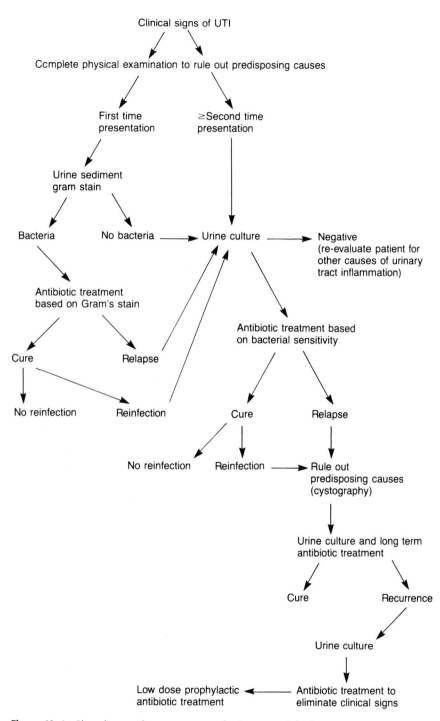

Figure 46–1. *Flow diagram for management of urinary tract infections.*

46-7). When antibiotic treatment is utilized for this period of time, long-term antibiotic side effects should be considered. Keratoconjunctivitis sicca and folate deficiency anemia may occur with long-term use of trimethoprim-sulfa, and nephrotoxicity is always a concern with aminoglycoside treatment, even for short-term treatment. If the infecting organism is highly resistant to antibiotics on Kirby-Bauer disc sensitivity (*e.g.*, susceptible only to aminoglycosides), minimum inhibitory concentration sensitivity testing should be utilized.

Many antibiotics are excreted by the kidneys; therefore, urine antibiotic concentrations are often much higher than serum and tissue antibiotic concentrations. Disk-diffusion techniques determine sensitivity based on typical serum concentrations of the antimicrobial drug. (One exception is nitrofurantoin, which uses urine concentrations.) A recent study showed that in vitro susceptibility testing (disk-diffusion) correctly predicted the outcome of ampicillin therapy in 173 of 187 (92.5%) of UTI caused by staphylococci, streptococci, *Proteus* organisms, *E coli*, and *Klebsiella* organisms. Likewise, disk-diffusion sensi-

tivity correctly predicted the outcome of trimethoprim-sulfa therapy in 239 of 283 (84%) of UTI caused by *E coli*, *Klebsiella* and *Proteus* organisms, streptococci, and staphylococci. However, due to differences in serum and urine concentrations of antibiotics, in vivo sensitivity may exist despite in vitro resistance if disk-diffusion sensitivity is used. When dealing with UTI, minimum inhibitory concentration sensitivity testing is often superior. For example, the minimum inhibitory concentration for penicillin for staphylococcal organisms, including penicillinase producing strains, is approximately 10 µg/ml. The average urinary concentrations of ampicillin at standard oral doses is greater than 300 µg/ml, whereas the expected serum concentration is 1 to 2 µg/ml. The high antibiotic concentrations in the urine frequently result in organism sensitivity even when the disk diffusion method indicates resistance. The general rule in interpreting minimum inhibitory concentration values is that if the minimum inhibitory concentration is less than 25% of the expected mean urine concentration (Table 46-8), the organism will be susceptible. However, with pyelonephritis or bladder infections with a thick-

Table 46–8 *Mean ± Standard Deviation Urine Concentrations of Selected Antimicrobial Agents Determined in Healthy Dogs with Normal Renal Function*

Antibiotic	Dose*	Route	Urine Concentration (µg/ml)	
Amikacin	5 mg/kg q 8 hours	SC	342	± 143
Amoxicillin	11 mg/kg q 8 hours	PO	202	± 93
Ampicillin	25 mg/kg q 8 hours	PO	309	± 55
Cephalexin	30 mg/kg q 12 hours	PO	805	± 421
Chloramphenicol	33 mg/kg q 8 hours	PO	124	± 40
Enrofloxacin	2.5 mg/kg q 12 hours	PO	43	± 12
Gentamicin	6 mg/kg q 24 hours	IM or SC	107	± 33
Hetacillin	26 mg/kg q 8 hours	PO	300.3	± 156.1
Kanamycin	6 mg/kg q 12 hours	IM or SC	530	± 151
Nitrofurantoin	4.4 mg/kg q 8 hours	PO	100	± ?
Penicillin G	40,000 U/kg q 8 hours	PO	294	± 211
Penicillin V	26 mg/kg q 8 hours	PO	148.3	± 98.5
Sulfisoxazole	22 mg/kg q 8 hours	PO	1466	± 832
Tetracycline	20 mg/kg q 8 hours	PO	138	± 65
Tobramycin	1 mg/kg q 8 hours	IM or SC	66	± 39
Trimethoprim-sulfa	15 mg/kg q 12 hours	PO	55	± 19

To determine antimicrobial efficacy of a drug, multiply the MIC by four. If the total is less than the mean urine concentration for that drug, the drug is expected to be efficacious.
* *Doses are the same for cats except: Chloramphenicol = 20 mg/kg q 8 hours for 1 week; Trimethoprim-sulfa dose for cats is unknown.*

ened bladder wall, tissue drug concentrations will be closer to serum concentrations than urine concentrations.

Fluoroquinolones are a new class of antibiotics that may prove to be useful for bacterial UTI and prostatitis in the dog. The FDA has recently approved enrofloxacin for veterinary use. Fluoroquinolones are bacteriocidal and act by inhibiting bacterial DNA gyrase. Enrofloxacin may be administered orally (2.5 mg/kg every 12 hours) and appears to have a broad spectrum of activity, including *E coli, Pseudomonas,* and *Staphylococcus aureus.*

The prognosis for complicated UTI is always guarded in comparison to uncomplicated UTI. The single most important treatment for a complicated UTI is correction of the underlying defect in the host immune system (Table 46-9). If predisposing factors cannot be corrected, antimicrobial therapy may have to be continued indefinitely. For animals with frequent infections that cannot be cured, low dose (one third to one half of the conventional daily dose) antimicrobial administration at bedtime may be recommended. This therapy allows the drug to be present in the bladder overnight and supplement the animal's defense mechanisms. For recurrences due to gram-positive bacteria, penicillins are recommended. For recurrences caused by gram-negative bacteria, trimethoprim-sulfa or cephalexin is recommended.

Urinary acidification (ammonium chloride) has been advocated as adjunctive therapy for lower UTI because acid urine provides a less favorable environment for bacterial growth. The antimicrobial activity of acidic urine, however, is inferior to that of antibiotics and should not be expected to eradicate infection; ammonium chloride should only be used in conjunction with other modes of therapy. Urinary acidification may also be effective adjunctive therapy in adjusting urine pH to optimize the value of certain antibiotics (*e.g.,* penicillin, ampicillin, carbenicillin, tetracycline, and nitrofurantoin). Ammonium chloride (66 mg/kg) should be given orally 3 times a day to maintain a constantly acid environment in the urinary tract; that is, urine pH should be maintained at less than 6.5.

Urinary antiseptics have been advocated as adjunctive therapy in the control or prophylaxis of lower urinary tract disease. Antiseptics are less effective than specific antimicrobial therapy in eradicating infections but are probably more effective than urinary acidifiers. Methenamine mandelate is a cyclic hydrocarbon, which is the most popular urinary tract antiseptic in use today. The oral dosage of methenamine mandelate for dogs is 10 mg/kg every 6 hours. In the presence of an acid environment (pH less than 6), methenamine hydrolyzes to form formaldehyde. Methenamine should be used in conjunction with ammonium chloride.

ADDITIONAL READING

Allen TA. Urinary tract infections. In: Breitschwerdt EB, ed. Nephrology and urology: Contemporary issues in small animal practice. New York: Churchill Livingstone, 1986: 89.

Allen TA, Jones RL, Purvance J. Microbiologic evaluation of canine urine: Direct microscopic examination and preservation of specimen quality for culture. J Am Vet Med Assoc 1987; 190:1289.

Barsanti JA, Chatfield RC, Shotts EB et al. Efficacy of cefadroxil in experimental canine cystitis. Journal of the American Animal Hospital Association 1985; 21:89.

Jang SS, Ling GV, Yamamoto R, Wolf AM. Mycoplasma as a cause of canine urinary tract infection. J Am Vet Med Assoc 1984; 185:45.

Lawler DF. New concepts of feline lower urinary tract disease. Compendium of Continuing Education 1988; 10:1015.

Lees GE, Rogers KS. Treatment of urinary tract infections in dogs and cats. J Am Vet Med Assoc 1986; 189:648.

Ling GV. Therapeutic strategies involving antimicrobial treatment of the canine urinary tract. J Am Vet Med Assoc 1984; 185:1162.

Table 46–9 *Reasons for Poor Therapeutic Response*

1. Use of ineffective drugs or ineffective duration of therapy.
2. Failure to administer prescribed dosage at proper intervals.
3. Impaired action of drugs either because bacteria are not multiplying or because they are sequestered in an inaccessible site.
4. Failure to recognize and eliminate predisposing causes.
5. Presence of mixed bacterial infections in which only one of the pathogens is eradicated by antimicrobial therapy.
6. Iatrogenic reinfection caused by catheterization.
7. Formation of drug-resistant bacteria.

Ling GV, Rohrich PJ, Ruby AL et al. Canine urinary tract infections: A comparison of in vitro antimicrobial susceptibility test results and response to oral therapy with ampicillin or with trimethoprim-sulfa. J Am Vet Med Assoc 1984; 185:277.

Osborne CA, Klausner JS, Lees GE. Urinary tract infections: Normal and abnormal host defense mechanisms. In: Osborne CA, Klausner JS, eds. Urinary tract infections. Vet Clin North Am [Small Anim Pract] 1979; 9:587.

Rohrich PJ, Ling GV, Ruby AL et al. In vitro susceptibilities of canine urinary bacteria to selected antimicrobial agents. J Am Vet Med Assoc 1983; 183:863.

Senior DF. Bacterial urinary tract infections: Invasion, host defenses, and new approaches to prevention. Compendium of Continuing Education 1985; 7:334.

Wilson RA, Keefe TJ, Davis MA et al. Strains of Escherichia coli associated with urogenital disease in dogs and cats. Am J Vet Res 1988; 49:743.

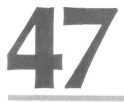

CANINE UROLITHIASIS

Gregory F. Grauer

The incidence of canine urolithiasis is between 0.4% and 2.8% in the United States, and similar incidence figures of 1.2% and 2.0% have been reported in the United Kingdom. Uroliths are most frequently observed in dogs between the ages of 3 and 9 years. In the United States, struvite uroliths are most commonly observed, accounting for approximately 69% of uroliths, followed by calcium oxalate (10%), urate (7%), silicate (3.5%) cystine (3.2%), and mixed urolith types (7%). Approximately 95% of the urolith weight is comprised of crystalline aggregates and as much as 5% may be comprised of an organic matrix made up of protein and mucoprotein complexes. The large majority of uroliths in dogs are found in the bladder or urethra, and only 5% to 10% are located in the kidneys or ureters.

CAUSES AND PATHOPHYSIOLOGY

Conditions that contribute to crystallization and urolith formation include a sufficiently high concentration of crystalloids in the urine, adequate time within the urinary tract (urinary retention of crystalloids), and a favorable urine pH for crystallization to occur. Theories concerning the pathogenesis of urolith formation include the precipitation-crystallization theory, which suggests that supersaturation of urine with crystalloids is the primary factor that initiates nidus formation and sustains growth of the urolith. Normal canine urine is supersaturated with several crystalloids. The greater the urine concentration of crystalloids and the less often voiding occurs (e.g., decreased water intake), the greater the chance of urolith formation. Supersaturated urine has a potential energy of precipitation or a driving force favoring crystal formation. The greater the magnitude of supersaturation, the greater the potential for crystallization. Conversely, undersaturated solutions have a potential energy of dissolution, resulting in crystal dissolution at a rate proportional to the degree of undersaturation.

Other theories of urolith formation suggest that substances in urine may promote or inhibit crystal formation. The matrix nucleation theory proposes that an organic matrix substance in urine promotes initial nidus formation. An immunologically unique protein, deficient in hydroxyproline, is thought to be present in many uroliths and has been termed matrix substance A. This proteinaceous matrix substance may allow crystallization to occur at a degree of supersaturation that would not ordinarily result in spontaneous crystallization. Another theory, the crystallization-inhibitor theory, suggests the absence of a critical inhibitor of crystal formation is the primary factor allowing initial nidus formation. Examples of crystallization inhibitors are citrates, glycosaminoglycans, and pyrophosphates. Decreased concentrations of these substances in urine may facilitate spontaneous crystallization and urolith growth. The extent that promoters and inhibitors of crystallization are involved in the pathogenesis of urolith formation is unknown. In all cases, however, supersaturation of urine with urolith constituents is essential for urolith formation.

Struvite or magnesium ammonium phosphate uroliths are the most common canine uroliths. Struvite uroliths also frequently contain small amounts of calcium phosphate or calcium carbonate. Urinary tract infections are an important predisposition for the formation of struvite uroliths, and *Staphylococcus aureus* and *Proteus* organisms are commonly associated pathogens. These organisms contain urease and are capable of splitting urea to ammonia, which increases urine ammonia concentrations, reduces hydrogen ion concentrations in urine, and results in increased urine *p*H. Alkaline urine decreases struvite solubility and facilitates crystal formation. Ammonia also damages glycosaminoglycans, which protect the urinary mucosa from bacterial pathogen adherence. Bacterial cystitis also increases the amount of organic debris available to serve as a surface for crystallization. Because of the high association with urinary tract infection, struvite uroliths are more frequent in female dogs; in fact, studies suggest that 97% of uroliths in female dogs are struvite.

The pathogenesis of struvite urolith formation in sterile urine is not known; however, struvite urolith formation in cats usually occurs in the absence of a urinary tract infection. Greater urine concentrating capacity and therefore a greater degree of urine supersaturation may be responsible for urolith formation in cats and dogs without urinary tract infections. Most canine diets are rich in minerals and protein and result in urine supersaturation with magnesium, ammonium, and phosphate. Struvite uroliths may occur in any breed; however, those commonly affected include: miniature schnauzers, Welsh corgis, dachshunds, poodles, beagles, and Scottish terriers. The high incidence of struvite uroliths in miniature schnauzers and poodles has led to the suggestion of a familial predisposition in these breeds.

Calcium oxalate uroliths are the most common type of urolith in humans; however, they are relatively rare in dogs. Calcium oxalate uroliths in dogs are usually the monohydrate (whewellite) rather than the dihydrate (weddellite) form. Factors involved in the pathogenesis of calcium oxalate urolithiasis in dogs are not well understood but frequently involve increased concentrations of calcium in the urine. In one study, three different groups of dogs with calcium oxalate urolithiasis were identified. The first and largest group of dogs had normal urine calcium excretion when fasted but had increased urinary calcium excretion postprandially. These dogs also had low to normal serum parathyroid hormone concentrations, suggesting the increased calcium excretion in urine was due to absorptive hypercalcemia. Another group of dogs with calcium oxalate urolithiasis had renal-leak hypercalciuria or defective tubular reabsorption of calcium, which was accompanied by increased parathyroid hormone concentrations. The third group of dogs had decreased urinary excretion of citrate, a calcium oxalate crystal inhibitor, when compared to normal dogs.

Approximately 70% of calcium oxalate uroliths are observed in male dogs; miniature schnauzers, miniature poodles, Yorkshire terriers, Lhasa apsos, and Shih Tzus are breeds that are commonly affected. Calcium oxalate uroliths frequently occur in older dogs (mean age 8–9 years) and concurrent urinary tract infection appears to be rare. Calcium oxalate solubility is increased in urine with a *p*H above 6.5, whereas a urine *p*H between 4.5 and 5.5 favors calcium oxalate crystal formation.

Most urate uroliths are composed of ammonium urate; 100% uric acid and sodium urate uroliths are rare in comparison. Supersaturation of urine with ammonium and urate ions is the primary cause of urate uroliths in dogs. Urate is derived from the metabolic degradation of endogenous purine ribonucleotides and dietary nucleic acids. Dalmatian dogs may have defective hepatic transport of urate compared to other dogs because urate conversion to allantoin is decreased in Dalmatian dogs even though hepatic uricase concentrations are adequate. Decreased production of allantoin in Dalmatian dogs results in increased urinary excretion of urate. Normally, allantoin is the major metabolite of purine metabolism and, in comparison to urate, allantoin is quite soluble in urine. In addition to decreased hepatic metabolism of urate, Dalmatian dogs have decreased proximal tubular reabsorption of urate and distal tubular secretion of urate, both of which augment urate concentrations in the urine. Urinary urate excretion in Dalmatian dogs is approximately ten times that of other dogs. Increased urinary excretion of urate is a predisposing factor rather than a primary cause, since all Dalmatian dogs excrete relatively high quantities of urate in their urine, but only a small percentage form urate stones. Absence of a crystallization inhibitor may facilitate urolith formation in some cases. Glycosaminoglycans in urine may combine with urate salts, resulting in an overall negative charge and reduced crystallization.

Ammonia, produced by renal tubular cells from glutamine, diffuses into the tubular lumen and serves as a buffer for secreted hydrogen ions forming ammonium ions. Ammonium ions are relatively lipid insoluble and therefore are trapped within the tubular lumen. Excretion of both urate and ammonium ions is increased secondary to protein ingestion.

Approximately 60% of urate uroliths occur in Dalmatian dogs and conversely 75% of the uroliths in Dalmatian dogs are urate uroliths. In addition to this breed predisposition, any dog with hepatic insufficiency (*e.g.*, hepatic cirrhosis, disseminated hepatic neoplasia, or a portosystemic shunt) may form ammonium urate stones because of increased renal excretion of ammonium urates. Portosystemic shunts are common in miniature schnauzers, Yorkshire terriers, and Pekingese dogs; therefore, ammonium urate uroliths are more common in these breeds. Uri-

nary tract infections, especially those with urease-producing bacteria, may facilitate ammonium urate crystallization by increasing urine ammonia concentrations. Urinary tract infection may also occur secondary to urolith-induced mucosal irritation. Urate crystallization is facilitated in acidic urine whereas an alkaline *p*H appears to favor ammonium urate crystallization.

Silicate uroliths were first reported in the United States in 1976 when crystallographic analysis of uroliths became available. Silicate uroliths frequently, but not always, have a jack-shape appearance, although not all jack-shaped stones are silicates (ammonium urate and struvite uroliths may also be jack-shaped). The etiology of silicate uroliths is unknown but may be related to dietary intake of silicates, silicic acid, or magnesium silicate. There appears to be a link between formation of silicate uroliths and consumption of large amounts of corn gluten or soybean hulls, which are high in silicates. Many of the reported silicate uroliths in this country have occurred in male German shepherd dogs. Alkaline urine appears to increase silicate solubility. Secondary urinary tract infections may occur due to mucosal irritation caused by the jack-shaped uroliths.

Cystine uroliths occur in dogs with cystinuria, an inherited disorder of renal tubular transport involving cystine and, in some cases, other amino acids (tubular reabsorption of cysteine, the immediate precursor of cystine, and lysine may also be decreased). Plasma cystine concentrations are normal in these dogs; however, plasma methionine, a precursor of cystine, may be increased. Plasma cystine is freely filtered through the glomerulus and is normally actively reabsorbed by proximal tubular epithelial cells. If it were not for the relative insolubility of cystine in urine and the potential for urolith formation, cystinuria would be of little consequence. Cystine is most soluble in alkaline solutions, and therefore cystine stones usually form in acidic urine. Not all dogs with cystinuria develop cystine uroliths; cystinuria is a predisposing rather than a primary causative factor. Cystinuria and cystine uroliths are most frequently observed in male dogs and principally dachshunds, but cystinuria has also been reported in basset hounds, English bulldogs, Yorkshire terriers, Irish terriers, and Chihuahuas. Cystine uroliths usually do not form in immature dogs; the average age at detection is between 3 and 5 years. The incidence of cystine urolithiasis in Europe has been reported to be approximately ten times that of the United States, probably because of the popularity of affected breeds in Europe. Urinary tract infections may occur secondarily; however, infection is not thought to play a primary role in the pathogenesis of cystine uroliths.

CLINICAL SIGNS AND DIAGNOSTIC APPROACH

Clinical signs associated with urolithiasis are dependent on the number, type, and location of the stones within the urinary tract. Inasmuch as most uroliths are located in the urinary bladder, clinical signs of cystitis (hematuria, pollakiuria, and stranguria or dysuria) are frequently observed. Uroepithelial irritation is relatively severe with jack-shaped uroliths compared to solitary, smooth stones; however, mucosal irritation and secondary urinary tract infection is possible with any urolith type or number. In male dogs, smaller uroliths may pass into the urethra causing partial or complete obstruction with signs of bladder distension and postrenal azotemia (depression, anorexia, and vomiting). Uroliths frequently lodge within the urethra at the caudal end of the os penis. Occasionally, the urinary bladder or urethra may be ruptured, resulting in ascites or subcutaneous perineal fluid accumulation and postrenal azotemia. Unilateral renal uroliths may be asymptomatic or associated with hematuria and chronic pyelonephritis. Bilateral renal uroliths, especially if associated with pyelonephritis, often lead to chronic renal failure. Ureteral uroliths may also be asymptomatic or associated with hematuria and abdominal pain. Unilateral obstruction of a ureter often results in unilateral hydronephrosis without evidence of decreased renal function.

Urinary bladder and urethral uroliths can often be palpated through the abdomen or rectum; however, a thickened, irritated bladder wall may obscure small uroliths. Palpation of the urinary bladder should be performed before and after voiding, as a full bladder may also obscure uroliths. In male dogs, the urethra should be palpated subcutaneously from the ischial arch to the os penis. Often plain or contrast radiographs of the urinary tract are necessary to confirm a diagnosis of urolithiasis. Calcium oxalate and struvite uroliths are the most radio-opaque stones, while urate uroliths are relatively radiolucent and often require contrast radiographs for diagnosis. Silicate and cystine uroliths have intermediate radiodensity.

Urinalysis findings in dogs with urolithiasis are often compatible with urinary tract inflammation (hematuria, pyuria, increased numbers of epithelial cells, and proteinuria). Urine pH varies depending on the stone type and presence or absence of a concurrent bacterial infection. In general, struvite uroliths are associated with alkaline urine (especially if urease-producing bacteria are present), cystine uroliths with an acidic urine, and oxalate, urate, and silicate uroliths with a variable urine pH. Crystalluria may be observed depending on urine concentration, pH, and temperature at which the urine was stored. Although crystalluria may exist without uroliths and uroliths may be present without crystalluria, if the two exist concurrently, the identity of the crystals is usually the same as the urolith (Figs. 47-1 through 47-5). Exceptions do exist, however; for example, urate or calcium oxalate uroliths may be complicated by a urease-producing bacterial infection, which could generate struvite crystals.

A bacterial urine culture and sensitivity should be performed in all cases of urolithiasis to rule out a concurrent urinary tract infection. Medical dissolution of uroliths is frequently ineffective if urinary tract infections are not appropriately treated. If a cystotomy is performed, a small piece of bladder mucosa should be submitted for bacterial culture, since the urine may be sterile in dogs that have been previously treated with antibiotics.

Whenever uroliths are passed or surgically removed, a quantitative analysis should be performed to identify the urolith type. Definitive diagnosis of urolith type allows the clinician to use

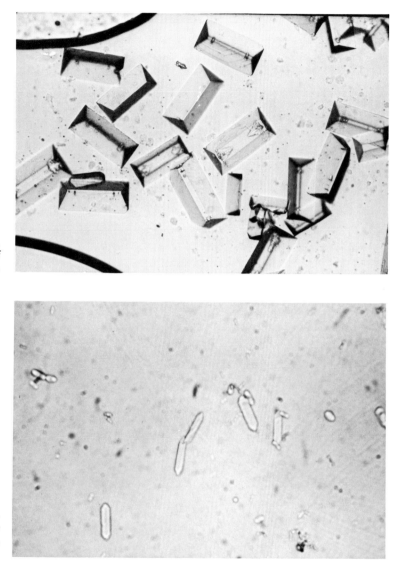

Figure 47–1. *Struvite crystals in urine sediment. These crystals are normally colorless. (Courtesy of Dr. Peter S. MacWilliams, University of Wisconsin).*

Figure 47–2. *Monohydrate calcium oxalate crystals in urine sediment. These crystals are normally colorless. (Courtesy of Dr. Peter S. MacWilliams, University of Wisconsin).*

specific measures for dissolution or prevention. Qualitative, commercial kit analysis of uroliths is not recommended since these kits will not detect silicate, frequently fail to detect calcium-containing uroliths, and give false-positive results for urates over half the time with cystine uroliths.

MANAGEMENT AND PATIENT MONITORING

General principles of treatment include relief of any urethral obstruction and decompression of the bladder if necessary. These treatments can

usually be accomplished by passage of a small bore catheter, cystocentesis, dislodgement of urethral calculi by hydropulsion (Figs. 47-6 and 47-7), or emergency urethrotomy. Fluid therapy should be initiated to restore water and electrolyte balance if postrenal azotemia exists. Hyperkalemia is a potentially life-threatening electrolyte disturbance that may occur with postrenal azotemia due to urethral obstruction or rupture of the urinary bladder or urethra. Bradycardia and ECG findings of flattened P waves, prolonged PR interval, widened QRS complexes, and tall or spiked T waves are suggestive of hyperkalemia

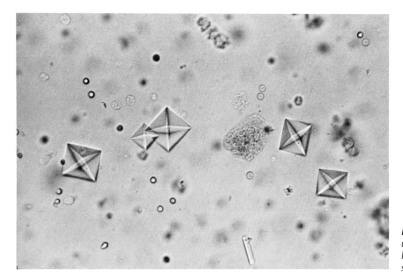

Figure 47–3. *Dihydrate calcium oxalate crystals in urine sediment. These crystals are normally colorless. (Courtesy of Dr. Peter S. MacWilliams, University of Wisconsin).*

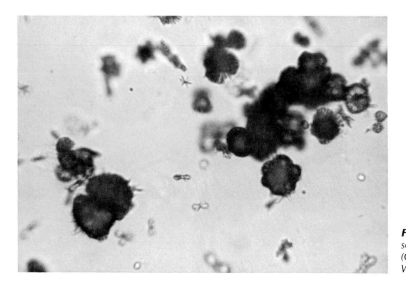

Figure 47–4. *Ammonium biurate crystals in urine sediment. These crystals are normally dark yellow. (Courtesy of Dr. Peter S. MacWilliams, University of Wisconsin).*

and warrant aggressive treatment. Isotonic saline and sodium bicarbonate or regular insulin followed by glucose should be administered intravenously to lower serum potassium concentrations (see Chapters 48 and 72).

Medical dissolution of struvite, urate, and cystine uroliths has been shown to be effective; however, the choice between surgical removal of uroliths and medical dissolution is not always clear (Table 47-1). Disadvantages of surgery include anesthesia, the invasiveness of the procedure, initial costs for anesthesia and surgery,

potential surgical complications, and the possibility of incomplete removal of uroliths. In addition, surgery does not decrease the rate of urolith recurrence. Medical treatment decreases the concentration of crystalloids in the urine, increases crystalloid solubility in urine, and increases urine volume, resulting in urine that is undersaturated with crystalloids. The major disadvantage of medical treatment of urolithiasis is the high degree of owner compliance required over several weeks to months. The cost of medical dissolution is comparable to the cost of surgery be-

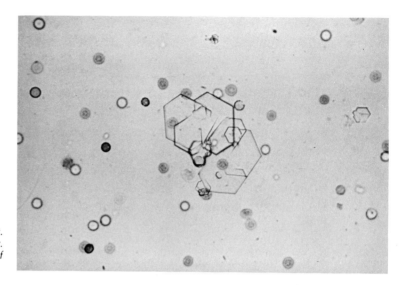

Figure 47–5. *Cystine crystals in urine sediment. These crystals are normally clear to light yellow. (Courtesy of Dr. Peter S. MacWilliams, University of Wisconsin).*

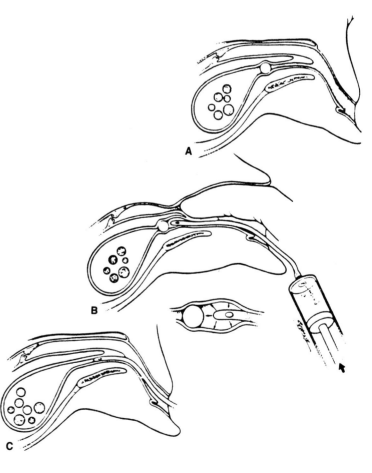

Figure 47–6. *Illustration of urethral hydropropulsion in a female dog with a solitary urolith, using a conventional catheter. (A) Urolith originating from the urinary bladder has lodged in the urethra. (B) The urethra distal to the urolith has been occluded by digital pressure through the vaginal wall (digital pressure may also be applied via rectal palpation in male and small female dogs) and the urethral lumen has been expanded by injection of saline through the catheter. (C) The urolith has been forced back into the urinary bladder and the urethral obstruction relieved. (From Osborne CA, Abdullhai S, Klausner JS et al. Nonsurgical removal of uroliths from the urethra of female dogs. J Am Vet Med Assoc 1983; 182:47.)*

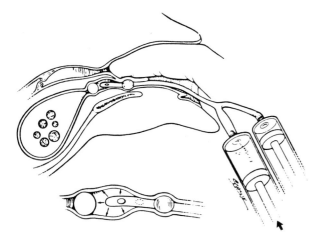

Figure 47–7. *Illustration of urethral hydropropulsion using a Foley balloon catheter. Inflation of the balloon with saline helps prevent reflux of saline solution out of the external urethral orifice. (From Osborne CA, Abdullahi S, Klausner JS et al. Nonsurgical removal of uroliths from the urethra of female dogs. J Am Vet Med Assoc 1983; 182:47.)*

cause multiple urinalyses, bacterial cultures, and radiographs are frequently required for follow-up.

General preventive measures that should be accomplished with surgery or medical manage-ment of uroliths, include induction of diuresis and eradication of urinary tract infections. Diuresis will lower urine specific gravity and the urinary concentration of crystalloids. The addition of 0.5 to 1.0 g salt (1 tsp. = 3.5 g NaCl) to the diet per day is usually recommended; however, exceptions to this recommendation exist. Hill's s/d diet contains high levels of salt and should not be further supplemented. Additionally, preventive treatment of calcium oxalate and cystine uroliths should include decreased dietary salt inasmuch as a natriuresis may increase urine calcium and cystine excretion. Maintenance of a urine specific gravity less than 1.020 is ideal, and dogs should be allowed frequent opportunities to urinate. The urine sediment and pH should be monitored routinely, and urinary tract infections should be treated quickly on the basis of bacterial culture and sensitivity.

Struvite uroliths can usually be dissolved by feeding a calculolytic diet (Table 47-1). Hill's s/d diet is severely restricted in protein, calcium, phosphorus, and magnesium, has a high salt content, and results in the production of acidic urine. Severe dietary protein restriction reduces hepatic

Table 47–1 *Treatment and Prevention of Canine Urolithiasis*

Urolith Type	Treatment Options	Prevention
Struvite	Surgical removal or dissolution: 1. Hill's s/d diet 2. Control infection 3. Urease inhibitor? Keep urine pH <6.5, blood urea nitrogen <10 mg/dl (<3.57 nmol/L) and urine specific gravity <1.015	Hill's c/d diet Monitor urine pH and urine sediment and treat any infections quickly and appropriately
Calcium oxalate	Surgical removal	Hill's u/d diet? Thiazide diuretics? Potassium citrate
Urate	Surgical removal or dissolution: 1. Hill's u/d diet 2. Allopurinol 7 to 10 mg/kg TID, PO 3. Control infection	Hill's u/d diet Allopurinol only if urate excretion is >10 mg/kg/day
Silicate	Surgical removal	Hill's u/d diet If necessary prevent consumption of dirt
Cystine	Surgical removal or dissolution: 1. Hill's u/d diet 2. D-penicillamine 15 mg/kg BID, PO or 3. N-(2-Mercaptopropionyl)-glycine (MPG) 15 to 20 mg/kg BID, PO	Hill's u/d diet Thiol-containing drugs if necessary to keep urine cystine <200 mg/L

production of urea and decreases urea concentrations in urine and in the renal medulla. The result is decreased substrate for bacterial urease and decreased medullary hypertonicity and therefore decreased urine concentrating ability. The average time for struvite urolith dissolution is approximately 12 weeks (range 2–28 weeks). Hill's s/d, however, cannot be fed routinely as a maintenance diet and should not be used during pregnancy, lactation, growth, or following surgery, as wound healing may be compromised by the ultralow protein intake. Additionally, due to its high salt content, s/d should not be fed to dogs with congestive heart failure or nephrotic syndrome. Hill's s/d should be fed for 30 days after the calculi are no longer palpable or visible radiographically. It should be noted that Hill's s/d diet will not dissolve nonstruvite uroliths and the diet will be ineffective if a urinary tract infection persists or anything in addition to the s/d diet is fed. Lack of the owner's compliance with dietary recommendations (instructions to feed s/d only) is suggested if serum urea nitrogen concentrations remain greater than 10 mg/dl (3.57 nmol/L).

In addition to decreasing the concentration of crystalloids in the urine, eradication of bacterial urinary tract infection is an essential part of medical treatment of struvite urolithiasis. In some cases, antibiotic treatment alone will result in struvite urolith dissolution. If infection is present at the start of treatment, antibiotics should be continued throughout the course of medical dissolution since bacteria may be liberated from the urolith as it dissolves. The choice of antibiotic should be made on the basis of urine culture and sensitivity. In cases of severe or persistent urinary tract infections caused by urease-producing bacteria, the urease inhibitor acetohydroxamic acid may be added to the treatment regime at an oral dosage of 12.5 mg/kg twice a day. Acetohydroxamic acid may help dissolve those struvite uroliths that are resistant to antibiotic and dietary treatment. Adjunctive treatment with urinary acidifiers (ammonium chloride 200 mg/kg divided three times a day, orally) should only be administered in conjunction with Hill's s/d if the diet fails to maintain the urine pH below 6.5. Medical treatment of sterile struvite uroliths is the same as above except antibiotics and

acetohydroxamic acid are not necessary. Dissolution of sterile struvite uroliths usually occurs more rapidly than those associated with urinary tract infections (2–6 weeks).

Measures to prevent struvite urolith recurrence include prevention and control of urinary tract infections, maintenance of an acidic urine pH, and decreased dietary intake of calculogenic crystalloids. Hill's c/d diet has been recommended as a maintenance diet to prevent struvite urolith recurrence, as it is moderately restricted in protein, magnesium, calcium, and phosphorus and results in an acidic urine pH. Inasmuch as the c/d diet is mildly restricted in sodium content, 0.5 gram of sodium should be supplemented on a daily basis to increase water consumption and urine production. In dogs with recurrent urinary tract infections, predisposing abnormalities (urachal remnant or bladder polyp, for example) should be ruled out with double contrast cystography. Occasionally, long-term prophylactic antibiotic treatment may be necessary to decrease recurrent urinary tract infections (see Chapter 46).

Medical treatment for the dissolution of oxalate urolithiasis has not yet been developed (see Table 47-1). Moderate restriction of protein, calcium, oxalate, and sodium with normal intake of phosphorus, magnesium, and vitamin D is recommended to prevent recurrence of calcium oxalate uroliths. Oral potassium citrate may be beneficial for preventing recurrence of calcium oxalate stones. Citrate complexes with calcium, decreasing the urine concentration of calcium oxalate, and potassium citrate results in urine alkalinization, which increases the solubility of calcium oxalate. The recommended oral dose of potassium citrate (Urocit-K) for humans is 60 mEq/day divided two or three times. Thiazide diuretics have also been recommended to decrease urinary excretion of calcium; however, studies in dogs have not shown consistent results, and long-term use of thiazides may increase serum calcium concentrations.

Medical dissolution of urate urolithiasis that are not associated with hepatic insufficiency (*e.g.,* portosystemic shunts) should include a diet low in protein and nucleic acids, alkalinization of the urine, xanthine oxidase inhibition, and elimination of urinary tract infections (see Table 47-1). Hill's u/d diet has reduced protein and purine content and results in alkaline urine and has been recommended for urate urolith dissolution and prevention. Similar to Hill's s/d diet, u/d decreases hepatic formation of urea and results in decreased renal medullary hypertonicity and decreased urine concentrating ability. Inasmuch as u/d diet is restricted in salt content, 0.5 to 1.0 gram of salt should be supplemented on a daily basis to increase water consumption and urine production. Additionally, allopurinol, a competitive inhibitor of the enzyme xanthine oxidase, which converts hypoxanthine to xanthine and xanthine to uric acid (Fig. 47-8), should be administered at an oral dosage of 30 mg/kg divided two or three times a day, and, if necessary, sodium bicarbonate or potassium citrate should be administered orally to maintain a urine pH of 7.0. Allopurinol should not be administered to dogs consuming normal or high protein diets, as this may result in xanthine urolith formation.

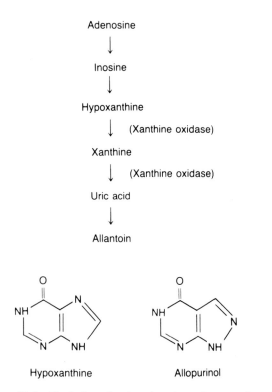

Figure 47–8. *Metabolism of purine adenosine and a comparison of the structures of hypoxanthine and allopurinol.*

Similar to the management of struvite uroliths, any urinary tract infection should be appropriately treated since urease-producing organisms will increase urine ammonium ion concentration and potentiate ammonium urate production. In dogs with urate urolithiasis secondary to severe hepatic insufficiency, the underlying disorder should be corrected if possible. If hepatic function can be improved and the urine becomes undersaturated with ammonium and urate ions, urolith dissolution may occur spontaneously. Since very low protein diets and alkalinization are not recommended for dogs with hepatic insufficiency, Hill's k/d diet should be fed to dogs with severe hepatic dysfunction.

Guidelines for medical dissolution of silicate uroliths are not yet available; however, recommendations to decrease recurrence after surgical removal include dietary change, augmentation of urine volume, and urine alkalinization (see Table 47-1). Hill's u/d diet may be beneficial as it contains low amounts of silicates and results in alkaline urine. Sodium chloride should be supplemented at a dose of 0.5 to 1.0 g/day. In certain regions, soil may contain high concentrations of silicate; therefore, consumption of dirt should be discouraged.

Recommendations for medical dissolution and prevention of cystine uroliths include reduction of dietary protein and methionine, alkalinization of urine, and administration of thiol-containing drugs (see Table 47-1). Hill's u/d diet is appropriate as it has a very low protein content, causes urine alkalinization, and decreases urine concentrating ability. Urine pH should be maintained at approximately 7.5 with oral potassium citrate. D-penicillamine (given orally at 15 mg/kg twice a day, with food to reduce likelihood of nausea and vomiting) forms a disulfide compound with cystine and therefore reduces the cystine content of the urine (Fig. 47-9). This disulfide compound is 50 times more soluble than cystine in the urine. D-penicillamine may interfere with surgical wound healing and should not be initiated until 2 weeks after surgery. Other side effects of d-penicillamine may include immune complex glomerulonephritis, fever, lymphadenopathy, and skin hypersensitivity. Another thiol-containing drug, n-(2-mercaptopropionyl)-glycine increases the

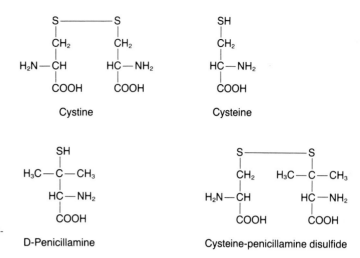

Figure 47–9. *Structures of cystine, cysteine, d-penicillamine, and cysteine-penicillamine disulfide.*

solubility of cystine in urine by a disulfide exchange reaction similar to d-penicillamine but with fewer toxic side effects. The dosage of n-(2-mercaptopropionyl)-glycine that has been recommended for dogs is 15 to 20 mg/kg twice a day. Thiol-containing drugs should be used for cystine urolith prevention if necessary to keep urine cystine concentrations less than 200 mg/L.

Whenever medical dissolution of uroliths is attempted, the patient should be re-examined at least monthly. A complete urinalysis should be performed and abdominal palpation or radiographs accomplished to assess urolith size. If urinalysis findings are suggestive of a urinary tract infection, a bacterial culture and sensitivity should be performed and antibiotic treatment initiated or adjusted accordingly. If urolith size is not decreased after 2 months of treatment, owner compliance, control of infection, and urolith type should be reassessed and surgical removal considered.

Recurrence rates of urolith formation in dogs of up to 25% have been reported (recurrences appear to be greatest in dogs with urate and cystine uroliths). Prior to the development of Hill's s/d, the recurrence rate for struvite uroliths was ap-

proximately 21%; however, this rate has dropped significantly with the appropriate use of s/d and c/d diets.

ADDITIONAL READING

Bovee KC, McGuire T. Qualitative and quantitative analysis of uroliths in dogs: Definitive determination of chemical type. J Am Vet Med Assoc 1984: 185:983.

Brown NO, Parks JL, Greene RW. Canine urolithiasis: Retrospective analysis of 438 cases. J Am Vet Med Assoc 1977: 170;414.

DiBartola SP, Chew DJ. Canine urolithiasis. Compendium of Continuing Education 1981: 3;226.

Lulich JP, Osborne CA, Parker ML et al. Canine calcium oxalate urolithiasis. In: Kirk RW, ed. Current veterinary therapy X. Philadelphia: WB Saunders, 1989: 1182.

Marretta SM, Pask AJ, Greene RW, Liu S. Urinary calculi associated with portosystemic shunts in six dogs. J Am Vet Med Assoc 1981: 178;133.

Osborne CA, Abdullahi S, Klausner JS et al. Nonsurgical removal of uroliths from the urethra of female dogs. J Am Vet Med Assoc 1983: 182;47.

Polzin DJ. Urocystolithiasis. In: Morgan RV, ed. Handbook of small animal practice. New York: Churchill Livingstone, 1988: 611.

48

FELINE LOWER URINARY TRACT INFLAMMATION

Susan L. Longhofer, Gregory F. Grauer

Feline lower urinary tract inflammation is characterized by one or more of the following: pollakiuria, hematuria, dysuria or stranguria, and partial or complete urethral obstruction. These clinical signs have historically been termed *feline urologic syndrome* (FUS); however, this syndrome is not a single disease entity. The definition of FUS has varied between studies and authors, and it is difficult to interpret the current literature without a broader definition that includes all feline lower urinary tract inflammation.

The incidence of feline lower urinary tract inflammation has been reported to be somewhere between 0.34% to 0.64% of all cats and is thought to be responsible for 4% to 10% of all feline admissions to veterinary hospitals. An equal incidence is found between male and female cats; however, overweight cats have a higher incidence of lower urinary tract inflammation. Indoor cats are also reported to have a greater predisposition for the syndrome than outdoor cats; however, the urination habits of indoor cats are more closely observed than those of outdoor cats. The majority of feline lower urinary tract disorders occur in cats

between 2 and 6 years of age, and increased risk of disease has been found in the winter and spring months. Between 30% and 70% of cats affected with one episode of feline lower urinary tract inflammation will have a recurrence.

The mortality rate of cats with lower urinary tract inflammation ranges from 6% to 36%; the extreme value may reflect an unwillingness of the people to repeatedly finance hospitalization for relief of urinary obstruction. Chronic renal disease secondary to ascending pyelonephritis is another possible long-term sequela or complication of feline lower urinary tract inflammation.

CAUSES AND PATHOPHYSIOLOGY

Bacterial cystitis or urethritis, neoplasia, trauma, irritant cystitis or urethritis, urolithiasis, urethral strictures secondary to scar tissue, prostatic lesions, extraluminal inflammation and masses, and neurologic disorders are potential causes of pollakiuria, hematuria, dysuria, and partial or complete urethral obstruction in cats. When these disorders have been eliminated from the differential list, the diagnosis of idiopathic lower urinary tract inflammation is made by exclusion.

Dietary magnesium content, dietary phosphorus content, Tamm-Horsfall glycoproteins, cell-associated herpesviruses, Manx virus, calicivirus, mycoplasmas, ureaplasmas, inadequate water intake, obesity, sedentary life styles, and decreased access to a litter box have all been implicated as factors in the pathogenesis of one or more aspects of idiopathic feline lower urinary tract inflammation. A combination of several of these factors may interact and contribute to development of the syndrome; however, the exact etiology or sequence of events has not been defined.

Frequently, inflammation of the feline lower urinary tract results from the presence of uroliths, microcalculi or crystals, which irritate the uroepithelium. The primary crystal type found in cats with spontaneously-occurring lower urinary tract inflammation is magnesium ammonium phosphate (struvite). As with canine urolithiasis, the formation of uroliths or crystals requires a sufficiently high concentration of urolith-forming constituents in the urine, a favorable pH for crystallization to occur, and adequate time in the urinary tract. The pH of the urine is an important determinant in the formation of struvite crystals. At a urine pH 6.4, magnesium ammonium phosphate is 100 times more soluble than at a urine pH 7.7. A post-prandial increase in urine pH of approximately one unit normally occurs 3 to 5 hours after cats eat a meal. Cats fed ad libitum have less fluctuation in urinary pH.

In addition to urine pH, dietary factors, especially high dietary magnesium, are currently thought to play a major role in the development of struvite crystals and uroliths. Diets with high ash content have also been incriminated in the past and are of major concern to owners; however, dietary ash consists of all noncombustible materials in the diet including magnesium, calcium, phosphorus, sodium, and chloride. Magnesium content is related to total ash content in dry and semi-moist foods, but not in canned foods. Despite owner concern, high dietary ash content would be beneficial if it were due to high calcium and salt content. In contrast, however, a low ash diet may enhance the development of crystalluria if the dietary magnesium concentration is high.

Dry cat foods have lower available energy density when compared to canned cat foods and contain more magnesium per kilocalorie than do canned or semi-moist foods. Additionally, most dry cat foods are higher in fiber and less digestible than canned or semi-moist foods, resulting in increased total intake of magnesium because most cats eat to meet their caloric needs. Another negative factor associated with consumption of dry food is the production of a larger quantity of feces with a corresponding larger volume of fecal water and decreased urine volume. Decreased urine volume increases the concentration of magnesium and other calculogenic substances in the urine.

Feline lower urinary tract inflammation is rarely observed in feral cats that normally eat small mammals and birds. A rat carcass contains approximately 64% protein and 0.085% magnesium on a dry matter basis, which is equivalent to 16 mg magnesium per 100 kcal metabolizable energy. Additionally, the high protein content found in small mammals acts to acidify urine; the average urine pH of cats fed mouse carcasses ranges from 6.0 to 6.3.

Uroliths are hard concretions of crystals, while urethral plugs are composed of a proteinaceous matrix with struvite crystals. Tamm-Horsfall glycoprotein, secreted by the renal tubules, is the major protein found in struvite calculi. The role of Tamm-Horsfall glycoprotein in the pathogenesis of urethral plugs is under investigation.

Urinary obstruction is more common in the male cat; the length and diameter of the urethra are significant factors in the propensity of male cats to become obstructed. Most obstructions are caused by urethral plugs that lodge in the penile urethra. Uroliths may lodge in any portion of the urethra, including sections proximal to fibrous connective tissue strictures from previous injuries. Local inflammation in response to urethral calculi or plugs may further exacerbate the condition by creating intraluminal urethral edema. Iatrogenic trauma created by urethral catheterization may also cause urethritis or inflammation of the periurethral tissue leading to urethral compression.

In a study of 143 cats with naturally occurring lower urinary tract inflammation, vesicourachal diverticula were observed in 23% of the cats. Vesicourachal diverticula may be congenital or acquired, and the acquired diverticula are seen primarily in cats older than 1 year with a mean age of 3.7 years. Male cats are twice as likely to develop the abnormality than female cats, and increased intravesicular pressure during urethral obstruction may play a major role in the pathogenesis of the acquired condition. While a urachal diverticula may be an incidental finding in an asymptomatic cat, hematuria and dysuria are frequently noted clinical signs. Vesicourachal diverticula are currently thought to develop secondary to feline lower urinary tract inflammation and are not thought to be an initiating factor. These lesions tend to resolve with successful treatment of the inflammation and diverticulectomy is not generally required.

Bacterial infection of the feline urinary tract, although rare in comparison to dogs, may be a cause of the clinical signs observed in cats with lower urinary tract inflammation. Urease-forming bacteria, primarily *Staphylococcus* species, create alkaline urine, which may exacerbate crystalluria and initiate the formation of cystic or urethral calculi. In the our experience, urinary tract infections in cats are frequently iatrogenic associated with urinary bladder catheterization. Concurrent use of urinary catheters and diuretic therapy significantly decreases host defense mechanisms that protect against urinary tract infection.

Irritation of the uroepithelium by struvite crystals may alter normal host defense and allow secondary bacterial colonization of the bladder or urethra. Complete voiding is a major host defense against bacterial infection, and anatomic abnormalities or partial obstructions increase urine residual volume after normal voiding. Chronic inflammation of the bladder may lead to fibrosis and thickening of the bladder wall, a condition that may also inhibit complete voiding or may create pollakiuria because the bladder is unable to distend normally.

Decreased urine volume and frequency of urination are thought to facilitate development of feline lower urinary tract inflammation. Possible causes of decreased urine volume and frequency of urination include a dirty or poorly available litter box, decreased physical activity (cold weather, castration, obesity, illness, and confinement), and decreased water consumption due to water taste, availability, or temperature. Stress may also contribute to the development of the clinical signs of urinary tract disease. While the role of stress is difficult to prove, it is often implicated; history from the owners frequently points out a recent association with stress (*e.g.*, boarding, a cat show, a new pet in the home, or vacation).

CLINICAL SIGNS

The clinical symptoms of feline lower urinary tract inflammation are dependent on the component of the disease complex present (Table 48-1). Unobstructed cats will usually present with pollakiuria, dysuria, microscopic or gross hematuria, and inappropriate urination, often in a

Table 48–1 *Clinical Signs Associated With Feline Lower Urinary Tract Inflammation*

CYSTITIS/URETHRITIS
Hematuria
Pollakiuria
Dysuria/stranguria
Licking at genitalia
Urination in inappropriate locations

PARTIAL OR COMPLETE URETHRAL OBSTRUCTION
Inability to urinate, straining in the litter box
Hiding
Vocalizing
Painful abdomen
Licking at genitalia
Congested penis extended from prepuce
Symptoms of postrenal uremia
  Depression
  Weakness
  Anorexia
  Emesis
  Dehydration
  Hypothermia
  Acidosis and hyperventilation
  Electrolyte disturbances (hyperkalemia)
  Bradycardia

bathtub or sink. These symptoms may be readily apparent in cats that live indoors or may be missed in cats that live primarily outdoors.

The presentation of a cat with urinary obstruction will depend on how long the obstruction has been present. Within 6 to 24 hours, most obstructed cats will make frequent attempts to urinate (which may be confused with constipation by the owners), pace, vocalize, hide under beds or behind couches, lick their genitalia, and display anxiety. If the obstruction is not relieved within 36 to 48 hours, symptoms characteristic of postrenal uremia including anorexia, emesis, dehydration, depression, weakness, collapse, stupor, hypothermia, acidosis with hyperventilation, bradycardia or sudden death may be present.

On physical examination, an unobstructed cat will be apparently healthy except for a small, easily expressed bladder. The bladder wall may be thickened, and palpation of the bladder may result in voiding. Abdominal palpation is usually not painful to the unobstructed cat in contrast to the obstructed cat, which resents manipulation of the caudal abdomen. The most significant finding on physical examination of the obstructed cat will be a turgid, distended bladder that is difficult or impossible to express. Care should be exercised in manipulation of the distended bladder since the wall has been injured by the increased intravesicular pressure and is vulnerable to rupture. The penis may protrude from the prepuce and may be congested. Occasionally a urethral plug will be observed extending from the urethral orifice, and, in some cases, the cat may lick the penis until it becomes excoriated and bleeds.

DIAGNOSTIC APPROACH

A history of acute onset of pollakiuria, dysuria, and hematuria and finding an apparently healthy cat on physical examination strongly suggests idiopathic lower urinary tract inflammation (Table 48-2, Fig. 48-1). The physical examination should include digital rectal palpation of the caudal bladder and urethra in an attempt to rule out masses and calculi. The perineal reflex and the bulbourethral reflex should be evaluated to determine the status of the pudendal nerve and the sacral plexus. Palpation of the bladder prior to

Table 48–2 *Diagnostic Plan for Feline Urinary Tract Inflammation*

1. Rule out postrenal obstruction; relieve obstruction if present.
2. Obtain urinalysis, by cystocentesis if possible, for evaluation of urine pH and urine sediment. Culture if evidence of urinary tract infection (pyuria, bacteriuria) exists.
3. Assess degree of hyperkalemia with an ECG and obtain blood urea nitrogen, serum creatinine, and potassium concentrations if cat is obstructed and depressed.
4. Management with diet containing <20 mEq magnesium/100 KCal and acidifying urine (between pH 5.9 and 6.4) with ammonium chloride or methionine if necessary.
5. If symptoms persist or recur, obtain urinalysis:
   If there is no evidence of urinary tract infection, radiograph the abdomen and/or obtain contrast radiographs of the bladder and urethra.
   If there is evidence of urinary tract infection, perform bacterial culture and sensitivity and treat with appropriate antibiotic.

and after voiding will help determine residual urine volume and the presence of intraluminal masses or uroliths.

The minimum data base should include a complete urinalysis (Table 48-3). Urine is preferably obtained by cystocentesis; however, manipulation of the bladder during abdominal palpation may result in voiding, and a sample obtained from a clean table top may be used to assess urine pH and to examine urine sediment.

An extensive diagnostic workup of the unobstructed dysuric cat is unwarranted, as most cases are bacteriologically sterile and respond to dietary therapy. If clinical signs persist beyond 7 to 10 days of dietary therapy, a second urinalysis with urine culture and sensitivity, survey radiographs of the abdomen, and a contrast cystogram or urethrogram should be considered. Additionally, ultrasonic examination of the bladder may be useful for detection of masses, cystic calculi, or thickening of the bladder wall (see Table 48-3).

MANAGEMENT

Management of a cat with lower urinary tract inflammation will depend on the clinical signs at presentation. Unobstructed cats with idiopathic dysuria and hematuria will often become asymp-

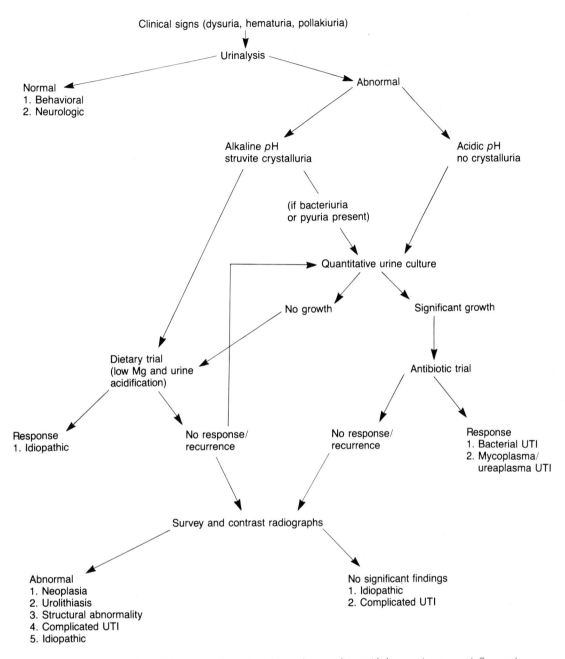

Figure 48–1. *Diagnostic and therapeutic flow chart for unobstructed cat with lower urinary tract inflammation.*

tomatic within 5 to 7 days of presentation without therapy. The empiric use of antibiotics is not indicated since the vast majority of cats with these symptoms have bacteriologically sterile urine. In cats presenting with severe dysuria or stranguria, propantheline bromide, diazepam, or aminopro-

prazine may be prescribed, but no controlled studies have proven the efficacy of these treatment modalities, and propantheline bromide was no more effective than lactated Ringer's solution in one controlled trial (Table 48-4).

The use of anti-inflammatory drugs (glucocor-

Table 48–3 *Laboratory Evaluation of Feline Lower Urinary Tract Inflammation*

Test	What to Check For
Urinalysis	Evidence of urinary tract inflammation: WBCs, RBCs, crystals, bacteria, proteinuria, alkaline *p*H Evidence of neoplasia: neoplasic cells Evidence of parasitic disease: ova of *Capillaria* species
Urine culture	Evidence of urinary tract infection: any organisms in cystocentesis samples, or >1,000 organisms/ml in catheterized samples, or >10,000 organisms/ml in voided urine sample
Serum creatinine, urea nitrogen, and potassium concentrations	Rule out postrenal obstruction
Abdominal radiographs	Rule out radiopaque cystic calculi
Ultrasound of bladder	Rule out mass lesions, urolithiasis, bladder wall thickening
Contrast cystogram and/or urethrogram	Rule out mass lesions, urolithiasis, bladder wall thickening, vesicourachal diverticula

ticoids) is controversial, and no controlled trials have been conducted to prove their efficacy. Decreasing inflammation and swelling within the urinary tract and stimulation of appetite, especially associated with diet change, are potential benefits of corticosteroids. In general, cats do not develop polyuria after administration of corticosteroids, and attempts to decrease urine specific gravity with corticosteroids are usually not successful. Intravesicular dimethyl sulfoxide has been advocated as a local anti-inflammatory therapy, but, once again, no controlled studies have been conducted to suggest this therapy is more efficacious than no therapy at all. Urinary antiseptics and analgesics such as phenazopyridine and methylene blue should not be administered to cats because of potential Heinz body anemias.

Several sources of fresh water should be made available to the cat. Increase fluid consumption by adding water to canned cat food, providing chicken or beef broth to drink, or lightly salting food may be attempted. Litter boxes should be cleaned frequently and should be placed in convenient locations.

If an alkaline urine *p*H with struvite crystal-

Table 48–4 *Drugs Used in the Pharmacologic Management of Feline Lower Urinary Tract Inflammation*

Drug	Action	Dosage
Aminoproprazine	Smooth muscle relaxant	2.0 mg/kg two times daily, IM
Ammonium chloride	Urinary acidifier	1 g once a day, PO
Bethanechol	Parasympathomimetic increased detrusor contractility	1.25 to 5 mg three times daily, PO
Diazepam	Skeletal muscle relaxant	2 to 5 mg three times daily, PO
Methionine	Urinary acidifier	0.2 to 0.5 g two times daily, PO
Prednisone	Anti-inflammatory	2.5 to 5 mg once daily, PO
Propantheline bromide	Anticholinergic decrease detrusor contractility	7.5 mg three times daily, PO

luria is observed on the initial urinalysis, Hill's prescription diet feline s/d should be fed as the sole diet for 1 to 3 months. This diet is magnesium restricted, high in salt content to cause increased water intake and urine output, and maintains an average urine pH less than 6.4. Urine culture and sensitivity should be performed and appropriate antibiotics administered if there is evidence of bacterial infection (for example, pyuria or bacteriuria).

To prevent recurrence of lower urinary tract symptoms after s/d diet treatment, a nutritionally adequate diet containing less than 20 mg magnesium per 100 kcal metabolizable energy should be fed. Examples include Hill's prescription diet feline c/d (canned or dry), and Science Diet Feline Maintenance (canned or dry).

Ideally, urine pH, measured 4 to 8 hours after feeding, should be maintained between 5.9 and 6.4. Feline prescription diet c/d, canned or dry, is metabolized to form acid ions that are excreted in the urine. If an acidic urine pH cannot be maintained with c/d, urinary acidifiers may be added to the treatment protocol. Ammonium chloride is the most effective urinary acidifier (1.0 g per day on food); however, diarrhea, emesis, and anorexia are potential side effects of ammonium chloride administration. If diarrhea persists after 7 to 10 day, methionine (200–500 mg, twice a day) may be substituted for the ammonium chloride.

If the initial urinalysis does not demonstrate struvite crystalluria or an alkaline urine pH, dietary management may not be beneficial. Some clinicians will recommend anti-inflammatory doses of prednisone for 3 to 5 days in these cases. If clinical symptoms are still present in 7 to 10 days, and if repeated urinalysis still reveals a urine pH less than 6.4 without struvite crystalluria, a urine sample should be obtained by cystocentesis for urine culture, and abdominal radiographs and contrast studies of the bladder and urethra should be performed.

In cats presented with urethral obstruction, the relative urgency for relieving urethral obstruction will depend on the physical status of the cat. Cats that are alert and not azotemic may be sedated for urethral catheterization without further diagnostics or treatment; however, in a depressed cat with urethral obstruction, an ECG rhythm strip should be assessed to determine the degree of hyperkalemia (Table 48-5) and an intravenous catheter placed for administration of normal saline in addition to establishing urethral patency.

If the ECG suggests hyperkalemia, the cat should be treated aggressively with 0.9% saline (dilutional therapy) and sodium bicarbonate (2–3 mEq/kg IV slowly). Bicarbonate therapy will drive potassium into cells in exchange for hydrogen ions. Most cats with postrenal uremia are moderately to severely acidotic, a condition that exacerbates hyperkalemia. Alternatively, dextrose and insulin may be administered to decrease the serum potassium concentration inasmuch as insulin facilitates cellular uptake of potassium. Regular insulin (0.5 units/kg) is administered intravenously followed by a bolus of dextrose (2 g/unit of insulin administered) to protect against hypoglycemia. If cardiac arrhythmias are life-threatening, calcium gluconate (0.5–1 ml/kg of 10% solution) may be administered intravenously. Calcium plays a cardio-protective role in hyperkalemia without decreasing serum potassium concentrations.

The degree of restraint required for urethral catheterization will depend on the patient's temperament and physical status. Physical restraint in a towel or cat bag with or without the use of topical lidocaine may be all the restraint required in a severely depressed cat. In cases requiring more restraint, ketamine hydrochloride (1–2 mg/kg IV) or an ultrashort-acting barbiturate (thiamylal sodium or thiopental sodium 1 mg/kg IV titrated to effect) may be used. Ketamine is eliminated by the kidney, and low intravenous doses (1/10 of the IM dose) are frequently adequate for restraint. Additional doses of ketamine should be avoided in severely uremic cats.

Relief of urethral obstruction may be accom-

Table 48–5 *Electrocardiographic Findings in Hyperkalemia*

Absent or flattened P waves
Prolonged PR interval
Widened QRS complex
Tented or spiked T waves
Bradycardia (not a consistent finding in cats)
Sinoatrial or ventricular arrhythmias

plished in some cases by penile massage and gentle expression of the bladder. If massage of the penis does not result in urine flow, palpation of the urethra per rectum may dislodge a urethral plug/calculi. Sterile isotonic saline should be used to hydropulse urethral plugs into the bladder through well-lubricated catheters or cannulae. A variety of cannulae and catheters may be used; however, nonmetal catheters with smooth open ends are preferred to prevent iatrogenic damage to the urethral mucosa. Adherence to strict aseptic technique is essential to prevent urinary tract infections. If difficulty is encountered catheterizing the bladder, cystocentesis (see Cystocentesis in Chapter 80) may decrease intravesicular pressure and allow the urethral obstruction to be flushed back into the bladder.

Questions frequently arise as to when indwelling urinary catheters are necessary in male cats that have just been unobstructed. The following are indications for the use of an indwelling urethral catheter: 1) an inability to restore a normal urine stream; 2) an abundance of debris, which cannot be lavaged or aspirated from the bladder; 3) evidence of decreased bladder muscle tone (detrusor atony) in situations where the bladder cannot be manually expressed four to six times a day; or 4) intensive care of critically ill patients when urine formation is being monitored as a guide to fluid therapy. When an indwelling urinary catheter is necessary, strict aseptic technique should be used during placement. A soft, red, rubber feeding tube (3 French) should be used, and placing the feeding tube in the freezer for 30 minutes prior to use facilitates its passage. The catheter should be inserted only as far as necessary to reach the neck of the bladder (6–8 cm), and ability to aspirate urine should serve as a guide to proper placement of the catheter. A closed urine collection system should be employed, and the catheter should be sutured to the prepuce and left in place for as short a period of time as possible. An Elizabethan collar or tape hobbles are needed to prevent the cat from chewing out the sutures and removing the catheter. Prophylactic antibiotics are not recommended; however, the urine sediment should be examined daily and urine cultured if necessary.

The degree of postrenal uremia should be as-sessed by measurement of blood urea nitrogen, serum creatinine, and serum potassium concentrations. Intravenous fluid therapy is indicated, especially in cats with uremia. Maintenance (60 ml/kg/day) and replacement therapy (percent dehydration × body weight [kg] × 1000 = milliliters) should be administered intravenously over 24 hours. Subcutaneous administration of a balanced electrolyte solution (5 ml/kg three times a day) is an acceptable mode of fluid therapy in some cases after the initial uremic crisis is under control. Large volume, post-obstructive diuresis develops in some cats, and measurement of urine volume every 2 to 4 hours will facilitate administration of correct replacement therapy. In cases with marked post-obstructive diuresis, intravenous fluid therapy is essential. Blood urea nitrogen, creatinine, and serum electrolyte concentrations should be reassessed as needed, depending on the degree of uremia and the response to treatment, to insure adequate recovery of renal function. If hematuria is severe, the hematocrit should be monitored once or twice a day.

Detrusor atony from disruption of smooth muscle tight junctions is fairly common in cats obstructed for more than 24 hours. If the bladder can be expressed four to six times a day, an indwelling catheter may not be necessary. If the bladder cannot be expressed at least four times a day, an indwelling catheter is indicated. Bethanechol (2.5 mg three times a day, orally) may be administered to stimulate detrusor contractility only after urethral patency has been assured by a wide urine stream or an indwelling urinary catheter.

Perineal urethrostomy is rarely required for emergency relief of urethral obstruction. If the urethral obstruction cannot be relieved by medical methods, uremic cats must be stabilized prior to surgery. Percutaneous prepubic urinary drainage or repeated cystocentesis should ideally be employed to keep the bladder empty until hyperkalemia, acidosis, and uremia are corrected. Elective perineal urethrostomies are occasionally recommended in male cats with recurrent obstructions to decrease the likelihood of death due to post renal uremia.

The dietary management of an obstructed cat is similar to management of unobstructed cat with struvite crystalluria and alkaline urine. Hill's prescription diet feline s/d should be fed as the sole diet for 1 to 3 months. Diets with less than 20 mg magnesium/100 kcal metabolizable energy should be fed thereafter to help prevent recurrences of lower urinary tract inflammation or obstruction.

PATIENT MONITORING

Probably the most important aspect of patient monitoring is ensuring that the owners recognize both the significance and the clinical signs of urethral obstruction. Owners with male cats with urinary obstruction must be warned of the risks of reobstruction, especially during the first 24 to 48 hours. Allowing the owners to palpate the distended bladder during the initial examination is a good step in teaching them to differentiate between pollakiuria or dysuria and obstruction. Any straining in the litter box should be cause for alarm in a male cat with a history of urethral obstruction, and careful observation for continued voiding of urine is essential to detect a recurrence early.

A follow-up urinalysis should be performed on all cats that have been catheterized to relieve urethral obstruction. Normal host defenses are bypassed when a catheter is introduced into the bladder, and urinary tract infections post catheterization, especially when an indwelling urinary catheter or diuresis therapy was utilized, are common. Dietary therapy designed to decrease urine specific gravity may further compromise host defense mechanisms, and early detection of urinary tract infection is important in these patients. All cats receiving corticosteroids should have a follow-up urinalysis and urine culture since corticosteroids may decrease immune function (and inflammatory urine sediment changes) and predispose cats to urinary tract infection.

Pyelonephritis is a significant concern with any urinary tract infection, and bacterial pyelonephritis is a possible complication of feline lower urinary tract inflammation.

Periodic urinalysis to measure *p*H are beneficial to cats on dietary management for prevention of recurrent episodes of dysuria. Urine *p*H measured 4 to 8 hours after eating should be 6.4 or less. Yearly urinalysis and culture are especially important in cats with perineal urethrostomies since the normal host defenses of the lower urethra have been surgically removed in these cats.

ADDITIONAL READING

Barsanti JA, Finco DR. Feline urologic syndrome. In: Breitschwerdt ED, ed. Contemporary issues in small animal practice. Volume 4: Nephrology and urology. New York: Churchill Livingston, 1986: 43.

Osborne CA, ed. Disorders of feline lower urinary tract. Vet Clin North Am 1984; 14.

Osborne CA, Johnston GR, Kruger JM et al. Etiopathogenesis and biological behavior of feline vesicourachal diverticula. Vet Clin North Am 1986; 17:697.

Osborne CA, Polzin DJ, Kruger JM et al. Relationship of nutritional factors to the cause, dissolution, and prevention of feline uroliths and urethral plugs. Vet Clin North Am 1989; 19:561.

Osborne CA, Kruger JM, Johnston GR: Feline vesicourachal diverticula: Biologic behavior, diagnosis, and treatment. In: Kirk RW, ed. Current veterinary therapy X. Philadelphia: WB Saunders, 1989: 1153.

Osborne CA, Lulich JP, Kruger JM, Polzin DJ et al. Medical dissolution of feline struvite urocystoliths. J Amer Vet Med Assoc 1990; 196:1053.

Osborne CA, Kruger JM, Polzin DJ et al: Medical dissolution and prevention of feline struvite urolithiasis. In: Kirk RW, ed. Current veterinary therapy IX. Philadelphia, WB Saunders, 1986: 1188.

Osborne CA, Polzin DJ, Kruger JM et al: Medical management of feline urologic syndrome. In: Kirk RW, ed. Current veterinary therapy IX. Philadelphia, WB Saunders, 1986: 1196.

THE SKIN

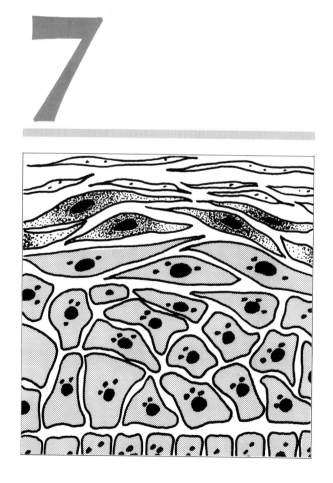

49

ALOPECIA

Edmund J. Rosser, Jr., Ann W. Sams

Alopecia is a general term meaning hair loss. In veterinary medicine, alopecia is used to describe a lack of hair compared to normal for a given animal. In this chapter, diseases are described whose primary, most common, or earliest manifestation is that of hair loss.

In normal, healthy dogs and cats, haired skin covers the entire body, except for the nose, footpads, and mucocutaneous junctions. While the colors, textures, lengths, and densities of hair coats differ, the basic anatomy of the hair follicle is similar in both dogs and cats.

The portion of the hair visible to the naked eye is called the shaft. It consists of three concentric layers, from outside to inside: the protective, lamellar cuticle; the strong, fibrillar cortex; and the vacuolated, sometimes absent, medulla. While the hair shaft is completely composed of dead, keratinized material, it is still susceptible to change or damage from the environment, and it continually reflects the overall body health.

The growing portion of the hair, below the level of the skin, is called the root. It consists of a proximal hair bulb, where proliferation of cells occurs, resulting in hair growth. Melanocytes, which donate pigment to the hair, are located in this area. An inner root sheath surrounds the growing part of the hair; an outer root sheath surrounds them both and is continuous with the surface epidermis. A non-cellular hyaline or glassy membrane (the basement membrane) connects the outer root sheath to the dermis and is surrounded by the connective tissue fibrous root sheath. The root sheaths are thought to support and nourish the growing hair, but their exact function is not known. A dermal papilla of fibroblast origin projects into the base of each hair bulb (Fig. 49-1). This papilla is responsible for regulating the growth cycle of hair follicles.

Hairs grow in a cyclic manner, with each hair following its own pattern of growth (anagen phase), involution (catagen phase), and senescence (telogen phase). Normally, most follicles are in anagen, a minute percentage are in catagen, and the rest are in telogen. The cycle is as follows: during anagen, the hair grows by cellular proliferation and maturation in the hair bulb region; in catagen, matrix cell proliferation from the bulb ceases; in telogen, the inactive hair remains in the follicle, and the base of the hair follicle remains as the secondary germ. When the next anagen period begins, the new hair grows up and pushes out the old, inactive hair.

The relative lengths of anagen and telogen may be modified by disease, including endocrine imbalances, nutrition, and so forth. When consider-

659

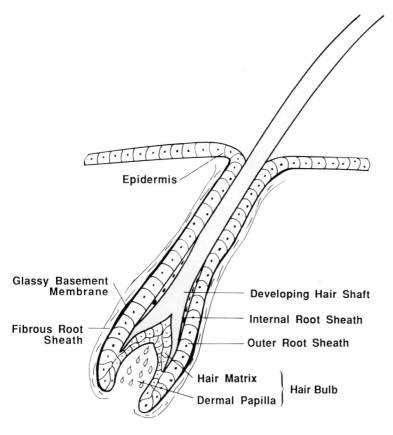

Epidermis

Glassy Basement
Membrane

Developing Hair Shaft

Internal Root Sheath

Fibrous Root
Sheath

Outer Root Sheath

Hair Matrix

Dermal Papilla — Hair Bulb

Figure 49–1. *Normal hair follicle in anagen phase.*

ing possible causes for alopecia, these changes in the follicular growth cycle often yield important diagnostic clues.

CAUSES

The causes of alopecia in small animals are listed in Table 49-1.

Canine Demodicosis

Pathophysiology

Demodicosis is an infestation of the hair follicles by mites of the genus *Demodex*. Many different species exist; they are specific for, and named for, the species that they affect (for example, *Demodex canis*).

In the dog, *Demodex* mites are acquired by neonates from the bitch in the first 2 to 3 days of life and are considered a normal resident of the skin in small numbers. Abnormal increases in mite population causes reversible damage to the hair follicle and resultant alopecia. Many attempts have been made to clarify the reason for this dramatic shift in mite population, but the pathophysiology of this condition is still not completely understood. However, it has been demonstrated that, as generalized demodicosis progressively worsens, one can detect the presence of a serum factor that subsequently suppresses the function of T lymphocytes. This phenomenon has been observed in advanced generalized demodicosis, generalized demodicosis with secondary pyoderma (due to coagulase positive staphylococci), and generalized pyoderma (due to coagulase positive staphylococci) alone. This serum suppressor phenomenon, however, is not the cause of the disease but a consequence of the disease and resolves when the primary disease is successfully treated. Generalized demodicosis is known to have a hereditary predisposition.

Table 49–1 *Causes of Alopecia*

I. Diseases Causing Hair to Fall Out (spontaneous alopecias)
   A. Canine Demodicosis
   B. Dermatophytosis
   C. Congenital/hereditary dermatoses
      1. Color mutant alopecia
   D. Endocrine dermatoses
      1. Hypothyroidism
      2. Hyperadrenocorticism (Cushing's syndrome)
      3. Canine ovarian imbalance type I (hyperestrogenism)
      4. Canine ovarian imbalance type II (hypoestrogenism)
      5. Sertoli's cell tumor
      6. Hypoandrogenism of male dogs
      7. Pituitary dwarfism
      8. Growth hormone-responsive dermatosis
      9. Castration-responsive dermatosis
II. Diseases Causing Hair to be Pulled Out or Broken (post-traumatic alopecias; see Chapter 51)
   A. Symmetrical alopecia on the ventral abdomen of cats (Feline Endocrine Alopecia, Feline Psychogenic Alopecia)

Clinical Signs

Localized demodicosis usually presents as circumscribed areas of alopecia, with varying degrees of erythema, scaling, and hyperpigmentation (Color Fig. 1). The lesions may or may not be pruritic. The disease usually affects the face and forelegs of dogs less than twelve months of age and is rarely observed in mature animals.

Generalized demodicosis often begins as the localized form, with coalescence of smaller lesions forming more diffuse lesions that can progress to affect the trunk and limbs. The clinical appearance includes alopecia, excessive scaling, erythema, hyperpigmentation, and lichenification. A superficial or deep secondary pyoderma is a common complication (Color Fig. 2).

Most cases of generalized demodicosis occur at less than 12 months of age and are called *juvenile onset demodicosis*. This form is an inherited condition that many consider to be an indication of excessive inbreeding.

Adult onset demodicosis is a rare form of generalized demodicosis and may be associated with immunosuppressive factors, such as immune-suppressant chemotherapy, hypothyroidism, neoplasia, and Cushing's syndrome (iatrogenic or spontaneous).

Pododemodicosis is a form of the disease affecting the feet. The history may indicate previous generalized disease that responded to therapy except for the foot lesions or foot lesions that were the only noted problem from the onset. Interdigital erythema, alopecia, and swelling can progress to secondary pyoderma (Color Fig. 3), even becoming tender enough to cause lameness.

Management

Localized demodicosis, if mild, seldom requires treatment. It often resolves with time. If desired, Goodwinol (1% rotenone) ointment may be applied to affected areas once daily for 21 days and then rechecked with a skin scraping. If the scraping is negative then treatment is discontinued. If the skin scraping is still positive then one should consider the possibility of a developing generalized demodicosis.

Although 25% to 50% of dogs with generalized infestation with *Demodex* mites undergo spontaneous remission, the remaining cases of generalized demodicosis can be difficult and involving to treat. Committed, compliant people are a necessity! In dogs, the current treatment of choice is an amitraz (Mitaban) rinse every 2 weeks until 2 successive skin scrapings are negative, when taken 2 weeks apart. Whole body clipping facilitates treatment and is mandatory in all but short-coated breeds of dogs. The Mitaban treatment protocol should be implemented in the following manner:

1. Put a protective ophthalmic ointment in both eyes (sterile petrolatum ophthalmic ointment).
2. Wash the entire dog with a degreasing and follicular flushing shampoo such as Oxydex, Sulf Oxydex or Pyoben shampoo and lather for 10 minutes prior to thorough rinsing.
3. Towel dry the dog.
4. Sponge the Mitaban solution over the entire dog. Apply in a well-ventilated area while wearing protective gloves (should take 10–15 minutes).
5. Place the dog in a cage with a dryer.

Due to the association of generalized demodicosis with secondary immunosuppression, corticosteroids are contraindicated. In most cases the pruritus is due to the secondary pyoderma, which responds well to appropriate systemic antibiotics (see Chapter 52). If pruritus persists, then antihistamines (see Chapter 51) or essential fatty acid dietary supplements (*e.g.*,

DVM Derm caps, EfaVet, Efa-Z Plus) may be used to bring a pruritic patient some relief. When the secondary pyoderma is deep or severe, the patient should be first treated for this only (see Chapter 52). This treatment usually requires 5 to 10 days before improvement is noted; then treatment with Mitaban can be started. Due to hereditary considerations, all dogs with generalized demodicosis should be neutered after being successfully treated.

Dermatophytosis (Ringworm)

Pathophysiology

Dermatophytes are fungi that affect keratinized structures of the body, which include hair, nails, and epidermis. Dermatophytes affect actively growing hairs (telogen hairs limit the source of nutrition to the fungus) without affecting the matrix. Therefore, when the fungal infection is eliminated, the hair will regrow.

Microsporum canis is responsible for the vast majority of cases of dermatophytosis observed in both dogs and cats, although *Microsporum gypseum* and *Trichophyton mentagrophytes* are also seen. Cats are often asymptomatic carriers of *M canis* and a source of infection for other animals and humans. All three species are zoonotic, and human exposure must be considered when the disease is present. *Microsporum gypseum* is also a geophilic fungus, and, therefore, the initial source of infection can be from the soil.

Elimination of an existing dermatophytosis problem can be frustrating because of the long duration of treatment and the difficulty in preventing recurrence. Persistence of fungal spores in the environment and presence of asymptomatic carriers have combined to make dermatophytosis a dreaded problem in catteries.

Proper cell-mediated immune function is important in limiting or eliminating the infection. Therefore, young or debilitated animals and immunosuppressed patients are at increased risk.

Clinical Signs

The most common presentation for dermatophytosis is that of focal alopecia and scaling, especially on the face and head. In the canine, the lesions are often initially annular (Color Fig. 4), but the peripheral margin of marked erythema associated with human ringworm lesions is rarely present. Annular lesions with marked erythema at the periphery are more typical for superficial pyodermas due to coagulase positive staphylococci (see Chapter 52) and seborrheic dermatitis (see Chapter 50). In the feline, the lesions are rarely annular and are most frequently irregular shaped areas of alopecia with mild erythema and scaling (Color Fig. 5). As many as 30% or more of cats may be asymptomatic carriers of the disease. In both the dog and cat, pruritus is usually absent.

In some cases the infection may become generalized, an occurrence that is most often associated with *T mentagrophytes*. The generalized form is usually pruritic and is often associated with the development of a concurrent superficial or deep pyoderma (Color Fig. 6).

Microsporum canis and *T mentagrophytes* are zoophilic fungi (adapted to animals) and show a lesser inflammatory component. *Microsporum gypseum* is geophilic (adapted to soil) and tends to result in marked erythema, hyperpigmentation, and scaling. Asymptomatic carriers may be an important reservoir for infection; this is most often encountered in mature cats.

The kerion form of ringworm has a slightly different appearance, as the affected areas show raised, erythematous, alopecic lesions with purulent, draining fistulas. In the early stages of development, these lesions often look clinically similar to the histiocytoma. This form may involve a hypersensitivity reaction of the host. The folliculitis form of ringworm can manifest as a papular, pustular skin disease clinically indistinguishable from pyoderma, with or without the presence of a concurrent bacterial infection. The pseudomycetoma form of ringworm begins as a folliculitis and furunculosis and progresses to a nodular and diffuse granulomatous dermatitis in the dermis and subcutaneous tissue with subsequent ulceration and drainage. It is more common in cats.

Management

It is important to remember that immune competent adult animals should be able to prevent or limit dermatophytosis. Therefore, in protracted or generalized adult cases, possible causes of decreased cell-mediated immunity should be explored: hypothyroidism, Cushing's syndrome, diabetes mellitus, or a primary T lymphocyte immunodeficiency.

Localized cases of dermatophytosis can resolve spontaneously. However, because of the zoonotic potential and the possible presence of infectious spores in nonlesional areas, ringworm patients should be treated both topically and systemically. The affected areas should first be clipped free of hair. For focal lesions the following topical imidazole creams are effective: miconazole (Conofite), clotrimazole (Veltrim, Lotrimin), and econazole (Spectrozole) creams. Very inflammatory lesions (such as the kerion) often respond more rapidly to treatment if the topical agent also contains a corticosteroid as in Lotrisone (clotrimazole and betamethasone) or Tresaderm (thiabendazole, neomycin, and dexamethasone). These products should be applied as a thin film twice daily for the duration of the systemic therapy (usually 4–6 weeks). For patients with multiple lesions or generalized ringworm, a whole body rinse preparation should be used. Effective products include: captan (2 tablespoons of 50% captan wettable powder per gallon of water) and chlorhexidine solution (15 ml of Nolvasan solution per gallon of water). These products should be applied as a whole body rinse once to twice weekly for 4 to 6 weeks. Tolnaftate preparations, not effective on *M canis* infections and poorly effective on *T mentagrophytes* infections in animals, work poorly on hair covered skin.

Griseofulvin (Fulvicin U/F) is the systemic treatment of choice. However, since its action is to inhibit fungal DNA synthesis, it is fungistatic and must be given for 4 to 6 weeks to be effective. The dosage of griseofulvin in dogs and cats is 50 to 100 mg/kg divided twice daily to be given with food and a source of fat (1/2 to 1 tablespoon of corn oil for dogs, 1/2 teaspoon of tuna oil for cats). The duration of treatment required is usually 4 to 6 weeks but should be continued for 2 weeks beyond the apparent clinical cure. Additional measures included in the management of dermatophytosis are: the initial isolation of the patient from other animals and people (especially the very young,

geriatrics, or immunocompromised individuals) and a thorough vacuuming (for households) and cleaning of the environment (such as kennels) with dilute chlorine bleach, chlorhexidine, or formalin. When the above measures have been followed, refractory cases of ringworm are a rarity. However, should a griseofulvin resistant case be encountered, then ketoconazole (Nizoral) may be tried. The oral dose of ketoconazole in dogs is 5 to 10 mg/kg once or twice daily and in cats is 5 to 10 mg/kg once daily to every 48 hours. Ketoconazole is best absorbed if given with food in an acid environment (such as tomato juice).

CONGENITAL OR HEREDITARY DERMATOSES: COLOR MUTANT ALOPECIA

Pathophysiology

Color mutant alopecia appears to be a hereditary follicular dysplasia and melaninization defect associated with dilute coat colors in various breeds.

Clinical Signs

The alopecia generally begins after puberty and affects the trunk first, generally sparing the head and extremities. Color dilutes of normal coat colors are affected and include: blue, fawn, red, and black Doberman pinschers, blue dachshunds, blue chow chows, blue Great Danes, blue whippets, blue standard poodles, blue Yorkshire terriers, fawn Irish setters and white-coated animals with bi-color and tri-color dilutions. Loss of hair in dilute-colored areas may be partial (a diffuse thinning or "moth-eaten" alopecia) or total. The hair coat in color dilute areas is dry and lusterless with excess scaling. Follicular plugging leads to formation of comedones, papules, and pustules. A common and recurrent problem is the development of a bacterial folliculitis.

Management

While this alopecia is usually permanent, some cases respond partially to treatment of coexisting hypothyroidism, when present. Symptomatic control of excessive scaling, comedones, and folliculitis by regular bathing once to twice weekly with an antiseborrheic and follicular flushing agent, such as Sulf-oxydex shampoo, is recommended. This shampoo should be followed by an emollient or conditioning rinse such as Humilac or Hy-lyt conditioner. For episodes of bacterial folliculitis, the concurrent use of systemic antibiotics may be necessary (see Chapter 52).

ENDOCRINE DERMATOSES: HYPOTHYROIDISM

Pathophysiology

In animals, thyroid hormones are known to affect basal metabolic rate, possibly at the sub-cellular level of the mitochondrion. While deficiency of thyroid hormones affect the entire body, the skin can serve as an early indicator of this disease because of its accessibility to inspection.

Triiodothyronine (T_3) is the active circulating thyroid hormone; tetraiodothyronine (T_4) is its immediate precursor. T_3 and T_4 are released from the thyroid gland in response to thyrotropin stimulating hormone from the anterior pituitary gland. In turn, this process is regulated by thyrotropin-releasing hormone from the hypothalamus. Certainly, many potential sites for breakdown exist in this pathway, and any of them may result in thyroid dysfunction (see Chapter 62).

It is currently believed that most cases of clinical hypothyroidism in small animals result from lymphocytic thyroiditis, idiopathic thyroid atrophy, or autoantibodies against circulating T_3 and T_4. Of equal importance are the instances where the T_3 and T_4 levels are artificially lowered and the change is not related to the true hypothyroid state. This condition is referred to as non-thyroid illness, or the euthyroid sick syndrome. Possible causes include: a chronic disease or illness not related to thyroid function, spontaneously occurring hyperadrenocorticism, and various drugs (*e.g.*, glucocorticoids, phenobarbital, phenylbutazone, o,p'-DDD, diazepam, sulfonylureas, salicylates, diphenylhydantoin, propranolol, propylthiouracil, quinidine and radiocontrast agents).

Clinical Signs

Hypothyroidism most commonly occurs in dogs that are middle-aged and older. Some breeds have recently been observed to be hypothyroid at less than 1 year of age, especially the golden retriever and the Chinese shar pei.

The most common dermatologic change observed is alopecia, which is usually bilaterally symmetrical or diffuse and "moth eaten" in appearance. The hair coat may be dull, dry, and brittle with easily epilated hairs. The skin may be hyperpigmented in the areas of alopecia, and comedones may be present. Less frequently encountered changes include a hair coat color change (usually to a lighter color) and retarded shedding or abnormally long hair coat. Secondary complications can include pyoderma, excessive scaling, seborrheic changes (keratinization

Table 49–2 Clinical Signs Associated with Hypothyroidism

System Affected	Clinical Signs
General metabolism	Lethargy
	Increased sleeping time
	Weight gain
	Decreased exercise tolerance
	Hypothermia/heat-seeking
Reproductive system	Decreased libido
	Infertility
	Diminished to absent estrus
	Testicular atrophy
Cardiovascular system	Bradycardia
Ocular system	Non-healing corneal ulcers
	Corneal lipidosis
Neuromuscular system	Facial palsy
	Laryngeal hemiplegia
	Megaesophagus
Integumentary system	Diffuse/moth-eaten alopecia
	Bilaterally symmetrical alopecia
	Dull, dry hair coat
	Brittle, easily epilated hairs
	Hyperpigmentation of skin
	Secondary pyoderma
	Excessive scaling (keratinization abnormality)
	Ceruminous otitis externa
	Myxedema

abnormality), and ceruminous otitis externa. Occasionally, the skin feels thick and puffy due to the development of myxedema.

Hypothyroidism can imitate many other diseases. While the classic picture of a hypothyroid individual would generally be that of an obese, heat-seeking animal with a sparse, dry, flaky hair coat, this picture often is not the case. Many possible symptoms exist, and a given patient may present with any one or a combination of them (Table 49-2). The diagnostic approach to hypothyroidism is outlined in Chapter 62.

Management

Once the diagnosis of hypothyroidism has been established, then replacement therapy with T_4 (sodium levothyroxine, L-thyroxine) is the treatment of choice. It is initiated at 0.02 mg/kg twice daily; some dogs can be maintained on once daily therapy. T_3 replacement therapy is available but is much more costly and usually unnecessary (most cases of low T_3 respond to oral T_4 supplementation). T_3 (Cytobin) is dosed at 4 μg/kg, three times daily.

If appropriate response to thyroid replacement (T_4 supplementation) has not been observed after 45 days of therapy, then a 6-hour post-pill measurement of thyroid levels should be evaluated.

Table 49–3 *Reasons for an Inadequate Response to Thyroid Hormones*

1. Wrong diagnosis.
2. Inadequate dosage of thyroid hormone replacement.
3. Inappropriate form of the drug; some generic forms of thyroid hormone replacement do not give good therapeutic responses.
4. Defect in peripheral conversion of T_4 to T_3; extremely rare, but patient may require T_3 supplementation rather than T_4 (see Chapter 62).
5. Poor compliance of the owner.
6. Poor gastrointestinal absorption.
7. Presence of autoantibodies to peripheral T_3 and T_4 which are affecting the absorbed replacement therapy.
8. An abnormally rapid metabolism or excretion of the replacement therapy.
9. Exogenous or endogenous drug interference, especially glucocorticoids.
10. Presence of a separate primary disease causing a non-thyroid illness.

The post-pill values for both T_3 and T_4 should fall well within the mid-range of normal (for each particular laboratory) for both hormones. If the values are well within normal but the original chief complaint has persisted, then one should reevaluate the initial diagnosis of hypothyroidism and consider the causes of non-thyroid illness. If the values have remained abnormally low, then one needs to systematically evaluate the patient for the source of the problem (Table 49-3). It is important to remember that one should not get caught up in trying to treat some "abnormally low numbers" on a piece of paper but should treat the patient's symptoms relative to the appropriate underlying disease.

Hyperadrenocorticism (Cushing's syndrome)

Pathophysiology

Hyperadrenocorticism is caused by an excess of glucocorticoids in the body. The most common causes include pituitary-dependent hyperadrenocorticism (usually a functional pituitary microadenoma excreting excess ACTH), bilateral adrenocortical hyperplasia, a functional adrenal neoplasia, and excessive exogenous corticosteroids (iatrogenic Cushing's syndrome). The major effects of excess glucocorticoids on the body are its catabolic effect on various metabolic pathways of the body involving protein metabolism (see Chapter 59).

Clinical Signs

Since glucocorticoids can affect nearly every tissue in the body, their effects are multiple and diverse (Table 49-4). Although canine Cushing's syndrome can affect any breed, the Boston terrier, poodle, dachshund, and boxer are most often affected. Usually, these dogs are middle-aged or older.

The dermatological changes that accompany Cushing's syndrome resemble other endocrinopathies, including: bilaterally symmetrical, diffuse, or moth-eaten alopecia that spares the extremities; thin, hypotonic skin that is easily

Table 49–4 *Clinical Signs Suggestive of Hyperadrenocorticism*

System Affected	Clinical Sign
Respiratory system	Increased panting
	Recurrent respiratory infections
Ocular system	Exophthalmos
	Indolent corneal ulcers
Integumentary system	Bilaterally symmetrical alopecia
	Moth eaten alopecia
	Hyperpigmentation
	Comedones
	Failure of shaved hair to regrow
	Dull, dry hair coat
	Keratinization abnormality (seborrhea)
	Thin, hypotonic skin
	Easy bruising, hematomas
	Poor wound healing
	Recurrent pyoderma
	Dermatophytosis
	Demodicosis
	Calcinosis cutis
Musculoskeletal system	Lameness
	Muscle weakness and atrophy, especially abdominal muscles, temporal muscles, and pelvic musculature
	Pot-bellied appearance
Reproductive system	Anestrus and clitoral hypertrophy
	Testicular atrophy
	Decreased libido
	Infertility
Neurologic system	Seizures
	Visual deficits
Cardiovascular system	Elevated blood pressure and hypertension
	Congestive heart failure

bruised and easily forms hematomas at venipuncture sites; easily epilated hair; poor wound healing; failure of clipped hair to regrow; increased susceptibility to infection (recurrent pyoderma, dermatophytosis); excess scaling (keratinization abnormality); follicular plugging and comedones; dull, dry hair coat; and change in color of hair coat (usually to a lighter shade). More unique to hyperadrenocorticism is calcinosis cutis (Color Fig. 7), which usually affects the dorsal midline, ventral abdomen, or inguinal region as symmetrical firm or gritty nodules that often ulcerate. An often frustrating complication of spontaneous or iatrogenic Cushing's syndrome is the opportunistic development of demodicosis.

Other problems associated with Cushing's syndrome may be noted concurrently. Polydipsia, polyuria, and polyphagia often alert the practitioner to suspect the diagnosis of Cushing's syndrome, but they need not be present. Muscle breakdown, fat redistribution, and hepatomegaly often lead to a typical appearance of a pot-bellied, lethargic, weak-muscled dog with fat over the hips and trunk but not legs. Palpable hepatomegaly may be present due to increased hepatic glycogen deposition.

Management

Treatment selected for the management of the dog with Cushing's syndrome depends on the etiology of the disease (see Chapter 59). The most common form is iatrogenic Cushing's syndrome; it is easily treated by cessation of the use of exogenous glucocorticoids (including oral, parenteral, and topical forms). When the glucocorticoids have been administered for a long time, the withdrawal should be gradual: in this case, the adrenal glands may atrophy because of the suppression of pituitary corticotropin, and sudden withdrawal can result in an Addisonian crisis.

When an adrenal tumor is present, the patient should first be radiographed to check for any evidence of metastasis; if absent, an exploratory laparotomy should be performed. Many of the adrenal tumors are unilateral, and unilateral adrenalectomy can be done. If the hyperadrenocorticism is pituitary-dependent, hypophysectomy can be performed, or the adrenal hyperplasia can be reduced with o,p'-DDD (Lysodren). Generally, Lysodren is initiated at 25 mg/kg once daily, or divided twice daily, orally for 5 to 12 days. As water consumption returns to normal, or as eosinopenia disappears, a maintenance dose of 25 to 50 mg/kg Lysodren is continued once weekly. Side effects of medical treatment include anorexia, vomiting, diarrhea, lethargy, weakness, depression, disorientation, head pressing, ataxia, transient or permanent hypoadrenocorticism, and a lower insulin requirement if concurrently diabetic. Dogs refractory to o,p'-DDD may benefit from treatment with ketoconazole (see Chapter 59).

Ovarian Imbalance Type I (Hyperestrogenism)

Pathophysiology

This form of ovarian imbalance includes the excessive production of one or more of the reproductive hormones in the female dog. Of the hormones evaluated to date (testosterone, estradiol, and progesterone), the most commonly elevated is estradiol. However, any of the aforementioned may be elevated. When the ovaries and uterus are removed and submitted for histopathological examination, the most common findings are cystic ovaries with endometrial hyperplasia or a functional ovarian tumor. This disease can occur in the iatrogenic form, due to excess exogenous estrogen administration used in the treatment of urinary incontinence, mismating, or hypoestrogenism.

Clinical Signs

The spontaneous form is usually observed in middle-aged and older intact female dogs. The bilaterally symmetrical alopecia begins in the perineal and perivulvar region and may progress anteriorly along the ventral trunk with time. In some cases, the alopecia may be confined to the flank areas and change in severity with the estrus cycle or changes in seasons. Unique to this endocrinopathy is the pruritus component, which may be noticed before the onset of secondary lichenification and hyperpigmentation. Keratinization abnormalities (seborrheic changes) and ceruminous otitis externa may be present; gynecomastia is common. History typically reveals abnormal estrus cycles, pseudopregnancies, and some owners may notice an exacerbation of signs during estrus.

Management

Ovariohysterectomy is the recommended treatment, and a response should be noted within 3 to 6 months. When secondary complications are present they need to be treated concurrently. Treatment includes the use of antiseborrheic shampoos for any keratinization abnormalities (see Chapter 50) and the appropriate use of otic preparations for ceruminous otitis externa.

Ovarian Imbalance Type II (Hypoestrogenism)

Pathophysiology

This disease is thought to be the result of decreased estrogen levels in dogs that have had an ovariohysterectomy early in life. However, this link has not yet been proven in the dog, although a majority of the dogs that have had their serum estradiol levels measured have a value near zero.

Clinical Signs

Clinically, the bilaterally symmetrical alopecia (perineal and perivulvar region, ventral trunk) is very similar in distribution to hyperestrogenism. However, pruritus and lichenification are not a feature of this condition, and hyperpigmentation is rare. Juvenile vulva and nipples may be noted on physical examination, and the dog may have a history of urinary incontinence, which is responsive to estrogen replacement or phenylpropanolamine (see Chapter 42).

Management

The recommended treatment is diethylstilbestrol (DES) at a dosage of 0.1 to 1.0 mg orally once daily for 3 to 4 weeks, then once to twice weekly thereafter as needed. In most cases, a complete response to therapy is observed within 3 months. Since exogenous estrogen treatment can cause bone marrow suppression, the complete blood count, including platelet numbers, should be monitored periodically (see Diethylstilbestrol, Appendix II).

Sertoli's Cell Tumor

Pathophysiology

The most common cause of hyperestrogenism in male dogs is a testicular Sertoli's cell tumor associated with an increased production of estrogens. An identical clinical syndrome can be seen with testicular interstitial cell tumors and seminomas. These tumors are most frequently noted in the retained testicles of cryptorchid patients but may occur in testicles located in the inguinal or scrotal region.

Clinical Signs

This condition is most frequently reported in boxers, Shetland sheepdogs, Cairn terriers, Pekingese, collies, and Weimaraners. The dogs are usually middle-aged and older.

Dermatologic signs are very similar to those observed in hyperestrogenism of females: bilaterally symmetrical alopecia, which begins in the perineal and genital region and may progress anteriorly along the trunk. Hyperpigmentation and lichenification may be noticed in the areas of alopecia. The development of a well-defined and linear area of erythematous macules or melanosis may be present along the ventral aspect of the prepuce. This condition, referred to as linear preputial dermatosis, is a skin change occasionally associated with the disease. Secondary keratinization abnormalities and ceruminous otitis externa may be noted.

The hyperestrogenism present in most cases results in a feminizing syndrome, with gynecomastia, lactation, pendulous prepuce, and the attraction of male dogs. The non-tumorous testicle is usually soft and atrophic; the tumor laden testicle is often palpable. The chronic estrogen stimulation may also result in prostatic hyperplasia or neoplasia, decreased libido and spermatogenesis, and bone marrow suppression.

Management

Bilateral castration is the recommended treatment, and a complete response to therapy is observed within 3 months. If prostatitis, bone marrow suppression, keratinization abnormalities, or ceruminous otitis externa are present, they will need to be specifically treated.

Hypoandrogenism of Male Dogs (Testosterone-Responsive Dermatosis)

Pathophysiology

This condition is thought to be the result of decreased testosterone levels in dogs that have been castrated at a young age. However, this link has not yet been proven in the dog, although a majority of the dogs that have had their serum testosterone levels measured have a value near zero.

Clinical Signs

The most common clinical sign of this disease is a bilaterally symmetrical alopecia affecting the perineal and genital regions that may progress to involve the caudomedial thighs and anterior ventral trunk. The hair coat may be dull and dry, with seborrheic changes and thin, hypotonic skin. Occasionally, the dog may also have a problem with urinary incontinence that is responsive to testosterone replacement therapy (see Chapter 42).

Management

The first treatment recommended is methyl-testosterone at 1.0 mg/kg orally every other day, not to exceed a total dose of 30 mg. This dosage is given for 1 to 3 months, then reduced to twice weekly. Occasionally, dogs may not respond to oral replacement but may respond to repositol testosterone injection: 2 mg/kg intramuscularly, not to exceed a maximum dose of 30 mg, given every 1 to 4 months. Since exogenous testosterone may cause hepatotoxicity, the patient should have serum alanine aminotransferase, aspartate aminotransferase, and alkaline phosphatase levels monitored periodically. Behavioral changes of increased aggression can occur.

Pituitary Dwarfism

Pathophysiology

Pituitary dwarfism is an inherited, simple autosomal recessive condition in which a cyst in the pituitary gland (cystic Rathke's cleft) is usually found resulting in pituitary insufficiency. The most common abnormality is a resultant growth hormone deficiency but a lack of follicle-stimulating hormone, luteinizing hormone, thyrotropin stimulating hormone, or corticotropin may occur.

Clinical Signs

This condition has a predilection for the German shepherd and Carnelian bear dog breeds. Affected individuals first become conspicuous when they are noticed to be smaller than their littermates by 2 to 3 months of age. The spectrum of clinical signs observed depends on the degree to which pituitary function is lacking with symptoms referable to a deficiency of follicle-stimulating hormone, luteinizing hormone, thyrotropin stimulating hormone, or corticotropin. However, cutaneous manifestations often show a typical syndrome of retention of puppy coat (secondary hairs), with primary hairs present on the face and distal extremities only. This may progress to bilaterally symmetrical alopecia, especially on the neck and caudomedial thighs, thin, hypotonic, scaly skin, and hyperpigmentation. Additional findings on the physical examination usually includes the retention of deciduous teeth and open fontanelles.

Management

Bovine growth hormone (GH) (10 IU subcutaneously every other day for 30 days) is recommended for treatment but is often very difficult to obtain. Generally, skin and hair coat show improvement in 6 to 8 weeks. Rapid closure of growth plates occurs, so the size of the patient generally does not change. Potential side effects include hypersensitivity reactions (anaphylactic type) to exogenous growth hormone, acromegaly, and diabetes mellitus.

Pituitary dwarfs generally have a shorter life expectancy than normal and frequently have concurrent hypothyroidism, adrenocortical insufficiency, and reproductive hormone abnormalities. For these reasons, the owners should be educated as to the chronic nature and poor prognosis of the problem prior to undertaking treatment.

Growth Hormone-Responsive Dermatosis

Pathophysiology

Although the pathogenesis is unknown, this condition is considered to be a result of a functional deficiency in growth hormone that develops after maturity.

Clinical Signs

Chow chows, keeshonds, Pomeranians, miniature poodles, and Siberian huskies appear predisposed; affected dogs are generally young (1–3 years of age), intact male dogs.

This condition is clinically very similar to castration-responsive dermatosis. Bilaterally symmetrical alopecia and hyperpigmentation may affect the perineal and genital regions, posterior and medial thighs, ventral abdomen, and neck. Where present, the hair coat can be dull, dry, and fuzzy; excess scaling and hair coat color changes may occur. Interestingly, a plug or line of hair may regrow at sites of full-thickness trauma to the skin (skin biopsy sites, lacerations).

Management

Some cases have responded to treatment with exogenous growth hormone, but results have been extremely variable. Clinical responses to growth hormone injections for this condition have included: no hair regrowth, partial hair regrowth, regrowth of hair at injection sites only, complete hair regrowth followed by subsequent loss of hair, and permanent hair regrowth. Bovine GH (2.5 IU for dogs less than 14 kg, 5 IU for dogs more than 14 kg) may be administered subcutaneously every other day for 10 injections. Response should be noted within 3 months and may last for 6 months to 3 years. Side effects include diabetes mellitus and acromegaly. Recently, human GH has also been used (0.15 IU/kg subcutaneously twice weekly for 6 weeks).

Castration-Responsive Dermatosis

Pathophysiology

Pathogenesis of this condition is unknown. Testicles of affected animals descend normally and are histologically normal, although a mild to moderate elevation of serum estradiol is usually present.

Clinical Signs

Breed predisposition and clinical signs are strikingly similar to growth hormone-responsive dermatosis. Intact male dogs of the Pomeranian, chow chow, miniature poodle, and keeshond breeds are most often affected. Bilaterally symmetrical alopecia and hyperpigmentation affect the neck (Fig. 49-2), perineal and genital regions, posterior and medial thighs, ventral abdomen, and tail. Hair coat is dull, dry, and fuzzy; excessive scaling and changes in hair coat color may be seen (Color Fig. 8). As in growth hormone-responsive dermatosis, a plug or line of hair may regrow at sites of full-thickness trauma to the skin (skin biopsy sites, laceration).

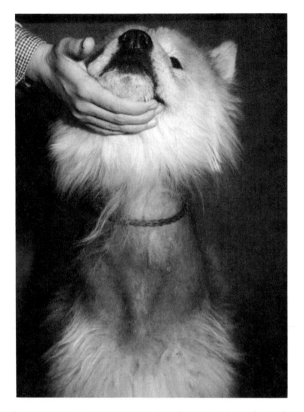

Figure 49–2. *Castration-responsive dermatosis in a chow chow with a band-like area of alopecia around the neck.*

Management

Bilateral castration results in resolution of signs within 2 to 3 months (Color Fig. 9).

Symmetrical Alopecia on the Ventral Abdomen of Cats (Feline Endocrine Alopecia, Feline Psychogenic Alopecia)

Pathophysiology

The presence of symmetrical alopecia on the ventral abdomen of cats (Fig. 49-3) is currently believed to be a clinical manifestation of several possible underlying diseases.

Feline endocrine alopecia, as a specific and distinct endocrine syndrome, is no longer believed to be a distinct entity in the cat. This belief stems from the observation that numerous attempts to define a specific endocrine abnormality have

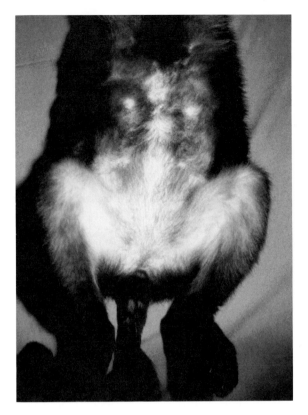

Figure 49–3. *Symmetrical alopecia on the ventral abdomen of a cat secondary to excessive licking.*

been unrewarding. Although the specific endocrine diseases of hypothyroidism and Cushing's syndrome may present with this pattern of alopecia, these diseases are extremely rare in the cat. Moreover, the majority of cases with this pattern of alopecia are now believed to be due to self trauma in the form of excess licking, with the "barbs" of the cat's tongue breaking the hair shafts.

Allergic disorders are believed to be responsible for a large number of cases. Some cats with this particular pattern of alopecia have shown positive intradermal skin tests for flea antigen or airborne allergens; the alopecia is believed to be a sign of the underlying flea allergy or atopy. Many of these cats have subsequently responded to flea treatment protocols or hyposensitization injection protocols for atopy. Other patients have responded to hypoallergenic diet trials suggesting their alopecia is a symptom of food allergy (see Chapter 51).

Feline psychogenic alopecia is named for its presumed cause, compulsive over-grooming. This disease is believed to be an anxiety neurosis of cats, since it is known to be precipitated by disturbing influences (*e.g.*, new baby in home, barking dogs, strange cats in the pet's perceived territory).

Very rarely, this pattern of alopecia may be associated with demodicosis or dermatophytosis. The condition is deemed idiopathic when all efforts to define an underlying etiology are unsuccessful.

Clinical Signs

Alopecia begins on the ventral abdomen (see Fig. 49-3) and may progress to involve the medial and caudal thighs and perineum. The underlying skin is usually not irritated nor inflamed. Diffuse thinning is more common than total alopecia.

Psychogenic alopecia may have a predilection for emotional breeds such as the Siamese and Abyssinian. Owners may or may not be aware of any excess grooming behavior as many cats are secret or nocturnal groomers.

Management

If skin scrapings are positive for *Demodex mites*, or fungal cultures positive for dermatophytes, then specific treatment is indicated. Accordingly, when a specific endocrine disorder can be documented, such as hypothyroidism or Cushing's syndrome, then the appropriate specific treatment is recommended. Elimination of an existing flea problem or hyposensitization injections are appropriate for cats that show positive reactions to intradermal skin testing. When the problem is present on a continual and non-seasonal basis and is responsive to a hypoallergenic diet trial, then lifelong dietary control measures are appropriate (see Chapter 51).

Anti-inflammatory dosages of prednisone or prednisolone should be tried next in the treatment of this condition (1.0 mg/kg twice daily for 7 days, then once daily for 7 days, then every other day for 7 days). When responsive to this mode of treatment, a primary underlying allergic cause should be considered, and additional effort put into identifying the probable allergy (with repeat skin test, or hypoallergenic diet trial).

When the above conditions have been ruled out and microscopic examination of hair shafts indicates the presence of a post-traumatic alopecia, then skin biopsies should be taken. If skin biopsies reveal the presence of histologically normal skin, then a tentative diagnosis of psychogenic alopecia can be made. If the cause of the anxiety can be identified and eliminated or changed, then that, ideally, is the treatment of choice; however, this process is often difficult to accomplish (see Chapter 65). One must keep in mind at this point that medical treatment does not have to be undertaken since the problem is primarily an aesthetic one and the excess grooming behavior may be serving as a psychological outlet or release. In most cases, it is then recommended to begin treatment with a mood-altering drug. This includes phenobarbital (1/8 grain twice daily, and gradually increasing the dosage until the cat becomes very sedated or stops excessively grooming); diazepam (1–2 mg three times daily); and, as a last resort, megestrol acetate (Ovaban, 2.5–5 mg every 48 hours until a response is noted, then every 7 days as needed). Ovaban should be reserved as a last resort because of its potential side effects, which include: polyuria and polydipsia (and urinary accidents or increased need to clean the litter pan), polyphagia and weight gain, mood change ("doormat" cat), infertility in males, pyometra in females, diabetes mellitus, Cushing's syndrome, suppression of pituitary corticotropin and adrenal suppression, and mammary gland hyperplasia or neoplasia.

The idiopathic form of the disease may be treated with combined androgen or estrogen injection (repositol testosterone, 12.5 mg; repositol DES, 0.625 mg). Other alternatives that have sometimes been successful include L-thyroxine (0.1 mg twice daily) and megestrol acetate (Ovaban, 2.5–5 mg every 48 hours until a response is noted, then every 7 days as needed).

DIAGNOSTIC APPROACH

In the diagnostic approach to a patient with alopecia, it must first be determined if the hair is falling out spontaneously (spontaneous alopecia) or if it is being broken off or pulled out from licking, rubbing, or chewing (post-traumatic alopecia) (Table 49-5). In the dog, this determination is easy since the history usually suggests one or the other, and broken canine hairs will feel coarse on examination. In the cat, however, the hairs are finer, and broken hairs often feel soft and don't appear to be broken. In addition, the cat may only be licking or chewing the hairs off when the owners are not home or nocturnally; the owners may not be aware of the trauma to the hair coat. At this time, the microscopic examination of plucked hairs from an area of partial alopecia is of the greatest value.

Microscopic Examination of the Hairs

Epilating several representative hairs and examining both ends microscopically may help determine whether spontaneous alopecia or post-traumatic alopecia exists.

In normal dogs and cats the majority of hairs are usually difficult to epilate, with the proximal ends in anagen and the distal ends smooth and tapered. If the majority of the hairs are easily epilated, with the proximal ends in telogen and the distal ends tapered (Fig. 49-4), the alopecia is considered to be spontaneous (as seen in endocrine alopecias). If the proximal ends are in anagen and the distal ends are broken or frayed (Fig. 49-5), it is likely that the animal is breaking the hairs off; the alopecia is then considered post-traumatic (as seen in pruritic disease and psychogenic alopecia). For a discussion of the causes of post-traumatic alopecia, see Chapter 51.

Pattern of Distribution

Many diseases can be suspected or eliminated as probable causes of alopecia by their pattern of distribution.

Of the spontaneous alopecias, some reproductive hormone abnormalities can have similar distribution patterns. A bilaterally symmetrical alopecia of the perineal and genital area that may extend forward to involve the inguinal area, abdomen, and trunk may be seen with any of the following endocrinopathies: ovarian imbalance

Table 49–5 Diagnostic Tests for Evaluation of Alopecia

Test	What to Look For
Microscopic exam of epilated hair shafts	Anagen bulbs with broken distal ends indicate posttraumatic alopecia Telogen bulbs with tapered distal ends indicate spontaneous alopecia
Skin scraping, Scotch tape preparation	Mites (*Demodex, Sarcoptes, Chelyletiella,* and *Notoedres* species)
Woods lamp examination	Apple-green fluorescence of hairs: only present in 50% of *Microsporum canis* infections
KOH prep	Ectothrix spores on proximal hairs: dermatophytosis
DTM fungal culture	Small, white fungal colony with media color change to red in 1–14 days: dermatophyte
Thyroid profile and TSH response test	Hypothyroidism
Dexamethasone suppression/ACTH response test, or low-dose dexamethasone suppression test	Hyperadrenocorticism
Urinary corticoid/creatinine	
Reproductive hormone assays	Excess or deficiency of estradiol, progesterone, or testosterone suggestive of endocrinopathies such as Sertoli's cell tumor, hyperestrogenism, hypoestrogenism, castration-responsive dermatosis, testosterone-responsive dermatosis
Growth hormone stimulation test	Growth hormone-responsive dermatosis
Skin biopsy	Parasites (especially demodicosis); dermatophytes; congenital disorders; changes suggestive of endocrinopathy

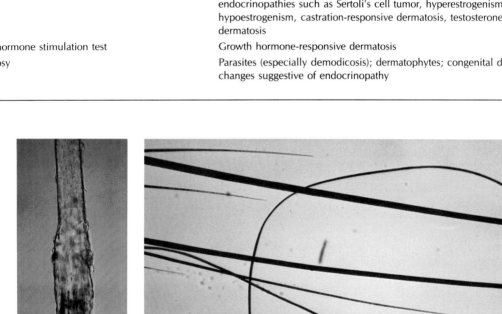

Figure 49–4. Microscopic appearance of epilated hairs from a cat. (A) Telogen bulb. (B) Normal tapered ends.

type I (hyperestrogenism) and II (hypoestrogenism), Sertoli's cell tumor, testosterone-responsive dermatosis, growth hormone-responsive dermatosis, and castration-responsive dermatosis. Hypothyroidism and Cushing's syndrome may present as bilaterally symmetrical truncal alopecia or generalized diffuse alopecia, which spares the extremities.

Some spontaneous alopecias may follow the pigmentation of the hair. Color mutant alopecia, may or may not show bilateral symmetry, according to the markings of the dog.

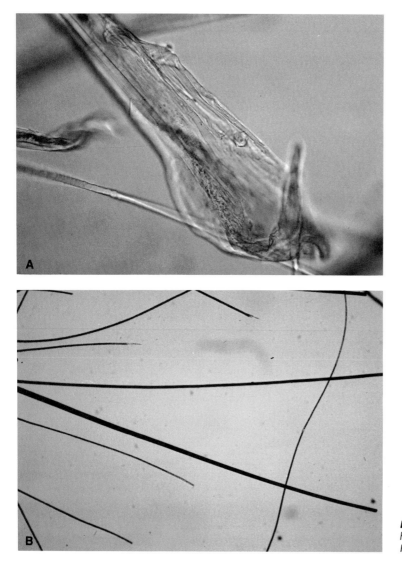

Figure 49–5. *Microscopic appearance of epilated hairs from a cat. (A) Anagen bulb. (B) "Blunted & Frayed" ends.*

Post-traumatic alopecias are usually bilaterally symmetrical when due to pruritus or a psychogenic phenomenon because most pruritic skin diseases itch symmetrically and most behavioral licking and chewing is symmetrical.

Other diseases may not present in as defined or symmetrical a pattern. These alopecias may be spontaneous, traumatic, or both. For example, demodicosis or dermatophytosis may present with variable patterns of alopecia: symmetrical, asymmetrical, generalized diffuse, or focal alopecia. Localized focal alopecias are also seen, especially in localized demodicosis, and early dermatophytosis, which tends to affect the head, face, and ears.

Symmetrical alopecias on the ventral abdomen of cats have similar distribution patterns, regardless as to whether they are of spontaneous or traumatic origin. Microscopic examination of the hairs is an important tool to differentiate among possible etiologies.

Skin Scraping, Scotch Tape Preparation

A skin scraping takes only minutes to perform and gives instant information. Because of the prevalence and treatment implications of many types of parasitic skin diseases, a skin scraping should be included in the diagnostic workup of all cases of alopecia.

A new #10 scalpel blade moistened with mineral oil should be used. When inspecting for *Demodex* mites, scrape several areas of skin, approximately 1 cm. in diameter. It is helpful to squeeze a fold of skin, to tighten the skin so it is easier to scrape, and to force *Demodex* mites toward the follicular opening. It is important to scrape until capillary oozing is observed, to insure that the skin scraping is deep enough. The debris collected is transferred to a microscope slide and mixed into a small amount of mineral oil. A cover slip is placed over the debris, and the slide examined for parasites.

When mites of the *Cheyletiella* and *Sarcoptes* species are suspected, the skin scrapings need not be as deep; however, several large areas should be scraped with as much debris collected as possible. Another excellent technique for demonstrating parasites is to take samples by pressing Scotch tape onto several shaved areas of skin to collect keratinous debris. Put a very thin film of mineral oil onto a microscope slide and place the piece of Scotch tape on the slide (sticky side down) for microscopic examination.

Woods Lamp Examination

About half of the cases of dermatophytosis caused by *Microsporum canis* will show bright apple-green fluorescence of affected hairs under a Woods lamp. The fluorescence is due to tryptophan metabolites unique to the fungus. This test is merely for screening, as many species of dermatophytes do not fluoresce. However, when positive, the test gives a quick answer. Dull green, yellow, or white fluorescence of hair or skin is not significant and some hair and keratinous debris should be submitted for a fungal culture if dermatophytosis is still suspected. Several hairs should also be plucked from the edge of a lesion and examined under the Woods lamp to observe for positive fluorescence of the proximal end of the hair shaft found within the follicle.

KOH Prep

Potassium hydroxide (KOH) is a strong base, which dissolves keratinized debris to allow more accurate inspection of the hairs. In this instance, we attempt to identify the presence of fungal spores as another method of diagnosis of dermatophytes.

Several hairs should be plucked from the edge of the suspected ringworm lesion and placed on a slide with several drops of KOH. The solution should be left in place for 30 minutes for clearing to occur. Alternatively, the slide may be gently heated over a Bunsen burner for 3 to 5 minutes (do not boil).

Almost all small animal dermatophytes have ectothrix spores. That is, the round spores may be seen clustered around the outside of the hair shaft (in contrast to endothrix spores, which would be seen in the medulla of the hair). Finding these round, refractile spores around the proximal end of the hair is diagnostic for ringworm.

Fungal Culture

When dermatophytosis is suspected and Woods lamp examination and KOH prep are negative, fungal culture is warranted.

Dermatophyte Test Media (DTM) is readily available to all practitioners. A few hairs and keratinous debris should be plucked from the edge of an alopecic area and placed on the surface of the test media. In cases where an absence of lesions occurs and one is suspicious of the presence of an asymptomatic carrier, a toothbrush sampling technique (MacKenzie brush technique) can be used. A sterile toothbrush is brushed over the entire animal's hair coat and the collected hair and keratinous debris is placed on the surface of the test media. The culture should be incubated at room temperature, preferably in a dark place, for 14 days. The cap should be loosened to allow for adequate oxygenation.

Dermatophyte Test Media kits contain a phenol indicator, which turns red in the presence of alkaline *p*H. Dermatophytes preferentially use the protein in the media, leaving alkaline metabolites, which turn the indicator red. This reaction usually occurs within the first 7 days, occasionally as early as the first 1 to 2 days. Simultaneous fungal growth is white in color and small in size. Saprophytic (contaminant) fungi preferentially utilize the carbohydrate in the media as an energy source, resulting in an acidic metabolite; the test media color remains yellow or am-

Table 49–6 *Findings Suggestive of Hypothyroidism*

Test	What to Check For
Hemogram	Borderline anemia: normocytic, normochromic, and nonregenerative
Serum biochemistry profile	Mild to severe increase in cholesterol Mild elevations in ALT, AST, Alk Phos
Urinalysis	Lower urinary tract infection
Basal TT_4, TT_3	Decreased resting serum TT_4 and TT_3
TSH response test	Decreased response of the thyroid gland in response to exogenous TSH

Key: ALT = alanine aminotransferase; AST = aspartate aminotransferase; Alk phos = alkaline phosphatase; TT = total thyroid hormone.

ber. However, even saprophytes may utilize the protein when the carbohydrate is depleted, and a color change may occur after 14 days. This change is not considered significant. In this case, the fungal colony is dark in color and large in size.

Assessment of Thyroid Function

The most common laboratory alterations suggestive of hypothyroidism are summarized in Table 49-6.

Specific assessment of the thyroid gland and diagnosis of hypothyroidism is made by measuring the circulating levels of T_3 and T_4. When the resting thyroid levels are borderline low or normal and hypothyroidism is still suspected, a thyrotropin stimulating hormone response test should be performed (Table 49-7). When the presence of autoantibody production directed against circulating T_3 or T_4 is suspected, a serum sample can be submitted to detect the presence of this form of the disease (see Chapter 62).

Table 49–7 *The TSH Response Test*

Step #1:	Resting serum sample
Step #2:	Intravenous administration* of aqueous TSH (Dermathycin): 0.2 IU/kg
Step #3:	Draw 6-hour post-TSH serum sample; doubling of T_4 value should be observed

* Note: If TSH has ever been administered previously, give dose intramuscularly and draw post-TSH sample 8–12 hours later to avoid anaphylaxis.

Adrenal Axis Testing

The most common findings suggestive of hyperadrenocorticism (Cushing's syndrome) are summarized in Table 49-8.

When hyperadrenocorticism is suspected, complete blood count, serum biochemistry profile, and urinalysis should be run to determine the extent of involvement of other systems. If evidence suggestive of Cushing's syndrome is found, specific adrenal axis testing is in order (see Chapter 59).

Gonadal Hormone Assays

Currently, assays for testosterone, progesterone, and estradiol are available. Interpretation of these results, however, may be difficult because of lack of documentation of expected values for various endocrinopathies. Elevated serum estradiol is generally present with ovarian imbalance type I, Sertoli's cell tumor, and castration-responsive dermatosis. Estradiol values near zero suggest ovarian imbalance type II, and testosterone values near zero suggest hypoandrogenism of male dogs.

Growth Hormone Response Test

The growth hormone response test is used to diagnose growth hormone-responsive dermatosis and, as one marker, to aid in the diagnosis of

Table 49–8 *Findings Suggestive of Cushing's Syndrome*

Test	What to Check For
Hemogram	Mild polycythemia or Anemia: normocytic, normochromic, nonregenerative Mature neutrophilia, lymphopenia, monocytosis, eosinopenia
Serum biochemistry profile	Lipemia Hypercholesterolemia Increased SAP, ALT, AST Elevated bile acids and BSP retention Increased amylase and lipase Hyperglycemia Below normal blood urea nitrogen
Urinalysis	Hyposthenuria Glucosuria Bacteriuria without evidence of inflammatory response Proteinuria
Radiographic abnormalities	Hepatomegaly Osteoporosis Enlarged or calcified adrenal gland Distended urinary bladder Dystrophic mineralization of soft tissues, especially lung and skin Pulmonary thromboembolism
Low-dose dexamethasone suppression test	Failure of exogenous corticosteroid to reduce endogenous cortisol levels
Combination test (Dexamethasone suppression/ACTH response test)	Failure of exogenous corticosteroid to reduce endogenous cortisol levels Failure of ACTH to increase endogenous cortisol levels is suggestive of iatrogenic hyperadrenocorticism or Addison's disease

pituitary dwarfism (Table 49-9). Normal dogs show an increase in serum GH levels in response to intravenous xylazine administration; pituitary dwarfs and dogs with growth hormone-responsive dermatosis have low baseline GH levels and a poor response to intravenous xylazine.

This test must be interpreted with caution. Animals with other endocrine abnormalities (especially castration-responsive dermatosis) and normal Pomeranian dogs can show low baseline GH levels and a poor response to xylazine. Therefore, patients should be carefully evaluated for other endocrine abnormalities before considering growth hormone inadequacy as an etiology for skin disease. If the patient is a young, intact male dog, then evaluation of serum estradiol levels should also be measured to rule out a possible castration-responsive dermatosis.

Skin Biopsy

Histopathology of alopecic areas may confirm a diagnosis, as in the case of dermatophytosis, demodicosis, and color mutant alopecia, or may suggest an etiology, such as endocrine disease (see Skin Biopsy in Chapter 80). When one is suspicious of an endocrine cause for an alopecia, the skin biopsy can usually support that contention. The histologic changes most frequently observed

Table 49–9 *Xylazine Response Test*

Step #1: Resting serum sample
Step #2: Give 0.1 mg/kg xylazine (Rompun) intravenously
Step #3: Serum samples at 15 and 30 minutes post-xylazine for GH

Table 49–10 *Additional Histologic Changes That May Be Observed in Certain Endocrine Skin Diseases*

Disease Suspected	Histological Change
Hypothyroidism	Myxedema Thickened dermis
Hyperadrenocorticism	Dystrophic mineralization (calcinosis cutis) Thin dermis Absence of arrector pili muscles Phlebectasia
Growth hormone-responsive dermatosis and castration-responsive dermatosis	Hypereosinophilic tricholemmal, keratinization ("flame follicles")

in an endocrine skin disease include: surface and follicular hyperkeratosis, epidermal atrophy and melanosis, follicular dilatation and atrophy, telogen hair follicles, and atrophy of sebaceous glands. These changes are also referred to as compatible with a non-scarring alopecia. In some instances, additional changes are noted that may suggest the presence of a specific endocrine disease (Table 49-10).

ADDITIONAL READING

Barta O, Waltman C, Oyelan PP et al. Lymphocyte transformation suppression caused by pyoderma: Failure to demonstrate it in uncomplicated demodectic mange. Comp Immunol Microbiol Infect Dis 1983; 6:9.

Foil CS. Antifungal agents in dermatology. In: Kirk RW, ed. Current veterinary therapy IX. Philadelphia: WB Saunders, 1986: 560.

Kwochka KW. Canine demodicosis. In: Kirk RW, ed. Current veterinary therapy IX. Philadelphia: WB Saunders, 1986: 531.

O'Neil CS. Hereditary skin disease in the dog and the cat. Compendium of Continuing Education 1981; 3:791.

Peterson ME. Symposium on endocrinology. Vet Clin North Am 1984; 14:4.

Scott DW, Farrow BRH, Schultz RD. Studies on the therapeutic and immunologic aspects of generalized demodectic mange in the dog. Journal of the American Animal Hospital Association 1974; 2:233.

Scott DW, Schultz RD, Baker E. Further studies on the therapeutic and immunologic aspects of generalized demodectic mange in the dog. Journal of the American Animal Hospital Association 1976; 12:203.

Thomas MLE, Scheidt VJ, Walker RL. Inapparent carriage of Microsporum canis in cats. Compendium of Continuing Education 1989; 11:563.

50

SCALING DERMATOSES

Edmund J. Rosser, Jr., Ann W. Sams

This chapter addresses those dermatologic conditions in which the first noted abnormality is an excessive amount of scaling, and, as the problem progresses, the excessive scaling remains the chief complaint. It is important to realize that most dermatologic disorders are capable of causing some changes in the normal keratinization process with a subsequent increase in the amount of noticeable scales. However, in these instances, the disease historically has some other symptom or lesion noted first (for example, papules, pustules, pruritus, alopecia), and these diseases will not be discussed in this chapter.

The normal process of keratinization within the epidermis is a progressive orderly maturation of epidermal cells that ultimately results in the death of the cells and then a shedding of these dead cells. This process begins with the deepest cells of the epidermis, which are the basal cells of the stratum basale. The process continues through the remaining layers of the epidermis to the spinous cells of the stratum spinosum, to the granular cells of the stratum granulosum, to the clear cells of the stratum lucidum, and finally the horny cells of the stratum corneum (Fig. 50-1). Normally, a relatively constant thickness of the epidermis is maintained by the continuous proliferation of cells from the stratum basale and a relatively constant rate of desquamation of cells from the outermost stratum corneum. In the normal individual, this loss of keratinocytes is not noticeable within the hair coat. However, certain diseases exert as their major influence a disruption of this orderly process, resulting in a keratinization abnormality with the appearance of varying amounts of scales noticeable within the hair coat (Table 50-1).

Keratinization Abnormalities (Canine Seborrheic Dermatoses)

Pathophysiology

This category of diseases is best referred to as primary keratinization disorders and not as seborrheic diseases. Over the years the term *seborrhea* has been loosely applied to a myriad of scaling, alopecic, dry-to-oily skin diseases without much attention to the definition of the word and its proper use. The word "seborrhea" refers to the flow of sebum and should be used to describe

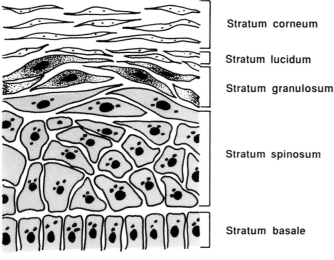

Stratum corneum

Stratum lucidum

Stratum granulosum

Stratum spinosum

Stratum basale

Figure 50–1. *Layers of the normal epidermis.*

Table 50–1 *Causes of Scaling Dermatosis*

I. Keratinization abnormalities (canine seborrheic dermatoses)
  A. Seborrhea sicca
  B. Seborrhea oleosa
  C. Seborrheic dermatitis
II. Nutritional skin diseases
  A. Dietary imbalances, fatty acid deficiencies
  B. Vitamin A-responsive dermatosis
  C. Zinc-responsive dermatosis
III. Parasitic skin diseases
  A. Cheyletiella dermatitis
IV. Endocrine skin diseases
  A. Hypothyroidism
V. Environmental skin diseases
  A. Heating with low humidity
  B. Excessive or inappropriate bathing
VI. Miscellaneous skin diseases
  A. Schnauzer comedo syndrome
  B. Sebaceous adenitis
  C. Epidermal dysplasia of West Highland white terriers

those conditions in which abnormalities in the flow of sebum have been documented. The many familial forms of seborrhea have not had the sebum flow measured to demonstrate if a specific abnormality in this area exists; current investigations suggest a primary keratinization disorder. The primary form of the disease is still considered to be idiopathic, but evidence suggests that the condition may be a genetically inherited epidermal defect. The defect is believed to have a more rapid epidermal turnover time of maturing keratinocytes from the stratum basale to the stratum

corneum. This process only takes 10 to 11 days in affected dogs compared to a normal dog with a turnover time of 21 to 22 days. If this belief is true, then it would help explain the clinical appearance of the patient and the chronic course of the condition (a condition that can be controlled but not cured).

In addition to the keratinization abnormality, it has been shown that the skin of these patients harbors greater than normal numbers of bacteria, especially coagulase positive staphylococci. This finding may help explain the high incidence of secondary bacterial folliculitis observed, particularly in the seborrheic dermatitis form of the disease.

Even though these keratinization disorders are not believed to have abnormalities in sebum production, three clinically distinct forms of this disease are referred to as seborrhea sicca (dry form), seborrhea oleosa (oily form) and seborrheic dermatitis (inflammatory form). One must keep in mind, however, that these clinical presentations may overlap in a given patient and are used exclusively to describe the clinical appearance of the patient and not a specific disease entity.

Diagnostic Approach

The diagnosis of a primary keratinization disorder must be considered when the many dermatologic diseases capable of causing the production of an excess amount of scale have been systematically ruled out. Virtually any skin disease can produce an excess amount of scaling at one point in time in the development of the disease. Therefore, close attention must be paid to the historical development of the condition, the breed affected, the type of lesions present on physical examination, and the distribution pattern of the lesions. When the history and physical examination are most suggestive of a primary pruritic skin disease; alopecic skin disease; or papular, pustular, or vesicular skin disease, the reader is referred to the appropriate accompanying chapters. A complete dietary history should be taken to look for the presence of a possible fatty acid deficiency or zinc-responsive dermatosis (see below, Nutritional Skin Diseases). The history should also include an evaluation of the type of shampoos used by the owners and the frequency of application, as well as the type of heat used in the home and the relative humidity (see below, Environmental Skin Diseases).

In assessing the patient with the chief complaint of excess scale formation, the following tests need to be considered: skin scrapings, Scotch tape prep, KOH prep, Wood's lamp examination, fungal cultures, bacterial culture and sensitivity, fecal flotation, dietary fat absorption tests, complete blood count, serum biochemistry profile, urinalysis, thyrotropin response test, cortisol function test, liver function test, and skin biopsies (Table 50-2).

Once the systematic evaluation of the patient with a scaling dermatosis has been completed, the skin biopsy (see Skin Biopsy in Chapter 80) is a very valuable tool. In some instances, the skin biopsy might establish the diagnosis of an overlooked underlying disease, causing the scaling dermatosis such as demodicosis, dermatophytosis, pyoderma, autoimmune skin disease (especially pemphigus foliaceus), neoplastic disease (especially mycosis fungoides) and vitamin A or zinc-responsive dermatosis (see below, Nutritional Skin Diseases). In other instances, the re-

Table 50–2 *Laboratory Assessment of Scaling Dermatoses**

Test	What to Check For
Skin scraping	*Demodex, Sarcoptes, Cheyletiella* mites
Scotch tape prep	*Cheyletiella, Sarcoptes* mites
KOH prep	Ectothrix spores of dermatophytes
Wood's lamp exam	Bright apple green fluorescence, suggests presence of *Microsporum canis*
Fungal culture	Dermatophytosis
Bacterial culture	Primary or secondary pyoderma, usually coagulase positive staphylococci
Fecal flotation	Endoparasites
Fat absorption	Malabsorption, maldigestion
Cell blood count	Stress leukogram, suggests chronic disease or hyperadrenocorticism Normochromic, normocytic, nonregenerative anemia, suggests chronic disease, hypothyroidism, or hyperadrenocorticism
Serum biochemistry profile	Look for evidence of a primary metabolic disease, such as hyperadrenocorticism, diabetes mellitus, or liver disease
Urinalysis	Look for support of a primary metabolic disease
TSH response test	Rule out hypothyroidism
Cortisol function tests	Rule out hyperadrenocorticism
Liver function tests	Rule out primary liver disease

* Note: See Chapters 49 and 51 for a discussion of the proper use of the above techniques.

sults may be suggestive of an underlying endocrine or allergic skin disease that has not yet been considered. At this point, the histopathological findings most suggestive (but not in themselves diagnostic) of a primary keratinization abnormality include a spongiotic or hyperplastic superficial perivascular dermatitis, moderate to marked hyperkeratosis and parakeratosis with follicular keratosis, and focal mounds of parakeratosis overlying the follicular ostia.

Seborrhea Sicca

Clinical Signs

The patient usually presents with a complaint of an overall dull and dry hair coat with focal to diffuse accumulations of white to gray scales. In most cases the dorsal and lateral trunk regions are first to be affected, and pruritus is either absent or mild. The breeds most predisposed to this form include the Irish setter, German shepherd, dachshund, and Doberman pinscher.

Management

The objective of the treatment of the patient with dry seborrhea is to moisturize and condition the hair coat. This is best accomplished by mild, hypoallergenic, moisturizing shampoos, such as Allergroom or HyLyt efa shampoo used once to twice weekly as needed. After the shampoo has been thoroughly rinsed, a conditioner such as Humilac or HyLyt efa should be applied as a spray or rinse. In some instances, the patient will additionally benefit from the use of an essential fatty acid containing supplement (Derm Caps, Efa Vet, Efa Z plus, Nutrisol) added to the diet on a daily basis.

Seborrhea Oleosa

Clinical Signs

The chief complaint of owners with a dog with seborrhea oleosa is the development of a undesirable odor and a hair coat that is greasy to the touch. Present is an accumulation of brownish-yellow, nit-like flakes of lipid material, which adheres to the skin and hair and which is most notable on the dorsal and lateral aspects of the trunk. The patient often has a concurrent bilateral ceruminous otitis externa. The breeds most predisposed to this form include the cocker spaniel, springer spaniel, Chinese shar pei and Basset hound.

Management

The objective of the treatment of the patient with oily seborrhea is to control the odor, remove the greasiness, remove the excess scales, and slow down the epidermal turnover time. This objective is best accomplished by the use of mild to moderate keratolytic and keratoplastic shampoos with some degreasing properties. The sulfur and salicylic acid containing shampoos in general are best for this, such as SebaLyt, Sebolux, and Sebbafon shampoo used once to twice weekly. Occasionally, a patient will benefit from a better degreasing effect with the use of a benzoyl peroxide containing shampoo, such as OxyDex, or Pyoben shampoo. A recently introduced product, SulfOxydex shampoo, combines both sulfur and benzoyl peroxide and has the potential of being an optimal shampoo for this type of keratinization disorder, but further evaluation is necessary. Most cases will additionally benefit from the use of a conditioning spray or rinse and the use of an essential fatty acid containing dietary supplement (see Seborrhea Sicca).

Seborrheic Dermatitis

Clinical Signs

This patient presents with various combinations of the above signs such as a dull, dry hair coat, malodor, greasiness, focal to diffuse accumulations of white to gray scales, brownish-yellow, nit-like flakes of lipid material that adhere to the skin and hair, and a bilateral ceruminous otitis externa. A unique feature of this form is the presence of individual lesions that present as circumscribed areas of alopecia, erythema, and a tightly adhered scale and crust with a margin of inflammation (Color Fig. 10). The lesions are typically located on the trunk, ventral neck, and chest region. In addition, these patients are moderately to severely pruritic, and often papules and pustules indicating the development of a secondary bacterial folliculitis are present. The breeds most predisposed to this form include the cocker spaniel, springer spaniel, West Highland white terrier and Basset hound.

Management

The objective of the treatment of the patient with inflammatory seborrhea is to decrease the pruritus and inflammation, decrease the odor and greasiness, remove the excess scales and crusts, and slow down the epidermal turnover time. This objective is best accomplished with potent keratolytic and keratoplastic shampoos, such as Allerseb T or LyTar shampoo used once to twice weekly. Most cases will additionally benefit from the use of a conditioning spray or rinse and the use of an essential fatty acid containing dietary supplement, as for seborrhea sicca and seborrhea oleosa.

Medications can also be used systemically to try to slow down the epidermal turnover time. Vitamin A and the retinoids have been used for this purpose. Vitamin A can be given at a dosage of 10,000 I.U. once a day for a trial period of 1 to 3 months. When the medication is beneficial, the frequency of bathing can usually be decreased, and on rare occasions medicated baths may no longer be necessary to control the condition. In refractory cases of seborrheic dermatitis, the recently introduced retinoids may be of benefit, but they have only been used on an experimental and limited basis. The preparations tried thus far include isotretinoin (Accutane) or etretinate (Tegison) at an oral dosage of 1 mg/kg once to twice daily. Most patients have tolerated the medication well with only minor side effects, which include lethargy and depression, anorexia, vomiting, cheilitis, erythema, pruritus, epiphora, conjunctivitis, and hyperactivity. Potentially more serious side effects include abdominal distention, swollen tongue, and collapse. These products are also known to be teratogenic. Evaluation of the hemogram and serum biochemistry profile has revealed occasional and reversible increases

in platelets counts, triglycerides, cholesterol, and liver enzymes (alanine aminotransferase and aspartate aminotransferase).

Patients with a concurrent bacterial folliculitis may need to be additionally bathed with a benzoyl peroxide containing shampoo, such as Oxydex or Pyoben shampoo, or the recently introduced sulfur and benzoyl peroxide containing product, SulfOxydex shampoo. When a secondary bacterial folliculitis is present, it is also indicated to place the patient on an appropriate systemic antibiotic for 21 consecutive days (see Chapter 52).

For the immediate relief of the inflammation and pruritus, the short-term use of corticosteroids is beneficial. This treatment can be accomplished with prednisone or prednisolone at 0.50 mg/kg of body weight twice daily for 7 days, then 0.50 mg/kg once daily for 7 days, 0.50 mg/kg every other day for 1 week, then discontinue the medication. It must be emphasized that long-term use of corticosteroids in the management of primary keratinization abnormalities is contraindicated because it can increase the formation of dry scales and predispose the patient to bacterial folliculitis; in addition, the short-term benefits of corticosteroids will be lost if they are used chronically. Therefore, the client must be appropriately educated about the proper long-term management of the patient with a keratinization abnormality; the goal of the treatments is to control and not cure the condition. With this approach, a satisfactory treatment regimen can usually be established.

NUTRITIONAL SKIN DISEASES

Dietary Imbalances

Pathophysiology

The most recognized cause of excess scaling due to a dietary imbalance is a deficiency of dietary fat. The skin of dogs and cats requires the following essential fatty acids: linoleic acid, linolenic acid, and arachidonic acid. In the dog, a dietary source of linoleic acid can be converted to linolenic and arachidonic acid. However, in cats, a lack of the active enzyme delta-6-desaturase responsible for conversion of linoleic acid to linolenic and arachidonic acid means these fatty acids need to be supplied in the diet. The types of diets occasionally believed to be associated with fatty acid deficiency include: semi-moist dog foods, dry foods stored for long periods of time, generic dog foods, and homemade diets. A fatty acid deficiency can also be observed due to a deficiency in the proper digestion, absorption, or metabolism of fats, as in maldigestion syndromes, malabsorption syndromes, and liver disease.

Clinical Signs

The patient usually presents with a history of a generalized dull, dry hair coat with excessive scaling. As the problem continues, the skin and hair coat may become greasy and malodorous.

Diagnostic Approach and Management

The history of the patient fed a semi-moist dog food, exclusively dry dog food or dry dog food stored for long periods of time, generic dog food, or a homemade diet should lead one to suspect the possibility of a fatty acid deficiency. At this point, the diet should be changed to a known and well-balanced diet. If the change alone is not effective, then supplementing the diet with an essential fatty acid supplement (Derm Caps, Efa Vet, Efa Z plus, Nutrisol) can be tried for 1 month. If the scaling dermatosis persists, then specific diagnostic tests and a systematic approach to the problem needs to be initiated.

Vitamin A-Responsive Dermatosis

Pathophysiology, Clinical Signs, Diagnostic Approach, and Management

The pathophysiology of vitamin A-responsive dermatosis is unknown. The features of this disease very closely resemble seborrheic dermatitis of cocker spaniels. At this point, one cannot be certain whether a patient with primary seborrheic dermatitis is benefiting from the ability of vitamin A to slow down epidermal turnover time or whether this entity is different and specific. Vitamin A-responsive dermatosis is suggested when a skin biopsy reveals the features compatible with a primary keratinization abnormality (see Keratinization Abnormalities) plus the additional change of marked follicular hyperkeratosis. Diagnosis is confirmed by response to vitamin A supplementation as used for seborrheic dermatitis.

Zinc-Responsive Dermatosis

Pathophysiology

Two separate forms of zinc-responsive dermatosis have been reported in the dog. Syndrome I is believed to be the result of a decreased absorption of dietary zinc from the intestines, resulting in decreased serum and/or hair zinc levels. Therefore, the problem is observed in dogs on a balanced commercial diet. Syndrome II occurs in rapidly growing puppies on a zinc deficient diet or a diet high in calcium or phytates, resulting in the binding of dietary zinc in the intestines and subsequent decreased absorption.

Clinical Signs

Syndrome I is usually observed in dogs near puberty or young adult dogs. The breeds most predisposed to this form include the Siberian husky, Alaskan malamute, Doberman pinscher, and Great Dane. The first noticeable changes are focal areas of erythema affecting any combination of the following areas: the commissures of the mouth, lip fold region, chin, periorbital region, pinnae, elbows, hocks, scrotum, prepuce, and vulva. Subsequently, alopecia is noted with the appearance of tightly adherent scales and crusts (Color Figs. 11 and 12). In some cases, only a thickening of the footpads with or without the formation of fissures is noted. Historically, the patient is usually on a well balanced commercial dog food diet.

Syndrome II is a rare form of the disease observed in growing puppies on zinc deficient diets or diets high in calcium or phytates. The patient develops thickened, circumscribed, crusted and scaling plaques that may affect the pressure point regions of the body, face, footpads, and virtually anywhere on the body. In addition to the skin lesions, the patient may be depressed, anorectic, and stunted with a peripheral lymphadenopathy.

Diagnostic Approach and Management

The history and physical examination alone should lead one to suspect the diagnosis of a zinc-responsive dermatosis. A skin biopsy usually reveals the presence of a hyperplastic superficial dermatitis with marked surface and follicular parakeratosis. Syndrome I can be treated with oral zinc sulfate at 100 to 220 mg twice daily and is usually required for life. Syndrome II can be treated by correcting the dietary problem alone or additionally supplementing the diet with zinc sulfate at 10 mg/kg once daily, stopping after maturity.

PARASITIC SKIN DISEASES

Cheyletiella Dermatitis

Pathophysiology

This parasitic skin disease is presented in this section on scaling dermatoses because scaling is usually the major or only clinical sign of infection with this ectoparasite in dogs and cats. The disease in dogs and cats is the result of an infection with any of the following three mites: *Cheyletiella yasguri*, *Cheyletiella blakei*, or *Cheyletiella parasitovorax*. This mite dwells on the surface of the stratum corneum, can complete its entire life cycle on the host, and attaches its eggs to the hairs with fine fibrillar strands. However, adult mites can be found living in the environment of the patient and may serve as a source of re-infestation. This mite is not species specific and is capable of parasitizing humans.

Clinical Signs

This disease is most frequently observed in kittens or puppies recently acquired from a breeder, private owner, pet store, or humane society. Endemic problems may also be encountered in certain catteries. The first sign noted is usually an excessive scaling along the dorsal midline that may become generalized over time. Younger animals tend to have more severe lesions with varying degrees of pruritus, while older animals have milder lesions with pruritus being minimal or absent with occasional asymptomatic carriers. Some cats may develop moderate to severe pruritus, papules, crusts, and excoriations (see Chapter 51). This disease is potentially contagious to other dogs and cats in the environment, which may be similarly affected, less severely affected, more severely affected, or completely unaffected. People in contact with these dogs or cats may or may not exhibit evidence of infection including pruritus, papules, macules, pustules, vesicles, crusts, and excoriations on the arms, trunk, and buttocks.

Diagnostic Approach

The physical findings and history of recent exposure to other animals first leads one to suspect the diagnosis of cheyletiella dermatitis. The diagnosis is further supported if other pets or people in the household are affected. Demonstration of this mite is best achieved by skin scrapings, Scotch tape preps, flea combing, vacuuming technique, and fecal flotation (see Chapter 51).

Management

In general, *Cheyletiella* mites are relatively easy to kill once the diagnosis is established. All dogs and cats in the environment should be powdered or sprayed twice weekly for 4 weeks with a pyrethrin or carbaryl containing product (Sectrol 2 way Pet Spray, Duocide L.A. Flea Spray, Diryl flea powder). The environment should be thoroughly vacuumed and the vacuum cleaner bag disposed of as well as disposal of any bedding. Very young or debilitated animals can be treated with lime sulfur containing rinses such as LymDyp or Orthorix applied once weekly for 4 weeks. Ivermectin may be useful in situations where large numbers of animals are affected and the above topical treatments are impractical. Ivermectin (Ivomec) can be given at a dosage of 200 to 300 μg/kg subcutaneously and repeated in 2 to 3 weeks. Ivermectin is contraindicated for the treatment of cheyletiella dermatitis in collies, Shetland sheepdogs, and any crossbreeds of collies or shelties. The disease is usually self-limiting in affected people once the pets and environment have been treated.

ENDOCRINE DERMATOSES

Hypothyroidism

Pathophysiology, Clinical Signs, Diagnostic Approach, and Management

The reason for alerting the practitioner or student to the possibility of hypothyroidism under scaling dermatoses is that, occasionally, the only symptom of hypothyroidism is a dull, dry hair coat with an increase in the amount of scales. In addition, hypothyroidism can imitate the primary keratinization disorders including seborrhea sicca, seborrhea oleosa, and seborrheic dermatitis. For further discussion, refer to Chapters 49 and 62.

ENVIRONMENTAL DERMATOSES

Heating With Low Humidity, Excessive or Inappropriate Bathing

Pathophysiology, Clinical Signs, Diagnostic Approach, and Management

These causes of excess scaling in dogs and cats are fairly straight forward but often easily overlooked. The patient that is sensitive to warm, dry heat usually presents with a history of excess scaling and a dull, dry hair coat most noticeable in indoor pets in the winter after the heat has been turned on (also called "winter heat syndrome"). The house is often heated with forced hot air with a low relative humidity. Adding a humidifier to the house is very beneficial but often impractical. Satisfactory treatment can be accomplished by using the treatments discussed under Seborrhea

Sicca. The history may also reveal that the owners' bathing of the pet is the cause of the excess scaling and may include the regular use of human shampoos (most of which are too irritating for dogs and cats), or overly frequent bathing of a normal dog (some people feel their pets should be bathed daily or every other day). In this case, the owners should be informed that the preferred method of grooming in dogs and cats is brushing and combing and that the normal pet need not be bathed more often than once monthly. For people who insist they must bathe their pet (some people find any animal odor offensive), the use of mild, hypoallergenic moisturizing shampoos such as HyLyt efa or Allergroom can be used every 1 to 2 weeks.

MISCELLANEOUS SKIN DISEASES

Schnauzer Comedo Syndrome

Pathophysiology

The pathophysiology of schnauzer comedo syndrome is unknown but is thought to be a hereditary developmental dysplasia of hair follicles with subsequent formation of comedones (blackheads).

Clinical Signs

This condition seems to occur exclusively in miniature schnauzers. The owner usually first notices small bumps (comedones and papules) with excess scaling along the dorsal midline. The comedones and papules are most apparent when petting the dog and may not be easily visualized in early cases. In chronic cases, often a thinning of the hair coat along the dorsum is found. The condition is usually non-pruritic unless a secondary bacterial folliculitis develops, and then additional papules and pustules can be observed.

Diagnostic Approach

The history and physical examination leads one to consider this diagnosis. The hair may be clipped over the dorsum in early cases to better visualize the lesions. A skin biopsy (see Skin Biopsy in Chapter 80) reveals the presence of dilated hair follicles with large keratin plugs. Additionally, a bacterial folliculitis or evidence of rupture of the hair follicle and development of a furuncle and foreign body reaction may be found.

Management

This condition tends to be a chronic problem for the rest of the dog's life once it develops; therefore, client education is very important. The patient should be initially bathed with a benzoyl peroxide containing shampoo, such as Oxydex or Pyoben shampoo, or a sulfur and benzoyl peroxide containing shampoo, such as SulfOxydex, twice weekly. Individual lesions should be additionally treated with a benzoyl peroxide containing gel, such as Oxydex or Pyoben gel, once to twice daily. If this treatment does not significantly improve the condition within 2 to 3 weeks, then daily alcohol rubs over the back may be necessary to dry up the lesions. Once a response is observed, then a maintenance program using the shampoo and gel should be established by gradually decreasing the frequency of applications. When the problem is nonresponsive to topical treatment, then an essential fatty acid containing dietary supplement, vitamin A, or the retinoids may be tried as discussed under Seborrheic Dermatitis.

Sebaceous Adenitis

Pathophysiology

The pathophysiology of sebaceous adenitis is unknown. The current hypotheses suggest that the sebaceous gland destruction is a developmental and genetically inherited defect or that the sebaceous gland destruction is an immune-mediated or autoimmune disease directed against a component of sebaceous glands.

Clinical Signs

From a clinical and histopathological standpoint, two slightly different forms of the disease occur.

The first type occurs in long-coated breeds of dogs, including the standard poodle, Akita and Samoyed. Initially, a partial and symmetrical alopecia with excess scaling is found with the formation of keratinous casts that adhere to the hair shafts. The scales present are tightly adherent to the skin and are either silver-white or yellow-brown in color. The areas affected include the dorsal planum of the nose, top of head, dorsal neck and trunk, tail, and pinnae (Color Figs. 13 and 14). In the early stages, the patient is non-pruritic or mildly pruritic with no offensive odor. As the condition progresses, these patients are prone to the development of secondary bacterial folliculitis, pruritus, and malodor.

The second type occurs in short-coated breeds of dogs, including the Vizsla and Weimaraner. Initially, a moth-eaten alopecia with mild scaling that primarily affects the trunk is found. As the condition progresses, the focal areas of alopecia coalesce, resulting in large alopecic areas. The condition is usually non-pruritic.

Diagnostic Approach

The history and physical findings suggest the possibility of this disease. A skin biopsy is the best method to confirm the diagnosis and reveals nodular to pyogranulomatous inflammation at the level of the sebaceous glands. In long-coated breeds of dogs, moderate to marked hyperkeratosis and keratinous follicular cast formation are found. In short-coated breeds of dogs, the hyperkeratotic changes are mild or absent. As the disease progresses, a complete loss of sebaceous glands replaced by fibrosis occurs, and in rare instances the entire hair follicle may be destroyed.

Management

The prognosis for complete recovery from this condition is poor, especially in the more chronic cases where the sebaceous glands have already been lost. The use of antiseborrheic shampoos, conditioners, and emollients have been of little benefit. The most effective symptomatic treatment is the use of 50% to 75% propylene glycol mixed with water and applied once daily as a spray to the affected areas. The propylene glycol acts as a hygroscopic lipid solvent that penetrates the horny layer and increases water content. In refractory cases, the retinoid isotretinoin (Accutane) may be effective at an oral dosage of 1 mg/kg once or twice daily. When a secondary pyoderma is present, the patient should be placed on an appropriate systemic antibiotic and antibacterial shampoo (see Chapter 52).

Epidermal Dysplasia of West Highland White Terriers

Pathophysiology

The pathophysiology of epidermal dysplasia is unknown, but it is considered to be a genetically inherited skin disease. One study revealed the presence of an elevation of basal serum bile acids and an increase in the clearance of bile acids after the intravenous administration of bile salts.

Clinical Signs

This condition seems to occur exclusively in West Highland white terriers. The first signs are usually noticed between several weeks to months of age and include pruritus, erythema, alopecia, and excess scaling. The initial areas affected are the feet, legs, and ventrum, but the condition rapidly progresses to a generalized form with chronic dermatitis and severe lichenification, hyperpigmentation, and scaling ("The Armadillo Syndrome of Westies") (Color Fig. 15).

Diagnostic Approach

The initial presentation of these patients is very similar to other known familial skin diseases of the Westie, and the initial differential diagnosis should include food allergy, atopy, seborrheic dermatitis, and scabies. However, these dogs have been nonresponsive to hypoallergenic diets trials, skin test negative, nonresponsive to scabicidal treatment, and nonresponsive to various symptomatic treatment regimens tried thus far. Skin biopsies reveal the presence of a hyperplastic perivascular dermatitis and epidermal dysplasia, which include keratinocyte hyperchromasia, abnormal aggregates of keratinocytes with increased mitosis, loss of palisading of basal cells, and the presence of epidermal "buds." Further measurement of resting and post-prandial bile acids may lead to a better understanding of this disease.

Management

The prognosis for most patients with this disease is poor, and the majority of the dogs affected with this condition have been euthanized. Until the pathophysiology of this frustrating dermatologic skin disease is understood, very little can be offered in terms of an effective treatment protocol.

ADDITIONAL READING

Kunkle GA. Zinc-responsive dermatoses. In: Kirk RW, ed. Current veterinary therapy VII. Philadelphia: WB Saunders, 1980: 472.

Kwochka KW. Retinoids in dermatology. In: Kirk RW, ed. Current veterinary therapy X. Philadelphia: WB Saunders, 1989: 553.

Miller WH. Nutritional considerations in small animal dermatology. Vet Clin North Am 1989; 19:497.

Rosser EJ, Dunstan RW, Breen PT, Johnson GR. Sebaceous adenitis with hyperkeratosis in the standard poodle: A discussion of 10 cases. Journal of the American Animal Hospital Association 1987; 23:341.

Scott DW. Granulomatous sebaceous adenitis in dogs. Journal of the American Animal Hospital Association 1986; 22:631.

51

PRURITUS

Edmund J. Rosser, Jr., Ann Washabaugh Sams

This chapter will address those dermatologic conditions in which pruritus is the initiating event and is a major feature as the disease progresses. The diseases addressed are those most commonly encountered in the practice situation; no attempt has been made to make this a treatise on pruritic skin diseases.

PATHOPHYSIOLOGY

The cutaneous perception of pruritus remains a controversial entity. It is still uncertain whether there are separate receptors for perception of itch vs. pain and whether there is a central pruritus center in the medulla. However, pruritus appears to be a primary cutaneous sensation elicited from the epidermis and upper dermis and mucous membranes. Stimuli of pruritus are transmitted by way of unmyelinated C fibers for diffuse burning itch sensation and through myelinated A delta fibers for sharp, well-localized itch. These fibers enter the dorsal route of the spinal cord, and the sensation ultimately is transmitted to the sensory portion of the cerebral cortex.

Controversy also exists as to what the biochemical initiator and mediator of pruritus is within the tissues. Most sources agree that histamine is not the main mediator of pruritus; cur-

rently proteolytic enzymes (*e.g.*, kallikrein, cathepsins, leukopeptidases, microbial proteases, plasmin) are thought to be one of the main mediators in dogs and cats. Proteolytic enzymes that initiate a pruritic response can be supplied from mast cells, bacteria, fungi, neutrophils, and lymphocytes involved in antigen–antibody reactions. Recent studies are examining the possible role of leukotrienes as a mediator of pruritus in dogs and cats.

Consideration of the role and response of the immune system is also essential to a complete understanding of pruritus and inflammation (Halliwell and Gorman, Additional Reading).

The major causes of pruritus will be considered in the categories of parasitic skin diseases and allergic and hypersensitivity disorders (Table 51-1).

PARASITIC SKIN DISEASES

Sarcoptic Mange (Canine Scabies)

Pathophysiology

Sarcoptic mange is an intensely pruritic and potentially contagious skin disease caused by the mite *Sarcoptes scabiei var. canis*. These mites are

Table 51–1 *Causes of Pruritus in Small Animals*

PARASITIC SKIN DISEASES

Sarcoptic mange
Notoedric mange
Otodectic mange
Fly bite dermatitis
Cheyletiellosis (see Chapter 50)
Canine demodicosis (see Chapter 49)

ALLERGIC AND HYPERSENSITIVITY DISORDERS

Flea allergy dermatitis
Tick bite hypersensitivity
Atopy
Food allergy
Irritant contact dermatitis
Allergic contact dermatitis
Acute moist dermatitis and pyotraumatic folliculitis
Staphylococcal hypersensitivity (see Chapter 52)

host-specific for dogs, but can cause lesions in the fox, cat, and human as well.

S. scabiei var. canis is a skin surface-dwelling mite, with the gravid female burrowing into the stratum corneum to lay her eggs. The entire life cycle is completed on the host and can occur within 3 weeks.

The initial cause of the pruritus is the burrowing of the mites into the epidermis. However, this in itself does not adequately explain the pruritus in all patients. In many instances, the patient has a severe and somewhat generalized pruritus that is responsive to scabicidal treatment even though the parasites are not demonstrable on skin scraping. This suggests the possibility of an immunologic hypersensitivity to the presence of an undetectable but small population of mites ("scabies incognito"). The immune response of the host is also believed to be important in controlling and limiting the degree of infestation. In support of this, immunosuppressed patients infected with *S. scabiei* var. *canis* have large numbers of mites that are readily found on skin scraping, and the degree of pruritus is much less severe than in nonimmunosuppressed patients (Norwegian scabies).

Proteinuria is often demonstrated in patients with canine scabies, leading to speculation about the occurrence of a type III hypersensitivity reaction and the development of immune complex deposition glomerulonephritis.

Clinical Signs

Intense, nonseasonal pruritus is the hallmark of sarcoptic mange. The ears, elbows, hocks, ventral abdomen, and chest are most commonly affected. Primary papules quickly progress to yellowish crusts with post-traumatic alopecia and excoriations. A generalized reactive peripheral lymphadenopathy and the development of pustules and a secondary pyoderma commonly occur.

Historically there may be evidence of the possible source of exposure to the mite, as with a pet obtained from the humane society or recently boarded, but in many cases the source of infection cannot be determined. To further challenge the clinician, only one pet may be affected, with all other pets and humans in the household being normal, or several pets and humans may be affected to various degrees. When people are affected they most commonly have papules and pruritus on the trunk and arms. Therefore, a lack of historical exposure to the mite and lack of pruritus in other animals does not preclude the possible diagnosis of scabies. The diagnosis must often be made based on the index of suspicion alone.

Management

Various parasiticidal dips are currently used to treat sarcoptic mange, with geographic differences in efficacy. Organophosphate, lindane, sulfurated lime topical solution, and amitraz dips may be effective; oral or subcutaneous ivermectin may be the most effective agent in some areas (Table 51-2). All contact dogs should be treated, whether symptomatic or not. Before choosing an agent one should consult with a dermatologist familiar with any scabicidal resistance problems that have been documented in the geographic area. Scabicidal resistance is a problem that is increasing throughout the world.

While mites are susceptible to dehydration and usually do not live well apart from the host, it is recommended that owners dispose of the pet's bedding and thoroughly vacuum the local environment. Recent evidence has indicated the ability of *S. scabiei* to survive in the environment and serve as a source of reinfection. This helps explain why on rare occasions the problem appears to have resolved after appropriate treatment, only

Table 51–2 Treatment Modalities for Canine Scabies

Agent	Trade Name	How Administered	Frequency/Duration
Organophosphate	Kill-a-mite	Dip	Once weekly for 4 to 6 weeks
Amitraz*	Mitaban	Dip	Every 2 weeks for three total treatments
Sulfurated lime topical solution	Lym Dyp	Dip	Once weekly for 4 or more weeks
Ivermectin†	Ivomec	200 to 400 µg/kg subcutaneously	Every 2 weeks for 2 total treatments

* Not approved for this use in dogs
† Not approved for this use in dogs and contraindicated in collies or Shetland sheepdogs or their crosses

to recur when treatment is stopped. Professional extermination of the environment as an adjunct to treatment is effective when this occurs. In most cases, if humans in the house have lesions they will undergo spontaneous remission within 4 weeks after the pets have been treated; only rarely do humans require scabicidal treatment.

Notoedric Mange (Feline Scabies)

Pathophysiology

This pruritic skin disease is caused by the mite *Notoedres cati*. Its life cycle is similar to the *Sarcoptes scabiei* that affects dogs. The mite is specific to cats, but may transiently infect humans, dogs, foxes, and rabbits. In contrast to canine scabies, the disease is highly contagious among cats. Typically, all contact cats are affected and large numbers of mites are demonstrated.

Clinical Signs

Feline scabies is a problem in certain endemic pockets throughout the world, but seems to be virtually nonexistent elsewhere. The chief complaint is intense pruritus that initially affects the ears and progresses to the face, eyelids, neck, and top of the head. The lesions start as small, crusted papules (miliary lesions). This stage is followed by post-traumatic alopecia, a thickening and wrinkling of the skin, and formation of thick yellow to gray crusts (Fig. 51-1). This disease represents one of the many causes of the miliary dermatitis reaction (which is a clinical sign and not a disease) in the cat. Contact cats in the environ-

ment usually develop similar lesions; dogs or humans in the environment may or may not be affected with pruritus and papules.

Management

The hair should be clipped near the affected areas and the cat bathed with a mild shampoo to facili-

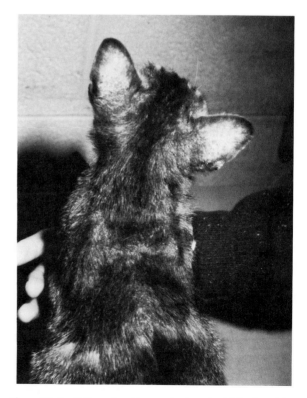

Figure 51–1. Pattern of post-traumatic alopecia, thickening of skin, and crust formation in a cat with notoedric mange.

tate the removal of any crusts. A sulfurated lime topical solution (Lym Dyp, Orthorix) is used as a whole-body rinse, and allowed to dry on the cat. This procedure should be repeated every 7 to 10 days for four total treatments. All cats in the environment should be treated, regardless of whether or not they have skin lesions or pruritus. Recently, both an amitraz solution used as a rinse and ivermectin given subcutaneously have been shown to be effective against *Notoedres cati;* however, neither is approved for use in the cat.

Otodectic Mange (Ear Mites)

Pathophysiology

Otodectes cyanotis is a surface-dwelling mite that feeds on epithelial debris. Their preferred environment is the external ear canal, but they occasionally can be found elsewhere on the body on the surface of the skin. They are not host-specific, but affect dogs, cats, and many other carnivores.

Clinical Signs

Pruritus of the ear area is the most common clinical presentation. Grossly, "coffee ground"-type debris is evident in the ear canal, and white mites may be seen on otoscopic examination. Secondary alopecia, excoriation, and even aural hematomas may be present. Mites and accompanying pruritus are not always limited to the ear canal, but may affect the surrounding head, neck, and even tail areas.

Management

Topical treatment with either Tresaderm or a mixture of one part Canex and three parts mineral oil is very effective. Ears should be treated twice daily for 10 consecutive days. The treatment is then stopped for 10 days, and followed by another 10-day treatment to eliminate any recently hatched mites that were not killed as eggs during the first 10 days of treatment. Secondary bacterial or yeast otitis externa should be addressed, and all contact animals (dogs and cats) should be treated. In recurrent cases it is recommended that animals be sprayed with pyrethrin flea sprays (Sectrol, Duo-cide L.A., SynerKyl) concurrently to eliminate mites that may not be in the ear canal.

Fly Bite Dermatitis (Fly Bite Ears)

Pathophysiology

Stomoxys calcitrans, the stable fly, is worldwide in distribution. Its rasping teeth and blades of labellae tear an opening in the skin, and its bite is painful and irritating to the host. Adult stable flies prefer strong light to shade and are more abundant in the summer and fall.

Clinical Signs

The face and ears of dogs are the most commonly affected areas. Lesions occur at the ear tips in erect-eared breeds of dogs, and at the folded edge of the ear in flop-eared breeds of dogs. Erythema, ulceration, and dark, hemorrhagic crusts from oozing blood and serum are evident. Historically, the dogs are usually housed outdoors and confined where they cannot escape the flies.

Management

Topical nonstinging antibiotic and steroid creams (Panalog, NeoPredef) help relieve pain and pruritus while the lesions heal. It is important to keep the dog indoors during early treatment to eliminate continued trauma from flies. Fly repellents are helpful in treatment as well as prevention, and insecticide treatment of manure and compost piles where flies reproduce may be necessary.

ALLERGIC AND HYPERSENSITIVITY DISORDERS

Flea Allergy Dermatitis

Pathophysiology

Flea allergy dermatitis is the most common pruritic dermatosis seen in both the dog and cat in small animal practice. The most common flea found on both dogs and cats is *Ctenocephalides felis*, and only on rare occasions is *Ctenocephalides canis* found. Some animals are so sensitized to the flea bite that a single bite every 10 to 14 days may be sufficient to keep the patient pruritic.

Flea allergy dermatitis represents a true hypersensitivity to the flea saliva that is injected into the skin during the biting and feeding process. More than one mechanism appears to be involved. This has been examined closely in the dog.

First, the flea saliva contains a salivary protein that by itself is not antigenic, referred to as a *hapten* (incomplete antigen). The hapten binds to collagen in the dermis and forms a complete antigen. This process has been associated immunologically with the type IV hypersensitivity reaction (delayed reaction) that occurs 24 to 48 hours after intradermal exposure to the salivary hapten (see Table 30-2).

Flea saliva also contains a protein that by itself is antigenic. It is associated immunologically with the type I hypersensitivity reaction (immediate reaction) that occurs within 15 to 20 minutes of intradermal exposure to the salivary antigen.

Two other immunologic reactions to a salivary antigen are believed to play a role in flea allergy dermatitis, namely, a late-onset immunoglobin E-mediated reaction and cutaneous basophil hypersensitivity. The role played by these reactions in the development of flea allergy dermatitis is not well understood.

Finally, flea saliva contains a heparinlike substance that allows the flea to feed by preventing blood coagulation at the site. It is important to note that in the nonflea-allergic patient, flea bites cause very little to no itch sensation. Subsequently, nonflea-allergic patients do not develop the clinical signs to be discussed in this chapter. This also helps explain why many households with several dogs and cats and known periodic flea exposure often have only one pet (the flea-allergic pet) with the clinical signs of a flea allergy and an absence of pruritus and lesions in the other pets (nonflea-allergic pets).

Adult fleas live on the dog and cat; controversy exists as to whether the adult fleas jump on and off of the host or remain on the host most of the time. However, what is certain is that all of the preadult and young adult developmental stages of the flea are spent off of the host in the host's environment. Fleas in these developmental stages account for a large percentage of the total flea population and serve as the source for new infestation and reinfestation. This is why treatment of the environment is so important in complete flea control. The eggs are laid on the host by the adult flea, and fall off into the house or yard, where they progress through larval and pupal stages before hatching into parasitic adults. In warm areas, fleas may cause problems all year; in colder areas, they may be limited to summer and fall. Fleas do not hatch well in cold weather, low humidity, or high altitude.

Clinical Signs

Flea allergy dermatitis is a warm-weather disease that is usually seasonal (late spring to early winter) in cold areas, and nonseasonal in warm areas. In both dogs and cats the chief complaint is pruritus. In the dog, the pruritus primarily affects the posterior one third of the body, including the rump, tail base, perineal region, posterior and medial thighs, inguinal and umbilical region, or entire abdomen (Fig. 51-2). In a given patient from one to all of these areas (any combination) may be affected. The primary lesion noted is the papule, followed by secondary lesions of post-traumatic alopecia, excess scaling, excoriation, and, possibly, formation of hot spots. With chronicity, hyperpigmentation and lichenification may occur. Additionally in some canine patients there may be pruritus of the axillae, face, ears, or feet. This is especially common in patients with chronic disease, severe type I hypersensitivity reactions (positive immediate intradermal skin test reactors), or concurrent atopy or food allergies. A common complication is the development of pustules or epidermal collarettes, especially in the inguinal and abdominal region, indicating the presence of a secondary pyoderma.

In the cat, the pruritus most frequently affects the posterior one third of the body (Fig. 51-3), the entire dorsum, or the head and neck region. The primary lesion present in most cases is a small crusted papule (miliary lesion), followed by evidence of post-traumatic alopecia and excoria-

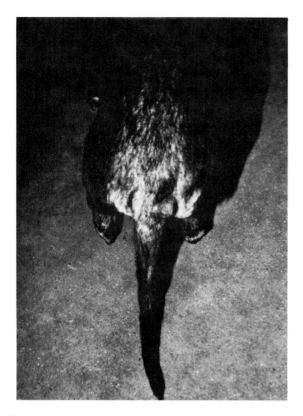

Figure 51–2. *Typical pattern of post-traumatic alopecia in a dog with flea allergy dermatitis.*

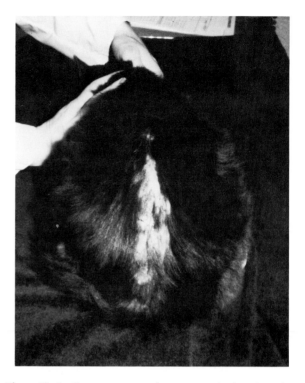

Figure 51–3. *Common pattern of post-traumatic alopecia and excoriations in a cat with flea allergy dermatitis.*

tions. For cats, flea allergy dermatitis is the number one cause of the miliary dermatitis reaction. In contrast to the dog, it is rare for the cat to develop hot spots, secondary pyoderma, hyperpigmentation, or lichenification. Occasionally, the only symptom is evidence of post-traumatic alopecia, especially of the ventral abdomen, flanks, or rump (see Chapter 49). In some patients there may be the formation of well-circumscribed, erythematous plaques on the ventral abdomen (Table 51-3 and Color Fig. 16).

Fleas and flea dirt (flea excrement) may or may not be obvious on the animal. Commonly (especially in cats), no evidence of fleas is found on the animal at the time of examination. The presence of *Dipylidium caninum* segments around the anus is an indication of past or present flea exposure, as the flea functions as the intermediate host for this tapeworm. However, pruritic alopecia of the posterior one third of the body should be considered flea allergy dermatitis until proven otherwise.

Once again, it is essential to realize that only the individuals (including all dogs, cats, and humans) in the same environment that are allergic to flea bites will show any significant pruritus or formation of primary lesions. The pet being presented to the veterinarian may indeed be the only one with a problem.

Table 51–3 *Skin Lesions That May Be Associated With Atopy, Flea Allergy Dermatitis, or Food Allergy in the Cat*

Lesion	Older Names for These Changes
Symmetrical alopecia on the ventral abdomen of cats	Feline endocrine alopecia Feline psychogenic alopecia
Papules with crusts, or "miliary" lesions	Miliary dermatitis
Indolent (rodent) ulcer, eosinophilic plaque, linear granuloma	Eosinophilic granuloma complex

Management

It is imperative that clients understand the flea life cycle so that they recognize the importance of eliminating the fleas in the pet's environment, not just on the pet itself. *Without exception*, flea treatment for an animal with flea allergy dermatitis *must* include treatment of the home, the affected pets, the unaffected dogs and cats in the environment, and often the yard as well. In warm areas, flea control or prevention will need to be continued throughout the life of the animal. Many different products are available for treatment of the pet and premises; treatment regimens may need to be tailored to fit the needs of the individual clients.

TREATING THE ANIMAL. The most commonly used flea products fall into two groups: carbamates or organophosphates (sustained action, higher potential for toxicity) and pyrethrins (short action, quick kill, low toxicity). Recently, the formulation of microencapsulated or stabilized synergized pyrethrins, and pyrethroids has offered the lower toxicity of pyrethrins and a more sustained duration of effect. When recommending a treatment program, clinicians must consider both duration of action and toxic potential of all products used; use of more than one product from the carbamate/organophosphate group on the same animal simultaneously is not recommended.

In cold climates, resistance to common flea products is not usually a problem. Therefore, most powders, sprays, and dips are adequate when used with adequate frequency and regularity. Animals with known flea allergy must be treated preventively for fleas during the appropriate seasons of every year, whether or not fleas are ever seen.

In warm climates, the flea population has developed resistance to many of the readily available flea chemicals. In these areas, regular dipping is the most effective way to control fleas on dogs; they may be dipped once every 3 to 4 weeks with an organophosphate dip. Organophosphate dips should not be used on cats; cats may be dipped with pyrethrin dips as directed by the manufacturer, or sprayed with pyrethrin and pyrethroid sprays twice weekly.

The following is a summary of available product modalities and their effectiveness:

Flea shampoos: These shampoos generally contain carbaryl or pyrethrins. These products should not be used in the treatment of the flea-allergic patient, since they have almost no residual action. However, bathing the pet does help soothe irritated skin, decreases seborrheic odor, and is useful on the first day of treatment in obviously flea-infected animals to remove the fleas for 1 to 2 days.

Flea dips: In most warm weather areas, flea dips are the basis of flea control. They often give the fastest and most complete flea elimination of all topical treatments. However, the duration of effectiveness of pyrethrin dips may be short, and the toxic potential of organophosphate dips is always a concern. Organophosphates are never used on cats.

Flea sprays: These are our treatment of choice for patients with flea bite hypersensitivity in cooler weather regions. While organophosphate sprays have the advantage of longer action, pyrethrin or pyrethroid sprays such as Sectrol and Duo-Cide L.A., SynerKyl have some degree of sustained activity, and they represent a very low toxic hazard. Therefore, with flea allergy dermatitis, in which more frequent spraying is desirable for a greater degree of protection, the pyrethrin/pyrethroid sprays are preferred. A light spraying is required every other day to twice weekly in dogs and twice weekly in cats during the entire flea season.

Flea powders: While they tend to be messy and impart a gritty texture to the haircoat, and dry the haircoat out with chronic use, flea powders may be preferred for some animals—particularly cats, who often object to the hiss of spray bottles and the wetting of their haircoat. Five-percent carbaryl powders should be applied every other day to twice weekly in dogs and twice weekly in cats. Diryl flea powder (5% carbaryl, 0.1% pyrethrin, 1% piperonyl butoxide) has been effective in this regimen. Powders are also useful for patients with a history of toxic reactions to various insecticides, as the powder vehicle allows minimal percutaneous or gastrointestinal absorption.

Percutaneous absorbable fenthion products: While these products (Pro-Spot, Spot-On) are effective in killing fleas and are widely used for flea treatment or prevention on nonallergic dogs, they are not the best alternative for flea-allergic dogs. These products are ingested by the flea as it takes a blood meal. Since the flea has to bite the dog in order to be killed, and since it is the flea saliva to which the dog is allergic, the patient will remain pruritic. Products that kill the flea prior to feeding are preferred for flea-allergic dogs. Only those products licensed for use in dogs should be used; these products should not be used on cats.

Flea collars: Flea collars (Escort) are acceptable for flea prevention in small dogs and cats. They are not strong enough and do not act quickly enough to treat an existing flea problem, nor are they effective in patients with a flea allergy. However, owners of small pets (less than 12 kg) find that they can avoid seasonal flea problems by prophylactically placing a fresh collar on their pets every 2 to 3 months from spring to early winter.

Oral flea products: Cythioate (Proban) flea pills are used successfully for flea prevention in some areas. Again, they do not work until the flea bites, so pets with flea allergy dermatitis will remain pruritic. Yeast, thiamine, and garlic products are not effective.

Electronic flea collars: Effectiveness in flea allergy dermatitis has not been demonstrated.

Hyposensitization: Based on studies and clinical experience, hyposensitization is insufficient as a sole method of treatment in the vast majority of cases. Therefore, it is only considered when all other types of management have failed.

TREATING THE HOUSE. Environmental treatment for fleas is just as important as treating the patient; pruritus will continue as long as fleas continue to hatch in the environment and pester pets. In cases of flea allergy dermatitis, the premises must always be treated for fleas. There are no exceptions! Since flea eradication is neither cheap nor easy, professional exterminators are often recommended. Clients should select an exterminator whose treatment methods affect adult, larval, and egg stages. One must be careful in selecting the exterminator to make certain that the chemicals used will not potentiate any toxicity of the flea products being used on the pets or the yard. In warm areas, treatment of the premises is often continued on a regular basis. Vacuuming is an important part of premise treatment. Vacuuming reduces the number of preadult fleas present, and facilitates eradication. Clients should dispose of vacuum bags immediately, or vacuum up a small amount of flea powder to kill fleas in the bag. Foggers and sprays can be effective if used in adequate amounts with appropriate frequency, but these require a diligent client to apply them, and the cost often approaches that of a professional exterminator.

TREATING THE YARD. During flea season it is recommended that small yards (those less than 1 acre in size and fenced) or outdoor kennels be treated with a yard and kennel spray (Sevin, Vet-Kem). These products are very effective but also very potent, and therefore the manufacturer's instructions should be followed carefully.

ADJUNCT SYMPTOMATIC THERAPY. Along with treatment related to eliminating and controlling the fleas themselves, most patients will initially require some symptomatic therapy to break the pruritus cycle. In dogs, prednisolone or prednisone can be given at an oral dosage of 0.5 mg/kg twice daily for 7 days, then 0.5 mg/kg once daily for 7 days, then 0.5 mg/kg every other day for 1 week, then stop and reevaluate response to flea treatment. If a secondary pyoderma or excess scaling is also present, then appropriate systemic antibiotics and antiseborrheic shampoos are also indicated (see Chapters 50 and 52).

For cats, prednisolone or prednisone can be given at a dosage of 1 mg/kg twice daily for 7 days, then 1 mg/kg once daily for 7 days, then 1 mg/kg every other day for 1 week, then stop and reevaluate response to flea treatment. If the owner cannot give the cat oral medication, a repositol corticosteroid can be used. Cats generally tolerate corticosteroids better than dogs, experiencing fewer harmful side-effects. Methylprednisolone acetate (Depo-Medrol) can be given once at a dosage of 2 to 3 mg/kg intramuscularly under these circumstances.

In summary, management of a patient with flea allergy dermatitis includes the following:

1. Extermination of fleas in the environment (house, basement, garage, dog house, kennel, yard, car), preferably by a professional exterminator
2. Regular application of an insecticide (spray, dip, or powder) on all contact dogs and cats, not just the allergic animal
3. Regular and thorough vacuuming of all floor surfaces and furniture

It is recommended that the veterinarian design a client education and flea treatment protocol sheet that can be handed to the owner, with specific instructions indicated for one's area.

Recurrence of a flea problem is usually immediately obvious, with return of the patient's pruritus. In most cases, preventive flea treatment is necessary for the entire flea season for the rest of the animal's life.

Tick Bite Hypersensitivity

Pathophysiology

Tick bites may result in a type III or IV hypersensitivity reaction. *Argasidae* (soft-bodied) ticks often infest premises occupied by the host, while *Ixodidae* (hard-bodied) ticks are acquired in open country and woods. Ticks are only moderately host-specific, and may affect dogs, cats, humans, wild mammals, and other domestic animals.

Clinical Signs

A hypersensitivity reaction to tick bites usually results in focal areas of ulceration and erythema, which may or may not form nodules. These lesions seem to be either painful or pruritic. Lesions may occur anywhere on the body, but most frequently occur interdigitally, at the base of the ear, in the external ear canal, or in the pinnae. Often, engorged female ticks or tiny seed ticks (nymphs) may be evident on the animal. Signs associated with tick paralysis, Lyme disease, Rocky Mountain spotted fever, ehrlichiosis, and babesiosis can be concurrent.

Management

For single or a few ticks, manual removal is sufficient. The tick should be soaked in alcohol to anesthetize it, then the mouth parts grasped close to the skin with a fine hemostat and the tick gently dislodged. Care should be exercised so as not to leave mouth parts embedded in the skin; infection may result. Ticks removed in this manner must be destroyed, or they will reinfest the environment. For severe or recurrent infestations, pyrethrin and organophosphate dips are available. Treatment of the inside environment and yard may be indicated (foggers or sprays), and

woods and open fields should be avoided. Control of wild host populations may be important in some instances.

Atopy (Allergic Inhalant Dermatitis, Atopic Dermatitis)

Pathophysiology

To state that the pathophysiology of canine atopy is currently undergoing reevaluation and is a very controversial subject would be an understatement. Even less is known about feline atopy. The most accepted theory is that canine atopy is a strikingly familial skin disease associated with immunoglobin E (IgE) production to various environmental allergens. The immunologic reaction involved in the development of atopy is believed to be the type I hypersensitivity reaction (immediate reaction). When a genetically predisposed dog is exposed to various environmental allergens, its immune system can become "sensitized," and specific IgE to that allergen is produced. The IgE is then bound to mast cells in connective tissue of the skin. After this has occurred, if a specific allergen finds its way to the allergen-specific IgE on the surface of a mast cell and bridges two adjacent IgE molecules, then degranulation of the mast cell occurs. At this time various preformed mediators of pruritus and inflammation are released, and initiation of the synthesis of additional mediators occurs. This reaction occurs within minutes of exposure to the antigen; it is the basis of how intra-skin testing is used to document the presence of a type I hypersensitivity reaction. How the allergen gains access to the IgE and mast cells in a dog is unknown, but absorption through the respiratory tract, skin, or gastrointestinal tract may be involved. Modifications of this reaction are believed to be involved in canine atopy, and include stimulation of mast cell degranulation by a subclass of immunoglobin G (IgGd) and a late-onset IgE-mediated reaction (occurring hours after exposure to a specific allergen rather than minutes). Other immunologic defects or mechanisms being investigated for their possible role in the development of canine atopy are defects in the population of suppressor and helper T lymphocytes involved in the initial processing of allergens, defects in the β-adrenergic surface receptors of mast cells, and defects in the enzymatic conversion of fatty acids (delta 6-desaturase defect).

An area of interest in human patients with atopic dermatitis is the documentation of increased adherence of staphylococci to the keratinocytes and the suppressed response of lymphocytes and neutrophils compared to the human patients without atopic dermatitis. If similar defects are found in canine patients with atopy, then this might help explain the frequent problem of recurrent secondary pyodermas observed in dogs with this disease.

Clinical Signs

The initial chief complaint of the canine patient with atopy is pruritus. This symptom usually occurs at between 1 and 3 years of age, and occurs with an increased frequency in females. Several breeds are predisposed to developing atopy: terriers (West Highland white, Cairn, Scottish, wirehaired fox, Boston), Dalmatians, Lhasa apsos, Irish setters, pugs, miniature schnauzers, English bulldogs, Labrador retrievers, and golden retrievers. Recent observations suggest that the Shar Pei, cocker spaniel, and German shepherd are at an increased risk. Another recent observation is the development of atopy in dogs younger than 1 year of age, especially in West Highland white terriers, golden retrievers, and Shar Peis.

Atopy typically presents as a warm-weather seasonal pruritus (spring, summer, fall); symptoms initially occur during pollen season in 75% to 80% of cases. This pattern is less apparent, however, in warmer climates, where pollination can occur on almost a year-round basis. The pattern often changes from a seasonal to a nonseasonal problem (or year-round problem), but exacerbation of pruritus is often still noticed in warmer weather (or times of increased pollination). The least common presentation for atopy is a nonseasonal (or year-round) pruritus from its onset.

The distribution pattern of pruritus in dogs with atopy includes the face, ears, feet, axillae, inguinal region, and anterior and proximal foreleg region (Color Fig. 17). Just one area may be affected, or any combination of these areas—up to all of them may be involved. For example, the only symptom of a patient with atopy might be a recurrent pruritic otitis externa, or a chronic foot-licking problem. Upon initial examination of the patient, especially in the early stages of the disease, the animal often appears to be free of lesions or mildly erythematous in the pruritic areas. As the pruritus continues, secondary lesions often develop, such as post-traumatic alopecia (Color Fig. 18), excoriations, hot spots, hyperpigmentation, lichenification, and salivary staining of the haircoat from excess licking (Color Fig. 19). Secondary complications of excess scaling (keratinization abnormality or seborrhea) and pyoderma are common. A change in the temperament of the dog may be noted, with the patient being more easily irritated. On rare occasions the patient may also have symptoms of sneezing or diarrhea that correspond to skin changes.

At this point in time, the possibility of feline atopy is under investigation. Various skin lesions in the cat and patterns of pruritus are not well understood. Skin tests are now being performed on cats more routinely. The goal is to look for documentation of a type I hypersensitivity reaction (intradermal skin testing) and then make a possible correlation of one's findings with the pathophysiology of pruritic skin diseases in the cat. Some of the pruritic problems in cats that may be initiated by a type I hypersensitivity reaction to environmental allergens are listed in Table 51-3. Current thoughts about these lesions in the cat are that they are only clinical signs, due to various underlying diseases. With this approach, diagnosis of the disease *miliary dermatitis* or *eosinophilic granuloma complex* based on the finding of a particular lesion is no longer valid. Not only cats with the lesion patterns described in Table 51-3, but those with facial, pinnal, pedal, or generalized pruritus are receiving intradermal skin testing and are being evaluated for the possibility of atopy as the underlying disease.

Management

Treatment of concurrent flea allergy dermatitis, secondary seborrhea, and secondary pyoderma must precede or coincide with the treatment of

Table 51–4 *Antihistamines Used for Control of Pruritus in the Dog*

Category	Generic Name	Brand Name	Oral Dosage
Ethanolamine	Diphenhydramine	Benadryl	2 mg/kg b.i.d.–t.i.d.
Alkylamine	Chlorpheniramine maleate	Chlor-Trimeton	0.5 mg/kg b.i.d.–t.i.d.
Piperazine	Hydroxyzine hydrochloride	Atarax	2 mg/kg b.i.d.–t.i.d.
Phenothiazine	Trimeprazine tartrate	Temaril	0.5 mg/kg b.i.d.
Piperidine	Cyproheptadine hydrochloride	Periactin	1 mg/kg b.i.d.–t.i.d.
Miscellaneous	Terfenadine	Seldane	4 to 10 mg/kg b.i.d.

atopy. Since these conditions independently produce pruritus, response to treatment cannot be evaluated while they are present.

Systemic corticosteroids form the basis of treatment for most seasonally atopic dogs. Most commonly recommended are prednisone or prednisolone at 0.5 mg/kg twice daily for 5 to 7 days, then 0.5 mg/kg once daily for 5 to 7 days, then 0.5 mg/kg every other day for 5 to 7 days, then tapering off to the lowest effective alternate-day dose. The dosage for cats is 1 mg/kg twice daily for 5 to 7 days, then 1 mg/kg once daily for 5 to 7 days, then 1 mg/kg every other day for 5 to 7 days, then tapering off to the lowest effective alternate-day dose. Longer-acting oral corticosteroids (dexamethasone, triamcinolone) and injectable corticosteroids (betamethasone, methylprednisolone acetate) are not recommended for long-term use due to their suppressive effects on the adrenal glands and their greater potential for inducing iatrogenic Cushing's syndrome (see Chapter 59 and Appendix II).

Many other symptomatic treatments are available for mild or short seasonal atopy problems. In the dog, fatty acid supplements (Derm Caps, EfaVet, Efa-Z Plus, NutriSol EFA) and antihistamines have shown some efficacy, and may be helpful as sole treatment or an adjunct to other treatments (Table 51-4 and Appendix II). We have observed the best responses to the use of Atarax and Temaril.

In cats, the most commonly used nonsteroidal anti-inflammatory agent is chlorpheniramine maleate, at a dosage of 2 to 4 mg twice daily.

Recently, fatty acid supplements have been examined for their possible antipruritic effects in cats; they have been observed to occasionally be of benefit.

The antipruritic value of baths, emollients, and rinses makes them useful in combination with other systemic treatments. They are also desirable when systemic medications are contraindicated owing to undesirable side-effects or during periods of drug withdrawal in preparation for intradermal skin testing. Bathing the pet with a mild shampoo in cool water, then spraying or rinsing with a coat conditioner often yields 1 to 3 days of an antipruritic effect (Table 51-5).

For patients with nonseasonal or uncontrollable pruritus due to atopy, hyposensitization therapy is recommended. Approximately 70% of canine patients benefit from hyposensitization therapy within 6 to 12 months.

Hyposensitization therapy is based on the theory of "blocking antibodies." It is believed that subcutaneous injections of antigen stimulate production of IgG antibodies, which bind the absorbed allergens before they can reach the IgE antibodies fixed to mast cells in the skin. Twelve

Table 51–5 *Topical Adjunct Antipruritic Therapy*

Hypoallergenic Shampoo	Conditioner	Rinse
Allergroom	Humilac	Colloidal oatmeal bath
HyLyt efa	HyLyt efa	(Aveeno—powdered form)

or fewer of the most significant allergens are selected, as indicated by the patient's history and intradermal skin test results. Owner compliance is very important, since the dog will usually need to have monthly injections for life. Figure 51-4 indicates the injection protocol we use, which utilizes aqueous allergens.

In general, the long-term goal is to give only 1 ml of allergens from the maintenance vial every 30 days for life. However, to achieve an optimum response to hyposensitization injections, this protocol often has to be modified for each individual.

The frequency of injections may need to be increased or decreased during different times of the year with different environmental allergen levels. The volume of allergen administered may also need to be decreased, especially if the injections result in exacerbation of clinical signs or cause untoward reactions (Table 51-6). When a patient has not responded optimally to a standard injection protocol, it is best to consult with a specialist experienced in hyposensitization of animals for recommendations on how to best modify the protocol. For patients whose response to hyposensi-

Vial #1 (200 PNU/ml)			Vial #3 (20,000 PNU/ml)		
Day	Date	Amount	Day	Date	Amount
0	_____	0.1 ml	20	_____	0.1 ml
2	_____	0.2 ml	22	_____	0.2 ml
4	_____	0.4 ml	24	_____	0.4 ml
6	_____	0.8 ml	26	_____	0.8 ml
8	_____	1.0 ml	28*	_____	1.0 ml

Vial #2 (2000 PNU/ml)			Maintenance Vial (Vial #3, 20,000 PNU/ml)		
Day	Date	Amount	Day	Date	Amount
10	_____	0.1 ml	35	_____	1 ml
12	_____	0.2 ml	42	_____	1 ml
14	_____	0.4 ml	56	_____	1 ml
16	_____	0.8 ml	70	_____	1 ml
18	_____	1.0 ml	91	_____	1 ml
			112	_____	1 ml
			142	_____	1 ml

Then 1 ml once monthly for life.

*Please schedule an appointment for reevaluation.

EXTRACTS MUST BE KEPT REFRIGERATED.

Observe for any abnormal reactions, such as swelling or redness at injection sites, worsening of itching, difficulties in breathing, or irritability.

Give injections subcutaneously.

Figure 51–4. *Aqueous hyposensitization protocol used by the authors. (PNU = protein nitrogen unit)*

Table 51–6 *Adverse Reactions Observed to Hyposensitization Injections in the Dog*

Reaction	Frequency
Exacerbation of previous clinical signs (especially pruritus)	Common—especially during the first month of hyposensitization
Local reaction (pain, pruritus, erythema, swelling) at injection site	Rare
Urticaria or angioedema	Rare
Vomiting or diarrhea	Rare
Nervousness or excitability	Rare
Anaphylaxis	Extremely rare

tization is incomplete, antihistamines, corticosteroids, fatty acid supplements, and topical adjuncts may be used concurrently.

Food Allergy

Pathophysiology

The definitive pathologic mechanisms involved in the development of a food allergy in dogs and cats is unknown. Type I hypersensitivity reactions to foods have been well documented in humans, and type III and IV reactions have been suspected of playing a role in some food-allergic patients. However, the involvement of these immunologic reactions in the development of food allergy in the dog and cat have not yet been demonstrated.

Numerous items are capable of inducing the allergic response, and the culprit is usually one or more of the items found in commercially prepared canned or dry diets. Since commercially prepared diets are a veritable potpourri of possible allergens, it is impossible to make an educated guess as to the offending agent. The offending allergen may be any of the sources of protein or carbohydrate in the diet or the variety of food additives and preservatives. These ingredients are common to most commercial dog and cat food products; accordingly, owners of food-allergic pets often report that the symptoms of hypersensitivity persist regardless of the brand of commercial diet fed. Furthermore, since prior sensitiza-

tion is required, it is not surprising that most owners report that their pets were eating the same diet for several years prior to the onset of signs.

Clinical Signs

There does not appear to be a sex predilection for the development of food allergy in the dog and cat, but we have observed an increased incidence of the disease in the Labrador retriever, cocker and springer spaniels, West Highland white terrier, collie, and miniature schnauzer, In the dog, the age of onset of the disease is usually less than 3 years. The clinical signs of food allergy are variable, and include pruritus or dermatitis only, diarrhea only, or both reactions simultaneously.

In the dog and cat, when dermatologic signs are present the chief complaint is pruritus that has been nonseasonal since the onset. This occurs due to the similar diet regimens usually fed throughout the year. The distribution pattern of pruritus and lesions in the dog is extremely variable, and can imitate the appearance of virtually any pruritic skin disease (especially scabies, atopy, recurrent bacterial folliculitis, and recurrent otitis externa). The most commonly affected areas include the ears (Color Fig. 20), inguinal and axillary region, proximal and anterior foreleg region, and face. The lesions present on physical examination are also quite variable. They may include any combination of the following: erythema, post-traumatic alopecia, hot spots, papules, hyperpigmentation, lichenification, or otitis externa. Less often observed is either urticaria or angioedema. On rare occasions, seizures or respiratory signs may also be a symptom associated with a food allergy. Secondary pyoderma in the form of bacterial folliculitis and secondary seborrhea (keratinization abnormality) are common features in dogs.

In the cat, the lesions present and the distribution pattern of pruritus is more predictable. Most commonly affected are the ears, face, and neck region, with varying degrees of papules with crusts (miliary lesions) and excoriations. A common feature is the development of papules and crusts in a symmetrical bandlike pattern between the base of the ears and the lateral canthus of the eyes (Color Fig. 21). Occasionally, a cat may show a somewhat generalized pruritus as well as the patterns mentioned in Table 51-3.

Management

Management consists of eliminating the offending allergens from the diet. Commercial "hypoallergenic" diets are available that lack beef, egg, poultry, soy, corn, and preservatives. The following diets may be considered for use as the treatment diet, but not as the elimination diet for establishing the diagnosis: Anergen Diet (Wysong), Hill's Prescription Diet d/d (canned or dry); Nature's Recipe lamb-based diet, Cornucopia natural pet foods, and Nutro Max Kibble dog food. Rarely, no suitable commercial diet is available and pets need to be maintained on home-cooked fresh food; it has been postulated that these pets are intolerant of some ingredient obtained during the processing of the food.

Pets must be kept on a diet free from offending allergens for life, with special attention paid to treats and table scraps. Occasionally, an animal will develop additional food allergies after being stabilized, requiring additional dietary changes over time. As always, any secondary pyoderma or seborrhea must be treated concurrently for optimum results.

Irritant Contact Dermatitis

Pathophysiology

Although this disease is not initiated by the immune system, the immune system certainly contributes to the reaction observed subsequent to contact of the skin with an agent. It is presented here for contrast with allergic contact dermatitis. Irritant contact dermatitis is caused by the irritant nature of an agent that comes in contact with skin, resulting in the dermatitis reaction. In contrast to allergic contact dermatitis, irritant contact dermatitis does not represent a hypersensitivity reaction. Therefore, it requires no prior exposure and has no hereditary component—any individual may experience skin irritation.

Commonly implicated agents include acids, alkalis, soaps, detergents, floor waxes, petroleum, fertilizers, insect sprays, and selenium disulfide.

Absolute primary irritants injure the skin immediately; relative irritants are less toxic, and may require repeated contact to manifest irritation.

Clinical Signs

Pain and pruritus are usually acute in onset. Erythema, exudation, and erosions (sometimes papules and vesicles) are evident on contact areas of the body, including the abdomen, chest, perineum, flanks, axillae, ventrum of tail base, scrotum or vulva, foot pads, interdigital spaces, and, occasionally, ears and chin.

Management

Treatment of irritant contact dermatitis consists of removal of the offending agent and symptomatic care for the injured skin. Immediate cleansing with a hypoallergenic shampoo (Allergroom, HyLyt efa) is important to halt irritation. Topical and systemic corticosteroids, astringents (Domeboro), and antibiotics are used as needed.

Allergic Contact Dermatitis

Pathophysiology

Allergic contact dermatitis represents a type IV hypersensitivity reaction (delayed reaction); it requires previous sensitization and subsequent challenge. In most cases, the offending agent is believed to be a hapten (incomplete antigen) that becomes antigenic when it combines with tissue protein. In humans, the complete antigen is then processed by the Langerhans' cells and presented to the T lymphocyte system, resulting in "sensitized" T lymphocytes. Upon subsequent exposure to the offending allergen, these sensitized T cells release various lymphokines, which attract lymphocytes and macrophages to the area of exposure to the contact allergen, with subsequent inflammation and tissue damage. This reaction occurs over a 24- to 72-hour time period. Contact allergic dermatitis occurs much less frequently in dogs and cats than in humans, and it is not certain whether the exact same immunologic mechanisms are involved. Some of the more commonly implicated agents include wool, nylon, cedar chips, flea collars, topical medications, leather and metal collars, cat litter, fertilizers, vinyl resins in food dishes, poison oak, poison ivy, pine needles, wandering Jew, jasmine blossoms, grasses and weeds, dips, sprays, powders, detergents, finishes, polishes, and cleansers.

Clinical Signs

The clinical signs and description to follow apply primarily to dogs with allergic contact dermatitis, as this disease is exceedingly rare in the cat. We have observed an increased incidence of this disease in Labrador retrievers.

Pruritus, erythema, papules, hyperpigmentation, and lichenification may be seasonal or nonseasonal, depending on the allergen. Secondary seborrhea or pyoderma are common. Contact areas, which may include any combination of the following areas, are affected: abdomen, chest, axillae, flanks, perineum, scrotum or vulva, ventrum of tail base, and, occasionally, ears and chin. Interdigital areas are often affected, but not the footpads. In contrast to many of the other pruritic skin diseases, severe hyperpigmentation and lichenification tend to occur frequently in a relatively short period of time.

Management

Avoidance is the key to resolving allergic contact dermatitis once the agent has been identified; hyposensitization is not successful. Topical or systemic corticosteroids and treatment of secondary pyoderma or seborrhea are indicated when initiating therapy.

Since a chronic dermatitis reaction and secondary pyoderma are common with this disease, the initial symptomatic treatment with steroids and antibiotics often needs to last for 4 to 6 weeks. When the offending allergen cannot be avoided, then lifelong and continuous symptomatic therapy is, unfortunately, the remaining alternative. Usually prednisone or prednisolone is given to dogs at a dosage of 0.5 mg/kg twice daily for 10 days, then 0.5 mg/kg once daily for 10 days, then 0.5 mg/kg every other day for 10 days; the dosage is then gradually decreased to the lowest possible effective dose and given on an alternate-day basis. It is not known how effective the nonsteroidal anti-inflammatory drugs are for this disease, but they are certainly worth considering before deciding to use corticosteroids for the life of the dog (see section on Atopy).

Acute Moist Dermatitis (Pyotraumatic Dermatitis, Hot Spots) and Pyotraumatic Folliculitis

Pathophysiology

Although this disease is not primarily mediated by the immune system, it is included in this section because it is most often seen in patients with allergic skin diseases. In most instances it is agreed that canine hot spots are acutely developing lesions that are the result of focal self-trauma due to an underlying pruritic or painful process. However, some discrepancies in this concept include the fact that many patients experiencing extreme pruritus and self-trauma never develop hot spots, and that occasionally a hot spot seems to occur spontaneously, without any observed self-trauma. The lesion is a superficial erosive, ulcerative, and inflammatory process with a surface colonization of typically coagulase-positive staphylococci (especially *Staphylococcus intermedius*) or a true hot spot. In some instances, lesions that look clinically like hot spots, but are refractory to conventional therapy, have been shown to be associated with a deeper pyogenic process. Such lesions involve a true bacterial folliculitis and furunculosis due to coagulase-positive staphylococci, and are referred to as *pyotraumatic folliculitis*.

Hot spots occur most commonly in thick- and long-coated breeds of dogs during hot, humid weather, suggesting that environmental factors may also play a role. In most cases, an underlying disease process can be identified as the initiating cause of the hot spot (Table 51-7), with the most common cause being flea allergy dermatitis.

Clinical Signs

True acute moist dermatitis occurs most frequently as a single lesion over the rump region in thick- or long-coated breeds of dogs such as the golden retriever, Labrador retriever, Saint Bernard, Old English sheepdog, collie, German shep-

Table 51–7 *Conditions That May Be Associated With the Development of Hot Spots*

Disease Category	Examples
Allergic skin diseases	Flea allergy dermatitis
	Atopy
	Food allergy
	Allergic contact dermatitis
	Staphylococcal hypersensitivity
Ectoparasites	Canine scabies
	Cheyletiellosis
Otitis externa	Allergic otitis externa
	Ceruminous otitis externa
Environmental causes	Irritant contact dermatitis
	Poor grooming
	Burs or plant awns in the skin or hair coat
Musculoskeletal disorders	Hip dysplasia
	Degenerative joint disease
	Potentially any arthritis
Anal sac problems	Impacted anal sacs
	Anal sacculitis

herd, and Newfoundland. The affected area is very pruritic or painful, and has a characteristic appearance of a circumscribed, thickened, erythematous, and erosive lesion with a thin exudative film over the surface, with the hairs being frequently matted into the lesion (Color Fig. 22). The lesion develops acutely, going from normal skin to a lesion within hours.

Pyotraumatic folliculitis occurs most frequently over the cheek region (unilateral or bilateral), and may extend over the top of the head. The breeds most often affected are golden retrievers, Saint Bernards, and Bouviers. The lesion develops in a similar fashion to the hot spot, and at first glance looks identical to a hot spot. Closer inspection after clipping usually reveals the presence of large follicular papules at the margins of the lesion.

Management

For either true acute moist dermatitis or pyotraumatic folliculitis, the lesion should first be gently clipped free of hair in and around the lesion. This may require sedation or anesthesia in some patients when the lesion is extremely painful. The lesion is then gently cleansed with water and an antiseptic shampoo such as Betadine sur-

gical scrub, and gently patted dry. An astringent such as Burows solution (Domeboro powder and water) or DermaCool is then applied, and the lesion is allowed to dry. Since there is much pain or pruritus associated with this lesion and since many of the underlying causes are allergic in nature, corticosteroids are indicated. For rapid relief, injectable prednisolone can be administered in the form of prednisolone sodium phosphate in aqueous suspension at a dosage of 0.5 mg/kg intramuscularly. This is then followed the next day with oral prednisolone at a dosage of 0.5 mg/kg twice daily for 5 to 7 days, then 0.5 mg/kg once daily for 5 to 7 days. A topical antibiotic or steroid cream (not an ointment, which is occlusive) such as Panalog cream may be applied to the lesion twice daily for 5 to 10 days.

When a pyotraumatic folliculitis is present, it is essential that appropriate systemic antibiotics be given simultaneously. This regimen is usually 21 days; it should be continued for 1 week beyond the apparent clinical remission.

Most hot spots are secondary to an underlying problem (see Table 51-7). These problems should be investigated thoroughly and treated simultaneously once identified.

DIAGNOSTIC APPROACH

Diagnosis of pruritic skin diseases can be frustrating for veterinarians and clients alike. Constant licking and scratching on the part of their pet can lead to impatience on the part of the owners. Time pressures and the intensive physical examination and history needed to identify subtle differences in distribution patterns can tempt veterinarians to reach for the cortisone bottle instead of the diagnostic workup sheet. However, it is in the best interest of all concerned to identify the underlying causes of the itch and begin specific treatment.

History

Perhaps nowhere else is the history as singularly important as in the diagnosis of pruritus. Determining the presence or absence of seasonality is of major importance. Owners may be unaware of a seasonal pattern even when one exists; excellent history-taking skills may be necessary to jog the client's memory (Table 51-8).

Progression of pruritus and skin lesions is also important. Specifically where it started, how it appeared, and how it spread must be ascertained. "She itches all over" is usually not an acceptable answer, as hardly any skin diseases are manifested in this manner (especially initially).

Treatments attempted, and response to those treatments, may add valuable clues and prevent duplication of effort. An important clue is that atopy in general is one of the most dramatically responsive diseases to antipruritic dosages of prednisolone or prednisone, especially when it is first treated. The other pruritic skin diseases share a less predictable response (Table 51-9). Therefore, if one has made a primary diagnosis of atopy but the response to corticosteroids is poor, one should immediately reevaluate the diagnosis. In recurrent pruritic skin diseases with a pyoderma component, it is essential to treat the patient with an appropriate systemic antibiotic alone (rather than steroids alone or steroids and antibiotics concurrently) and to observe the response for clues to the likely underlying disease (see Chapter 52).

Involvement of other animals or humans in the household should be questioned, and when present one should consider contagious skin diseases such as sarcoptic mange, notoedric mange, and cheyletiellosis.

Table 51–8 *History of Pruritus*

Description of Pruritus	What to Look For
Initial seasonal pruritus that may or may not become nonseasonal over time	Flea allergy dermatitis Atopy Tick bite hypersensitivity Allergic contact dermatitis Fly bite dermatitis
Nonseasonal pruritus from the onset	Food allergy Sarcoptic mange Cheyletiellosis Notoedric mange Demodicosis Allergic contact dermatitis Staphylococcal hypersensitivity
Pruritus developing in an animal younger than 6 months of age	Sarcoptic mange Cheyletiellosis Notoedric mange Demodicosis Otodectic mange Food allergy
Severe pruritus	Sarcoptic mange Notoedric mange Allergic contact dermatitis

Table 51–9 *Summary of Some Common Canine Pruritic Skin Diseases*

Diagnosis	Distribution Pattern	Breed Predisposition	Age of Onset	Seasonality	Response to Corticosteroids
Flea allergy dermatitis	Caudal one third of the body	All breeds	1 to 3 years	Usually initially a warm weather seasonal problem	+/−
Atopy	Face, feet, ears, axillae, abdomen, proximal and anterior foreleg	Many, especially terriers	1 to 3 years	75% to 80% are initially a warm weather seasonal problem	+++
Food allergy	Any, but often affects ears, feet, inguinal and axillary region, proximal and anterior foreleg, and face	Any breed, especially Labrador retriever, Cocker and Springer spaniel, West Highland white terrier, Collie and Miniature Schnauzer	Usually less than 3 years	Nonseasonal from the onset	+/−
Scabies	Margins of pinnae, elbows, hocks	Any	Young (or any age)	Nonseasonal from the onset	+/−
Allergic contact dermatitis	Abdomen, axillae, scrotum or vulva, perianal or perineal region, ventrum of tail base, interdigital skin	Labrador retriever	Any	Depends on allergen (a grass vs. an indoor carpet)	+/−

(+ = responds to corticosteroids; − = does not respond to corticosteroids.)

Pattern of Distribution

In determining the pattern of distribution of pruritus, important clues include historical observations and the distribution of primary and secondary lesions (especially post-traumatic alopecia and salivary staining of the hair) at the time of the examination.

Flea allergy dermatitis is the most common cause of pruritus. In dogs, this is usually most severe over the caudal and dorsal one third of the body (rump and tailhead; may include the inguinal region and medial thighs). In cats, a similar pattern is usually observed, and the head and neck area may also be involved (see Table 51-3). This distribution pattern of pruritus is very important, as fleas or flea dirt may or may not be present at the time of examination. Pruritus of this area should be considered flea allergy dermatitis until proven otherwise.

Atopy in the dog may be manifest as pruritus in any or all of the following areas: feet, face (muzzle and periocular), ears, axillae, inguinal area, and anterior and proximal foreleg region. These areas are collectively referred to as the *type I hypersensitivity distribution pattern*. Of course, other type I hypersensitivities (*e.g.*, food allergy) may follow the same distribution pattern. For patterns in the cat see Table 51-3 and the Atopy section, earlier, under Clinical Signs.

Food allergy in the dog has traditionally been considered to have that elusive distribution pattern called "any." However, we have noted a tendency for canine food allergy to affect the ears, feet, inguinal and axillary region, proximal and anterior foreleg region, and face. Feline food allergy most often affects the ears, head, and neck region (see Table 51-3).

Allergic contact dermatitis and irritant contact dermatitis affect areas that contact causative agents (usually some combination of the abdomen, axillae, feet, vulva or scrotum, perianal area, ventrum of tail base, chin, and ears). As a rule, allergic contact dermatitis spares the footpads and affects interdigital skin, while irritant contact dermatitis involves the footpads.

Canine scabies initially involves the margins of the ear pinnae, elbows, and hocks; left untreated, it may progress to involve the entire ventrum.

Pruritus associated with *Otodectes* mites is not necessarily confined to the ear area; mites and pruritus may be found on the neck or trunk, as well. See Table 51-9 for a summary of some of the more common canine pruritic skin diseases.

Physical Examination

A thorough physical examination can confirm several causes of pruritus. Fleas or flea dirt are most commonly found in the rump area, but may be beneath the tail or in the inguinal area as well. Flea dirt may be distinguished from other dark granules by placing it on a moist paper towel; flea dirt "runs red," since it is composed of digested blood.

Ticks may be present, especially in ears, poorly haired areas, and interdigital areas.

Cheyletiellosis may present as flaking of the dorsal midline ("walking dandruff") or pruritic skin disease (see Chapter 50).

Otodectes mites may be visible on otoscopic examination; they are often associated with brown, "coffee ground" exudate in the ear canal.

"Fly bite ears" have a characteristic appearance. Alopecia and dark, hemorrhagic crusts are present at the tips of the ear pinnae or at the folded edge in flop-eared breeds.

Hot spots are identified on physical examination by their characteristic appearance and history. These circumscribed areas of erythema and exudation are fiercely pruritic or painful, may be alopecic, and may contain areas of matted hair.

Diagnostic Tests

Skin Scraping

Microscopic examination of skin scrapings may show mites or eggs of *Cheyletiella*, *Notoedres*, or *Sarcoptes* parasites. While *Notoedres* and *Cheyletiella* mites are relatively easy to find, *Sarcoptes* mites are relatively difficult; therefore, a high index of suspicion warrants treatment for scabies whether or not mites are found on skin scrapings. The diagnosis may be confirmed by response to treatment (see Chapter 49).

Ear Scratch Test

Dogs suspected of having pruritic pinnae should have the ear pinna folded over on itself and the two edges rubbed together to observe for a scratching response of the dog's hind leg. This *positive ear scratch test* is considered suggestive of scabies, but can also be observed in diseases such as atopy, food allergy, otodectic mange, and fly bite dermatitis.

Scotch Tape Prep

This technique is especially helpful for *Cheyletiella* mites, which are the most superficial dwellers of the skin mites. A 10 × 10 cm area of hair is clipped along the dorsum in a region of excessive scaling. A piece of clear Scotch tape (not the frosted type) is repeatedly pressed over the area, sticky side down, to collect flakes and mites. The scotch tape is then placed on a thin film of mineral oil, debris-side down, on a microscope slide, and examined for mites and eggs.

Vacuum Technique

This is a good concentrating technique for detection of fleas and surface-dwelling parasites. Using a vacuum cleaner with an extension hose, a piece of standard filter paper is placed between the attachment parts (nozzle) and the hose. Then the pet is vacuumed well. Debris collected is scraped into a centrifuge tube with a standard fecal flotation solution and centrifuged. Mites, fleas, and eggs will float to the top, and can be transferred to a microscope slide for identification.

Fecal Analysis

Routine fecal analysis may be helpful in the diagnosis of pruritic skin disease. Intestinal parasites, including hookworms, roundworms, and whipworms, may be associated with intestinal parasite hypersensitivity reactions. *Dipylidium caninum* eggs or segments indicate past or present flea infestation, and fleas or flea eggs may occasionally show up in the stool. Other parasites that may occasionally be noted in the stool (due to ingestion by the pet licking or biting at pruritic skin) include *Cheyletiella*, *Sarcoptes*, and *Notoedres* eggs and mites.

Intradermal Skin Test

Intradermal skin testing is used to diagnose atopy and flea allergy dermatitis. At this time, successful testing with food antigens has not been demonstrated in animals. Injection of various allergens tests intradermally for the presence of IgE to the particular allergens in an animal's skin. If allergen-specific IgE is present, the formation of a wheal will occur due to the degranulation of mast cells. The patient should be taken off of any antipruritic drugs for an adequate length of time before intradermal skin testing is performed (Table 51-10).

Using saline as a negative control (0) and histamine as a positive control (4+), graded responses (0 to 4+) are determined for each antigen. Responses of 2+ or greater are considered potentially significant; they are evaluated in light of the patient's historical development of the problem and sources of possible exposure to the allergen. Spring allergens (trees), late spring and early summer allergens (grasses), summer and fall allergens (weeds, especially ragweed), and non-

Table 51–10 *Recommendations on Drug Withdrawal Times Before Performing Intradermal Skin Testing*

Drug	Recommended Minimum Withdrawal Time
Antihistamines, aspirin, essential fatty acid supplements	14 days
Progesterones, estrogens, and testosterones	
Oral form	30 days
Repositol injections	90 days
Oral corticosteroids	30 days
Injectable corticosteroids	
Dexamethasone (Azium)	30 days
Triamcinolone (Vetalog)	30 days
Methylprednisolone acetate (Depo-Medrol)	90 days
Betamethasone sodium phosphate (Betasone)	90 days
Topical corticosteroids	30 days

seasonal allergens (molds, housedust, and other indoor allergens) are considered significant only if they meet both of the following criteria: their wheal is 2+ or greater and their seasonality fits with the history of the patient's pruritus. If either criterion is missing, additional workup should be pursued for other possible sources of pruritus.

Because of the expense of testing allergens, their short shelf life, and the technical expertise required to supervise skin testing and hyposensitization, intradermal skin testing is not economically feasible for most private practices. Exceptions include practices with large caseloads and referral situations. Therefore, it is advantageous if a veterinarian with training in this area can work with other local veterinarians on a referral basis and concentrate his or her time in this specialty.

For owners who experience difficulty in accepting the reality and degree of the pet's allergy to fleas, a positive "mini" skin test of only saline, histamine, and flea antigen may help reinforce the significance of unseen fleas to their pets. The flea skin test site should be observed at 15 to 20 minutes (immediate reaction) and over the next 48 hours (delayed reaction) after the test is performed.

RAST and ELISA Tests

The radioallergosorbent test (RAST) and the enzyme-linked immunosorbent assay (ELISA) are in vitro tests for determination of IgE levels to inhalant, food, and insect antigens. While the technique used is appealing due to the ease of performance (serologic tests mailed to a laboratory), consistency and reliability of the results are currently hindering the tests' widespread use. While the results may be used in combination with intradermal skin testing and accurate dietary trials, the RAST and ELISA are not recommended as sole diagnostic methods at this time.

Elimination Diet

At this time, an elimination diet trial is the most accurate way to diagnose food allergy in dogs and cats. An elimination diet is severely restricted, and generally consists of rice or potatoes and a protein source to which the animal has never been exposed (usually lamb, rabbit, or venison). The diet is not well balanced, and it is not intended for long-term or maintenance use. It should not be fed to animals younger than 6 months of age due to its poor mineral balance. During the trial nothing should pass the animal's lips except the elimination diet and water. This requires cessation of the feeding of table scraps, pet treats, chewable heartworm preventive medication, chewable vitamin and mineral supplements, fatty acid dietary supplements, and rawhide chew toys. If a favorable response to the diet occurs (cessation in pruritus), then refeeding of the original diet is recommended for 7 days. This usually results in a return of the pruritus within 2 to 3 days, which confirms that food was the cause of the pruritus.

The most commonly used elimination diet in dogs is home-cooked lamb (rabbit or venison may be used if the patient has eaten lamb before) and white rice (not instant) in a 50:50 mixture (boil each until cooked in plain water with no salt or seasoning; the amount fed should approximate in volume what the patient would eat in commercial food). For cats the best diet is home-cooked lamb or rabbit alone, since cats will rarely eat rice. No taurine supplementation is necessary, as these freshly prepared meats have adequate taurine levels.

The elimination diet trial should be set up to run for up to 60 days. The animal should be rechecked or the client contacted for a progress report after 1 week, 30 days, and 60 days of the trial. Possibly due to the variability of immunologic mechanisms involved in a food allergy in a given patient, the animal may show a noticeable decrease in pruritus after 1 week, 3 weeks, 4 to 6 weeks, or 7 to 8 weeks of the diet trial. We have observed three instances in a dog and one instance in a cat where complete cessation of pruritus was not observed until the diet had been fed for 10 weeks!

When improvement is seen with the elimination diet, individual ingredients may be added back to the diet, one at a time, at a rate of one new allergen per week. The patient's sensitivity profile is outlined in this manner (add back beef one week, chicken one week, corn one week, and so on).

It is often important to explain to the client the difference between the elimination diet and a hypoallergenic diet. The elimination diet is a diagnostic tool used to identify the presence of a food allergy. Once the diagnosis is made, different types of diets that are hypoallergenic for the individual patient may be fed. These diets omit various ingredients, according to the pet's individual hypersensitivity (*e.g.*, preservatives, beef, poultry, egg, wheat, corn, soy, fish, dairy products). Switching commercial diets is not sufficient for diagnosis of food allergy due to the large numbers of ingredients and the similarity of ingredients among different brands. Furthermore, processed diets formulated from lamb and rice are not sufficient in the diagnostic phase, since some patients will improve on a home-cooked diet that will not benefit from the same ingredients when they come out of a can or a bag.

Patch Test

Patch testing is the diagnostic method of choice for allergic contact dermatitis. Difficulties in gathering sufficient samples from the environment of allergic pets and the technical difficulty involved in keeping multiple allergens in close contact with a designated area of the dog's skin have limited its widespread use. However, with a little ingenuity and persistence, patch testing can be performed. The owner collects small samples from the environment (both indoor and outdoor) that the animal is known to come in contact with. Both sides of the chest are shaved and the samples taped to the skin under individual Telfa pads. A chest wrap of gauze and tape is then secured.

The samples are kept in place for 72 hours and then removed to look for evidence of erythema, papules, vesicles, and edema. Recently, a commercial kit has become available (Finn Chambers on Scanpor and allergens supplied by Hermal Labs) that may standardize the tests and facilitate ease of performance. This kit uses small aluminum reservoirs fixed on hypoallergenic adhesive patches to hold petrolatum-based allergens in contact with the shaved lateral thorax for 48 hours; positive results of erythema, edema, induration, and vesiculation are read 30 minutes after removal of reservoirs and adhesive.

Environmental Deprivation and Challenge Testing

Dusts and molds can be irritating when injected intradermally for allergy testing, potentially giving false-positive reactions. Therefore, when they appear to represent the only hypersensitivity responsible for a case of pruritus, after food allergy has been ruled out, confirmation of the diagnosis is recommended.

The environmental deprivation and challenge test is based on the observation that patients with suspected and skin test-positive dust and mold allergies showed decreased pruritus when hospitalized and that pruritus was exacerbated when they returned to the home environment. It was postulated that the continuous cleaning with fungistatic agents and the smooth, nonupholstered surfaces found in hospital situations created an environment with decreased dust and mold spore concentrations.

In this test, patients are hospitalized for 7 days. If dust and mold allergies are indeed the source of the problem, the animal's pruritus is usually markedly decreased within 3 to 5 days, and acute exacerbation occurs within minutes of returning to the home environment. If the remission–exacerbation pattern does not occur, reevaluation of the diagnosis is recommended. It is important that the patient be fed its usual diet during this trial.

When these rapid changes are observed it is our opinion that a contact allergic dermatitis reaction is unlikely to be the cause of the problem. In general, patients with contact allergic dermatitis have chronic dermatitis reactions; they do not show a noticeable change in pruritus within 7 days and the pruritus takes hours to days to become exacerbated when reentering the home.

ADDITIONAL READING

Halliwell REW, Gorman NT, eds. Veterinary clinical immunology. Philadelphia: WB Saunders, 1989.
MacDonald JM, Miller TA. Parasiticide therapy in small animal dermatology. In: Kirk RW, ed. Current veterinary therapy IX. Philadelphia: WB Saunders, 1986: 571.

Reedy LM, Miller WH. Allergic skin diseases of dogs and cats. Philadelphia: WB Saunders, 1989.

Reinke SJ, Stannard AA, Ihrke PJ, Reinke JD. Histopathologic features of pyotraumatic dermatitis. J Am Vet Med Assoc 1987; 190:57.

Rosser EJ. Antipruritic drugs. Vet Clin North Am [Small Anim Pract] 1988; 18:1093.

White SD. Food hypersensitivity in 30 dogs. J Am Vet Med Assoc 1986; 7:695.

52

PAPULAR/PUSTULAR, VESICULAR/BULLOUS, AND EROSIVE/ULCERATIVE DERMATOSES

Edmund J. Rosser, Jr., Ann Washabaugh Sams

This chapter will address dermatologic diseases that have as their first symptom the presence of a primary lesion such as a papule, pustule, vesicle, or bulla. In many of the diseases to be discussed these primary lesions are often a transient event. However, after they have ruptured, a hallmark of their previous existence will be evident in the presence of an erosion, ulcer, crust, or epidermal collarette. At this point it is important to describe and define these terms as they will be used throughout this chapter.

Papule: A solid, elevated lesion up to 1 cm in diameter caused by an infiltrate of inflammatory cells and associated edema. Papules are usually reddish in color.

Pustule: A circumscribed and elevated, purulent, fluid-filled cavity within the epidermis that is less than 0.5 cm in diameter. The area around the base of the pustule is often erythematous.

Papule/pustule: A papule with a pustule located at the very tip of the lesion (these pustules are often only the size of a pinpoint)

Bullous pustule: A pustule greater than 0.5 cm in diameter

Vesicle: A circumscribed, clear, fluid-filled cavity formed within or beneath the epidermis that is less than 1 cm in diameter

Bulla: A vesicle greater than 1 cm in diameter

Hemorrhagic bulla: A reddish to purplish bulla caused by the influx of erythrocytes into the cavity. These lesions are most often located within the dermis (Color Fig. 23).

Erosion: A defect caused by the partial loss of the epidermis. Because it does not extend below the basement membrane zone, healing can occur without scarring.

Ulcer: A defect caused by the complete loss of the epidermis. Because it extends below the basement membrane zone into the underlying dermis, scarring usually occurs.

Epidermal collarette: An accumulation of scale or crust arranged in a circular pattern (Color Fig. 24). The center of the lesion may show varying degrees of hyperpigmentation, and the margin of the lesion may be erythematous (Color Fig. 25). It is most often an indication of a previously existing pustule.

Crust: A dried exudate, primarily in the stratum corneum epidermis, composed of a mixture of serum, blood, degenerate neutrophils, and scales. Crusts are usually formed as the result of a ruptured pustule, vesicle, or bulla.

Of the primary lesions to be discussed, the papule, pustule, and papule/pustule are by far the most commonly encountered. Recognition of these lesions is very important in veterinary dermatology, as they are usually an indication of bacterial skin disease (pyoderma) (Table 52-1). These lesions are most often observed in canine dermatoses, and may represent the presence of a primary pyoderma or the much more prevalent problem of a secondary pyoderma. The pustule can also indicate the presence of an autoimmune skin disease in the dog or cat, such as pemphigus foliaceus or pemphigus erythematosus, but these diseases are relatively rare when compared to the incidence of pyodermas.

The presence of vesicles or bullae on the skin or mucous membranes of the dog or cat are much less commonly encountered. These lesions may be observed in patients with relatively rare auto-immune skin diseases such as pemphigus vulgaris, bullous pemphigoid, and the lupus skin diseases.

BACTERIAL SKIN DISEASES

This discussion will be limited to bacterial skin diseases of the dog, since the development of a pyoderma is an extremely rare event in the cat. Bacteria that are isolated from the skin of the dog are divided into three categories: resident organisms, transient organisms, and common pathogenic organisms. Resident bacterial organisms can be routinely and repeatedly isolated and cultured from the surface of the skin or hair coat of the dog. Under normal circumstances these bacteria live on the skin without causing any clinical disease. The resident bacteria of canine skin include coagulase-negative staphylococci (*Staphylococcus epidermidis, S. hominis, S. haemolyticus, S. cohnii, S. saprophyticus, S. capitis, S. warneri, S. xylosus, S. simulans, and S. sciuri*), coagulase-positive staphylococci (*S. intermedius*), *Micrococcus* organisms, α-hemolytic streptococci, and *Acinetobacter* organisms. The resident bacteria of canine hair are coagulase-positive staphylococci. In early bacterial isolation studies the most prevalent coagulase-positive staphylococci isolated in the dog were believed to be *S. aureus*. However, more recent studies utilizing improved technology have indicated that the most prevalent coagulase-positive staphylococci isolated from the skin, hair, or pyodermas in the dog are actually *S. intermedius*.

Transient bacterial organisms are not routinely or repeatedly isolated and cultured from the skin and hair coat of the dog. Under normal circumstances these organisms do not multiply on the patient; however, they occasionally become pathogens by secondary invasion. The bacteria in this category include *Escherichia coli, Proteus mirabilis, Pseudomonas aerugenosa*, corynebacteria, and bacillus sp.

Primary pathogenic organisms are capable of invading tissue and creating disease by themselves. They are usually coagulase-positive staphylococci (*S. intermedius, S. aureus, S. hyicus*).

Table 52–1 *Causes of Papular/Pustular, Vesicular/Bullous, and Erosive/Ulcerative Skin Diseases*

I. Bacterial skin diseases (pyodermas)
  A. Impetigo (puppy pyoderma)
  B. Superficial folliculitis
  C. Deep folliculitis and furunculosis
  D. Recurrent pyodermas
  E. Unique pyodermas
    1. Staphylococcal hypersensitivity (pruritic superficial pyoderma)
    2. Nasal pyoderma
    3. Canine acne (muzzle folliculitis and furunculosis)
    4. Juvenile pyoderma (puppy strangles, juvenile cellulitis)
    5. Cell-mediated immunodeficiencies with secondary pyoderma
II. Autoimmune skin diseases
  A. Pemphigus complex
    1. Pemphigus foliaceus
    2. Pemphigus erythematosus
    3. Pemphigus vulgaris
    4. Pemphigus vegetans
  B. Bullous pemphigoid
  C. Systemic lupus erythematosus
  D. Discoid lupus erythematosus

Of these organisms, *S. intermedius* is the most common isolate from canine skin infections.

Recent attention has been directed to the importance of anaerobic bacteria in the development of canine pyodermas, specifically deep pyodermas and cellulitis. These bacteria are readily isolated and cultured from fecal material, which may serve as source of secondary infection. The anaerobic bacteria isolated from deep skin infections of the dog include clostridia, *Peptostreptococcus* organisms, bacteroides, fusobacteria, and *Propionibacterium* organisms.

The ability of any of these organisms to be involved in a disease process is dependent on numerous factors. These will be specifically addressed for each disease topic.

Impetigo (Puppy Pyoderma)

Pathophysiology

This disease is a superficial pyoderma caused by coagulase-positive staphylococci. In humans impetigo is associated with potentially contagious streptococcal organisms; however, it is a noncontagious phenomenon in dogs. This infection is considered to be an opportunistic or secondary pyoderma in young dogs, and is most frequently associated with poor nutrition, a dirty environment, viral infections, ectoparasites, and intestinal parasitism.

Clinical Signs

Impetigo most often affects young dogs before the age of puberty. The disease is associated with the formation of superficial pustules (which do not involve hair follicles) located in the abdominal or inguinal and, occasionally, the axillary region. Usually the lesions are an incidental finding by the owner or are noticed on routine physical examination, since the lesions tend to be nonpruritic.

Management

The owners of a puppy with impetigo should be routinely questioned about their pet's current diet and environment. Recommendations should be made accordingly. A fecal sample should be obtained for routine fecal flotation, and the dog given an anthelmintic if any intestinal parasites are found. In many cases this is all that is necessary; the pustules will spontaneously resolve. However, a more rapid resolution of the pustules can be easily achieved with the daily use of an antibacterial shampoo. Effective shampoos include povidone–iodine (Betadine, Weladol), benzoyl peroxide (Oxydex, Pyoben), and chlorhexidine (Nolvasan) shampoos.

Superficial Folliculitis

Pathophysiology

This condition represents a bacterial infection within the superficial portion of the hair follicle, usually due to *S. intermedius*. This condition can be primary in origin, in which case the reason for its occurrence in the first place is not well understood. However, many animals develop this type of pyoderma, and when recognized as such and appropriately treated, the condition resolves and does not recur (see Recurrent Pyodermas).

Clinical Signs

The initial presentation of a dog with a superficial folliculitis is similar to a puppy with impetigo, except that the dog is usually past puberty. The lesions include pustules, papules, and papule/pustules affecting hair follicles (one can often see a hair shaft protruding through the center of the lesion) located in the abdominal or inguinal and axillary regions. As the disease progresses, epidermal collarettes form, with varying degrees of central hyperpigmentation and marginal erythema. Additional areas affected may include the lateral aspects of the trunk and ventral chest. In some patients a more generalized trunkal form of the disease occurs (with the same lesions as described above), with the most striking change being the presence of a diffuse, trunkal moth-eaten alopecia, (especially in short-coated breeds of dogs; Color Fig. 26). In most cases there is some degree of pruritus present.

Management

The treatment for superficial folliculitis needs to be more aggressive than that for impetigo; it requires both topical and systemic treatment. Treatment is initiated with twice-weekly bathing using a benzoyl peroxide shampoo, chosen for both its antibacterial properties and its unique "follicular flushing" action. Effective shampoos include Oxydex, Pyoben, and Sulf Oxydex. If the hair coat is excessively dry, with excess scale formation, then a conditioner or emollient should be used after each bath (see Chapter 50 under Seborrhea Sicca).

Systemic antibiotic therapy needs to be chosen wisely, since one cause of recurrent bacterial folliculitis is inappropriate selection or inadequate use of antibiotics. The antibiotic should be chosen based on results of a culture and sensitivity (rarely necessary on a first visit) or on the knowledge of antibiotics proven empirically to be highly effective against coagulase-positive staphylococci in one's geographic location (see Recurrent Pyodermas). The total treatment time should be 7 days beyond the complete clinical remission. This usually requires a minimum total treatment time of 21 days.

When a patient with a superficial bacterial folliculitis shows an initial response to treatment but the condition recurs shortly after stopping the therapy, it is imperative that some sort of a systematic approach be established to attempt to rule out and identify any underlying disease process (see Recurrent Pyodermas).

Deep Folliculitis and Furunculosis

Pathophysiology

This disease usually begins as a superficial bacterial folliculitis, but the infection extends deeper into the hair follicle, causing a deep folliculitis. If the process is not arrested at this stage, the inflammatory process breaks through the wall of the hair follicle. This results in the release of bacteria, follicular keratinocytes, and hair shaft material (all of which act as foreign bodies) into the surrounding dermis, and a subsequent pyogranulomatous inflammatory response. The resultant lesion is referred to as a *furuncle* (boil), and the process is called *furunculosis*. In chronic cases this can lead to the formation of a more diffuse inflammatory process, causing cellulitis or panniculitis. With the deeper penetration of bacteria the patient is also predisposed to the development of bacteremia and septicemia.

The bacteria most often involved initially are *S. intermedius,* but as the disease progresses, *Pseudomonas aerugenosa, Proteus mirabilis,* and *Escherichia coli* may act as pathogens. Recently, an emphasis has been placed on the role of anaerobic bacteria and coagulase-negative staphylococci as added pathogens in deep pyodermas. Invariably, these deeper infections are associated with an underlying disease process or the use of an inappropriate or inadequate antibiotic. Therefore, a systematic approach for assessing the patient is necessary even at the first presentation (see Recurrent Pyodermas). This should include a history of all previously tried antibiotics and the body-weight dosage, frequency of administration, and consecutive number of days the drug was administered.

Clinical Signs

The lesions initially observed include papules, pustules, papule/pustules, and epidermal collarettes, followed by the presence of exudation, crust formation, and deep draining tracts (or fistulas). As the process of folliculitis and furunculosis formation continues and the lesions coalesce, areas may become nodular and indurated or a cellulitis may develop (Color Fig. 27). Another lesion occasionally observed in these patients is a hemorrhagic bulla (see Color Fig. 23), which has a blood-blisterlike appearance. Lesions may begin in the inguinal or abdominal and axillary regions, followed by involvement of the entire ventrum, and may eventually become a generalized process. Occasionally, the lesions are most severe over the pressure and wear areas of the body such as the elbow, lateral aspects of the stifle, hip, and chest region (Color Fig. 28). In most cases the lesions seem to be pruritic or painful.

Signs of systemic involvement may be evident,

including anorexia, depression, weight loss, lethargy, and fever. These signs often indicate the development of bacteremia or septicemia. A peripheral lymphadenopathy is also a common finding. Certain breeds of dogs seem predisposed to the development of these deeper infections, including the Doberman pinscher, dalmatian, boxer, bull terrier, Great Dane, German shepherd, golden retriever, and Irish setter.

Management

Because multiple bacteria are frequently found, and because of the depth of the infection and its potential seriousness (bacteremia, septicemia, and death), systemic antibiotic therapy in deep pyodermas should always be based on a culture and sensitivity. The patient can be placed on a broad-spectrum antibiotic for the first 1 or 2 days, pending results of the test, and then placed on the most appropriate antibiotic after reviewing the results. The total duration of continuous antibiotic therapy should be for at least 2 weeks beyond the complete clinical remission. This usually requires a total minimum treatment time of 6 to 8 consecutive weeks. For recommended dosages, see Recurrent Pyodermas.

The initial topical treatment needs to be aggressive, with whole-body clipping for long-coated breeds of dogs and bathing or whirlpooling once to twice daily with povidone–iodine preparations (Weladol shampoo or Betadine whirlpool concentrate). As the patient improves, the frequency of bathing can be decreased to daily, then twice weekly.

Recently, increased problems with resistant strains of *Pseudomonas* have surfaced. This has lead to the need for use of the potent and broad-spectrum family of antibiotics, the fluorinated quinolones (see Appendix II). These antibiotics should only be chosen when a culture and sensitivity indicates that they are necessary and that no other antibiotic would be effective. Recommended fluorinated quinolones for resistant infections include norfloxacin (Noroxin) at 22 mg/kg orally twice daily, ciprofloxacin (Cipro) at 11 mg/kg orally twice daily, and enrofloxacin (Baytril) at 2.5 mg/kg orally twice daily. Recent

evaluations of enrofloxacin for more resistant *Pseudomonas* infections have revealed some therapeutic failures at a dosage of 2.5 mg/kg orally twice daily, and higher dosages of 5 mg/kg (or even higher in some instances) orally twice daily may be necessary. The fluorinated quinolones have been well tolerated at the above recommended dosages in the dog. They are contraindicated in growing dogs (in which it is associated with the development of an arthropathy and cartilage damage) and pregnant animals (it may be associated with abortion and teratogenic effects). A topical preparation very useful as an adjunct to systemic therapy for resistant *Pseudomonas* organisms is a 1% silver sulfadiazine (Silvadene) cream, which may be applied once to twice daily.

Since development of a deep folliculitis and furunculosis is usually associated with an underlying disease process, attempts must be made to establish the primary diagnosis or diagnoses (see Recurrent Pyodermas). This is necessary to prevent the disease from recurring after all of the above effort.

Recurrent Pyodermas

Pathophysiology

Recurrent pyodermas usually occur in the form of a superficial or deep folliculitis and furunculosis; therefore, one should review those sections before proceeding. In most cases, the pathogen involved is a coagulase-positive staphylococcus (usually *S. intermedius*). The possible reasons for the recurrent nature of a pyoderma are numerous (Table 52-2), and will be discussed under Diagnostic Approach. In these instances the bacterial skin infection is actually an opportunist to the cutaneous, metabolic, or immunologic changes induced by the primary disease, and therefore the pyoderma is only a secondary problem. One must also make certain that a recurrent pyoderma is not iatrogenic in nature. Iatrogenic recurrent pyodermas may be due to previous attempted drug therapy, including inappropriate antibiotic selection; inadequate dosage, frequency, and duration of antibiotic therapy; and the chronic use

Table 52–2 *Diseases Commonly Associated With the Development of a Secondary Pyoderma*

Allergic and hypersensitivity disorders
  Flea allergy dermatitis
  Atopy
  Food allergy
  Allergic contact dermatitis
Parasitic diseases
  Demodicosis
  Scabies
  Pelodera dermatitis
Metabolic diseases
  Hypothyroidism
  Cushing's syndrome
  Diabetes mellitus
Keratinization abnormalities
  Seborrhea complex (especially seborrheic dermatitis)
  Schnauzer comedo syndrome
Congenital and hereditary diseases
  Color-mutant alopecia
Miscellaneous diseases
  Sebaceous adenitis

of corticosteroids as an adjunct to the treatment of a pyoderma.

Clinical Signs

See Superficial Folliculitis, Deep Folliculitis and Furunculosis, and Staphylococcal Hypersensitivity.

Diagnostic Approach

The first step in diagnosing a patient with a pyoderma is to recognize the various lesions that indicate its presence. One of the most misinterpreted lesions on dermatologic examination is the epidermal collarette, especially when its margins are erythematous. It is often inappropriately thought to indicate a ringworm infection, but should be viewed as a superficial pyoderma until proven otherwise. The presence of papules in patients with pruritus is frequently thought to be associated with primary allergic skin diseases; thus such papules are often treated solely with a corticosteroid. However, in most cases closer inspection reveals a pinpoint pustule on top of the papule or a hair shaft exiting the center of the papule, which indicate the presence of a pyoderma. If one is uncertain whether the lesion indi-

cates a bacterial skin disease, then a skin biopsy should be performed.

In approaching an antibiotic-responsive but recurrent pyoderma, the first step is to make sure that the antibiotic selected is appropriate. A culture and sensitivity and cytology of a pustule or exudate should always be used to help select the best antibiotic when starting the "new" treatment for a recurrent pyoderma (see Diagnostic Approach at the end of this chapter).

The next step involves using the patient's response to therapy as an aid to the definitive diagnosis. In a majority of patients with a recurrent pyoderma, some degree of pruritus is present. However, at this stage of the workup, pruritus is not an indication for the use of a corticosteroid (or any other antipruritic drug). If a patient is pruritic but the lesions present on physical examination are consistent with a pyoderma, one must resist the temptation to use corticosteroids concurrently. At this stage the patient is placed on the appropriate antibiotic and shampoo therapy only, usually for a period of 3 to 4 consecutive weeks, at which point the animal is reevaluated.

On reevaluation, usually one of two things has become apparent. The first possibility is that the pyoderma is responding to treatment but the pruritus persists. One must inform the client that this outcome is possible, but that noncorticosteroid therapy is necessary in the attempt to establish the primary disease. In most cases, the clinical appearance of the dog is noticeably improved and a partial decrease in pruritus has occurred. The owner must be alerted to observe the dog for the areas of the body where the pruritus is persisting or is most severe. If the appropriate antibiotic resolves the pyoderma, but the pruritus is persisting, the following diseases should be ruled out (Table 52-3): flea allergy dermatitis, atopy, food allergy, scabies, demodicosis, cheyletiellosis, allergic contact dermatitis, and keratinization abnormalities (seborrheic dermatitis).

The second possible response to the therapy is that as the pyoderma responds to treatment, the pruritus also resolves (without the concurrent use of a corticosteroid). At this point in the systematic approach it is necessary to prove that the pyoderma is truly recurrent. The appropriate antibiotic and shampoo therapy should be contin-

Table 52–3 *Primary Pruritic Skin Diseases Commonly Associated With a Recurrent (or Secondary) Pyoderma*

Disease	Distribution Pattern	History of Pruritus	Method of Diagnosis
Flea allergy dermatitis	Caudal one third of the body	Usually initially a warm weather seasonal problem	History and physical examination Intradermal skin testing Response to flea treatment
Atopy	Face, feet, ears, axillae, abdomen, proximal and anterior foreleg	75% to 80% are initially a warm weather seasonal problem	History and physical examination Intradermal skin testing
Food allergy	Any, but often affects ears, feet, inguinal and axillary regions, and proximal and anterior foreleg, and face	Nonseasonal from the onset	History and physical examination Elimination diet trial
Scabies	Margins of pinnae, elbows, hocks	Nonseasonal from the onset, possible pruritus of other pets or people in the household	History and physical examination Skin scrapings Response to parasite treatment
Demodicosis	Face, feet, anywhere on body	Nonseasonal from the onset	History and physical examination Skin scrapings
Seborrheic dermatitis	Seborrheic plaquelike lesions on ventral neck, chest, and trunk	Nonseasonal from the onset	History and physical examination Systematic rule-outs Skin biopsy
Allergic contact dermatitis	Abdomen, axillae, scrotum or vulva, perianal or perineal region, ventrum of tail base, interdigital skin	Depends on allergen (a grass vs. an indoor carpet)	History and physical examination Patch testing
Cheyletiellosis	Scaling on the dorsal midline	Nonseasonal from the onset	History and physical examination Skin scrapings and scotch tape preps

ued for a total treatment time of 8 weeks. Approximately 50% of the infections treated this way will resolve permanently. If the pyoderma recurs after this treatment, in which an antibiotic alone resolved both the lesions of pyoderma and the pruritus concurrently, then the following diseases should be ruled out (Table 52-4): hypothyroidism, Cushing's syndrome, diabetes mellitus, demodicosis, cheyletiellosis, food allergy, staphylococcal hypersensitivity, and cell-mediated immunodeficiency (see Diagnostic Approach at the end of this chapter). The inclusion of food allergy as an underlying nonpruritic skin disease may seem a bit odd. However, on rare occasions the only symptom of a food allergy may be a recurrent pyoderma, and the pruritus may be apparent only when the pyoderma develops.

Management

The key to successful management of a patient with a recurrent pyoderma is identifying the primary disease and instituting specific treatment. Without accomplishing this goal, the recurrent nature of the disease is inevitable.

The other aspect of successful treatment is the proper selection and use of systemic antibiotics. The sensitivity of coagulase-positive staphylococci (especially *S. intermedius*) to certain antibiotics has been evaluated for various geographic locations throughout the world; this information is helpful for empirical selection of an agent to

Table 52–4 *Primary Nonpruritic Skin Diseases That May Be Associated With a Recurrent (or Secondary) Pyoderma*

Hypothyroidism
Cushing's syndrome
Diabetes mellitus
Demodicosis
Cheyletiellosis
Cell-Mediated immunodeficiency
Food allergy

treat a pyoderma. The following antibiotics are those we have found to be most useful in our practice in Michigan; of course, one must keep in mind that subtle differences exist from one part of the world to another. Antibiotics that have exhibited a high sensitivity rating for their effectiveness against *S. intermedius* (Table 52-5) are oxacillin, erythromycin, chloramphenicol, cephadroxil, and cephalexin. Of these, oxacillin and erythromycin are best for empirical selection, as they have a narrower spectrum of activity. Chloramphenicol, cephadroxil, and cephalexin, which are broad-spectrum in activity, should be reserved for mixed infections or more resistant infections, which are selected based on results of a culture and sensitivity. The next group of antibiotics has exhibited only a moderate sensitivity rating for its effectiveness against *S. intermedius* (Table 52-6): lincomycin, trimethoprim–sulfadiazine, and amoxicillin–clavulanate. It is best not to use these antibiotics based on empirical selection only, but they are usually very effective when selected based on the results of a culture and sensitivity. The last group of antibiotics has exhibited a very poor sensitivity rating for their effectiveness against *S. intermedius*: penicillin, ampicillin, amoxicillin, tetracycline, and the sulfonamides (nontrimethoprim-potentiated). These antibiotics should not be used for the treatment of pyodermas due to coagulase-positive staphylococci based on either empirical selection or a culture and sensitivity, as the in vivo response to these antibiotics is generally poor.

The selection of an antibiotic should always be guided by interpretation of the cytology of a pustule or exudate. It is important to compare the morphologic features of the predominant organism on cytology to the organisms isolated through culture, and to select the best antibiotic for the

Table 52–6 Antibiotics With a Moderate Sensitivity Rating for Staphylococcus intermedius *in Dogs*

Lincomycin: 15 to 22 mg/kg t.i.d. PO
Trimethoprim–sulfadiazine: 30 mg/kg b.i.d. PO
Amoxicillin–clavulanate: 13.75 mg/kg b.i.d. PO

predominant organism on cytology (and therefore the most likely primary pathogen).

In some instances, such as chronic, recurrent, or refractory pyodermas; pyodermas that have recently been treated with various antibiotics; deep pyodermas; and anaerobic infections, the selection of an antibiotic should always be partially based on the results of a culture and sensitivity.

For recommendations on the duration of antibiotic therapy and appropriate adjunct topical therapy, see Superficial Folliculitis and Deep Folliculitis and Furunculosis.

Staphylococcal Hypersensitivity (Pruritic Superficial Pyoderma)

Pathophysiology

The pathophysiologic mechanisms involved in the development of a primary staphylococcal hypersensitivity remain one of the more controversial issues in veterinary dermatology. According to some of the studies performed to date, Types I and III hypersensitivity reactions to staphylococci may be involved in the pathogenesis of this disorder; however, their specific role in the development of this disease remains to be proven.

Clinical Signs

The initial presentation of a patient with staphylococcal hypersensitivity is clinically similar to patients with a primary allergy (flea allergy, atopy, food allergy, or contact allergy) and a secondary pyoderma. There is usually moderate to marked pruritus that is nonseasonal in nature. On physical examination there are papules, pustules, papule/pustules, epidermal collarettes

Table 52–5 Antibiotics With a High Sensitivity Rating for Staphylococcus intermedius *in Dogs*

Oxacillin: 22 mg/kg t.i.d. PO
Erythromycin: 11 mg/kg t.i.d. PO
Chloramphenicol: 30 to 50 mg/kg t.i.d. PO
Cephalexin: 30 mg/kg b.i.d. or 22 mg/kg t.i.d. PO
Cephadroxil: 22 mg/kg b.i.d.–t.i.d. PO

(with varying degrees of central hyperpigmentation, crusting, and marginal erythema), crusts, and scales (see Color Figs. 24 and 25). The initial areas affected are the inguinal–abdominal and axillary regions. The lesions may advance to involve the entire ventrum and lateral aspects of the chest. As the disease progresses, the expanding nature of the epidermal collarettes may result in coalescence of several lesions, causing large circumscribed areas of alopecia (especially in long-coated breeds of dogs). In some patients, a more generalized, trunkal form of the disease occurs, with the development of a moth-eaten alopecia (especially in short-coated breeds of dogs).

The historical response to various treatments is useful in leading one to suspect this disease (see Recurrent Pyodermas). A typical historical response includes a poor or partial response to the use of corticosteroids alone, resolution of the pyoderma and pruritus simultaneously with appropriate antibiotic therapy alone, and rapid relapses after stopping short-term antibiotic therapy.

Management

The specific treatment of staphylococcal hypersensitivity involves the use of the staphylococcal bacterin Staphage Lysate (Table 52-7). This product has been well tolerated by most dogs, and very few side-effects have been reported (Table 52-8). The idea behind the use of this product for this disease is that if a patient that it is believed to be hypersensitive or "allergic" to its own resident staphylococci is presented with staphylococcal antigens, it will form blocking antibodies and become hyposensitized. This is based on the theory of the formation of increased levels of aller-

Table 52–8 Side-effects or Reactions to Staphage Lysate Injections

Pruritus, pain, or swelling at injection site
Lethargy
Shivering
Fever
Polyarthritis
Proteinuria

gen-specific (staphylococcal) immunoglobulin G (IgG). This immunoglobulin class may bind to staphylococcal antigens in the circulation and prevent them from binding to allergen-specific IgE, which is already bound to mast cells in the skin. This would subsequently prevent the degranulation of mast cells if a Type I hypersensitivity reaction is involved in the pathogenesis of this disease.

The goal of this treatment is to prevent recurrence of the disease and not to induce the initial remission of the disease by itself. Therefore, as an adjunct to this treatment the patient needs to be put on an appropriate antibiotic for 4 to 6 weeks to induce the remission of the recurrent pyoderma (see Recurrent Pyodermas).

Topical therapy should include bathing of the patient twice weekly for the first 4 weeks of treatment using a benzoyl peroxide shampoo (Oxydex, Pyoben, or Sulf Oxydex). Thereafter, the dog should be bathed every 1 to 2 weeks for life as an adjunct to the Staphage Lysate injections.

Cases that have been refractory to the above treatment may benefit from the use of cimetidine (Tagamet), at a dosage of 6 to 8 mg/kg orally three times daily, as a replacement for the Staphage Lysate injections (see Appendix II).

When the above treatments have been tried and "all else has failed," then the patient is a candidate for life-long, once-daily antibiotic therapy. This is to be considered only after one has thoroughly reviewed the systematic approach to recurrent pyodermas. The patient should be placed on appropriate full-dosage antibiotic therapy one more time to induce a complete remission of the pyoderma, followed by the once daily administration of that antibiotic for life. One of the more useful antibiotics for this purpose, in our experience, is oxacillin.

Table 52–7 Staphage Lysate Injection Protocol

Week	Volume
1	0.25 ml
2	0.50 ml
3	0.75 ml
4	1.00

Follow this protocol with 1 to 2 ml every 3 to 21 days as needed to prevent recurrence of the pyoderma. Injections are given subcutaneously.

Nasal Pyoderma

Pathophysiology

The pathophysiology of nasal pyoderma is unknown, but it is associated with the presence of coagulase-positive staphylococci and a painful and localized folliculitis and furunculosis reaction. In our experience, the appearance of a nasal pyoderma has often been preceded by an angioedemic reaction on the muzzle related to exposure to various antigens (especially insect bites). This suggests the possibility of an underlying Type I hypersensitivity reaction and helps explain the need for the use of corticosteroids in addition to antibiotics in the treatment of this pyoderma.

Clinical Signs

The dolichocephalic breeds of dogs are most commonly affected, especially German shepherds, collies, German short-haired pointers, and other hunting breeds of dogs. The disease is peracute in onset (occurring within hours), and may begin as an angioedema of the muzzle region. The lesions that develop are a combination of papules, pustules, papule/pustules, nodules, erosions, ulcers, exudation, and crusts, and affect the bridge of the nose, the area around the nostrils, and, occasionally, the lip region (Color Fig. 29). Scar formation may be a sequela to severe reactions or overzealous topical treatment. This condition is usually only a one-time event in a patient, and recurrences are rare.

Management

Treatment is initiated by gently washing the area to remove any exudate and crusts, using a povidone–iodine shampoo (Weladol or Betadine). The area should then be dried with a mild astringent such as Burow's Solution (Domeboro powder and water) applied as a compress with gauze pads and then allowed to air dry.

An appropriate systemic antibiotic (see Recurrent Pyodermas) should be administered for 7 days beyond the complete clinical remission, which usually means at least 21 days of treatment. The use of systemic corticosteroids greatly reduces the time required for complete recovery. Prednisone or prednisolone can be given at a dosage of 0.5 mg/kg orally twice daily for the first 7 to 10 days of treatment. This treatment can be supplemented by the daily topical application of a steroid or antibiotic cream (not an ointment, which is occlusive) such as Panalog.

Canine Acne (Muzzle Folliculitis and Furunculosis)

Pathophysiology

The pathophysiology of canine acne is unknown. It is associated with the presence of coagulase-positive staphylococci and the formation of folliculitis in mild cases and furunculosis in severe or chronic cases. Because of the anatomic location of the lesions and the young age of most dogs when this disease occurs, deep skin scrapings should be performed on all cases to rule out the possibility of demodicosis as an underlying disease.

Clinical Signs

Short-coated breeds of dogs, including boxers, Doberman pinschers, bulldogs, Great Danes, weimaraners, mastiffs, and pointers, are predisposed to developing canine acne. The disease often occurs between 3 and 12 months of age, with the development of papules, pustules, and papule/pustules on the chin and, occasionally, lip regions. In younger dogs the condition may be mild and heal spontaneously after sexual maturity. If the disease is present after 1 year of age, the problem tends to be more chronic in nature, and nodules and draining tracts may develop (Color Fig. 30).

Management

Mild cases in young dogs may spontaneously resolve by 1 year of age. Milder cases may also be treated initially with once-to-twice daily washing with a benzoyl peroxide shampoo (Oxydex or Pyoben) for the first few days, followed by the once-to-twice daily application of benzoyl peroxide gels (Oxydex or Pyoben) as needed. For more severe or chronic cases the initial treatment is the same as for nasal pyoderma. Once the condition is brought under control, the basis of maintenance treatment is the regular use of benzoyl peroxide shampoos and gels.

Juvenile Pyoderma (Puppy Strangles, Juvenile Cellulitis)

Pathophysiology

The pathophysiology of juvenile pyoderma is unknown. When the early lesions of edema, pustules, vesicles, or cellulitis are cultured or examined histologically, they are initially sterile. The histopathology of early-developing lesions may reveal an inflammatory infiltrate directed toward the panniculus or sebaceous glands, suggesting the possibility of a hypersensitivity reaction to lipidlike structures. As the disease progresses and these lesions rupture to the surface of the skin, coagulase-positive staphylococci often become opportunists; however, staphylococci do not appear to be the cause of the disease. These observations may help explain why severe cases of juvenile pyoderma are usually unresponsive to treatment with antibiotics alone and require aggressive corticosteroid therapy.

Clinical Signs

This disease most commonly occurs in puppies younger than 4 months of age, and may affect one pup, several pups, or all pups (to varying degrees) in a litter. Golden retrievers and dachshunds seem to be predisposed to developing this disease. An acute swelling of the face and lips (often resembling an angioedema) is the most common initial presentation, but the ears, anus, prepuce, vulva, and feet may also be affected. This may be followed by the development of pustules and vesicles, then exudation and crust formation. In severe cases there may be several deep draining tracts in the skin, and the entire external ear canal may fill up with a purulent exudate. There is usually a submandibular and prescapular lymphadenopathy, and in severe cases these areas may also ulcerate and drain. Depending on the severity of the case, the puppy may also be febrile, with signs of systemic disease. The potential exists for the development of bacteremia or septicemia.

Management

Treatment should be initiated using prednisone or prednisolone at 1 mg/kg twice daily for the first 10 to 14 days; the dosage is then gradually tapered off as the puppy improves. Broad-spectrum antibiotics such as cephalexin (22 mg/kg orally three times daily for 2–3 weeks, or 7 days beyond the complete clinical remission) should also be given to prevent secondary bacterial invasion. Topical therapy includes the use of Burow's Solution (Domeboro powder and water) applied as a wet compress and allowed to air dry. Systemically ill and anorexic puppies may also require initial supportive fluid therapy.

Cell-Mediated Immunodeficiencies With Secondary Pyoderma

Pathophysiology

Primary cell-mediated immunodeficiency as a cause of recurrent pyodermas in the dog is extremely rare. It is often easy to assume that a patient with recurrent infections has a malfunction of the immune response. However, the many diseases discussed in the section Recurrent Pyodermas all have the potential to secondarily suppress the cell-mediated immune response. With these, treatment of the primary disease (such as atopy or Cushing's syndrome) allows the immune response to return to normal. The use of an immune stimulant is inappropriate, does not correct the primary problem, and does not elicit any favorable response from the patient.

Of the cells responsible for the cell-mediated immune response in the dog, the lymphocyte has been studied the most. The primary defects of lymphocytes that can occur have been in either the number of cells available to fight an infection or their functional ability to respond to an infection or both. In some patients there is a persistent and reproducible, absolute lymphopenia present during the infectious process or even while the patient is on antibiotics and is clinically free of disease. In other patients there may or may not be an absolute lymphopenia, but the lymphocytes are incapable of mounting an appropriate response to antigenic challenge when assessed by in vitro mitogen stimulation (or in vitro lymphocyte blastogenesis). The reason for the development of this lymphocyte dysfunction is unknown.

Clinical Signs

See Deep Folliculitis and Furunculosis and Color Figures 27 and 28. An increased incidence of lymphocyte deficiency as the primary cause for a recurrent deep pyoderma has been observed in the German shepherd and Dalmatian.

Management

The specific treatment of a dog with a primary lymphocyte deficiency consists of the use of an immune-stimulating agent. In our experience the most effective product has been the staphylococcal bacterin Staphage Lysate (see Table 52-7). This product has been very well tolerated by most dogs, and very few problems with side-effects have been reported (see Table 52-8). Staphylococcal antigens are used to directly stimulate the lymphocyte population, with the goal of improving the absolute number of lymphocytes to fight infection or improving their functional ability. This treatment is designed to prevent recurrence of the disease and not to induce the initial remission of the disease by itself. Therefore, as an adjunct to this treatment the patient needs to be put on an appropriate bactericidal antibiotic for 4 to 6 weeks to induce the remission of the recurrent pyoderma (see Recurrent Pyodermas).

For additional recommendations on the treatment of a patient with a lymphocyte deficiency and secondary pyoderma, see Deep Folliculitis and Furunculosis. Patients refractory to these treatment recommendations may benefit from the use of cimetidine or once-daily antibiotic therapy, as discussed in the section Staphylococcal Hypersensitivity.

Another potential immune stimulant that can be considered when the above measures have failed is levamisole (Levasole) at 2 mg/kg orally three times weekly. This drug should be only used as a last resort, as levamisole in certain patients can cause lymphopenia and a resultant immunosuppression (see Appendix II).

AUTOIMMUNE SKIN DISEASES

The following section addresses some of the rarer skin diseases observed in the dog and cat. These are certainly some of the most interesting and challenging skin diseases encountered in veterinary dermatology. The autoimmune skin diseases in general are best described as diseases that involve a lack of recognition of self antigens. That is, for reasons unknown in most instances, the patient's immune system begins forming antibodies directed against various components of the epidermis or dermis.

Pemphigus Complex

Pathophysiology

Four autoimmune skin diseases share a common pathophysiology. Pemphigus foliaceus, pemphigus erythematosus, pemphigus vulgaris, and pemphigus vegetans are all examples of a Type II hypersensitivity reaction that does not require the activation of complement for lesions to occur.

The first step in the formation of a lesion is the development of an autoantibody (pemphigus antibody), which is usually of the IgG class (IgM, IgA, and complement [C3] may also be involved). The specific antigen (pemphigus antigen) that the pemphigus antibody binds to remains uncertain, but is believed to be a keratinocyte cell surface antigen. However, some studies also suggest the possibility of a desmosomal surface antigen or antigen within the intercellular cement substance.

The next step is the activation and release of a proteolytic enzyme from within the keratinocytes (plasminogen activating factor, or pemphigus acantholytic factor) into the intercellular spaces.

This results in the loss of the cohesion between keratinocytes and the formation of an intraepidermal pustule or vesicle. This process is called *acantholysis*, and the freed-up keratinocytes within the blister (which are now round in shape rather than polyhedral or spindle-shaped) are called *acantholytic cells*.

In the diseases pemphigus foliaceus and pemphigus erythematosus, this process occurs within the most superficial layers of the epidermis, just beneath the stratum corneum, resulting in subcorneal pustules. In pemphigus vulgaris and pemphigus vegetans, this process occurs within the deeper layers of the epidermis, just above the stratum basale, resulting in a suprabasilar vesicle or bulla.

The role of ultraviolet light exposure in the pathophysiology of these diseases is uncertain, but they have often been noticed to be exacerbated by an increased exposure to ultraviolet light.

Pemphigus erythematosus is one of the more interesting of the diseases in the pemphigus complex in that it shares immunologic features observed in both the pemphigus complex and the lupus erythematosus diseases. The additional changes sometimes observed include the presence of immunoglobulins and complement at the basement membrane zone and circulating antinuclear antibodies.

Pemphigus Foliaceus

Clinical Signs

Pemphigus foliaceus has been reported in both the dog and cat. In dogs, the Akita, chow chow, dachshund, bearded collie, Newfoundland, Doberman pinscher, and schipperke appear to be predisposed. The initial lesions are pustules, which are often transient in nature. These pustules are clinically indistinguishable from those observed in cases of pyoderma. They usually occur only periodically, in a wavelike manner, and develop and subsequently rupture within hours. This is followed by epidermal collarettes (with varying degrees of central hyperpigmentation and marginal erythema), erythema, erosions, alopecia, and marked crust and scale formation (Color Fig. 31).

The areas most commonly affected are the face (especially the bridge of the nose and the periorbital region) and ears (Color Fig. 32). The disease is usually gradual in onset, and over time many cases take on a more generalized appearance. The footpads may also be affected, with either sloughing of a portion of the pads, leaving behind an erosion or ulcer, or a hyperkeratotic and fissuring process. On rare occasions only the foot pads are affected. The lesions are usually painful or pruritic, and a generalized peripheral lymphadenopathy is common. Severely affected animals may have signs of systemic illness, including lethargy, depression, anorexia, and fever. The more chronically affected animal may develop a secondary pyoderma. Some patients will also develop pitting edema of the limbs. Historically, many of these patients are often initially diagnosed as having a pyoderma, but show a poor response to systemic antibiotic therapy.

Management

To induce the initial remission of this disease, the treatment of choice is immunosuppressive dosages of corticosteroids. Prednisone or prednisolone is given at 1 to 3 mg/kg orally twice daily in the dog, and 2 to 6 mg/kg orally twice daily in the cat. These dosages need to be continued until the patient has shown a complete clinical remission; then the dosage is gradually decreased to establish the lowest possible dosage to keep the disease in remission. The patient should be closely monitored for any evidence of new lesions for 2 weeks following each slight decrease in dosage. If new lesions are noticed, then the patient is immediately put back on the dosage that was previously controlling the disease. In the dog the side-effects include any or all of the signs observed in Cushing's syndrome (see Chapter 59) and an increased susceptibility to infections (especially lower urinary tract infections, pyodermas, dermatophytosis, candidiasis, and respiratory infections). Since the dosage of steroids required to control this disease in dogs is frequently associated with unacceptable side-effects, these drugs are rarely used alone for long-term control and management. In cats, however, side-effects to steroid use are much less common and less severe. This has allowed many cats with pemphigus foliaceus to be successfully controlled on steroids alone.

In dogs, the most widely used adjunct therapy to corticosteroids are the chemotherapeutic purine analogs. Either azathioprine (Imuran) or mercaptopurine (Purinethol) is given at a dosage of 2 mg/kg orally once daily as an induction dosage. Several weeks of administration are required before clinical signs of immunosuppressive effects are seen. The long-term goal is to establish a maintenance dosage of 1 mg/kg orally every other day. This medication has been well tolerated by most dogs, but potential side-effects include gastrointestinal toxicity (anorexia, vomiting), hepatotoxicity (jaundice, increased liver enzymes), and bone marrow suppression. Therefore, a hemogram and platelet count, plus alanine aminotransferase, aspartate aminotransferase, and serum alkaline phosphatase levels, should be evaluated periodically during treatment. These drugs are generally not recommended for use in the cat because of its increased sensitivity to toxic reactions, including severe leukopenia and death.

In cats, where corticosteroids alone cannot control the disease or the cat develops unacceptable side-effects, the most widely used adjunct therapy is chrysotherapy (gold therapy). The most frequently used form of gold salt is sterile aurothioglucose suspension (Solganal), which is administered intramuscularly. Injections are given once weekly, with an initial test dose of 1 mg IM. This is done to observe for the possibility of an anaphylactoid reaction to the product (which can be a problem in humans but has not yet been reported in cats). The induction dosage is then 1 mg/kg IM once weekly for up to 12 weeks, as gold salts require several weeks to exert their immunosuppressive effects. Once a favorable response is observed, the maintenance dosage is 1 mg/kg IM every 2 to 4 weeks. This medication has been well tolerated by most cats, but potential side-effects include mucosal and cutaneous reactions (oral ulcers, stomatitis, pruritus, erythema, and toxic epidermal necrolysis), renal toxicity (proteinuria and glomerulonephritis), and bone marrow suppression (thrombocytopenia). Therefore,

the owner should be informed to observe for mucosal or cutaneous reactions, and there should be periodic monitoring of the hemogram, platelet count, and urinalysis.

If either a dog or cat is refractory to the above recommendations, an additional adjunct to corticosteroid therapy is the use of an alkylating agent. The most commonly used form is chlorambucil (Leukeran) at an induction dosage of 0.1 mg/kg orally once daily in dogs, and 0.1 mg/kg orally every other day in cats. Once a favorable response to treatment has been observed, the maintenance dosage of chlorambucil in dogs is 0.1 mg/kg orally every other day and in cats is 0.05 mg/kg every other day. This medication has been well tolerated in both dogs and cats, but potential side-effects include a decrease in new hair growth and bone marrow suppression. Therefore, a hemogram and platelet count should be monitored periodically during treatment.

The major effect of all of these medications is suppression of the immune system. The part of the body most susceptible to secondary infection while undergoing this type of treatment is the lower urinary tract. Therefore, a urinalysis looking for evidence of a lower urinary tract infection followed by a urine culture and sensitivity is recommended every 3 to 4 months. These infections, when discovered early, are responsive to appropriate antibiotic therapy (see Chapter 46).

Pemphigus Erythematosus

Clinical Signs

Pemphigus erythematosus has been reported in both the dog and cat. In dogs, the collie and German shepherd appear to be predisposed. The lesions formed initially are similar to those observed in pemphigus foliaceus. The major difference is that the lesions usually remain localized to the face and ears. In addition, the nose is often depigmented (Color Fig. 33), as seen in cases of discoid lupus erythematosus. Of the pemphigus diseases, it shows the most severe exacerbations upon exposure to ultraviolet light. Signs of systemic illness have not been reported, and this disease is often referred to as a benign or abortive form of pemphigus foliaceus.

Management

The initial treatment of choice for this disease in dogs is a water soluble form of vitamin E (d,l-alpha tocopherol acetate) at a dosage of 400 to 800 IU orally twice daily given 2 hours prior to or after feeding. This is recommended since any inorganic iron (which is present in essentially all commercial diets) will interfere with the gastrointestinal absorption of vitamin E. In dogs that show a partial response to this treatment, a capsule can be opened and its contents applied topically to the lesions once to twice daily; this often results in an additional improvement. A complete response to therapy often requires 2 to 3 months of observation before the desired effect is obtained. Vitamin E is well tolerated in dogs, and the only known side-effect to date was the changing of the hair coat color of a tricolored collie, with the black portion of the hair coat changing to white. To date, we have not tried vitamin E therapy in the cat.

For dogs that are unresponsive or only partially responsive to vitamin E, prednisone or prednisolone may be added to the treatment regimen, as described for pemphigus foliaceus. The treatment of choice for pemphigus erythematosus in the cat is prednisone or prednisolone (see Pemphigus Foliaceus).

An important adjunct to the above recommendations includes avoidance of ultraviolet light exposure during daylight hours. When this is not possible, topical sunscreens can be applied to the affected and depigmented areas three times daily. Effective sunscreens include Sundown 30 (Johnson & Johnson) and Photoplex (Herbert Laboratories).

Pemphigus Vulgaris

Clinical Signs

Pemphigus vulgaris is the most severe form of the pemphigus diseases in the dog and cat. The initial lesions are vesicles or bullae, which are often transient in nature. This is followed by erythema, alopecia, erosions, and ulcers, with some crust formation at the margin of the erosions and ulcers. The lesions most commonly occur at mu-cocutaneous junctions, the base of the nails, footpads, and the inguinal and axillary skin. The erosions and ulcers present in the inguinal or axillary area are often angular and sharply delineated. Vesicles, bullae, erosions, and ulcers are also observed to affect mucosal surfaces in most patients, with a majority of the cases showing lesions in the oral cavity. The lesions are usually pruritic or painful, and the patient frequently presents with signs of systemic illness. On occasion the disease has been fatal.

Management

Pemphigus vulgaris is the most difficult of the diseases in the pemphigus complex to treat successfully. Therefore, the client should be informed that there is a guarded prognosis for the long-term management of this disease. The recommended treatment is the same as that described for pemphigus foliaceus.

Pemphigus Vegetans

Clinical Signs

This is the rarest of the diseases in the pemphigus complex, and has only been reported in three dogs to date. The disease is believed to be a benign or abortive form of pemphigus vulgaris. The disease has been described as a vesicular and pustular disease, with erosions and ulcers that rapidly formed crusts and vegetative and papillomatous lesions. There was no evidence of systemic illness, and the lesions appeared to be pruritic or painful.

Management

Based on so few cases, no strong recommendation can be made for the treatment of this disease. However, the basic principles described in the section Pemphigus Foliaceus can be tried.

Bullous Pemphigoid

Pathophysiology

Bullous pemphigoid is a pemphiguslike disease, but is not a part of the pemphigus complex. It is another example of a Type II hypersensitivity reaction, but, in contrast to the pemphigus complex, it requires the activation of complement for lesions to be formed. The first step is the development of an autoantibody (pemphigoid antibody), which is usually of the IgG class (IgM and IgA may also be involved). The specific antigen (pemphigoid antigen) that the pemphigoid antibody binds to remains uncertain, but is believed to be an antigen located within the basement membrane zone, which includes antigens on the hemidesmosomes of basal epidermal cells or the laminin within the lamina lucida. This results in the activation of complement, and the subsequent chemotaxis of neutrophils and eosinophils and release of proteolytic enzymes. The result is the loss of dermoepidermal cohesion and the formation of a subepidermal vesicle or bulla.

Clinical Signs

Bullous pemphigoid has not been reported in the cat; in the dog, the collie and Doberman pinscher seem to be predisposed. The clinical presentation of the patient is often identical to that of pemphigus vulgaris (see Pemphigus Vulgaris and Color Fig. 34).

Management

The recommended treatment in the dog is the same as that for pemphigus foliaceus).

Systemic Lupus Erythematosus

Pathophysiology

Systemic lupus erythematosus is one of the most complex immune-mediated diseases. It involves the production of various autoantibodies that are directed against different tissues of the body. Factors that can play a role in the development of the disease include a genetic predisposition, suppressor T lymphocyte deficiency, B lymphocyte hyperactivity, viral infection, hormonal factors, and exposure to ultraviolet light. The pathophysiology of systemic lupus erythematosus for all possibly involved organ systems is beyond the scope of this chapter. Therefore, the remainder of this discussion will concentrate on the proposed mechanism of the development of skin lesions.

It is currently believed that a genetic predisposition for lupus and exposure to ultraviolet light are important features in the development of skin lesions. Upon exposure to ultraviolet light, damage to basal keratinocytes can occur. This may entail either a denaturing of nuclear DNA, which is subsequently extruded below the basal lamina, or a change in basal keratinocyte surface antigens. In either case this would result in the formation of antibodies against these altered, non–self antigens. The result is the deposition of autoantibodies to the altered non–self antigens, and damage to basal keratinocytes and the basement membrane zone, with subsequent inflammatory cell infiltrates directed toward this region, tissue damage, and possible subepidermal blister formation.

Clinical Signs

Because of the many possible tissues affected in the development of systemic lupus erythematosus, this disease is often appropriately referred to as the "great imitator." This disease has been reported in both the dog and cat. In dogs, the collie, Shetland sheepdog, and German shepherd seem to be predisposed. The skin lesions that develop are extremely variable, and include various combinations of erythema, alopecia, scaling, crusts, depigmentation, vesicles, bullae, erosions, and ulcers. Lesions may occur on the skin, mucous membranes, nose, and footpads. One of the key features that leads one to suspect systemic lupus erythematosus is evidence of multiple organ system disease. Some of the more common organ system diseases are immune complex deposition glomerulonephritis, autoimmune hemolytic anemia, immune-mediated thrombocytopenia, and immune-mediated polyarthritis. Other less commonly documented features include pericarditis, polymyositis, myocarditis, pneumonitis, pleuritis, seizures, meningitis, myelitis, psychosis, and polyneuropathy. The disease is often markedly exacerbated by exposure to ultraviolet light.

Management

The initial treatment of choice for cutaneous involvement in both dogs and cats is prednisone or prednisolone, as described for the treatment of pemphigus foliaceus. Refractory cases may be adjunctly treated with either azathioprine or chlorambucil (see Pemphigus Foliaceus). The overall prognosis and treatment regimens for each patient with this disease need to be catered to the individual according to the additional organ systems involved.

Discoid Lupus Erythematosus

Pathophysiology

Discoid lupus erythematosus is considered a benign variant of systemic lupus erythematosus, with the absence of multiple organ system involvement. It primarily affects only the skin and mucous membranes. The exact pathophysiology of this variant is unknown, but many of the same immunodermatologic features observed in systemic lupus are seen in discoid lupus. This disease is markedly exacerbated by exposure to ultraviolet light, and a genetic predisposition is believed to be important.

Clinical Signs

This disease has been reported in the dog but not the cat; collies, Shetland sheepdogs, German shepherds, and Siberian huskies are predisposed. The skin lesions noted are more predictable in this variant of lupus. The lesions most commonly occur on the nose and the bridge of the nose. One of the earliest changes is a loss of the cobblestone architecture of the nasal planum into a smooth surface, with a change in pigmentation from black to slate gray (Color Fig. 35). This is often followed by complete depigmentation, erythema, erosions, and ulcers (Color Fig. 36). Other areas that may be affected are the periorbital region, ears, distal limbs, genitalia, lips, and oral cavity. Scar formation and permanent depigmentation may be a sequela. Evidence of systemic illness is not a feature of this disease.

Management

The treatment recommendations for this disease are the same as for pemphigus erythematosus.

DIAGNOSTIC APPROACH

History and Physical Examination

As always, the initial evaluation of a patient with a dermatologic disease requires a thorough history and physical examination. The type of lesions present, their distribution pattern (Tables 52-9 and 52-10), and responses to attempted treatments should be noted. For a review of how to use the response to antibiotic treatment in the systematic approach to recurrent pyodermas and how to recognize the types of lesions present see Recurrent Pyodermas and the introduction to this chapter.

When considering the diagnosis of one of the autoimmune skin diseases discussed, certain observations are important. Many of these diseases often have waxing and waning cycles of activity, which seem to occur in spite of therapeutic efforts and not because of these efforts. The episodes of pustules or vesicles often occur in a wavelike fashion, appearing rapidly and then rupturing in a matter of hours. They are unresponsive to treatment with systemic antibiotics and poorly or only partially responsive to treatment with anti-inflammatory dosages of corticosteroids.

Cytology

Cytologic examination of pustules, vesicles, bullae, and exudates is easily performed and gives very rapid information. A useful stain prior to microscopic examination of the material on a slide is the Diff Quik stain. A pustule of bacterial origin usually contains bacterial cocci and inflammatory cells (neutrophils, eosinophils, and mononuclear cells). In cases of pyoderma that are refractory to a seemingly appropriate antibiotic, the cytology may reveal bacterial cocci and rods or bacterial rods only; these findings should be correlated with the organisms isolated on bacte-

Table 52–9 Bacterial Skin Diseases

Disease	Lesion	Distribution Pattern
Impetigo	Pustules	Abdominal or inguinal region Occasionally axillae
Superficial folliculitis	Pustules, papules, papule/pustules Hair shaft may be present in center of lesion Epidermal collarettes Moth-eaten alopecia, especially in short-coated breeds of dogs	Abdominal, inguinal, and axillary regions Occasionally ventral chest and lateral thorax Generalized on trunk
Deep folliculitis and furunculosis	Papules, pustules, papule/pustules Epidermal collarettes Nodules Cellulitis Hemorrhagic bullae Draining tracts	Abdominal, inguinal, and axillary regions Pressure points and wear areas of body Generalized
Staphylococcal hypersensitivity	Erythematous epidermal collarettes Pustules, papules, papule/pustules Moth-eaten alopecia, especially in short-coated breeds of dogs	Abdominal, inguinal, and axillary regions Entire ventrum and lateral chest Generalized on trunk
Nasal pyoderma	Pustules, papules, nodules, erosions, ulcers Exudation and crust formation	Bridge of nose, around nostrils, upper lips
Canine acne	Pustules, papules, papule/pustules Nodules and draining tracts in chronic cases	Chin Occasionally upper lips
Juvenile pyoderma	Angioedema Pustules and vesicles Draining tracts	Face, lips, and ears Occasionally anus, prepuce, vulva, and feet

rial culture before selecting the most appropriate antibiotic. The cytology may reveal that all of the bacteria are intracellular only, and an antibiotic capable of killing intracellular bacteria may be required (*e.g.*, erythromycin or rifampin). The findings on cytology of other diseases are summarized in Table 52-11.

Culture and Sensitivity

Intact pustules that appear cytologically to be bacterial in origin are best sampled in the following manner. Alcohol should be gently wiped over the lesions and allowed to air dry. Pinpoint pustules should be gently ruptured with a sterile 25- or 26-gauge needle and their contents transferred from the needle to a Culturette. Larger pustules can be ruptured in a similar manner and their contents sampled directly using a Mini-Tip Culturette.

Draining and fistulous tracts and closed small abscesses should be sampled in the following manner. The area should first be thoroughly cleaned, as recommended for the surgical preparation of an area. The lesion should be surgically opened to its depths, using sterile technique. A sample can then be taken from the deepest portion of the lesion using a Culturette.

Intact nodular lesions can be cultured by excising them surgically, after proper surgical preparation, using sterile technique. The entire nodule can then be placed in a sterile container and submitted for a macerated tissue culture.

Table 52–10 *Autoimmune Skin Diseases*

Disease	Lesion	Distribution Pattern
Pemphigus foliaceus	Pustules	Bridge of nose, periorbital region, ears
	Epidermal collarettes, erythema, erosions, alopecia	Generalized
	Crusts and scales	
	Pitting edema	Limbs
	Hyperkeratosis, fissures, ulcers	Footpads
Pemphigus erythematosus	Pustules	Bridge of nose, periorbital region, ears
	Epidermal collarettes, erythema, erosions, alopecia	
	Crusts and scales	
	Depigmentation	
Pemphigus vulgaris	Vesicles, bullae	Mucous membranes, mucocutaneous junctions, base of nails
	Erosions and ulcers	Inguinal and axillary skin
		Foot pads
Pemphigus vegetans	Vesicles, pustules	Too few cases reported to determine pattern
	Erosions and ulcers	
	Crusts	
	Vegetations and papillomatous lesions	
Bullous pemphigoid	Vesicles, bullae	Mucous membranes, mucocutaneous junctions, base of nails
	Erosions and ulcers	Inguinal and axillary skin
		Foot pads
Systemic lupus erythematosus	Extremely variable	Extremely variable
	Erythema, alopecia, scaling crusts, depigmentation, vesicles, bullae, erosions, ulcers	
Discoid lupus erythematosus	Loss of cobblestone architecture on nose	Nose, bridge of nose, periorbital region, ears
	Depigmentation, erythema, erosion, ulcers	

By using these techniques, the organisms isolated are more likely to truly represent the primary pathogen involved in the disease process. This will result in a more favorable response to the antibiotic chosen, based on the sensitivity pattern. When the disease process is a deep pyoderma, refractory pyoderma, or chronic recurrent pyoderma, then the samples submitted should be submitted for both aerobic and anaerobic bacterial culture and sensitivity and fungal culture.

Histopathology

For proper use of the skin biopsy see Skin Biopsy in Chapter 80. The histopathologic interpretation of skin biopsies is one of the most important tools utilized in establishing a diagnosis in veterinary dermatology. However, to obtain useful information it is mandatory that samples be submitted only to an individual known to be proficient in veterinary dermatohistopathology. When selecting a lesion for biopsy, a primary lesion, when present, is often the most useful. This includes papules, pustules, papule/pustules, nodules, hemorrhagic bullae, vesicles, and bullae. When considering the diagnosis of staphylococcal hypersensitivity, an additional lesion to biopsy is the inflammatory margin of an epidermal collarette. Tables 52-12 and 52-13 are a summary of the histopathologic changes observed for the diseases covered in this chapter.

Immunologic Tests

In establishing the diagnosis of the autoimmune skin diseases discussed, several adjunct tests are available. Direct immunofluorescence testing can be performed on skin biopsies preserved in a suitable media (such as Michel's Fixative). However, results have varied greatly from one laboratory to another, often adding to the confusion rather than clarifying the diagnosis. We do not currently recommend use of this technique. Table 52-14 lists the expected findings on direct immunofluorescence of several autoimmune skin diseases. Indirect immunofluorescence testing can be performed on serum from a patient suspected of having an autoimmune skin disease. However, in contrast to humans, the results of this test are usually negative when performed in the dog and cat. This occurs in confirmed cases of autoimmune skin disease, and therefore this test is not recommended. When considering the diagnosis of systemic lupus erythematosus with cutaneous involvement, the following tests may be helpful in confirming the diagnosis: antinuclear antibody (ANA), lupus erythematosus cell preparation (LE prep), Coomb's test, and platelet factor 3.

Complete Blood Count, Serum Biochemistry Profile, and Urinalysis

These tests are most useful in screening for evidence of an underlying metabolic disease (see Chapter 49 and Tables 49-5 and 49-7), especially in cases of recurrent pyoderma, and in looking for evidence of systemic involvement in autoimmune diseases (Table 52-15). The complete blood count is useful in assessing the patient with a recurrent pyoderma. When considering the possibility of a cell-mediated immunodeficiency, the two most important cell populations to quantitate are the lymphocytes and neutrophils. A persistent and reproducible lymphopenia or neutropenia is strong evidence in support of such a deficiency (see Chapter 76). However, it is important that these changes be noted both in the face of an active pyoderma and after the patient has been on antibiotics for several weeks and is temporarily free of clinical disease.

Table 52–11 Cytology of Pustules and Vesicles

Disease	Lesion	Cytology
Bacterial diseases	Pustules, draining tract	Usually cocci, occasionally rods Numerous neutrophils Variable numbers of eosinophils and mononuclear cells
Pemphigus foliaceus or erythematosus	Pustules, erosions	Acantholytic keratinocytes Numerous neutrophils Variable numbers of Eosinophils
Pemphigus vulgaris	Vesicles, bullae, erosions, ulcers	Acantholytic keratinocytes
Bullous pemphigoid	Vesicles, bullae, erosions, ulcers	Relatively acellular Eosinophils may be present

Table 52–12 Major Histopathologic Changes Observed for Various Bacterial Skin Diseases

Disease	Lesion	Histopathology
Impetigo	Pustules	Subcorneal pustules with bacteria, neutrophils, and eosinophils and mononuclear cells
Superficial folliculitis	Pustules, papules, papule/pustules	Neutrophilic infiltrate into superficial portion of hair follicles plus bacteria
Deep folliculitis and furunculosis	Pustules, papules, papule/pustules Nodules Hemorrhagic bullae	Neutrophilic infiltrate into deeper portion of hair follicles plus bacteria Perifolliculitis Rupture of follicular wall Foreign body reaction Pyogranulomas
Staphylococcal hypersensitivity	Erythematous epidermal collarettes	Variable, often shows hyperkeratosis with numerous cocci, spongiotic pustules, and mild to moderate superficial perivascular dermatitis with varying numbers of eosinophils and neutrophils

Table 52–13 Major Histopathologic Changes Observed for Various Autoimmune Skin Diseases

Disease	Lesion	Histopathology
Pemphigus foliaceus	Pustules	Subcorneal pustules with acantholytic cells, neutrophils, and eosinophils Micropustules in wall of hair follicles
Pemphigus erythematosus	Pustules	Subcorneal pustules with acantholytic cells, neutrophils, and eosinophils Micropustules in wall of hair follicles
	Depigmented areas	Hydropic degeneration of basal epidermal cells, thickened basement membrane, pigmentary incontinence Lichenoid cellular infiltrate Dyskeratotic cells Mononuclear cells and plasma cells around vessels, hair follicles, and sebaceous and apocrine glands
Pemphigus vulgaris	Vesicles, bullae	Suprabasilar vesicle or bulla with acantholytic cells
Pemphigus vegetans	Vegetations, papillomatous lesions	Epidermal hyperplasia, papillomatosis, intraepidermal microabscesses with eosinophils and acantholytic cells
Bullous pemphigoid	Vesicles, bullae	Subepidermal vesicle or bulla
Discoid lupus erythematosus	Depigmented areas	Hydropic degeneration of basal epidermal cells, thickened basement membrane, pigmentary incontinence Lichenoid cellular infiltrate Dyskeratotic cells Mononuclear cells and plasma cells around vessels, hair follicles, and sebaceous and apocrine glands

Table 52–14 *Patterns of Direct Immunofluorescence That May Be Observed for Several Autoimmune Skin Diseases*

Disease	Pattern
Pemphigus foliaceus	Intercellular spaces of epidermis May be limited to upper epidermis
Pemphigus erythematosus	Intercellular spaces of epidermis May be limited to upper epidermis Basement membrane zone—usually an irregular linear band
Pemphigus vulgaris	Intercellular spaces of epidermis May be limited to deeper epidermis
Pemphigus vegetans	Intercellular spaces of epidermis May be limited to deeper epidermis
Bullous pemphigoid	Basement membrane zone—usually a smooth linear band
Lupus erythematosus	Basement membrane zone—usually an irregular linear band

Table 52–15 *Changes Present in the Hemogram and Urinalysis That May Suggest Systemic Involvement in Autoimmune Disease*

Test	What to Check For	Possible Cause
Hemogram	Normochromic, normocytic, nonregenerative anemia	Chronic disease state Early autoimmune hemolytic anemia
	Regenerative anemia, spherocytes, nucleated red blood cells, reticulocytes	Autoimmune hemolytic anemia
	Thrombocytopenia	Immune-mediated thrombocytopenia
Urinalysis	Proteinuria	Immune complex deposition glomerulonephritis

Mitogen Stimulation

This test has not been widely used in veterinary dermatology due to its limited availability. However, it can be helpful in assessing the functional performance and response of the lymphocyte population to various antigens and the lymphocytes' subsequent ability to undergo appropriate blastogenic transformation and mitotic division. The test is used to establish the diagnosis of lymphocyte deficiencies within the cell-mediated immune response. When performed properly, it can differentiate between primary defects in the lymphocytes themselves (a rare phenomenon) and defects contained within the serum of patients that are secondarily suppressing the lymphocytes' response. It is critical that this differentiation be determined, since immune stimulants are ineffective with serum-related suppressive factors. In addition, a serum-related lymphocyte suppressor factor usually indicates the presence of a another disease process, and does not support the diagnosis of a primary cell-mediated immunodeficiency.

ADDITIONAL READING

Berg JN, Wendell DE, Vogelweid C, Fales WH. Identification of the major coagulase-positive *Staphylococcus* sp. of dogs as *Staphylococcus intermedius*. Am J Vet Res 1984; 45:1307.

Halliwell REW, Gorman NT. Veterinary clinical immunology. Philadelphia: WB Saunders, 1989: 212.

Medleau L, Long RE, Brown J, Miller WH. Frequency and antimicrobial susceptibility of *Staphylococcus* species isolated from canine pyodermas. Am J Vet Res 1986; 47:229.

Muller GH, Kirk RW, Scott DW. Bacterial skin disease. In: Small animal dermatology. Philadelphia: WB Saunders, 1989: 244.

Rosenkrantz W. Immunomodulating drugs in dermatology. In: Kirk RW, ed. Current veterinary therapy X. Philadelphia: WB Saunders, 1989: 570.

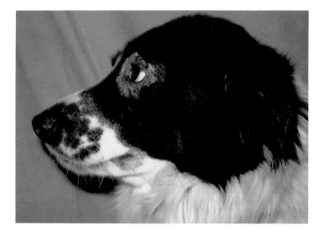

Color Figure 1. Localized demodicosis in a dog with focal areas of alopecia, erythema, and early hyperpigmentation.

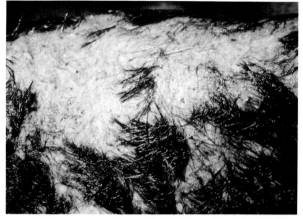

Color Figure 2. Generalized demodicosis with secondary deep pyoderma.

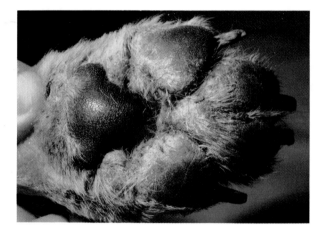

Color Figure 3. Pododemodicosis with secondary deep pyoderma.

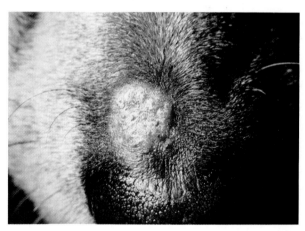

Color Figure 4. Localized dermatophytosis (due to infection with Microsporum canis) in a dog with annular alopecia and scale formation on the dorsal planum of the nose.

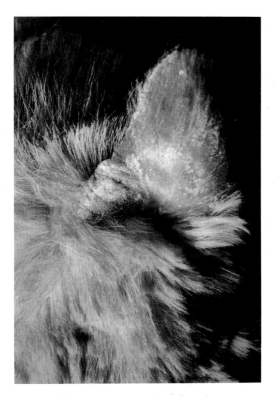

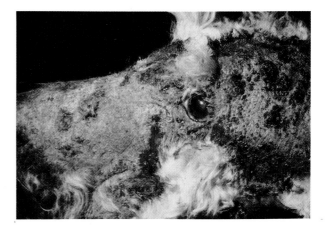

Color Figure 6. *Generalized dermatophytosis in a dog due to infection with* Trichophyton mentagrophytes *with a concurrent deep pyoderma.*

Color Figure 5. *Typical dermatophyte reaction (due to infection with* Microsporum canis*) in a cat with an irregularly shaped area of alopecia and mild erythema and scale formation.*

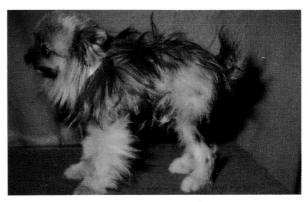

Color Figure 8. *Castration-responsive dermatosis in a Pomeranian with alopecia and haircoat color changes.*

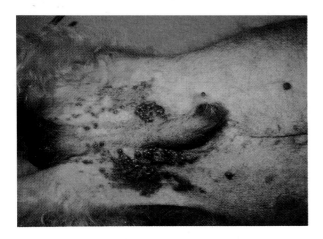

Color Figure 7. *Calcinosis cutis in the inguinal region of a dog. Lesions are usually symmetrical and firm or gritty upon palpation.*

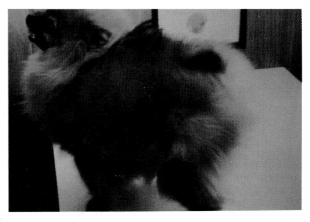

Color Figure 9. *Castration-responsive dermatosis (same patient as in Color Figure 8) 3 months following castration.*

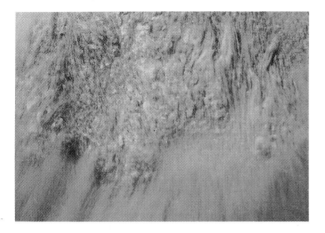

Color Figure 10. *Circumscribed lesion of seborrheic dermatitis in a cocker spaniel, showing tightly adherent yellowish scales and crusts with erythema.*

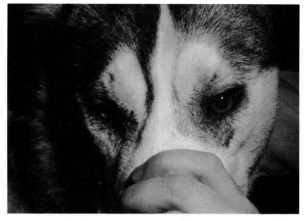

Color Figure 11. *Zinc-responsive dermatosis, Syndrome I. Note the focal areas of erythema and tightly adherent scales and crusts at the periorbital region.*

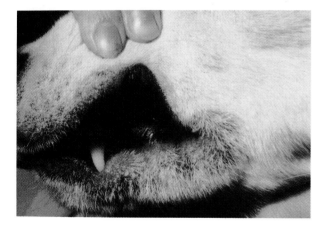

Color Figure 12. *Zinc-responsive dermatosis, Syndrome I. Note focal areas of erythema and tightly adherent scales and crusts at the lower lip.*

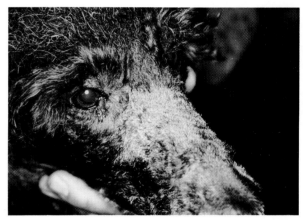

Color Figure 13. *Sebaceous adenitis in a standard poodle. Note tightly adherent silvery white scales over the dorsal planum of the nose. (From Rosser E. Sebaceous adenitis with hyperkeratosis in the standard poodle: A discussion of ten cases. Journal of the American Animal Hospital Association 1987; 23:342.)*

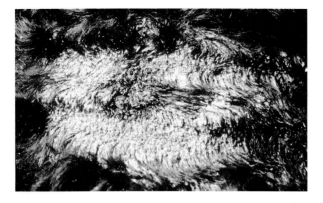

Color Figure 14. *Sebaceous adenitis in a standard poodle. Note tightly adherent silvery white scales over the dorsal planum of the dorsal trunk region. (From Rosser E. Sebaceous adenitis with hyperkeratosis in the standard poodle: A discussion of ten cases. Journal of the American Animal Hospital Association 1987; 23:342.)*

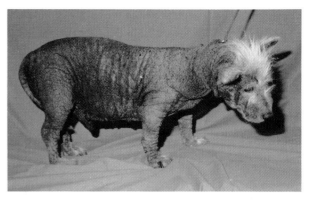

Color Figure 15. *Generalized epidermal dysplasia in a West Highland white terrier.*

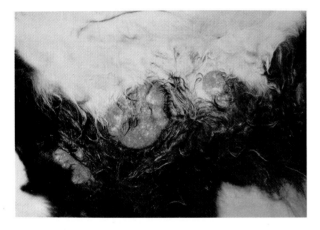

Color Figure 16. *Eosinophilic plaque lesion in a cat with flea allergy dermatitis.*

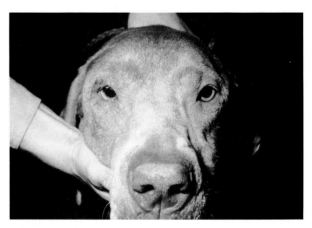

Color Figure 17. *Periorbital erythema and alopecia in a dog with atopy.*

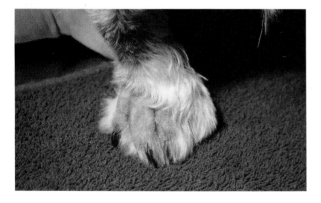

Color Figure 18. *Post-traumatic alopecia and erythema of the dorsal aspect of the foot in a dog with atopy.*

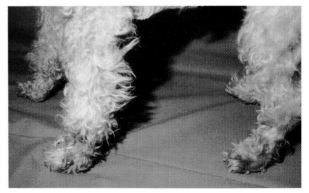

Color Figure 19. *Salivary staining of the hair on all four feet from excessive licking in a dog with atopy.*

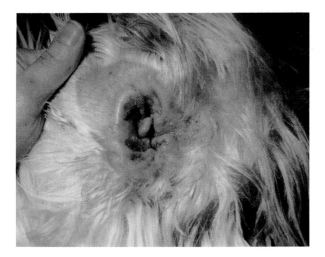

Color Figure 20. *Erythema and early proliferative changes of the pinnae and external ear canal in a dog with so-called "allergic otitis externa" due to a food allergy.*

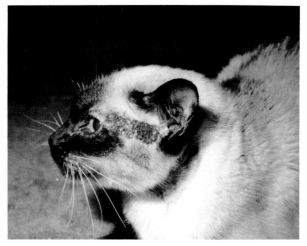

Color Figure 21. *Papules, crust formation, and excoriation in the preaural region of a cat with food allergy.*

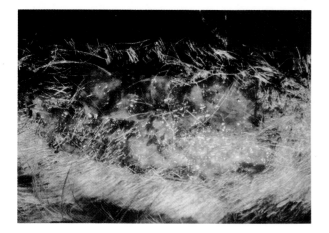

Color Figure 22. *Typical appearance of a hot spot over the tail base region in an dog with flea allergy dermatitis.*

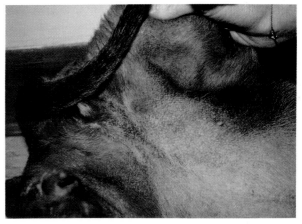

Color Figure 23. *Hemorrhagic bulla in a dog with recurrent deep folliculitis and furunculosis.*

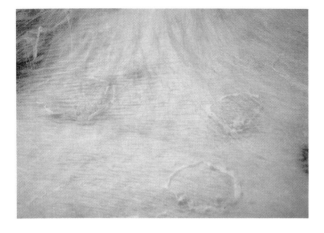

Color Figure 24. *Epidermal collarettes in a dog with a recurrent superficial pyoderma due to staphylococcal hypersensitivity.*

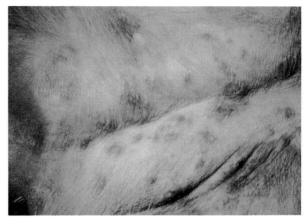

Color Figure 25. *Epidermal collarettes in a dog with marked erythema peripherally and hyperpigmentation centrally.*

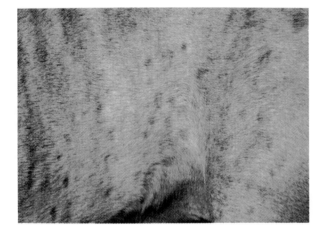

Color Figure 26. *Moth-eaten alopecia pattern on the trunk of a dog with recurrent superficial folliculitis secondary to hypothyroidism.*

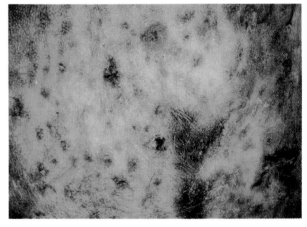

Color Figure 27. *Generalized deep folliculitis and furunculosis in a dog with papules, pustules, hemorrhagic bulla, and crust formation.*

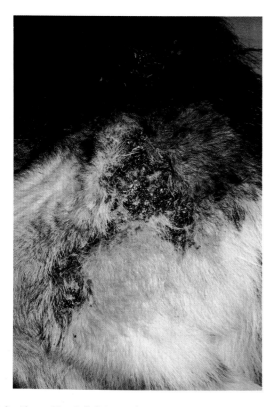

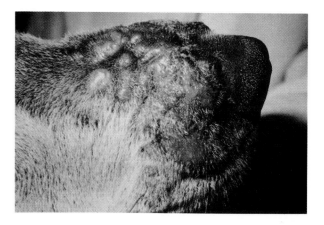

Color Figure 29. Nasal pyoderma in a dog with papules, nodules, and erosions over the bridge of the nose and nostril region.

Color Figure 28. Cellulitis-type lesion over lateral aspect of the hip region in a dog with a recurrent deep pyoderma due to a T lymphocyte immunodeficiency.

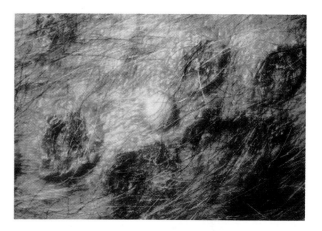

Color Figure 31. Pemphigus foliaceus in a dog with pustules, very inflamed epidermal collarettes, and crust formation.

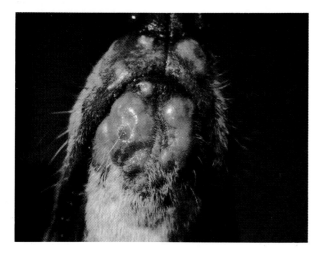

Color Figure 30. Chronic canine acne with development of severe folliculitis and furunculosis.

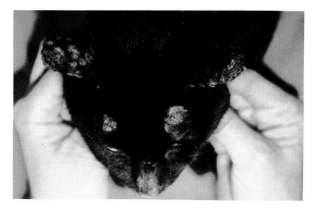

Color Figure 32. Pemphigus foliaceus in a cat with symmetrical crust formation over the bridge of the nose, ears, and periorbital regions.

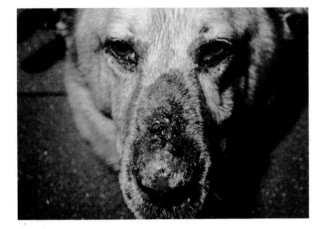

Color Figure 33. *Pemphigus erythematosus in a dog with depigmentation and ulceration of the nose and crust formation over the bridge of the nose.*

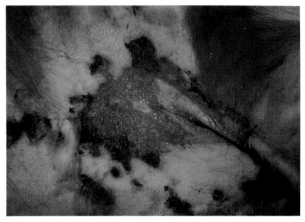

Color Figure 34. *Bullous pemphigoid in a dog with ulcers and crust formation in the axillary region.*

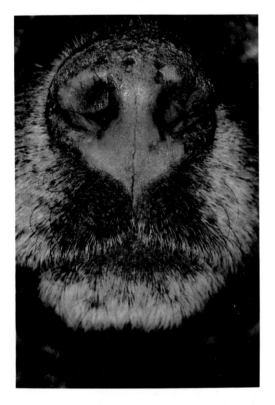

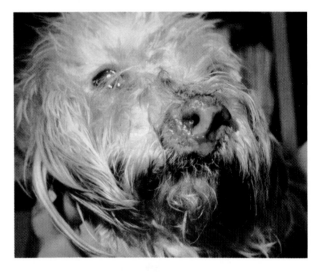

Color Figure 36. *Discoid lupus erythematosus in a dog with chronic changes of complete depigmentation, erosions, and ulcers of the nose.*

Color Figure 35. *Discoid lupus erythematosus in a dog with early depigmentation and slate gray coloration of the nose.*

THE NERVOUS SYSTEM

8

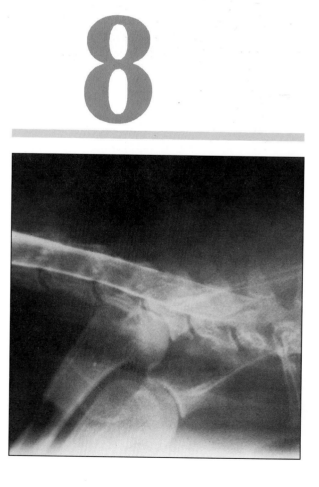

53

SEIZURES

Joane M. Parent, Susan M. Cochrane

Seizures represent one of the most common problems in small animal neurology. The prevalence of seizure activity in canine and feline patients is approximately 0.5% to 1%. The diagnosis and long-term management of seizure disorders can be a frustrating problem for both veterinarian and pet owner.

CAUSES

Seizures may be caused by intracranial or extracranial disorders. Regardless of the specific etiology, seizure activity originates from the thalamocortex.

A number of causes of seizures in dogs and cats have been reported in the veterinary literature. Table 53-1 lists these causes; this checklist may prove useful for assuring that all appropriate possibilities have been considered when establishing the diagnostic plan. In the present text, emphasis will be placed on the most common causes of seizures in the dog and cat.

Extracranial disorders usually produce generalized tonic–clonic motor seizures. Intracranial disorders can result in either generalized or partial seizures. Partial seizures are characterized by clinical signs such as unilateral facial twitching and tonic–clonic contractions of a limb, which can be localized to the affected portion of the thalamocortex. Partial seizures have a tendency to generalize as the disease progresses.

In both the dog and cat seizures are more frequently associated with intracranial causes. Idiopathic epilepsy, which is a functional disorder of the thalamocortex, is the more common cause of seizures in the dog. In contrast, the majority of seizures in the cat occur secondary to structural brain diseases such as encephalitis or neoplasia. Idiopathic epilepsy is rarely encountered in the cat.

Seizures observed with metabolic encephalopathies are usually the generalized motor type, without any localizing signs. While seizures have been associated with hepatic encephalopathy, these are relatively uncommon in the dog. Waxing and waning periods of depression, stupor, dementia, head pressing, and ataxia are more common neurologic signs of hepatic encephalopathy in the dog (see Chapter 40). In the cat, hepatic encephalopathy is more likely to result in seizure activity, irritability, and frequent bouts of salivation. Generalized tonic–clonic motor seizures secondary to hypoglycemia may be the only presenting complaint of a beta cell tumor in the dog (see Chapter 77).

Table 53-1 *Causes of Seizures in the Dog and Cat*

I. Extracranial causes
  A. Metabolic
    1. Hepatic encephalopathy*
    2. Hypoglycemia
    3. Cardiac arrhythmias*
    4. Renal failure
    5. Hypocalcemia
    6. Hyperlipidemia
  B. Toxic
    1. Lead
    2. Organophosphates
    3. Chlorinated hydrocarbons
    4. Ethylene glycol
    5. Strychnine
    6. Metaldehyde
    7. Mycotoxins
    8. Metrizamide
    9. Chocolate
    10. Caffeine
    11. Aspirin
II. Intracranial causes
  A. Idiopathic epilepsy
  B. Inflammatory
    1. Infectious
      a. Viral: feline infectious peritonitis, canine distemper virus, rabies
      b. Mycotic: cryptococcosis, blastomycosis
      c. Protozoal: toxoplasmosis
    2. Noninfectious: granulomatous meningoencephalitis
  C. Neoplastic
    1. Primary tumors: meningioma, glioma
    2. Secondary tumors: hemangiosarcoma
  D. Degenerative
    1. Feline ischemic encephalopathy
    2. Storage diseases
  E. Nutritional: thiamine deficiency
  F. Head trauma
    1. Acute injury
    2. Chronic injury
  G. Anomalies or malformations
    1. Hydrocephalus
    2. Lissencephaly/pachygyria
    3. Porencephaly

* *Seizures are more commonly seen in the cat with these diseases.*

In the cat cardiac arrhythmias can be associated with seizures, whereas in the dog the usual manifestation is syncope (see Chapter 5).

Toxin-related seizures occur more frequently in dogs than cats because of their less discriminating eating habits. Consequently, poisoning should be considered in any young dog presented with abnormal behavior or generalized seizures. Muscle fasciculations and hyperexcitability often precede toxin-related seizures, and the seizure activity usually continues until appropriate therapy is administered.

PATHOPHYSIOLOGY

Seizure activity originates from the thalamocortex. Seizures arise from a focus of neurons in the thalamocortex that exhibit a spontaneous paroxysmal discharge of abnormal electrical activity. Intracranial causes can give rise to partial or generalized seizures, while extracranial causes of seizures tend to lead to generalized seizures.

The most common type of seizure in the dog is the generalized motor seizure. In some cases, seizure activity may be limited to a focus in the brain, resulting in a partial seizure. A partial seizure may help to localize the lesion by displaying features characteristic of the area of the cerebral cortex involved (*e.g.*, a right facial twitch indicates a lesion of the left motor cortex). With spread of the electrical activity from the initial focus, a partial seizure may become generalized. Seizures of intracranial origin may be associated with other neurologic abnormalities, such as circling, abnormal behavior, or postural reaction deficits. However, seizure activity is often the only clinical abnormality.

A seizure, when short in duration, does not appear to be detrimental to neurons. However, seizures occuring in clusters (a group of seizures occurring close together, in which the animal does not fully recover from one seizure before going into the next) or as status epilepticus result in neuronal death. Status epilepticus is a life-threatening condition because of both the ensuing brain damage and the biochemical effects on the body, including hyperthermia, lactic acidosis, and hypoxia.

CLINICAL SIGNS

Since the seizure is often very short in duration and is over by the time the patient is presented, the veterinarian rarely is able to observe the event. Consequently, the veterinarian must rely on the description of the seizure provided by the owner.

The generalized motor seizure is often described as having an aura, ictus, and postictal period. The aura is the period that precedes the generalized motor activity, when the dog may exhibit abnormal behavior such as attention-seeking, fear, or anxiety. The aura is often short and may go unnoticed. The ictus is characterized by one or more of the following abnormalities: loss of consciousness, lateral recumbency with rigidity or paddling movements of the limbs, chomping of the jaw, salivation, pupillary dilation, and, in many cases, urination and defecation. This phase usually lasts for 30 to 90 seconds. The post-ictal phase is characterized by compulsive pacing, restlessness, staggering, polydipsia and polyphagia, apparent blindness, and decreased responsiveness to stimuli. This phase varies in severity and may last from a few minutes to a few days. The severity of the post-ictal phase, however, does not necessarily correlate with the apparent severity of the clinical signs observed during ictus.

DIAGNOSTIC APPROACH

The age and breed of the patient and the type and frequency of the seizures must be considered in any dog or cat that is presented for evaluation of seizure activity. On presentation, physical, neurologic, and ophthamologic examinations should be performed (Fig. 53-1). The minimum data base for any patient with seizures should include a complete blood count, a serum biochemistry profile, and urinalysis.

In the dog, the most common cause of seizures is idiopathic epilepsy. This is a functional disturbance of the thalamocortex in which no primary histologic lesion exists. The aim of the diagnostic approach presented here is to differentiate id-

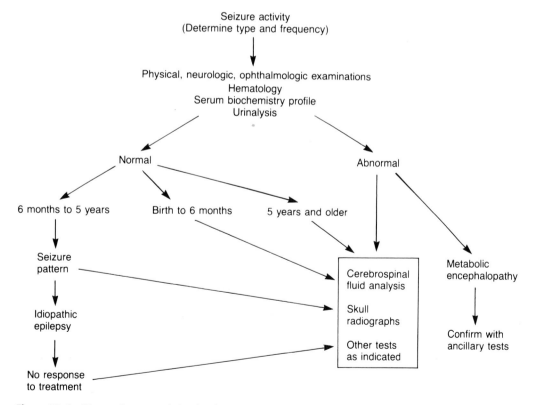

Figure 53–1. *Diagnostic approach for the dog presented with seizures.*

iopathic epilepsy from other diseases that cause seizures (see Table 53-1).

The age and breed of the dog and the seizure pattern are the most important factors in differentiating idiopathic epilepsy from other causes of seizures. In idiopathic epilepsy, the onset of seizure activity typically occurs between 6 months and 5 years of age. Therefore, a dog whose seizures begin when it is younger than 6 months or older than 5 years of age is unlikely to have idiopathic epilepsy. While idiopathic epilepsy can occur in any breed of dog, certain breeds are predisposed to this disorder (Table 53-2). In idiopathic epilepsy, the seizures are usually of the generalized motor type. In all breeds of dog with idiopathic epilepsy, seizures are typically infrequent at the onset. In small breeds, the seizures may remain infrequent, whereas in the larger breeds they tend to become more frequent and severe with time. The patient presenting with frequent, severe, or partial seizures at the onset is less likely to have idiopathic epilepsy.

The physical examination in patients with idiopathic epilepsy is normal. If abnormalities, such as weight loss have accompanied the development of seizures, the diagnostic approach should be directed toward an extracranial or structural intracranial etiology rather than idiopathic epilepsy.

Table 53–2 *Breeds of Dogs Predisposed to Idiopathic Epilepsy*

Beagle
Belgian Tervuren
Cocker spaniel
Collie
Corgi
Dachshund
Dalmatian
Irish setter
Keeshond
German shepherd
Golden retriever
Labrador retriever
Poodle
Nova Scotia duck tolling retriever
Saint Bernard
Siberian husky
Shetland sheepdog
Springer spaniel
Wirehaired fox terrier

The neurologic examination in patients with idiopathic epilepsy should be normal unless the dog is in the postictal phase, in which case transient neurologic deficits may be present. Abnormalities detected on neurologic examination, such as ataxia or compulsive behavior, that are not immediately associated with a seizure event eliminate idiopathic epilepsy as a cause of the seizures. These deficits may help to localize the lesion if a structural intracranial disorder is present.

The ophthalmologic examination is an important part of the initial evaluation. Since the optic nerve extends directly from the brain and is surrounded by cerebrospinal fluid, certain central nervous system disorders can result in abnormalities, such as optic neuritis, that can be detected by ophthalmologic examination. Several organisms that infect the central nervous system, such as canine distemper virus, *Toxoplasma gondii*, and the disseminated fungal agents, may cause a chorioretinitis as part of their multisystemic disease. Such abnormalities on ophthalmologic examination of a dog would rule out idiopathic epilepsy as a cause of the seizures.

The minimum data base, which includes a complete blood count, a serum biochemistry profile, and urinalysis, provides the next step in the diagnostic approach to a dog with seizures. The minimum data base is an especially important indicator of extracranial diseases, such as hepatic disorders or pancreatic islet cell neoplasia. The patient with idiopathic epilepsy will have a normal minimum data base. Since many patients with seizures will receive anticonvulsant therapy, the minimum data base also provides evaluation of major organ function, such as the liver and kidneys, prior to treatment.

In summary, the history, initial examinations, and minimum data base provide information that is important in determining whether or not idiopathic epilepsy is a likely cause of the patient's seizures. It is important to remember, however, that while the majority of extracranial and structural intracranial causes of seizures demonstrate abnormalities in the initial evaluation, this is not always the case.

If idiopathic epilepsy is not considered a likely cause of the seizures, an extended data base should be pursued. Depending on the individual case, this extended data base may involve cerebrospinal fluid analysis (see Cerebrospinal Fluid Collection in Chapter 80), including immunoglobulin evaluation and possibly microbial culture and viral titers. Skull radiographs and brain imaging techniques (*e.g.*, magnetic resonance imaging, computed tomography) may also be indicated. In certain geographic locations, specific serum titers for diseases such as *Erhlichia canis* and Rocky Mountain spotted fever may be indicated (see Chapter 79). If a metabolic disturbance is suspected based on the minimum data base, appropriate specific testing, such as serum ammonia and bile acid determinations for hepatic encephalopathy, should be pursued.

Many dogs that are suspected to have idiopathic epilepsy do not have a cerebrospinal fluid analysis performed. This procedure should, however, be considered in breeding or performance dogs, including guide dogs, as it is important to document the existence of idiopathic epilepsy in such cases. In addition, cerebrospinal fluid analysis should be performed in dogs that are originally suspected to have idiopathic epilepsy but whose seizure pattern is unusual or response to appropriate therapy is poor. These dogs may be suffering from another disorder, such as viral encephalitis, granulomatous meningoencephalomyelitis, or neoplasia. An extended data base will help to differentiate these cases from severe refractory idiopathic epileptics, for which satisfactory long-term control is poor. Idiopathic epilepsy is said to be refractory when adequate anticonvulsant serum levels have been achieved and the seizures are still poorly controlled. Refractory idiopathic epilepsy occurs more often in the larger breeds of dogs (*e.g.*, German shepherds).

The diagnostic approach to a cat with seizures is similar to that described for the dog, with a few important exceptions. Structural disorders such as viral encephalitis, vascular disease, or neoplasia are much more common than idiopathic epilepsy in this species. Therefore, the cat with seizures will usually require an extended data base, including cerebrospinal fluid analysis, to determine the cause of the seizures.

Clinical impressions suggest that cats with cardiac disease may present for seizurelike episodes. Therefore, a thorough cardiac evaluation is recommended in cats with a history of seizures.

In the evaluation of serum titers for viral disorders such as feline infectious peritonitis and feline leukemia virus, it is important to recognize that these titers may be negative in cases in which the disease is predominantly located within the central nervous system (see Chapter 79). Cats with hepatic vascular anomalies such as portosystemic shunts are more likely to have seizure activity as the only presenting neurologic sign than are dogs. Another abnormality observed in cats with hepatic encephalopathy that is not a feature in the dog is excessive salivation.

MANAGEMENT

Anticonvulsant medication should be initiated in the following circumstances: when seizures occur more often than once every 4 to 6 weeks, when there is more than one seizure per day (even if this is an infrequent occurrence), or in the case of status epilepticus. A minimum data base, including a complete blood count, serum biochemistry profile, and urinalysis, should be performed prior to starting anticonvulsant therapy. These data will provide a baseline for subsequent assessment of any adverse effects of the medication (see Appendix II). The data will also help to establish the presence of preexistent disease, especially of the liver or kidneys in the older patient, that might influence drug metabolism. The duration of anticonvulsant therapy will depend on the specific etiology of the seizure activity in the individual case.

The pharmacokinetics of many anticonvulsant drugs are known for the dog. Since this information is not as extensively available for the cat, anticonvulsants in this species have been used on more of an empirical basis. In the dog, oral phenobarbital is well recognized as the anticonvulsant of choice for maintenance therapy. Phenobarbital raises the threshold for seizure activity and helps limit the spread of activity from the seizure focus. Other maintenance anticonvulsant drugs used with some success in the dog include primidone, longer-acting benzodiazepines (clonazepam), and, more recently, potassium bromide. In the cat, the preferred anticonvulsants for maintenance therapy are phenobarbital and diazepam.

Following 2 to 3 weeks of continued phenobarbital therapy in the dog, steady-state serum drug levels should be measured. An initial dose of 1 to 2.5 mg/kg twice daily may be adjusted accordingly to attain therapeutic drug levels. The therapeutic range suggested for phenobarbital in the dog is 70 to 170 μmol/L (15 to 40 mg/dl). Serum drug levels should also be determined 2 weeks following alterations in the phenobarbital dose. The serum sample for phenobarbital determination is usually collected just prior to a treatment. In the cat an oral dose of phenobarbital of 4 mg/kg once daily or divided twice daily has been recommended.

Phenobarbital therapy should never be abruptly discontinued, as this may precipitate severe seizure activity. While phenobarbital is a relatively safe anticonvulsant, hepatotoxicity has been documented following chronic treatment at serum drug levels in the upper therapeutic range.

Clonazepam has been used in the dog mainly as an adjunct therapy in dogs that are unresponsive to phenobarbital therapy alone. It is given orally in conjunction with phenobarbital at a dose of 0.1 to 0.3 mg/kg three times daily. Unfortunately, the drug is expensive and tolerance often develops within a few months of administration. There are no data available for the use of this drug in the cat.

Primidone (Mysoline) is still widely used as an anticonvulsant in the dog. It has the advantage over phenobarbital of not being a controlled drug. The anticonvulsant action of primidone is derived from the parent compound primidone and the metabolites phenobarbital and phenylethylmalonide (PEMA). Since the half-lives of primidone and PEMA are short, three times a day treatment is required. Even with this therapeutic regime, approximately 85% or more of the anticonvulsant activity of primidone is derived from the metabolite phenobarbital. The risk of hepatotoxicity and subsequent hepatic cirrhosis is high with chronic primidone administration. Based on these facts, phenobarbital is the preferred maintenance anticonvulsant. The safety of primidone

in the cat has been questioned. While it may not be as toxic in this species as originally suspected, it does not appear to offer any advantages over phenobarbital and diazepam.

The pharmacokinetics of phenytoin (Dilantin) make this drug unsuitable for use in the dog and cat. Effective serum phenytoin concentrations are difficult to achieve because of the drug's short half-life in the dog. This drug is not recommended for use in the cat because toxicity results from the very long half-life in this species.

The short half-life of diazepam (Valium) in the dog makes it unsuitable for use as an oral maintenance anticonvulsant. Diazepam is, however, the drug of choice for ongoing seizures such as cluster seizures or status epilepticus. Following an intravenous bolus (5 to 20 mg, repeated up to three times) to control the major motor activity, diazepam is best administered as a constant-rate intravenous infusion at 5 to 20 mg/hour. In the occasional difficult case, phenobarbital at a dose of 3 to 6 mg/hour can be added to the diazepam infusion. Since these two drugs potentiate each other, phenobarbital must be added cautiously to avoid cardiac and respiratory depression. When intravenous administration is not possible, 5 to 20 mg of diazepam can be administered either intramuscularly or rectally by the owner to stop the cluster seizures and to allow for transport to a veterinary clinic.

In the cat the half-life of diazepam is longer than in the dog. As a result, this drug can be effectively used as an oral maintenance anticonvulsant in the cat at a dose of 2 to 5 mg twice daily.

Potassium bromide is an anticonvulsant recently recommended for use in the dog. This drug is thought to act by influencing chloride conductance. The half-life is extremely long, and the biochemical toxicities in the dog are not well established. The recommended dose is 10 to 20 mg/kg orally twice daily. The owner should be aware that the potential side-effects, especially with long-term therapy, are not known. Potassium bromide is used in conjunction with phenobarbital when phenobarbital therapy alone has been unable to adequately control the seizures. The serum levels should be maintained between approximately 1 and 3 mg/ml (9–15 mmol/L). Care should be taken in handling the product, since bromide toxicity is a concern in humans (see Appendix II).

PATIENT MONITORING

The majority of dogs and cats that exhibit recurrent seizure activity will require long-term treatment. For the well-controlled patient on a low- to mid-therapeutic serum level of phenobarbital, an evaluation of the complete blood count, serum biochemistry profile (especially the liver enzymes), and serum drug level should be performed at the time of annual vaccination. The patient that requires higher therapeutic levels of phenobarbital or multiple drug therapy should be evaluated every 3 to 6 months.

It must be remembered that idiopathic epilepsy is an incurable disease and that even if the patient is doing well, therapy is usually required for the life of the patient. In all cases, the owner should be aware that rapid withdrawal of any anticonvulsant may precipitate serious seizure activity. Possible drug interactions must be considered when therapy for another disorder is initiated in a patient already receiving anticonvulsant drugs. The most common interactions to be avoided are phenobarbital combined with chloramphenicol or cimetidine, since both of the latter drugs interfere with the metabolism of phenobarbital, potentially resulting in toxic levels of this anticonvulsant.

ADDITIONAL READING

Frey HH, Löscher W. Pharmacokinetics of antiepileptic drugs in the dog: A review. J Vet Pharmacol Ther 1985; 8:219.

Oliver JE. Seizure disorders and narcolepsy. In: Oliver JE, Horlein BF, Mayhew IG, eds. Veterinary neurology. Philadelphia: WB Saunders, 1987: 285.

Parent JM. Clinical management of canine seizures. Vet Clin North Am [Small Anim Pract] 1988; 18:947.

54

ATAXIA AND PARESIS

Susan M. Cochrane, Joane M. Parent

The evaluation of gait for ataxia can be a challenging aspect of the neurologic examination. Ataxia is defined as a lack of coordination of muscular function that results in irregular muscle movements and staggering. In veterinary medicine the three types of ataxia observed are sensory, cerebellar, and vestibular. This chapter will specifically address sensory ataxia, with comparisons made to the ataxias of cerebellar and vestibular disease origin. Sensory ataxia is differentiated from the other types of ataxia from the concomitant presence of paresis. This chapter discusses the sensory ataxia and paresis associated with spinal cord disorders.

CAUSES

Spinal cord sensory ataxia in the dog and cat originates from disorders of the vertebral column or spinal cord (Table 54-1). Diseases primarily involving the vertebral column are more common and include degenerative disorders (*e.g.,* intervertebral disk disease), trauma (*e.g.,* fracture, luxation), infection (*e.g.,* osteomyelitis, discospondylitis), congenital malformation, and neoplasia (*e.g.,* osteosarcoma, fibrosarcoma, chondrosarcoma). The sensory ataxia associated with disorders of the vertebral column originate from compression of the spinal cord.

Diseases that are restricted to the meninges of the spinal cord do not typically result in sensory ataxia. The classic signs of inflammation of the meninges (meningitis) include neck pain, cervical rigidity, stiff gait, and, in some cases, fever. It is only when the meningeal infiltration of inflammatory cells (*e.g.,* feline infectious peritonitis) or neoplastic cells (meningioma) invades the underlying spinal cord parenchyma and forms a space-occupying mass that a sensory ataxia develops.

Disorders primarily affecting the spinal cord parenchyma include inflammatory, neoplastic degenerative, and anomalous, diseases. Inflammatory disorders can be either infectious or noninfectious. Infectious myelitis may be present with viral (*e.g.,* canine distemper virus, feline infectious peritonitis), bacterial, fungal (*e.g.,* cryptococcosis, blastomycosis), or protozoal (*e.g.,* toxoplasmosis, *Neospora caninum*) disorders.

Primary neoplasms of the spinal cord parenchyma (intramedullary tumors) are uncommon. While gliomas usually occur in the older dog, spinal cord blastomas typically occur in the young (6 months to 3 years) large-breed dog (especially the German shepherd). They are exclusively located from T-10 to L-3.

Primary or secondary extramedullary neoplasms are encountered in the dog and cat. In the cat, lymphosarcoma is a common cause of ataxia and paresis. Although nerve sheath tumors origi-

Table 54–1 *Most Common Causes of Ataxia and Paresis or Tetraparesis in the Dog* by Spinal Cord Region*

Disease	Breeds More Frequently Affected	Typical Age	Site Most Commonly Involved	Hyperpathia
C-1– C-5‡				
Intervertebral disk disease	Chondrodystrophic breeds and other breeds	3 to 6 years	C-2–C-6	+
Fibrocartilaginous embolic myelopathy	Large breeds	Young–middle aged	Any Asymmetric	−
Cervical vertebral instability	Doberman pinschers	3 to 8 years	C-5–C-7	− / +
Diskospondylitis	Large breeds	Middle-aged	C-5–C-7	+
Bacterial meningitis	Large breeds	<2 years		+
Granulomatous meningoencephalomyelitis	Small breeds	1 to 10 years		+
Atlantoaxial subluxation	Toy breeds	6 to 18 months	C-1–C-2	+
Meningioma	Any	Older	C-1–T-2	− / +
C-6–T-2				
Fibrocartilaginous embolic myelopathy	Large breeds	Young–middle aged	Asymmetric	−
Intervertebral disk disease	Chondrodystrophic breeds and other small breeds	3 to 6 years	Does not occur at T-1–T-2	+
Nerve sheath tumor	Any	Older	Originates from spinal nerve or root	− / +
Road trauma	Any	Any	Asymmetric, avulsion of roots with cervical intumescence swelling	−
T-3–L-3				
Intervertebral disk disease				
Type I	Chondrodystrophic breeds and other small breeds	3 to 6 years	T-11–L-2	+
Type II	Large breeds	Older	T-11–L-2	+
Fibrocartilaginous embolic myelopathy	Large breeds	Young	Usually asymmetric	−
Degenerative radiculomyelopathy	German shepherds	>7 years	Thoracic/lumbar	−
Spinal cord blastoma	Large breeds especially German shepherds	6 months to 3 years	T-10–L-3	−
L-4 to caudal				
Trauma	Any	Any	Lumbosacral junction	+
Fibrocartilaginous embolic myelopathy	Large breeds	Young–middle aged	Usually asymmetric throughout region	−
Intervertebral disk disease	Large breeds	3 to 6 years	L-4–S-1	+
Diskospondylitis	Large breeds	Middle-aged to older	Lumbosacral junction	+
Lumbosacral stenosis	Large breeds	Middle-aged to older	Lumbosacral junction	+
Malformation	English bulldogs	Birth	Sacral and caudal segments	−

* No particular disease entity is defined as a common occurrence in the feline spinal cord. See text for specific entities.
(+ = present; − = not present)
‡ Or C1–C7 white matter alone.

nate outside of the vertebral column, these tumors often extend proximally up the spinal nerve and root to become intimately associated with the spinal cord. Spinal cord infiltration or compression by the nerve root tumor results in signs (often ipsilateral, initially) of sensory ataxia and paresis.

Spinal cord diseases occur more commonly in the dog due to the high incidence of intervertebral disk disease (IVDD). In contrast, IVDD is an uncommon occurrence in the cat.

Diseases of the brain stem may also interfere with the ascending proprioceptive and descending upper motor neuron pathways, resulting in a sensory ataxia and paresis. Other neurologic abnormalities, such as cranial nerve deficits, changes in mentation, or cerebellar signs, are usually present, aiding in localization of the lesion to the brain stem. Inflammatory and neoplastic etiologies most commonly affect the brain stem. In the cat, feline infectious peritonitis is the most common infectious disease to affect this region. Granulomatous meningoencephalomyelitis (GME) is a noninfectious inflammatory and idiopathic disease of the dog that is documented to affect the brain stem in either the disseminated, or focal form.

PATHOPHYSIOLOGY

Sensory ataxia results from a disturbance in sensory information as it ascends the spinal cord white matter to the brain stem and cerebral cortex. This system of general proprioceptive pathways provides the cerebral cortex with information regarding the spatial arrangement of the limbs and trunk. Since the general proprioceptive tracts cross to the contralateral side in the brain stem, the sensory information from the spinal cord is received by the contralateral cerebral cortex (*e.g.*, a left cerebral cortical lesion results in right-sided postural reaction deficits). Although the sensory information is initially perceived by the peripheral receptors located in the skin, tendons, and joints, and ascends through peripheral nerves to the spinal cord, peripheral nerve disease primarily results in paresis alone without ataxia.

The upper motor neuron (UMN) pathways descend from the sensorimotor area of the cerebral cortex to the spinal cord white matter, where they influence the lower motor neurons (LMN). The major descending UMN pathways in domestic animals cross to the contralateral side in the midbrain of the brain stem, such that unilateral lesions of the cerebral cortex produce motor deficits (paresis) in the limbs on the contralateral side of the body. Lesions in these UMN tracts caudal to this crossing produce ipsilateral paresis or paralysis.

The major role of the descending UMN pathways is to transmit motor information to the LMN, thereby regulating the reflex activity of the LMN. The LMN consists of the cell body located in the ventral gray column of the specific spinal cord segment and the associated ventral root, spinal nerve, peripheral nerve, and neuromuscular junction. The reflex arc is completed by the sensory portion of the peripheral nerve, dorsal root, and dorsal root ganglion.

Since the descending UMN pathways are closely associated with the ascending sensory tracts within the spinal cord, paresis accompanies the sensory ataxia of lesions in the spinal cord.

Many spinal cord disorders involve compression of the spinal cord parenchyma. The signs of ataxia and paresis seen with compressive lesions (*e.g.*, IVDD) are usually bilateral. There may, however, be an asymmetry to the deficits if the lesion is unilateral, especially if the disease is slowly progressive (*e.g.*, a nerve root tumor extending into the spinal canal) or vascular in origin (*e.g.*, fibrocartilaginous embolic myelopathy). Even with very asymmetrical lesions, subtle deficits are usually detected in the limb(s) on the opposite side of the body.

The degree of sensory and motor deficits with a spinal cord disorder can, in many cases, be used to determine the severity of the lesion. The order in which functions are lost is based on their position, and, hence, their relative protection within the spinal cord parenchyma and their fiber size. With increasing severity of spinal cord compression, neurologic abnormalities appear in the following order: sensory ataxia (ascending general proprioceptive pathways), paresis to paralysis (descending UMN pathways), loss of sphincter control for urination and defecation, and, finally, absence of pain perception. Since the pain pathways are the smallest and most resistant fiber type in the spinal cord, loss of this function suggests the most severe of spinal cord insults and is associated with a grave prognosis for recovery. When recovery from spinal cord disorders does occur, function returns in the reverse order to which it was lost.

CLINICAL SIGNS

One of the most challenging aspects of the neurologic examination is to differentiate ataxia or incoordination from paresis. Once the presence of ataxia has been established, sensory ataxia must be differentiated from cerebellar and vestibular ataxia.

Cerebellar ataxia is not associated with paresis, since the descending UMN pathways are intact. The cerebellum acts as a regulator rather than an initiator of movement. As a result, limb movements associated with cerebellar disease lack fine control and are incoordinated, spastic, and often hypermetric, but normal limb strength is preserved. There may also be other signs of cerebellar disease, such as an absent menace response, intention tremor, or abnormal nystagmus.

The salient feature of vestibular ataxia is a head tilt. If the lesion is bilateral, wide excursions of the head may be present, especially in the cat. The incoordination is one of dysequilibrium or imbalance. The animal may lean, fall, or circle toward the affected side. The deficits in proprioception and paresis observed with sensory ataxia may accompany central vestibular disturbances, but are not a feature of peripheral vestibular disease (see Chapter 55).

Sensory ataxia is the most common type of ataxia in the dog. Sensory ataxia is less common in the cat, and tends to be more difficult to diagnose in this species because of their smaller body size and naturally more cautious and controlled movements.

The clinical signs associated with sensory ataxia vary depending on the location and severity of the disorder. The incoordination is usually associated with paresis. This is especially the case with lesions of the spinal cord itself. Coordination is best evaluated by observing placement of the feet in relation to the axis of the body when the animal is walking slowly.

Postural reaction deficits such as delayed or absent proprioceptive positioning or poor hopping become evident as the lesion increases in severity. With more severe lesions, the animal may spontaneously knuckle over onto the dorsum of the paw when ambulating.

Once a sensory ataxia is recognized, the lesion must be localized based on the clinical signs present. Localization of the lesion within the spinal cord itself is based on noting which limbs are affected and evaluating the spinal reflexes (Fig. 54-1). Focal lesions in the cervical region of the spinal cord (C-1–C-5) tend to produce deficits in

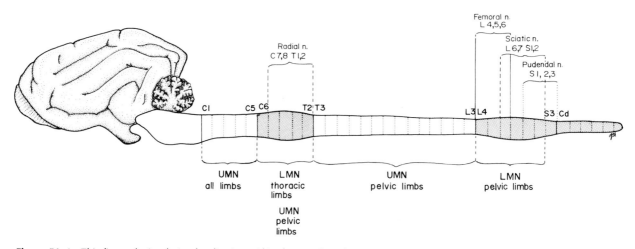

Figure 54–1. *This figure depicts lesion localization within the spinal cord.*

the thoracic limbs that are less severe than in the pelvic limbs, but the difference in degree of gait deficit should not be dramatic. If the deficits in the thoracic and pelvic limbs differ dramatically in severity, multifocal disease should be suspected. A focal thoracic or lumbar lesion would be expected to produce ataxia and paresis of only the pelvic limbs.

Since the descending UMN pathways regulate the LMN reflex arcs, disturbance of these tracts and subsequent release from UMN control usually results in increased muscle tone and normal to increased reflexes. If the pathologic process in the spinal cord also affects the segmental gray matter, LMN signs may be present. The classic signs of LMN disease that may accompany spinal cord gray matter pathology include decreased to absent reflexes, decreased to absent muscle tone, muscle atrophy, and flaccid paresis to paralysis. The LMN deficits are most useful for lesion localization in the intumescences of the brachial (C-6–T-2) and lumbar (L-4–S-3) spinal cord segments, where spinal cord reflexes can be elicited. The most valuable reflexes that reflect specific spinal cord gray matter segments are the patellar (femoral nerve, L-4, 5, 6 segments) and flexor reflexes (sciatic nerve, L-6, 7, S1, 2 segments) in the pelvic limb and the flexor reflex (C-6, 7, 8, T-1, 2 segments) and extensor function (radial nerve, C-7, 8, T-1, 2 segments) in the thoracic limb. Therefore, in addition to the signs of ataxia and UMN paresis suggesting spinal cord pathology, the identification of specific spinal cord gray matter segments by the presence of LMN deficits can be extremely helpful in lesion localization.

The sensory ataxia and paresis resulting from a lesion in the spinal cord is usually more profound than the sensory ataxia of a lesion in the cerebral cortex. This principle is based on the fact that in domestic animals, the major motor nuclei (red nuclei) are located in the midbrain of the brain stem. With lesions in the brain stem, tetraparesis may be quite severe; however, generally other signs, such as depression and cranial nerve deficits, help to differentiate a brain stem lesion from a spinal cord lesion.

The presence of pain or hyperpathia on manipulation of the vertebral column can also help localize focal spinal cord or vertebral column lesions. Hyperpathia is most consistently present with lesions involving the meninges, dorsal roots, or vertebrae. Signs of discomfort with lesions such as discospondylitis, IVDD, and some tumors may precede the development of a spinal cord ataxia.

Abnormalities detected on general physical and ophthalmologic examinations, such as fever, hepatomegaly, diarrhea, poor body condition, and chorioretinitis, when combined with the neurologic abnormalities may provide support for multisystemic disease.

DIAGNOSTIC APPROACH

The initial step in the approach to a dog or cat with an abnormal gait is the documentation of a detailed history. Features such as the environment, onset of signs, rate of progression, presence of discomfort, and the owner's description of the gait are especially important.

Evaluation of the gait should then be performed as part of the neurologic examination (Fig. 54-2). The most important and often most difficult step in this evaluation is determining whether or not the animal is ataxic. To aid in assessment of the gait, the patient should be walked slowly back and forth, with frequent changes in direction. In larger patients, circling may help to demonstrate gait abnormalities. The presence of abnormal head or body posture should be noted. In the absence of ataxia, musculoskeletal (see Chapter 63) or neuromuscular disorders should be considered as potential causes of the abnormal gait.

A complete neurologic examination should be performed to determine the type of ataxia present (sensory, vestibular, or cerebellar).

Once the presence of a sensory ataxia has been established, determination of the degree of paresis, along with the spinal reflex and cranial nerve examinations, will help localize the lesion within the central nervous system. The main purpose of lesion localization is to determine the presence of focal, multifocal, or disseminated disease.

The possibility of multisystemic disease is investigated by a complete blood count, a serum biochemistry profile, and urinalysis. In the presence of multifocal or disseminated disease, a cerebrospinal fluid (CSF) analysis should be per-

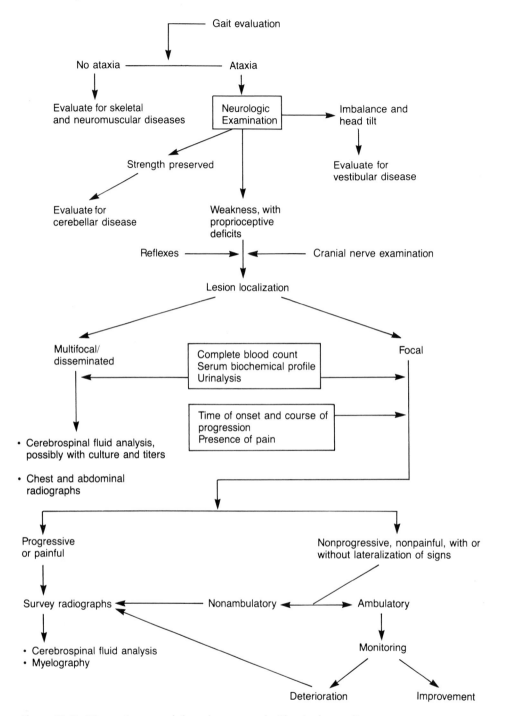

Figure 54–2. *Diagnostic approach for a dog presented with gait abnormality.*

formed (see Cerebrospinal Fluid Collection in Chapter 80). In certain cases, the CSF analysis will confirm a specific diagnosis (*e.g.,* observation of bacterial, fungal, or protozoal organisms). In other cases, it will strongly support a diagnosis (*e.g.,* a markedly elevated protein level with feline infectious peritonitis). Based on the results of the CSF analysis, specific cultures (*e.g.,* bacterial, fungal) and titers (*e.g.,* protozoal, fungal, rickettsial, viral [see Chapter 79]) should be submitted.

Focal spinal cord disorders are the most common causes of sensory ataxia and paresis or paralysis in small animal practice (see Table 54-1). The signalment, onset, and progression of disease and the presence of hyperpathia will help in establishing a list of differential diagnoses and selecting the appropriate diagnostic steps (see Fig. 54-2). In the presence of a nonpainful, nonprogressive spinal cord lesion (*e.g.,* fibrocartilaginous embolic myelopathy), a conservative approach may be selected initially. This is especially relevant to, but not restricted to, the ambulatory patient. If the patient's status deteriorates or the neurologic signs are severe, an extended diagnostic workup should be pursued (CSF analysis, myelography).

In the patient that demonstrates progressive spinal cord deficits and/or pain on palpation of the vertebral column, the extended diagnostic workup should include survey radiographs, CSF analysis, myelography, and possibly biopsy of the affected tissue. Spinal radiographs for the evaluation of intervertebral disk disease should be taken under general anesthesia to allow for adequate relaxation and positioning of the patient. In the case of vertebral lesions such as discospondylitis, neoplasia, or fracture or luxation, an initial radiograph taken with manual restraint or sedation alone may be diagnostic.

If, based on the neurologic deficits and survey radiographs, myelography is indicated, it is recommended that a CSF analysis be performed (nucleated cell count and protein estimation are adequate as a premyelographic screen, with the cell differential and quantitative protein level to follow) prior to dye injection. In the case of an inflammatory process (*e.g.,* septic meningitis), contrast agents may severely exacerbate the neurologic deficits. An exception to this recommendation of performing a CSF analysis before myelography would be when the signalment, history, neurologic examination, and survey radiographs are strongly suggestive of intervertebral disk disease and lumbar myelography is planned.

MANAGEMENT

The management of an animal exhibiting sensory ataxia and paresis due to a spinal cord lesion depends on the specific etiology. In general, the management of these patients is extremely intensive, especially if the animal is nonambulatory.

The majority of multifocal or diffuse diseases of the spinal cord are inflammatory (infectious or noninfectious) or degenerative processes. Many have a poor prognosis. In the case of myelitis secondary to infection by viruses such as canine distemper virus and feline infectious peritonitis, the prognosis is usually grave despite intensive supportive and symptomatic therapy. Fungal infections of the central nervous system (*e.g.,* cryptococcosis) carry a poor prognosis in both the dog and cat. The clinical signs of these disseminated fungal organisms usually reflect multiple organ involvement. Further, the toxicity of antifungal agents such as amphotericin B and the poor passage of ketoconazole across the blood–brain barrier complicate the therapeutic approach to the problem.

Similarly, the prognosis for recovery from central nervous system infection with protozoal agents such as *Toxoplasma gondii* and, more recently in the dog, *Neospora caninum* is poor. There is often evidence on physical examination of multisystemic disease with these protozoal infections. The recommended therapies include pyrimethamine and either the sulfonamides or clindamycin.

In contrast, bacterial infection of the central nervous system is usually associated with a much more favorable prognosis. Bacterial meningitis is encountered most often in the young, large-breed dog. The most consistent clinical signs reflecting inflammation of the meninges include fever and cervical pain and rigidity. In general, the prognosis for recovery with appropriate treatment is good. Usually, involvement of the spinal cord parenchyma (myelitis) with bacterial meningitis is not sufficient to cause a sensory ataxia and paresis. In the presence of signs suggestive of a bacterial encephalomyelitis, the prognosis is not as good.

Bacterial culture of CSF in the dog is usually unrewarding. Selection of the antibiotic is therefore usually based on spectrum of activity and passage across the blood–brain barrier. In the case of a specific organism that is not identified by culture, initial therapy with trimethoprim–sulfadiazine (15 mg/kg orally twice daily) is usually recommended; treatment lasts for 4 to 8 weeks. Another antibiotic group that has been documented to cross the blood–brain barrier and is used extensively in children are the third-generation cephalosporins (see Appendix II). Unfortunately, the cost is often prohibitive in veterinary medicine. Bacterial meningitis or meningoencephalomyelitis is a rare occurrence in the cat.

The most common noninfectious diffuse cause of myelitis in the dog is GME. Following confirmation of this diagnosis by CSF analysis, steroid therapy is instituted (see Chapter 55). The prognosis for GME is extremely variable. In general, steroid therapy is required for the life of the patient, and long-term control of this idiopathic disorder is often poor.

Focal spinal cord lesions resulting in a transverse myelopathy are more common. It should be remembered that inflammatory disorders (*e.g.,* feline infectious peritonitis, GME) can produce focal neurologic deficits, often by granuloma formation. The management of focal spinal cord lesions depends primarily on the location of the lesion (extradural or intradural). In the case of extradural compression, the prognosis for recovery with appropriate treatment is usually better with acute spinal cord compression (Type I IVDD) than with chronic compression (*e.g.,* neoplasia, vertebral stenosis, Type II IVDD), since chronic compression is more likely to result in irreversible axonal injury.

Management of extradural lesions often involves surgical decompression of the spinal cord and removal of the compressive lesion. This is usually performed by completing a ventral slot in the cervical spinal cord, or by dorsal or hemilaminectomy in the thoracolumbar spine. In the case of IVDD, prophylactic fenestration is often performed at the time of decompression or at a later date. In the presence of vertebral column instability such as fracture or luxation, stabilization techniques must be employed in addition to decompression. Neurologic recovery is not generally as extensive when the inciting cause involves instability, especially since perfect reduction and alignment of the vertebral column is difficult. In some traumatic vertebral column injuries in which instability and compression are minimal or purposeful movements of limbs distal to the site are present, a conservative approach of strict cage rest may be selected.

Extradural spinal cord compression may also occur in cases of diskospondylitis. The majority of cases of diskospondylitis are initially managed medically. Surgical decompression is only utilized if the signs of spinal cord or nerve root involvement are severe and rapidly progressive at the time of diagnosis or if the neurologic deficits worsen despite appropriate therapy (*e.g.,* due to bone remodelling during the healing process). Antibiotic selection is usually based on culture results from blood, urine, or disk material and bone. If no organism is cultured, therapy is directed toward *Staphylococcus aureus*, since this is the most common cause of diskospondylitis in the dog. Antibiotics such as the first-generation cephalosporins and cloxacillin are often recommended (see Appendix I and II).

In general, neoplasms of the vertebral column or associated nervous tissue have a poor prognosis. This is especially the case for primary vertebral neoplasia, such as osteosarcoma, fibrosarcoma, and chondrosarcoma. Tumors originating from the meninges and nerve sheath can potentially be removed surgically, but these tumors have usually resulted in chronic and irreversible compression of the spinal cord parenchyma by the time of diagnosis. Intramedullary neoplasms (*e.g.,* gliomas) are not surgically resectable, since they originate from and are intimately associated with the spinal cord parenchyma.

In the presence of an acute external or internal injury to the spinal cord with inflammation and edema, the use of anti-inflammatory medication is recommended. The most commonly used anti-inflammatory agents are the corticosteroids (*e.g.,* prednisone, dexamethasone). The diagnostic workup should rule out infectious etiologies prior to their use, since corticosteroid therapy in these cases would generally be contraindicated. In many cases, such as IVDD, anti-inflammatory agents are used as an adjunct to surgical decompression.

Regardless of specific etiology, nursing care in the presence of spinal cord disease is very important. If the patient is ambulatory, frequent short walks are recommended to help maintain some degree of muscle strength. In the paralyzed patient there is often loss of sphincter control, resulting in either a UMN (spastic) or LMN (flaccid) bladder (see Chapter 42). In both instances, bladder evacuation is crucial to prevent overstretching of the detrusor muscle. Initially this is best accomplished by an indwelling catheter and a closed urinary collection system. Some clinicians prefer intermittent (four–five times a day) catheterization of the urinary bladder. Culture of the urine should be performed when the catheter is removed, and appropriate antibiotic therapy instituted if necessary (see Chapter 46). Manual expression of the UMN bladder can be difficult initially due to the extreme spasticity of the urinary sphincter. In the case of the LMN bladder, expression is usually easy, but urine dribbling and subsequent urine scaulding often occur.

Protection of the musculoskeletal system is especially important in the nonambulatory patient. Muscle mass may decrease, making pressure sores a problem, especially with LMN disease, in which neurogenic atrophy occurs. Soft, dry bedding should be provided, and passive manipulation of the joints should be performed four to six times a day to prevent muscle contraction and tendon fixation. A whirlpool provides excellent physical therapy for the patient whose surgical incision, if present, has healed and whose vertebral column is stable (no history of fracture or luxation).

PATIENT MONITORING

In the presence of an inflammatory disorder, repeat CSF analysis is usually required to evaluate the response to therapy.

In patients recovering from spinal cord lesions, regular monitoring of neurologic status is recommended to evaluate the progress of the disease. Upon discharge from the hospital, frequent monitoring is recommended to evaluate neurologic progress and to monitor possible secondary complications, such as urinary tract infection.

ADDITIONAL READING

Barber DC, Oliver JE, Mayhew IG. Neuroradiology. In: Oliver JE, Hoerlein BF, Mayhew IG, eds. Veterinary neurology. Philadelphia: WB Saunders, 1987: 65.

Brown NO, Helprey ML, Prata RG. Thorocolumbar disk disease in the dog: A retrospective analysis of 187 cases. Journal of the American Animal Hospital Association 1977; 13:665.

de Lahunta A. Veterinary neuroanatomy and clinical neurology. Philadelphia: WB Saunders, 1983: 175.

Levine SH, Caywood DD. Recurrence of neurological deficits in dogs treated for thoracolumbar disk disease. Journal of the American Animal Hospital Association 1984; 20:889.

Seim HB, Prata RG. Ventral decompression for the treatment of cervical disk disease in the dog: A review of 54 cases. Journal of the American Animal Hospital Association 1982; 18:233.

55

HEAD TILT

Joane M. Parent, Susan M. Cochrane

Head tilt is a common neurologic abnormality encountered in small animal practice. Head tilt indicates a disturbance of the vestibular system. The approach to the problem must differentiate between central and peripheral vestibular disease.

CAUSES

Central vestibular disturbances originate from diseases predominantly affecting the vestibular nuclei, located in the rostral medulla of the brain stem. The causes of central vestibular disease are the same as those that affect other regions of the brain, and include degenerative, anomalous, neoplastic, inflammatory, traumatic, and toxic disorders (Table 55-1). The central vestibular system can be affected by these disorders primarily, or secondarily by extension of the pathologic process from adjacent nervous tissue.

In the dog and cat, the most common causes of a central vestibular system disturbance are the inflammatory diseases. Canine distemper virus encephalitis and granulomatous meningoencephalomyelitis (GME) are disseminated diseases that often affect the central vestibular system in dogs. Feline infectious peritonitis is the most common inflammatory cause of central ves-

tibular disease in the cat. Neoplasia is also a common cause of central vestibular disease. Tumors such as meningioma, nerve sheath tumor, and choroid plexus papilloma may compress the nervous tissue in the region of the central vestibular pathways. Parenchymal central nervous system tumors such as the gliomas may also damage these pathways. Head trauma, which can occasionally affect the central vestibular pathways, is usually associated with other serious brain stem abnormalities, such as tetraparesis and an abnormal level of consciousness.

The peripheral vestibular system is composed of the vestibular nerve (cranial nerve VIII) and the receptors within the ear. Peripheral vestibular disease occurs more frequently than central vestibular disease, and has been well described in both dogs and cats. Otitis media-interna is a common cause of peripheral vestibular disease. In the cat, it is often secondary to mite infestation of the external ear canal. In both species, an idiopathic peripheral vestibular syndrome has been described. Idiopathic canine geriatric vestibular syndrome is encountered primarily in the old dog. In cats, the idiopathic syndrome is not associated with a specific age group, but does tend to occur more frequently in the summer and early fall. Both syndromes are peracute in onset and often incapacitating. The aminoglycoside antibi-

Table 55–1 *Common Causes of Vestibular Disease in the Dog and Cat*

	Central Vestibular Disease	Peripheral Vestibular Disease
Inflammatory	Viral (canine distemper virus, feline infectious peritonitis) Fungal (cryptococcosis) Bacterial Protozoal (toxoplasmosis) Granulomatous meningoencephalomyelitis	Otitis media-interna
Neoplastic	Glioma Neoplasia of associated bony structures Choroid plexus papilloma Meningioma	
Idiosyncratic		Aminoglycoside antibiotics
Idiopathic		Feline idiopathic vestibular syndrome Canine geriatric vestibular syndrome
Nutritional	Thiamine deficiency	
Metabolic		Hypothyroid neuropathy
Traumatic	Brain stem injury	Tympanic bulla injury
Anomalous		Congenital vestibular abnormalities

otics can cause degeneration of vestibular receptors, resulting in a head tilt. Cats are particularly sensitive to the streptomycin. Fracture of the petrosal bone following road injury may also cause peripheral vestibular signs.

Since the facial nerve is closely associated with the vestibular nerve, facial nerve paresis or paralysis sometimes occurs in conjunction with inflammatory or neoplastic disorders of the peripheral vestibular system. Hypothyroidism has also been associated with bilateral or unilateral facial nerve and/or vestibular nerve deficits. In a few cases of peripheral vestibular and facial nerve deficits, no specific etiology was documented. Cranial nerve polyneuropathy, including a peripheral vestibular disturbance, may rarely be observed as a paraneoplastic disorder in the dog. An idiopathic polyneuritis limited to the cranial nerves is also occasionally seen in the dog.

PATHOPHYSIOLOGY

The central vestibular system is composed primarily of the vestibular nuclei located in the rostral medulla. Other important components of the central nervous system situated in the rostral medulla include the reticular formation, the nuclei of cranial nerves V (sensory), VI, and VII, the ascending proprioceptive pathways, and the descending upper motor neuron pathways for all four limbs. Since the rostral medulla is anatomically closely associated with the cerebellum and pons, this area is often referred to as the *pontocerebellomedullary angle*. Disorders affecting the central vestibular system often produce neurologic defects that can be localized to this area. Since the reticular formation is an important structure in the brain stem and is responsible for the state of consciousness of the animal, depression is a common clinical sign associated with central vestibular disease.

The basic function of the vestibular system is to maintain equilibrium by coordinating movements of the head with the eyes, trunk, and limbs. The peripheral vestibular system comprises the vestibular receptors in the semicircular canals of the inner ear and the vestibular portion of the vestibulocochlear nerve. Head movements stimulate the receptors in the ear, and this information is carried to the vestibular nuclei in the rostral medulla by the vestibular nerve. The information is then distributed by way of the medial longitudinal fasciculus to the extraocular muscles, which are innervated by cranial nerves III, IV, and VI, to the trunk and limbs by way of the vestibulospinal tracts, to the cerebellum (flocculonodular lobe), and to the vomiting center in the reticular formation. These pathways continuously coordinate movements of the eyes, trunk, and limbs with movements of the head. Failure of this system results in abnormal posture (head or body tilt), ataxia (loss of equilibrium), and abnormal eye movements (nystagmus) and position (vestibular strabismus).

CLINICAL SIGNS

The salient feature of both central and peripheral vestibular disease is the presence of a head tilt, which is usually directed toward the side of the lesion. The vestibular ataxia present in many cases of central or peripheral vestibular disease may also cause the animal to lean, fall, or circle toward the affected side.

An inappropriate or abnormal nystagmus may be present with vestibular disease. Nystagmus is an involuntary rhythmic movement of the eyes. In a healthy animal a normal or physiologic nystagmus is observed when the head is moved from side to side. In vestibular disease the nystagmus can be resting (seen when the head is at rest in a normal position) or positional (induced by holding the head in full lateral or dorsal flexion). The direction of the nystagmus can help differentiate peripheral from central vestibular disease. With peripheral vestibular disease the direction of the abnormal nystagmus can be horizontal or rotatory, and should not change direction with changes in head position. The fast phase of the horizontal nystagmus is directed away from the side of the lesion. The eyelids may close rhythmically with the eye motion. In contrast, the nystagmus associated with central vestibular disease can be horizontal, rotatory, or vertical, and can change direction with changes in head position (Table 55-2).

A ventral deviation of the eye or vestibular strabismus that is exacerbated upon extension of

Table 55–2 *Differentiation of Central and Peripheral Vestibular Disease Based on Neurologic Signs*

	Central Vestibular Disease	*Peripheral Vestibular Disease*
Head tilt*	+	+
Circling, rolling, or falling	+	+
Nystagmus		
Horizontal	+	+
Rotatory	+	+
Vertical	+	−
Alters with position of head	+	−
Vestibular nystagmus	+	+
Ataxia (vestibular)	+	+
Course of disease	Usually static or progressive	Usually improves
ASSOCIATED NEUROLOGIC ABNORMALITIES		
Paresis	+	−
Proprioceptive deficits	+	−
Depression	+	−
Horner's syndrome	−	+
Facial nerve paresis or paralysis	+	+
Other cranial nerve deficits (e.g., deficits of cranial nerve V, VI, or VII)	+	−

* *With bilateral vestibular disease, wide excursions of the head may be present rather than a head tilt.*
(+ = may be present; − = not present)

the head is often present on the side of the vestibular disturbance. This eye deviation differs from the strabismus seen with lower motor neuron lesions of cranial nerves III, IV, or VI, since the vestibular strabismus can be corrected by moving the head. Lower motor neuron strabismus is a permanent deviation of the affected eye that is not altered by head position.

On rare occasions, a bilateral peripheral vestibular disturbance occurs. This event is more commonly seen in the cat than the dog. In these cases, instead of a definite head tilt to one side, the head keeps moving in wide excursions from side to side. Usually no normal or physiologic nystagmus can be elicited. The animal crawls, or if ambulatory, falls to either side. A mild head tilt may also be present, and is directed toward the side with the most severe damage.

Paradoxical vestibular disease is an interesting central nervous system phenomenon that results from a lesion in the cerebellum and its connection to the brain stem. Clinically, it is characterized by a head tilt directed away from the side of the lesion. If a horizontal nystagmus is present, the fast phase may be directed toward the side of the lesion. The most reliable feature to identify the side of the lesion is the presence of postural reaction deficits on the side ipsilateral to the lesion, which result from disturbance of the ascending general proprioceptive pathways. This syndrome has only been observed in dogs.

With otitis media-interna, an ipsilateral facial nerve paresis or paralysis and/or Horner's syndrome may accompany the peripheral vestibular abnormalities. These deficits result from the close association of the facial and vestibulocochlear nerves in the petrosal bone, and passage of the sympathetic nerve through the middle ear in the dog and cat.

Acute diseases of the vestibular system are more incapacitating than chronic disorders. The animal can often compensate well for ataxia and nystagmus due to unilateral peripheral vestibular dysfunction, since the other side of the vestibular system is intact. However, the head tilt may persist (although it is usually milder than at the onset of the disorder). With general anesthesia or an unrelated illness, a transient decompensation may occur. Unilateral central vestibular disease has a good prognosis for recovery if the disease is treatable. However, in most cases of central vestibular disease the nature of the pathologic process is such that it carries a poor prognosis.

DIAGNOSTIC APPROACH

The most important step in the diagnostic approach is to differentiate central from peripheral vestibular disease (see Table 55-2 and Fig. 55-1). Clinical signs will help to do this, although the case may not always be straightforward. As an example, a nerve sheath tumor of the vestibular nerve may, at the onset, have all the features of a peripheral vestibular syndrome. As the neoplasm increases in size it may extend centrally to compress the rostral medulla, resulting in clinical signs characteristic of a central vestibular disturbance.

Physical, neurologic, and otoscopic examinations should be performed. In some patients, sedation or general anesthesia will be required to adequately visualize the tympanic membranes. If the neurologic deficits, such as head tilt, ataxia, and nystagmus, support a peripheral vestibular disturbance and the otoscopic examination suggests an ear infection, a workup for otitis media-interna should be pursued. Ipsilateral facial paresis or paralysis and/or Horner's syndrome associated with head tilt represent the classic picture of otitis media-interna. Under general anesthesia, oblique and open-mouth radiographic views of the tympanic bullae should be taken. The otitis should be treated based on culture and sensitivity results. If the radiographs indicate osseous involvement of the bullae, a biopsy may be necessary to differentiate tumor from infection. Most of these cases will necessitate drainage of the affected bullae, making biopsy and cultures readily available.

In the case of acute peripheral vestibular disease in which no evidence for pathology is present in the ear canal, idiopathic vestibular disease should be suspected. This syndrome occurs most often in the geriatric dog, and in any age of cat. Electrodiagnostic evaluation of the cochlear portion of the vestibulocochlear nerve by means of a brainstem auditory evoked response (BAER) and tympanometry can be used to assess the status of

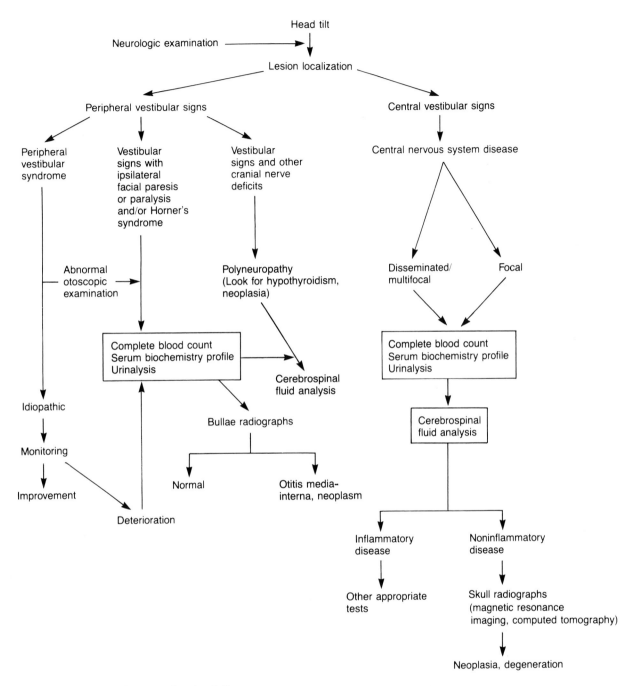

Figure 55–1. *Diagnostic approach to head tilt.*

the auditory apparatus and to help in lesion localization and differential diagnosis. If the cochlear portion of the vestibulocochlear nerve is affected, the disease is not likely to be an idiopathic syndrome.

Occasionally, dogs are encountered that exhibit both peripheral vestibular signs and facial paresis or paralysis without abnormalities on otoscopic or radiographic assessment of the ear canal. In these cases, evaluation for hypothyroidism should be considered, especially if there is evidence on physical examination or hematologic and biochemical evaluation to support this endocrine neuropathy (see Chapter 62). Even if hypothyroidism is diagnosed and thyroid replacement initiated, the deficits may persist due to the neuropathy already present. Based on human literature, thyroid supplementation may avoid further deterioration.

In those rare cases of multiple cranial nerve involvement in which a polyneuropathy is suspected, a cerebrospinal fluid (CSF) analysis should be performed to establish the presence of ganglioradicular diseases (see Cerebrospinal Fluid Collection in Chapter 80) and a thorough metabolic workup for a paraneoplastic or endocrine disorder should be performed.

If central vestibular disease is suspected, an attempt should be made to establish the presence of a focal, disseminated, or multifocal disorder. In the case of a focal lesion such as a neoplasm, feline infectious peritonitis in the cat, or the focal form of granulomatous meningoencephalomyelitis in the dog, clinical signs referrable to the pontocerebellomedullary angle may be present. In focal, disseminated, or multifocal disorders, the initial diagnostic step involves a complete blood count, serum biochemistry profile, and urinalysis, followed by CSF collection and analysis. It should be kept in mind that animals with space-occupying lesions in the caudal brain stem or severe inflammation with alterations in CSF pressure are at increased risk of brain herniation following CSF collection. The CSF analysis will help differentiate inflammatory diseases such as granulomatous meningoencephalomyelitis, feline infectious peritonitis, and canine distemper virus from noninflammatory diseases. It should be noted that the CSF associated with a meningioma may also demonstrate an inflammatory picture, due to irritation of surrounding brain parenchyma and overlying bone.

Skull radiographs are indicated when focal lesions of the central vestibular system are suspected. In the absence of skull trauma, however, radiographs are unlikely to be rewarding for the diagnosis of lesions in this area of the brain. Imaging techniques such as computed tomography or magnetic resonance imaging are much more likely to demonstrate focal pathology in the pontocerebellomedullary area.

In the presence of an inflammatory disorder, serum viral, fungal, and rickettsial titers and cultures should be pursued, depending on the specific CSF analysis and geographic location (see Chapter 79).

MANAGEMENT AND PATIENT MONITORING

Specific management of a vestibular disorder will depend on the suspected etiology. In the case of the idiopathic peripheral vestibular syndromes in both the cat and dog, no specific therapy is required. Supportive nursing care is often required; this is especially important in the geriatric patient, in which dehydration can be a serious sequela to the incapacitation of the disease. Occasionally, sedation is required to stop injury induced by the constant rolling. In all cases of idiopathic peripheral vestibular disease, improvement should be observed within 7 to 10 days.

Otitis media-interna is usually initially treated medically. A culture can be obtained from the middle ear by aspiration through the tympanic membrane. Systemic antibiotics should be administered for 4 to 6 weeks. If a sample for culture cannot be obtained, trimethoprim-sulfadiazine is recommended (15 mg/kg orally twice daily for 4 weeks). If there is radiographic indication for osseous involvement of the tympanic bullae, surgical drainage through bulla osteotomy is advocated. Biopsy and culture can be obtained at the time of surgery. Topical drugs should not be administered into the ear canal if the tympanic membrane is perforated. The ears can be gently flushed with sterile saline, and a dilute disinfecting agent added.

If a metabolic or paraneoplastic disorder is diagnosed as the cause of the peripheral vestibular disease, then the specific underlying disorder should be addressed.

The etiology of inflammatory polyneuropathies and ganglioradiculoneuropathies limited to the cranial nerves is unknown. If an infectious etiology cannot be demonstrated, anti-inflammatory drugs such as dexamethasone (0.1 mg/kg orally once daily) should be considered. A response to treatment should be observed by the end of the first week of therapy. If improvement is seen, then a 6- to 12-week course of prednisone (0.5–1 mg/kg orally once daily, decreasing to alternate day treatment) is instituted.

In general, diseases of the central vestibular system have a poorer prognosis for complete recovery. If a neoplasm is suspected, an oncologist should be consulted regarding the therapeutic possibilities. Tumors in the pontocerebello-medullary angle are generally not amenable to surgical removal.

The prognosis for inflammatory diseases causing a central vestibular disturbance varies depending on the specific etiology. In the case of feline infectious peritonitis and canine distemper virus, the prognosis for recovery even with intensive management is poor. For the noninfectious inflammatory disorders such as the focal or disseminated form of granulomatous meningoencephalomyelitis in the dog, dexamethasone is the anti-inflammatory drug of choice. A dose of 0.25 mg/kg orally three times daily is recommended for the first day, followed by 0.25 mg/kg twice daily for approximately 3 days, then 0.25 mg/kg once daily for 3 days. Depending on the response, either dexamethasone can be continued at a dose of 0.1 mg/kg once daily for 2 weeks, then decreased to alternate day therapy, or prednisone therapy (0.5–1 mg/kg orally daily) can be initiated. Some cases do not respond as well to prednisone and require longer-term dexamethasone therapy (starting at 0.1 mg/kg/day and decreasing to alternate day doses). A repeat CSF analysis is recommended before major changes in the dose are made. Mild inflammation may still be present on CSF analysis despite clinical improvement in the vestibular signs. The majority of steriod-responsive meningoencephalitides require steriod treatment for many months, and usually for the life of the patient, with the long-term prognosis being quite variable.

ADDITIONAL READING

de Lahunta A. Veterinary neuroanatomy and clinical neurology, 2nd ed. Philadelphia: WB Saunders, 1983: 238.

Oliver JE, Lorenz MD. Handbook of veterinary neurologic diagnosis. Philadelphia: WB Saunders, 1983: 223.

Shell LG. Otitis media and otitis interna: Etiology, diagnosis and medical management. Vet Clin North Am [Small Anim Pract] 1988; 18: 885.

THE REPRODUCTIVE SYSTEM

9

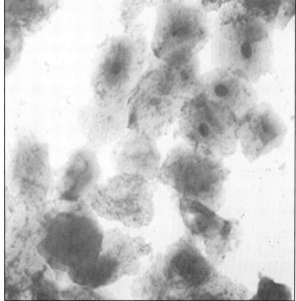

56

VULVAR DISCHARGE

Stefano E. Romagnoli, Shirley D. Johnston

A vulvar discharge can occur in normal bitches and queens or in those with underlying disease. After collection of information from the signalment, history, and physical examination, establishment of the cytologic character and organ of origin of the discharge should be the first steps leading to diagnosis and therapy. Fluids discharged from the vulva may originate from the vestibule, urinary tract, vagina, or uterus. This chapter presents a diagnostic algorithm (Fig. 56-1) for vulvar discharge in the bitch, with comments on the queen. As a presenting complaint, vulvar discharge can be due to many different diseases. Therefore, management of the vulvar discharge will vary depending on its cause. See Table 56-1 for the causes of vulvar discharge.

DATA BASE FOR STEPS IN THE ALGORITHM

The following data base should be collected for any bitch or queen presented with the complaint of vulvar discharge.

History

Is she intact? Is she prepuberal?

In the bitch, puberty occurs at between 6 and 24 months of age. The average age at first estrus is 10 to 12 months. The season of the year has no statistically significant influence on onset of estrus in the bitch, except in a few breeds, such as the basenji and dingo, which cycle annually. Small bitches may achieve their puberal estrus earlier than large bitches. Puberal heats are frequently split or false heats, characterized by proestrual bleeding for 2 to 5 days; after this the signs recede, and true estrus begins within a few weeks. The queen enters her puberal estrus at 4 to 12 months of age. Increasing day length from January to June helps induce earlier estrus. The queen does not, in contrast to the bitch, show presence of a vulvar discharge when she comes into heat.

If she is postpuberal, what is the average interval between her past estrus cycles, what is the date of onset of her last proestrus, and what are the dates of previous breedings and parturitions, if known?

In the bitch, the average duration of proestrus is 9 (range is 3–17) days. Vaginal epithelial cornification is complete late in the course of proestrus, about 4 days prior to the onset of standing heat. The average duration of estrus is 9 (range is 3–21) days. Maximal vaginal epithelial cornification is present throughout this phase until the first day of diestrus, when the percentage of cornified cells suddenly drops to less than 50%. Due to the wide range of duration of both proestrus and estrus, a bitch may have a 38-day cycle (proestrus plus estrus) and still be normal. It is important to collect a careful history in order to

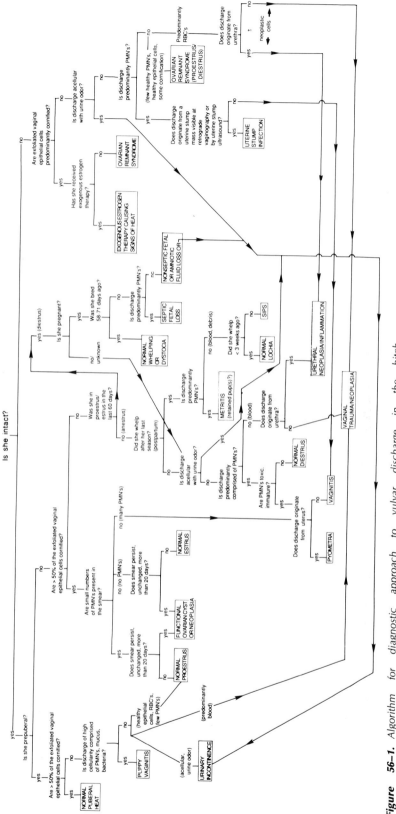

Figure 56–1. Algorithm for diagnostic approach to vulvar discharge in the bitch. (PMN = polymorphonuclear leukocyte; RBC = red blood cell; SIPS = subinvolution of placental sites)

Table 56–1 *Causes of Vulvar Discharge*

INTACT, PREPUBERAL FEMALE

Normal puberal estrous cycle
Puppy vaginitis
Urogenital trauma
Urogenital neoplasia
Urinary incontinence

INTACT, POSTPUBERAL, NONPREGNANT FEMALE

Normal estrous cycle
Functional ovarian cyst or ovarian neoplasia
Pyometra
Vaginitis
Urogenital trauma
Urogenital neoplasia
Urinary incontinence

INTACT, POSTPUBERAL, PREGNANT FEMALE

Fetal loss (septic or nonseptic)
Normal placental fluid discharge at whelping
Lochia
Subinvolution of placental sites
Metritis
Urogenital trauma
Urogenital neoplasia
Urinary incontinence

OVARIECTOMIZED FEMALE

Exogenous estrogen therapy
Ovarian remnant syndrome
Vaginitis
Uterine stump infection
Urogenital trauma
Urogenital neoplasia
Urinary incontinence

rule in an abnormal length of the estrous cycle, such as may be present with a functional ovarian cyst or neoplasm.

The serum progesterone concentration can be an important aid in detecting failure to ovulate, which may be associated with prolonged proestrus plus estrus. In the cycling bitch, the serum progesterone concentration increases to more than 2 ng/ml about 2 days prior to ovulation. It reaches a concentration of about 4 to 8 ng/ml on the day of ovulation, and then peaks at between 10 to 80 ng/ml during the first month of pregnancy. A serum progesterone concentration of less than 2 ng/ml more than 30 days after the onset of proestrous sanguinous vulvar discharge indicates a failure or delay of ovulation. Such a bitch should be followed with intermittent serum pro-

gesterone assays to determine whether or not she ovulates and maintains a normal luteal phase.

Another important piece of information that the veterinarian should collect from the owner is the approximate date of onset of the luteal phase. A nonpregnant bitch with a purulent vulvar discharge in diestrus (serum progesterone concentration more than 2 ng/ml) is a high-risk candidate for pyometra; the risk increases if the bitch is older than 6 years of age or has (in the last 8 weeks) received an injection of estrogen to prevent a pregnancy. Most middle-aged to older bitches have asymptomatic cystic endometrial hyperplasia, which may develop into pyometra when the bitch undergoes the 2-month period of progesterone influence after each season. Cystic endometrial hyperplasia, followed by acute endometritis, can be induced in normal bitches by administering progesterone, and withdrawal of progesterone in experimental cases of acute endometritis is followed by relief of clinical signs. Therefore, it is important to know whether or not a bitch is under the influence of progesterone. If the bitch is in diestrus and has a purulent vulvar discharge, pyometra is the first rule-out and, if pyometra is diagnosed, action must be taken quickly to preserve the bitch's life and reproductive potential.

A presumptive diagnosis of diestrus can be made from the history, without having to wait for progesterone assay results, by carefully interpreting the owner's observations. The question "When was she in heat?" makes the owner focus his or her attention on either the first day of the bitch's season or the first day she was bred. This often leads to an incomplete answer, and incorrect assessment by the veterinarian. Instead, by interpreting the owners' answers to questions such as "When did you first notice a sanguinous vulvar discharge?" (first day of proestrus: first serum progesterone rise to more than 2 ng/ml is 3–30 days later); "When did she become receptive to breeding for the first time?" (first day of estrus: first serum progesterone rise is less than 5 days to more than 9 days later); and "When did she refuse mating for the first time?" (about the first day of diestrus: first serum progesterone rise was approximately 8 days earlier), the veterinarian can gain a better idea of when the bitch's luteal phase began.

Is she pregnant?

Pregnancy usually can be detected by transabdominal palpation of fetal vesicles at between 28 and 32 days after ovulation. Because the day of ovulation cannot be determined accurately based on mating behavior, and because fetal vesicles are best palpated at between 28 and 32 days after ovulation, examinations 28 to 32 days after the first breeding of the bitch may not be an accurate way of estimating pregnancy. If no fetal vesicles are palpated at this time, the examination should be repeated in 1 week. Pregnancy can be diagnosed by ultrasonography as early as 24 days after ovulation; if not pregnant at 24 days, the bitch or queen should be rechecked at 35 days in order to confirm the nonpregnant state. Fetal skeletons become calcified at about day 42 after ovulation, or 43 to 54 days from the first breeding in the bitch. If diagnosed as not pregnant, the bitch should be rechecked by ultrasonography 55 days after the first breeding in order to rule out the presence of dead fetuses. If the bitch is pregnant and it is considered a high-risk pregnancy (she is old, her previous litters were small, or there was loss of a previous pregnancy), fetal viability should be checked at 55 days from the first breeding by radiography or ultrasonography. A bitch may whelp 58 to 71 days after a single breeding, due to the long life spans of ova and spermatozoa. Therefore, a vulvar discharge in a bitch bred 58 to 71 days earlier may indicate a fetal loss, normal parturition, or dystocia. If the bitch was bred less than 58 days ago and has a vulvar discharge, rule-outs are septic or nonseptic fetal loss, vaginitis (rare), or urinary incontinence.

Has she received exogenous estrogen therapy?

Estrous behavior in a spayed female may be caused by the administration of exogenous estrogens to treat signs of estrogen insufficency (urinary incontinence, alopecia, atrophic vaginitis), which may develop after an ovariectomy. Administration of such drugs must be ruled out when dealing with a spayed female showing signs of estrus.

What is the duration, color, volume, and consistency of the vulvar discharge? Does she have a history of other urogenital abnormalities, such as dysuria or pollakiuria, dystocia, or previous pyometra?

Physical Examination

General physical examination of patients with vulvar discharge should include determination of rectal temperature, inspection of the vulva for signs of hypoplasia or infolding of the mucocutaneous junction, and examination of the mammary glands for signs of lactation. The color, consistency, odor, and amount of vaginal discharge should be observed and recorded. The uterus or uterine stump should be palpated per abdomen, if possible, in order to determine uterine size. Digital examination of the vestibule and vagina should be performed in the bitch, following vaginal cytology and culture, in order to rule out masses or congenital structural abnormalities of the vagina. A digital examination of the canine vagina per rectum allows the clinician to check vaginal size and the presence of vaginal masses in the pelvis.

Special Diagnostic Techniques

Cytology of the Vulvar Discharge

A cotton-tipped swab (canine) or an ear-nose-throat (ENT) swab (Calgiswab [Hardwood Products]; feline), a glass slide, and a cytology stain are necessary to perform a cytologic examination of the vulvar discharge. Many cytology stains are satisfactory; our choice for a rapid, versatile stain for clinical practice use is Diff-Quik (American Scientific Products). To collect the specimen, moisten the cotton-tipped swab with a few drops of physiologic saline or tap water; while the female's tail is held aside, part the labia and insert the swab into the dorsal commissure of the vulva, directing it craniodorsally so as to avoid the clitoral fossa ventrally. In the bitch, advance the swab gently toward the vertebral column until it goes over the ischial arch, and then direct it cranially. The swab should be inserted at least 10 cm deep in the average bitch, and 1 to 2 cm deep in the queen, to avoid collecting a sample of squamous epithelial cells from the vestibule, which would not be representative of estrus status. After insertion, gently scrape the moistened swab against the dorsal vaginal mucosa (to avoid accidental trauma to the ventral urethral orifice), withdraw the swab, and roll it onto a clean glass slide. Do not smear the swab across the slide, or cells will be damaged. Let the slide air dry, and then stain it.

Evaluation of exfoliative vaginal cytology allows the clinician to determine whether a patient is under the influence of estrogen and to verify the presence of an inflammatory exudate, if any. The vaginal epithelium is cuboidal and noncornified during anestrus. As the bitch approaches proestrus and serum estrogen concentrations increase, the vaginal epithelium becomes 20 to 30 cell layers thick. In anestrus and early proestrus, exfoliated vaginal epithelial cells are predominantly ovoid, with a large nucleus : cytoplasm ratio (parabasal and intermediate cells); as serum estradiol increases, these cells become larger with angular borders, their nuclei become pyknotic, and keratin is incorporated into their cytoplasm (superficial cells). Superficial cells with nuclei that do not take up stain are referred to as *anuclear squames* (Fig. 56-2). Superficial and squame cells are dead cells, incapable of further change.

Under the influence of estrogen, red blood cells (RBCs) enter the uterine and vaginal lumens by diapedesis; therefore, these cells may be found in the smear during proestrus, estrus, and early diestrus. No standard correlation has been reported between the presence of RBCs in the vaginal smear of the bitch and morphologic changes in the vaginal epithelial cells.

Polymorphonuclear leukocytes (PMNs) migrate from the subepithelial vasculature through the vaginal epithelium, and are released into the vaginal lumen, where they may be found during most stages of the estrous cycle of the bitch and queen. During late proestrus and estrus the increased layers of stratified squamous epithelium block the migration of PMNs, which are thought to accumulate in the submucosa at this time. At a constant interval after ovulation (generally 6 days) the keratinized epithelium is sloughed, and an abrupt change from predominantly cornified to predominantly noncornified vaginal epithelium can be observed on the vaginal epithelial smear. Due to the sloughing off of the vaginal epithelium, PMNs can again reach the vaginal lumen, and are observed on the smear in early diestrus (Fig. 56-3). Neutrophils with engulfed bacteria are often present in high quantities in early diestrus smears, but their numbers decrease sharply after about a week. Large numbers of PMNs persisting more than 1 week after the onset of diestrus, or the presence of toxic or immature (band) forms of PMNs, indicates the presence of inflammation (Fig. 56-4).

Bacteria are present in the normal canine vagina at all stages of the estrous cycle, and are usually observed in vaginal smears. Bacteria are often most prominent during peak estrus, when they may be observed adhering to the surface of cornified epithelial cells.

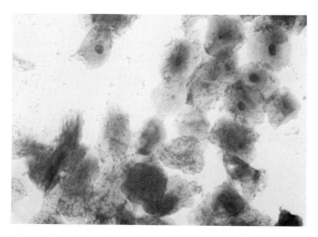

Figure 56–2. Vaginal smear from a bitch in estrus. All of the epithelial cells are completely cornified (hematoxylin–eosin stain, original magnification × 100).

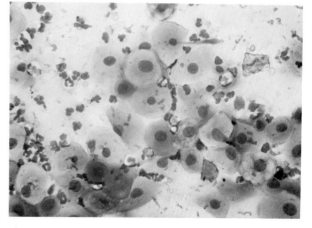

Figure 56–3. Vaginal smear from a bitch that has just entered diestrus. The majority of cells are not cornified, and polymorphonuclear leukocytes are present (hematoxylin–eosin stain, original magnification × 100).

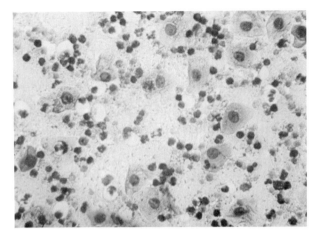

Figure 56–4. Vaginal smear from a bitch with a purulent vulvar discharge. Note the high percentage of leukocytes, and also the presence of toxic polymorphonuclear leukocytes and band cell (hematoxylin–eosin stain, original magnification × 100).

Shortly before the delivery of pups by the pregnant bitch, an acellular clear vulvar discharge consisting of amniotic fluid and placental breakdown products occurs. The greenish pigment uteroverdin is often seen in the vulvar discharge from a periparturient bitch or queen; this pigment is released after placental separation, and can be observed in a vulvar discharge during parturition and in lochia for up to 4 weeks postpartum. For up to 3 to 4 weeks after parturition a green to red–brown vulvar discharge, *lochia*, an acellular discharge consisting of uterine fluid, mucus, and RBCs, is observed.

Culture of the Vulvar Discharge

Culture of the vulvar discharge or of the cranial vagina should be obtained whenever inflammatory disease of the reproductive tract is diagnosed, since identification of the causative agent allows the veterinarian to choose appropriate antibiotic therapy. A variety of microorganisms can be cultured from the vagina of normal females. Therefore, one must be careful in associating disease with a positive bacterial culture. Aerobic bacteria can be cultured from the cranial vagina of more than 50% of normal bitches and from the caudal vagina of almost all normal bitches. Isola-

tion of bacteria from the vagina in the absence of other signs of disease is not enough evidence for a diagnosis of reproductive disease. Conversely, organisms responsible for infertility, abortion, stillbirth, or neonatal death (*e.g.*, herpesvirus, *Brucella canis*, feline leukemia virus) necessitate special culture techniques and do not grow easily in culture. Therefore, a negative vaginal culture does not rule out the presence of disease of the reproductive system.

Vaginal culture results can be a useful aid in the diagnosis and treatment of abnormal vulvar discharge in the bitch and queen. Bacteria that are normally present may infect reproductive tissues if uterine or vaginal defense mechanisms are altered, as in the diestrous uterus under progestational influence (especially if cystic endometrial hyperplasia is present); the postpartum uterus following prolonged labor, retained puppies, or retained placentas; the vagina in which urine or vaginal secretion pooling occurs because of congenital structural abnormalities; or the vagina undergoing mechanical irritation from clitoral hypertrophy or foreign bodies.

Aerobic bacteria can be isolated from the vagina of most normal bitches and queens. The type of organisms isolated may vary with age. A higher percentage of coagulase-positive staphylococci is found in the vagina of prepuberal than postpuberal bitches. The stage of the estrous cycle does not seem to influence the type of bacteria cultured from the canine vagina, but proestrus and estrus appear to be characterized by an increased number of bacteria in the vagina. The presence of high numbers of bacteria on the vaginal smear of estrous bitches is not an abnormal finding unless it is accompanied by signs of vaginitis (inflamed vaginal mucosa, purulent or foul-smelling vulvar discharge, pollakiuria, licking of the vulva) and unless many toxic PMNs and band cells are present.

Anaerobic organisms, such as *Bacteroides melaninogenicus* and other *Bacteroides* organisms, corynebacteria, *Haemophilus aprophilus*, anaerobic enterococci, and peptostreptococci, and other organisms, such as *Mycoplasma* and *Ureaplasma* organisms, have been isolated from healthy and infertile bitches. No correlation has been established between the presence of anaerobic bacteria and *Mycoplasma* or *Ureaplasma* organisms and infertility in the bitch.

Vaginoscopic Examination

Vaginoscopy can be useful in the bitch for detecting or inspecting congenital abnormalities and abnormal or traumatic conditions causing vaginal discharge, such as ectopic ureters, vaginitis, tumors, trauma, and pyometra. Fiberoptic endoscopes are ideal for viewing the canine vagina because they are generally flexible and provide cool lighting and good visualization. Rigid instruments such as human proctoscopes and sigmoidoscopes can also be used; these are generally cheaper. These instruments magnify and insufflate the vagina. Insufflation of the vagina and distention of the vaginal wall eliminates mucosal infoldings, which may preclude complete visualization of the entire vaginal mucosal surface. Nasal specula, otoscopes, and cystoscopes can be used in small bitches and occasionally in sedated queens; in medium-sized to large bitches these instruments allow visualization of the vestibule, clitoris, and caudal to midvagina only. Since lubricants are often required to insert the vaginoscope, cytologic or culture specimens should be collected before performing a vaginoscopic examination. Also, digital palpation of the vagina should precede vaginoscopic examination to check for the presence of strictures, persistent hymen, or vaginal masses.

Vaginoscopic instruments should be sterile, and the use of a sterile aqueous lubricant may be necessary, depending on the degree of natural lubrication of the vaginal mucosa. In order to avoid trauma, rigid instruments should always be inserted craniodorsally until they have passed over the pelvic brim. Normal vaginal mucosa is light pink and smooth. A mild erythema may result from prolonged exposure of the vaginal mucosa to air; therefore, an opinion on vaginal mucosa conditions should be noted early in the course of the examination. In patients with vaginitis, the vaginal mucosa may be bright to dark red in color, may be edematous and bleed easily into the lumen, and may be associated with enlarged vestibular lymphoid follicles.

Abdominal Radiography or Ultrasonography to Determine Uterine Size and Content

Survey abdominal radiography can be used to assess the presence of uterine enlargement. In the normal, nonpregnant adult female the uterus is $1/2$ to 1 cm in diameter and cannot be distinguished from a loop of small intestine, due to similarities in size and soft-tissue density. If the uterus is only slightly enlarged, abdominal compression with a plastic or wooden spoon may separate and distinguish the colon, uterus, and urinary bladder. As the uterus enlarges during pregnancy or during endometrial inflammation with fluid accumulation, it becomes more easily distinguishable from small intestine loops due to its thickened walls. At mid- to late gestation, or when fluid accumulation has caused uterine enlargement, the canine uterus generally can be palpated and seen radiographically in the midventral to posteroventral abdomen. Enlargement of the uterus at this site causes craniodorsal displacement of the small intestine, dorsolateral displacement of the descending colon, and ventral compression of the urinary bladder. In the bitch and queen, early fetal mineralization can be seen radiographically 45 days after ovulation. Pregnant females should be rechecked with a lateral abdominal radiograph at 55 days of pregnancy to check for the number of pups present and their degree of mineralization.

B-mode gray-scale ultrasonography is the most reliable way to determine the presence of uterine enlargement, measure uterine diameter, diagnose pregnancy, and assess fetal viability. Both uterine diameter and uterine wall thickness should be determined, and the presence of fluid within the uterine lumen should be noted. In the case of moderate uterine enlargement without inflammation, as in an early pregnancy or hydrometra or mucometra, the uterus can be differentiated from a small intestine loop simply by keeping the transducer in place while waiting for a peristaltic wave. If no peristaltic movement appears and the transducer is placed in an area of the caudal abdomen compatible with the presence of uterine horns, the structure examined is likely to be the uterus. Later in the course of pregnancy, the fetus becomes visible by uterine ultrasonography. Heart beats can be distinguished from about day 28 to 32 after ovulation. Visualizing fetal heart beats is the most reliable means of assessing fetal viability; this should be performed routinely 55 days after breeding. Ultrasonography is also important for monitoring changes in uterine diameter when a bitch with open pyometra is undergoing treatment with prostaglandins. Uterine size should be measured every 2 to 3 days to make sure that the therapy is having the desired effect of uterine evacuation.

Brucella canis, *Canine Herpesvirus, and Feline Leukemia Virus Serology*

In the bitch, brucellosis due to *Brucella canis* is responsible for fetal death, abortion of live fetuses at or near term, and purulent vulvar discharge. *Brucella canis* is not part of the normal canine uterine or vaginal flora. Serologic tests are available for the practitioner to check suspected animals for the presence of antibodies against *B. canis* (see Chapter 79). A rapid slide agglutination test (RSAT; Pitman-Moore) should be performed in every such case. The RSAT has high sensitivity, but low specificity. Therefore, false-positive results are possible. A negative RSAT is generally considered reliable; a positive test should be followed with a tube agglutination test. Probably the most accurate serologic test for *B. canis* is radial immunodiffusion. *Brucella canis* can also be grown in culture, although this is a very difficult procedure, since *B. canis* is inhibited by carbon dioxide, and takes 48 to 72 hours to grow in enriched media. Although canine brucellosis can be diagnosed based on clinical signs and persistent high titers, the diagnosis can only be confirmed by culture of the organism. The RSAT is a good test for a general screening of suspected cases. All RSAT-positive dogs should be rechecked with a tube agglutination test or radial immunodiffusion. Attempts to isolate *B. canis* from blood, lymph node aspirates, and bone marrow aspirates should be done on dogs with positive tube agglutination test or radial immunodiffusion titers. Isolation of *B. canis* is difficult, and infected animals may not always be bacteremic. Therefore, while isolation of the organism is diagnostic, a negative blood or vaginal culture cannot rule out a diagnosis of canine brucellosis.

Canine herpesvirus infection is responsible for reproductive failure, placental infection with subsequent fetal death, abortion of live fetuses at or near term, stillbirths, and also upper respiratory tract infection, conjunctivitis, balanoposthitis, and vaginitis. A laboratory diagnosis is necessary to rule out the presence of canine herpesvirus in bitches presented for reproductive failure or urogenital lesions. If a bitch has a vulvar discharge, cranial cervical swabs should be collected aseptically coincident with clinical signs and shipped chilled to a laboratory for viral isolation. Following experimental oronasal inoculation, canine herpesvirus can be cultured from the vagina of infected bitches for up to 2 weeks. Following natural infection, canine herpesvirus can be cultured for up to 18 days after whelping. Viral isolation is difficult and time-consuming, and a negative culture may not rule out infection.

Viral infection can also be diagnosed by demonstrating a four-fold or greater increase in antibody titer. Paired serum samples should be submitted for detection of neutralizing antibodies. The first serum sample should be collected at the time clinical signs are manifested or as soon afterward as possible; a 2-week interval should elapse between drawing the first and second samples. This is important because canine herpesvirus, as with herpesviruses in general, induces a weak humoral immune response, with antibody titers rising and falling rapidly (for 8–20 weeks) following exposure.

Feline leukemia virus has been incriminated as a cause of pregnancy loss in the queen; a negative test should be demonstrated in cats presented for pregnancy loss.

Serum Progesterone Concentrations

Measurement of serum or plasma progesterone concentrations can be used to confirm and time ovulation, diagnose ovulation failure, detect the presence of a progesterone-secreting ovarian cyst or neoplasm, and detect and follow the luteal phase (in patients with an ovarian remnant following ovariohysterectomy). In the bitch, nonluteal phase baseline progesterone concentrations are less than 1 ng/ml. Serum progesterone rises to 1.6 +/− 0.2 ng/ml on the day of the luteinizing hormone surge (48 hours before ovulation) and to 2.6 +/− 0.2 ng/ml on the day after the surge. Therefore, if blood for progesterone assay is drawn on a day estimated to be close to the day of ovulation (day 12 from onset of standing heat in the average bitch), serum progesterone results can fall into three different categories:

1. Less than 1 ng/ml: The bitch has not ovulated yet.
2. Between 1 and 2 ng/ml: The bitch is having her luteinizing hormone peak, and ovulation will occur in approximately 48 hours; she can be bred at or 2 days after ovulation and will whelp about 65 days from now.
3. More than 2 ng/ml: It is near or after the time of ovulation and, if the bitch is bred, she will whelp 58 to 71 days from now.

If the bitch has already ovulated (serum progesterone higher than 4 ng/ml), she should be bred immediately, since conception can occur from breeding up to only about 5 days after ovulation. Determining the day of ovulation is important for establishing the day of parturition, and therefore managing possible high-risk pregnancies (bitches with a history of dystocia or one pup litters). Also, timing ovulation is essential when performing artificial insemination using a single dose of frozen semen, since conception rates may be low if the bitch is not inseminated 1 to 4 days after ovulation.

To confirm a diagnosis of prolonged estrus, behavioral proestrus plus estrus lasting for more than 38 days should be observed, with serum progesterone concentrations never exceeding 2 ng/ml. When dealing with an ovarian remnant syndrome, estrus should be confirmed cytologically, and serum progesterone concentrations should be higher than 2 ng/ml 3 to 4 weeks after the occurrence of estrus.

Biopsy of Vaginal Masses

Vaginal masses may be epithelial in origin, such as those due to a transmissible venereal tumor or transitional cell carcinoma of the urethra spreading into the vagina, or they can be intramural,

such as leiomyomas. Exfoliating cells from an epithelial vaginal mass is relatively easy, and can be done with the tip of a moistened cotton swab. The swab is twisted against the mass to pick up a sample of cells and rolled onto a clean glass slide; the slide is then stained with a cytology stain. With intramural masses, incisional biopsy is necessary. Transmissible venereal tumors and transitional cell carcinomas may have a friable tumor surface that permits the grasping and removal of a small piece of tissue using an alligator forceps per vagina. Once the tissue sample has been collected, it should be blotted onto a glass slide and stained; the tissue can then be fixed and prepared for histology.

MANAGEMENT OF VARIOUS CAUSES OF VULVAR DISCHARGE

Intact, Prepuberal Female

Normal Puberal Estrous Cycle

The puberal estrus of the bitch includes the stages of proestrus (follicular phase: the bitch is attractive to males but not receptive to mating), estrus (transition between the follicular and luteal phases: the bitch is receptive to mating), and diestrus (luteal phase: the bitch is no longer receptive to mating), followed by anestrus. When compared with bitches undergoing later seasons, the puberal bitch may have milder vulvar swelling, less sanguinous vulvar discharge, and ovulation nearer the beginning of behavioral estrus (receptivity to mating) than the 2- to 3-day (receptivity to ovulation) interval observed in postpuberal bitches. The diagnosis of onset of puberal estrus in a bitch with sanguinous or clear vulvar discharge is done by examining vaginal cytology samples every few days and observing the progressive increase in the percentage of cornified cells. Queens in puberal estrus do not show a vulvar discharge.

Puppy Vaginitis

Prepuberal or puppy vaginitis may occur in bitches of any breed prior to their first estrus. It is a poorly understood disorder that is thought to be due to vaginal immaturity or poor vaginal mucosal tone due to the absence of ovarian steroid (estradiol or progesterone) stimulation. Puppy vaginitis generally will resolve spontaneously at or after the first estrus. Therefore, if the discharge is mild and the bitch does not show extreme discomfort, treatment may be withheld. If the discharge is heavy or if the owner is especially concerned, a 4-week course of specific antimicrobial therapy may be started. Occasionally, if the problem persists, a 3- to 4-week course of estrogen therapy (oral diethylstilbestrol, 0.5–2 mg orally once daily) may provide improved vaginal tone and resolution of the signs.

Urogenital Trauma

Vaginal trauma is very uncommon in prepuberal bitches, and is not always associated with vulvar discharge. If present, vulvar discharge is composed of RBCs, mucus, debris, macrophages, and small numbers of PMNs.

Urogenital Neoplasia

Neoplasms of the vagina and vestibule are very rare in the prepuberal bitch, and represent 2.5% to 3% of all tumors in the adult dog. The leiomyoma and transmissible venereal tumor are the most common vaginal tumors in the bitch. Other vaginal tumors, such as the fibroma, fibrosarcoma, neurofibroma, reticulum cell sarcoma, squamous carcinoma, and lymphosarcoma, may occur, but are less common. Clinical signs such as bulging of the perineal region, prolapse of tumor tissue from the vulva, dysuria, pollakiuria, tenesmus, difficult defecation, constipation, and urinary tract infection may be present in females with vaginal neoplasia. Vulvar discharge may be noticed in some cases of necrotic leiomyosarcoma, but is especially common in bitches with urethral carcinomas invading the vagina. Vulvar discharge is associated with the transmissible venereal tumor, and often includes neoplastic cells.

A sanguinous vulvar discharge is a common presenting sign of a transmissible venereal tumor. Diagnosis is based on clinical signs and the presence of space-occupying masses in the vestibule or vagina, which may be identified by digital palpation and vaginoscopy. Vaginal cytology should be used to characterize the vulvar discharge, if present; otherwise, a cotton-tipped swab could be used to collect a cytologic sample from the tumor, if the tumor itself is superficial. The presence of tumor cells on the smear may help establish a diagnosis. The diagnosis of a tumor is confirmed on histopathologic examination following excisional biopsy.

The transmissible venereal tumor is a naturally occuring transplantable neoplasm characterized by the presence of nodules on the genital and oronasal mucosa of the dog. Single or multiple nodules may develop into pedunculated, ulcerated cauliflowerlike masses. Growth patterns of the transmissible venereal tumor depend on the immune system of the host; in healthy adult dogs tumors tend to undergo spontaneous regression within a few months, while in immunosuppressed animals tumors may grow and metastasize widely. Transmission occurs at mating when tumor cells exfoliating from nodules or masses implant onto the vaginal or oronasal mucous membranes or the skin. Since transmission occurs at mating, vaginal or vestibular transmissible venereal tumor is more frequent in younger bitches than other vaginal tumors. No breed predisposition has been demonstrated. In general, vaginal tumors should be excised surgically, after the presence of thoracic and abdominal metastatic disease is ruled out by survey radiographs. The transmissible venereal tumor can be treated successfully by surgical excision, chemotherapy with intravenous vincristine sulphate alone, orthovoltage radiotherapy, or immunotherapy.

Surgical excision is easily performed, but recurrence is common. Recurrence may be caused by intraoperative tumor cell transplantation, and the rate of recurrence seems to be lower if electrosurgery is used. Chemotherapy with vincristine sulfate (Oncovin solution; 0.025 mg/kg [not to exceed 1 mg] intravenously once weekly until there is no more evidence of disease) has a high cure rate, especially with metastatic disease. Side-effects include vomiting and a transient leukopenia. A hemogram should be performed prior to each treatment. Orthovoltage radiotherapy (total dose of 1000–3000 rads administered one to six times) is also reported to be successful with most dogs. Immunotherapy has been reported to be successful in experimental studies, but has not been evaluated clinically.

Vaginal tumors (leiomyomas) in the queen have been reported only occasionally in isolated literature reports, and are therefore considered to be rare. Affected queens may show signs of constipation due to compression of the rectum. Clinical signs and treatment of vaginal tumors in the queen are the same as in the bitch.

Urinary Incontinence

Urinary incontinence may be misinterpreted as vulvar discharge originating from the reproductive tract. Urine leakage may be observed while the animal is at rest or awake. Sometimes urine pools in the vagina, where it can cause a mild vaginitis. Diagnosis of urinary incontinence is based on the presence of a yellowish, urine-smelling vulvar discharge that is cytologically acellular; scarce neutrophils may be present if urine pooling is causing vaginitis. Vaginoscopy and contrast radiographic studies of the vagina, urethra, kidney, and ureters may help confirm the diagnosis and localize abnormalities such as urethral obstructive lesions (calculi, neoplasms, strictures, space-occupying masses in the periurethral tissue) or ectopic ureters. Urinary incontinence may also develop in a small percentage of ovariohysterectomized females. The pathogenesis of this condition is poorly understood, but it is thought to be caused by hypoestrogenism affecting the vesicourethral sphincter tone (see Chapter 42). Urinary incontinence is rare in the queen.

Intact, Postpuberal, Nonpregnant Female

Normal Estrous Cycle

The typical estrous cycle of the postpuberal bitch includes a 9-day sanguinous vulvar discharge during proestrus (RBCs, few PMNs, progressive vaginal epithelial cornification), a 9-day straw-colored or sanguinous vulvar discharge during estrus (receptivity to mating, cornified vaginal epithelial cells), and a 3- to 10-day scant vulvar discharge during early diestrus, which may be clear, red, or brown in color (noncornified epithelial cells, PMNs, RBCs). Many normal bitches, however, will show stages that are much more variable in length than these, and the color of the discharge (sanguinous, straw-colored, clear) varies tremendously in individual animals; for example, some bitches have a heavy blood-tinged discharge throughout proestrus, estrus, and early diestrus, whereas others may show very little bloody discharge, even at the onset of proestrus. The way to diagnose the presence of a normal postpuberal estrous cycle is to follow vaginal cytology throughout the course of the discharge (to see progressive cornification of epithelial cells, followed by an abrupt increase in noncornified cells) and to measure serum progesterone after the suspected day of ovulation (usually about 12 days after the onset of proestrus) to confirm (by a progesterone rise to more than 2 ng/ml) the occurrence of ovulation. Queens in estrus usually do not have a vaginal discharge.

Functional Ovarian Cyst or Ovarian Neoplasia

Bitches or queens with functional ovarian cysts may be asymptomatic, may have estrous cycle irregularities, or may show signs of proestrus or estrus lasting more than 38 days from the onset of a sanguinous vulvar discharge (onset of proestrus). Ovarian cysts, which appear as spherical space-occupying masses in the caudal abdomen, often are not functional in dogs and cats, and can be found incidentally at ovariohysterectomy or necropsy, or by palpation, radiography, or ultrasonography.

While acquiring the history, the client's observation of vulvar discharge or attraction of males at estrus should be evaluated carefully in order to ascertain the actual length of the estrous cycle. Physical signs resemble those of a normal estrus (vulvar swelling, blood-tinged or straw-colored vulvar discharge in the bitch, and attraction of males). The vulvar discharge contains RBCs and cornified epithelial cells; small numbers of PMNs may be present in some females. The diagnosis is based on the presence of persistent signs of estrus and vaginal epithelial cornification. Normal estrus must be ruled out by repeated examination of the patient; persistent estrus is confirmed by serial vaginal cytology and serial serum progesterone assays. Serum estradiol concentrations may be measured if a radioimmunoassay laboratory is available, but results are difficult to interpret unless the bitch is bled on a regular basis more than once a day, since estradiol is released in pulses. Abdominal radiography or ultrasonography may reveal regular or irregular spherical masses caudal to the kidneys.

Induction of ovulation of normal follicles in the bitch can be accomplished using one of the following treatments administered once:

Gonadotropin releasing hormone, 50 μg IM in dogs (25 μg in cats)
Human chorionic gonadotropin, 1000 IU, half IV and half IM in dogs (500 IU in cats)

If these treatments are not effective in taking the female out of heat within 7 to 10 days, and if the patient is not to be used for breeding, she should be ovariohysterectomized.

Pyometra

Pyometra may occur in intact bitches and queens as young as 1 year of age, although most affected animals are older than 5 years and were in estrus 1 to 12 weeks earlier. In a female with a purulent vulvar discharge, uterine infection should be suspected if the patient received a mismate injection (diethylstilbestrol or estradiol cypionate) at her last season, if she has been treated recently with progestogens to suppress her heat, or if the purulent vulvar discharge starts during diestrus. Diagnosis of pyometra is based on the presence of high numbers of PMNs (which are often toxic or immature) in the vulvar discharge, on establishing that the vulvar discharge originates from the uterus, and (usually) on the presence of an enlarged uterus. Although uterine size can be estimated by abdominal palpation during physical examination, the most reliable way to measure uterine size is by ultrasonography, and by radiography if ultrasonography is not available. Both uterine diameter and uterine wall thickness should be determined, if possible, and the presence of fluid within the uterine lumen should be noted. A high circulating white blood cell count and a nonregenerative normocytic, normochromic anemia may be observed in some cases, but in bitches with a recent onset of uterine infection, the complete blood count may be normal.

The treatment of choice for bitches not intended for reproduction, older than 7 years, or having a closed-cervix pyometra is ovariohysterectomy with supportive fluid and antibiotic administration. A broad-spectrum antibiotic such as ampicillin should be used initially, and then changed as needed when culture results become available.

If a bitch or queen is a valuable breeding animal and has an open-cervix pyometra (diagnosed by the presence of a purulent vulvar discharge), medical therapy can be used to lyse the corpus luteum (if functional) and evacuate the uterus. Uterine size should be determined by ultrasonography (or palpation and radiography if ultrasonography is not available) at the beginning of therapy, and monitored throughout the treatment period. Culture and sensitivity of the vulvar discharge should be performed, and the bitch or queen treated for 4 weeks with specific antibiotic therapy. Prostaglandin $F_{2\alpha}$ ($PGF_{2\alpha}$, Lutalyse) may then be used at a dosage of 0.25 mg/kg subcutaneously once daily for 2 to 7 days. Only natural prostaglandins should be used at this dose; analogs are much more powerful, and their use at this dose may result in shock and possibly death. This treatment regimen should cause myometrial contraction and uterine evacuation. If the bitch is more than 5 days into diestrus (based on history or serum progesterone assay) the same dose used twice daily will lyse the corpus luteum, thus blocking the undesirable effect of progesterone on the bitch's uterus. Side-effects of $PGF_{2\alpha}$ administration in most bitches include restlessness, hypersalivation, and panting; many bitches will also develop transient abdominal discomfort, tachycardia, fever, vomiting, or defecation. Side-effects are typically less pronounced with each dose, and are usually minor or absent by the end of therapy. Vaginal discharge may persist for up to 1 month. At the next proestrus, a cranial vaginal culture should be obtained and the bitch should be treated with specific antibiotics for 3 weeks. The bitch should be bred at that season, since pyometra tends to recur during subsequent luteal phases. Although bitches can conceive and carry a pregnancy to term following PGF$_{2\alpha}$ treatment, the fertility rate at the cycle immediately following luteolysis with PGF$_{2\alpha}$ has not yet been assessed, and probably depends on the severity of the endometrial pathology present. The queen, which does not undergo a spontaneous ovulation and luteal phase, may be allowed to cycle without being bred following treatment for pyometra. Once her reproductive life has ended, the affected bitch or queen should be spayed. Prostaglandin F$_{2\alpha}$ is not approved for use in the dog or cat.

Vaginitis

Inflammation of the vagina (vaginitis) is often associated with infection caused by normal vaginal bacterial flora following compromise of host defense mechanisms. The canine vaginal mucosa can be irritated and predisposed to inflammation by conditions such as immaturity (puppy vaginitis), congenital vaginal anomalies (*e.g.*, strictures, vaginal hypoplasia, a persistent hymen or wall of tissue bifurcating the vagina), vaginal irritation due to infolding of the mucocutaneous junction, clitoral hypertrophy or foreign bodies, vaginal masses, or vaginal atrophy following ovariectomy. Primary vaginitis is not usually caused by an infectious agent, although *Brucella canis*, canine herpesvirus, feline rhinotracheitis virus, and possibly *Mycoplasma* and *Ureaplasma* infections may be exceptions to this rule. Bitches may harbor mycoplasmas as normal vaginal flora, so a positive culture for these organisms does not constitute a definitive diagnosis of inflammation.

Bitches with vaginitis may be asymptomatic (with signs of inflammation found only on routine vaginal smears), or the owner may report signs such as the presence of a vaginal discharge (which may be associated with attraction of males), increased licking at the vulva, and occasionally, dysuria or pollakiuria. Close examination of the conformation of the vulva may reveal infolding and irritation of the vulvar mucosa by the cutaneous surface. A digital examination may reveal the presence of strictures.

Hyperemia of the vaginal mucosa, which may or may not be associated with a discharge, is a common finding on vaginoscopy. Vesicular lymphoid follicles are often observed in the vaginal mucosa of affected bitches. A vaginal smear should be performed to support the diagnosis (a high PMN count is diagnostic) and to stage the estrous cycle. Establishing the stage of the estrous cycle will prevent the diagnostician from being led astray by a bitch in early diestrus whose PMN count is normally higher for up to a week after the first day of diestrus. Other cell types, such as macrophages and lymphocytes, which are not normally found on vaginal smears from healthy females or females with acute vaginitis, may be observed on vaginal smears from patients with chronic vaginitis. Culture for aerobic bacteria, mycoplasmas, and *Ureaplasma* organisms should be performed on a sample of the vulvar discharge (if the discharge is copious) or on a cranial vaginal swab (if the discharge is scant) in order to determine the best antimicrobial therapy. The bitch should then be started on a broad-spectrum antibiotic (*e.g.*, ampicillin) until the culture results become available. Uterine size should always be checked to rule out pyometra, and, if signs of dysuria or pollakiuria are present, the urethra or bladder should be checked to rule out the lower urinary tract as the source of the discharge.

Adult vaginitis is often refractory to therapy. If all other problems have been ruled out (strictures, infolding of the vulva that can be corrected surgically, pyometra) a 4-week course of specific antibiotic therapy should be started. Sometimes estrogen therapy (diethylstilbestrol at 1 mg/day orally for bitches larger than 10 kg) for 1 to 4 weeks (depending on the age and general health of the bitch and the results of hemogram monitoring) may have a beneficial effect in improving vaginal mucosal tone, especially in spayed bitches. Vaginitis is rare in the queen, and the use of diethylstilbestrol in the queen for this purpose has not been reported.

Urogenital Trauma

In the postpuberal bitch and queen, urogenital trauma such as vaginal tears may occur at whelping following the use of surgical instruments to manage dystocia, or by forced mating of a bitch not in physiologic estrus, when refusal of the bitch to stand is wrongly attributed to temperament. A bloody vaginal discharge may lead to the observation of vaginal tears or blood clots in the vaginal lumen during vaginoscopy. Most vaginal tears heal spontaneously, provided that the bitch is given antibiotic treatment. Healing may take several weeks, and another vaginoscopic examination should be performed prior to the next mating. Surgical repair should be performed in the case of rectovaginal fistulas resulting from complete perforating tears of the vaginal wall.

Urogenital Neoplasia

See under Intact, Prepuberal Female.

Urinary Incontinence

See under Intact, Prepuberal Female.

Intact, Postpuberal, Pregnant Female

Fetal Loss (Septic or Nonseptic)

Fetal loss should be suspected in a pregnant bitch presented with a vulvar discharge before day 58 from the first breeding. The incidence of fetal loss in the bitch and queen is unknown due to the lack of a pregnancy-specific gonadotropin, which could be used early on to diagnose pregnancy. Fetal loss in the bitch and queen can be due to chromosomal and developmental abnormalities of the fetus, infectious agents, maternal endocrine abnormalities, trauma, exogenous drugs, uterine torsion, and dystocia. The following abnormalities of the canine and feline karyotype (78,XX or 78,XY; 38,XX or 38,XY) have been reported in association with fetal death or stillbirth: autosomal trisomy (39,XY + 11), triploidy (117,XXX), and mosaicism (117,XXY/156,XXYY and 78,XY/156,XXYY). In addition, monosomy and translocations, associated with fetal death in other species, have been reported in the dog and cat. Other causes of fetal loss include abnormalities due to congenital defects, inbreeding, lethal traits, or hereditary traits not detectable by karyotyping.

While karyotyping of the aborted or stillborn fetus is necessary to rule in a chromosomal abnormality, a normal karyotype may not allow one to rule out the presence of hereditary traits. Reportedly, hybrid or mongrel dogs have a lower incidence of neonatal puppy mortality than purebred dogs, suggesting that inbreeding contributes to poor reproductive performance.

The infectious agents most commonly regarded as responsible for fetal loss are canine herpesvirus, *B. canis*, and feline leukemia virus. Although relatively uncommon, *B. canis* infection should be suspected in every bitch with a purulent vulvar discharge. *Brucella canis* bacteremia is present for 2 to 4 weeks after oral ingestion of the organism, and dogs may be infected for more than 5 years. Following the initial bacteremia, *B. canis* is commonly found in reticuloendothelial tissues and in the gravid uterus. Fetuses may be invaded through the placenta or by fetal ingestion of amniotic fluid. In the bitch, *B. canis* infection is responsible for failure to conceive due to early embryonic death and resorption, undiagnosed early abortion, or abortion between 30 and 57 days of gestation. Following an abortion, a mucoid to sanguinous vulvar discharge may be present for up to 6 weeks. This discharge is highly infectious to other dogs. Antibiotic treatment (minocycline hydrochloride at 25 mg/kg orally twice daily for 14 days, given with streptomycin at 10 mg/kg IM twice daily for 7 days) may cause a transient decline in *B. canis* titers. No treatment has been proven to eliminate *B. canis* from the bitch permanently.

Canine herpesvirus can cross the canine placenta and cause infection of the puppy in utero. Fetal mummification or abortion of live puppies occurs in bitches if canine herpesvirus is inoculated intravenously at between 30 and 40 days of gestation, whereas spontaneous delivery of infected puppies occurs if canine herpesvirus is inoculated intravenously at between 47 and 53 days of gestation.

Other infectious agents less commonly reported to cause fetal loss and whose incidence and mechanism of action on the fetus is unknown are canine distemper virus, *Campylobacter jejuni*, *Escherichia coli*, salmonellae, streptococci, and mycoplasmas. *Escherichia coli* has been isolated from vaginal swabs and uterine exudate collected at cesarean section from a bitch with vulvar hemorrhage at 38 days of pregnancy followed by abortion at 41 days and delivery of live and dead pups at 61 days. *Campylobacter jejuni* and salmonellae have been isolated from a few cases of aborted or stillborn puppies. Abortion of streptococci-infected puppies has been reported in bitches following experimental intravenous or oral inoculation of suspensions of streptococci.

The role of the corpora lutea and thyroid gland in spontaneous abortion or resorption in the dog and cat is unclear. Abnormal luteal function or thyroid insufficiency leading to naturally occurring pregnancy termination in these species has never been documented, although queens commonly abort at the time (42–45 days of gestation) when placental progesterone starts to replace ovarian progesterone in pregnancy maintenance. Maternal trauma during pregnancy may increase the incidence of premature placental separation. However, hysterotomy performed in bitches supported with progesterone administration does not cause abortion. Drugs such as bromocriptine, dexamethasone, estradiol cypionate, estradiol benzoate, $PGF_{2\alpha}$, antineoplastic agents (cyclophosphamide, vincristine, procarbazine), griseofulvin, and choramphenicol are reported to cause fetal death at some stages of pregnancy in the dog.

A purulent or sanguinous vulvar discharge may indicate the presence of septic fetal loss; nonpurulent watery vulvar discharge may be due to amniotic fluid loss, which is indicative of nonseptic fetal loss. Blood samples should be drawn immediately from the mother to check for *B. canis*, herpesvirus, or feline leukemia virus antibodies. The vulvar discharge should be cultured, and antibiotic therapy started. The therapy may be changed, if necessary, when culture results become available. Aborted puppies, if present, should be saved and sent to a diagnostic laboratory for histopathology and microbiologic culture.

The following antibiotics are reported to be safe for use in pregnancy: amoxicillin, ampicillin, cephalothin, chloramphenicol (in the last half of pregnancy only), clindamycin, dicloxacillin, kanamycin, lincomycin, penicillin, and the sulphonamides. In general, once signs of abortion occur, fetal compromise is already present, and trying to stop abortion might result in harm to the dam. In patients with recurrent abortion in which the only abnormality is low serum progesterone (less than 2 ng/ml) in midgestation, progesterone administration (1.1–2.2 mg/kg intramuscularly, not to exceed 25 mg, once weekly starting 1 week prior to the expected date of fetal loss and continued until 1 week before the expected date of parturition) may be considered. However, progesterone may induce pyometra and masculinize fetuses that survive the treatment. If signs of shock are present during pregnancy (due to trauma or disease), glucocorticoids can be administered (prednisolone is preferred to dexamethasone); however, they may cause death and resorption of fetuses. An ovariohysterectomy can be performed if the uterus is infected. When treating a pregnant female, one should always try to be conservative, in order to avoid damage to remaining viable fetuses.

Normal Placental Fluid Discharge at Whelping

In a near-term female, amniotic fluid is generally passed from the vulva shortly before the onset of whelping. Amniotic fluid appears as an acellular, watery, nonmalodorous discharge, prior to which a water-filled sac protruding from the vulva may be observed.

Lochia

In the postpartum bitch, a nonpurulent vulvar discharge comprised predominantly of erythrocytes and debris is suggestive of normal lochia if it occurs less than 3 weeks after whelping, and of subinvolution of placental sites if it occurs more than 3 weeks after whelping.

Subinvolution of Placental Sites

Subinvolution of placental sites (SIPS) is a postpartum disorder of dogs that is associated with severe postpartum hemorrhage or persistent postpartum lochial vulvar discharge. Lochial discharge persists in the normal bitch for 3 to 4 weeks postpartum. Subinvolution of placental sites usually occurs in young dogs (younger than 3 years of age), and the incidence is high in bitches whelping their first litter. One or more of the placental attachment sites in the uterus may be affected. Bacterial infection is not usually present, nor are the typical signs of metritis (fever, depression, anorexia, malodorous vulvar discharge). There is no reported influence of SIPS on subsequent fertility; bitches with SIPS have been shown to conceive at the next season, deliver a normal litter, and undergo normal uterine involution.

A vulvar discharge ranging from serosanguinous to frank hemorrhage with blood clots and persisting more than 4 weeks postpartum is the typical presenting complaint in bitches with SIPS. The discharge is variable in quantity and may persist until the onset of the next proestrus. Cytologically, the discharge is composed of RBCs and debris. Bitches with SIPS usually have a normal attitude, appetite, temperature, pulse, and respiratory rate. Abdominal palpation may reveal a normal uterus, or some spherical enlargements (up to 3 times the normal diameter) may be palpated. Subinvolution of placental sites should be differentiated from metritis, vaginal inflammation or trauma, endogenous or exogenous estrogen influence, or uterine or vaginal neoplasia. The diagnosis is based on cytologic examination of the vulvar discharge and determination of the source of the discharge by endoscopy. Uterine size should be evaluated by radiography or ultrasonography. A complete blood count should be performed to rule out metritis (characterized by neutrophilia) and to monitor changes in the hematocrit due to the effect of chronic hemorrhage. *Brucella canis* serology is indicated as well.

The diagnosis of SIPS is based on the presence of a nonpurulent sanguinous discharge from the uterus lasting more than 4 weeks postpartum in a bitch with noncornified vaginal epithelium and no signs of systemic illness. The diagnosis can be confirmed by histologic examination of the placental attachment sites on the endometrium at excisional uterine biopsy. Treatment of SIPS is supportive, and the prognosis for future breeding is usually good. Some bitches with SIPS after one parturition are normal thereafter. Oxytocin injection, ergonovine maleate, and $PGF_{2\alpha}$ have been used in bitches with SIPS, but have not been tested critically. Patients with SIPS that are not needed for breeding should be ovariohysterectomized. Breeding bitches should be treated supportively, as indicated by laboratory data.

Metritis

Metritis is a bacterial infection of the postpartum uterus; it may follow delivery with or without obstetric manipulation, abortion, or fetal infection. Bitches or queens with metritis typically have a foul-smelling vulvar discharge and are anorexic, depressed, neglectful of pups, and febrile. If proper treatment is not administered, septicemia, toxemia, and shock may occur. The hemogram generally shows the presence of an immature neutrophilia. The vulvar discharge should be cultured in order to choose the appropriate antibiotic treatment; gram-negative Enterobacteriaceae are common findings in these discharges. Abdominal palpation, radiography, or ultrasonography should be performed to rule out a retained fetus or placenta. The diagnosis is based on the history and the presence of a thick, bloody to purulent, foul-smelling vulvar discharge that is characterized by high numbers of PMNs, circulating neutrophilia, and systemic signs of illness.

Initial broad-spectrum antibiotic treatment followed by specific therapy based on culture results, when they become available, should be used. Uterine evacuation with prostaglandins may be indicated if the uterus is large and the cervix is still open (see Pyometra, under Intact, Postpuberal, Nonpregnant Female). If medical therapy is not successful in evacuating the uterus, surgical intervention and lavage may be necessary. Puppies should be removed from the dam when metritis is diagnosed. They can be returned to the mother after she is started on therapy if no signs of toxemia are present.

Urogenital Trauma

See under Intact, Prepuberal Female.

Urogenital Neoplasia

See under Intact, Prepuberal Female.

Urinary Incontinence

See under Intact, Prepuberal Female.

Ovariectomized Bitch

Exogenous Estrogen Therapy

See under History.

Ovarian Remnant Syndrome

Ovarian remnant syndrome is marked by signs of estrus in a spayed female due to the presence of remnant ovarian tissue. The condition results from failure to remove all of a normal ovary at ovariohysterectomy or from the presence of a fragment of ovary that becomes partially or completely separated during development. Such fragments are not uncommon, especially in the queen, and are generally located near the ovary in the broad ligament.

Ovarian remnant syndrome is more common in the queen, but can also occur in the bitch. The diagnosis is based on the presence of a cornified vaginal smear and high (more than 2 ng/ml) plasma progesterone concentrations 3 to 4 weeks following ovulation. Spayed queens in estrus should be induced to ovulate, using an intramuscular injection of 25 mg of gonadotropin releasing hormone. Bitches are spontaneous ovulators, and therefore a progesterone increase will occur spontaneously in affected bitches without the need to induce the ovulation. Exploratory surgery and removal of retained or accessory ovarian tissue at both ovarian stumps is the treatment of choice.

Vaginitis

See under Intact, Prepuberal Female.

Uterine Stump Infection

The pathogenesis and clinical signs of infection of the uterine stump after hysterectomy closely resemble those of pyometra. Therefore, uterine stump infection is the first rule-out in a spayed bitch showing signs of pyometra (polyuria, polydipsia, purulent vulvar discharge). The diagnosis is confirmed by cytologic characterization of the vulvar discharge and by radiographic or ultrasonographic evidence of a mass at the uterine stump. Infection or abscess of the uterine stump is characterized radiographically as a mass between the colon and the bladder. Surgical removal is the recommended treatment.

Urogenital Trauma

See under Intact, Prepuberal Female.

Urogenital Neoplasia

See under Intact, Prepuberal Female.

Urinary Incontinence

See under Intact, Prepuberal Female.

ADDITIONAL READING

Dow C. The cystic hyperplasia–pyometra complex in the bitch. Vet Rec 1958; 70:1102.

Holst PA. Vaginal cytology in the bitch. In: Morrow DA, ed. Current therapy in theriogenology. Philadelphia: WB Saunders, 1986: 457.

Johnston SD. Subinvolution of placental sites. In: Kirk RW, ed. Current veterinary therapy X. Philadelphia: WB Saunders, 1986: 1231.

Johnston SD, Raksil S. Fetal loss in the dog and cat. Vet Clin North Am [Small Anim Pract] 1987; 17:535.

Olson PN, Jones RL, Mather EC. The use and misuse of vaginal cultures in diagnosing reproductive diseases in the bitch. In: Morrow DA, ed. Current therapy in theriogenology. Philadelphia: WB Saunders, 1986: 469.

Papich MG. Effects of drugs on pregnancy. In: Kirk RW, ed. Current veterinary therapy X. Philadelphia: WB Saunders, 1989: 1291.

Wykes PM. Diseases of the vagina and vulva in the bitch. In: Morrow DA, ed. Current therapy in theriogenology. Philadelphia: WB Saunders, 1986: 476.

57

PROSTATIC DISEASE

Laine A. Cowan, Jeanne A. Barsanti

Although the exact role of the prostate gland is unknown, it is thought to play a role in sperm transport, nutrition, and function by production of seminal fluid, and protection of the lower urinary tract against bacterial pathogens by secreting immunoglobulins and an antibacterial factor. Although many domestic species have a prostate gland, prostatic disease is rare in all except the dog. In the dog, the prostate gland lies in the pelvic or caudal abdominal cavity and surrounds the urethra just caudal to the urinary bladder.

Clinical manifestations of canine prostatic disease are usually associated with alterations in prostatic fluid, which may be reflected in the urine (hematuria, pyuria) or in a urethral discharge independent of urination. When the canine prostate gland increases in size, it usually expands outwardly. When prostatomegaly is marked, deviation or impingement of the colon or rectum frequently occurs (Fig. 57-1), resulting in rectal tenesmus. Diseases of the prostate gland can be divided into noninfectious (benign prostatic hyperplasia, prostatic and paraprostatic cysts, prostatic neoplasia) and infectious (acute bacterial prostatitis, chronic bacterial pros-

tatitis, prostatic abscess) categories. Although the underlying etiology, pathophysiology, and therapy of each may be different, the basic diagnostic approach to prostatic diseases is the same.

DIAGNOSTIC APPROACH TO PROSTATIC DISEASE

History, physical examination, clinical pathology, microbiology, radiography, ultrasonography, and histology may all play a role in the diagnosis of canine prostatic disease. Historical findings that may suggest a problem involving the prostate gland may include a history of recurrent urinary tract infections in an intact male dog, fluid dripping from the urethra independent of urination, infertility, rectal tenesmus, stiff or weak hind limb gait, or systemic illness.

On physical examination, palpation of the scrotal contents (testicles and spermatic cord) and caudal abdomen, digital rectal palpation of the urethra, prostate gland, and sublumbar lymph nodes, and examination of the penis and prepuce, are essential in detection and evaluation of prostatic disease. Prostatic contour, size, sym-

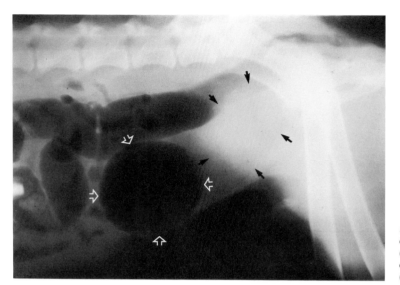

Figure 57–1. *Caudal abdominal radiograph of a dog with rectal tenesmus. A pneumocystogram (open arrows) was utilized to help identify the caudal abdominal mass as an enlarged prostate gland (closed arrows).*

metry, texture, mobility, and tenderness should be noted.

A urinalysis and complete blood count are generally part of the minimum data base in evaluating a dog with suspected prostatic disease. A serum biochemistry profile is recommended when the dog is systemically ill or when neoplasia, acute bacterial prostatitis, or prostatic abscesses are suspected. Hematuria, pyuria, bacteriuria, or,

occasionally, neoplastic cells may be present in urine samples collected from patients with prostatic disease. However, a normal urine sediment does not rule out a prostatic problem. Table 57-1 summarizes historical and physical examination findings in dogs with prostatic disease.

Prostatic fluid evaluation (cytology and quantitative culture) is important in localizing the problem to the prostate gland and in identifying

Table 57–1 *Common History and Results of Physical Examination Associated With Canine Prostatic Diseases*

	History or Clinical Findings	Urinary Tract Signs*	Rectal Tenesmus	Systemic Illness†	Rear Limb Weakness or Stiffness
Benign prostatic hypertrophy	May be none Hematuria	− / + +	− / +	Absent	Absent
Paraprostatic cyst	Abdominal distention	+ + +	+ / + +	− / +	Absent
Prostatic adenocarcinoma	Prostate gland may be painful Weight loss	+ + +	+ +	+ / + + +	+ +
Acute bacterial prostatitis	Prostate painful on digital examination	+ +	+ +	+ + +	Absent
Chronic bacterial prostatitis	May be none Recurrent urinary tract infections	+ + +	+	− / +	Absent
Prostatic abscess	Prostate gland may be painful	+ +	− / + +	+ +	Absent

* *Includes urethral discharge, hematuria, dysuria, pyuria, and urinary incontinence*
† *Includes anorexia, lethargy, and fever (+ = 10% to 30% of cases; + + = 30% to 60% of cases; + + + = greater than 60% of cases; − = absent)*

the underlying etiology. Prostatic fluid can be obtained by collecting the third fraction of an ejaculate or by prostatic massage (see Prostatic Massage, Urethral Brush Technique, and Ejaculation in Chapter 80). Specimens obtained by either means may be contaminated with nonprostatic fluid. The testicle, epididymis, vas deferens, and urethra may contribute to an ejaculate, and bladder and urethral contamination may occur when obtaining prostatic fluid by way of massage. Compared to prostatic massage samples, prostatic fluid collected by ejaculation has increased sensitivity in detecting chronic bacterial prostatitis. In theory, the advantage of prostatic massage samples is the ability to more accurately localize an infection to the prostate gland. This is accomplished by comparing the fluid obtained from flushing the bladder prior to prostatic massage (sample 1) to the fluid obtained after digital prostatic massage (sample 2). If sample 2 contains a factor of 10^2 more organisms per milliliter than sample 1, the infection is likely to be of prostatic origin. The massage technique is unable to identify a bacterial prostatitis when a urinary tract infection is present, since most laboratories will not quantitate bacterial colonies when they are greater than 10^5 per milliliter. The best technique for obtaining prostatic fluid for evaluation of noninfectious prostatic problems has not been investigated.

If no cytologic evidence of septic inflammation or neoplasia is present upon prostatic fluid evaluation, further evaluation of the dog may be indicated to rule out a prostatic neoplasm. Thoracic and abdominal radiographs and, where available, a nuclear bone scan may used as to screen for metastatic disease. Fine needle aspiration cytology or a prostatic biopsy may be necessary for confirmation of prostatic neoplasia. A prostatic biopsy can usually be readily obtained by a perineal, abdominal percutaneous, or intraoperative route (see Prostatic Biopsy in Chapter 80). If a biopsy is taken without ultrasonic guidance or direct visualization, fine needle aspiration should be done first to diagnose cavitary lesions. Ultrasonographic guidance can be used for aspiration of a cavitary lesion or for a directed percutaneous biopsy. Ultrasonographic guidance has the advantage (vs. blind percutaneous biopsy) of increasing the likelihood of obtaining a sample of a focal lesion. False-negative results are possible with biopsies, especially those taken percutaneously, since the small sample size may miss focal or multifocal lesions.

Survey abdominal radiographs may be helpful in quantitating the degree of prostatomegaly and detecting sublumbar lymphadenopathy or vertebral or pelvic bony lesions suggestive of prostatic neoplasia. Ultrasonographic evaluation of the prostate gland is helpful in determining prostatic parenchymal architecture, and is particularly useful in distinguishing cavitary from noncavitary prostatic and periprostatic diseases.

NONINFECTIOUS DISEASES OF THE PROSTATE GLAND

Benign Prostatic Hypertrophy

Benign prostatic hypertrophy (BPH) is the most common prostatic disease of intact adult male dogs. In one study, 50% of dogs had BPH by 5 years of age, with 90% of dogs affected by 8 years of age. Although BPH is a common morphologic finding, uncomplicated BPH is not commonly associated with clinical signs.

Causes and Pathophysiology

Canine BPH is a benign alteration of the prostate gland characterized by diffuse hypertrophy and hyperplasia of the prostatic glandular epithelium, and mild stromal proliferation. These microscopic changes are usually reflected in a symmetrical, nonpainful enlargement of the prostate gland, which can be detected on digital rectal palpation. Benign prostatic hypertrophy can be subdivided histologically into simple and complex forms. In simple BPH, the hyperplasia and hypertrophy of the glandular epithelium results in an increased size of the prostatic alveoli and lobules. In complex BPH, areas of glandular hyperplasia are interspersed with dilated alveoli and ducts, resulting in small intraparenchymal cysts. Since the incidence of complex BPH increases with the age of the dog and the incidence of simple BPH decreases with advancing age, the complex or cystic form has been considered an advanced form of simple glandular BPH.

The intraprostatic estrogen:androgen ratio and advancing age are thought to play essential roles in the development of canine BPH. Naturally occurring BPH is dependent on the presence of testicular hormones, since it does not occur in dogs previously castrated. With advancing age, the relative increase of intraprostatic estrogen concentration primarily acts to stimulate stromal proliferation and increase prostatic sensitivity to androgens. These androgens then stimulate epithelial proliferation.

Clinical Signs

The majority of dogs with BPH do not have clinical signs related to the disease. When BPH does cause a clinical problem it is usually related to a hemorrhagic urethral discharge, independent of urination, or rectal tenesmus.

Diagnostic Approach

As in most prostatic diseases, initial evaluation of the prostate gland includes palpation, assessment of the prostatic fluid (cytologically, and aerobic bacterial culture), and radiographic or ultrasonographic evaluation of prostatic architecture. An easily movable, symmetrical, nonpainful, enlarged prostate is consistent with BPH. Cytologic evaluation of the prostatic fluid may show it to be within normal limits or hemorrhagic. Radiographically, prostatomegaly is observed (Fig. 57-2), and ultrasonographically, symmetrical prostatomegaly with or without focal or diffuse hyperechoic parenchyma and with or without small cavitary lesions (Fig. 57-3) may be observed.

Management

Castration, by removing the primary site of androgen production, causes involution of the prostate gland (detectable by 1–2 weeks, and maximal by 3 months, after castration) and resultant resolution of BPH. Experimentally, antiandrogens have the same effect, and potentially may be used to treat BPH. However, since a dose of

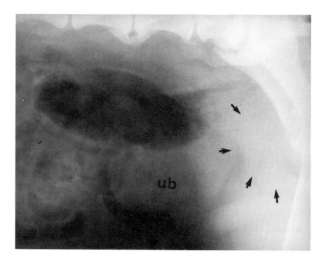

Figure 57–2. *Prostatomegaly (arrows) is the most common radiographic finding in dogs with benign prostatic hypertrophy. (ub = urinary bladder)*

antiandrogens only temporarily suppresses androgens, continual administration of the drugs would be necessary. Progestational compounds, luteinizing hormone releasing hormone agonists, drugs that block the action of testosterone in the prostate gland, and estrogens have been experimentally used (with variable success and variable side-effects) to reduce the size of the canine prostate gland. Estrogen administration can cause the potentially serious side-effects of bone marrow suppression and squamous metaplasia of the prostatic epithelium, the latter of which can predispose the dog to bacterial prostatitis or prostatic cysts. None of the drugs with antiandrogen actions have been approved for use in dogs with prostatic disease.

Squamous Metaplasia

In squamous metaplasia, the normal cuboidal and columnar epithelium lining the prostatic ducts and alveoli is transformed to a flattened (squamous) epithelium. These alterations may result in partial occlusion of the prostatic ducts and subsequent cystic intraprostatic accumulation of prostatic fluid.

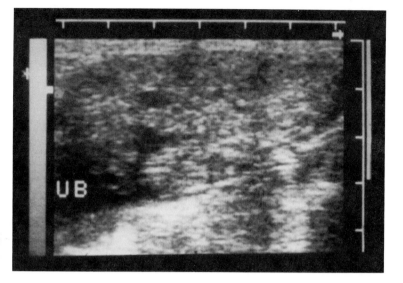

Figure 57–3. *Ultrasonogram of cystic benign prostatic hypertrophy with prostatomegaly and small multifocal hypoechoic (cavitary) foci. (UB = urinary bladder)*

Causes and Pathophysiology

Excess estrogen is responsible for the metaplastic changes observed in this condition. The estrogenic hormones may be the result of exogenous administration or endogenous excess production, as from a Sertoli's cell tumor. The exact amount or concentration of estrogen needed to elicit this change has not been determined; probably individual variation exists in the sensitivity of the prostate gland to metaplastic effects of estrogen. As with any cavitary prostatic problem, although bacteria do not contribute to the pathophysiology of the disease, secondary bacterial infection can occur.

Clinical Signs

Clinical signs associated with squamous metaplasia in the prostate gland are similar to what is expected with prostatic cysts. In addition, some dogs may have palpable testicular abnormalities or systemic signs (gynecomastia, hyperpigmentation, alopecia, bone marrow suppression), which are suggestive of hyperestrogenism.

Diagnostic Approach

Squamous metaplasia is a histologic diagnosis that may be suspected in a dog with cavitary prostatomegaly with historical or clinical findings compatible with hyperestrogenism.

Prostatic Cysts

Cystic prostatic disease has been reported in 11% to 25% of dogs with prostatic disease. Cystic lesions associated with the prostate gland include intraparenchymal cysts, which usually are multiple microscopic cysts associated with complex benign prostatic hyperplasia, and paraprostatic cysts, which are commonly large and singular. Discrete intraparenchymal prostatic cysts, calcified prostatic cysts, and multiple intraparenchymal cysts associated with squamous metaplasia have also been reported.

Causes and Pathophysiology

True retention cysts are thought to result from obstruction of the prostatic ducts by inflammation, hyperplasia, or neoplasia; however, in an individual dog, the underlying etiology often remains undetermined. In cysts associated with BPH and squamous metaplasia, the prostatic ducts are patent, and the cysts that develop are likely a result of alterations in the glandular epithelial morphology and secretion. Although not always anatomically proven, paraprostatic cysts are thought to involve distention of embryologic remnants, such as the uterus masculinus, which may or may not have a patent opening into the urethra, and have variable attachment to the prostate gland.

Clinical Signs

Most prostatic cysts are asymptomatic until they become large enough to cause physical impingement of the colon, urinary bladder, or urethra. In one study, 7 of 12 dogs with paraprostatic cysts had presenting clinical signs associated with the lower urinary tract (see Table 57-1) and 6 of 12 dogs had signs associated with fecal tenesmus (one dog had urinary and intestinal signs). Multiple intraprostatic cysts associated with BPH may be asymptomatic or may result in hematuria or rectal tenesmus (see Benign Prostatic Hypertrophy).

Diagnostic Approach

A nontender, enlarged, asymmetrical, fluctuant prostate gland may be palpable on rectal or abdominal palpation in dogs with prostatic or paraprostatic cysts. However, most paraprostatic cysts are located craniolateral to the prostate gland in the caudal abdomen, and digital pros-

tatic palpation (per rectum) may be normal. Radiographically, prostatic cysts usually appear as a smooth, large, soft-tissue mass in the caudal abdomen (Fig. 57-4). In a minority of dogs with paraprostatic cysts, smooth calcification around the periphery of the cyst may be apparent radiographically. Asymmetrical prostatic enlargement due to intraprostatic cysts has also been observed. Ultrasonographically, fluid-filled parenchymal or paraprostatic cavities are seen with prostatic (Fig. 57-5) or paraprostatic cysts. Since prostatic abscesses cannot be differentiated ultrasonographically from prostatic cysts, cytologic examination of prostatic fluid is necessary to differentiate between the two types of lesions. If the prostatic fluid is noninflammatory, the cavitary lesions may not be infected (*e.g.,* prostatic cyst), or the infected cavitary lesion (abscess) may not communicate with the urethra. When no evidence of prostatic fluid inflammation is present, aspiration of the cyst may be indicated.

Management

Complete surgical excision of prostatic and paraprostatic cysts, although ideal, may not be possible if cysts are intraprostatic or if multiple attachments of the cyst to the urinary bladder, urethra, or prostate gland are present. Although marsupialization is the treatment of choice for para-

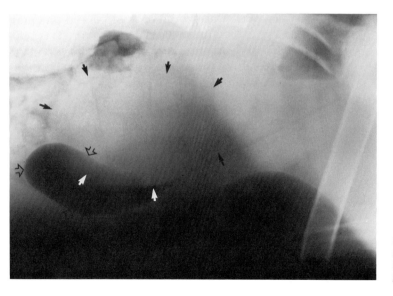

Figure 57–4. *Caudal abdominal radiograph utilizing a negative contrast cystogram (open arrows) to help identify the caudal abdominal mass as a periprostatic cyst (closed arrows).*

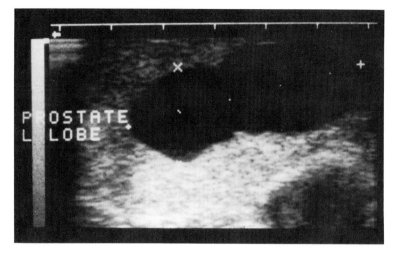

Figure 57–5. *Ultrasonogram of a prostrate with a large intraprostatic cyst.*

prostatic cysts when complete excision is not possible, it is not a procedure without potential serious complications (*e.g.*, ascending infection).

Prostatic Neoplasia

Prostatic neoplasia is relatively uncommon in the dog, with an estimated occurrence of 0.29% to 0.6% in all male dogs, and 11.5% to 15.7% in dogs with clinically evident prostatic disease. Dogs with malignant prostatic neoplasms tend to be older (mean age of 8.5–10.1 years) and medium to large sized. Of the primary prostatic neoplasms reported, more than 90% have been adenocarcinomas. Prostatic leiomyomas, fibromas, and sarcomas have been infrequently reported.

Causes and Pathophysiology

Unlike most types of prostatic disease, and in contrast to human prostatic carcinoma, canine prostatic neoplasia appears to be independent of testicular hormones. Recent reports have demonstrated that previous castration did not prevent the development of prostatic carcinoma, and no clinical response was detected following castration or estrogen therapy. Although as yet unproven, some authors have suggested that the lack of response of canine prostatic neoplasms to castration is due to the persistence of adrenal androgenic hormones. Commonly, by the time of

diagnosis, local infiltration and metastatic spread to the regional lymph nodes, urinary bladder, paraprostatic tissue, lungs, and bone (lumbar vertebral bodies, pelvis, proximal femur) has occurred (Fig. 57-6).

Clinical Signs

Weight loss, hind limb weakness, lumbar pain, urinary signs (predominantly dysuria), and rec-

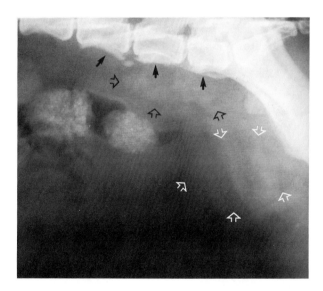

Figure 57–6. *Prostatomegaly with an irregular border (open white arrows), calcified sublumbar lymphadenopathy (open black arrows), and lumbar vertebral bony reaction (closed black arrows) are present in this dog with prostatic adenocarcinoma.*

tal tenesmus are common presenting problems in dogs with prostatic neoplasia. On rectal examination, the gland usually is enlarged, firm, nodular, asymmetrical, and less movable than normal, and may be tender. Occasionally, enlarged sublumbar lymph nodes may be palpable. Neutrophilia, hematuria, pyuria, and proteinuria have been present in some dogs with prostatic adenocarcinoma. Survey radiographic findings in dogs with prostatic or prostatic urethral neoplasms may include prostatomegaly, an irregular prostatic outline, parenchymal mineralization, decreased caudal abdominal contrast, sublumbar lymphadenopathy, and osteoproliferative lesions. Ultrasonographically, prostatic parenchymal asymmetry, echogenic foci (potentially coalescing), and disruption of the prostatic capsule are present in some dogs with prostatic or prostatic urethral neoplasia. Since many of the clinical, radiographic, and laboratory parameters are not specific for neoplasia, and since prostatic neoplasia may be complicated by prostatic cysts or infection, prostatic cytology or biopsy is essential, especially in cases lacking radiographic evidence of metastases (see Prostatic Massage, Urethral Brush Technique, and Ejaculation and Prostatic Biopsy in Chapter 80).

Management

Prostatectomy has been the recommended treatment for prostatic neoplasia, as long as local invasion and metastases have not occurred. In dogs with localized prostatic adenocarcinoma, intraoperative radiotherapy has been able to prolong survival several months after diagnosis and may be a viable alternative to prostatectomy. However, since metastases and local invasion are common by the time of diagnosis and reports of effective chemotherapeutic protocols are lacking, the prognosis for prostatic carcinoma is very poor, and most dogs are euthanized within 1 month of surgery or diagnosis.

INFECTIOUS DISEASES OF THE PROSTATE GLAND

Bacterial infection of the prostate gland has been estimated to be a contributing factor in up to 20% to 74% of dogs with clinical prostatic disease.

Prostatic infections can cause local or systemic signs, or may complicate other prostatic problems, such as BPH, prostatic cysts, or neoplasia. Bacterial infection of the prostate gland can be subdivided into acute bacterial prostatitis (ABP), chronic bacterial prostatitis (CBP), and prostatic abscess. Fungal organisms have been isolated from the prostate glands of dogs with systemic blastomycosis and cryptococcosis.

Causes and Pathophysiology

Ascending migration of urethral bacteria is considered the most common source of prostatic pathogens in humans, although hematogenous, lymphatic, or direct extension of infection into the prostate gland may also occur. Similar routes of infection are expected in the dog. Potentially, any condition that increases bacterial numbers in the periprostatic urethra or urinary bladder or that decreases the local or systemic resistance of the host may increase the likelihood of a prostatic infection. Strictures, masses, calculi, or other anatomic abnormalities involving the lower urinary tract may predispose the dog to lower urinary tract infections by preventing complete emptying of the urinary bladder or altering the normal urethral flora, which decreases the host's resistance to bacterial pathogens. The most common bacterial pathogens in canine prostatitis include *Escherichia coli*, Proteus sp., staphylococci, and streptococci.

Management

Treatment of bacterial prostatitis in the dog is aimed at the elimination of any predisposing factors and selection of an antimicrobial drug to which the bacteria are susceptible that reaches an adequate concentration in the prostate gland. Surgical drainage and adjunctive therapy may be indicated in some cases.

In CBP, achievement of therapeutic concentrations at the site of infection is limited by the blood–prostatic barrier. The blood–prostatic barrier is the anatomic and functional barrier of the prostatic epithelium's bilipid membrane, which limits the penetration of antimicrobial agents from the plasma into the prostatic secretion. Since antimicrobial agents penetrate this membrane only by passive diffusion, the lipid solubility of the antimicrobial is a major determinant influencing the concentration achieved by the drug in the prostatic fluid. The lipid solubility of a drug at any given time depends on the degree of ionization, which in turn is dependent on the pKa of the drug and the pH of the fluid compartment.

Most antimicrobials are weak acids or weak bases. Weak acids, such as ampicillin, tend to be ionized at plasma pH; weak bases, such as trimethoprim, on the other hand, tend to be less ionized at a pH of 7.4. Since the prostatic fluid of dogs with bacterial prostatitis is usually more acidic than plasma, weak bases with low pKas are better able to enter the prostate gland lumen in therapeutic concentrations. After entering the prostatic secretions, the acidic pH increases the degree of ionization of the weak bases. This results in an ionized, lipid-insoluble drug that is "trapped" in the prostatic secretory side of the prostatic epithelium and cannot readily cross the epithelial membrane back into the plasma compartment. So, in CBP, antimicrobials with basic pKas or antimicrobials that do not ionize to an appreciable extent are the drugs of choice. Currently available antibiotics that are known to diffuse into the prostate gland and attain therapeutic concentrations, are listed in Table 57-2.

If the elimination of factors that may predispose the patient to infection and appropriate antimicrobial therapy are incapable of resolving the ABP or CBP in a timely fashion (within 4–6 weeks), adjunctive therapy is indicated to augment host resistance or decrease the size of the prostate gland. Hormonal manipulation is the predominant adjunctive therapy utilized to decrease prostatic mass. More specifically, surgical castration is the most commonly used method to decrease prostatic size in the canine patient. In an experimental model of canine CBP, castration augmented resolution of prostatic infection. Since in prostatic abscesses surgical drainage usually is an essential component of therapy, castration is often performed in the same surgery. However, the ideal time to castrate these patients has not been investigated.

Acute Bacterial Prostatitis

Diagnostic Approach

Dogs with ABP may be systemically ill or may just have signs related to the lower urinary tract (urethral discharge independent of urination). The prostate is usually tender, and may be mildly enlarged or "boggy" on rectal palpation. Usually, pyuria and bacteriuria are present. Examination of prostatic fluid may be difficult, as often these dogs are unwilling to ejaculate (due to discomfort or systemic illness), and prostatic massage samples may be difficult to interpret in the presence of bacteriuria. Abdominal radiographs may be normal or may demonstrate decreased caudal abdominal detail. Ultrasonography of the prostate gland is helpful in ruling out a prostatic abscess or an infected cyst, which will need surgical drainage. A leukocytosis with a left shift may be present.

Management

In ABP the primary concern is choosing an antimicrobial agent to which the organism is susceptible, although initiation of therapy should not be delayed while awaiting sensitivity results, especially if the dog is systemically ill. The antimicrobial drug should be administered for at least 3 weeks. To be certain that the infection has

Table 57–2 *Penetration of Antimicrobial Drugs Into the Noninflamed Canine Prostate Gland*

ANTIMICROBIAL AGENTS CAPABLE OF ENTERING THE PROSTATE GLAND

Trimethoprim-sulfa
Chloramphenicol
Fluroquinolones (enrofloxacin, norfloxacin ciprofloxacin)
Erythromycin
Minocycline
Doxycycline
Clindamycin

ANTIMICROBIAL AGENTS THAT DO NOT ENTER THE PROSTATE GLAND IN THERAPEUTIC CONCENTRATIONS

Penicillins
Cephalosporins
Aminoglycosides

resolved, prostatic fluid should be submitted for bacterial culture 3 to 5 days and 30 days after discontinuing therapy. Therapy may be curative, or the ABP may progress to a prostatic abscess or chronic bacterial prostatitis.

Chronic Bacterial Prostatitis

Diagnostic Approach

Dogs with CBP may have a history of recurrent urinary tract infection, or they may have clinical signs related to prostatic disease, such as a urethral discharge. The dogs are usually not systemically ill, and digital rectal examination of the prostate gland may be unremarkable. Pyuria, bacteriuria, and hematuria may be present. Since a bacterial infection can coexist with hyperplasia or neoplasia, the prostate gland may be large, irregular, or normal in size (CBP alone probably does not cause prostatomegaly.) Prostatic fluid evaluation (culture and cytology) is essential for the diagnosis of CBP.

Management

In CBP, achieving therapeutic concentrations at the site of infection is limited by the blood–prostatic barrier. The antimicrobial agent used should be based on culture and susceptibility testing of the prostatic fluid and on the known penetrability of the drug into the prostate gland. A minimum of 4 weeks of systemic therapy is considered appropriate for adequate control of the infection, although the optimal duration of treatment is unknown. Prostatic fluid samples should be cultured 5 to 7 days after discontinuing therapy, and again in 30 and 60 days.

Prostatic Abscess

Diagnostic Approach

Detection of an abscess in a dog with bacterial prostatitis is essential, since prostatic abscesses require surgical treatment. The presence of a tender, fluctuant, enlarged prostate gland on rectal

Table 57–3 *Summary of Therapeutic Management of Canine Prostatic Diseases*

	Medical	Surgical	Comments, Problems, Complications
Benign prostatic hypertrophy		Castration	In the absence of clinical signs, no therapy is needed
Paraprostatic cyst		Excision or drainage Marsupialization	May become infected secondarily
Prostatic adenocarcinoma	Radiation therapy*	Prostatectomy*	Usually has metastasized by time of diagnosis Incontinence is common following prostatectomy
Acute bacterial prostatitis	Antimicrobial therapy		May progress to chronic bacterial prostatitis or abscess
Chronic bacterial prostatitis	Antimicrobial therapy (long-term)	Castration†	May have recurrent infection or abscessation
Prostatic abscess	Antimicrobial therapy (long-term)	Surgical drainage Prostatectomy Castration‡	Recurrent or chronic infection or abcess is common Urinary incontinence may occur (especially with prostatectomy)

* In the absence of metastases
† As adjunctive therapy; decreasing prostatic size may increase the rate of resolution of infection

palpation is suggestive of a prostatic abscess. However, if the abscess is not superficially and caudally located within the prostate gland, the surface of the gland may be undulant or normal on palpation. Most dogs will be systemically ill, and they may have clinical signs related to abnormalities of urination or defecation. A leukocytosis with a left shift may be present, especially if the abscess ruptures. Elevation of alkaline phosphatase and alanine aminotransferase levels and hyperbilirubinemia occur in approximately 30% of dogs with prostatic abscesssses, and may be more common in dogs with ruptured abscesses. Release of endotoxin or bacteria from the prostate gland is thought to be responsible for the liver dysfunction.

In dogs with bacterial prostatitis, ultrasonographic evaluation of the prostate gland may be especially helpful in detecting focal areas of intraprostatic fluid accumulation, which, in the presence of an inflammatory or septic prostatic fluid, are indicative of prostatic abscessation.

Management

In prostatic abscesses, as in CBP, selection of antimicrobials that penetrate the prostatic epithelium and to which the organisms are sensitive is important. However, medical management alone is inadequate, and surgical drainage or removal is essential for elimination of the infection. Several surgical options are available (drainage, marsupialization, prostatectomy), all of which may have postsurgical complications, such as recurrent abscess formation, chronic urinary tract infection, and urinary incontinence.

For a summary of the management of prostatic disease in the dog, see Table 57-3.

ADDITIONAL READING

Barsanti JA, Finco DR. Evaluation of techniques for diagnosis of canine prostatic diseases. J Am Vet Med Assoc 1984; 185:198.

Barsanti JA, Prasse KW, Crowell WA et al. Evaluation of various techniques for diagnosis of chronic bacterial prostatitis in the dog. J Am Vet Med Assoc 1983; 183:219.

Basinger RR, Barsanti JA. Urodynamic abnormalities associated with canine prostatic diseases and therapeutic intervention. In: Kirk RW, ed. Current veterinary therapy X. Philadelphia: WB Saunders, 1989: 1151.

Cowan LA, Barsanti JA. Chronic bacterial prostatitis in the dog. In: Kirk RW, ed. Current veterinary therapy X. Philadelphia: WB Saunders, 1989: 1243.

Feeney DA, Johnston GR, Klausner JS et al. Canine prostatic disease—comparison of radiographic appearance with morphologic and microbiologic findings: 30 cases (1981–1985). J Am Vet Med Assoc 1987; 190:1018.

Feeney DA, Johnston GR, Klausner JS et al. Canine prostatic disease—comparison of ultrasonographic appearance with morphologic and microbiologic findings: 30 cases (1981–1985). J Am Vet Med Assoc 1987; 190:1027.

Hardie EM, Barsanti JA, Rawlings CA. Complications of prostatic surgery. Journal of the American Animal Hospital Association 1984; 20:50.

Hargis AM, Miller LM. Prostatic carcinoma in dogs. Compendium of Continuing Educucation 1983; 5:647.

Hornbuckle WE, MacCoy DM, Allan GS et al. Prostatic disease in the dog. Cornell Vet 1978; 68:284.

Obradovich J, Walshaw R, Boullaud E. The influence of castration on the development of prostatic carcinoma in the dog. Journal of Veterinary Internal Medicine 1987; 1:183.

Turrel JM. Intraoperative radiotherapy of carcinoma of the prostate gland in ten dogs. J Am Vet Med Assoc 1987; 190:48.

Weaver AD. Discrete prostatic (paraprostatic) cysts in the dog. Vet Rec 1978; 102:435.

Weaver AD. Fifteen cases of prostatic carcinoma in the dog. Vet Rec 1981; 109:71.

THE ENDOCRINE SYSTEM

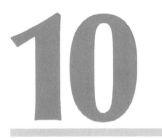

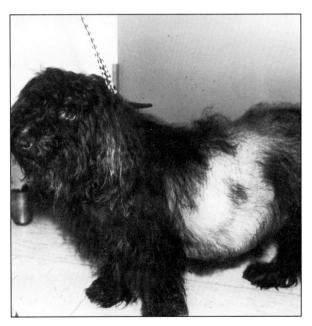

58

DIABETES MELLITUS

Margarethe Hoenig, Duncan C. Ferguson

Diabetes mellitus is a disease state characterized by an absolute or relative deficiency of insulin or lack of its action.

Spontaneous diabetes mellitus has been reported in many species. Diabetes is a major health problem and one of the leading causes of death in humans. In dogs, it is also a relatively common disease with an incidence of approximately 0.2%, while it is less frequently seen in the cat.

Diabetes mellitus is characterized by a generalized derangement of carbohydrate, lipid, and protein metabolism, the most demonstrable clinical abnormality being hyperglycemia.

Diabetes in humans can be broadly divided into two main categories: insulin-dependent diabetes mellitus (IDDM), also called Type I or juvenile onset diabetes; and non–insulin-dependent diabetes (NIDDM), also called Type II or maturity-onset diabetes. Insulin-dependent diabetes is characterized by insulin deficiency. This type of diabetes is usually of sudden onset, and severe hyperglycemia, ketoacidosis, and death follow if it remains untreated. The non–insulin-dependent diabetics are usually able to survive in the absence of insulin treatment and do not exhibit ketoacidosis. This type has a slow onset and usually occurs in obese people.

Diabetes in dogs, as in humans, can be classified into more than one type based on the results of exogenous glucose tolerance testing. Using this test, it was found that diabetic dogs can be classified into three main categories. Group I included dogs which had a high basal blood glucose concentration and were unable to respond to a glucose challenge with release of insulin, similar to Type I diabetes in humans. This is the most common form in the dog. Group II consisted of dogs with a high basal blood glucose concentration and a normal or high basal insulin concentration with no further increase in response to glucose. Using the classification for diabetes in humans, these dogs resemble Type II diabetics. Group III consisted of dogs with mildly elevated blood glucose concentrations and normal basal insulin concentrations. These dogs were able to respond to the glucose challenge with either a normal or delayed insulin response.

When glucose tolerance tests were performed in diabetic cats, most of them were unable to release insulin in response to the glucose challenge and were, therefore, similar to Type I diabetics. In some cats the early insulin response was abnormal, while the second phase of insulin release was normal. This response is similar to early changes seen in Type I diabetics. A third group had glucose-stimulated insulin responses similar to those of controls.

The highest incidence of canine diabetes mellitus occurs in the poodle and dachshund breeds while German shepherd dogs, cocker spaniels, collies, and boxers show a significantly decreased risk. Lines of keeshonds and golden retriever dogs have been identified in which diabetes mellitus is inherited in an autosomal recessive manner. In cats it has been shown that males have an equal incidence of diabetes compared to females, while the Siamese breed seems more frequently affected than other breeds. Diabetes in the dog and cat usually occurs in older animals (5–12 years); however, it also has been described in dogs less than one year old. Intact and neutered female dogs are more frequently affected than males.

CAUSES

Although the etiology and pathogenesis of diabetes mellitus is unknown, it has become apparent that diabetes is not one disease but comprises a heterogeneous group of syndromes which are influenced by a variety of genetic and environmental factors.

The clinical onset of insulin-dependent diabetes in humans is associated with a specific loss of the β-cells in the islets of Langerhans, and autoimmune phenomena may play a role in the pathogenic process. A majority of newly diagnosed diabetic patients have antibodies directed against β-cells (either islet cell surface or cytoplasmic antibodies). In fact, the appearance of islet cell antibodies may precede the clinical onset of diabetes in man by several years. Using immunofluorescent staining for anti-islet cell antibodies, it was found that diabetes in humans does not have an acute onset but is characterized by a latent period of several months or years which precedes the onset of overt diabetes. Recent studies have suggested the importance of these antibodies in humans. It has been shown that

serum or immunoglobulin fractions containing islet-cell antibodies from Type I diabetics suppress glucose-induced insulin release in vitro from mouse, human, and rat islets. Such species nonspecificity implies that the serum antibodies inhibit islet function at a site or sites which have been retained in phylogenetic development. These antibodies are directed against a human islet cell protein. The antibodies seem to be organ-specific and have not been found in people with other autoimmune or endocrine disorders.

The detection of antibodies several years before the diabetes is clinically manifest lends support to the concept that an autoimmune attack on β-cells may start long before the clinical onset. As has been shown in experiments in mice that a critical loss of 80% to 90% of β-cells is needed before clinical symptoms of diabetes develop, it is possible that a similar progressive loss of β-cell function over a long period of time has also occurred before the clinical onset of diabetes in dogs. However, the extent of the analogy between human and canine diabetes mellitus is not known. Recently, antibodies were demonstrated in dogs with diabetes mellitus, hypo- and hyperadrenocorticism, hypothyroidism, and pancreatitis; however, the tissue specificity was not tested.

Other factors may influence β-cell function. Excessive secretion of counter-insulin hormones and administration of these hormones or of drugs antagonizing insulin release or action frequently lead to secondary diabetes. In fact, it seems that secondary diabetes is a major form of diabetes in the dog. Most frequently this type of diabetes is caused by glucocorticoid excess. Growth hormone excess plays a major role in the female dog during diestrus and possibly in the cat. The diabetogenic effect of these hormones or drugs leads to constant overstimulation of the pancreas followed by exhaustion of the β-cell. The deleterious effect of high glucose concentrations on β-cell function has been well documented in vivo and in vitro. Insulin release cannot be sustained under these conditions. Much is still to be learned, and basic questions about the regulation of insulin release need to be answered before identification of the cause or causes of diabetes in dogs or cats is possible.

PATHOPHYSIOLOGY

Insulin is an anabolic hormone. It increases the synthesis of glycogen, protein, and fat. It enhances glucose oxidation and increases the transport of glucose into most cells except for erythrocytes and most brain cells. The main metabolic defects in diabetes are related to alterations in carbohydrate, protein, and lipid metabolism, the most demonstrable clinical abnormality being hyperglycemia. In diabetes, glucose production in the liver is increased. Insulin is not required for glucose uptake in the liver. This process is contrary to the situation in many peripheral tissues, where insulin deficiency leads to a decrease in utilization of glucose. The result is an increase in plasma glucose concentrations which soon exceed the renal threshold (blood glucose greater than 180–220 mg/dl or 9.9–12.1 mmol/L in dogs and greater than 200–300 mg/dl or 11.1–16.7 mmol/L in cats) for maximal reabsorption of glucose. An osmotic diuresis ensues with concomitant loss of large amounts of water and salt. Unless water and electrolytes are adequately replaced, a vicious cycle occurs: intravenous volume depletion leads to poor perfusion of the kidneys, resulting in decreased clearance of glucose and an increase in stress hormones, causing a further rise in plasma glucose concentrations.

With insulin deficiency, the kidney increases excretion of nitrogen due to increased gluconeogenesis. Insulin deficiency and glycogen excess also accelerate lipolysis from fat depots and increase delivery of free fatty acids (FFA) to the liver. In the liver, FFA are either re-esterified or oxidized. In diabetes, fatty acid oxidation is enhanced, resulting in the production of large amounts of acetyl-CoA that are converted to acetoacetate, β-hydroxybutyrate, and acetone. Since the liver cannot utilize these ketone bodies, they are released into the bloodstream and rapidly dissociate, thereby causing an increase in arterial hydrogen concentration. In addition, utilization of ketones by peripheral tissues is impaired in diabetes mellitus. The resulting ketoacidosis leads to a decrease in the serum bicarbonate concentration and a widening of the anion gap. As organic anions, keto acids bind both sodium and potassium. They are excreted by the kidneys together with sodium and potassium, thereby contributing to the electrolyte and water loss in diabetic ketoacidosis and aggravating hypovolemia and dehydration. As systemic acidosis develops, a compensatory hyperventilation may develop (Kussmaul's breathing), and persisting acidosis may ultimately lead to a depression of the respiratory center. The events following insulin deficiency are summarized in Figure 58-1.

CLINICAL SIGNS

The most common historical findings in diabetic dogs and cats are listed in Table 58-1. Polydipsia and polyuria are most frequently noticed by the owner. Diabetes mellitus leads to an osmotic diuresis. The increased water loss into the urine results in a compensatory polydipsia. Glycosuria, decreased peripheral tissue glucose utilization, and the catabolic effect of insulin deficiency on muscle and adipose tissue contribute to weight loss in the chronic, uncontrolled diabetic animal. The sensation of hunger is governed by the amount of plasma glucose that enters the satiety center located in the hypothalamus. The more glucose that enters these cells, the less the sensation of hunger. The concentration of glucose in this area of the brain is under the influence of plasma insulin. In the insulin deficient animal, glucose does not readily enter the satiety center, the sensation of hunger is not suppressed, and polyphagia may be seen in a limited number of animals clinically (Feldman and Nelson, 1987, Additional Reading). Rarely, severe weakness or acute blindness are the only reasons for dog owners to seek veterinary help. Most diabetic animals are not brought to the veterinarian at the onset of clinical signs but usually have been sick for over a month before professional help is sought. Taking into consideration that the onset of diabetes is insidious, these animals may have had metabolic derangements for quite a long period of time.

There are no pathognomonic findings in the diabetic dog or cat on physical examination except for the characteristic sweet odor of ketones found in the ketoacidotic animal (ketone breath). Note that some individuals are more capable

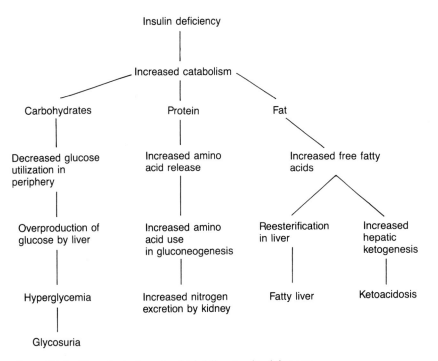

Figure 58–1. *Flow chart of events which follow insulin deficiency.*

than others of detecting ketone breath. Frequently, the animals are in good physical condition, and the clinician may not appreciate the weight loss as much as the people because many of the diabetics have been obese. Hepatomegaly is found in the majority of dogs and cats. Cataracts are detected in about one third of all diabetic dogs on presentation. They have not been reported in diabetic cats. Icterus is a common finding in the diabetic cat.

Table 58–1 *Historical Findings in 89 Diabetic Dogs and 18 Diabetic Cats*

Findings	% of Dogs	% of Cats
Polydipsia	85	100
Polyuria	82	100
Decreased food intake	50	56
Vomiting	49	16
Weight loss	45	66
Increased food intake	27	33
Diarrhea	17	6
Weight gain	9	6
Blindness	6	—
Severe weakness	6	—

The physical examination is important for the assessment of the clinical condition of the dog, but also to look for complications associated with diabetes, such as peripheral or autonomic neuropathy, state of the reproductive cycle in the female, infections such as pyometra, and to examine for the presence of other diseases. Other endocrine problems may have a very similar presentation.

DIAGNOSTIC APPROACH

The diagnosis of overt diabetes mellitus is made based on findings on routine laboratory evaluation (Table 58-2). It is, therefore, important to obtain a complete blood cell count, serum biochemistry profile, and urinalysis at the time of admission in order to avoid alterations of laboratory tests by drugs and, especially, by fluid therapy.

The hematologic findings are usually normal. In about one third of diabetics a mild decrease in the hematocrit is found. The white blood cell

Table 58–2 *Laboratory Assessment of Diabetes Mellitus*

Test	What To Check For
Complete blood cell count	Neutrophilia Left shift
Serum biochemistry profile	Hyperglycemia Increased alanine aminotransferase Increased alkaline phosphatase Electrolyte abnormalities Acid-base abormalities Increased anion gap Increased serum urea, creatinine Hypercholesterolemia Increased serum lipase
Urinalysis	Glucosuria Proteinuria Ketonuria Pyuria Bacteriuria Casts

count is increased in about 60% of the cases. In most cases, this increase is due to a mature neutrophilia; in fewer cases, a left shift is seen indicating the presence of an infectious process. It has also been shown in dogs and other species that neutrophil function is abnormal in diabetes and may predispose diabetics to the development of infections. Increased platelet aggregation and increased concentration of coagulation factors together with diminished fibrinolytic activity have been described in humans but have not been studied in companion animals. They may lead to disseminated intravascular coagulation.

The glucose concentration is abnormally high in all diabetics and generally ranges from 200 mg/dl (11.1 mmol/L) to values greater than 1000 mg/dl (55.5 mmol/L). In some cases, the glucose may range from the upper limit of normal (usually 120 mg/dl or 6.7 mmol/L) to values less than 200 mg/dl or 11.1 mmol/L. In some cases, these mild elevations may be the result of a postprandial increase after a meal high in sugar. More often, however, this kind of glucose intolerance is seen with other endocrine diseases such as hyperthyroidism or hyperadrenocorticism. Correction of the primary problem will often lead to the normalization of the blood glucose concentration.

In cats a stress-induced hyperglycemia is common and very high serum glucose concentrations (even up to 500 mg/dl or 27.6 mmol/L) may be encountered. Glycosuria may also be present. In order to make a correct diagnosis of diabetes mellitus in these cases, it is necessary to take the history into consideration and test blood and urine glucose concentrations several times, preferably after the cat has been hospitalized and has become acquainted with the new environment. Owners may also be able to test urine glucose in the home environment.

Serum alanine aminotransferase and alkaline phosphatase are increased in approximately one half of diabetic dogs and cats. In animals with concomitant hyperadrenocorticism, alkaline phosphatase concentrations are generally higher and abnormalities occur in a larger number of animals because of enzyme induction caused by hypercortisolism. In the diabetic, the abnormalities in liver enzymes are due to fatty infiltration of the liver.

Serum sodium concentrations may be low, normal, or high. Several factors affect serum sodium levels in diabetes mellitus. Hyperglycemia and hyperosmolarity lead to a dilutional hyponatremia which is the result of transferral of water from the intracellular to the extracellular space. Insulin increases tubular reabsorption of sodium, whereas glucagon is a natriuretic hormone; therefore, the lack of insulin and excess of glucagon associated with diabetes results in an increased loss of sodium into the urine. In ketoacidosis the osmotic diuresis, together with the excretion of keto acids in forms of sodium salts, may also lower the serum sodium concentration. However, since water is usually lost in excess of sodium in diabetes, this action tends to increase rather than decrease serum sodium concentrations. A spurious lowering of the serum sodium concentration (pseudohyponatremia) may occur if the animal is hyperlipemic. Although the sodium concentration in plasma water remains normal, the sodium concentration, expressed as milliequivalents per total volume of serum (which in ketoacidosis contains a large nonaqueous phase), is low.

Serum potassium concentrations are usually normal in diabetics, but very low or high levels may be seen. The serum potassium concentrations do not reflect the status of the body stores. Body potassium stores are commonly depleted in diabetic ketoacidosis as a consequence of the acidosis, diuresis, and vomiting. Serum potassium concentrations, however, may be increased as a result of volume contraction and acidosis. A low or normal serum potassium concentration is therefore almost always indicative of total body potassium depletion.

Serum phosphorus concentrations may range from very low to very high but are usually normal or elevated. Again, as is true for potassium, serum phosphorus levels are not representative of body stores, and phosphorus depletion may occur in diabetic ketoacidosis as a consequence of the acidosis and osmotic diuresis.

The total carbon dioxide (TCO_2) concentration is normal in about 60% of diabetics but may be low. The anion gap has been found to be high in the majority of diabetic dogs and cats due to the increase in plasma keto acids.

The blood urea nitrogen (BUN) is usually normal, but may be elevated due to prerenal azotemia. Renal failure is not a common complication of diabetes in the dog and cat as it is in human diabetics.

An increase in serum cholesterol concentrations is a frequent finding in diabetics because of the catabolic effect of insulin deficiency on fat metabolism.

The serum lipase concentration is increased in the majority of diabetic dogs. It may be increased as a result of concomitant or inciting pancreatitis, or the result of prerenal or renal azotemia.

Urine should preferably be obtained by cystocentesis (see Cystocentesis in Chapter 80). Glucosuria, ketonuria, and proteinuria are frequent findings in diabetics. Urine sediment examination may show pyuria and bacteriuria. Fine or coarse granular casts are also commonly seen. Ketonuria does not imply that the animal needs to be treated automatically as a complicated diabetic. Rather, the overall clinical presentation will dictate the treatment requirements.

It is usually assumed that diabetic dogs and cats are insulin deficient and require insulin treatment. Insulin measurements are, therefore, rarely done. However, in order to gain more infor-

mation about possible classifications of diabetes in dogs or cats, it would be advisable to test each newly diagnosed diabetic for glucose tolerance with an IV glucose tolerance test and insulin response. Since this necessitates a controlled environment, it may best be done at referral institutions. The information obtained from a single insulin measurement is limited.

MANAGEMENT

Treatment of diabetes mellitus must be adjusted to the clinical presentation of the animal. Usually two forms can be differentiated:
1. Uncomplicated diabetes mellitus
2. Complicated diabetes mellitus
   a. Ketoacidosis
   b. Nonketotic hyperosmolar coma

Treatment of Uncomplicated Diabetes Mellitus

The uncomplicated diabetic is treated with insulin. Several preparations are available, which are classified as intermediate (*e.g.*, NPH, Lente) or long-acting (*e.g.*, PZI, Ultralente) insulin preparations. The species source of the insulin can be pork, beef, or a combination of both. The strength can be U40 (40 units/ml) or U100 (100 units/ml). The initial treatment is best performed in the hospital. A baseline blood glucose determination is done, and insulin is given subcutaneously in the flank area at a fixed time every day, (*e.g.*, 8 AM). At the same time one fourth to one half of the daily amount of food is fed. The recommended initial insulin dose (NPH) is 1.1 U/kg in the dog. The duration of NPH insulin in cats is generally short, causing wide fluctuations in blood glucose concentrations. Protamine zinc (PZI) and ultralente insulin are preferred by some clinicians in this species. Of the two, ultralente appears to have a more consistent and longer duration of action (Nelson, Additional Reading). Both preparations are given once or twice daily as required, and the average cat is started on 1 to 3 units. Blood glucose concentrations are monitored every 2 hours to follow the insulin action. Monitoring can be performed at longer intervals as soon as the insulin effect decreases, (the blood glucose concentration rises). The rest of the daily food requirement should be given about 2 hours before the anticipated peak of insulin action occurs (the blood glucose reaches the lowest level) to allow sufficient time for digestion and absorption.

Initially, one assumes that the peak action time of NPH and Lente in the dog is about 6 to 8 hours and that of the long-acting insulins (PZI and Ultralente) is about 8 to 12 hours after injection. However, it must be kept in mind that action times vary. The goal of insulin treatment is to keep the blood glucose in a range of 140 to 180 mg/dl (7.8–10 mmol/L) for most of the day. This range seems to be safe for avoiding the dangers of hypoglycemia (weakness, seizures, or insulin-induced hyperglycemia, also called Somogyi rebound) and alleviating the signs of hyperglycemia. Oral hypoglycemic agents are not beneficial in most cases of diabetic animals because most diabetics are truly insulin deficient. However, it seems possible that those diabetics with normal or high endogenous insulin concentrations may benefit from treatment with oral hypoglycemic agents. These agents not only lower blood glucose by increasing insulin release from the pancreas, they may also increase the sensitivity of peripheral tissues to the effects of glucose.

Dietary management is an important aspect of the treatment of a diabetic dog and cat. In general, food administration should follow a strict schedule. A diet high in fiber and complex carbohydrates and low in fat content should be given (*e.g.*, Hill's prescription diet w/d or r/d), in the same quantity and at the same time each day. The best feeding time has to be preferably established with a glucose response curve which determines the peak time of insulin action. The caloric requirement is approximately 50 to 75 kcal/kg/day.

If a peak of insulin action is seen with a particular insulin preparation early after injection and the animal is hyperglycemic for most of the day, the insulin preparation used obviously does not provide the desired effect and should either be changed to a different preparation or given twice daily to better control blood glucose concentra-tions. However, it should be remembered that it usually takes a few days to observe a consistent response to a given insulin preparation; therefore, changes should not be made hastily. If different preparations are chosen, it cannot be predicted whether an intermediate or long-acting preparation would be preferable because every animal reacts differently to a given insulin preparation. Glucose monitoring can be done by visual inspection of glucose-impregnated strips (*e.g.*, Dextrostix, Ames; Chemstrip bG, Bio Dynamics). Very accurate glucose measurements can be achieved by reading the test strips with a reflectance colorimeter (*e.g.*, Dextrometer, Ames).

It is frequently difficult to accurately measure a small dose of insulin. In these cases, insulin can be diluted, preferably with the proper diluent for the particular type of insulin used, which can be obtained from the company. The initial regulation of the diabetic animal often requires patience since it is not uncommon to require several days before a consistent response to a given insulin preparation is seen and the animal can be discharged. The owners can monitor urine glucose and ketone concentrations and adjust the insulin dose at home (Table 58-3). Since glucose determinations of the urine are not as accurate as a blood glucose determination, the diabetic should be rechecked by the veterinarian at regular intervals (every 2–4 months), preferably at the assumed time of peak insulin action. The owners also should be made aware of the signs of hypoglycemia and hyperglycemia in order to be able to monitor the animal at home. Corn syrup or honey can be given orally by the owners in a

Table 58–3 *Treatment of the Uncomplicated Diabetic*

	Insulin Dose Adjustment	
	Small Dog (<15 kg)	**Large Dog**
AM **Urine Glucose**		
2%* (2000 mg/dl)	↑ 1 unit	↑ 2 units
0.5% to 1% (500 to 1000 mg/dl)	↑ ½ unit	↑ 1 unit
0.1% to 0.25% (100 to 250 mg/dl)	— no change —	
Negative**	↓ 1 unit	↓ 2 units

* If consistently high for more than 3 days, notify veterinarian.
** If consistently low for more than 3 days, notify veterinarian.

hypoglycemic crisis. Since treatment of a diabetic is complicated and requires much understanding and patience from the owners, communication is of utmost importance. For best results, the owners should not only monitor clinical signs and urine glucose in the diabetic animal in the morning but also at the assumed time of peak insulin action.

A common complication in the treatment of diabetes is the occurrence of the Somogyi rebound effect. This effect is caused by an overdose of insulin leading to hypoglycemia. The low blood glucose in turn stimulates stress hormone release with a subsequent rise in the blood glucose concentrations. This sequence of events illustrates the importance of frequent monitoring of the diabetic by the owner. Insulin-induced hypoglycemia should be considered in diabetic animals when persistent morning glycosuria (greater than 1 g/dl), persistent polyuria and polydipsia, weight loss, or signs of hypoglycemia at the time of insulin peak (weakness, seizure) occur.

Decreased insulin sensitivity is another commonly encountered problem in the diabetic and is seen with excessive secretion of counter-insulin hormones (*e.g.*, cortisol in Cushing's syndrome or growth hormone in the cycling bitch) or with the administration of these hormones. Decreased insulin sensitivity can also be seen with acute illnesses and is due to an increased stress hormone release.

Treatment of Complicated Diabetes Mellitus

Ketoacidosis may develop in a previously well controlled diabetic secondary to systemic illness (bacterial infections often involving the urinary system, pulmonary system or skin), chronic stress, proestrus (estrogen-induced insulin antagonism), or diestrus (progesterone-induced insulin antagonism). The ketoacidotic animal presents with more severe metabolic disturbances than the uncomplicated diabetic and usually is dehydrated, vomiting, moderately to severely acidotic, and weak. Some animals may actually present in coma. The nonketotic hyperosmolar animal is not ketoacidotic, but these animals are severely dehydrated and show extremely high blood glucose concentration. The complicated diabetic state, therefore, has to be treated aggressively, since it constitutes an acute life-threatening condition. Therapy should consist of fluid and electrolyte replacement and insulin administration (Table 58-4). The initial fluid replacement needed to correct the dehydration deficit is calculated according to the formula:

Fluid deficit (ml) = percent dehydration × kg body weight × 1000. (Example: A 10 kg dog whose dehydration deficit is estimated to be ~10% would need 0.1 × 10 × 1000 = 1000 ml of fluids to replace the deficit)

The replacement can be given at a rate of 20 to

Table 58–4 *Low-dose, Continuous IV Infusion Protocol for the Treatment of Diabetic Ketoacidosis*

1. Place intravenous catheter.
2. Start fluid therapy. (NaCl, 0.9% consider replacement and maintenance fluid requirements.)
3. Insert urinary catheter and attach to a closed monitoring system.
4. Add regular insulin to the saline solution (2.2units/kg/day in the dog; 1.1unit/kg/day in the cat). Change insulin/saline solution every 6 hours. Use pediatric infusion set or infusion pump for accurate administration.
5. Monitor blood glucose concentrations every 1 to 2 hours.
6. Monitor urinary output.
7. Monitor electrolytes (K^+ twice daily; others). Adjust if necessary.
8. Change saline solution to 2.5% dextrose in 0.45% saline or in lactated Ringer's or to 5% dextrose solution when blood glucose reaches 250 mg/dl (13.8 mmol/L). Continue to administer regular insulin.
9. Keep animals on this regimen until they are able to eat without vomiting.
10. Stop insulin infusion in PM. Start treatment of the uncomplicated diabetic the next morning.

40 ml/kg/hour. The patient should be monitored carefully for any signs of fluid overload. If possible, central venous pressure (see Central Venous Pressure in Chapter 80) should be monitored. It is also advisable to monitor urine output, which can be best done by inserting a urinary catheter. This technique is especially important in the nonketotic hyperosmolar patients in which oliguric and anuric renal failure are common. Maintenance fluid therapy after correction of the dehydration is 50 to 60 ml/kg daily; however, the rate has to be increased if the animal is vomiting or urinating excessively. Initially, isotonic saline is recommended as replacement fluid; once the animal is well rehydrated and insulin therapy has been initiated, Ringer's or lactated Ringer's solution can be used. The most common electrolyte disturbances found in ketoacidosis include hypokalemia and hypophosphatemia. They can be corrected by adding 20 to 40 mEq of potassium chloride or (in the case of hypophosphatemia) potassium phosphate per liter of fluids after adequate urine production has been established. The rate should not exceed 0.5 mEq/kg/hour. It is not recommended to treat the acidosis routinely with sodium bicarbonate because of its side effects (tissue hypoxia, paradoxical central nervous acidosis, alkalosis occurring after correction). The acidotic state will usually be corrected with proper fluid and insulin therapy.

As soon as fluid therapy is being administered and a diagnosis of complicated diabetes mellitus is made, treatment with regular insulin should be initiated. Regular insulin is a fast-acting insulin that can be administered intravenously, intramuscularly, or subcutaneously. Different treatment methods have been described. In the authors' hands the best results are usually obtained using a continuous low-dose insulin infusion method. The initial dose for dogs is 2.2 units/kg/day, and for cats it is 1.1 units/kg/day. The insulin is added to the fluids and best delivered with a pediatric intravenous set to allow for accurate administration. The glucose concentration is monitored every 1 to 2 hours.

Once the glucose concentration reaches 250 mg/dl (13.8 mmol/L) the intravenous fluids should be changed to a dextrose-containing solution (either 2.5% dextrose in 0.45% saline or 5% dextrose in water). Insulin is again added to the fluids. It is important to provide continuous substrate for insulin in the absence of oral caloric intake to avoid hypoglycemia and to aid in the regulation of normal metabolism. Once the animal is stable and able to eat without vomiting, the low-dose insulin infusion can be terminated and the animal can be treated with an intermediate or long-acting insulin preparation as outlined for the uncomplicated diabetic. If the animal shows insulin resistance, the rate of the continuous insulin infusion should be increased until blood glucose concentrations decrease to less than 250 mg/dl (13.8 mmol/L). For example, if a significant decrease in glucose levels is not seen after 4 to 6 hours of intravenous regular insulin and fluid therapy, the infused insulin dose should be increased by 25%; if the response is still minimal after another 4- to 6-hour period, the dose is increased by 50% above the original insulin dose. The goal of treatment is to increase the dose as needed to obtain effective insulin concentrations within a reasonable period of time.

Conversely, in animals that develop hypoglycemia during the continuous intravenous infusion, the insulin infusion should be temporarily stopped, and the animal should be maintained on a dextrose-containing solution until the blood glucose concentration again increases to greater than 250 mg/dl (13.8 mmol/L). The insulin infusion can then be measured with a lower dose.

Other treatment regimens have been described for the complicated diabetic: the low-dose intramuscular method and the high-dose bolus method. With the first method, the protocol for dogs weighing less than 10 kg consists of the administration of 2.0 units of regular insulin per dog or cat initially, with hourly injections of 1.0 U/hour thereafter. In larger dogs, the initial dose is 0.25 U/kg followed by hourly injections of 0.1 U/kg. As soon as the blood glucose concentrations fall below 250 mg/dl (13.8 mmol/L), regular insulin is administered subcutaneously (0.1–0.4 U/kg) every 6 hours. Once the animals are stabilized and eat without vomiting, they are treated as an uncomplicated diabetic. The high-dose bolus method consists of subcutaneous bolus injections of regular insulin at 6-hour intervals. This method leads to poor control of the diabetic state and is not recommended in the initial acute condition of complicated diabetes.

Avoiding hypoglycemia is as important as treating hyperglycemia. A common reason for hypoglycemia in diabetic ketoacidosis is the use of excessive insulin doses because of persisting ketonuria during treatment. However, adjustment in insulin dosages should be based on the plasma glucose concentration and not on that of ketones bodies. With proper insulin and fluid therapy ketone bodies will be cleared from the plasma, albeit slowly for some.

PATIENT MONITORING

Treatment of a diabetic animal is always challenging; not many diseases require the veterinarian and the owners to work so closely together. The veterinarian needs to spend much time on the owners' education before the diabetic dog or cat is discharged; otherwise, the home treatment will be frustrating for both the owners and the veterinarian.

The owners should be well aware of the possible side effects of insulin and should know how to monitor insulin action (*e.g.*, clinical signs of hyperglycemia and hypoglycemia, urine glucose testing). Insulin requirements do change and adjustments must be made accordingly.

The owners should also know the practical aspects of insulin administration, which include knowledge about the differences in insulin preparations and strength and the differences in insulin syringes (U40 vs. U100). The owners should give one or several subcutaneous injections under supervision in the hospital.

The prognosis for the treatment of the uncomplicated diabetic is good if the owners and the veterinarian communicate effectively. The prognosis of the complicated ketoacidotic dog is guarded and depends on the response to treatment within the first few days of hospitalization. The nonketotic hyperosmolar diabetic has a poor prognosis.

As the etiology of diabetes mellitus is still not known, no curative treatment is available. Progress has been made in humans with the transplantation of islets cells using the immunosuppressive agent cyclosporine A. Islets have been isolated from the dog pancreas and have been transplanted into immunosuppressed diabetic dogs. While the feasibility of such a treatment regimen for the diabetic animal will depend on many factors, such as survival of islet allografts, toxicity of cyclosporine A, and yield of islets obtained from pancreases, the transplantation of islets is an attractive consideration for the future treatment of diabetes.

ADDITIONAL READING

Alejandro R, Feldman EC, Shienvold FL, Mintz DH. Advances in canine diabetes mellitus research: Etiopathology and results of islet transplantation. J Am Vet Med Assoc 1988; 193:1050.

Chastain CB, Nichols CE. Low dose intramuscular insulin therapy for diabetic ketoacidosis in dogs. J Am Vet Med Assoc 1981; 178:561.

Chastain CB. Intensive case of dogs and cats with diabetic ketoacidosis. J Am Vet Med Assoc 1981; 179:972.

Fajans SS, Cloutier MC, Crowther RL. Clinical and etiologic heterogeneity of idiopathic diabetes mellitus. Diabetes 1982; 27:1112.

Feldman EC, Nelson RW. Insulin induced hypoglycemia in diabetic dogs. J Am Vet Med Assoc 1982; 180:1432.

Feldman EC, Nelson RW. Diabetes mellitus. In: Feldman EC, Nelson RW, eds. Canine and feline endocrinology and reproduction. Philadelphia: WB Saunders, 1987: 229.

Duffell SJ. Some aspects of pancreatic disease in the cat. Journal of Small Animal Practice 1975; 16:365.

Hoenig M. Diabetic ketoacidosis. In: Kirk RW, ed. Current veterinary therapy IX. Philadelphia: WB Saunders, 1986: 987.

Kaneko JJ, Mattheeuws D, Rottiers RP, Vermeulen A. Glucose tolerance and insulin response in diabetes mellitus of dogs. Journal of Small Animal Practice 1977; 18:85.

Kruth SA, Cowgill LD. Renal glucose transport in the cat. Proceedings of the American College of Veterinary Internal Medicine (abstr) 1982: 78.

Lebovitz HE, Feinglos MN. Mechanism of action of second generation sulfonylurea glipizide. Am J Med 1983; 75:46.

Lockwood DL, Maloft BL, Novak SM, McCaleb ML. Extrapancreatic effects of sulfonylureas: Potentiation of insulin action through post-binding mechanisms. Am J Med 1983; 74:102.

Marmor M, Willeberg P, Glickman LT et al. Epizootiologic patterns of diabetes mellitus in dogs. Am J Vet Res 1982; 43:465.

Mattheeuws D, Rottiers R, Kaneko JJ. Diabetes mellitus in dogs: Relationship of obesity to glucose tolerance and insulin response. Am J Vet Res 1984; 45:98.

Moise NS, Reimers JJ. Insulin therapy in cats with diabetes mellitus. J Am Vet Med Assoc 1983; 182:158.

O'Brien TD, Hayden DW, Johnson KH, Stevens JB. High dose intravenous glucose tolerance test and serum insulin and glucagon levels in diabetic and nondiabetic cats: Relationships to insular amyloidosis. Vet Pathol 1985; 22:250.

Nelson RW. Feline diabetes mellitus. Proceeding of the ACVIM 199; 189.

Schaer M. A clinical survey of thirty cats with diabetes mellitus. Journal of the American Animal Hospital Association 1977; 13:23.

Schaer M. Insulin treatment for the diabetic dog and cat. Compendium of Continuing Education 1983; 5:579.

Schall WD, Cornelius LM. Diabetes mellitus. Vet Clin North Am [Small Anim Pract] 1977; 7:613.

Unger RH, Foster DW. Diabetes mellitus. In: Wilson JD, Foster DW, eds. Textbook of endocrinology. Philadelphia: WB Saunders, 1985: 1018.

Williams MD, Gregory R, Schall W et al. Characterization of naturally occurring diabetes in a colony of golden retrievers. Federation Proceedings 1981; 40:740.

59

HYPERADRENOCORTICISM
Margarethe Hoenig, Duncan C. Ferguson

In 1932 Harvey Cushing described a clinical syndrome of central obesity, cutaneous striae, osteoporosis, weakness, hypertension, diabetes mellitus, and hirsutism in connection with basophil adenomas of the pituitary gland. It was, however, felt at the time that not only a pituitary lesion was responsible for the syndrome, but that the adrenal cortex played a role also in the pathogenesis of this syndrome. Ten years later, Cushing's syndrome was attributed to an excess secretion of the adrenocortical "sugar hormone." At the same time, the structures of several steroids from the adrenal cortex were identified. Among them, cortisol and cortisone were shown to have biological activity, and an adrenocorticotropic hormone (ACTH), isolated from the pituitary gland, was shown to stimulate the adrenal cortex.

It was demonstrated that an excess of cortisol was the common denominator of all cases of Cushing's syndrome. The term *Cushing's syndrome*, therefore, does not differentiate the cause for the hypercortisolemia, while the term *Cushing's disease* is used when the hypercortisolemia is caused by inappropriate secretion of corticotropin by the pituitary as originally described by Cushing.

Cushing's syndrome is one of the most common endocrine diseases in the dog but is very rare in the cat. The majority of cats and dogs (about 80%–85%) with naturally occurring hyperadrenocorticism have the pituitary-dependent form (pituitary-dependent hyperadrenocorti-

cism [PDH]) of the disorder; only about 15% of dogs and cats have functional adrenal tumors. A third form, iatrogenic hyperadrenocorticism caused by exogenous glucocorticoid administration, is a well-recognized and common problem in the dog, but it is rare in the cat (cats are more resistant to the effects of these drugs).

Hyperadrenocorticism occurs mostly in middle-aged to older dogs and cats; however, PDH also has been described in dogs less than 2 years of age. Poodles, dachshunds, boxers, and beagles seem to be at increased risk to develop PDH. While no breed predilection has been seen in dogs with adrenal tumors, adrenal tumors seem to be more frequent in the female dog. Most cats with hyperadrenocorticism are domestic shorthairs.

CAUSES

Figure 59-1 shows the hypothalamic pituitary-adrenal axis in the normal dog. This figure will be used to facilitate the understanding of changes seen in the different forms of hyperadrenocorticism. Causes of hyperadrenocorticism are listed in Table 59-1.

Primary Hyperadrenocorticism

Primary adrenal tumors, adenomas, or carcinomas, arise spontaneously and lose their dependence on ACTH. Secretion of cortisol becomes

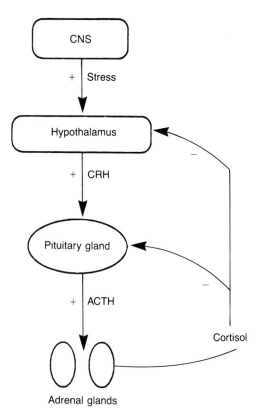

Figure 59–1. *The hypothalamic-pituitary-adrenal axis in the normal dog.*

autonomous, and as the cortisol concentration increases above normal, ACTH secretion from the pituitary gland decreases or ceases because of negative feedback inhibition. Typically, because of the autonomous nature of cortisol secretion,

Table 59–1 *Causes of Hyperadrenocorticism*

PRIMARY HYPERADRENOCORTICISM
Adrenal adenoma
Adrenal carcinoma

SECONDARY HYPERADRENOCORTICISM
Pituitary microadenoma
Pituitary macroadenoma
Corticotroph hyperplasia

IATROGENIC HYPERADRENOCORTICISM
Exogenous glucocorticoids

these tumors do not respond to ACTH with stimulation or to high doses of glucocorticoids such as dexamethasone with suppression. However, some tumors will maintain responsiveness to ACTH and may show suppression with high doses of dexamethasone.

Secondary Hyperadrenocorticism

Inappropriate secretion of ACTH by the pituitary gland leads to hypercortisolism (PDH, Cushing's disease). In the majority of dogs, the excessive ACTH secretion appears to be caused by microadenomas of the pars distalis and pars intermedia. In the cat, a pituitary lesion also seems to occur more frequently than an adrenal tumor. In approximately 10% of cases of PDH, macroadenomas are seen. Macroadenomas are large pituitary tumors (greater than 1 cm diameter) that extend into the area of the hypothalamus and may be associated with depression, anorexia, lethargy, or behavioral changes. A few cases have been reported with diffuse hyperplasia of pituitary corticotroph cells indicative of increased release of corticotropin-releasing hormone (CRH), which in turn stimulates ACTH release. The excessive ACTH release in PDH stimulates the adrenal glands to synthesize and secrete excessive amounts of cortisol. However, whereas most adrenal tumors have lost responsiveness and cortisol release cannot be suppressed with large amounts of glucocorticoids such as dexamethasone, in PDH the adrenal secretory activity is at least partially suppressible with large amounts of glucocorticoids. The ACTH secretion in PDH, although inappropriately high, is not autonomous. Rather, it seems to be regulated at a higher set point. Some or all tumors arising from the pars intermedia, however, may also be nonsuppressive with dexamethasone.

Iatrogenic Hyperadrenocorticism

Excessive administration of exogenous glucocorticoids is as harmful as the excessive release of endogenous glucocorticoids. Exogenous glucocorticoids mimic the action of cortisol and act as negative feedback regulators on the hypothalamus and pituitary gland, causing a decreased release of ACTH. This results in decreased stimulation of the adrenal cortex with loss of endogenous cortisol release and atrophy of adrenocortical cells. The animal becomes unable to respond to stress, and, if the exogenous glucocorticoids are withdrawn, the animal is in a potentially life-threatening situation identical to that of naturally occurring secondary hypoadrenocorticism.

Ectopic ACTH Syndrome

This syndrome has not yet been described in the dog or cat. It stems from the production of ACTH by a nonpituitary neoplasm. About 20 tumors, mostly carcinomas, have been described in humans as sources of ectopic ACTH.

PATHOPHYSIOLOGY

Hypercortisolism affects every tissue in the body because cortisol has multitudinous actions.

Hypercortisolism leads to increased glucose production from amino acids and reduces the incorporation of amino acids into protein (catabolic action). Both insulin and glucagon concentrations may rise in response to high cortisol concentrations. Eventually the pancreatic β-cells may become exhausted and overt diabetes mellitus may be seen (see Chapter 58). Muscle wasting is not uncommon and can lead to profound weakness. Fatty acids are mobilized from adipose tissue under the influence of high cortisol levels and often distributed in a peculiar way. Redistribution of fat from the limbs to the abdomen contributes, together with abdominal muscle weakness, to the abdominal distention seen in Cushing's syndrome.

High cortisol concentrations induce sodium retention and potassium excretion leading to hypertension and possibly hypokalemia. However, in addition to increasing extracellular fluid volume, cortisol also increases the glomerular filtration rate, initiating a diuresis. It has been suggested that the polyuria in hypercortisolism is due to decreased release of vasopressin; however, an interference with the action of vasopressin on the distal tubule is also possible (see Chapter 9).

Excess cortisol concentrations inhibit inflammatory reactions at multiple points. They stabilize lysosomal membranes, appear to block the increased permeability of capillaries induced by acute inflammation, and inhibit the migration of leukocytes and granuloma formation. They also suppress the immune system. The most important effect seems to be the suppression of leukocyte accumulation at sites of inflammation.

In addition to their diabetogenic effect, high concentrations of cortisol suppress secretion of thyrotropin (TSH), growth hormone (GH), prolactin, and luteinizing hormone (LH), as well as follicle-stimulating hormone (FSH). Suppression of TSH is a likely, although unproven, mechanism causing low total thyroxine concentration in a large percentage of dogs with Cushing's syndrome.

Hypercortisolism leads to many other changes, including stimulation of hematopoiesis, mental effects, stimulation of appetite, osteoporosis, and induction of enzymes such as alkaline phosphatase.

CLINICAL SIGNS

Cushing's syndrome is slowly progressive in most cases and the owner may notice a change in the animal only when hair loss, polydipsia and polyuria, or abdominal distention and weakness become obvious. It is, therefore, often difficult to assess the duration of the illness.

Physical examination of dogs and cats with hyperadrenocorticism will often confirm the clinician's suspicion of the presence of the disease, and additional signs can often be found that the owners may not have noticed, such as hepatomegaly, testicular atrophy, clitoral hypertrophy, or muscle wasting. However, sometimes the animals do not show obvious clinical signs or only show mild changes, which makes the clinical diagnosis of Cushing's syndrome more difficult. Some dogs also have been described as having intermittent clinical signs with periods of remission and relapse. The occurrence of clinical signs

Table 59–2 *Clinical Findings in 300 Dogs and 18 Cats With Hyperadrenocorticism*

Findings	% of Dogs	% of Cats
Polyuria/polydipsia	82	94
Pendulous abdomen	67	94
Hepatomegaly	67	56
Hair loss	63	72
Lethargy	62	N/A
Polyphagia	57	89
Muscle weakness	57	N/A
Anestrus (69 females)	54	N/A
Obesity	47	61
Muscle atrophy	35	67
Comedones	34	N/A
Increased panting	31	N/A
Testicular atrophy (128 males)	29	N/A
Hyperpigmentation	23	N/A
Calcinosis cutis	8	N/A
Facial nerve paralysis	7	N/A
Infection	N/A	39
Weight loss	N/A	11
Diarrhea	N/A	11

N/A = Not available.

of dogs and cats with hyperadrenocorticism is listed in Table 59-2.

Over 80% of dogs with Cushing's syndrome are polyuric and polydipsic. The polyuria is the primary problem, while the polydipsia is a compensatory response. It is unknown why hyperadrenocorticism leads to polyuria. It has been suggested that hypercortisolism may lead to an abnormality in the release or action of vasopressin. Glucocorticoids also appear to increase glomerular filtration rate and inhibit tubular water reabsorption.

A potbellied appearance is present in the majority of dogs and cats with hyperadrenocorticism. Muscle atrophy and fat redistribution together with a frequently prominent enlargement of the liver contribute to the development of the classic pot-bellied appearance. The increase in liver size is due to glycogen infiltration caused by excessive concentrations of glucocorticoids.

The hair loss in hyperadrenocorticism is typically bilateral and symmetrical and cannot be differentiated from alopecia seen in other endocrine disorders (Fig. 59-2). The hair loss is due to atrophy of hair follicles and the pilosebaceous apparatus (see Chapter 49).

It is difficult to assess whether the lethargy seen in hyperadrenocorticism is a primary disorder caused by direct effects of hypercortisolism or whether it is secondary to muscle wasting caused by the protein catabolic effect of cortisol.

Increased appetite is seen in a majority of dogs and cats and may be due to a direct effect of hypercortisolism.

Muscle wasting and muscle weakness are usually mild to moderate and are signs of protein wasting.

Hypercortisolism leads to a decrease in pituitary gonadotropin secretion (luteinizing hor-

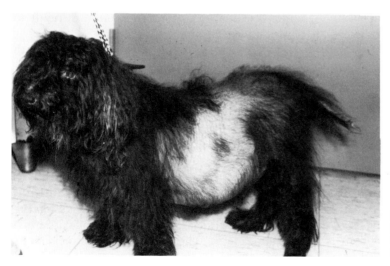

Figure 59–2. *This 8-year-old poodle with pituitary-dependent hyperadrenocorticism illustrates alopecia, a poor haircoat, and abdominal enlargement ("pot-bellied").*

mone and follicle-stimulating hormone). Testicles become small and soft, and in the female estrous cycling ceases. Some female dogs with hypercortisolism have an excess of adrenal androgen secretion, which may result in clitoral hypertrophy.

Fat redistribution, obesity, hepatomegaly, and weakness of the respiratory muscles are likely causes of panting seen in dogs with hypercortisolism.

Acute respiratory distress can be seen in dogs with pulmonary thromboembolism, which is a potential complication of hypercortisolism (see Chapter 24).

Thin skin is a sequela of the protein catabolism. Frequently dogs present with skin ulcerations that seem to heal poorly (Fig. 59-3). The skin may be wrinkled and the animal may bruise easily. In addition, keratin-plugged follicles are found and the skin may be hyperpigmented. Skin infections are common because of the suppressed immune system associated with hypercortisolism. Calcium deposition, *calcinosis cutis*, in the skin is a characteristic lesion in the dog with hypercortisolism.

Pseudomyotonia, a myopathy characterized by the persistence of active muscle contraction after cessation of the stimulative effort, has been described in dogs with hyperadrenocorticism. Some affected dogs have a stiff, stilted gait with hyperextended limbs. Rarely, central nervous signs are seen. Unilateral or bilateral paralysis of the cranial nerve VII has been described. In dogs with enlarging pituitary tumors, seizures, ataxia, nystagmus, tetraparesis, and other signs related to compression of the hypothalamus may be seen.

DIAGNOSTIC APPROACH

A diagnosis of hyperadrenocorticism cannot be definitively made on findings of routine laboratory examination and certainly should not be excluded based on these data alone. However, as in any sick animal, a thorough evaluation of the clinical status of the animal should include a complete blood cell count, serum biochemistry profile, and urinalysis. Preferably, blood and urine should be obtained at the time of admission. Results from these tests may support the clinical diagnosis, and they will help to recognize concomitant medical problems that may exist unassociated with the primary disease.

The hematologic findings are inconsistent. Because of the stimulating effect of cortisol on the bone marrow, a mild to moderate erythrocytosis may be found. A mature leukocytosis with eosinopenia and lymphopenia ("stress" leukogram) may be seen. The most reliable change in the white blood cells seems to be the low eosinophil count. Table 59-3 shows hematologic findings in dogs and cats with hyperadrenocorticism.

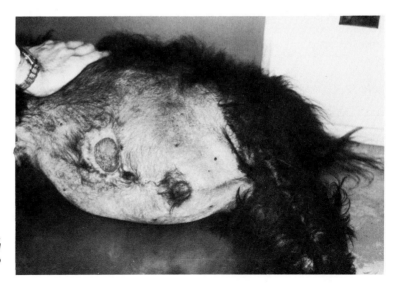

Figure 59–3. *Close-up of the dog in Figure 59–2, showing a large ulcer on the ventral abdominal wall which had not healed despite several attempts to close the wound.*

Table 59–3 *Hematologic Findings in 300 Dogs and 18 Cats With Hyperadrenocorticism*

Findings	% of Dogs	% of Cats
Erythrocytosis	17	N/A
Mature leukocytosis	32	42
Lymphopenia	14	67
Eosinopenia	84	58

N/A = Not available.

The most common abnormalities found in serum biochemistry profiles are listed in Table 59–4.

The alkaline phosphatase enzyme may be elevated (5–40 times above normal mean) due to induction of a specific isoenzyme. This finding is one of the most reliable indicators of hyperadrenocorticism in the dog; however, only about one third of cats with Cushing's syndrome show an increase in this enzyme.

The alanine aminotransferase enzyme is usually only mildly elevated (about twofold) in the dog and is due to hepatocellular necrosis commonly seen with hypercortisolism.

A common finding in Cushing's syndrome in the dog and cat is lipemia and hypercholesterolemia from the mobilization of fatty acids from adipose tissue.

Cortisol is an anti-insulin hormone. It appears to induce a state of insulin resistance. Some animals will compensate and respond with increased insulin release to maintain euglycemia. However, some dogs and all cats described with hypercortisolism are unable to maintain this re-sponse and become hyperglycemic. Usually mild hyperglycemia (less than 200 mg/dl or 11 mmol/L) is seen, but overt diabetes may occur.

A low phosphate concentration (hypophosphatemia) has been seen in the dog and has been attributed to decreased renal tubular absorption.

An increase in total carbon dioxide (TCO_2) has been described in the dog and may be caused by respiratory alkalosis seen in some dogs.

The urinalysis frequently shows a low specific gravity and aids in confirming polydipsia and polyuria. Glucosuria may be seen if the glucose concentration exceeds the renal threshold. Frequently, a cystitis is present because the animal's immune system is suppressed. Glucose provides an ideal medium for bacteria in those animals that are diabetic or borderline diabetic (see Chapter 46). Only a few white blood cells may be seen in the urine because the high cortisol concentration inhibits the appropriate inflammatory response.

Chest and abdominal radiographs are indicated. Calcification of tracheal rings, principal bronchi, skin, and vasculature can be seen in some animals with hyperadrenocorticism. Osteoporosis may be seen in the thoracic vertebrae. Lung metastases are infrequently seen in dogs with adrenal carcinomas.

Hepatomegaly, osteoporosis, and calcification of the skin and subcutaneous tissue are findings in hyperadrenocorticism. In about 25% to 50% of dogs with adrenal tumors, calcification can be seen in the area of the adrenal gland.

A majority of dogs (57%–82%) with hyperadrenocorticism appear to be hypertensive with elevations of both systolic and diastolic pressures. It has been suggested that the high blood pressure is caused by increased levels of angiotensinogen (see Chapter 24).

Frequently, animals with suspected hyperadrenocorticism will undergo thyroid function testing. It is not possible on physical examination and routine blood analysis to exclude hypothyroidism, especially in animals that present with bilateral alopecia as their sole problem. The effect of spontaneous hyperadrenocorticism on serum thyroid concentrations has been examined in a large number of dogs. Basal serum thyroxine (T_4) and triiodothyronine (T_3) are decreased in the majority of dogs. Some of these also have a de-

Table 59–4 *Serum Biochemistry Findings in 300 Dogs and 18 Cats With Hyperadrenocorticism*

Findings	% of Dogs	% of Cats
Increased alkaline phosphatase	86	36
Increased alanine aminotransferase	53	N/A
Hypercholesterolemia	48	86
Hyperglycemia	45	100
Hypophosphatemia	38	N/A
Increased total CO_2	33	N/A

N/A = Not available.

crease in free thyroxine (free T_4) concentrations. In people, this decrease is due to a decrease of TSH secretion by the pituitary. Due to the lack of a TSH assay, this decrease has not been evaluated in the dog. Administration of TSH increases serum T_4 concentration in dogs in a manner parallel to increases in normal dogs; however, the total concentration of T_4 is less for the basal and the 6-hour concentration after TSH. The laboratory assessment of hypercortisolism is summarized in Table 59-5.

Specific Evaluation of Pituitary-Adrenal Function: Screening Tests

Screening tests will help in the differentiation between a normal animal and an animal with hyperadrenocorticism. They will in most cases not provide any information about the cause of the hyperadrenocorticism (primary vs. second-

ary). Figure 59-4 shows a flow chart of the diagnostic approach for the specific evaluation of pituitary-adrenal function.

Resting Plasma Cortisol Concentrations

Single basal plasma cortisol concentrations do not allow differentiation of normal animals and animals with hyperadrenocorticism because frequent fluctuations of plasma cortisol concentrations occur in both.

ACTH Stimulation Test

This test is probably the most frequently used test to screen dogs for hyperadrenocorticism. It is a simple test that can be completed within a short time period. A blood sample is taken for basal cortisol concentrations, and another sample is taken at various times after the injection of ACTH. Table 59-6 shows the various protocols for the

Table 59–5 *Laboratory Assessment of Hyperadrenocorticism*

Test	What to Check For
Complete blood cell count	Erythrocytosis Leukocytosis Neutrophilia Lymphopenia Eosinopenia
Serum biochemistry profile	Increased alkaline phosphatase Increased alanine aminotransferase Increased cholesterol Increased glucose Low phosphate Increased total CO_2
Urinalysis	Low specific gravity Glucosuria Urinary tract infection
Chest radiographs	Calcification (tracheal rings, principal bronchi, skin, vasculature) Osteoporosis (vertebrae) Metastases
Abdominal radiographs	Hepatomegaly Osteoporosis Calcification (skin, adrenal tumor)
Blood pressure (dogs)	Increased systolic and diastolic pressure
Thyroid function tests	Low T_4/T_3 Lower pre-TSH and post-TSH total serum T_4 concentration. Increase parallel to increase in normal dogs in response to TSH.

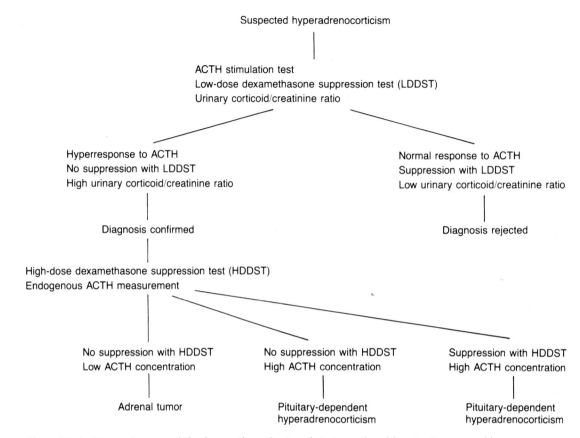

Figure 59–4. *Diagnostic approach for the specific evaluation of pituitary-adrenal function in suspected hyperadrenocorticism.*

ACTH stimulation test. The sampling time after ACTH administration is shorter with the synthetic ACTH preparation (Cortrosyn, Organon Pharmaceuticals) than with the natural porcine ACTH (Cortigel-40, Savage Laboratories); however, the porcine gel preparation is less expensive.

Normal values need to be established for each laboratory. For most laboratories the basal cortisol concentration ranges between 0.5 and 6.0 μg/100 ml (13.8–165.5 nmol/L), and the cortisol concentration after ACTH lies between 8 and 15 μg/100 ml (220.7–413.9 nmol/L). Values above 20 μg/100 ml (551.8 nmol/L) are considered diagnostic. The majority of dogs and cats with PDH and approximately one half of dogs with adrenal tumors will show an exaggerated cortisol response to ACTH. It must be cautioned, however, that stressed or ill animals also may show an abnor-mally high cortisol response. In these patients, the test should be done once the animal is stabilized.

The ACTH stimulation test is a good test to diagnose iatrogenic hyperadrenocorticism. Usually, a low basal cortisol concentration is seen with little or no response to exogenous ACTH because the secretory capacity of the adrenal glands has been suppressed by the excessive concentrations of exogenous glucocorticoids. Clinical signs and changes in the complete blood cell count and the serum biochemistry are suggestive, however, of hyperadrenocorticism. If the animal received glucocorticoids (except dexamethasone) within 24 hours of ACTH testing, one may see an apparently high initial cortisol concentration due to cross reactivity of hydrocortisone, cortisone, prednisolone, or prednisone in most cortisol immu-

Table 59–6 *ACTH Stimulation Test Protocols*

ACTH Preparation	Dose	Route of Administration	Sampling Time After ACTH
Synthetic ACTH (Cortrosyn)	0.25 mg/dog	IM/IV	30 min
	0.125 mg/cat	IM/IV	30 and 60 min
ACTH gel (Cortigel)	2.2 units/kg (dog or cat)	IM	dog: 120 min cat: 60 and 120 min

noassays. The cortisol concentration after ACTH administration may actually be lower because of metabolism of the drug.

Low-Dose Dexamethasone Suppression Test (LDDST)

This is a sensitive test for the diagnosis of hyperadrenocorticism. A small amount of dexamethasone sodium phosphate (0.015 mg/kg) is injected intramuscularly (Table 59-7). In a normal animal this small dose will lead to suppression of endogenous cortisol secretion because of negative feedback inhibition on pituitary ACTH secretion. At 8 hours after dexamethasone injection, cortisol in the normal dog or cat will be suppressed to a concentration at the lower limit of the cortisol assay used, which for most laboratories is less than 1 μg/100 ml (27.6 nmol/L). In dogs and cats with hyperadrenocorticism, the small amount of dexamethasone injection will not affect pituitary ACTH secretion because the pituitary gland in dogs and cats with hyperadrenocor-

ticism is less sensitive to the suppressive effect of glucocorticoids. It also has been shown that dogs with hyperadrenocorticism clear dexamethasone faster from their plasma than do normal dogs. At 8 hours after injection, therefore, cortisol concentrations will be higher than those in normal animals. False positive and false negative results caused by stress, illness, or medication may occur.

High-Dose Dexamethasone Suppression Test (HDDST)

This test is used to determine if the animal has a pituitary disorder or an adrenal tumor causing hypercortisolism. It is the preferred screening test for hyperadrenocorticism in the cat. The protocol is similar to that of the LDDST (see Table 59-7). The dose used in the dog is 1.0 mg/kg, given intravenously or intramuscularly; in the cat it has been suggested to use 0.1 mg/kg. Samples are collected before and 2, 4, 6, and 8 hours after administration of dexamethasone. The most im-

Table 59–7 *Protocol For Low- and High-Dose Dexamethasone Suppression Test*

LOW DOSE

Take sample for baseline cortisol.
Inject 0.015 mg/kg dexamethasone IM.
Take samples for cortisol at 2, 4, 6, 8 hours after injection (the 6- and 8-hour samples are the most important if cost of all 5 samples is prohibitive).

HIGH DOSE

Take sample for baseline cortisol.
Inject 1.0 mg/kg dexamethasone IM (dog).
Inject 0.1 mg/kg dexamethasone IM (cat).
Take samples for cortisol at 2, 4, 6, 8 hours after injection (the 6- and 8-hour samples are the most important).

portant samples are the 6- and 8-hour samples because the degree of suppression is greatest at that time. About 80% of dogs with PDH will show suppression at 8 hours. Suppression is defined at the cortisol concentration at the lower limit of the cortisol assay used. A combined dexamethasone suppression and corticotropin stimulation test has been described. This test is not recommended because the test results are not diagnostic in most cases.

About 15% of dogs will show various degrees of suppression at 2 and 4 hours but have increased concentrations at 6 and 8 hours, and about 5% will not show any suppression at all. Some of these animals will show suppression at 8 hours when the dose of dexamethasone is increased to 2 mg/kg; however, frequently endogenous ACTH measurement of concentrations is necessary to make an accurate diagnosis. Dogs with adrenal tumors may show some initial suppression, but clearly cortisol concentrations are not suppressed at 8 hours.

Urinary Corticoid : Creatinine Ratio

In dogs the determination of corticoid : creatinine ratios in two consecutive morning urine samples has been shown to have a high predictive value in the diagnosis of hyperadrenocorticism. Ratios exceeding 10×10^{-6} are regarded as compatible with hyperadrenocorticism. For the urinary corticoid : creatinine ratios, the corticoid measurements can be performed in a routine cortisol assay. About 90% of urinary corticoids is free cortisol. Most of the remainder are cortisol metabolites. Therefore, the level of crude, nonpurified corticoid seems to give a meaningful assessment of cortisol secretion. Further studies in different laboratories are needed to assess the value of this test. The initial studies indicate that this may be the method with the highest diagnostic value. False positive results, however, may occur in dogs with severe nonadrenal illness. No data are available in the cat.

Plasma ACTH Determinations

In dogs with pituitary disorders, the secretion of ACTH is inappropriately high for the high circulating cortisol concentrations, indicating a defect in negative feedback inhibition of the pituitary gland. Dogs with adrenal tumors, however, have a normally functioning pituitary gland. Therefore, in these cases ACTH concentrations will be low or undetectable because the high cortisol concentrations inhibit ACTH secretion by negative feedback inhibition. Measuring ACTH concentrations can be an effective aid to differentiate the cause of hyperadrenocorticism. However, it is often difficult to find a laboratory with an assay validated for the dog. In addition, ACTH is rapidly degraded; samples must be processed quickly on ice and shipped on dry ice. Samples also should not be processed in glass containers, as ACTH binds to glass.

The combination of a high-dose dexamethasone suppression test and endogenous ACTH measurement probably provides the best diagnostic approach to the diagnosis of the cause of hyperadrenocorticism.

ACTH measurements have been done in a few cats; further studies are needed to determine their usefulness in this species.

MANAGEMENT

Pituitary-Dependent Hyperadrenocorticism

The majority of cats and dogs with naturally occurring hyperadrenocorticism have the pituitary-dependent form of the disorder. It can be treated surgically or medically.

Surgical Treatment

The surgical treatment includes hypophysectomy or bilateral adrenalectomy. Both surgeries lead to deficiencies in several hormones and are not the treatment of choice in the dog. Because of the difficulty of technique, they should only be performed by surgeons with expertise with the procedures. In the cat, where medical treatment has not been proven successful, surgical adrenalectomy at this time seems to be the best treatment.

Medical Treatment

Most cases of PDH in the dog are treated medically. The drug o,p'-DDD (mitotane) is the most widely used in this disorder. Although the exact mechanism of action of o,p'-DDD has not been elucidated, it is well established that administration of the drug leads to selective necrosis of the zona fasciculata and reticularis of the adrenal cortex. The zona glomerulosa rarely becomes damaged and signs of mineralocorticoid deficiency are rare.

The protocol for the treatment of PDH with o,p'-DDD is well established. The drug is given at 50 mg/kg/day for a 10-day period. The goal of this so-called loading period is to decrease the capacity of the adrenal cortex to a degree where cortisol secretion becomes minimal and the animal is unable to respond to exogenous ACTH with an increase in cortisol secretion. After a successful loading period, plasma cortisol will usually be at the lower limit of the cortisol assay, which is approximately 1 μg/100 ml (27.6 nmol/L) in most laboratories. Figure 59-5 shows a flow chart for

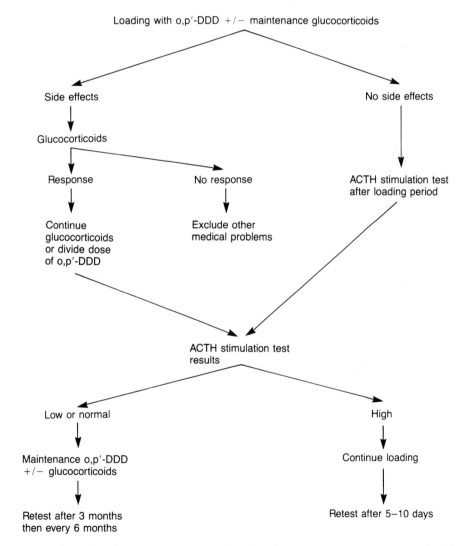

Figure 59–5. *Flow chart for the management of pituitary-dependent hyperadrenocorticism (PDH) with o,p'-DDD.*

the management of PDH with o,p'-DDD. It has been recommended to use 35 mg/kg of o,p'-DDD per day in diabetic animals with PDH to lessen the dangers of hypoglycemia. (Diabetic animals with concomitant PDH show insulin resistance because of cortisol's anti-insulin effect. Serum cortisol levels decrease with o,p'-DDD treatment, and the animal becomes more sensitive to insulin.) If after the 10-day loading period, the ACTH stimulation test indicates little or no response to the drug and cortisol concentrations are low, the dog is kept on the same dose of o,p'-DDD. However, now the dose is given once weekly only. To reduce side effects of the drug, it is advisable to divide the dose and give it over a 2-day period. Many owners like to give the drug on the weekend in order to be able to observe the dog for immediate side effects.

If after the loading period the ACTH stimulation test indicates a normal or exaggerated response, then treatment with o,p'-DDD is continued and the dog retested at 5- to 10-day intervals until the desired response is obtained.

The most common side effects of o,p'-DDD are lethargy, weakness, vomiting, and anorexia. Side effects develop mostly during the loading period; however, they can often be reduced by dividing the dose. In some dogs, maintenance therapy with glucocorticoids becomes necessary to minimize or eliminate adverse effects of the drug (Table 59-8). If adverse signs persist, then the drug should be stopped and the dog should be evaluated for other medical problems.

Some dogs need glucocorticoid replacement therapy for the rest of their lives, while other dogs do well without it. However, all treated dogs need 5 to 10 times the physiologic replacement dose in times of stress.

o,p'-DDD treatment during the loading period can be successfully administered at home by the owners as long as they realize the potential dangers of the treatment and are made fully aware of the drug's side effects. The owners also should have glucocorticoids at hand. If o,p'-DDD treatment is carried out at home, the clinician should contact the owners daily and inquire about the status of the dog.

While on maintenance therapy, the dog should be re-evaluated after 3 months. An ACTH stimulation test is done at that time together with a complete physical examination, complete blood count, serum biochemistry profile, and urinalysis. The ACTH stimulation test should show no or little cortisol response. If the test results are satisfactory, the animal can then be examined every 6 months. If the ACTH stimulation test shows normal or exaggerated cortisol response, the animal should undergo "loading" again with o,p'-DDD for 3 to 10 days. In some cases, it is necessary to increase the dose of o,p'-DDD by 50% or more to achieve the desired response.

A more radical approach to the treatment of PDH with o,p'-DDD in the dog has been taken by some clinicians. The aim is the complete destruction of the adrenal cortices rather than a selective destruction. o,p'-DDD is given for 25 days at a dose of 50 to 75 mg/kg body weight daily, divided in 3 to 4 portions and administered with food. The dogs need to receive replacement therapy with glucocorticoids and mineralocorticoids for the rest of their lives (see Chapter 60). It has been claimed that fewer relapses occur with this method; however, more dogs on this treatment regimen need to be evaluated. The disadvantage of this method is the resulting glucocorticoid and mineralocorticoid deficiency.

It is important to realize that o,p'-DDD treatment is not a curative treatment in PDH. It does not eliminate the cause, that is, the inappropriately high ACTH secretion. On the contrary, the low cortisol levels after o,p'-DDD treatment will actually stimulate the increases in pituitary and ACTH release. This stimulation may lead to complications in some cases, in which pituitary tumors increase in size and lead to neurologic signs.

Treatment with o,p'-DDD has been of questionable success in the cat and only led to adrenocortical suppression in a few cases. Because cats gen-

Table 59–8 *Physiologic Replacement Therapy With Glucocorticoids in Dogs on o,p'-DDD (Mitotane) Therapy*

Drug	Dose
Prednisolone	0.2 mg/kg/day PO
Prednisone	0.2 mg/kg/day PO
Cortisone	0.2 to 1.0 mg/kg/day PO
Hydrocortisone	0.2 to 1.0 mg/kg/day PO

erally are sensitive to chlorinated hydrocarbons, the use of o,p'-DDD has not been recommended. Further studies are needed to evaluate this drug in the feline.

Ketoconazole

Ketoconazole, an imidazole derivative and antifungal agent, is used as an alternative medical treatment of hyperadrenocorticism in the dog. It is not effective for this purpose in cats. Ketoconazole inhibits steroidogenesis and affects not only glucocorticoid synthesis but also testosterone and estrogen synthesis. It apparently has little effect on aldosterone secretion. The inhibition of steroidogenesis is reversible. Ketoconazole is very expensive and the owners' financial constraints may limit its use. It has been suggested to administer ketoconazole orally with food at 10 mg/kg twice a day for 7 to 10 days. The drug should be discontinued for 1 to 2 days if adverse reactions occur. Most commonly anorexia and vomiting are seen. An ACTH stimulation test is performed after the 7- to 10-day period. Cortisol concentrations should be low before stimulation with little or no response after ACTH administration. If the response is normal or exaggerated, the dose of ketoconazole is increased to 15 mg/kg twice a day, and the animal is re-evaluated 7 to 10 days later. The dose of ketoconazole is maintained once satisfactory control has been achieved. Twice daily administration is necessary because of the transient effect of the drug.

Ketoconazole treatment is indicated in dogs with severe adverse effects to o,p'-DDD treatment or in dogs showing resistance to the drug.

Adrenal Tumors

The treatment of choice in most cases of adrenal tumors is surgery. The surgical treatment and its possible complications will not be discussed. The long-term prognosis for dogs with resectable adenomas is good to excellent.

Medical Treatment

The response of adrenal tumors to o,p'-DDD has been variable. Some dogs do not respond to this therapy, some show a poor response even with administration of high amounts of the drug, and few dogs may respond well. Generally it is felt that adrenal tumors (adenomas and carcinomas) are relatively resistant to the effect of o,p'-DDD.

Ketoconazole

Ketoconazole is indicated in the treatment of dogs with inoperable adrenal tumors or metastatic disease and in cases where the owners decline surgical treatment. Ketoconazole is indicated also in the preparation of a dog for surgery. It has been suggested to administer ketoconazole for 4 to 8 weeks before surgery to reduce the anesthetic, surgical, and postsurgical complications associated with hypercortisolism.

Iatrogenic Hyperadrenocorticism

Animals with iatrogenic hyperadrenocorticism are managed by gradually tapering down the dose of glucocorticoid over a period of time to alternate day maintenance therapy (i.e., 0.5 mg/kg for prednisone), after which time efforts may be made to discontinue the drug altogether. The time required to achieve maintenance drug levels depends on the type of glucocorticoid used (short-acting vs. long-acting), the duration of drug used, and the dose used. No well established guidelines are available in veterinary medicine; however, with anti-inflammatory doses of prednisone (1.1 mg/kg divided twice daily, orally), rapid recovery (approximately 2 weeks) of adrenal function may be expected. Long-acting glucocorticoids must be tapered more gradually. During this time animals should be monitored for clinical signs of glucocorticoid deficiency (*e.g.*, vomiting, diarrhea, weakness). If these signs do occur, the dose of glucocorticoid should be increased to a level that controls these signs.

PATIENT MONITORING

The prognosis of dogs with PDH treated with o,p'-DDD is guarded. Forty to fifty percent of dogs relapse and require loading with o,p'-DDD again. An average life expectancy of 2 years has been reported. The prognosis of cats treated with bilateral adrenalectomy is good to excellent with proper replacement therapy.

Client education and compliance play a major role in the success of medical treatment. Frequently, owners are well aware of the treatment schedule and some side effects of o,p'-DDD. However, they are not aware of the inability of their dog to deal with stress and the need for glucocorticoid therapy, should their animal be stressed. Treatment with ketoconazole is often not a choice for the owners because of the expense of the drug.

The prognosis of dogs with adrenal tumors depends on the nature of the tumor, that is, the occurrence of metastases. The prognosis of dogs without metastases that underwent successful surgery is excellent, and a difference does not seem to be found in the life expectancy of dogs with adenomas or carcinomas of the adrenal gland. The average life expectancy of dogs with unilateral adrenalectomy was 18 months in a study by Emms (Emms, Additional Reading). If medical treatment is chosen, the prognosis is guarded. The response to o,p'-DDD treatment is generally poor, and long-term ketoconazole treatment is frequently declined because of the expense of the drug.

ADDITIONAL READING

Emms SG, Johnston DE. Adrenalectomy in the management of canine hyperadrenocorticism. Journal of the American Animal Hospital Association 1987; 23:557.

Feldman EC. Comparison of ACTH response and dexamethasone suppression as screening tests in canine hyperadrenocorticism. J Am Vet Med Assoc 1983; 182:506.

Feldman EC. Distinguishing dogs with functioning adrenocortical tumors from hyperadrenocorticism. J Am Vet Med Assoc 1983; 183:195.

Feldman EC. Evaluation of a combined dexamethasone suppression ACTH stimulation test in dogs with hyperadrenocorticism. J Am Vet Med Assoc 1985; 187:49.

Feldman EC, Nelson RW. Hyperadrenocorticism. In: Feldman EC, Nelson RW, eds. Canine and feline endocrinology and reproduction. Philadelphia: WB Saunders, 1987: 137.

Nelson RW, Feldman EC. Hyperadrenocorticism in cats: Seven cases. J Am Vet Med Assoc 1988; 193:245.

Nelson RW, Ihle SL, Feldman EC. Pituitary macroadenomas and macroadenocarcinomas in dogs treated with mitotane for pituitary dependent hyperadrenocorticism: 13 cases (1981-1986). J Am Vet Med Assoc 1989; 194:1612.

Penninck DG, Feldman EC, Nyland TG. Radiographic features of canine hyperadrenocorticism caused by autonomously functioning adrenocortical tumors: 23 cases. J Am Vet Med Assoc 1988; 192:1604.

Peterson ME. Endocrine disorders in cats: Four emerging diseases. Compendium of Continuing Education 1988; 10:1355.

Peterson ME. o,p'-DDD (Mitotane) treatment of canine pituitary dependent hyperadrenocorticism. J Am Vet Med Assoc 1983; 182:527.

Rijnberk A, van Wees A, Mol JA. Assessment of two tests for the diagnosis of canine hyperadrenocorticism. Vet Rec 1988; 122:178.

Sarfaty D, Carillo JM, Peterson ME. Neurologic, endocrinologic and pathologic findings associated with large pituitary tumors in dogs: 8 cases (1976-1984). J Am Vet Med Assoc 1988; 193:854.

60

HYPOADRENOCORTICISM

Margarethe Hoenig, Duncan C. Ferguson

Adrenal insufficiency was first reported by Addison in 1855. The clinical picture he described is that of a person "gradually falling off in general health, . . . the appetite is impaired or entirely lost, . . . there is occasionally actual vomiting, . . . disturbed cerebral circulation. The body wastes . . . the pulse becomes smaller and weaker. . . . " One year later it was shown that, indeed, the adrenal glands are essential to life. However, it was not until almost 100 years later that the structure of the adrenal hormones was elucidated and these compounds were synthesized.

Adrenocortical insufficiency in the dog was first reported in 1953 by Hadlow. It has since been well documented in the dog and recently in the cat. Adrenocortical insufficiency is not a common endocrine disease in the dog and is extremely rare in the cat. It seems to occur more frequently in the female dog, while male and female cats seem to be equally affected. Although it has been described in all age groups, it occurs most frequently in middle-aged animals. No breed predilection has been described in the dog. All cats reported to date with adrenal insufficiency have been domestic short hairs.

CAUSES

Adrenal insufficiency can occur as a result of a primary adrenal abnormality that impairs the capacity of the adrenal glands to secrete glucocorticoids (mainly cortisol) and mineralocorticoids (mainly aldosterone) in response to adrenal stimulators (*primary adrenal insufficiency*). Glucocorticoid deficiency can also occur as a consequence of adrenocorticotropin (ACTH) deficiency (*secondary adrenal insufficiency*). The reduced secretion of ACTH by the pituitary gland may be caused by destructive lesions in the pituitary gland or hypothalamus or the exogenous administration of glucocorticoids. Long-acting corticosteroids such as dexamethasone, betamethasone, and flumethasone are especially potent suppressors of the pituitary-adrenal axis, particularly when chronically administered.

Primary Adrenal Insufficiency

Destruction of the adrenal cortex leads to *hypoadrenocorticism*. According to one study, at least 90% of the adrenal cortex needs to be destroyed

821

Table 60–1 *Causes of Hypoadrenocorticism*

PRIMARY ADRENAL INSUFFICIENCY

Idiopathic (autoimmune?)
Granulomatous diseases (histoplasmosis, blastomycosis, tuberculosis)
Hemorrhagic infarction
Tumor metastasis to adrenal glands
Amyloidosis of adrenal cortices
Treatment with o,p'-DDD (mitotane)

SECONDARY ADRENAL INSUFFICIENCY

Glucocorticoids
Megestrol acetate (cats)
Medroxyprogesterone (cats)
Ketoconazole (dogs)

before adrenocortical failure becomes evident. A primary deficiency of glucocorticoids leads to a compensatory increase in the production of ACTH. The clinical signs are due to the lack of mineralocorticoids and glucocorticoids. When Addison described the disease, the most common cause of adrenal gland destruction was due to tuberculosis. Immune-mediated destruction of the glands is now the most common cause in humans and may also be the major cause of adrenocortical failure in the dog and cat (Table 60-1). All layers of the adrenal cortex are damaged in idiopathic or immune-mediated adrenal insufficiency, while the destruction of the adrenal cortex seen in granulomatous diseases, with infarction

or metastasis, may be localized or generalized. Treatment with the adrenolytic drug o,p'-DDD (mitotane) usually only leads to destruction of the zona fasciculata and reticularis of the adrenal gland, which secrete glucocorticoids, and, therefore, only a glucocorticoid deficiency is seen. However, a destruction of the zona glomerulosa is possible, although rare, and animals will then develop hypoadrenocorticism with mineralocorticoid and glucocorticoid deficiency.

Secondary Adrenal Insufficiency

ACTH deficiency results in decreased stimulation of the adrenal cortex, mainly the zona fasciculata, leading to decreased synthesis and release of glucocorticoids. A deficiency of mineralocorticoids is not seen because ACTH only exerts a permissive effect on aldosterone secretion. Spontaneous ACTH deficiency can be the result of destructive lesions in the pituitary or hypothalamic region; ACTH deficiency can also be secondary to iatrogenic corticosteroid administration. While spontaneous ACTH deficiency is rare in the dog, and has not yet been described in the cat, iatrogenically induced ACTH deficiency, secondary to the administration of exogenous corticosteroids, is a common and serious problem in veterinary medicine (Table 60-2). Adrenocortical suppression has also been reported in cats given megestrol ace-

Table 60–2 *Adrenocortical Suppressive Effects of a Single Injection of Various Glucocorticoids in Dogs*

Drug	Dose and Route	Duration of Adrenocortical Suppression
Dexamethasone	0.01 mg/kg IV or	less than 24 hours
	0.1 mg/kg IV	32 hours
Dexamethasone alcohol	1 mg/kg IM	24 to 48 hours
Dexamethosone sodium phosphate	0.1 mg/kg IV or 0.01 mg/kg IV	less than 24 hours
Dexamethasone 21-isonicotinate	0.1 mg/kg IM or	up to 10 days
	1 mg/kg IM	up to 4 weeks
Methylprednisolone acetate	2.5 mg/kg IM	up to 5 weeks
Prednisone	2.2 mg/kg IM	None
Triamcinolone acetonide	0.22 mg/kg IM	up to 4 weeks

(From Romatowski J. Iatrogenic adrenocortical insufficiency in dogs. J Am Vet Med Assoc 1990; 196:1144.

tate. Adrenal suppression is greater and more prolonged than that seen with prednisolone. Medroxyprogesterone has similar effects. In the dog, ketoconazole causes adrenal suppression.

PATHOPHYSIOLOGY

The most potent mineralocorticoid is aldosterone, which accounts for most of the mineralocorticoid activity, while desoxycorticosterone and corticosterone show only slight activity. Aldosterone exerts its major effects on the kidney where it stimulates tubular sodium reabsorption. It also acts in a similar manner on sweat and salivary glands and promotes intestinal sodium absorption. Sodium reabsorption by the renal tubular cells is accompanied by the reabsorption of an equivalent amount of water, which may increase the total extracellular fluid volume. Aldosterone also affects the regulation of potassium excretion. As sodium is transported into the peritubular fluid and reabsorbed, potassium is transported in the opposite direction and secreted into the urine. Aldosterone also stimulates H^+-ion transport.

Several factors influence mineralocorticoid secretion and action: the potassium ion concentration of the extracellular fluid; the renin-angiotensin system; the quantity of total body sodium; and the level of plasma ACTH. High serum potassium concentrations stimulate aldosterone secretion directly. A decrease in sodium also leads to aldosterone secretion through a direct effect on the zona glomerulosa cells. It has also been suggested that a decrease in sodium leads to a decrease in extracellular fluid volume and renal perfusion, which stimulates angiotensin formation and in turn stimulates aldosterone release. ACTH has a permissive effect on aldosterone secretion, that is, a minimal amount of ACTH is sufficient to allow full regulation of aldosterone secretion.

Without mineralocorticoids, the animal cannot conserve sodium and is unable to excrete potassium. A decrease in extracellular fluid volume leads to decreased cardiac output, hypotension, and decreased renal blood flow resulting in prerenal azotemia, weakness, and shock. A lack of aldosterone also leads to hyperkalemia and mild acidosis. The hyperkalemia affects the heart most prominently. A decrease in myocardial excitability and slowing of cardiac conduction is seen, followed by ventricular asystole or ventricular fibrillation and death.

The most potent and prevalent glucocorticoid in dogs and cats is cortisol. Cortisol has several metabolic effects. Together with other hormones, it stimulates gluconeogenesis by the liver leading to glycogen deposition in the liver cells. It also decreases glucose utilization by cells through several mechanisms. The increased rate of glucose production together with the decreased rate of glucose utilization and a possible direct negative effect on pancreatic insulin secretion lead to a mild increase in blood glucose. Cortisol also affects protein and fat metabolism. Cortisol enhances protein catabolism. The increased amino acids are primarily transported into liver cells where they are metabolized further, converted to glucose, or used for protein synthesis. Cortisol enhances fat metabolism in a similar way, leading to increased fatty acid mobilization from adipose tissue.

Cortisol, particularly in supraphysiologic quantities, prevents the development of inflammation or reverses its effects. It blocks the factors causing or maintaining inflammation by suppressing leukocyte accumulation at the site of inflammation, stabilizing lysosomal membranes, stabilizing capillary membranes and maintaining microcirculation, and inhibiting the functional capacity of macrophages and monocytes. Some of the anti-inflammatory effects are specific; however, most of the effects are nonspecific. Cortisol increases the production of red blood cells by an unknown mechanism. It also affects electrolyte and water balance and the glomerular filtration rate and ability of the kidney to dilute urine.

Cortisol directly affects the heart by positive chronotropic and inotropic actions and is necessary for maximal catecholamine sensitivity, therefore contributing to the maintenance of vascular tone. Cortisol has marked effects on the psyche and can lead to mental and physical dependence.

The great importance of cortisol lies in its effect and function in mental or physical stress. Cortisol levels rise in stressful situations, and, although the exact mechanism for its beneficial role in stress is not understood, cortisol is essential for an animal's survival of stressful situations. Lack of cortisol secretion affects most tissues in the body leading to anorexia, vomiting, abdominal pain, and weight loss. The mental state of the animal may be abnormal (lethargy, depression) as well as the physical appearance because of severe changes in metabolism. Often destruction of the adrenal gland progresses slowly, and clinical signs may only be obvious when the animal is stressed, indicating the importance to recognize changes associated with cortisol deficiency in the early diagnosis of the disease. As the adrenal reserve diminishes, clinical signs become more prominent.

CLINICAL SIGNS

The information provided by people who have animals with adrenal insufficiency is often vague because, depending on the degree of adrenal destruction, signs may be very mild or only become obvious in stressful situations. The signs associated with the disease, for example, anorexia, vomiting, diarrhea (sometimes with melena), depression, and weakness, are not very specific and can be seen with many other diseases. There are no pathognomonic signs for adrenal insufficiency. The course of the disease often has a "waxing-waning" nature that may go unrecognized by owners. Often, however, the owners sought help of a veterinarian, and the animal received fluid therapy or corticosteroids and promptly responded favorably for a variable period of time. Therefore, the clinician must maintain a high degree of suspicion in order to diagnose this disease. Adrenal insufficiency should be included in the differential diagnosis in all cases of episodic illness in young or middle-aged dogs and in cats. The degree of suspicion increases in the more advanced stage of the disease when electrolyte abnormalities become prominent. Table 60-3 lists the most common historical abnormalities of dogs with adrenal insufficiency. The clinical signs reported in cats are similar. A thorough physical examination is important in the evaluation of any patient. Animals with adrenal insufficiency usually have vague clinical signs. Although one might gain additional information from the physical examination, in most cases, it only indicates the severity of the problem. The most commonly noted findings on physical examination in the dog and cat are listed in Table 60-4.

DIAGNOSTIC APPROACH

The laboratory assessment of animals with hypoadrenocorticism is shown in Table 60-5.

In adrenal insufficiency, a mild normocytic, normochromic, nonregenerative anemia is usually seen in the dog and cat because the stimulative effect of glucocorticoids on the bone marrow is lacking. This anemia may not be evident in

Table 60–3 Historical Findings in Dogs and Cats With Adrenal Insufficiency

Sign	% of Dogs (n = 100)	% of Cats (n = 10)
Anorexia	77	100
Vomiting	68	40
Lethargy/Depression	64	100
Weakness	38	—
Weight Loss	23	90
Diarrhea	22	—
Shaking/Shivering	21	—
Polyuria (± Polydipsia)	15	30
Waxing-Waning course of disease	10	40
Sensitive abdomen	9	—

Table 60–4 Findings on Physical Examination in Dogs and Cats With Adrenal Insufficiency

Sign	% of Dogs	% of Cats
Hypothermia	—	80
Sensitive abdomen	11	10
Shaking/Shivering	19	—
Slow capillary refill time	21	50
Bradycardia	26	20
Dehydration	32	90
Weak pulse	37	50
Weakness	45	90
Depression	74	100

Table 60–5 *Laboratory Assessment of Animals With Hypoadrenocorticism*

Test	What to Check For
Complete blood cell count	High hematocrit (before rehydration)
	Low hematocrit (after rehydration)
	Eosinophilia
	Lymphocytosis
Serum biochemistry profile	Hyponatremia, hyperkalemia
	Sodium: Potassium ratio <27:1
	Hypercalcemia, hypoglycemia
	Elevated serum urea
Urinalysis	Low specific gravity
Chest radiographs	Small heart
	Decreased size of aorta and posterior vena cava
	Esophageal dilation
Electrocardiogram	Esophageal dilation
	Small P wave, spiked T wave, prolonged P–R and QRS intervals, bradycardia, ventricular asystole or fibrillation

many patients on presentation because they are dehydrated and hemoconcentrated. Following adequate rehydration, the anemia becomes apparent.

Wide variations in the white blood cell count have been reported in the dog. Although one might expect to see a lymphocytosis and eosinophilia with glucocorticoid deficiency, it is not always present. Therefore, one cannot exclude adrenal insufficiency based on a normal leukogram. However, if one finds a high eosinophil count or lymphocyte count, adrenal insufficiency should be included as a differential diagnosis. Lymphocytosis and eosinophilia have been described in the cat with adrenal insufficiency.

The major abnormalities seen with adrenal insufficiency are a decrease in the sodium : potassium ratio, prerenal azotemia, hypoglycemia, hypercalcemia, and a mild metabolic acidosis.

Lack of aldosterone leads to an increased excretion of sodium accompanied by chloride. In secondary adrenal insufficiency, this abnormality is not seen because mineralocorticoid secretion remains adequate. Electrolyte changes, therefore, are always indicative of primary adrenal failure. The increased sodium excretion leads to increased water excretion, and the patient soon becomes hypovolemic and may actually be presented in shock. Concomitant with the increase in sodium loss, potassium is reabsorbed, as are hydrogen ions, leading to hyperkalemia and mild acidosis. A low serum sodium concentration is not diagnostic for hypoadrenocorticism, nor is a high serum potassium concentration. Renal disease, gastrointestinal disease, heart failure, liver cirrhosis, hyperproteinemia, and the chronic administration of diuretics also are associated with hyponatremia. In addition, vomition and diarrhea may decrease the serum sodium concentration, and the osmotic effect of glucose in diabetes mellitus is also associated with hyponatremia. Pseudohyponatremia, a spurious lowering of the serum sodium concentration, may occur if the animal is hyperlipemic (see Chapter 72). Although the sodium concentration in plasma water in this case remains normal, the sodium concentration, expressed as milliequivalents per total volume of serum (which now contains a large nonaqueous phase) is low.

Hyperkalemia is frequently seen with primary acute renal failure, urethral obstruction, and severe metabolic and respiratory acidosis. It has also been described in dogs with primary gastrointestinal disease. Severe tissue breakdown following crush injuries or extensive surgery will also increase serum potassium concentration (see Chapter 72). It is obvious from the above discussion that a diagnosis of hypoadrenocorticism cannot be based on a change of the sodium : potassium ratio alone. If hypoadrenocorticism is suspected, however, it is mandatory to check the serum electrolytes. Likewise, if an animal shows electrolyte changes compatible with hypoadrenocorticism, it would be prudent to treat accordingly until a final diagnosis is reached.

Blood urea nitrogen (BUN) concentrations are usually elevated because of hemoconcentration and hypovolemia, leading to a decrease in renal perfusion (prerenal azotemia). The BUN concentrations are usually only mildly to moderately elevated, but severe increases have been observed. On rehydration of the animal, the BUN concentration will usually return to normal unless primary renal disease occurs concomitantly.

Hypercalcemia has been described in about 30% of dogs with hypoadrenocorticism. As in humans, it seems that hypercalcemia develops in cases with severe clinical and biochemical abnormalities. The exact cause of hypercalcemia in hypoadrenocorticism is unknown. It has been suggested that it may be due to increased intestinal calcium absorption, increased parathyroid hormone concentrations, hyperproteinemia resulting from hemoconcentration, or diminished renal excretion of calcium. Hypocalciuria and enhanced renal calcium absorption have been reported in adrenalectomized dogs and, therefore, may be important factors in the development of hypercalcemia. Many of the signs of hypercalcemia, for example, vomiting, weight loss, anorexia, depression, dehydration, and polyuria, are similar to those seen in animals with hypoadrenocorticism not associated with hypercalcemia and similar to those of hypercalcemia associated with other diseases. These similarities show the importance of carefully screening a dog with hypoadrenocorticism and also show the necessity to include hypoadrenocorticism in the differential diagnosis of hypercalcemia.

Hypoglycemia has been reported in some cases of hypoadrenocorticism; most often, however, the glucose concentration is normal. Low glucose concentrations are usually seen in severe cases.

A low urine specific gravity (less than 1.030 dogs, less than 1.035 cats) in the face of dehydration is often seen in dogs and cats with hypoadrenocorticism. The exact cause of the decrease in renal concentrating ability is not understood.

It has been suggested that renal medullary washout caused by the increased sodium loss in hypoadrenocorticism may be a contributing factor; however, other factors may be involved.

There are no specific radiographic findings in animals with hypoadrenocorticism. The degree of abnormalities seen is caused by the degree of hypovolemia. A frequent finding is a decreased heart size accompanied by a decreased diameter of the descending aortic arch and the posterior vena cava. Esophageal dilatation has also been seen. It is unclear whether electrolyte abnormalities are causing the motility disorder or if other factors are involved.

The electrocardiogram (ECG) is a valuable tool to detect and monitor hyperkalemia. The severity of ECG abnormalities found, however, is not related to the severity of the electrolyte disturbance, and the absence of ECG abnormalities does not rule out an altered plasma Na^+/K^+ ratio. With increasing potassium concentration, there tends to be a peaking of the T wave and a prolongation of the QRS interval. The P wave amplitude decreases, the P–R interval increases, and, as impulse conduction decreases even more with high potassium concentrations, the animal develops bradycardia. Eventually, ventricular asystole or ventricular fibrillation may occur. In spite of the hyperkalemia documented in cats with hypoadrenocorticism, electrocardiographic changes are uncommon.

Marked hyperkalemia (more than 7 mEq/L or 7 mmol/L) mandates emergency treatment regardless of the cause.

If the history, physical examination, and the initial laboratory assessment support the suspicion of hypoadrenocorticism, more definitive diagnostic tests are indicated. The most frequently used test is the ACTH stimulation test. Exogenous administration of ACTH in a normal dog leads to an increase in plasma cortisol concentrations that are at least two to three times higher than basal levels and should be within a range established for normal dogs or cats for a given laboratory. Animals with hypoadrenocorticism have low or normal basal cortisol concentrations and show no increase or only a small increase in cortisol concentrations after administration of

Table 60–6 *ACTH Stimulation Test Protocols*

ACTH Preparation	Dose	Route of Administration	Sampling Time After ACTH
Synthetic ACTH (Cortrosyn)	0.25 mg/dog	IM/IV	30 min
	0.125 mg/cat	IM/IV	30 and 60 min
ACTH gel (Cortigel)	2.2 units/kg (dog or cat)	IM	dog: 120 min cat: 60 and 120 min

ACTH. Table 60-6 shows the various protocols for the ACTH stimulation test. The sampling time after ACTH administration is shorter with the synthetic corticotropin preparation Cortrosyn (Organon Pharmaceuticals) than with the natural porcine ACTH Cortigel-40 (Savage Laboratories); however, the porcine gel preparation is less expensive.

The procedure for an ACTH stimulation test is simple. A sample for the determination of basal cortisol concentration is collected and the ACTH preparation injected. One post-ACTH sample is collected in the dog after 30 minutes (synthetic ACTH) or 120 minutes (ACTH gel), while in the cat, 2 samples are taken at 30 and 60 minutes (synthetic ACTH) or 60 and 120 minutes (ACTH gel) to ensure detection of the peak cortisol response. It has been cautioned to compare test results in the cat with established reference values obtained in normal cats, because cats seem to respond to ACTH with a smaller increment in serum cortisol concentration than that found in the dog.

Other tests that have been described to diagnose hypoadrenocorticism are basal plasma cortisol concentrations and plasma ACTH measurements. Neither test assesses the adrenal reserve capacity and, therefore, should not be used solely to make a diagnosis.

Most of the glucocorticoids, for example, prednisone, prednisolone, and cortisone, cross react in the assay used for the detection of cortisol. Dexamethasone has no influence on the measurement. It is, therefore, important to discontinue interfering glucocorticoid preparations at least 24 hours before a cortisol determination is made to avoid falsely elevated results.

MANAGEMENT

Acute Crisis

Animals with severe clinical signs require immediate attention. Often these animals present in shock. Before therapy is instituted, blood, for a complete blood cell count and a serum biochemistry profile, and urine should be obtained for analysis, and an intravenous catheter should be placed. Blood also should be checked with reagent strips for glucose and urea concentration. An electrocardiogram may aid in the diagnosis of hyperkalemia and be a valuable tool to the monitoring of successful treatment in the dog (see Chapter 72).

As hypovolemia and hypotension are the most serious problems in the dog with hypoadrenocorticism, fluid therapy should be initiated as soon as possible. Normal saline (0.9% NaCl) is the fluid of choice. The fluid rate varies depending on the severity of clinical signs. Rapid replacement therapy is in order in the acute crisis situation. This process requires careful monitoring of cardiac and renal function, and it is advisable to place a catheter for central venous pressure measurement (see Central Venous Pressure in Chapter 80) and urine collection. The rate during the first 1 or 2 hours can be as high as 80 ml/kg/hour in the dog or 60 ml/kg/hour in the cat. The infusion rate is then reduced to cover replacement and maintenance fluid needs. One should make sure that the fluid given is isotonic, because the rapid rate of infusion may otherwise cause shifts in the intracellular and extracellular fluid compartments. If laboratory results are available or if a quick assessment of blood glucose using a reagent strip indicates hypoglycemia, glucose may be administered at 0.5 g/kg (1 ml/kg/50% dextrose slowly intravenously).

Once the animal is on fluid therapy, blood for basal cortisol determination is collected and an ACTH stimulation test is performed. Dexamethasone does not interfere with the cortisol measurement and can be given during the test period. If the animal has already received a glucocorticoid preparation other than the dexamethasone, the animal cannot be tested at this time. The preparation should be changed to dexamethasone, then the dog or cat can be tested 24 hours later.

After fluid therapy has been initiated and the ACTH stimulation test has been completed, the animal can receive intravenous hydrocortisone sodium succinate or prednisolone sodium succinate at 5 to 20 mg/kg given over a period of 2 to 4 minutes and repeated in 2 to 6 hours. Both preparations are very fast acting, although of short duration. Dexamethasone, which has a slightly slower onset but longer duration, can be given at the same time (0.5–2 mg/kg IV) and repeated every 4 to 6 hours. In this case, the expensive hydrocortisone or prednisolone sodium succinate preparations are no longer needed.

As discussed above, if glucocorticoid administration is necessary during the ACTH testing period, dexamethasone can be administered with no direct influence on results of the test. If the animal is in severe shock requiring the administration of a rapid-acting glucocorticoid initially, the ACTH test should be postponed, as hydrocortisone and prednisolone preparations interfere with the cortisol assays.

If rapid evaluation of blood electrolyte concentrations is not possible, the ECG is a valuable tool to assess potassium concentrations. If changes compatible with hyperkalemia are seen, therapy needs to be instituted rapidly. In most cases with hypoadrenocorticism, infusion of normal saline alone will lower the potassium concentration within the first few hours. Although rarely necessary, the following emergency protocols are recommended for normalizing electrolytes:

1. Glucose can be added to the saline infusion at 0.5 g/kg, which increases potassium uptake into cells.

2. Sodium bicarbonate can be administered, which will also increase the movement of potassium into cells. The dose is calculated according to the formula: deficit (mEq/l) = body weight (kg) × 0.3 × base deficit.

3. Insulin has also been recommended to transfer potassium into cells; however, its use is dangerous and the potassium lowering effect can usually be safely obtained with saline and glucose.

Desoxycorticosterone acetate (DOCA) is the treatment of choice for the mineralocorticoid deficiency in primary adrenal failure. It is given intramuscularly. The dose, 0.2 mg/kg daily in the dog and 0.1 mg/kg daily in the cat, initially, needs to be adjusted by 0.05 mg to 0.1 mg/day according to the electrolyte concentrations for subsequent treatments. In animals that are not vomiting, fludrocortisone acetate may be used. It is administered orally at a dose of 0.1 to 0.5 mg per dog divided twice a day. Although the vigorous initial fluid therapy and the small mineralocorticoid activity of the glucocorticoids administered will alleviate the severe electrolyte imbalance, complete regulation of the electrolytes is not possible without mineralocorticoid administration.

Maintenance Therapy

Fortunately, most dogs with hypoadrenocorticism respond rapidly to appropriate therapy, and after the first day the animals can usually be offered water. If no vomiting is observed, small amounts of bland food can be offered and the animal can eventually be taken off fluids completely. As soon as the animal is clinically normal, the mineralocorticoid preparation is changed to either desoxycorticosterone pivalate (DOCP), a long-acting injectable mineralocorticoid preparation, which can be obtained from Ciba-Geigy on request, or fludrocortisone acetate, which is given daily per os. The dose of 1 mg/day of DOCA is equivalent to 25 mg/3 to 4 weeks of DOCP, since DOCP releases 1 mg of the hormone per day. Therefore, if a dog was stabilized on 1 mg of DOCA per day during the acute phase, it will need 25 mg of DOCP every 3 to 4 weeks.

Fludrocortisone acetate must be administered

daily for the treatment of hypoadrenocorticism. The dose is 0.1 to 0.5 mg per dog divided twice a day initially depending on the size of the animal and 0.1 mg per cat divided twice a day. The dose may have to be adjusted based on weekly electrolyte determinations. Once the animal is stable, rechecks should be made on a monthly basis. Dogs metabolize this drug rapidly and high doses may be necessary even for less than optimal results. In such cases, changing the preparation to DOCP may be advantageous. Salt supplementation (1–5 g per day) may help in some cases to reduce unusually high doses of fludrocortisone and is advocated by some clinicians as routine supplemental treatment.

In addition to proper mineralocorticoid replacement, replacing glucocorticoids is of equal importance, particularly in times of stress. Under normal conditions, glucocorticoid replacement therapy plays a lesser role; about 50% of dogs with hypoadrenocorticism do well without it. However, no animal with hypoadrenocorticism should be discharged without glucocorticoids, and the owners should be instructed to give glucocorticoids when the animal seems ill or when the animal experiences stressful situations (*e.g.,* boarding). The maintenance dose for glucocorticoids is listed in Table 60-7. Prednisone, prednisolone, and cortisone are most commonly used. In times of stress, the dose should be increased fivefold to tenfold. As dogs with glucocorticoid deficiency (secondary hypoadrenocorticism) and most dogs on o,p'-DDD therapy do not exhibit mineralocorticoid deficiency, these animals only need glucocorticoid therapy to alleviate clinical signs of hypoadrenocorticism. Again, a physiologic replacement dose is sufficient under normal conditions. In times of stress, the dose needs to be increased fivefold to tenfold.

PATIENT MONITORING

The prognosis for dogs and cats with hypoadrenocorticism is excellent with proper mineralocorticoid with or without glucocorticoid replacement. While dogs usually respond to therapy quickly, clinical signs may persist in cats for several days. Dogs and cats need to be mon-

Table 60–7 *Treatment of Hypoadrenocorticism*

ACUTE CRISIS

1. 0.9% sodium chloride
   dog: 80 ml/kg/hour
   cat: 60 ml/kg/hour
2. Hydrocortisone sodium succinate or prednisolone sodium succinate
   5 to 20 mg/kg/IV once
   and/or dexamethasone
   0.5 to 2 mg/kg/IV, repeated every 4 to 6 hours
3. Desoxycorticosterone acetate
   dog: 0.2 mg/kg IM
   cat: 0.1 mg/kg IM
   rarely needed:
   glucose: (0.5 g/kg slowly IV)
   sodium bicarbonate (deficit in mEq/l = body weight in kg × 0.3 × base deficit)

MAINTENANCE THERAPY

1. Desoxycorticosterone pivalate or fludrocortisone acetate
2. Prednisone 0.2 mg/kg PO
   or prednisolone 0.2 mg/kg PO
   or cortisone 1.0 mg/kg PO

itored and have weekly determinations of serum electrolyte concentrations initially. Once the animal is stabilized, the animal should be checked every 3 to 4 months. Most problems arise if the owners or clinicians are unaware of the need for glucocorticoids in high doses during times of stress, may it be a mild illness or an elective surgery. These problems are most frequent in animals maintained without glucocorticoids under normal circumstances.

ADDITIONAL READING

Chastain CB, Madsen RW, Franklin RT. A screening evaluation for endogenous glucocorticoid deficiency in dogs: A modified Thorn test. Journal of the American Animal Hospital Association 1989; 25:18.

DiBartola SP, Johnson SE. Clinicopathologic findings resembling hypoadrenocorticism in dogs with primary gastrointestinal disease. J Am Vet Med Assoc 1985; 187:60.

Eichenbaum JD, Macy DW, Servin GA, Paulsen ME. Effect in large dogs of ophthalmic prednisolone acetate on adrenal gland and hepatic function. Journal of the American Animal Hospital Association 1988; 24:705.

Feldman EC, Nelson RW. Hyperadrenocorticism. In: Feldman EC, Nelson RW, eds. Canine and feline endocrinology and reproduction. Philadelphia: WB Saunders, 1987: 137.

Golden DL, Lothrop CD. A retrospective study of aldosterone secretion in normal and adrenopathic dogs. Journal of the American College of Veterinary Internal Medicine 1988; 2:121.

Middleton DJ, Watson ADJ, Howe CJ, Caterson ID. Suppression of cortisol responses to exogenous adrenocorticotrophic hormone and the occurrence of side effects attributable to glucocorticoid excess in cats during therapy with megestrol acetate and prednisolone. Am J Vet Res 1987; 51:60.

Peterson ME. Endocrine disorders in cats: Four emerging diseases. Compendium of Continuing Education 1988; 10:1355.

Peterson ME, Feinman J. Hypercalcemia associated with hypoadrenocorticism in 16 dogs. J Am Vet Med Assoc 1982; 181:802.

Peterson ME, Greco DS, Orth DN. Primary hypoadrenocorticism in ten cats. Journal of the American College of Veterinary Internal Medicine 1989; 3:55.

Rakick PM, Lorenz MD. Clinical signs and laboratory abnormalities in 23 dogs with spontaneous hypoadrenocorticism. Journal of the American Animal Hospital Association 1984; 20:647.

Rogers W, Straus J, Chew D. Atypical hypoadrenocorticism in three dogs. J Am Vet Med Assoc 1981; 179:155.

Willard MD, Schall WD. Canine hypoadrenocorticism: Report of 37 cases and review of previously reported cases. J Am Vet Med Assoc 1982; 180:59.

Willard MD, Schall WD. Hypoadrenocorticism following therapy with op'-DDD mitotane for hyperadrenocorticism in four dogs. J Am Vet Med Assoc 1982; 180:638.

61

FELINE HYPERTHYROIDISM

Duncan C. Ferguson, Margarethe Hoenig

Hyperthyroidism, caused by excessive concentrations of the circulating thyroid hormones thyroxine (T_4) and triiodothyronine (T_3), is the most common endocrine disorder in the cat. Unlike the condition in the cat, hyperthyroidism in the dog is rare and is usually associated with thyroid malignancy. The management of the canine disorder will not be discussed here; however, the diagnostic considerations and therapeutic management of the metabolic derangements in the hyperthyroid dog are similar to those in the cat.

The vast majority of feline cases of hyperthyroidism are the result of hyperplastic or benign adenomatous thyroid glands. The clinical syndrome of feline hyperthyroidism was first described in 1978. The recognition of hyperthyroidism in cats has steadily increased since these reports; increased awareness of the disease and an increase in the average lifespan of cats certainly have contributed to the numbers of diagnoses; however, compelling evidence indicates that hyperthyroidism within the cat population has dramatically increased. Since 1977, both the prevalence of thyroid pathologic abnormalities and the associated clinical state of hyperthyroidism have been detected at a markedly increasing frequency. Although speculation about regional differences in the real incidence of the disease exists (*e.g.*, higher incidence on the East and West Coast of the United States), these suspicions have not yet been confirmed by controlled epizootiologic studies.

CAUSES

Although much has been learned in the last decade about the clinical diagnosis and management of feline hyperthyroidism, little is known about the cause of this generally benign (98%–99%) and bilateral (70%) enlargement of the thyroid associated with thyroid hypersecretion (Table 61-1). The enlarged thyroid lobes contain one or more well discernible foci of hyperplastic tissue, sometimes forming nodules ranging in diameter from less than 1 mm to 3 cm. Thyroid carcinoma, the primary cause of canine hyperthyroidism, rarely causes hyperthyroidism in the cat with a prevalence of approximately 1% to 2%.

Hypotheses have suggested that nutritional factors, such as iodine in the diet, and environ-

831

Table 61–1 *Causes of Feline Hyperthyroidism*

Thyroid hyperplasia or adenoma (Toxic nodular goiter)
(98% to 99%)
Thyroid follicular carcinoma (1% to 2%)

mental factors, such as toxins or goitrogens, may interact to cause thyroid pathology in the cats over time (Fig. 61-1). The presentation is similar to toxic nodular goiter in man, the incidence of which increases with age. Circulating thyroid function stimulating immunoglobulins, as found in human Graves' disease, do not appear to cause feline hyperthyroidism; however, increased amounts of thyroid growth stimulating immunoglobulins have been measured in affected cats. Despite the possibility of circulating stimulators, the tissue appears to function autonomously when studied outside the host animal by transplantation into immunodeficient mice.

PATHOPHYSIOLOGY

All of the signs of feline hyperthyroidism can be related to the excess of thyroid hormones observed in all cats. In excess, thyroid hormone increases the basal metabolic rate, increasing the oxygen and metabolic substrate demand of most tissues. Table 62-2 outlines the pathophysiologic

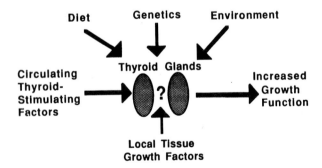

Figure 61–1. *Possible variables leading to the development of toxic nodular goiter in human and cats. Although presently under investigation, virtually all of these mechanisms are hypothetical causes of benign thyroid enlargement in elderly cats. (From Ferguson. New perspectives on the etiology, diagnosis, and treatment of feline hyperthyroidism. In: Small animal geriatrics: Viewpoints in veterinary medicine. Alpo Symposium on Geriatrics, 1989)*

mechanisms associated with hypothyroidism. For the most part, the pathophysiology of thyroid hormone excess can be understood as the opposite end of the spectrum.

Through direct effects on the nervous system, excess thyroid hormones cause hyperactivity, restlessness, pacing, or irritability in many affected cats. Changes that developed gradually in the cat may be more obvious to the veterinarian than to the owners. Completion of a physical examination can be a challenge, as hyperthyroid cats may be intractable and may resist restraint. In severely affected cats, generalized muscle wasting contributes to weight loss.

Increased appetite and food intake are common signs of feline hyperthyroidism and are clearly the result of increased caloric demand imposed by the condition. In most cats, however, compensation is inadequate, and mild to severe weight loss also develops. Although the cause is unclear, about 10% of hyperthyroid cats also have periods of decreased appetite, which usually alternate with periods of normal to increased appetite (see Apathetic Hyperthyroidism, below).

Vomiting, diarrhea, increased frequency of defecation, and increased volume of feces are also seen in feline hyperthyroidism. Vomiting may result from a direct action of thyroid hormone on the chemoreceptor trigger zone or from overeating. Intestinal hypermotility appears to be responsible for the increased frequency of defecation and diarrhea. Malabsorption with increased fecal fat excretion also develops in some cats with hyperthyroidism, possibly the result of reduced pancreatic exocrine secretion or excessive fat intake associated with polyphagia.

Although concurrent primary renal disease contributes to polyuria and polydipsia in some cats with hyperthyroidism, these signs also occur in many cats without evidence of renal dysfunction, and resolution of the polyuria and polydipsia usually occurs after treatment of hyperthyroidism. The exact cause of these signs in hyperthyroidism is unknown. The hyperthyroid state may, however, impair urine concentrating ability by increasing total renal blood flow and thereby decreasing renal medullary solute concentration; medullary washout may therefore cause polyuria with secondary polydipsia. In cats with normal renal concentrating ability, a hypothalamic disturbance caused by thyrotoxicosis may produce compulsive polydipsia with secondary polyuria.

The hyperthyroid state can produce multiple alterations in respiratory function, including decreased vital capacity, decreased pulmonary compliance, and an increase in respiratory rate, the results of respiratory muscle weakness and increased carbon dioxide production. Hyperthyroidism results in a high-output cardiac state in which vascular resistance is low and cardiac output is high because of increased tissue metabolism and oxygen requirements. Volume overload is created by low peripheral vascular resistance and by reflex renal mechanisms that conserve fluid. In addition, thyroid hormones act directly on heart muscle and increase activity of the sympathetic nervous system, which results in an increase in work demand of the heart.

The principal cardiac compensatory mechanisms in high-output states such as hyperthyroidism are dilatation and hypertrophy. Tachycardia, systolic murmurs, gallop rhythm, arrhythmias, and signs of congestive heart failure (*e.g.*, dyspnea, rales, muffled heart sounds, ascites) are common. Electrocardiographic abnormalities may include tachycardia, increased R wave amplitude in lead II, atrial and ventricular arrhythmias, and intraventricular conduction disturbances. Left ventricular hypertrophy, thickening of the interventricular septum, left atrial and ventricular dilatation, and myocardial hypercontractility have been documented by echocardiography. Hyperthyroidism, therefore, may induce a hypertrophic or, less commonly, a dilative type of cardiomyopathy. Either form may result in congestive heart failure, but severe cardiac failure is more common in hyperthyroid cats with dilated cardiomyopathy. The hypertrophic form of thyrotoxic cardiomyopathy is usually reversible on correction of the thyroid status.

CLINICAL SIGNS

Feline hyperthyroidism occurs in middle- to old-aged cats, with a reported range of 4 to 22 years (mean age, approximately 12–13 years). There is no breed or sex predilection.

Table 61-2 lists the most common historical and clinical signs recorded in cats with hyperthyroidism. Many of the signs of hyperthyroidism can be confused with primary diseases affecting a variety of organ systems, in particular, gastrointestinal, respiratory, and cardiac. Table 61-3 lists diseases that are often in the differential diagnosis of hyperthyroidism as well as the historical

Table 61–2 *Clinical Signs in Feline Hyperthyroidism**

Weight loss
Hyperactivity/Nervousness
Polyphagia
Tachycardia
Polyuria/Polydipsia
Cardiac murmur
Vomiting
Diarrhea
Increased fecal volume
Decreased appetite
Lethargy
Increased respiratory rate (panting)
Muscle weakness
Muscle tremor
Dyspnea

* *From highest to lowest incidence; all observed in greater than 10% of cases.*

Table 61–3 *Differential Diagnosis for Hyperthyroidism*

Condition	Signs Common With Hyperthyroidism
Diabetes mellitus	PU/PD, anorexia, weight loss
Kidney disease	PU/PD, anorexia, weight loss
G.I. disease	Diarrhea, weight loss, anorexia, vomiting
Heart disease and failure	Tachycardia, respiratory distress, cardiomegaly, arrhythmias
Respiratory disease	Respiratory distress, panting

or physical findings that overlap with hyperthyroidism. Before the recognition of feline hyperthyroidism as a clinical entity and the documentation of its secondary effects, it is possible that hyperthyroid cats were misdiagnosed as having primary diseases of these organ systems.

Because the cats generally remain bright and alert and have good appetites, many animals are not presented to the veterinarian for a year or more following the onset of signs. At this stage, weight loss is a common complaint, and the animal may have lost 50% of its original body weight. The most common clinical signs associated with hyperthyroidism are weight loss in spite of ravenous appetite, hyperactivity, polydipsia, polyuria, diarrhea, and periods of respiratory distress.

In about 10% of cases, hyperthyroid cats present in a way similar to what has been called "apathetic hyperthyroidism." Weight loss remains a common clinical sign but is usually accompanied by lethargy and anorexia rather than hyperactivity and an increased appetite. This form may represent an end-stage form of hyperthyroidism, and these cats also frequently have cardiac abnormalities, including arrhythmias and congestive heart failure.

Cats with the classic form of hyperthyroidism may be thin, nervous, mildly febrile, and show symptoms of cardiovascular disease such as tachycardia and dyspnea. Often the cats shed excessive amounts of hair and have a tendency to groom themselves excessively, resulting in matting of the hair coat. One should bear in mind when handling a hyperthyroid cat that they tend to have impaired tolerance to stresses.

Although the history and clinical presentation are usually highly suggestive of feline hyperthyroidism, a presumptive diagnosis can usually be made by palpation of the ventrolateral cervical region. Enlargement of one or both thyroid lobes can be detected in the majority of cases; sometimes one or both thyroid glands may even be visibly enlarged. In contrast, the thyroid gland is not usually palpable in the normal cat. As the thyroid glands of the cat are loosely attached to the trachea, they can be quite movable and may be found near the thoracic inlet. It should also be remembered that accessory thyroid tissue can be found along the trachea and in the cranial mediastinum. A useful method of palpation of the thyroid gland in a cat is to approach the cat from behind and to extend the neck gently. With the thumb, index, and middle fingers, the length of the neck should be palpated for soft and usually movable tissue masses. Although palpation of thyroid enlargement (goiter) in a cat with signs consistent with hyperthyroidism allows a presumptive diagnosis of thyrotoxicosis (thyroid hormone excess), it is occasionally recognized that elderly cats with no clinical or biochemical evidence for hyperthyroidism may also have palpable goiter. Such cats usually eventually develop overt thyrotoxicosis, presumably after further growth and oversecretion of the thyroid nodules.

DIAGNOSTIC APPROACH

Screening laboratory tests should always be performed in a cat suspected of having hyperthyroidism. Beyond providing evidence for the hyperthyroid condition, routine screening tests are prudent in an elderly cat as they may reveal the presence of a concurrent disorder not directly related to the hyperthyroid state. Table 61-4 reviews common laboratory findings in feline hyperthyroidism.

In hyperthyroidism an increase in erythropoiesis is triggered by the increased tissue oxygen demand. Therefore, hematocrit, hemoglobin, and red blood cell count may be increased (high-normal to high). Although less consistent, a mature leukocytosis and eosinopenia may also be found.

Elevation of alanine aminotransferase (ALT), aspartate aminotransferase (AST), alkaline phosphatase (SAP) and lactic dehydrogenase (LDH) are the most common biochemical abnormalities in hyperthyroidism. Elevations in serum creatinine and phosphate concentrations may also be found, indicative of concurrent renal insufficiency commonly associated with aging. Following correction of the hyperthyroid state and reduction of cardiac output and renal diuresis, further deterioration of renal function is possible. Increased renal tubular absorption of phosphate and increased bone resorption and muscle catabolism result in hyperphosphatemia of hyper-

Table 61–4 *Laboratory Assessment of Hyperthyroidism*

Test	What to Check For
Complete blood cell count	Increased PCV, RBC, and Hb Stress neutrophilia, eosinopenia
Serum biochemistry profile	Increased ALT, AST, SAP Increased LDH Increased serum phosphorous Slightly increased creatinine, glucose
Urinalysis	Variable SG R/O diabetes, urinary tract infection
Chest radiographs	Cardiac enlargement (especially left ventricle) Pulmonary edema (in CHF) Pleural effusion (in CHF)
ECG	Sinus tachycardia (>240 bpm) Increased R wave amplitude Atrial premature contractions Left axis deviation Widened QRS complex
Echocardiography	Thickened ventricular walls & hyperdynamic wall motion = hypertrophic cardiomyopathy
Hormonal	Elevated total and free T_4, total and free T_3 Elevated rT_3 Post-T_3 divided by Pre-T_3 serum T_4 > 0.5 or Post-T_3 serum T_4 < 1.5 μg/dl (20 nmol/L) Post-TSH T_4 minus Pre-TSH T_4 < 2.5 μg/dl (30 nmol/L)
Blood pressure	Elevated
Scintigraphic scan	Thyroid/salivary gland uptake ratio > 1 Enlarged thyroid gland or glands

(Key: ALT = alanine aminotransferase; AST = asparate aminotransferase; CHF = congestive heart failure; Hb = hemoglobin; LDH = lactic dehydrogenase; PCV = packed cell volume; RBC = red blood cell count)

thyroidism even in hyperthyroid cats without overt renal insufficiency. Slight elevations of serum glucose may be observed in nondiabetic cats, and cats with concomitant diabetes may be difficult to manage with insulin. Presumably due to insulin-resistance in peripheral tissues, glucose tolerance is reduced in nondiabetic hyperthyroid cats.

Most hyperthyroid cats show cardiac abnormalities, and, therefore, a complete cardiologic examination including electrocardiogram, chest x-ray, and if possible an echocardiogram should be performed. Symmetric hypertrophic cardiomyopathy is observed in more than 80% of cases. About 20% of cats may have congestive heart failure as evidenced by pleural effusion and pulmonary edema. Electrocardiographic findings may reveal sinus tachycardia, left ventricular dilata-tion, increased R wave amplitude, and premature atrial or ventricular beats. Echocardiograms show a high incidence of left ventricular wall thickening and an increased left ventricular fractional shortening. Hyperthyroid cats have also been shown to have a high incidence of systolic and diastolic hypertension.

Definitive Diagnosis

Figure 61-2 outlines a flow chart for the definitive diagnosis of hyperthyroidism in cats.

The definitive diagnosis of hyperthyroidism is, in the vast majority of cases, made based on the observation of an elevated serum T_4 concentration. Serum T_3 concentrations and free T_4 concentrations are also elevated in most cases. However,

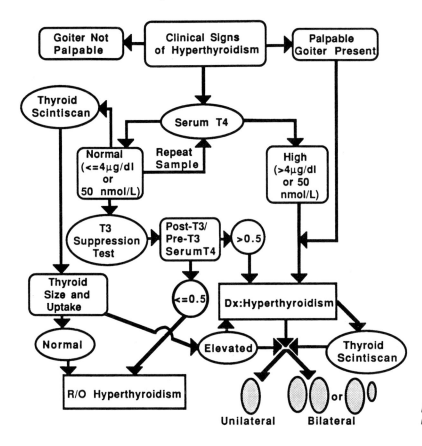

Figure 61–2. *Flow chart for the definitive diagnosis of hyperthyroidism.*

cats with clinical signs of hyperthyroidism but normal or high-normal serum total T_4 concentrations have also been observed. Because severe nonthyroidal illness reduces serum thyroid hormone concentrations into the subnormal range in euthyroid cats, concomitant hyperthyroidism should not be ruled out in an older cat with a nonthyroidal illness if serum T_4 and T_3 concentrations are normal or high-normal. Serum thyroid hormone concentrations will increase above the normal range on successful treatment of the nonthyroidal condition. Furthermore, it has been shown that mildly hyperthyroid cats may have serum thyroid hormone concentrations that fluctuate into and out of the normal range. Therefore, when in doubt, the cat should be observed for the development of more severe signs, or a blood sample should be taken at a later point in time (2 to 8 weeks) for the measurement of serum T_4 concentration. Alternatively, scintigraphy or the dynamic tests described below can be employed.

Occasionally, when baseline serum T_4 concentrations are borderline or even normal, it is useful to employ dynamic tests of the thyroid axis. Figure 61-3 illustrates the basis of the two tests described below.

Triiodothyronine (T_3) Suppression Test

Exogenous thyroid hormone, through negative feedback inhibition, inhibits endogenous serum thyrotropin (TSH) and, secondarily, serum T_4 concentrations. In borderline cases of hyperthyroidism, it may be of value to test the thyroid for autonomy from these regulatory mechanisms. In hyperthyroidism, endogenous serum TSH is already suppressed by the excess thyroid hormone secretion of the adenoma.

The protocol for the T_3 suppression test is as follows:

1. Draw blood for pre-T_3 serum T_4 determination.
2. Administer exogenous T_3 (Cytomel, Smith Kline

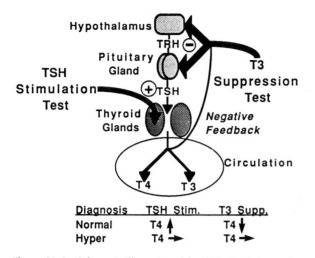

Figure 61–3. *Schematic illustration of the TSH stimulation and T3 suppression tests. When administered in pharmocologic doses, T3 will suppress endogenous TSh and secondarily serum T4 concentrations in normal cats but not in cats with autonomously functioning goiters. When bovine TSH is administered in the TSH stimulation test, normal but not adenomatous thyroid tissue will respond with an increase in serum T4 concentration.*

and French; Cytobin, Norden) at a dose of 25 μg every 8 hours for 2 days, giving a seventh dose on the morning of the third day.

3. Draw blood for post-T_3 serum T_4 determination 4 hours after the last T_3 dose.
   Interpretation: Post-T_3 serum T_4 divided by pre-T_3 serum T_4 concentration
   Normal: less than 0.5 (or serum T_4 less than 1.5 μg/dl, 19 nmol/L)
   Hyperthyroid: greater than 0.5 (usually little to no suppression)

Thyrotropin (TSH) Stimulation Test

In general, autonomously functioning adenomas do not respond to stimulation by exogenous thyrotropin. The protocol for the TSH stimulation test is as follows:

1. Draw a blood sample for pre-TSH serum T_4 determination.
2. Administer 1 U/kg bovine TSH intravenously.
3. Draw a blood sample for serum T_4 determination 6 hours after TSH administration.
   Interpretation: Post-TSH minus pre-TSH T_4 concentration
   Normal: 2.5 μg/dl (25 ng/ml or 32 nmol/L)
   Hyperthyroid: less than 2.5 μg/dl (25 ng/ml or 32 nmol/L)

When feasible, the T_3 suppression test is recommended over the TSH stimulation test for discrimination of borderline cases of hyperthyroidism. Assuming compliance by the owners, the doses of T_3 can be given at home on an outpatient basis with an office visit 4 hours after the last dose. The T_3 suppression test, because it is performed over a longer period of time, is more reliable than TSH stimulation. The TSH stimulation test requires 1 day of hospitalization, and bovine TSH is expensive, making its purchase difficult to justify in some practice situations.

Thyroid Radionuclide Scanning

Although palpation generally allows the diagnosis of goiter, it does not allow the distinction of unilateral and bilateral thyroid enlargement. Furthermore, the establishment of functional "normalcy" of tissue is not possible even at surgery. Therefore, where available at referral institutions, thyroid imaging is performed using radioactive iodine or ^{99m}Tc (technetium). Because of its rapid uptake (by mechanisms identical to iodide) and increased safety, technetium can be given in higher diagnostic doses and provides a better image than radioiodine. Technetium scanning is useful to document thyroid enlargement in cats with normal or high normal T_4 concentrations. A semiquantitative comparison of technetium uptake to that of the salivary glands, which also take up iodide can be used to assess increased uptake. Imaging is particularly useful in the diagnosis of the 30% of cases that are unilateral; in these cases, the function and size of the contralateral lobe is suppressed. Thyroid imaging is also useful in cats with adenomas that have slipped into the mediastinum or the 1% to 2% of cats with adenocarcinomas, which have a tendency to metastasize by extension into the the mediastinum. Figure 61-4 shows technetium scintigrams from a normal cat and a cat with bilateral adenomatous goiter.

MANAGEMENT

Three general modalities exist for the treatment of hyperthyroidism in cats: (1) thyroid ablation by radioactive iodine (^{131}I), (2) bilateral or uni-

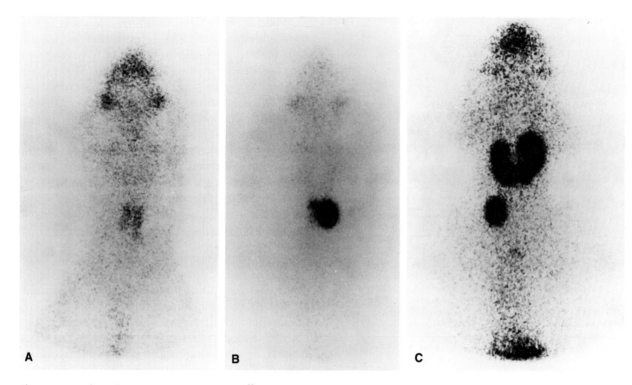

Figure 61–4. *Thyroid scintiscans with technetium (⁹⁹ᵐTc). (A) Ventrodorsal view of a scintiscan of a normal cat. Note the equal density and size of the thyroid glandular isotope uptake and compare t othe salivary glands at the top of the picture. The thyroid/salivary gland ratio is approximately. (B) Ventrodorsal view of a scintiscan of a cat with unilateral thyroid enlargement. Note that the isotope uptake on the contralateral side is suppressed. Note that the thyroid/salivary gland ratio is much greater than 1. (C) Ventrodorsal view of a scintiscan of a cat with bilateral thyroid enlargement and a separate area of enlargement closer to the thoracic inlet. This scan illustrates the value of scintiscans, as the ectopic thyroid enlargement may have been missed at surgery, and disease is likely to have recurred following removal of the two lobes in the standard location. The density at the bottom of the photograph is isotope in the cardiac lumen. (Courtesy of Dr. Barbara Selcer, University of Georgia Veterinary Teaching Hospital, Athens, GA)*

lateral surgical thyroidectomy, and (3) the administration of antithyroid drugs. In Figure 61-5, each of the treatment options are illustrated. Radioiodine ablation and surgery have the potential to result in a cure of this nonmalignant condition. When a unilateral condition has been documented with a thyroid scan, surgical therapy is preferred so that destruction of normal thyroid tissue will not be risked.

Antithyroid drugs, while indicated in cats with complications or in particularly poor condition, have no irreversible toxic effects on the thyroid gland and only temporarily ameliorate the signs of disease.

The following factors should be considered when planning therapy for hyperthyroidism:

1. The patient's general health and nutritional status: Medical therapy may be indicated when the animal requires time to improve body condition or the owners require evidence that the cat can improve with curative therapy. Anesthetic difficulties are minimized if euthyroidism is medically induced prior to surgery.

2. The owners' desire for a cure: Only radioiodine and surgery have curative potential in benign adenomatous goiter.

3. Owner compliance and economic factors: Antithyroid drugs generally must be administered two to three times a day for the remainder of the animal's life. However, medical therapy over the remainder of the life of an already elderly cat could be less expensive than the curative treatments.

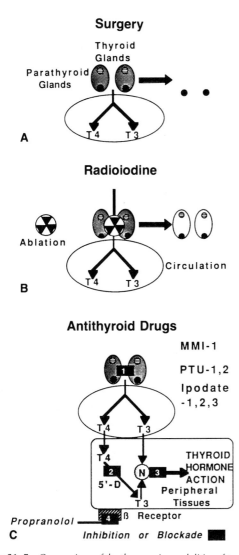

Surgery

Radioiodine

Antithyroid Drugs

MMI-1

PTU-1,2

Ipodate
-1,2,3

Propranolol

C   *Inhibition or Blockade* ■

Figure 61–5. *Comparison of the three main modalities of treatment of feline hyperthyroidism. (A) Surgery, performed properly, can spare two external parathyroid glands. (B) Radioiodine therapy can normalize thyroid function without damage t othe parathyroid glands. (C) The antithyroid drugs may reversibly block thyroid hormone secretion (site 1), block the 5'-deiodinationm of T4 and T3 (site 2), block the action of thyroi hormone (site 3), or block some aspect of thyroid hyperfunction (site 4). (From Ferguson. New perspectives on the etiology, diagnosis, and treatment of feline hyperthyroidism. In: Small animal geriatrics: Viewpoints in veterinary medicine, 1989).*

4. The practitioner's surgical skill in performing a thyroidectomy and the hospital's capacity to provide the necessary postoperative care: Postoperative hypocalcemia requiring intravenous calcium therapy is not unusual (see Chapter 72).

5. The availability of facilities for radioiodine ther-

apy and the owners' willingness to leave the cat in the hospital for the period required by radiation safety regulations. Radioiodine therapy is an option only available at certain referral institutions.

Medical Management of Hyperthyroidism

All available antithyroid drugs must be administered continuously two to three times daily to maintain suppression of serum thyroid hormone concentrations. Serum thyroid hormone concentrations rebound above the normal range on withdrawal of drugs and symptoms of disease may arise again. The thiourylene drugs propylthiouracil (PTU) and methimazole (MMI, Tapazole, Lilly) are the most commonly used antithyroid drugs in cats. Both inhibit the thyroidal synthesis of hormone (see Figure 61-5). After the initiation of daily therapy, there is usually a delay of several days before the fall of serum thyroid hormone concentrations. During this period, glandular hormone stores, which are unaffected by the drugs, are becoming depleted. The drug PTU has the additional beneficial effect of blocking the conversion of T_4 to the more active T_3 in peripheral tissues like the liver and kidney. Therefore, serum T_4 may fall following both PTU and MMI therapy, but with MMI, due to autoregulatory mechanisms in the peripheral tissues, serum T_3 is usually maintained within the normal range even when T_4 is quite low. As a result of this mechanism, it is rare to see a cat on MMI develop clinical signs of hypothyroidism.

However, PTU has fallen out of favor because of its serious side effects. Both PTU and MMI can result in anorexia, vomiting, lethargy, and the development of positive antinuclear antibody titers. Although autoimmune disease is observed with PTU and MMI, PTU was associated with an unacceptable incidence of autoimmune hemolytic anemia and immune-mediated thrombocytopenia. As these complications are particularly onerous in an animal being prepared for surgery, PTU can no longer be recommended for routine use in the hyperthyroid cat.

Methimazole is now the antithyroid medication of choice in the cat. The administration of 5 mg three times daily will generally bring the serum T_4 concentrations down into the normal range within 2 to 3 weeks. The daily dose of MMI should then be adjusted upward or downward in 2.5 mg ($^1/_2$ tablet) intervals until the serum T_4 concentration falls within the normal range. As mentioned, even cats with very low serum T_4 concentrations may not become hypothyroid because the serum T_3 concentration stays normal. Once a satisfactory therapeutic effect is seen, many cats can be maintained on once daily therapy because MMI's thyroid tissue residence time is longer than its serum residence time. Cats on chronic MMI therapy should be checked every 3 to 6 months to draw blood for serum T_4 measurement and to monitor for signs of MMI toxicity (see below). The therapeutic goal should be identification of the lowest MMI dose that maintains the serum T_4 concentration in the low-normal range (generally 1–2 µg/dl = 10–20 ng/ml = 13–26 nmol/L).

Mild clinical signs have been observed in about 15% of cats on MMI, but most signs are associated with gastrointestinal upset, are transient, and resolve despite continued therapy. Pruritus around the face, ears, or neck with self-induced excoriations have also been observed early in the course of therapy. The lesions are glucocorticoid-responsive; however, as with any drug allergy, therapy must be discontinued before complete relief is observed. The life-threatening side effects of MMI include drug-induced hepatopathy (less than 2%), thrombocytopenia, and agranulocytosis. During MMI therapy, serum antinuclear antibodies (ANA) are observed in a high percentage of cats, the incidence of which appears to be dependent on the size of the dose (more common in cats on 15 mg/day MMI) and the duration of therapy (incidence about 50% when duration 6 months). However, no signs consistent with lupus erythematosus, such as skin, joint, kidney disease or hemolytic anemia, have been observed. Withdrawal of MMI and institution of standard care for thrombocytopenia (*e.g.*, blood transfusion) or agranulocytosis (*e.g.*, prophylactic bacteriocidal antimicrobial drugs) generally result in resolution of the drug reaction. Cross-sensitivity to the thiourylenes MMI and PTU is common; therefore,

when it develops, the curative forms of therapy should then be utilized.

Other classes of drugs, such as the iodinated radiocontrast agents, are presently under investigation in humans and cats for their antithyroid effects. In the hyperthyroid individual, these drugs may act by inhibiting peripheral conversion of T_4 to T_3, by blocking nuclear receptors for T_3, by blocking thyroid hormone secretion (directly, by inhibition of synthesis and, indirectly, as they are metabolized through the release of inorganic iodide), and possibly by blocking the uptake of thyroid hormones into tissue. Due to problems with hypersensitivity and poor tolerance to the thiourylene drugs PTU and MMI, antithyroid drugs with alternative structures or actions are of particular interest for development as therapy for feline hyperthyroidism.

Radioactive Iodine (^{131}I) Therapy

Although generally only available at referral institutions, radioiodine is the most effective and appropriate cure for bilateral toxic goiter in the cat because it selectively destroys the functioning thyroid tissue without risking damage to the nearby parathyroid tissue responsible for regulating serum calcium. Iodine 131 has a half-life of 8 days and produces both τ and β radiation. The β particles serve to produce most of the local tissue destruction. The calculation of the appropriate ablative dose can be attempted following quantitation of uptake of a tracer amount of isotope. However, compared to the experience with human patients, a surprisingly low rate of recurrence of hyperthyroidism (underdosing) or induction of permanent hypothyroidism (overdosing) has been experienced with radioiodine treatment in cats. Therefore, a pragmatic approach is taken at many institutions: all cats receive 1 to 5 mCi of ^{131}I. This single-treatment regimen has been associated with a high rate of success (eventual euthyroidism in greater than 80%), possibly attributable to the recrudescence of extracervical thyroid tissue normally present in cats. Higher radioiodine doses are employed in metastatic thyroid follicular carcinomas (1%–2% of cases), with a much poorer prognosis. Following a therapeutic dose of ^{131}I (generally 1–5 mCi), the serum T$_4$ and T$_3$ concentrations will normalize within 1 to 2 weeks. The functionally normal (but originally suppressed) thyroid tissue remaining is usually able to eventually restore euthyroidism, and thyroid replacement therapy is generally unnecessary. When radioiodine therapy is to follow a period of MMI therapy, the MMI should be discontinued for at least 3 to 7 days prior to treatment. The efficacy of radioiodine is reduced by recent antithyroid medical therapy, as these drugs reduce the long-term incorporation of iodine into the thyroid gland and reduce radioiodine's therapeutic effect.

No matter what the dose of radioiodine, the major disadvantage of radioiodine therapy is that certain radiation safety precautions must be taken. Radioiodine is secreted in saliva and excreted in urine and feces. Unlike human patients who may receive therapeutic doses on an outpatient basis, radioiodine-treated cats must be hospitalized for periods of 1 to 4 weeks depending on the dose administered and the local radiation safety regulations. Despite these disadvantages, radioiodine therapy is the least invasive cure for bilateral adenomatous goiter, having no hypoparathyroidism or toxicity associated with it. Furthermore, radioiodine can be administered without anesthesia or sedation, an important consideration in the elderly cat with other medical problems.

Surgical Thyroidectomy

The only curative treatment available to private practitioners is surgical thyroidectomy. However, hyperthyroid cats, because of their advanced age and cardiovascular and metabolic complications, face increased anesthetic and surgical risks. Before preparation for thyroidectomy, all cats with hyperthyroidism should be evaluated for overt cardiac disease (hypertrophic cardiomyopathy and congestive heart failure) and treated appropriately. In a series of 85 cats treated surgically at the Animal Medical Center in New York City, 8 (9.4%) died. Of these animals, 6 out of 8 had no

preoperative medical therapy to return them to a euthyroid metabolic status.

The use of antithyroid drugs for a period before surgery is recommended until the serum T$_4$ concentration is within the normal range (usually 1–3 weeks). Methimazole, as described above, is presently the drug of choice for the preoperative preparation of a hyperthyroid cat. With medical induction of euthyroidism, the anesthetic and surgical risks are considerably reduced. The last dose of methimazole should be administered on the morning of surgery.

In cats that poorly tolerate MMI or PTU, preoperative propranolol or potassium iodide (50–100 mg/day for 1–2 weeks in gelatin capsules to improve tolerance) can be administered. Large amounts of iodide rapidly but transiently and incompletely reduce thyroid hormone release from the thyroid gland. Ideally, this therapy should be accompanied by a β-blocker such as propranolol (2.5–5 mg three times a day, 1–2 weeks before surgery) to minimize the tendency for intraoperative ventricular cardiac arrhythmias.

The reader is referred to detailed reviews (Peterson; Black and Peterson, Additional Readings) of anesthetic and surgical techniques associated with thyroidectomy in cats. The principles of this management are summarized here.

Because hyperthyroid cats are prone to cardiac disease and because hyperthyroidism predisposes the animal to cardiac arrhythmias and hypertension, the anesthetic plan should attempt to minimize the use of agents that are arrhythmogenic and hypertensive. Many, if not all, of these concerns can be waived if medical therapy has achieved euthyroidism before surgery. At all times, concerns of anesthesia in the elderly patient should apply.

Premedication with a phenothiazine (*e.g.,* acetylpromazine) serves to reduce the effect of circulating catecholamines and to counter arrhythmias induced by thiobarbiturates and inhalant anesthetics. Conversely, ketamine should be avoided because it leads to an increase in catecholamine release. Xylazine is also contraindicated because it potentiates the development of cardiac arrhythmias induced by inhalation or barbiturate anesthesia. Atropine can be omitted because it stimulates adrenergic activity and may induce tachycardia and arrhythmias. Glycopyrrolate is the antimuscarinic drug of choice because it has less effect on cardiac rate and rhythm than atropine. Thiobarbiturates are acceptable induction agents because they possess antithyroid activity and do not stimulate catecholamine secretion. Methoxyflurane and halothane, although commonly used, have the property of sensitizing the heart to catecholamine-induced arrhythmias.

Intraoperative monitoring of body temperature, electrocardiogram, and respiratory pattern is extremely important. In a metabolically hyperthyroid cat, the oxygen consumption is much greater and the risk of hypoxia greater. In general, the anesthetic requirements are high in hyperthyroidism. Ventricular arrhythmias are often observed, particularly in animals that are still hyperthyroid. Management of such arrhythmias should include an increase in the oxygen flow rate and propranolol (0.1 mg IV).

Thyroidectomy

UNILATERAL. In Figure 61-5, thyroidectomy is compared schematically with the other modes of treatment for feline hyperthyroidism. Unilateral thyroidectomy is the preferred treatment for unilateral disease (~30% of cases). However, even with visualization at surgery, definitive evaluation of the normalcy of a thyroid lobe is difficult (one gland may be only slightly enlarged and appear normal). Thyroid isotopic imaging is the most reliable method for establishment of the normalcy of a thyroid lobe. If thyroid imaging is not available, but the involvement appears unilateral at surgery, the obviously enlarged lobe should be removed while not disrupting the associated external parathyroid gland. If the other lobe develops gross enlargement (generally within 9 months) and surgery is again necessary, the risk of hypocalcemia is small.

BILATERAL. The goal of a bilateral thyroidectomy is to remove all thyroid tissue while maintaining viability of at least one, if not two of the external parathyroid glands. Two general surgical techniques are being used: intracapsular and extracapsular. The main advantage of the extracapsular, as compared to the intracapsular, technique is that the incidence of relapse is much less because the entire thyroid capsule is removed together with the thyroid lobe.

PATIENT MONITORING

Postoperative Considerations

Postoperative complications of bilateral thyroidectomy include hypocalcemia (~15% of cases), Horner's syndrome, and laryngeal paralysis due to disruption of the vagosympathetic trunk. Symptomatic hypocalcemia occurs only after all parathyroid glands have been removed or damaged. The true danger of hypoparathyroidism is that it may develop immediately or as late as 3 days after surgery (presumably after scar tissue starts to develop). The clinical signs of hypocalcemia may range from weakness, muscle tremors, and tetany to sudden death. Many cats may have mild hypocalcemia (less than 7 mg/dl or 1.75 mmol/L) without clinical signs. Severe hypocalcemia associated with clinical signs should be managed with intravenous calcium. Once the cat will eat, oral calcium supplementation (up to 750 mg/kg/day calcium gluconate or 600 mg/kg/day calcium lactate) may be used. In addition, vitamin D therapy should be instituted with dihydrotachysterol (Hytakerol liquid, Winthrop; tablets, Philips-Roxane), a synthetic vitamin D analogue that is active in hypoparathyroidism. A loading dose of 0.03 mg/kg/day orally for 3 to 4 days followed by a maintenance dose of 0.01 to 0.02 mg/kg/day, if effective, will increase the serum calcium 4 to 5 days after initiation of therapy. Although hypoparathyroidism may remain in some cats, others will be able to regulate serum calcium again beginning weeks to months after surgery.

Following a successful unilateral or bilateral thyroidectomy, the serum T_4 will generally fall into the subnormal range by 1 to 2 weeks after surgery and remain there for 2 to 3 months. Clinical signs of hypothyroidism rarely develop. However, after bilateral thyroidectomy, it may be wise to start thyroxine supplementation (0.1–0.2 mg daily in single or divided doses) beginning 1 to 2 days after surgery. In most cases, however, it is likely that after recrudescence of normal extracervical thyroid tissue, cats can maintain normal serum T_4 concentrations. All cats treated by thyroidectomy or radioiodine should have serum T_4 monitored once or twice yearly for evidence of a return to hyperthyroidism. When recurrence following bilateral surgery is documented by a high serum T_4 concentration, retreatment with nonsurgical modalities is preferred because the incidence of hypoparathyroidism increases greatly with repeat surgeries.

Hyperthyroidism is a disease of elderly cats, and concurrent nonthyroidal illnesses are not uncommon. However, the prognosis for a return to normalcy of an uncomplicated case of adenomatous goiter is excellent following definitive therapy. Often, this is difficult for cat owners to appreciate when decisions as to therapy are being made. Therefore, the more inexpensive palliative antithyroid drugs may allow the owners to see the degree to which the disease signs can regress before committing to curative therapy such as surgery or radioiodine.

ADDITIONAL READING

Black AP, Peterson ME: Thyroid biopsy and thyroidectomy. In: Bojrab MJ, ed. Current techniques in small animal surgery. Philadelphia: Lea and Febiger, 1983: 388.

Feldman EC, Nelson RW, eds. Hyperthyroidism and thyroid tumors. In: Canine and feline endocrinology and reproduction. Philadelphia: WB Saunders, 1987: 91.

Ferguson DC. New perspectives on the etiology, diagnosis, and treatment of feline hyperthyroidism. Alpo Symposium proceedings. Small animal geriatrics: Viewpoint in veterinary medicine, 1989: 23.

Peterson ME. Considerations and complications in anesthesia with pathophysiologic changes in the endocrine system. In Short CE, ed. Veterinary anesthesiology. Baltimore: Williams and Wilkins, 1987: 251.

Peterson ME. Treatment of feline hyperthyroidism. In: Kirk RW, ed. Current veterinary therapy X. Philadelphia: WB Saunders, 1989: 1002.

Peterson ME, Ferguson DC. Thyroid Diseases. In: Ettinger SJ, ed. Textbook of veterinary internal medicine, 3rd ed. Philadelphia: WB Saunders, 1989: 1632.

Peterson ME, Keene B, Ferguson DC, Pipers F. Electrocardiographic findings in forty-five cats with hyperthyroidism. J Am Vet Med Assoc 1982; 18:934.

Peterson ME, Kintzer PP, Cavanagh PG et al. Feline hyperthyroidism: Pretreatment clinical and laboratory evaluation of 131 cases. J Am Vet Med Assoc 1983; 183:103.

Peterson ME, Kintzer PP, Hurvitz AI: Methimazole treatment of 262 cats with hyperthyroidism. Journal College of Veterinary Internal Medicine 1988; 2:150.

62

HYPOTHYROIDISM

Duncan C. Ferguson, Margarethe Hoenig

Hypothyroidism is one of the more common endocrinopathies of the dog and yet is a rare disorder in the cat. Defined as the lack of thyroid hormone secretion or action, hypothyroidism is most often the result of reduced thyroid hormone secretion by the thyroid glands. The resultant clinical picture is quite variable, and almost any organ system may be involved. However, the recognition of hypothyroidism frequently follows presentation for complaints relating to the skin and hair coat. Although dysfunction anywhere in the hypothalamic-pituitary-thyroidal axis may result in thyroid hormone deficiency, greater than 95% of clinical cases of hypothyroidism appear to result from destruction of the thyroid gland itself (primary hypothyroidism).

Although hypothyroidism is rarely, if ever, a diagnostic or therapeutic emergency, it is important to maintain a high degree of clinical suspicion for syndromes associated with thyroid insufficiency, as it may be the underlying cause of hematologic abnormalities, recurrent infections, musculoskeletal disorders, and gastrointestinal and reproductive abnormalities. Conversely, careful attention should be paid to the accurate diagnosis of this disorder, as other illnesses also influence thyroid function tests. Following careful diagnostic procedure, the treatment of affected animals with thyroid replacement medication is generally rewarding.

CAUSES

The two most common causes of canine adult-onset primary hypothyroidism are lymphocytic thyroiditis and idiopathic atrophy of the thyroid gland (Table 62-1). These each account for about one half of the cases of hypothyroidism. Other rare forms of canine hypothyroidism include iatrogenic conditions, neoplastic destruction of thyroid tissue, and congenital (or juvenile-onset) hypothyroidism (cretinism).

Lymphocytic thyroiditis is characterized histologically by a diffuse infiltration of the gland by lymphocytes, plasma cells, and macrophages, resulting in progressive destruction of follicles and secondary fibrosis. Clinical signs of hypothyroidism are generally associated with destruction of over three fourths of the thyroid tissue. Lymphocytic thyroiditis is probably an immune-mediated disease, as suggested by the morphology of the thyroid lesions and the frequent occurrence of circulating antibodies directed against thyroglobulin, a thyroid-specific protein. The clinical presentation of thyroiditis in the dog may vary considerably depending on the time of presentation during the natural course of disease. A dog with acute thyroiditis may have transient signs of polyuria and polydipsia, possibly referable to thyroid hormone release into the circulation, but no signs of inflammation such as pain or

Table 62–1 *Causes of Hypothyroidism*

Type	Causes
Primary	Cretinism
	Lymphocytic thyroiditis
	Idiopathic atrophy
	Goitrogens
	Iodine deficiency
	Neoplastic destruction
Secondary	Pituitary destruction
	Pituitary suppression

fever are generally observed. Eventually, these animals will present with signs referable to thyroid hormone deficiency.

Idiopathic atrophy of the thyroid gland is the second major histologic form of canine primary hypothyroidism. Histologically, loss of thyroid parenchyma occurs with replacement by adipose tissue. The cause of idiopathic thyroid atrophy is not known. Although this follicular atrophy may represent the end-stage form of lymphocytic thyroiditis, it is unlikely because of the lack of an inflammatory cell infiltrate in this form of hypothyroidism. Idiopathic follicular atrophy is most likely a primary degenerative disorder of the thyroid gland affecting individual follicular cells.

Hypothyroidism appearing in neonates or animals less than 1 year of age is most likely associated with a congenital defect causing thyroid aplasia or the absence of key enzymes involved in the thyroidal synthesis of thyroid hormones. The incidence of congenital or juvenile-onset primary hypothyroidism in the dog appears to be extremely rare. It is likely that congenital hypothyroidism usually results in early death of the puppy and is rarely diagnosed.

Hypothyroidism may result from an impaired ability of the pituitary gland to secrete. thyrotropin (TSH), resulting in secondary follicular atrophy. In the dog, secondary hypothyroidism accounts for less than 5% of clinical cases of hypothyroidism. Causes could include pituitary tumors, congenital pituitary malformation, isolated TSH deficiency, or a sequelae of the treatment of pituitary tumors with surgery or irradiation.

Although the deficient production or release of thyrotropin-releasing hormone (TRH) also has been reported to cause hypothyroidism in man, this type of hypothyroidism has not been documented in the dog. Until a valid TSH assay is available for the dog, it will be difficult to prove such an etiology.

An inability to convert thyroxine (T_4) to triiodothyronine (T_3) by peripheral tissues (caused by a selective absence or reduction of 5'-deiodinase activity), although considered by some to be a possible cause of canine hypothyroidism, has yet to be documented to produce a hypothyroid state in any species. The finding of low serum T_3 concentrations in conjunction with normal serum T_4 concentrations is most likely the result anti-T_3 antibodies (see below).

In an attempt to establish an underlying cause, it is not uncommon for adult obese cats to be suspected of having primary hypothyroidism. However, spontaneous adult-onset primary hypothyroidism has not yet been documented in an adult cat. Congenital or juvenile-onset hypothyroidism has been described in the cat. However, as in the dog, this condition likely results in early death in affected kittens and is rarely diagnosed.

The most common cause for the development of feline hypothyroidism is the surgical and radioiodine treatment of hyperthyroidism. This condition is often transient because previously nonfunctional extracervical thyroid tissue becomes functional and restores normal thyroid hormone levels. Although antithyroid drug overdosage could also produce hypothyroidism, this outcome appears to be rare with methimazole (Tapazole).

PATHOPHYSIOLOGY

Critical to the understanding of the disorder, its diagnosis, and its treatment is an understanding of the physiology of thyroid hormone secretion and action.

Although direct species-specific information is lacking in the dog and cat, similarities between the hypothalamic-pituitary-thyroid-extrathyroid (HPTE) axis in other species suggest a scheme similar to that in Figure 62-1. The hypothalamus

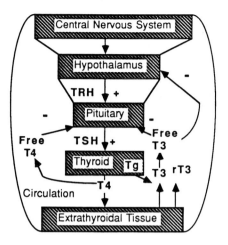

Figure 62–1. *Thyroid hormone secretion. (From Peterson ME, Ferguson DC. Thyroid diseases. In: Ettinger, SJ, ed. Textbook of veterinary internal medicine, 3rd ed. Philadelphia: WB Saunders, 1989: 1646.)*

secretes the tripeptide TRH into the hypophyseal portal system, which extends to the pituitary. Thyrotropin releasing hormone stimulates TSH secretion by the pituitary. The synthesis and secretion of TSH is regulated primarily through negative feedback at the pituitary and hypothalamus by plasma T_4 and T_3 in the free or unbound form. Episodic but no circadian rhythm of thyroid hormones has been observed in the dog.

The metabolically active thyroid hormones are the iodothyronines L-thyroxine (L-T_4), and L-3,5,3'-triiodothyronine (L-T_3). Thyroxine is the main secretory product of the normal thyroid gland; however, T_3, which is about 3 to 5 times more potent than T_4, and smaller amounts of L-3,3',5'-triiodothyronine (rT_3), an inactive product, are also secreted by the canine thyroid.

Although all T_4 is secreted by the thyroid, a considerable amount (40%–60% in the dog) of T_3 is derived from extrathyroidal enzymatic 5'-deiodination of T_4. Therefore, although it also has intrinsic metabolic activity, T_4 has been called a *prohormone*, and its "activation" to the more potent T_3 is a step regulated individually by peripheral tissues. The vast majority of reverse T_3 (~90%) is derived from extrathyroidal sources in the dog. Except for T_3 and T_4, the other metabolites do not have thyromimetic activity. A number of nonthyroidal illnesses and drugs may influence the local tissue regulation of thyroid hormone deiodination and serum thyroid hormone concentrations.

The circulation of thyroid hormones in plasma is dependent on specific and nonspecific binding by plasma proteins, some of which serve to "buffer" hormone delivery into tissue and provide a hormone reservoir (Fig. 62-2). The dog has approximately 15% of the thyroxine binding globulin in plasma compared to humans, while the cat does not appear to have this high affinity binder. In the healthy euthyroid dog or cat, therefore, about 0.1% of total serum T_4 is unbound or free, whereas about 1% of T_3 is free. It is clinically important to recognize that thyroid hormones are highly bound to plasma proteins, as this binding relationship may change in response to drugs or illness. Most evidence suggests that the free hormone fraction predicts the amount of hormone that is available to tissues at equilibrium. Although clinical measurements of serum concentrations of thyroid hormone are limited to the plasma compartment, approximately 50% to 60% of the body's T_4 and 90% to 95% of the T_3 is intracellular. Therefore, because T_3 is primarily an intracellular hormone and a significant amount is derived from extrathyroidal sources, the isolated measurement of its serum concentration is a less meaningful estimate of thyroid function than is the measurement of serum total T_4 concentration.

The proportion of free hormone is a primary determinant of the rate of fractional metabolic and excretory turnover. Humans have a greater amount of thyroxine binding globulin in plasma compared to the dog, and the fractional free T_4 is one-third to one-fifth that of the dog. In the dog, the plasma half-life of T_4 has been estimated to be between 10 to 16 hours, compared to about 7 days in humans, and the plasma half-life of T_3 in the dog is estimated to be 5 to 6 hours. It should be emphasized that these figures reflect plasma disappearance and do not necessarily indicate extent or duration of biologic action.

Thyroid hormones have a wide range of effects on metabolism and function; therefore, hypothyroidism shares signs with many other disease entities. The correction of signs of hypothyroidism following treatment with thyroid hormone

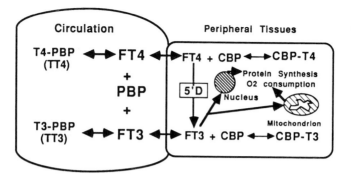

Figure 62–2. *Overview of site and mechanism of cellular thyroid hormone action. Thyroid hormone (T_3 has the highest potency) acts at the nucleus of most tissues to regulate protein synthesis, the mechanism by which most long-term or delayed effects are mediated. More rapid effects on cellular oxygen consumption are likely mediated via direct or indirect mitochondrial oxygen consumption. Circulating thyroid hormones are carried bound noncovalently to plasma binding proteins (PBP). In the normal dog, only about 0.1% of T_4 and 1% of T_3 are free from protein binding (FT_4 and FT_3). Thyroxine is converted to T_3 by the 5'-deiodinase enzyme (5'D), the activity of which is regulated, in peripheral tissues. Within the tissue, a large proportion of hormone is also noncovalently bound to cellular thyroid hormone binding proteins (CBP) which serve as a hormone reservoir within the cells. (From Ferguson DC. Hypothyroidism: Many presentations, on e treatment. Small animal geriatrics: Viewpoints in veterinary medicine. Proceedings of the 1989 Alpo symposium on geriatrics, 1989:31.*

can be related to the cellular action of thyroid hormones (primarily but not exclusively due to T_3). Figure 62-2 shows a general scheme for the cellular actions of thyroid hormone. Immediate effects (within hours) include increased calorigenesis, oxygen consumption, and increased mental activity. These effects are generally mediated by actions at subcellular organelles such as the mitochondria and plasma membrane. Delayed effects (within days to weeks) include hair regrowth. Such effects are generally mediated by binding to the nuclear thyroid hormone receptor followed by protein synthesis.

CLINICAL SIGNS

Table 62-2 lists the clinical signs associated with hypothyroidism and their associated pathogenetic mechanisms. Special mention will now be made of the pathophysiology underlying the following clinical presentations of hypothyroidism.

Lethargy and heat-seeking are directly related to reduced cellular metabolism. This results in

the development of mental dullness, lethargy, and an unwillingness to exercise. Obesity may develop in some dogs despite a normal appetite and caloric intake. The reduced basal metabolic rate results in hypothermia (temperature less than 38°C) in some dogs. Hypothyroid dogs may seek heat for this reason.

People with hypothyroid dogs commonly first seek veterinary care when dermatologic problems develop. Dryness of the hair coat, excessive shedding, and retarded regrowth of hair are early signs. Alopecia, present in about two thirds of affected dogs, is usually bilateral and symmetrical in distribution, is most obvious over points of friction, such as the ventral trunk and neck, axilla, and tail ("rat-tail" appearance) (Fig. 62-3), but also is common in the perineal area and the dorsum of the tail and nose. The alopecia is classically nonpruritic unless secondary seborrhea or dermatitis has developed (see Chapter 49). Thyroid insufficiency results in an increased percentage of telogen (inactive) hair follicles and an increase in keratin and sebum production. Thickening of the skin or the development of myx-

Table 62–2 *Pathogenesis of Clinical Signs in Hypothyroidism*

Site of Action	Effect of Deficit	Clinical Signs
Calorigenesis Thermoregulation	Decrease in BMR and O_2 consumption	Lethargy, weakness Distal extremity hypothermia Heat-seeking
Growth and Maturation	Deficit particularly critical to CNS	Mental retardation of cretin and dullness in adults Neuropathies
Carbohydrate Metabolism	Decreases in glycogenolysis and glycolysis Increased sensitivity to insulin	Obesity despite normal or decreased appetite
Protein Metabolism	Decreased synthesis and degradation	Muscle weakness Poor hair coat and regrowth
Dermatologic	Increased telogen hairs Increased sebum & keratinization Accumulation of mucopolysaccharides in dermis	Bilateral symmetrical alopecia Hyperkeratosis Myxedema
Cardiovascular	Alteration of cardiac muscle enzymes Decreased β-receptor numbers	Decreased heart rate, pulse pressure, and cardiac output
Neuromuscular	Accumulation of mucopolysaccharides in and around nerves Hypertrophy of slow-twitch and atrophy of fast-twitch fibers	Polyneuropathy, muscle atrophy Weakness, stiffness, myotonia
Gastrointestinal	Reduction of electrical activity of GI smooth muscle, reduced segmentation	Diarrhea or constipation
Reproductive	Diminished function	Female: anestrus, irregular cycles, galactorrhea, still-birth Male: azospermia; lack of libido
Immunologic	Suppressed humoral and cell-mediated immunity	Recurrent infections (particularly pyodermas)
Hematologic	Reduced bone marrow stimulation Reduced Factor VIII and VIIIAg	Nonresponsive anemia Possible bleeding tendency
Endocrine	Decreased secretion of growth hormone, gonadotropins, cortisol Increased secretion of prolactin	Secondary growth hormone deficiency Galactorrhea

BMR = basal metabolic rate; CNS = central nervous system; GI = gastrointestinal
(Modified from: Ferguson DC. Hypothyroidism: Many presentations, one treatment. Small animal geriatrics: Viewpoints in veterinary medicine. Proceedings of the 1989 Alpo Symposium on Geriatrics 1989: 30.)

edema (subcutaneous accumulation of gly-cosaminoglycans), develops in some cases. Myx-edema is most prominent in the facial features, which may take on a puffy or "tragic" appearance (Fig. 62-4).

Myopathies have also been associated with hy-pothyroidism both in humans and the dog. Se-vere muscle weakness and delayed reflexes may be the clinical manifestation, or the signs may be vague such as stiffness, reluctance to move, and muscle wasting. The myopathy in hypothyroid-ism is not inflammatory in nature, and in humans creatine phosphokinase (CPK) is generally ele-vated; however, this observation is inconsistent in the dog and CPK may be normal. An association between hypothyroidism and megaesophagus has been postulated but not proven.

Facial muscle and eyelid weakness (lip and lid droop) attributable to cranial nerve VII paralysis or paresis has been observed in hypothyroid peo-ple and dogs. Also, head tilt may be observed consistent with vestibular nerve disruption (see Chapter 55). These changes are likely due to the swelling of and around the dural sheath of the facial, vestibular, and cochlear nerves as they pass through bony foramina in the facial bones. Bilateral laryngeal paralysis has been associated with hypothyroidism in dogs as well. The pa-

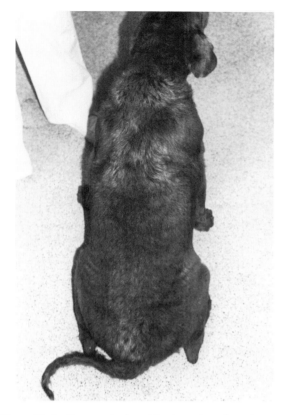

Figure 62–3. *Dorsum of a dog with primary hypothyroidism illustrating the "rat-tailed" appearance.*

thophysiology of polyneuropathies associated with hypothyroidism is poorly understood but may be due to altered neuronal metabolism. Segmental demyelination and axonopathy have also been shown. Alternatively, compressive neurologic abnormalities may be the result of tissue swelling (myxedema) surrounding the spinal cord or peripheral nerve. Clinically and electrodiagnostically, the polyneuropathy is indistinguishable from those caused by other diseases with hyporeflexia, slow nerve conduction velocities, fibrillation potentials, and positive sharp waves on electromyography. Although extremely rare, central nervous system (CNS) signs of seizures, disorientation, and circling also have been reported in hypothyroid dogs with cerebrovascular atherosclerosis caused by the hyperlipidemia associated hypothyroidism. Severe mental obtundation can be also observed in the syndromes of cretinism and myxedema coma (see Special Presentations of Hypothyroidism below).

The cardiac muscle is rapidly and extensively affected by severe hypothyroidism. The strength of cardiac contraction is reduced. On an electrocardiogram, the most common abnormalities observed in hypothyroid dogs are low voltage and inverted T waves. A weak apex beat may be aus-

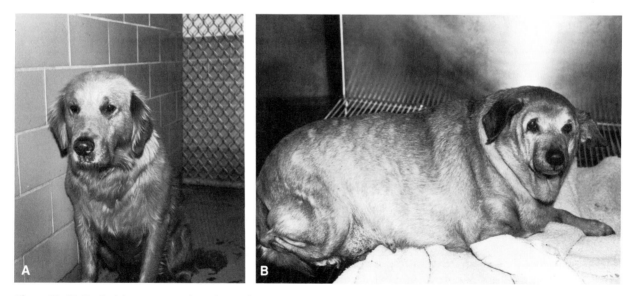

Figure 62–4A, B. *Facial appearance of two dogs with profound primary hypothyroidism, illustrating the "tragic expression" associated with facial myxedema.*

culted. It has been proposed that some cardio-myopathies in large breed dogs may be secondary to hypothyroidism and that thyroid supplementation aids therapy. However, a study of 13 Doberman pinschers with congestive cardiomyopathy showed that 12 responded normally to TSH, making hypothyroidism as a primary cause unlikely. The distinction of low serum T_4 due to a cardiac nonthyroidal illness (see below) secondary to hypothyroidism is important, as the administration of thyroid hormone may lead to further cardiac decompensation by rapidly increasing the tissue demand for oxygen delivery.

Hypothyroidism has been associated with a variety of reproductive disturbances. In breeding bitches, persistent or sporadic anestrus, infertility, abortion, and high puppy mortality have been observed. Galactorrhea is a rare sign of hypothyroidism that develops in some intact female dogs whose mammae have been primed for lactation. Hyperprolactinemia, perhaps resulting from the excessive stimulation of prolactin-secreting pituitary cells by TRH, appears to be the cause of galactorrhea in susceptible bitches and may be at least partially responsible for the infertility associated with canine hypothyroidism. Lack of libido, testicular atrophy, hypospermia, or infertility can be seen in the male. A careful study of the incidence of these abnormalities in breeding animals has not been reported.

Studies in hypothyroid dogs have demonstrated a decrease in the intestinal and gastric electrical and motor activity. Although hypothyroid dogs usually have normal bowel movements, constipation and diarrhea have been also observed.

Any dog with a recurrent infection, particularly of the skin, should be evaluated for hypothyroidism. Pyoderma, which is unresponsive or only temporarily responsive to appropriate antibacterial agents, may be exacerbated by the reduced phagocytic function of white blood cells in hypothyroidism. Most dogs with pyoderma, however, have normal thyroid function (see Chapter 52).

A cause and effect relationship between canine hypothyroidism and the development of an acquired coagulation defect (von Willebrand's disease) has been postulated. Similarly, in dogs with von Willebrand's disease treated with thyroid hormone, a rise in factor VIII antigen has been described even when little evidence of primary hypothyroidism exists (see Chapter 16). The mechanism of action of T_4 in these circumstances is uncertain, but may reflect the nonspecific action of thyroid hormone on protein synthesis. It has been shown that factor VIII : Ag is lower than normal in experimental models of canine hypothyroidism and higher than normal in a model of hyperthyroidism. Since the breed incidence of von Willebrand's disease and hypothyroidism overlap (*e.g.*, Doberman pinscher, golden retriever, miniature schnauzer), it is critical to rule out the coexistence of these conditions in individual dogs where hypothyroidism may unmask a subclinical bleeding tendency.

Adult-Onset Primary Canine Hypothyroidism

Table 62-3 summarizes the clinical signs, which may be observed in adult-onset canine hypothyroidism.

As illustrated in Figure 62-5, hypothyroidism is a disorder that develops most commonly in middle-aged dogs. It is more common in mid- to large-size breeds of dogs, while hypothyroidism is rare in toy and miniature breeds of dogs. The incidence of hypothyroidism is higher in the

Table 62–3 *Clinical Signs in Adult-Onset Canine Hypothyroidism*

Lethargy/Mental dullness
Alopecia/Hair loss
Weight gain/Obesity
Dry hair coat/Excessive shedding
Facial swelling (myxedema)
Hyperpigmentation/Skin thickening
Cold intolerance/Hypothermia
Bradycardia/Decreased pulse pressure
Constipation or diarrhea
Proprioceptive defects
Laryngeal or Nerve VII paralysis
Polyneuropathy/Myopathy
Secondary infections
Anestrus
Galactorrhea (female)
Lack of libido (male or female)

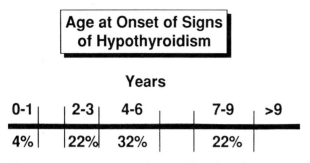

Age at Onset of Signs of Hypothyroidism				
Years				
0-1	2-3	4-6	7-9	>9
4%	22%	32%	22%	

Figure 62–5. *Age at onset of signs of hypothyroidism in 3026 cases. (From Milne KL, Hayes HM. Epidemiological Features of canine hypothyroidism. Cornell Vet 1981;71:3.)*

Great Dane, old English sheepdog, Irish setter, Doberman pinscher, dachshund, miniature schnauzer, golden retriever, and boxer (Fig. 62-6). This incidence suggests a genetic predilection. In fact, Great Danes, Irish setters, old English sheepdogs and Doberman pinschers have been shown to have a significantly greater occurrence of antithyroglobulin antibodies than other breeds including mixed-breeds. There does not appear to be a sex predilection, but spayed female dogs appear to be at a higher risk for the development of hypothyroidism than intact females.

Because the historical and physical findings in dogs with hypothyroidism may be vague and variable and the manifestations wide-reaching, the animal should be carefully examined and the owners carefully questioned. Significant attention should be paid to those aspects of the history and physical examination, which are more easily documented. For example, if the owner complains that the animal is gaining weight despite a normal appetite, records of the animal's weight, if available, should be examined, and the owners should be asked about the dog's normal diet and caloric intake (including snacks).

When examining the animal, any findings consistent with a reduced rate of metabolism should be considered to be consistent with hypothyroidism (*e.g.,* reduced body temperature and heart rate, mental dullness, or general lethargy). As it is common (but not universal) to observe alterations in the skin and hair coat, bilateral symmetrical alopecia, easily epilated coarse hairs, and hyperpigmentation, particularly in areas of friction, are consistent with hypothyroidism. Recurrent infections of the skin and of other organ systems that respond poorly to appropriate antibiotic therapy (particularly if bacteriostatic agents are used) should also be considered to be possibly secondary to hypothyroidism and its associated state of immune deficiency.

Special Presentations of Hypothyroidism in the Dog

Cretinism

Thyroid hormones are crucial for growth and development of the skeleton and CNS. Therefore, in addition to the well-recognized signs of adult-onset hypothyroidism, disproportionate dwarfism and impaired mental development (cretinism) are prominent signs of congenital and juvenile-onset hypothyroidism. With primary congenital hypothyroidism, enlargement of the thyroid gland (goiter) is also often observed. Cre-

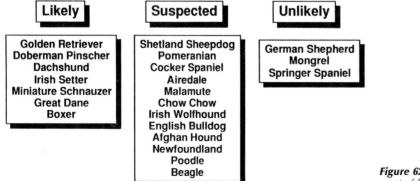

Likely	Suspected	Unlikely
Golden Retriever	Shetland Sheepdog	German Shepherd
Doberman Pinscher	Pomeranian	Mongrel
Dachshund	Cocker Spaniel	Springer Spaniel
Irish Setter	Airedale	
Miniature Schnauzer	Malamute	
Great Dane	Chow Chow	
Boxer	Irish Wolfhound	
	English Bulldog	
	Afghan Hound	
	Newfoundland	
	Poodle	
	Beagle	

Figure 62–6. *Breed predisposition for the development of hypothyroidism.*

tinous puppies are behaviorally dull and less active and may have a shuffling gait and a poor appetite. On neurologic examination, the affected pup is often weak, hyporeflexic, or hyperreflexic (if there is muscle tremor or spasticity) and may lack conscious proprioception. Radiographic signs of underdeveloped epiphyses, shortened vertebral bodies, and delayed epiphyseal closure are common. These animals can generally be distinguished from those with pituitary dwarfism (congenital hypopituitarism), as the latter animals have proportionate dwarfism. Usually, these animals (cretins) are diagnosed by 2 months of age when the clinical signs become obvious to the owners.

Myxedema Coma

There have been reports of "myxedema coma" in the dog. Classically, this syndrome, usually seen in elderly profoundly hypothyroid people, is characterized by severe mental obtundation terminating in coma and hypothermia. The course, which can develop rapidly, is often one of lethargy progressing to stupor and coma. The more common signs of hypothyroidism are usually present but hypoventilation, hypotension, bradycardia, and profound hypothermia are usually observed as well. These animals may have an elevated blood PCO_2, decreased PO_2, and low plasma sodium and glucose concentrations. Often, these events are triggered by an anesthetic episode, and the results can be fatal. While the incidence is rare, great care should be taken in anesthetizing or tranquilizing a dog that you suspect or know to be hypothyroid.

Adult-Onset Secondary Canine Hypothyroidism

Dogs suspected of having secondary hypothyroidism should also be evaluated for other endocrine abnormalities and neurologic disorders that may be associated with pituitary tumors. However, dogs with primary hypothyroidism also tend to have diminished concentrations of basal and stimulated (with xylazine, clonidine, or growth hormone releasing factor) growth hormone concentrations, without pituitary or hypothalamic pathology.

Clinical Signs of Hypothyroidism in Cats

In contrast to dogs, primary hypothyroidism, which may develop in an adult cat following treatment for hyperthyroidism, does not generally present with bilateral symmetrical alopecia, poor hair regrowth, or obesity. These animals may simply be lethargic and have a nonpruritic seborrhea sicca. Alopecia, if it does develop, is most common over the pinna of the ears. The cats may have a generally unkempt look because they may not be grooming themselves regularly.

DIAGNOSTIC APPROACH

The importance of having a suspicion for hypothyroidism when beginning diagnostic tests cannot be overemphasized. There is no hematologic or biochemical test that is conclusive for hypothyroidism (Table 62-4). Even hormonal tests must be interpreted carefully in light of historical and physical findings.

Well-recognized clinical and pathologic abnormalities are associated with hypothyroidism, the severity of which usually correlates with the severity and chronicity of the hypothyroid state. It is important to remember that these alterations are non-specific and may be associated with many other diseases in the dog. Their presence, however, adds supportive evidence for a diagnosis of hypothyroidism in a dog with appropriate clinical signs.

A normocytic, normochromic, nonregenerative anemia is classically found (see Table 62-4). This nonresponsive "physiological" anemia associated with hypothyroidism is the result of decreased tissue oxygen consumption resulting in decreased erythropoietin production. Thyroid hormone lack may also directly reduce proliferation of bone marrow stem cells.

Although certainly not unique to hypothyroidism, hypercholesterolemia occurs in about three fourths of dogs with hypothyroidism (see Table 62-4). Serum triglyceride concentrations may also be increased. Both hypercholesterolemia and hypertriglyceridemia result from decreased metabolism and clearance of these substances from the blood. Serum CPK may also be elevated, the result of reduced plasma enzyme turnover.

Table 62–4 *Laboratory Assessment of Hypothyroidism*

Test	What to Check For
Complete blood cell count	Normocytic, normochromic anemia
Serum biochemistry profile	Increased cholesterol Increased creatine phosphokinase
Urinalysis	Non-specific changes: secondary urinary tract infections
Chest radiographs	Non-specific changes: thoracic or abdominal effusion, increased abdominal fat
ECG	Bradycardia, low R wave amplitude, inverted T waves
Hormonal	Reduced concentrations of: TT_4, TT_3, FT_4, FT_3 (non-specific) Reduced TT_4 increment following bovine TSH or TRH: post-TSH concentration < 4 µg/dl (51 nmol/L)

There are no changes in the urinalysis that are pathognomonic for hypothyroidism. However, due to the tendency for secondary infection in affected animals, a complete urinalysis is recommended to rule out a urinary tract infection.

As discussed before, in severe hypothyroidism, low amplitude and inverted T waves may be observed on the electrocardiogram. Bradycardia may also be documented in affected animals. None of these changes are specific for hypothyroidism and may reflect concomitant cardiac disease.

Although not specific for hypothyroidism, radiographic evidence of thoracic or abdominal effusion may be observed in certain cases. Cardiomegaly and pulmonary edema may be present in dogs with concurrent congestive cardiomyopathy (see Chapter 21).

Specific Thyroid Function Tests

Figure 62-7 shows a flow diagram for the diagnosis of hypothyroidism. When using this diagram, the clinician should recognize the following theoretical goals of thyroid function testing. Tests of thyroid hypofunction should:

1. Preferably follow and confirm the observation of clinical signs consistent with hypothyroidism;
2. Have the proven ability (in that species) of distinguishing the hypothyroid animal from the healthy euthyroid and the sick euthyroid animal; and
3. Ultimately be judged by their ability to predict a successful response to subsequent thyroid hormone replacement therapy.

The practitioner should be careful not to treat an animal for hypothyroidism based only on a laboratory result outside the normal range. This tendency would appear to be rising as biochemistry screening tests being offered by some diagnostic laboratories now include basal serum T_4 measurement for dogs and cats. This is not to say that the availability of this information has no place for the early detection of thyroid disease. It simply should be recognized that the observation of a low serum T_4 concentration may also be consistent with a nonthyroidal disorder (Figs. 62-8 through 62-10). With regards to principle 2, no single test has yet satisfied this criterion. The final principle might appear to be common sense, as the real value of any diagnostic test is in its indication of the proper therapeutic pathway. Presently, the TSH stimulation test is the only test that has been assessed by this criterion.

The available and practical thyroid function tests will be described individually in approximately the order of their availability and utility in the diagnosis of hypothyroidism.

Serum Total T₄ Concentration

The determination of basal serum total T_4 concentration by radioimmunoassay (RIA) may provide important information to a diagnosis of hypothyroidism. As T_4 is produced only from the thyroid gland, dogs with hypothyroidism can, in most cases, be distinguished from normal dogs on the basis of a low serum T_4 concentration. However, nonthyroidal conditions on the list of differential diagnoses and certain drugs may also lower

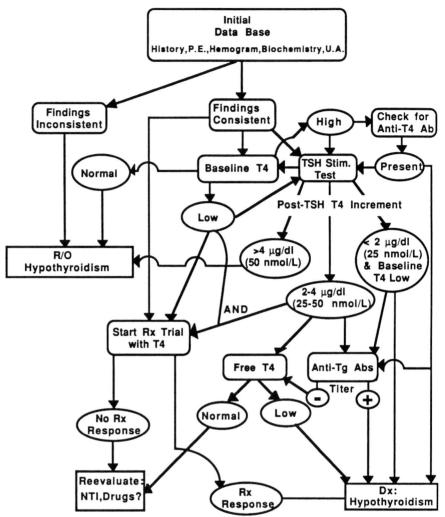

Figure 62–7. *Diagnostic approach to cases with suspect hypothyroid disease.*

baseline serum T_4 concentrations (see Figs. 62-8 through 62-10). Even when historical and physical findings do not suggest the presence of other factors that would lower serum T_4, it is wise to confirm the diagnosis of hypothyroidism with a dynamic thyroid function test (see TSH and TRH stimulation tests).

Serum Total T_3 Concentration

Because T_3 is the most potent thyroid hormone at the cellular level, it would seem logical to measure its concentration for diagnostic purposes. Indeed, when used alone, the serum T_3 concentration is about as good a discriminator between normal and hypothyroid dogs as is the serum T_4 concentration. However, in hypothyroidism and in canine nonthyroidal illness, a lowering of serum T_3 usually follows a lowering of serum T_4 (see Nonthyroidal Factors Altering Thyroid Function Tests in the Dog below). Elevations in serum T_3 concentration relative to T_4 may be indicative of anti-T_3 antibodies or of the tendency of the failing thyroid gland to increase the synthesis and secretion of the hormonally more active T_3. The serum carries only 5% to 10% of the body's T_3 content; the majority of this intracellular hormone resides in tissues such as muscle and skin, which exchange T_3 with serum only very slowly. Therefore, the observation of a reduced basal serum T_3 con-

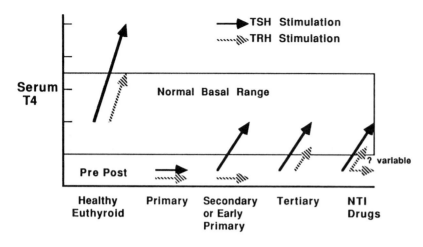

Figure 62–8. *Serum T4 responses to TSH and TRH in various conditions. The arrows indicate the classical response of serum T₄ concentrations to optimal doses of TRH and TSH. (NTI = nonthyroidal illness)*

Condition	TT4	FFT4	FT4	TT3	TrT3	TSH Stim.	TRH Stim.
Neonate	↑						
Aging	↓	↓then↑	↓then↑	↓then↑	↓then↑	↓	
Pregnancy	↑						
Fasting	N to↓			↓	N		
Obesity	↑			↑			
Time of Day	N or↓			N or↓			

Figure 62–9. *The effect of physiologic conditions on thyroid function tests. (Blank spaces indicate lack of information.)*

Condition	TT4	FFT4	FT4	TT3	TrT3	TSH Stim.	TRH Stim.
Cushing's	N or↓	N or↑	N or↓	N or↓	N or↓	N	N or↓
Sertoli Cell	N			N		↓	
Diabetes	N,↓			↑,↓	↑	N or↓	
Addison's	N or↓					N or↓	
Kidney Dis.	↓	N or↑	N or↓	N,↓	N,↑		
Liver Dis.	N or↓			N	↑		
I.C.U.	↓			↓			
Surg/ Anes	↓			↓	↓		

Figure 62–10. *The effect of disease on thyroid function tests. (Blank spaces indicate lack of information.)*

centration without other confirmatory evidence is of questionable value in the diagnosis of hypothyroidism.

Thyrotropin (TSH) Stimulation Test

The administration of exogenous bovine TSH followed by the measurement of serum T_4 or T_3 provides important information in the diagnosis of hypothyroidism because it tests thyroid secretory reserve.

At this time, the TSH stimulation test continues to be the most definitive noninvasive test for the diagnosis of primary hypothyroidism, which constitutes the vast majority of cases.

Protocols for this test vary widely. Although the TSH dose and serum sampling times are often dictated by practical and economic considerations, it seems logical that the TSH stimulation test should utilize the lowest TSH dose required to give a maximal thyroidal T_4 response, and a blood sample should be obtained at the time of the peak T_4 concentration. The response of serum T_3 concentration to TSH tends to be less consistent. In the dog and cat, increasing the TSH dose administered generally delays the time of the T_4 peak and, up to a limit, results in a higher serum T_4 response and a plateau, which is maintained for a longer period of time. The route of administration may be intravenous, intramuscular, or subcutaneous; however, the most consistent and rapid response is seen after intravenous dosing. For the dog, we suggest drawing a baseline blood sample for serum T_4 determination, the administration of 0.1 U/kg TSH intravenously (maximum dose 5 U), followed by a blood sample at 6 hours after TSH. In the cat, the serum T_4 increment above the baseline concentration 6 hours after TSH administration was found to increase up to the highest dose examined, 1 U/kg intravenously. If cost is a factor, considerably more value is found in a single determination after TSH T_4 than a baseline T_4 determination. The TSH stimulation test may be performed concurrently with the ACTH stimulation test for hypoadrenocorticism or hyperadrenocorticism without significant effects on the results of either test.

In Figure 62-8, the various possibilities for results of TSH and TRH stimulation tests (see next section) are summarized. The diagnosis of hypothyroidism in the dog is usually confirmed when the serum T_4 concentration after TSH is below the normal range for basal T_4 (usually less than 1.0 μg/dl or less than 13 nmol/L) and rarely increases above the baseline (greater than 0.2 μg/dl or greater than 2.6 nmol/L). In hypothalamic (tertiary, TRH deficiency) and pituitary (secondary, TSH deficiency) hypothyroidism, the thyroid gland should remain responsive to TSH. With the TSH stimulation test, depression of baseline serum T_4 concentrations due to drugs and illness may be distinguished from advanced primary hypothyroidism but not from secondary or tertiary hypothyroidism or from earlier stages of primary hypothyroidism. In the former cases, a significant and parallel response to TSH is seen. The rare cases of long-standing secondary (pituitary) or tertiary (hypothalamic) hypothyroidism with subsequent thyroid atrophy may require two or three consecutive daily doses of TSH to eventually demonstrate thyroid responsiveness.

A study of normal dogs evaluated the predictive value of blood sampling times after 5 units of intravenous TSH: in 80% of the animals, a doubling of the serum T_4 concentration was not achieved by 4 hours but was achieved in all cases by 6 hours after TSH. Judgment of the normalcy of the TSH response must also be tempered by the knowledge that the maximum T_4 increment decreases linearly from a mean of about 4 μg/dl (51 nmol/L) in 2-year-old dogs to about 2 μg/dl (26 nmol/L) in 15-year-old dogs. One study has shown that the animals that responded favorably to thyroid replacement therapy had, on the average, virtually no increase in serum T_4 concentration following TSH. Variation in basal T_4 and T_3 concentrations has been demonstrated throughout the day in euthyroid healthy animals and euthyroid animals with dermatopathies or nonthyroidal illness. As a result, the post-TSH to pre-TSH T_4 concentration ratio is also quite variable. An advantage of the TSH stimulation test is that T_4 concentrations after TSH tend to be less variable because the thyroid is maximally stimulated. In general, to rule out hypothyroidism using the dose of TSH recommended above, the T_4 concentration after TSH should exceed the normal range of basal T_4 concentrations (generally ~4 μg/dl or 51 nmol/L).

Thyrotropin-Releasing Hormone (TRH) Stimulation Test

The TRH stimulation test, as it is used diagnostically in the diagnosis of human pituitary and thyroid disease, is designed to evaluate the pituitary's responsiveness to TRH as manifested by the change in serum TSH concentration. In primary thyroid gland failure, the pituitary response to TRH is increased, and, in hyperthyroidism, it is decreased. As a valid homologous canine TSH radioimmunoassay (RIA) is not yet widely available, application of the TRH stimulation test requires the measurement of serum T_4 concentrations. In theory, the administration of TRH should lead to an increase in T_4 only if the pituitary-thyroid axis is intact (see Fig. 62-7). Therefore, responsiveness to TRH should only be observed in tertiary (hypothalamic) thyroid insufficiency, a condition not yet documented in the dog.

Several studies have examined a range of TRH doses for use in the dog. In general, increasing the TRH dose increased the duration of the response. Side effects were more significant at dosages greater than 0.1 mg/kg; salivation, urination, defecation, vomiting, miosis, tachycardia, and tachypnea were observed. The recommended protocol for the TRH stimulation test is the administration of 0.1 mg TRH/kg intravenously with the collection of serum for T_4 measurement at 0 and 6 hours after TRH. Using this protocol in normal dogs, at least a 50% increase in serum T_4 was observed in 90% of dogs, and all dogs had an increase of at least 0.5 μg/dl (6.4 nmol/L) above baseline. With the lower dose of 0.2 mg TRH per dog, serum T_4 was shown to be maximal 4 hours after TRH administration. Perhaps the main limitation of the TRH stimulation test is that little information has been published on the effects of drugs and nonthyroidal illness.

Serum Free T_4 (FT$_4$) and T_3 (FT$_3$) Concentrations

The FT_4 concentration reflects the hormone available to cells at equilibrium and is the moiety that correlates best with the tissue thyroid status. Furthermore, the free T_4 concentration is not as likely to be affected by nonthyroidal illness or by drug therapy, although this statement has not been verified for many conditions in the dog or cat. The free fraction of T_4 by equilibrium dialysis is about 0.1% in the healthy euthyroid dog. The absolute concentration of FT_4 is very similar among species.

Two general methods are available for the determination of the FT_4 concentration. The standard technique involves the determination of the FT_4 fraction (% FT_4) by equilibrium dialysis and the total T_4 (TT$_4$) concentration by RIA. The absolute FT_4 concentration is then calculated as follows: FT_4 (ng/dl) = % FT_4 × TT_4 (μg/dl) × 10. Equilibrium dialysis, considered to be the method of choice for free hormone measurements, requires special dialysis chambers and, at this time, is not performed routinely by veterinary diagnostic laboratories. Commercial FT_4 kits, which theoretically measure the FT_4 concentration directly by RIA, are available and are being used by some veterinary diagnostic laboratories. Methodological idiosyncrasies (including steps requiring serum dilution) with these kits may result in artificially reduced or inaccurate values, particularly in the presence of serum hormone binding inhibitors (such as with nonthyroidal illness and drugs). Until proven useful in these situations in the dog and cat, these direct methods for FT_4 measurement should be interpreted with caution. Although when used alone, they are likely to provide at least the diagnostic information of TT$_4$ measurement. It is not yet clear if any or all methods will provide accurate FT_4 measurements when the serum binding of hormone is altered. Free T_3 measurements, performed by some diagnostic laboratories, have the same methodological problems as the commercial FT_4 measurements and have dubious diagnostic value for the same reasons as TT$_3$ concentrations.

Serum Total rT$_3$ Concentration

Reverse T_3, the inactive product of T_4 deiodination, may also be measured by specific RIA and is available in certain diagnostic and research laboratories. Reverse T_3 concentrations are best interpreted along with serum T_4 and T_3 concentrations. As virtually all circulating rT_3 is derived from T_4 secreted from the thyroid gland, a low serum rT_3 concentration provides confirmatory evidence for low amounts of free or available T_4. The usefulness of a rT_3 determination comes in the distinction of nonthyroidal causes of low serum total T_4 and T_3 from hypothyroidism; in certain nonthyroidal illnesses, a fall in serum T_3 is accompanied by a reciprocal increase in serum rT_3.

Circulating Antibodies to Thyroglobulin

Antibodies to thyroglobulin are often generated early in the course of thyroidal destruction associated with lymphocytic thyroiditis. Although only reported as a research tool, anti-thyroglobulin antibodies have been detected by enzyme-linked immunosorbent assay methods in 59% of hypothyroid dogs and potentially could provide a tool for the early diagnosis of lymphocytic thyroiditis. The clinical significance of positive anti-thyroglobulin titers must still be established. It is not clear whether autoantibodies are the cause or effect of the disease. However, because their incidence is significantly higher in hypothyroid dogs, routine measurement is likely to have clinical value particularly in following dogs in the early stages of the disease.

The incidence of antibodies to thyroglobulin in normal dogs was 13%, and higher incidence than normal has been seen in dogs with other autoimmune diseases. Measurement of anti-thyroglobulin antibody may have value for early recognition of autoimmune thyroiditis and for purposes of genetic counseling.

SPECIAL CASE-ANTIBODIES AGAINST THYROID HORMONES. In a subset of human and canine patients with anti-thyroglobulin antibodies, the thyroglobulin acts as a hapten to immunize the animal against thyroid hormone itself. When high autoantibody titers are reached, they have the potential for interfering with the hormone immunoassay measurements. This situation should be suspected in a dog with an apparently extremely high value of T_4 or T_3 in the face of clinical and historical evidence of hypothyroidism. Apparent elevations in serum thyroid hormones can be seen in certain assays, and other methodologies will result in an undetectable or very low result. For reasons that are not clear, the incidence or recognition of anti-T_3 antibodies appears to be greater than for anti-T_4 antibodies. The clinical significance of anti-thyroid hormone antibodies is primarily in their indication of the diagnosis of lymphocytic thyroiditis and the confusion they create for the interpretation of thyroid function tests. It appears clear now that dogs with normal serum T_4 concentrations (before or after levothyroxine treatment) and undetectable serum T_3 concentrations were not "poor converters" of T_4 to T_3 as had been suggested; they were dogs with anti-T_3 autoantibodies whose serum T_3 was measured in an assay in which the presence of autoantibodies results in an artifactually low result. In most situations, the presence of antibodies has no influence on the choice of thyroid medication because the capacity of the antibodies is small and is easily saturated.

Endogenous Serum TSH Concentrations

The measurement of basal endogenous serum TSH and TSH following TRH administration has proven to be extremely important for the early diagnosis of hypothyroidism in humans. Basal and TRH-stimulated serum TSH concentrations are invariably elevated in primary hypothyroidism. Humans with secondary and tertiary hypothyroidism and low serum T_4 concentrations generally have low serum TSH concentrations. Because TSH is a species-specific glycoprotein, attempts to use commercially available anti-human TSH RIA kits have generally failed to measure anything of diagnostic usefulness, and a valid canine-specific TSH assay is not yet commercially available.

Simultaneous Analysis of Multiple Tests in the Diagnosis of Hypothyroidism

Formulae combining the results of multiple single tests have been proposed to improve the diagnostic accuracy of a single blood sample. In a study that examined total T_4, free T_4 by direct RIA, total T_3, cholesterol, triglycerides, and pre-

TSH and post-TSH T_4 concentrations, the best accuracy in the diagnosis of hypothyroidism, based on the success in predicting a response to replacement therapy, was obtained by the following relation: $K = 0.5 \times$ basal T_4 concentration (nmol/L) + T_4 increment following TSH (nmol/L) (or $K = 6.4 \times$ basal T_4 concentration (μg/dl) + $12.9 \times T_4$ increment following TSH (μg/dl)). All dogs with a K value less than 15 were considered hypothyroid. Dogs with a K value greater than 30 were considered euthyroid. In dogs with a K value between 15 and 30, the results were equivocal. Other diagnostic tests, such as a valid free T_4 measurement, scintigraphy, or a therapeutic trial, might be indicated. Of the combination of static tests, the following relation between free T_4 and cholesterol was found to give the highest diagnostic accuracy as a screening test: $0.7 \times$ free T_4 (pmol/L) − cholesterol (mmol/L) or $9 \times$ free T_4 (ng/dl) − $0.027 \times$ cholesterol (mg/dl). Values less than -4 virtually confirmed hypothyroidism, while values greater than $+1$ ruled it out. With intermediate values, a TSH stimulation test was performed to aid in confirming the diagnosis. These formulae should be established for each laboratory's normal range.

Thyroid Radionuclide Uptake and Imaging

While only available at certain referral institutions, quantitation thyroidal radioiodine uptake using external γ camera imaging evaluates the functional capacity of the thyroid, including the endogenous secretion of TSH and the dietary iodine intake. Even in the absence of dietary factors, thyroid radioiodine uptake measurement can be a relatively insensitive diagnostic test for hypothyroidism and is impractical for routine clinical use. Therefore, thyroid uptake determinations are no longer used as a general screening test for canine hypothyroidism but are reserved as an aid in characterizing congenital defects of thyroid hormone synthesis.

Thyroid Biopsy

While not often practical, the histologic examination of a biopsy of the thyroid gland obtained at surgery is a definitive means of differentiating the primary and secondary forms of hypothyroidism. In primary hypothyroidism, there is loss of thyroid follicles resulting from either lymphocytic thyroiditis or thyroidal atrophy. In dogs in which the hypothyroid state is secondary to TSH deficiency, the thyroid follicles become distended with colloid and the lining epithelial cells become flattened.

Therapeutic Trial for Diagnosis of Hypothyroidism

The institution of thyroid replacement therapy in the absence of confirmatory laboratory evidence (serum T_4 or TSH stimulation test) has been suggested as a valid diagnostic step in an animal suspected to be hypothyroid. Although the major factor cited in defense of this practice is the cost of the diagnostic testing for the owners, it should be emphasized to the owners that replacement therapy is generally necessary for the remainder of the animal's life. Therefore, an incorrect diagnosis can also be quite expensive, a delayed diagnosis of another disease could be detrimental, and diagnostic procedures following a therapeutic trial with equivocal results can be quite difficult to interpret because secretion of the normal thyroid gland is inhibited by this procedure. Retesting of thyroid function with a TSH stimulation test should not be performed prior to 6 to 8 weeks following discontinuation of replacement therapy.

If a therapeutic trial is to be attempted, the following guidelines are suggested: (1) Make every attempt to rule out nonthyroidal illnesses using history, physical examination, routine laboratory, and other appropriate testing. (2) Decide on a criterion by which the success of the therapy will be judged (for example, greater than 50% regrowth of hair on flanks). (3) Decide on the manner and time when the therapy will be reevaluated according to the criteria chosen (for example, at 4 and 8 weeks). (4) Administer an appropriate dosage of levothyroxine using a brand name preparation twice daily (see Treatment below). (5) Decide on the next course of action if therapy is unsuccessful or only partially successful.

Nonthyroidal Factors Altering Thyroid Function Tests in the Dog

The diagnosis of thyroid hypofunction has become more complicated with the recognition that basal serum total concentrations of the thyroid hormones T_4 and T_3 may be profoundly lowered by nonthyroidal illnesses. At the very least, these changes are clinically relevant when the diagnosis of hypothyroidism is being considered. However, they may also be important as protective phenomena associated with the body's response to illness and nutritional state and, therefore may help prognosticate survival of serious illness.

The effects of nonthyroidal illness on thyroid hormone metabolism (the euthyroid sick syndrome) are less well characterized in the dog than in humans. A lowering of serum TT_3 alone (the low T_3 syndrome) is less likely to be observed than is the lowering of both TT_4 and TT_3 (the low T_4 state of medical illness) where the low TT_3 occurs secondary to a lowered TT_4 from which it is derived. Although no information is available in the dog, reductions in serum TT_4 concentration in severe medical illness predict a higher mortality rate.

Figures 62-8 through 62-11 summarize the effects of various physiological, pathophysiologic, and pharmacologic factors on the available tests of thyroid function in the dog. Most of the time, a careful history, physical examination, laboratory screening tests, and common sense will allow one to distinguish nonthyroidal illness from hypothyroidism. In most species, reductions in thyroid hormone concentrations in nonthyroidal illness appear to serve as a protective mechanism against the catabolism of illness. Therefore, until further information is available in the dog, thyroid replacement therapy of nonthyroidal illness is not recommended and may be contraindicated.

Recommendations for Routine Performance of Thyroid Function Tests

In the absence of a valid canine TSH RIA, the ideal test or combination should: (1) take into consideration valid (or at least predictive) measurement of the free T4 concentration in order to factor out the binding effects of drugs and nonthyroidal illness, and (2) assess thyroid functional reserve. Although not proven, the measurement of basal free T_4 (free fraction by equilibrium dialysis and total T_4 by RIA or by a validated direct RIA) and a serum total T_4 concentration after TSH should provide the most useful diagnostic combination of tests now available (see Fig. 62-7).

Diagnosis of Hypothyroidism in the Cat

Tentative diagnosis in suspected adult cats should be based on the clinical signs described above together with a history of surgical thyroidectomy or treatment with radioiodine for hyperthyroidism. For the same reasons as in the dog, the definitive diagnosis of iatrogenic or spontaneous feline hypothyroidism should be confirmed by the finding of a subnormal resting serum T_4 concentration that fails to rise adequately 6 hours after administration of bovine TSH (1.0 IU/kg, IV, maximum 5 U). A normal response is a T_4 concentration after TSH that either is 2.0 to 3.0 µg/dl (26–39 nmol/L) higher than the basal serum T_4 value or exceeds the normal normal range of basal T_4 concentrations (~4 µg/dl or 51 nmol/L in most laboratories). In kittens with documented hypothyroidism, other procedures (*e.g.*, thyroid scanning, thyroid biopsy) should be considered to identify the etiology of thyroid insufficiency.

MANAGEMENT

Once the clinical presentations are recognized and the diagnosis is made, the treatment of this disorder is very straightforward. The goal of hormone administration in an endocrine deficiency state is the reversal of the pathophysiologic effects of deficiency in a manner that mimics the natural pattern of secretion and metabolism of that hormone. Care should be taken in initially confirming the diagnosis because inappropriate therapy, while relatively benign, may delay an accurate diagnosis. Furthermore, therapy in virtually all cases is lifelong and, considered over that time frame, may be expensive.

Thyroid hormone preparations can be classified into the following groups: crude hormones prepared from animal thyroid, synthetic levothyroxine, synthetic triiodothyronine, and synthetic combinations of L-T_4 and L-T_3. Each group will be discussed individually with recommended or reported treatment protocols.

Crude Thyroid Products

Thyroid hormone products derived from thyroid tissue from hog, sheep, or cattle are available in the forms of desiccated thyroid. There appear to be no good reasons to continue to use these products for replacement therapy. Problems that include a highly variable content of T_4 and T_3, unphysiologically high ratios of T_3/T_4, and short shelf-life, outweigh the lower cost of these products.

Synthetic Levothyroxine

Thyroxine is the thyroid hormone replacement compound of choice for virtually all indications. It is generally formulated and used as levothyroxine sodium for oral administration. Injectable forms are also available for the rare indication of myxedema coma (see below). Thyroxine is the treatment of choice for hypothyroidism for the following reasons: levothyroxine is the main secretory product of the thyroid gland; and levothyroxine is the physiological prohormone. Administration of levothyroxine does not bypass the cellular regulatory processes controlling the production of the more potent T_3 from T_4. When starting an animal on a thyroid replacement product, it is recommended to start with a brand-name product with which broad experience has been obtained and use this product until a distinct clinical response has been seen. If no response is seen at a reasonable dose after a period of at least 4 to 6 weeks, and normal serum T_4 concentrations are achieved after administration, then the diagnosis should be reevaluated.

The reported oral replacement doses for levothyroxine sodium (*e.g.*, Synthroid, Soloxine, Levothroid, Levoid, Noroxine, Thyro-Tab) range from a total dose of 0.02 mg/kg to 0.04 mg/kg daily.

It has also been proposed that dosage be calculated according to body surface area (0.5 mg/M^2), which is proportional to the metabolic rate. When dosed on a body weight basis, large breed dogs have a greater tendency to develop thyrotoxicosis or at least elevated serum T_4 concentrations. It is common practice to administer T_4 in single or divided doses. As thyroid replacement therapy is begun in a hypothyroid animal, a common practice is the division of the oral daily dose (*e.g.*, 0.02 mg/kg twice a day). Because of the significant intracellular capacity for storage of T_4, the initial oral doses of thyroid hormone may be substantially distributed into tissue stores. Eventually,

DRUG	TT4	FFT4	FT4	TT3	TrT3	TSH Stim.	TRH Stim.
Steroids	↓			↓	↑then↓	N	
PTU	N or↓			↓	↓		
Contrast Dyes	↑			↓	N		
Antiepileptics	↓	↑(DPH)		N	N	N	
Furosemide		↑					
Phenylbutazone	↓					N	
Fatty Acids		↑					
Propranolol	N			N	N	N	

Figure 62–11. The effect of drugs on thyroid function tests. (Blank spaces indicate lack of information.)

some hypothyroid animals may be maintained on once-daily T_4 therapy despite the fact that the serum half-life for T_4 in normal dogs is 10 to 16 hours. Although the serum T_4 concentration might be high at one time of the day and low at another, the tissue response reflects the average concentration. It is also important that once-daily administration leads to greater compliance by the owners.

In an animal that has responded to twice-daily therapy, the reappearance of clinical signs of hypothyroidism on a once-daily regimen should be a signal to return to the successful twice-a-day regimen.

Gradual introduction of hormone is ideal, particularly in individuals with decreased ability to metabolize T_4 and increased risk to the development of thyrotoxicosis, such as hypoadrenal, aged, cardiac, or diabetic patients. In these groups, it is recommended to use divided dose protocols and to increase the daily dose in 20% to 25% increments (*e.g.*, 0.1 mg/M^2, 0.2 mg/M^2, 0.3 mg/M^2, 0.4 mg/M^2, 0.5 mg/M^2 divided twice a day) over a period of 4 to 8 weeks. Glucocorticoid replacement should begin prior to thyroid replacement therapy in patients with concomitant hypoadrenocorticism (*e.g.*, hypopituitarism). This therapy assures steroid replacement prior to the increase in metabolic demand for endogenous steroids, which follows correction of hypothyroidism. In all cases, because the metabolism of thyroid hormone changes with correction of hypothyroidism, dosage regimens should be reassessed by clinical or laboratory criteria after at least 4 weeks of initial therapy.

As in the dog, the recommended treatment for feline hypothyroidism is daily administration of levothyroxine, using an initial dose of 0.1 to 0.2 mg/day. This dosage should subsequently be adjusted on the basis of the cat's clinical response and post-pill serum T_4 evaluation (as described below under Monitoring for the dog). Complete resolution of clinical signs can usually be expected in cats with adult-onset iatrogenic hypothyroidism. However, the mental dullness and dwarfism that develops in kittens with hypothyroidism usually persist because of delayed period of time from onset to diagnosis in these cats.

Synthetic L-Triiodothyronine

Although T_3 is the active intracellular hormone, there are few valid reasons to use this product for replacement therapy and some good reasons not to use it. Triiodothyronine "replacement" is not physiological and bypasses the final cellular regulatory step of 5'-deiodination of T_4. At the present time, it cannot be recommended that T_3 therapy be instituted in the low T_3 syndrome associated with nonthyroidal illness. Because of its higher oral bioavailability, it may be used to improve the clinical response in an animal with demonstrated or suspected poor T_4 absorption in which post-therapy serum T_4 and T_3 concentrations are low despite increases in the oral T_4 dose. Triiodothyronine therapy may be indicated when thyroid replacement is necessary with the simultaneous administration of drugs that inhibit the conversion of T_4 to T_3, such as with glucocorticoids.

Anecdotal reports suggest that a small fraction of hypothyroid dogs do not respond to levothyroxine therapy because they convert T_4 to T_3 poorly. Triiodothyronine or combination T_4/T_3 therapy has been recommended in these cases as an adjunct to T_4 or as sole therapy. The most likely cause of apparently low serum T_3 concentrations and normal or high T_4 concentrations following T_4 therapy is the presence of anti-T_3 antibodies. As previously discussed, this observation is an artifact: it is recommended that the levothyroxine dose be increased until a clinical response is seen and that the serum T_3 concentration be ignored.

A divided oral dose regimen for L-T_3 (Cytobin, Cytomel) of 4 to 6 µg/kg three times a day or possibly twice a day appears necessary to maintain serum T_3 concentrations without high peaks, which appear to be associated with signs of thyrotoxicosis.

Synthetic Combinations of L-T_4 and L-T_3

The use of commercial combinations of synthetic L-T_4 and L-T_3 has little rational basis in human or veterinary medicine. These preparations, containing a 4 : 1 mixture of T_4 and T_3, were designed to mimic the ratio of T_4/T_3 in thyroidal secretion.

A variety of dosage schemes have been proposed, but the most common suggests dosing according to the T_4 content and division of the dose to account for the shorter serum half-life of T_3. Administration of these preparations will commonly lead to a low normal to normal serum T_4. Increasing the dose to normalize serum T_4 can result in high serum T_3 concentrations and can potentially produce thyrotoxicosis due to the T_3 content. These preparations share the disadvantages of the T_3 preparations: increased cost, increased complexity of dosing regimes, and a higher incidence of thyrotoxic signs.

Treatment of Myxedema Coma

Because of the extremely high mortality associated with untreated myxedema coma, it is essential that treatment be instituted promptly and vigorously as soon as the diagnosis is made. Treatment should include an intravenous dose of levothyroxine prepared for injection (100–200 µg), passive rewarming (wrapping in blankets, etc.), and mechanical respiratory support as needed. Therapy for shock must include glucocorticoids and fluid and electrolyte replacement (see Chapter 4). Oral T_4 therapy can be instituted when the animal stabilizes.

Side Effects (with Overdose)

Except for financial reasons, the concern about mild overreplacement is minimal in most cases as the dog is very resistant to the development of thyrotoxic signs. This resistance to iatrogenic thyrotoxicosis is the result of the dog's capacity to efficiently clear thyroid hormone through biliary and fecal excretion. Animals on replacement therapy, particularly with a T_3 containing product, can develop signs of thyrotoxicosis; however, the incidence at recommended doses is rare. Animals should be monitored for signs suggesting an overdose including polyuria, polydipsia, nervousness, weight loss, increase in appetite, panting, and fever. Diagnosis is confirmed by elevated serum

T_4 or T_3 concentrations and the amelioration of signs by temporary discontinuation of therapy.

PATIENT MONITORING

The success of thyroid replacement therapy should first and foremost be judged on the presence or lack of clinical improvement. Before therapy is begun, the clinician and the owners should have a clear idea of the goals of therapy and the time frame over which they can reasonably be expected to be achieved. The reversal of changes in hair coat and body weight should be assessed only after a period of 1 to 5 months on therapy. In cases in which clinical improvement is marginal or signs of thyrotoxicosis are seen, the clinical observations can be supported by therapeutic monitoring of serum thyroid hormone concentrations, also called "post-pill testing." Clearly, the documentation of distinctly elevated serum T_4 concentrations following T_4 administration and elevated serum T_3 concentrations following T_3 administration, concomitant with signs of thyrotoxicosis, confirm an overdose. The interpretation of "post-pill" serum thyroid hormone concentrations in cases of suspected underdosing can be more complicated because the timing of sampling may be critical to the proper interpretation. Ideally, therapeutic monitoring should not be attempted until steady-state conditions are reached, minimally 1 month after the initiation of therapy. With once daily T_4 administration, the peak serum concentrations of T_4 generally should be in the normal to high normal range 4 to 8 hours after dosing and should be low normal to normal 24 hours after dosing. Given the dog's resistance to signs of thyrotoxicosis, it may be reasonable and adequate to check the serum T_4 concentration 24 hours after the previous day's dose, expecting it to still be in the normal range. Animals on twice daily administration probably can be checked at any time, but peak concentrations can be expected at the middle of the dosing interval (4–8 hours), and the nadir just prior to the next dose. Once the animal's dose is stabilized, once or twice yearly checks of serum T_4 (with or without

T3) concentrations will guard against impending therapeutic failure or toxicosis.

If serum T_3 concentrations are to be measured following T_4 administration, something not routinely recommended, they should be interpreted carefully together with the serum T_4 results and, most importantly, the clinical response. Low serum T_3 and T_4 concentrations, together with a poor clinical response, suggest an underdose or inadequate bioavailability (absorption). With T_3 administration, serum concentrations are reported to peak 2 to 3 hours after administration. Serum T_4 concentrations are routinely low or undetectable; remaining endogenous thyroidal T_4 secretion is inhibited because of the suppression of pituitary TSH secretion by T_3.

If clinical signs of hypothyroidism remain despite the use of reasonable doses of thyroid hormone, the following possibilities must be considered in approximate order of likelihood: (1) the dose or frequency of administration is improper; (2) the owners are not complying with instructions or are not successfully administrating the product; (3) the animal may not be absorbing the product well or is metabolizing or excreting it too rapidly; (4) the product is outdated; or (5) the diagnosis is incorrect.

If the condition is treated appropriately, the prognosis for resolution of all clinical signs is excellent. Thyroid hormone replacement therapy is invariably a life-long requirement.

ADDITIONAL READING

Feldman EC, Nelson RW, eds. Hypothyroidism. In: Canine and feline endocrinology and reproduction. Philadelphia: WB Saunders, 1987: 55.

Ferguson DC. Effect of nonthyroidal factors on thyroid function tests in the dog. Compendium of Continuing Education 1988; 10:1365.

Ferguson DC. Hypothyroidism: Many presentations, one treatment. Small animal geriatrics: Viewpoints in veterinary medicine. Proceedings of the 1989 Alpo Symposium on Geriatrics, 1989: 30.

Ferguson DC. Thyroid function tests in the dog. Vet Clin North Am [Small Animal Pract] 1984; 14:783.

Ferguson DC. Thyroid hormone replacement therapy. In: Kirk RW, ed. Current veterinary therapy IX. Philadelphia: WB Saunders, 1986: 1018.

Lothrop CD, Tamas PM, Fadok VA. Canine and feline thyroid assessment with thyrotropin releasing hormone response test. Am J Vet Res 1984; 45:2310.

Larsson MG. Determination of free thyroxine and cholesterol as a new screeening test for canine hypothyroidism. Journal of the American Animal Hospital Association 1988; 24:209.

Milne KL, Hayes HM. Epidemiological features of canine hypothyroidism. Cornell Vet 1981; 71:3.

Peterson ME, Ferguson DC. Thyroid diseases. In: Ettinger SJ, ed. Textbook of veterinary internal medicine, 3rd ed. Philadelphia: WB Saunders, 1989: 1632.

THE MUSCULOSKELETAL SYSTEM

11

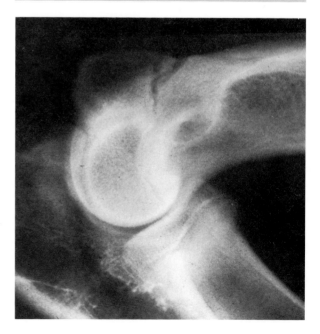

63

LAMENESS

David L. Holmberg

Animals are commonly presented to the practicing veterinarian with the owners' complaint of limping or lameness. Occasionally, a specific history of trauma is known, but more frequently the onset of signs will be reported to have occurred over a period of days, often without a clear indication of which leg is involved. In these situations, it is essential that the clinician be able to localize the problem based on signalment, history, and physical examination. Further, the practitioner must understand the type of injuries that may occur in the different anatomic locations and form a plan that efficiently confirms the diagnosis.

It is not the function of this chapter to be an exhaustive review of all of the causes of lameness in the small animal patient. Volumes have been written on the diagnosis and treatment of orthopedic injuries and disease. Only the most common diseases will be cited. Similarly, only a few well-established modes of therapy will be suggested. Treatments for the specific diseases will vary depending on financial constraints of the owners, equipment availability, and the development of new surgical techniques. It is the goal of this chapter to assist the clinician in developing their own unique but logical "lameness plan of attack" that suits their practice situation.

CAUSES

The most common etiology of lameness in the small animal patient (especially the cat) is trauma. Seen in animals of all ages, this can be the result of an impact with a moving object (the bumper of a car), collision with a stationary surface (jumping from a height), or dynamic forces acting on an internal structure (rotation, distraction, or hyperextension of a joint). This type of injury can cause any combination of soft tissue bruising or laceration, bone fracture, luxation/subluxation of a joint, or rupture of the surrounding ligamentous structures (Table 63-1).

Developmental problems can result from a variety of growth disturbances in the immature animal. These disturbances can either directly effect the cartilage and subchondral bone of young dogs (osteochondritis dissecans, fragmented coronoid process and Legg-Calvé-Perthes), result from the failure of ossification centers to unite (ununited anconeal process), or occur because of asynchronous growth in two adjacent bones (radius curvus). Developmental problems with conformation can also lead to lameness both directly (hip dysplasia) and secondarily (patellar luxation).

Inflammatory lesions of the bone or soft tissue

Table 63–1 *Clinical Signs Associated With the Common Causes of Lameness*

Causes	Signs
Arthrosis	Stiff, painful gait, often worse following rest, or during cold, damp weather Lameness initially improves with activity Crepitus palpable in joint
Fractures	Non-weight-bearing lameness Local pain and swelling Abnormal mobility or angular deformity of the limb Crepitus palpable in area
FCP, UAP, or OCD of the distal humerus	Forelimb lameness which worsens with activity Elbow is circumducted during advancement Crepitus palpable in elbow joint Joint effusion
Hip dysplasia or Legg-Calvé-Perthes Disease	Progressive lameness in hindleg(s) Pain/crepitus elicited during palpation of the hip joint Subluxation of hip joint during palpation "Ortolani sign" (hip dysplasia)
Hypertrophic osteodystrophy	Single or multiple limb involvement Warm, painful swelling of the metaphysis of the affected bone Fever and anorexia are variable with severity of disease
Infraspinatus muscle contracture	Tenderness in shoulder area following strenuous activity Nonpainful lameness by the time abnormal leg carriage is noted Adduction of the elbow and external rotation of leg Atrophy of infraspinatus muscle
Luxations and ligamentous injury	Abnormal mobility of the affected joint Abnormal anatomic relationships of the adjacent bones Pain and crepitus elicited by palpation of the joint Local swelling and joint effusion in acute cases Thickening of the joint capsule in chronic cases
Neoplasia or osteomyelitis	Weight-bearing or non-weight-bearing lameness Local pain and swelling Infections may be associated with fever and local drainage
Osteochondritis dissecans	Shortened stride in the affected leg Pain elicited on palpation of the affected joint Joint effusion in acute cases Thickening of the joint capsule in chronic cases
Panosteitis	Shifting leg lameness lasting days to weeks Severe pain elicited by deep palpation of the affected bone Fever and general malaise
Patellar luxation	Normal gait with occasional lameness, "skipping" Non-weight bearing lameness associated with ligamentous damage Bowlegged stance with toes internally rotated (medial luxation) Knock-knee stance with toes externally rotated (lateral luxation) Palpation of luxating patella, most noticeable with leg extended
Radius curvus	Lateral deviation of the carpus External rotation of the carpus Anterior bowing of the radius Distal subluxation of the ulna in the elbow joint

can be either septic or sterile. Septic problems are almost always secondary to surgical manipulations or foreign body penetration. Sterile inflammation of the joints may be immune-mediated (see Chapter 64), the result of poor bone and cartilage development or acute mechanical stresses. Osteoarthrosis, or degenerative joint disease (DJD), is a common complication of joint damage and is caused by chronic instability or abnormal cartilage wear. This damage may be primary, as a result of day-to-day wear on articular cartilage, or secondary from abnormal joint conformation or laxity. Typically DJD infrequently causes acute lameness but rather is characterized by chronic discomfort and osteophyte production.

Neoplasms of the appendicular skeleton are a less common cause of lameness and affect middle-aged to older animals. These tumors can be either primary or metastatic lesions from distant parts of the body and are typically located in the metaphyseal region of the long bones. This etiology should be considered in any mature animal presented with an acute lameness that has no previous history of skeletal problems.

PATHOPHYSIOLOGY

With few exceptions, all diseases or conditions that result in lameness do so by causing pain. Pain of bone origin is created by the stimulation of sensory neural tissue associated with the periosteum, endosteum, or surrounding soft tissues. This pain can be humorally-mediated secondary to inflammation or be caused directly by mechanical stimulation or damage to the neural structures associated with the bone or joint. For clarity, the pathophysiology of some of the causes of lameness listed in Table 63-1 will be addressed individually.

Arthrosis, or, more correctly, degenerative joint disease (DJD), starts when stresses applied to the cartilage result in the exposure of collagen and the release of degradative enzymes. This process results in an inflammatory synovitis and joint effusion. When abnormal forces are applied to the joint and cause tension on its surrounding ligamentous structures, the response is the development of periarticular osteophytes. Although

these osteophytes are usually not a primary source of pain, they can become large enough to rub against the inner surface of the joint and create more irritation. The exact mechanism of osteophyte production is unclear, but they are probably the most commonly recognized radiographic finding with joint disease in small animals (Fig 63-1).

Fractures, generally speaking, occur when the external forces applied to a bone are greater than its structural strength. These forces can usually be divided into components of compression, distraction, rotation, and angular deformity (Fig. 63-2). Depending on the combination of stresses, the resultant fracture will either be complete or a fissure; transverse, oblique, or spiral; simple, comminuted, or multiple; open or closed. The anatomic location or acknowledgement of specific forces responsible for the injury can further characterize fractures such as physeal, intercondylar, compression, or avulsion. The presence of certain "weak points" can predispose a bone to fracture. Such weaknesses would include actively growing physes, poor mineralization, or neoplasia.

Fragmented coronoid process (FCP) is most commonly seen in the large and giant breeds of dogs. Although it may occur by itself, FCP is often associated with osteochondritis of the distal medial condyle of the humerus and may itself be a form of this condition. As such, the etiopathogenesis of FCP is probably related to a phenotypic predilection for the disease and brought to fruition by over nutrition and trauma to the newly developing joint.

Hip dysplasia (HD) is a conformational defect commonly seen in the larger and chondrodystrophoid breeds of dogs. Because HD results from a combination of congenital malformation and environmental stresses, its incidence varies greatly between breeding populations. Basically, HD is a problem associated with a disparity between skeletal growth and muscle development, which results in an instability of the hip joint. Components of the condition are: poor fitting of the femoral head into the acetabulum; a shallow acetabulum, which gives minimal coverage of a flattened femoral head; valgus deformity and thickening of the femoral neck; and secondary DJD. Because HD develops during the first years

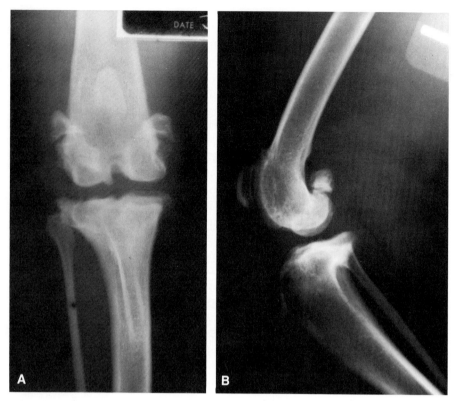

Figure 63–1. *A–P (A) and lateral (B) views of a stifle with DJD. Roughening of the periarticular surfaces is due to the presence of osteophytes.*

of the dog's life, it is not considered a true congenital defect.

Hypertrophic osteodystrophy (HOD) is a disease that occurs during the rapid growth phase of young, large breed dogs. The etiology is unknown, but abnormal vitamin C metabolism has been suggested. The disease is also seen in animals whose diets have been oversupplemented with protein, minerals, and vitamins. Presenting clinical signs are pyrexia, lameness of one or more limbs, and warm, painful swelling of the metaphyseal area of the affected long bones. Radiographic changes of HOD are enlargement and mottled density of the metaphyseal region. Ab-

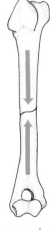
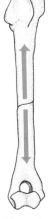
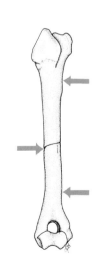

Compression   Distraction   Rotation   Angular deformity

Figure 63–2. *Graphic depiction of forces acting on normal bone that, when excessive, can cause fractures.*

normal subperiosteal and extraperiosteal new bone development is seen in some cases.

Infraspinatus muscle contracture is a condition seen in working or sporting dogs. The exact etiology is unknown, but traumatic rupture of the muscle followed by inflammation, fibrosis, and contracture have been suggested. Although painful in the early stages, most animals presenting with this are lame because of the mechanical restrictions it causes in the shoulder joint. This type of contracture has also been reported to occur, less frequently, in the supraspinatus and semitendinosus muscles.

Legg-Calvé-Perthes disease, also called avascular necrosis of the femoral head, is a disease of unknown etiology that occurs exclusively in young, small breed dogs. Starting as a necrosis of the bone within the femoral head, weight bearing results in the collapse of the femoral head or fracture of the femoral neck (Fig 63-3). Joint incongruity and instability causes progressive DJD.

Ligamentous injury and subluxation can occur without complete disruption of the integrity of the joint. An example of this occurrence is rupture of the anterior cruciate ligament (RACL), which is one of the most common orthopedic injuries seen in small animal practice. Usually caused by either hyperextension of the stifle or forceful internal rotation of the tibia, RACL occurs in dogs of all ages and breeds. Most commonly it is a disease of obese, adult dogs. It is rare in cats. It has been postulated that an underlying degeneration of the ligaments or joint instability is responsible for predisposing to the injury as frequently both anterior cruciate ligaments will rupture within months of each other. The stifle instability created by the RACL leads to DJD, thickening of the joint capsule, and osteophyte production within weeks of the injury. Tearing of the medial meniscus often occurs concurrently with the RACL when the tibial plateau moves forward relative to the femoral condyles (Fig. 63-4). Rupture of the

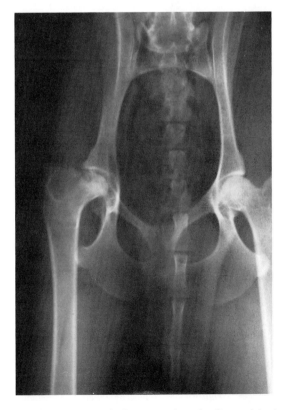

Figure 63–3. *Radiograph showing unilateral collapse of the femoral head in an animal with Legg-Calvé-Perthes disease and secondary arthritic changes.*

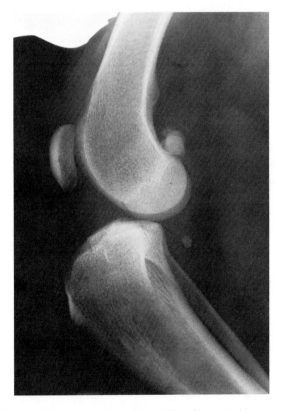

Figure 63–4. *Lateral radiograph of a stifle with a RACL, demonstrating abnormal displacement of the proximal tibia relative to the femoral condyles.*

medial collateral ligament is also reported but much less frequently. Medial patellar luxation is also a common finding with RACL in small dogs, although it is not known which disease occurs first.

Luxations, like fractures, are the result of excessive force, this time being applied to a joint. Complete rupture of the normal stabilizing ligamentous structures usually occurs, as does damage to the joint capsule and articular cartilage. Because of the anatomic configuration and direction of the normally applied external forces, joints tend to luxate in consistent ways. The femoral head is generally displaced craniodorsal out of the acetabulum. Tearing of the teres ligament or avulsion of a portion of the femoral head are common sequelae (Fig. 63-5). The humeral head most often luxates laterally in larger breeds and medial to the glenoid in small dogs. The elbow nearly always luxates lateral to the distal humerus. Carpal injuries are usually caused by hyperextension and therefore end with the distal radius anterior to the carpal bones. Luxations of the hock joint are variable depending on the forces applied during the injury and are usually accompanied by fracture of one or both malleoli.

Because articular cartilage requires normal weight bearing to force nutrients throughout its thickness, articular cartilage will be replaced by less functional fibrocartilage if left outside of an intact joint for more than 7 days. This fibrocartilage is less able to withstand the rigors of weight bearing and is usually associated with the development of DJD.

Osteochondritis dissecans (OCD) is characterized by the separation of articular cartilage from its subchondral bone. Although the exact etiology is unknown, the rapidly growing cartilage becomes too thick for the efficient diffusion of nutrients through its deeper portions. Similarly, the subchondral bone outgrows its endosteal blood supply and a line of cleavage forms between the two degenerating layers. With the normal trauma associated with daily life, a flap of cartilage may form on the articular surface. Formation of this flap will cause inflammation within the joint, and it may break free to become a joint mouse. Seen in young, rapidly growing large breed dogs, OCD is commonly associated with overnutrition and hypersupplementation. Often bilateral, OCD is most commonly found on the caudal aspect of the humeral head (Fig. 63-6) but also occurs on the medial aspect of the lateral femoral condyle, medial trochlear ridge of the hock, and the medial humeral condyle. Affected dogs should be screened for other developmental defects such as hip dysplasia.

Panosteitis is a disease of unknown etiology

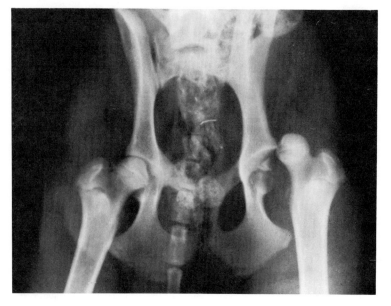

Figure 63–5. Typical radiographic appearance of a dorsally luxated femoral head with avulsion of a bone fragment at the insertion of the teres ligament.

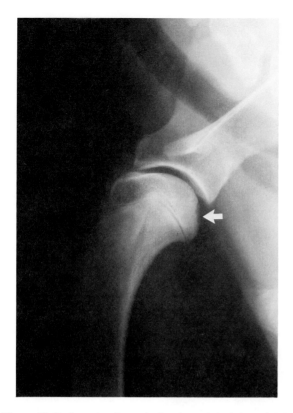

Figure 63–6. *Lateral radiograph showing a lytic lesion of OCD (arrow) on the caudal articular surface of the humeral head.*

that results in a shifting leg lameness in large and giant breed dogs. Seen only in young rapidly growing dogs, panosteitis typically resolves in one site, is followed by a period of normalcy, and recurs in another limb. Although no reason has been found for the pain, new bone formation within the medullary cavity of affected bones is characteristic of the disease.

Patellar luxation begins with a varus or valgus deformation of the femoral neck, which causes an abnormal pull of the quadriceps muscle on the tibial crest. This traction will result in rotation of the crest towards the side of the tension and malalignment of the patella with the trochlear groove. In small breed dogs (varus hip deformation) this displacement will be medial, while lateral luxation is more common in the large breeds (valgus hips) (Fig. 63-7). The affected animals are often graded 1 to 4, depending on the severity of the luxations, secondary changes to the tibia and distal femur, and the clinical signs. Traumatic

luxation can also occur either medially or laterally, and medial luxation has been seen secondary to RACL or hip luxation.

Radius curvus is a condition that follows the traumatic closure of the distal ulnar physis. Because of its conical shape, the distal ulnar physis is unable to slip sideways along its layer of hypertrophying cells as can the flattened physis of the distal radius. The result is that any overt stresses to the radius and ulna will cause a compression injury (Salter-Harris V fracture) and cessation of growth in the distal ulnar physis (Fig. 63-8). As the radial physes continues to produce bone, the ulna forms a "bowstring" effect, forcing the anterior bowing, external rotation, and valgus deviation of the distal radius and carpus (Fig. 63-9). Radius curvus has been reported to occur following 25% of all fractures involving the radius and ulna.

Ununited anconeal process (UAP) occurs because of failure of the anconeal process' center of ossification to unite with the rest of the ulna by 5 months of age (Fig. 63-10). The result is an increase in joint instability, trauma to the articular cartilage, and DJD. Although the etiology of UAP isn't known, its frequent occurrence in German shepherds, basset hounds, and Saint Bernards suggests a genetic predisposition.

CLINICAL SIGNS

As would be expected, the most common clinical sign shown by the lame animal is a lack of full weight bearing on one or more of its legs. In the extreme case, this lack will result in carrying of the leg. More frequently, the discomfort will result in gait abnormalities, such as a shortening of the limb's anterior swing phase during the stride, raising of the patient's head when the affected forelimb is supporting the weight, or dropping of the hip when the affected hindlimb is weight bearing. Occasionally, the lameness will be subtle enough that exacerbation of the problem with forced exercise such as running or climbing stairs is necessary. Conversely, many arthritic problems improve with moderate activity, and the animals will in fact have "warmed out" of the

(Text continues on page 878)

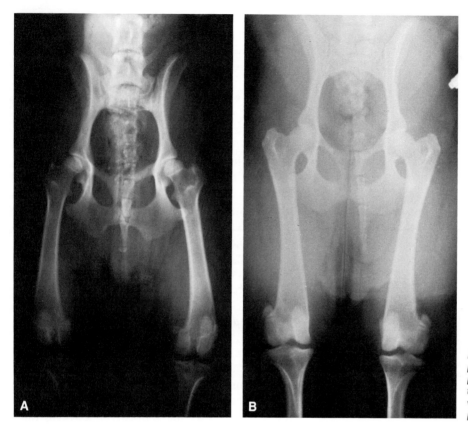

Figure 63–7. Radiographs comparing a mildly dysplastic dog (A, patellas seated on lateral surface of trachlear groove) with those of a dog with hips having varus deformity (B, patellas positioned medially).

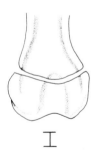

I

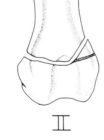

II

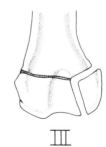

III

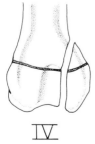

IV

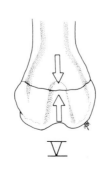

V

Figure 63–8. Graphic depiction of the Salter-Harris classification of physeal fractures 1–5.

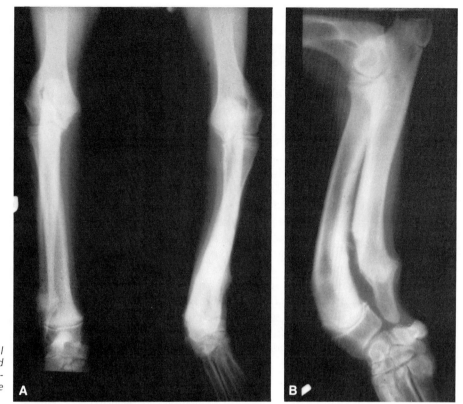

Figure 63–9. A–P (A) and lateral (B) radiographs of a dog affected with unilateral radius curvus secondary to premature closure of the distal physis of the left ulna.

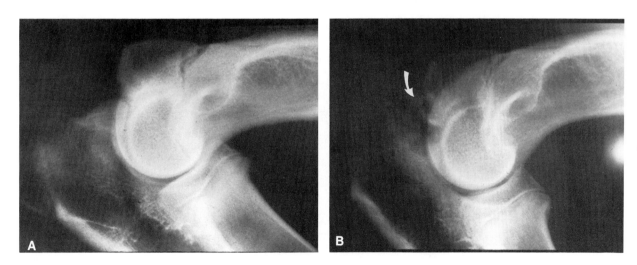

Figure 63–10. Lateral radiographs comparing a normal elbow (A) and one affected with UAP (B, arrow).

lameness by the time they reach the veterinary practice. This improvement is also true with a mild lameness that the patient may choose to ignore in favor of the distractions attendant with the examination.

Local pain, swelling and abnormal mobility are classic signs of acute diseases affecting a bone or joint. Conversely, disuse atrophy of the muscles of the affected leg and stiffness of affected joints are more common with chronic conditions. Difficulties arise when dealing with the athletic dog or very stoic animal. Abnormalities that may be difficult to detect in the examination room can become significant in the "high performance" dog required to run at great speeds or for long distances. Further, well-trained animals may not react to the same stimulus that sends a less accommodating patient into fits of screaming and biting. It therefore behooves the clinician to consider the animal's lifestyle and personality during the examination and observe it closely during palpation of the affected part for the more subtle signs

of discomfort such as changes in breathing patterns and pupillary dilation.

Rarely, a disease that results in a lameness will become so severe that the animal becomes debilitated or anorexic. These signs usually accompany inflammatory conditions and are associated with a fever or elevated white blood cell count (see Table 63-1).

DIAGNOSTIC APPROACH

Signalment should be the first information considered when presented with a lame animal. Often this process will eliminate many diseases from the list of possible differentials (Fig. 63-11). Adult animals are, for example, not commonly affected by developmental defects, nor are juveniles often bothered with neoplasia. Similarly, toy breeds are not candidates for developing hip dysplasia, and larger dogs do not get Legg-Calvé-Perthes disease. Some conditions, such as RACL, affect animals of all age groups and breed.

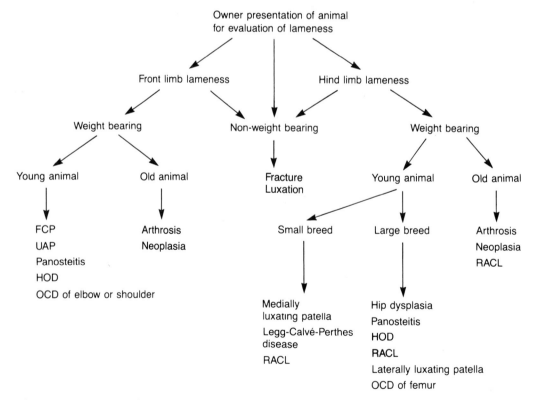

Figure 63–11. *History and signalment of an animal presented for lameness.*

An accurate history regarding the clinical course of the lameness will assist in narrowing the list of differentials as well as preparing the clinician for the type of physical examination findings to expect. A shifting leg lameness, for example, is not a common complaint and would be highly suggestive of panosteitis in the young dog. Further, a clinician examining a patient presented with a hindleg lameness of a month's duration should not expect to find the typical anterior drawer motion found in a stifle with a RACL.

It should be noted that no hard and fast rules exist when considering the history of lameness. As with the clinical signs, a stoic animal may have no history of pain associated with a developmental defect until later in life when its DJD becomes severe. Likewise, a timid dog may carry its leg long after a relatively minor injury has healed. The owners' relationship with the dog must also be considered when taking a history. Lack of a previously observed lameness may not be significant if the animal is newly acquired or is allowed to roam freely.

Physical examination is mandatory for the evaluation of the lame animal and should cover all major body systems. No doubt, a consistent approach to the lameness examination, which includes the palpation of all muscles, bones, and joints and tests the major appendicular neural reflexes and sensation, is the most useful tool available for localization of these injuries. It is especially important in the multiple trauma patient in which obvious damage, such as a fracture, may mask the signs of other important injuries, such as a luxation. It is always a good idea to examine all normal limbs prior to palpation of the injured portion. This act will serve not only to instruct the clinician as to what is normal for that animal but will help to put the patient at ease and make the evaluation of the painful area more informative. For example, when palpating a dog's stifle, forceful contraction of the quadriceps muscles due to apprehension can mask any evidence of an anterior drawer sign in a strong dog. Figure 63-12 is a flow diagram of the physical examination findings associated with some of the common causes of lameness in small animals.

Radiographic evaluation of the localized lesion will usually be indicated to confirm the tentative diagnosis, determine the prognosis, and form a rational plan of treatment. Some form of sedation or anesthesia is recommended to position the patient adequately. This action will reduce the expense incurred by repeating less than optimal films and will allow completion of the radiographic study without risking undue radiation exposure to the clinical staff. A minimum of two views of each suspected area are required and the same views of the normal opposite limb are useful for comparison. These "control" radiographs are especially useful when dealing with the developmental defects in young animals.

Fractures, luxations, and some of the developmental defects have obvious radiographic changes that are diagnostic for the specific condition (Table 63-2). The most common radiographic changes seen in the lame animal are bony remodelling and osteophyte production secondary to inflammation and the application of abnormal stresses to joints. While no good correlation is found between the radiographic appearance of arthritic changes and clinical signs, extensive secondary DJD generally worsens the prognosis for the surgical correction or medical management of the disease.

Arthrocentesis (Chapter 80) is not a routine part of a lameness examination and should only be performed in patients that have already had complete physical and radiographic examinations. Indications for joint aspiration are evidence of multiple joint involvement, joints that show gross evidence of inflammation (local heat and swelling), systemic illness associated with the lameness, or radiographic signs consistent with immune-mediated disease (Chapter 64).

MANAGEMENT

Treatments for the diseases that cause lameness are aimed at total correction (fracture repair), minimizing ongoing damage (stabilization of a RACL), or salvage of an abnormal but functional limb (excision arthroplasty). The following is a brief summary of the current treatments and prognosis for some of the common causes of lameness in small animals.

(Text continues on page 882)

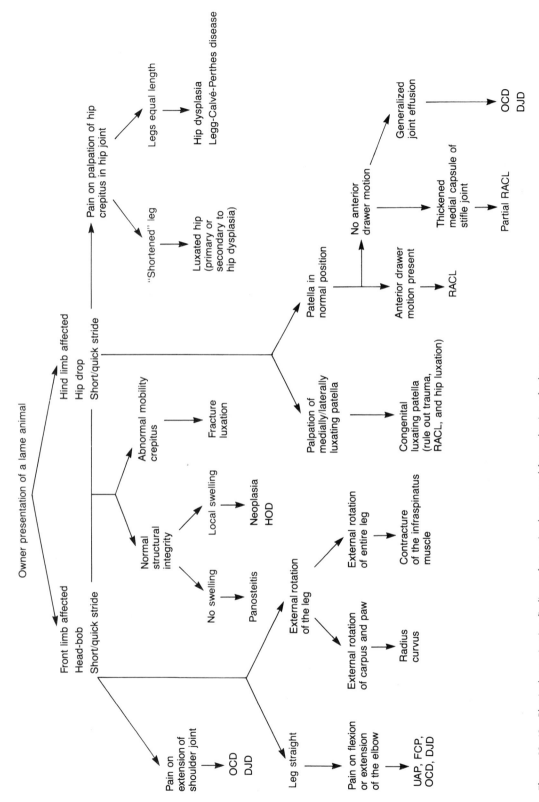

Figure 63–12. *Physical examination findings of an animal presented for evaluation of a lameness.*

Table 63–2 Radiographic Changes Associated With the Common Causes of Lameness

Causes	Radiographic Changes
Arthrosis	Sclerosis of the subcondral bone
	Roughening of the periarticular areas due to osteophyte production
	Joint effusion suggested by soft tissue swelling and prominence of intra-articular fat pad
Fractures	Loss of normal bone architecture and cortical integrity
FCP, UAP, or OCD of the distal humerus	All three conditions result in signs consistent with arthrosis (see above)
	UAP, additional finding of open anconeal physis after 20 weeks of age
	OCD, additional findings consistent with that disease (see below)
Hip Dysplasia	Subluxation and poor congruency of coxofemoral joint
	Shallow acetabulum with less than 60% coverage of the femoral head
	Flattened fremoral head and thickened femoral neck
	Periarticular osteophyte production
Legg-Calvé-Perthes Disease	Poor congruency of the coxofemoral joint
	Lucency within the femoral head and neck
	Flattening of the femoral head and collapse of the femoral neck
Hypertrophic osteodystrophy	Enlargement of the metaphysis
	"Granular" density in the metaphysis
	Abnormal subperiosteal and extraperiosteal new bone formation
Infraspinatus muscle contracture	No radiographic evidence of disease
Luxations and ligamentous injury	Abnormal anatomic relationships between the adjacent bones
	Avulsion fractures associated with ligamentous attachments
	Joint effusion and local soft tissue swelling
Neoplasia	Proliferation and destruction of bony tissues
	Most commonly localized in metaphyseal areas of long bones
	Does not involve or cross joints
Osteomyelitis	Periosteal proliferation with calcification
	Mottled lucency indicating bone destruction, most often around implants
	Local soft tissue swelling and loss of fascial detail
	Can extend throughout bone lengths and may involve joints
Osteochondritis dissecans	Flattening/dishing of the subcondral bone
	Dystrophic calcification of cartilage flap
Panosteitis	Blurring of trabecular patterns
	Loss of contrast between cortical bone and medullary cavity
	Mottled, increased density in the medullary cavity
	In the early stages of the lameness, no changes may be apparent
Patellar luxation	Medial* or lateral† displacement of the patella
	Varus* or valgus† deformity of the hip
	Distal third of the femur bowed medially* or laterally†
	Proximal third of the tibia bowed laterally* or medially†
	Relative medial* or lateral† deviation of the tibial crest
Radius curvus	Closed distal ulnar physis in the presence of an open distal radial physis
	Lateral deprivation of the carpus
	External rotation of the carpus
	Anterior bowing of the radius
	Distal subluxation of the ulna in the elbow joint

Arthrosis

The initial treatment of DJD is generally aimed at reducing the ongoing stresses on the joint by weight reduction and moderation of the exercise requirements of the animal. The medical control of the joint pain will do nothing to reverse the degenerative process but rather is aimed at managing the patient's discomfort. Analgesics should only be used after a diagnosis of DJD has been made. Removing the animal's discomfort makes it increasingly difficult to localize a lesion, and the ongoing damage to an unstable joint will become worse with the increased weight bearing. Many analgesics are available and the exact product prescribed will depend largely on the clinician's own preferences (Table 63–3). Currently, the systemic nonsteroidal anti-inflammatory drugs are the most common type used. The injection of intra-articular steroids is to be strongly condemned as they have been shown to speed the destruction of articular cartilage.

When an animal becomes refractory to analgesics, some form of surgical salvage may be needed. Excision arthroplasty can be done to prevent contact between the two sides of the joint, the goal being a non-painful pseudoarthrosis. The implantation of artificial joints is an option in some animals but is expensive and usually limited to larger dogs. Arthrodesis or joint fusion can be used successfully to stop pain from a degenerating joint but is generally not widely applicable in working or sporting dogs because of stress and break-down of the fused bones, implants, or adjacent joints.

Fractures

A discussion covering the surgical repair of fractures is not within the scope of this book. Suffice it to say, in deciding what technique to use, the veterinarian must assess the type of fracture, equipment, available expertise, personality, and future lifestyle of the patient.

Fractures that are comminuted, in which bone is missing, open fractures and fractures involving joints should be treated with internal fixation or external pin splintage. Conversely, fissures or fractures that involve only one bone of two bone systems (*e.g.,* radius and ulna) can usually be handled with a cast or other form of coaptation splintage.

Generally, external coaptation splinting entails less equipment for its application but requires greater postoperative monitoring than internal fixation. Animals that are expected to return to heavy work or high performance will probably benefit from the improved anatomic reduction and early return to function, which is usually achieved with internal fixation. Further, an animal that is difficult to handle, consistently chews off any form of coaptation, or that cannot be closely supervised after fracture repair should not be treated with a cast. Financial considerations do not play a great role in determining the

Table 63–3 *Commonly Used Analgesic Drugs for the Control of Pain Due to Degenerative Joint Disease*

Drug	Dose, Route and Frequency
Acetylsalicylic acid **Aspirin**	Dog: 10 to 25 mg/kg PO, b.i.d.–t.i.d. Cat: 10 mg/kg PO, q 48 hours
Phenylbutazone **Butazolidin**	Dog: 10 mg/kg PO, t.i.d. (max, 800 mg daily) Cat: Not recommended
Ibuprofen **Advil or Amersol**	Dog: 15 mg/kg divided PO, t.i.d. Cat: Not recommended
Piroxicam **Feldene**	Dog: 20 mg/kg PO, t.i.d. Cat: Not recommended
Efa-Z Plus	Dog and cat: See Appendix II

technique to be used for fracture repair. While the initial outlay for internal fixation is greater, the more frequent required rechecks and replacements of the external supports makes the long-term cost similar.

Fragmented Coronoid Process

The surgical treatment of FCP involves the removal of loose or damaged cartilage from the elbow via a medial arthrotomy. Early treatment will slow the progression of signs, but ongoing DJD may pose problems in working or sporting breeds.

Hip Dysplasia

The young animal with hip dysplasia should be restricted in its activity to minimize the trauma done to the articular cartilage secondary to subluxation. Physical conditioning, using non-concussive exercise such as swimming, may help muscle development and promote better seating of the femoral head into the acetabulum. Generally, the very young dog will go through a very painful period from 6 to 10 months of age. During this time, general joint laxity potentiates the pathologic luxation of the hips. Analgesics will help reduce the dog's pain but must be used conservatively so as not to remove all discomfort and promote ongoing trauma.

Corrective surgical procedures, such as triple pelvic osteotomy and varus osteotomy of the proximal femur, have been reported as techniques that can improve the congruency between the femoral head and acetabulum. Both procedures must be done while the animal is young enough to remodel the articular surfaces easily and before DJD has become extensive. Excision arthroplasty and total hip replacement are salvage procedures reserved for the animal that is no longer responsive to medical management of the DJD. Excision arthroplasty will have its best results when done in mature dogs less than 30 kg body weight. Young animals with active periosteum are more prone to exuberant callus pro-

duction and complications associated with rubbing between the bony surfaces causing pain. Giant breed dogs and very active working or sporting breeds may be candidates for total hip replacement. This procedure is currently very popular in certain facilities but the long-term results tend to be variable. Breakage of the implant and loosening at the implant bone interface are complications yet to be completely resolved.

Hypertrophic Osteodystrophy

Although self-limiting, symptomatic treatment with aspirin or corticosteroids (prednisone 0.5 mg/kg twice daily, orally) of the HOD patient may be indicated if the animal is febrile, incapacitated, or anorexic. Variable results have been achieved with vitamin C supplementation (500 mg daily, orally). The diet should be controlled in all cases, and supplementation with added protein, vitamins, and minerals should be discontinued. Recovery may take weeks but should be uneventful.

Infections

The successful treatment of osteomyelitis must entail the surgical removal of all devitalized tissue, loose foreign material, or bone fragments; culture and antibiotic sensitivity testing of the organism responsible; and the long-term use of appropriate systemic antibiotics. In my experience, the use of closed suction and continuous lavage have not made significant improvements in the treatment of these cases.

Infraspinatus Muscle Contracture

Transection and removal of a portion of the tendon of the infraspinatus muscle is curative for this condition. No appreciable residual lameness persists although the atrophy of the infraspinatus muscle is somewhat cosmetically objectionable in short-haired dogs.

Legg-Calvé-Perthes Disease

The early stages of this disease may be treated by strict rest and non-weight-bearing bandaging of the affected leg. Often, however, this treatment merely postpones surgical intervention as collapse of the femoral head, fracture of the femoral neck, and DJD usually necessitates excision arthroplasty. More consistently good results are achieved with early excision before significant muscle atrophy takes place and the animal becomes used to not walking on the affected leg(s).

Ligamentous Injury

Uncomplicated strains of muscles and tendons or sprains of ligaments are usually treated by strict rest and the application of heat to reduce the pain of muscle spasm. When the injury includes damage to the bony attachments or results in gross instability of the associated joint, some form of internal repair or stabilization is indicated. The most common injury of this type is the RACL. While it has been shown that small breeds of dogs can often achieve adequate stability and return to function without veterinary intervention, larger dogs with a RACL generally require some form of surgical repair. In spite of the multitude of reported techniques for the stabilization of the stifle, DJD will still progress in the affected joint due to the presurgical trauma to the articular cartilage and supporting structures.

Luxations

Replacement of a luxated joint should be performed as soon as the patient's general condition permits. Articular cartilage will only survive outside of an intact joint for approximately 7 days before being replaced with fibrocartilage. Also, the muscle contracture and fibrosis that occurs will make reduction progressively more difficult with time. Closed reduction of the luxation should be attempted whenever possible. Associated fractures or avulsion of the ligamentous structures surrounding the luxation generally necessitate open reduction and some form of internal stabilization. Postoperative external coaptation or sling bandaging is recommended

following either form of reduction. Prognosis is dependent on duration of the luxation and the attendant damage to the articular cartilage and the surrounding ligamentous structures.

Neoplasia

Currently, no curative treatment exists for bone cancer. Some long-term control and remission of primary bone tumors, however, has been achieved using a combination of amputation and chemotherapy (*e.g.*, cisplatin). Neoplasms metastatic to bone are currently not controllable and are generally an indication for euthanasia.

Osteochondritis Dissecans

Removal of the cartilage flap and debridement of the sclerotic subchondral bone is the treatment of choice for OCD. The long-term goal is that granulation tissue and later fibrocartilage will fill in the defect resulting in a pain-free articular surface. Depending on the location, the long-term prognosis for OCD ranges from good (humeral head), fair (elbow and hock), to poor (distal femur).

Panosteitis

No specific treatment exists for panosteitis. It is a self-limiting condition and will resolve with no lasting effects as the animal matures. Occasionally, symptomatic treatment with aspirin or corticosteroids may be indicated if the animal is febrile, incapacitated or anorexic.

Patellar Luxation

The technique used for correction of congenital patellar luxation is dependent on the severity of the deformity. Transplantation of the tibial crest is usually done to realign the patella with the trochlear groove. Deepening of the trochlear groove is also recommended if it is too shallow. Correctional osteotomies of the femur and tibia have been reported for those animals that have severe tilting of the tibial plateau, but arthrodesis of the stifle joint may be more efficient in these cases.

Acute traumatic luxation of the patella may be treated effectively by closed reduction and bandaging. In chronic conditions or if reluxation occurs, open reduction and imbrication of the joint capsule and associated retinaculum is indicated. Occasionally, retention sutures from the patella to the appropriate fabella are needed to prevent reluxation in chronic cases.

Radius Curvus

Presuming closure of the distal ulnar physis is the cause of the deviation, osteotomy of the ulna has been reported to be an effective treatment. The goal is to permit continued longitudinal development of the radius; as such this procedure is limited to those dogs in which the distal radial physis is still open. Surgical closure of the medial side of the radial physis has also been performed in an attempt to encourage straightening of an already deviated limb. In animals that have a significant deformity and minimal continued growth potential, a correctional osteotomy of the radius is needed. This procedure must take into account the lateral deviation and external rotation of the carpus, anterior bowing of the radius, attempt to realign the carpal and radiohumeral joints, and permit proper articulation of the often subluxated proximal ulna.

Ununited Anconeal Process

Treatment of UAP may take two forms. Stabilization of the anconeal process by interfragmentary screw fixation, which attempts to maintain the normal anatomy of the elbow joint, has been reported. The more common approach is removal of the loose fragment. Progressive DJD is unavoidable with either treatment, but most dogs retain limb function with some loss in joint mobility.

PATIENT MONITORING

The long-term success of the treatment of lameness depends on the accuracy of the diagnosis, specificity of the treatment, client education, and long-term monitoring of the condition. Most of the diseases that have been discussed result, more or less, in the development of degenerative changes within the joint. If not appropriately handled, this unavoidable progression can, at best, result in the owners' dissatisfaction and, at worst, result in euthanasia of the patient. Good education for the owners is needed to ensure that they understand the natural history of the disease and that, if the changes become clinically significant, medical management of the problem can be approached in a stepwise fashion. Further, it is important to stress that this treatment is often a control situation so the owners do not become frustrated by the lack of a cure.

ADDITIONAL READING

Alexander JW. Pathogenesis and biochemical aspects of degenerative joint disease. Compendium of Continuing Education 1980; 11:961.

Alexander JW, Richardson DC, Selcer BA. Osteochondritis dissecans of the elbow, stifle and hock—A review. J Amer Anim Hosp Assoc 1981; 17:51.

Arnoczky SP. The cruciate ligaments: The enigma of the canine stifle. J Small Anim Pract 1988;29:71.

Barr A, Houlton J. Clinical investigation of the lame dog. J Small Anim Pract 1988; 29:695.

Berzon JL, Howard PE, Covell SJ et al. A retrospective study of the efficacy of femoral head and neck excisions in 94 dogs and cats. Vet Surg 1980; 9:88.

Bohning RH, Suter PF, Hohn RB, Marshall J. Clinical and radiologic survey of canine panosteitis. J Amer Vet Med Assoc 1970; 156:870.

DeCamp CE, Hauptman J, Knowlen G et al. Periosteum and healing of partial ulnar ostectomy in radius curvus of dogs. Vet Surg 1986; 15:185.

Fox SM, Bloomberg MS, Bright RM. Developmental anomalies of the canine elbow. J Amer Anim Hosp Assoc 1983; 19:605.

Lust G, Rendano VT, Summers BA. Canine hip dysplasia: Concepts and diagnosis. J Amer Vet Med Assoc 1985; 187:638.

Olmstead ML, Hohn RB, Turner TM. A five-year study of 221 total hip replacements in the dog. J Amer Vet Med Assoc 1983; 183:191.

Paatsama S, Rokkanen P, Jussila J et al: A study of osteochondritis dissecans of the canine humeral head using histological, OTC bone labelling, microradiographic and microangiographic methods. J Small Anim Pract 1971; 12:603.

Salter RB, Harris WR. Injuries involving the epiphyseal plate. J Bone Joint Surg 1963; 45:587.

64

IMMUNE-MEDIATED JOINT DISEASE

Stephen A. Kruth

The most common joint abnormality in the dog is degenerative joint disease, a condition associated with daily wear and tear on the joint and minimal inflammation (*arthrosis*). Inflammatory joint disease (*arthritis*) occurs less frequently and is mediated by both infectious and non-infectious mechanisms. Infectious arthritis can be either secondary to penetrating trauma to the joint or associated with systemic infection. In our experience, arthritis due to the hematogenous spread of organisms is usually confined to one (monoarticular) or a few (pauciarticular, less than five) joints and tends to involve the large joints of the hip, shoulder, and intervertebral discs. Recently, systemic infections with *Borrelia burgdorferi* and *Ehrlichia canis* have been associated with polyarthritis (more than five joints affected) in dogs.

The second, more common group of inflammatory arthropathies is thought to be mediated by immunologic disturbances, which lead to inflammation of the synovial membrane; these disorders are the focus of this chapter. Although infectious agents may supply the initiating antigen in these disorders, they cannot be recovered from the joints. Immune-mediated arthritis tends to affect the distal appendicular joints and is often polyarticular.

Some types of inflammation lead to destruction of the articular cartilage; this is termed *erosive arthritis*. Joint inflammation that does not cause destruction of the articular surface is called *non-erosive arthritis*. A classification of inflammatory joint disease is given in Table 64-1.

The incidence of immune-mediated joint disease is unknown but appears to be relatively low. Non-erosive joint disease is much more common than erosive disease; both forms are well documented in the dog and cat.

CAUSES

In non-infectious arthritis, joint inflammation is the result of an immune response. The inciting cause is usually not identified but is thought to be one of the following: viral infection (*e.g.*, feline syncytia-forming virus), bacterial infection (usually chronic, such as bacterial endocarditis), mycotic infection, parasitic infestation (such as heartworm disease), vaccine antigen, or drug related (*e.g.*, trimethoprim sulfadiazine).

Polyarthritis has also been described in cats. The non-erosive form is usually idiopathic but has been associated with systemic lupus

887

Table 64–1 *Classification of Arthritis*

INFECTIOUS ARTHRITIS
(ORGANISMS RECOVERABLE FROM JOINTS)

BACTERIAL
Penetrating wound
Hematogenous spread from infected focus
Mycoplasma
Borrelia burgdorferi (dog)
Ehrlichia canis (dog)

NON-INFECTIOUS (IMMUNE-MEDIATED) ARTHRITIS

EROSIVE
Rheumatoid-like arthritis

NON-EROSIVE
Immune-complex deposition leading to inflammation. Possible antigenic sources include:
    Infectious organisms
      Viral: feline calicivirus
      Bacterial: endocarditis, diskospondylitis, urinary tract
      infection, pyometra, severe periodontitis, and others
      Fungal: deep mycoses
      Parasitic: *Dirofilaria immitis*
    Vaccines
    Drugs (Trimethoprim-sulfadiazine)
    Neoplasia
    Chronic inflammatory bowel disease
    Systemic lupus erythematosus
    Idiopathic (most common)

erythematosus (SLE), respiratory tract infections, enteritis, and myeloproliferative disorders. Feline syncytia-forming virus has been associated with *feline chronic progressive polyarthritis,* a rheumatoid-like disorder.

PATHOPHYSIOLOGY

The non-erosive polyarthropathies are thought to be caused by immune-complex deposition in the synovium. Immune complexes activate the complement cascade, which in turn acts as a recruitment signal to neutrophils. Inflammation within the joint follows.

The erosive polyarthropathies appear to have a somewhat different pathophysiology. Native immunoglobulin (usually IgG) reacts with a triggering antigen, is altered, and becomes antigenic in turn. An immune response (usually IgM) is directed at the newly antigenic IgG, leading to immune complex formation and synovitis. Cell-mediated immunity also plays an important role in joint inflammation through the elaboration of a variety of cytokines.

A fibrovascular extension of the perichondrial synovial membrane (termed *pannus*) grows over the articular cartilage and invades the cartilage matrix. Inflammation at the cartilage-pannus junction leads to erosion of the articular cartilage and eventual collapse of subchondral bone. Periarticular structures may also become involved, with tenosynovitis, bursitis, and subcutaneous cysts developing.

In both types of arthritis, pain and stiffness result from joint inflammation. Systemic signs of inflammation, such as fever and malaise, often follow. Other organs and cells, such as muscle, kidneys, brain, spinal cord, red blood cells, and platelets, may also undergo immune-mediated injury.

CLINICAL SIGNS

Non-erosive polyarthritis may affect any breed and age of dog or cat. In dogs, it tends to occur more frequently in medium and large breeds. Erosive polyarthritis occurs more frequently in small and toy breeds, with an average age of onset of 4 to 5 years (range of 8 months to 13 years). A relatively mild form of erosive polyarthritis has been described in greyhounds but has not been well documented.

The clinical signs of non-erosive polyarthritis are sometimes non-specific. Anorexia and depression may be the only change noted by the owners. Vague, sometimes shifting or cyclic lameness may occur. There may be a history of recent vaccination, medication, or illness; the remaining history may be unremarkable.

The physical findings may also be non-specific. Fever is usually present, and signs of an underlying disorder (*e.g.,* endocarditis, neoplasm, heartworm disease) may be found. A stiff gait and reluctance to move may be present. Lymphadenopathy and muscle wasting are less frequent findings.

Distended joints are not always present, although joints may feel warmer than other areas of the limb and may be painful when manipulated.

Erosive arthritis is often associated with soft tissue swelling around the distal appendicular joints, and crepitus and reduced range of motion may be found. The conformation of the animal is usually normal except in advanced rheumatoid arthritis, where marked limb angulation secondary to joint collapse may develop.

A steroid-responsive suppurative meningitis associated with non-erosive polyarthritis has been described in dogs. In addition to the signs mentioned above, these animals may have cervical rigidity and spinal pain.

The findings of malaise, stiff gait, and fever are suggestive of polyarthritis. It may be difficult to establish a short list of differential diagnoses at this point; it may not even be possible to narrow the abnormality to the musculoskeletal system. Many of the patients that we have seen have been treated with antibiotics for non-specific infectious disorders, usually without effect. Because many of these animals are febrile for no apparent cause, they are often referred to our clinic for diagnosis of fever of unknown origin (see Chapter 6). Some animals are referred for neurologic evaluation; others have received steroids, usually with improvement occurring, only to have signs recur when the steroid is withdrawn.

DIAGNOSTIC APPROACH

The goals of the clinical evaluation of an animal with the above signs are to establish if polyarthritis is present, to determine if it is erosive or not, and to identify an underlying cause. The workup should include a complete blood cell count (CBC), serum biochemistry profile, urinalysis, test for heartworm disease, chest radiographs, multiple arthrocenteses, and radiographs of the joints. Serologic testing for *Borrelia burgdorferi* and *Ehrlichia canis* should be requested if the dog was at risk for exposure to these organisms (see Chapter 79).

Hematologic abnormalities may include varying degrees of leukocytosis and occasionally a non-responsive anemia of chronic inflammatory disease. A Coombs positive anemia may be present, although this finding is uncommon in our experience. Fibrinogen levels are usually elevated, as is the erythrocyte sedimentation rate (ESR). Abnormalities in serum biochemistry may reflect primary disorders; no abnormalities are specific for any form of polyarthritis. Proteinuria may occur if the glomeruli have been damaged by immune complex disease (see Chapter 45). The CBC, biochemistry profile, and urinalysis are important baseline data to collect because the drugs used to manage immune-mediated polyarthritis are often associated with bone marrow and liver toxicity.

We have seen several dogs with non-erosive polyarthritis that were positive for heartworm disease (see Chapter 25). The parasite may be the source of antigen in these patients and should be eliminated. Chest radiographs will aid in the diagnosis of heartworm disease and other chronic infectious and neoplastic conditions.

Arthrocentesis (see Arthrocentesis in Chapter 80) is the key diagnostic procedure for these patients. This procedure is safe and simple to perform and can often be done without sedation. We aspirate both carpi and both stifles routinely; other joints should be aspirated if they appear to be involved. The extended analysis of synovial fluid is presented in Table 64-2; however, the finding of greater than 5% neutrophils is diagnostic for joint inflammation. Absolute cell counts are often not performed because of the small amount of fluid collected. A non-septic inflammatory response in the synovial fluid does not differentiate non-erosive from erosive joint disease. The presence of LE cells is diagnostic for SLE.

Although bacterial polyarthritis is uncommon, it must be ruled out. Organisms and neutrophils with toxic changes can usually be seen on synovial fluid smears. Synovial fluid culture is usually positive in these cases, although culture of synovial biopsy tissue appears to be more sensitive. The inability to demonstrate a primary focus of infection elsewhere in the animal is probably the most important evidence against this disorder.

Because chronic bacterial infections, such as bacterial endocarditis and pyelonephritis, may act as sources of antigen leading to immune-complex disease (as opposed to causing hematogenous showering of joints with bacteria and development of bacterial polyarthritis), it may be

Table 64–2 *Joint Fluid Analysis*

Condition	Clarity	Mucin Clot*	Nucleated Cells/μl	% PMN†
Normal	clear	good	0 to 3000	0 to 6
Degenerative joint disease	clear	good–fair	0 to 5000	0 to 12
Non-erosive forms	turbid	good–poor	4500 to 375,000	15 to 95
Erosive forms	turbid	fair–poor	3000 to 87,000	17 to 95
Septic arthritis	turbid, bloody	poor	40,000 to 270,000	43 to 99

* *Joint fluid gels and returns to liquid form on gentle shaking. Spontaneous clotting is suggestive of inflammation. Mucin is a glycoprotein found in joint fluid; the mucin clot test evaluates the quality of mucin. One drop of joint fluid is mixed on a slide with three drops of 2% acetic acid solution and left to stand for one minute. A "good" score is given is there is a tight ropy clump in clear fluid. A "fair" score is given to a soft clot in slightly cloudy solution, and a "poor" score is given if there are only a few flecks of precipitate in a cloudy solution.*
† *PMN = polymorphonuclear leukocyte*

prudent to obtain blood and urine cultures prior to instituting immunosuppressive therapy. While the majority of animals do not have an underlying infection, we have had to manage the occasional dog that became septic after immunosuppressive therapy was initiated.

Usually, no radiographic changes are found in non-erosive disease, even after several months of clinical signs. Radiographs of joints with erosive arthritis may be normal at initial presentation; however, a variety of lesions will become apparent with time. Periarticular soft tissue swelling, periarticular osteophyte production, and a decrease in epiphyseal trabecular bone density are usually present, as are subchondral cysts. Eventually, joint collapse may occur.

If polyarthritis is found and an underlying problem cannot be identified, autoimmune disease should be suspected. The anti-nuclear antibody (ANA) titer should be evaluated, and a rheumatoid factor (RF) test performed. Rheumatoid factor is the antibody directed toward the altered immunoglobulin; a positive RF test is present in approximately 40% to 70% of cases of rheumatoid arthritis. We have found markedly elevated ANA titers in several patients, suggesting SLE. The sensitivity, specificity, and positive predictive values for these tests are not known in veterinary medicine. Also, the normal values for both ANA and RF tests vary widely between laboratories. It has been reported that the latex fixation RF test used in humans is not applicable to dogs, while the sheep red blood cell agglutination (Rose-Waaler) test is useful.

Synovial biopsy may be helpful in arriving at a tentative diagnosis of immune-mediated joint disease. In erosive arthritis, villous hyperplasia of the synovium and stromal lymphoid infiltrates are found. In non-erosive disease, mild to moderate inflammation without villous hyperplasia occurs.

In humans, specific clinical, radiographic, and laboratory criteria must be met before the diagnosis of rheumatoid arthritis is made. Bennett and others (Bennett, Additional Reading) have proposed similar schemes based on those used in people; however, their utility in dogs and cats has not been evaluated. Table 64-3 presents one set of proposed criteria.

MANAGEMENT

The prognosis for the patient with non-erosive immune-mediated polyarthritis is variable and difficult to predict. If caused by a drug or vaccine, the prognosis for return to normalcy may be excellent. If caused by an underlying chronic disease, the prognosis depends more on the prognosis for that disorder. Some dogs with SLE respond to prednisone alone, while others are non-responsive to aggressive therapy with prednisone and cytotoxic drugs. The prognosis for dogs with idiopathic polyarthritis is variable; some dogs return to normal function with a relatively short course of prednisone therapy, while some require long-term management with high levels of prednisone and cytotoxic drugs to control the signs.

Table 64–3 *Criteria for the Diagnosis of Canine Rheumatoid Arthritis*

1. Stiffness after rest
2. Pain or tenderness in at least one joint
3. Swelling (not bony overgrowth alone) in at least one joint
4. Swelling of at least one other joint within 3 months
5. Symmetrical joint swelling
6. Subcutaneous nodules over bony prominences, on extensor surface or in juxta-articular regions
7. Destructive radiographic changes typical of rheumatoid arthritis
8. Positive test for rheumatoid factor
9. Poor mucin clot from synovial fluid
10. Characteristic histopathologic changes in the synovial membrane
11. Characteristic histopathologic changes in nodules

Classical *rheumatoid arthritis is diagnosed when seven criteria are satisfied;* definite *rheumatoid arthritis when five are satisfied. Two of criteria 7, 8, and 10 must be satisfied in all cases.*

Dogs with rheumatoid arthritis have a poor prognosis for return to normal function, and joint collapse is likely to occur. In our experience, these dogs are not candidates for arthrodesis because many joints are involved. The most common reason for euthanasia of patients requiring long-term management is probably the owners' dissatisfaction with the side effects of the drugs.

The first goal of management is to control any underlying disorder that may be causing the inflammation. Any drug that was started before the arthritis developed should be withdrawn, and infectious and neoplastic disorders must be managed.

The next goal of management is to control joint inflammation. In our experience, dogs with immune-mediated polyarthritis do not respond adequately to nonsteroidal anti-inflammatory drugs.

Prednisone, due to its potent anti-inflammatory action and moderate immunosuppressive effects, is the cornerstone of therapy for these patients. Many animals show rapid and dramatic clinical improvement when given 2 to 4 mg/kg daily. We continue this dose for 2 weeks and then evaluate synovial fluid cytology. If it has returned to normal, we begin to taper the dose. We usually go directly to alternate day therapy and re-evaluate synovial fluid in 2 weeks. If the cytology is still normal, we taper the dose over 2 to 3 months, depending on how well the animal tolerates the drug.

If the animal does not respond to prednisone, or if it requires levels of prednisone that cause unreasonable side effects for long-term management, a cytotoxic drug should be started. These drugs are immunosuppressive, altering humoral and cell-mediated immunity, and also have some anti-inflammatory actions. The drugs that have been used most frequently in the dog and cat are cyclophosphamide and azathioprine. Some authors suggest that the cytotoxic drug should be stopped after the animal responds, and then the prednisone can be decreased. Because many of our patients are started on cytotoxic drugs due to their intolerance of prednisone, we follow the opposite strategy of tapering the steroid and continuing the cytotoxic drug. If long-term cytotoxic drugs are required, we use azathioprine because it is associated with fewer side effects than cyclophosphamide.

Combination therapy with prednisone and cyclophosphamide is the current induction management of choice for animals with rheumatoid arthritis. After the signs have stabilized, an attempt should be made to substitute azathioprine for cyclophosphamide.

Chrysotherapy (gold salt therapy) is effective in humans with rheumatoid arthritis; however, its indications, efficacy, and safety have not been thoroughly evaluated in dogs and cats. The mechanism of action of gold salts is not known, although they appear to have an immunoregulatory action on helper T lymphocytes. Anti-inflammatory, anti-enzymatic, and immunosuppressive effects have also been documented.

These drugs are given by weekly injection, making therapy difficult for some of the owners. An oral preparation (triethylphosphine gold), which may make chrysotherapy easier to deliver, has recently become available (Serra, Additional Reading).

The management of immune-mediated polyarthritis is summarized in Tables 64-4 and 64-5.

PATIENT MONITORING

The goals of patient monitoring in dogs with immune-mediated arthritis are to monitor the progression of the disease and to monitor for signs of treatment-induced problems.

The monitoring of the disease process is somewhat complicated by the fact that dogs may show dramatic clinical improvement when therapy is started, yet synovial cytology may still be abnormal. For this reason, we evaluate synovial fluid periodically.

Reduction in the level of a positive ANA titer can be followed, although it is rare for it to become negative.

The complications of steroid therapy are many and well known. Iatrogenic Cushing's syndrome is monitored by physical examination and periodic serum biochemistry profiles (see Chapter 59). Dogs receiving glucocorticoids are at risk for the development of urinary tract infection (and possible sepsis) without the development of clinical signs; periodic urine culture is therefore recommended (see Chapter 46).

The main complication arising from the use of cytotoxic drugs is bone marrow suppression, especially of the myeloid cell line. Periodic white blood cell counts are recommended; if the count falls below 2,500 cells/μL (or 2.5×10^9/L), the drug should be discontinued until the count returns to normal, then resumed at 75% of the original dose. Cyclophosphamide metabolites may induce a sterile hemorrhagic cystitis, which may be difficult to control if allowed to progress. The owners should be instructed to discontinue the drug if hematuria occurs, and azathioprine should be substituted.

Table 64–5 *Management of Erosive Polyarthritis*

CYTOTOXIC DRUGS

Prednisone and cyclophosphamide are started together. Once in remission, it may be safer to discontinue cyclophosphamide and switch to azathioprine. Doses are given in Table 64–4.

GOLD SALTS

Triethylphosphine gold (Auranofin, Smith Kline): 0.05 to 0.2 mg/kg b.i.d. to a maximum of 9 mg/day PO until remission, then taper dose.

Side effects (incidence not known): dermatitis, stomatitis, thrombocytopenia, anemia, leukopenia, proteinuria, diarrhea.

The indications, toxicities, and response to gold salts are not well described in the dog and cat.

Table 64–4 *Management of Nonerosive Polyarthritis*

Drug	Dosage
Prednisone	2 to 4 mg/kg daily PO, taper dose after remission is achieved
Cyclophosphamide	2.5 mg/kg/day PO to animals less than 10 kg; 2.0 mg/kg/day PO for dogs 10 to 35 kg; 1.5 mg/kg/day PO for dogs more than 35 kg
	Give for 4 consecutive days, followed by 3 days rest. Continue cycles until remission achieved.
	Side effects: bone marrow suppression, sterile hemorrhagic cystitis
Azathioprine	2.0 mg/kg daily PO until signs are controlled, then every other day
	Side effects: bone marrow suppression (usually less than that associated with cyclophosphamide)

Note: long-term low-dose exposure to cytotoxic drugs may be teratogenic and carcinogenic. These drugs should be handled accordingly (Swanson, Additional Reading).

Complications reported in humans receiving parenterally administered chrysotherapy include cutaneous reactions, stomatitis, proteinuria, and hematologic complications. Oral gold therapy appears to be less toxic, with diarrhea being the major side effect. A CBC, platelet count, serum biochemistry profile, and urinalysis should be monitored periodically.

ADDITIONAL READING

Beal KM. Azathioprine for treatment of immune-mediated disease of dogs and cats. J Am Vet Med Assoc 1988; 192:1316.

Bennett D. Immune-based erosive inflammatory joint disease of the dog: Canine rheumatoid arthritis. I. Clinical, radiological and laboratory investigations. Journal of Small Animal Practice 1987; 28:779.

Bennett D, Nash AS. Feline immune-base polyarthritis: A study of thirty-one cases. Journal of Small Animal Practice 1988; 29:501.

Bennett D, Taylor DJ. Bacterial infective arthritis in the dog. Journal of Small Animal Practice 1987; 29:207.

Cowell RL, Tyler RD, Clinkenbeard K, Meinkoth JH. Ehrlichiosis and polyarthritis in three dogs. J Am Vet Med Assoc 1988; 8:1093.

Fernandez FR, Grindem CB, Lipowitz AJ, Perman V. Synovial fluid analysis: Preparation of smears for cytologic examination of canine synovial fluid. J Am Anim Hosp Assoc 1983; 19:727.

Gorman NT, Werner LL. Immune-mediated diseases of the dog and cat. IV. Therapy and immunodiagnosis. Br Vet J 1986; 142:498.

Kornblatt AN, Urband PH, Steere AC. Arthritis caused by *Borrelia burgdorferi* in dogs. J Am Vet Med Assoc 1985; 186:960.

Long RE. Potential of chrysotherapy in veterinary medicine. J Am Vet Med Assoc 1986; 188:539.

Medleau L, Miller WH. Immunodiagnostic tests for small-animal practice. Compendium of Continuing Education 1983; 5:705.

Meric SM. Canine meningitis: A changing emphasis. Journal of the College of Veterinary Internal Medicine 1988; 2:26.

Pedersen NC, Pool RR, O'Brien T. Feline chronic progressive polyarthritis. Am J Vet Res 1980; 41:522.

Romatowski J. Comparative therapeutics of canine and human rheumatoid arthritis. J Am Vet Med Assoc 1984; 185:558.

Serra DA, White SD. Oral chrysotherapy with auranofin in dogs. J Am Vet Med Assoc 1989; 194:1327.

Stanton ME, Legendre AM. Effects of cyclophosphamide in dogs and cats. J Am Vet Med Assoc 1986; 188:1319.

Swanson LV. Potential hazards with low-dose exposure to antineoplastic agents. Part II. Recommendations for minimizing exposure. Compendium of Continuing Education 1988; 10:616.

Werner L, Bright JM. Drug-induced immune hypersensitivity disorders in two dogs treated with trimethoprim sulfadiazine: Case reports and drug challenge studies. J Am Anim Hosp Assoc 1983; 19:783.

BEHAVIOR

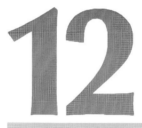

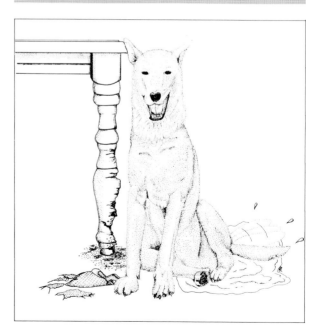

65

PRINCIPLES OF BEHAVIORAL DIAGNOSIS AND TREATMENT

Amy R. Marder

Behavior is essentially what an animal does. Most people keep pets because they like the way they behave. When a pet's behavior becomes objectionable to the owners, however, problems arise. The behavior of a pet is just as important to most people as its physical well-being, and unacceptable behavior all too often results in euthanasia or abandonment. Proper behavioral counseling given to the owners early in a pet's life helps to prevent the development of many behavioral problems. Successful treatment of an already existing problem can save an animal's life.

CAUSES

Behavior may be influenced by a variety of factors, including genetic predisposition, early experience, learning, physiologic state, and specific environmental stimuli. For example, a pit bull terrier may be genetically predisposed to display aggression to other dogs but may not express the aggression fully unless it receives training and exposure to other dogs. A female cat may spray only during estrus or, if spayed, only when her territory is invaded by other cats.

Behaviors and behavioral problems have been classified in several ways. The most useful, and therefore the most common method employed by veterinary behavioral consultants, is classification by function or motivation (Table 65-1). A functional classification scheme is based on an analysis of the sequences and patterns of behaviors and the circumstances in which they occur. This method is objective and allows the clinician to determine an animal's motivation and the stimuli that elicit the behavior.

Many people view animals with behavioral problems as abnormal. However, most pets that exhibit problem behaviors are not abnormal. They are merely exhibiting normal species typical behaviors, which are incompatible with the behaviors of the owners.

CLINICAL SIGNS

When approaching a behavioral problem, it is important to realize that the owners' presenting complaint is not the diagnosis; it is only the equivalent of a clinical sign. Owners who complain that their dog barks excessively may have a

Table 65–1 *Classification of Behavioral Problems*

Presenting Complaint	Behavioral Rule-outs
Dogs	
Aggression to family	Dominance-related aggression
	Fear-induced or defensive aggression
	Pain-induced aggression
	Redirected aggression
	Possessive aggression
	Parental aggression
	Play aggression
Aggression to strangers	Protective aggression
	Territorial aggression
	Fear-induced aggression
	Pain-induced aggression
	Parental aggression
	Dominance-related aggression (rare)
	Predatory aggression
	Play aggression
Intraspecific aggression	Intermale aggression
	Interfemale aggression
	Dominance-related aggression
	Territorial or protective aggression
	Redirected aggression
	Fear-induced or defensive aggression
	Possessive aggression
	Parental aggression
Destruction	Separation anxiety
	Play destruction
	Loud noise phobia
Inappropriate elimination	Housebreaking
	Submissive urination
	Excitement urination
	Separation anxiety
	Marking
	Fear-induced
	Loud noise phobia
Barking	Stimulus induced
	Separation anxiety
	Play behavior
	Attention-getting or reinforced
Self-mutilation	Displacement activity
	Stereotypic or obsessive behavior
Cats	
Interfeline aggression	Territorial aggression
	Fear-induced aggression
	Redirected aggression
	Intermale aggression
Aggression to people	Play aggression
	Redirected aggression
	Fear-induced aggression
	Territorial aggression
	Aggression while being petted
	Pain or punishment-induced aggression

(continued)

Table 65–1 (continued)

Presenting Complaint	Behavioral Rule-outs

Inappropriate elimination	Inappropriate elimination
	    Location preference
	    Substrate preference
	    Location aversion
	    Substrate aversion
	    Marking
	    Separation anxiety

Destruction and ingestive problems	Scratching Wool chewing Displacement activity Redirected behavior Plant eating
Vocalization	Attention seeking "Old cat" nighttime howling
Self-mutilation	Displacement activity Stereotypic or obsessive behavior

dog that is suffering from separation anxiety, is merely very sensitive to external stimuli, or has learned in the past that barking receives attention, just as a dog that is coughing may be in congestive heart failure, have bronchitis, pneumonia, or any other disease that results in the clinical sign of coughing. A list of behavioral rule-outs should be made as is done for any medical or surgical problem (see Table 65-1).

DIAGNOSTIC APPROACH

Many organic problems are manifested by behavioral changes. For example, hyperthyroid cats often display hyperactive behavior and vocalize excessively. Therefore, before considering a strictly behavioral etiology for a behavioral problem, all possible medical causes must first be ruled out.

After medical causes have been eliminated, a behavioral diagnosis may be pursued. In order to make a proper behavioral diagnosis, a complete, accurate, and detailed history must be obtained, through a special behavioral interview (Table 65-2). The initial interview may last from one to several hours and should include all relevant family members and the pet. Although the interview is probably best done at the owner's home, time constraints may make this unfeasible. If the interview takes place at the office, it should not be done in a typical examination room. The owners and the pet will be more relaxed if the waiting room or private office is used. The atmosphere of the interview should be congenial, relaxed, and, above all, non-judgmental.

It is important for the owners to understand that behavioral problems originate from a combination of factors involving the owners and the pet. In other words, the problem is not solely the owners' fault. It is also important for the veterinarian to understand that most people keep problem pets because they are emotionally attached to them, not because they themselves have psychological problems. In general, when taking a behavioral history, one should try to determine how the problem initially developed, the stimuli and circumstances that elicit the behaviors, and their immediate consequences. The owners should first be allowed to describe the problem at their own pace without direction. More specific questions may then be asked. First, the corrections the people have tried and the results of these, then a detailed description of the most recent events and their consequences is obtained. The first time the owners noticed the behavior must be discussed, as well as the duration of the behavior and its frequency. The pet's general life style, including sleeping area, diet, exercise, play, time spent with the owners, and general management is then covered. At some point, questions

Table 65–2 *Sample Behavioral Interview*
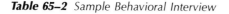

Client information (name, address, phone number)
Pet information (name, date of birth, species, breed, sex; if neutered, declawed, age performed and reason)
Place pet obtained, age obtained, reason for getting pet, previous pets, reason for getting rid of, any behavioral problems
Behavior of parents and littermates if known
Time spent outdoors, general management (tied, fenced yard, etc.)
Diet
Medical problems (present, past, medication)
Presenting behavioral complaints
Duration
Frequency
Corrections tried and results (including obedience, drug therapy)
Development of problem, chronology
Recent incidents (last, next to last, third to last)
Typical 24-hour day (including sleeping area, walks, play, exercise, feeding, who does caretaking)
Owners thoughts about giving pet up, general seriousness of problem, and euthanasia
Tentative Diagnosis
More specific questions pertaining to specific problem (for example, litter type, type of litter box, how often cleaned, location)
Diagnosis
Prognosis
Treatment

pertaining to genetic predisposition, such as behavior of parents and littermates, are asked as well as questions as to the reason for obtaining the pet so that the owners' expectations are clear. The degree of attachment of each family member to the animal and whether or not euthanasia has been considered must always be addressed. At this point, a tentative diagnosis can be made and more specific questions asked concerning the individual behavioral problem in question. After all the pertinent information is obtained, a physical examination is performed if it has not already been done. Only then can the diagnosis be discussed with the owners. The prognosis is always discussed prior to setting up a treatment plan, because some people will opt not to treat, especially when dealing with aggression.

MANAGEMENT

As a behavior may be influenced by numerous internal and external variables, behavioral problems may be treated by one or a combination of the following methods: environmental alteration, physiologic manipulation through pharmaco-

logic or surgical intervention, or behavioral modification utilizing learning principles.

Alteration of a pet's environment is often used in the treatment of behavioral problems primarily to change or prevent exposure to some of the stimuli that elicit the problem behavior. For example, a cat may spray less if he is prevented from seeing outdoor cats by merely keeping the window shades closed. A dog may cease eliminating in a certain area if the owners make the area the dog's feeding place or prevent the dog from gaining access to the area. Techniques of environmental modification are among the easiest and least invasive of all treatment methods and are usually used before trying other methods or at the same time that the other methods are utilized.

The two methods commonly used to change an animal's physiologic state are surgery and drug therapy. The most common surgery that is performed in an attempt to change an animal's behavior is neutering. Castration of adult male dogs and cats affects only the typically male behaviors. In dogs these include intermale aggression, urine marking in the house, mounting of other dogs or people, and roaming. It is the clinical impression of most veterinary behaviorists that castration also helps reduce the frequency and intensity of dominance-related aggression. As territorial aggression occurs equally in both males and females, it is not a typically masculine trait and is not likely to be affected by castration. In cats, castration has been shown to reduce or eliminate fighting, urine spraying in the house, and roaming. Studies indicate that the effects of castration are the same no matter the age at which it is performed.

It has not been shown that ovariohysterectomy has any significant effect on the behavior of a female dog or cat, unless the exhibition of a behavior is correlated with the estrus cycle. Spraying in female cats while in estrus will likely be modified by spaying, as will aggressive behavior associated with pseudocyesis or estrus in dogs. Drug therapy is still in its infancy. At this time, no good controlled studies of the effectiveness of psychotropic drugs for the treatment of behavioral problems in dogs and cats have been done, and very little is known about optimum drug dosages, therapeutic blood levels, and side effects (Table 65-3). Drug therapy should be considered experimental, and until we are able to learn more, it should not be relied on as the sole treatment for a behavioral problem. Psychotropic drugs can be helpful adjuvants to a behavioral modification program but are not often curative alone. Quite frequently, effects seen while on a drug may not transfer to the non-drugged state.

When prescribing drug therapy to help change the behavior of a pet, the owners must be informed that most of the psychotropic drugs are not approved for use in animals and that behavioral drug therapy is still experimental. Also, as there is both species and individual variability in response to each drug, people should arrange to have someone observe the animal the first time the drug is given for any serious side effects until the drug wears off. In addition, the veterinarian should be thoroughly familiar with all potential side effects (see Appendix II).

The greatest, and usually the most important, part of most treatment programs utilizes behavioral modification techniques. The most common methods utilized by animal behavioral consultants to change the frequency of a behavior employ the principles of reinforcement, extinction, shaping, punishment, counterconditioning, systematic desensitization, and flooding.

Positive reinforcement is the application of a stimulus or event (a positive reinforcer or reward) after a response that increases the probability

Table 65–3 *Drugs Commonly Used to Treat Behavior Problems*

Generic	Trade	Dosage	Uses
DOGS			
Diazepam	Valium	.55 to 2.2 mg/kg as needed PO	Noise phobias
Clorazepate dipotassium	Tranxene-SD	11.25 to 22.5 mg/dog PO s.i.d.–b.i.d.	Noise phobias
Amitriptyline HCl	Elavil	2.2 to 4.4 mg/kg, PO s.i.d.	Separation anxiety
Megestrol acetate	Ovaban Megace	2.2 to 4.4 mg/kg, PO s.i.d. for 2 weeks, ½ dose q 2 weeks	Typically masculine behaviors Dominance aggression
Medroxyprogesterone acetate	Depo-Provera	11 mg/kg, SC, IM, PRN	Same as megestrol acetate
CATS			
Diazepam	Valium	1 to 2 mg/cat, PO b.i.d.	Marking, anxiety
Amitriptyline HCl	Elavil	5 to 10 mg/cat, PO s.i.d.	Anxiety, spraying, excessive grooming
Chlorpheniramine	Chlor-Trimeton	1 to 2 mg/cat, PO b.i.d.	Excessive grooming
Megestrol acetate	Ovaban	2.5 mg, PO SID for 7 days, then 2.5 mg weekly	Marking, aggression, anxiety
Medroxyprogesterone	Depo-Provera	10 to 20 mg/kg SC, IM PRN	Same as megestrol acetate

that the response will occur again. A reward is most effective when given a half second after the response occurs. The owners often inadvertently use positive reinforcement and actually "teach" their pet to perform a problem behavior. To take a simple example, the dog that jumps up on people when they arrive home is often petted or kneed. Petting is an obvious positive reinforcer, but many dogs also consider kneeing a positive reinforcer as well for it closely resembles play behavior. Within treatment programs, positive reinforcement is often used to teach a dog an alternative behavior; for example, eliminating outside in a housebreaking program, teaching a dog to sit and stay in an aggression program.

Behaviors that are acquired or enhanced through reinforcement extinguish or reduce in frequency when the reinforcement ceases. Take the jumping dog again. If the owners were advised to stop petting the dog and ignore the dog unless it was in a sitting position, the jumping up behavioral problem would be extinguished, while the sit would be reinforced.

Shaping (or successive approximation) is a technique whereby approximations of a desired behavior are reinforced successively until ultimately only the precise desired response is reinforced. A type of shaping is used in the treatment of litter box problems. If during the interview and initial treatment it has been determined that a cat prefers to eliminate on soft surfaces such as towels (but the people would prefer that the cat uses cat litter), the behavior may be shaped as follows. The cat may at first be offered a towel without a litter box. Then once the cat is using the towel, a box is added. Again, after the cat has used the towel in the box for a period of time, then litter may be added. Litter is gradually added until the time that the cat is using the litter regularly. Then the towel may be removed. Shaping is also often used by animal trainers to teach complicated tricks.

Punishment is the application of an aversive stimulus or event that stops or prevents a behavior from occurring. It is often difficult to administer effectively and may result in undesirable side effects, such as anxiety and aggression. For punishment to be effective, it should be of appropriate intensity and be administered immediately and every time the animal begins to engage in the undesirable behavior. In addition, when punishment is used, it is best when the animal has a clear and appropriate alternative behavior. Punishment after the fact is generally not an effective method of punishment. Again, consider the jumping dog. The punishment the owners were using (kneeing) was ineffective because it was of insufficient intensity to stop the behavior, it was misinterpreted by the dog as a game, and it was not used every time. The dog also did not have a clear, acceptable alternative until it was taught to sit. Fearful dogs often become defensively aggressive when physically punished, while dominant-aggressive or protective-aggressive dogs often escalate their aggression when physically punished. Punishment is contraindicated in the treatment of purely fear-related behaviors and may be very dangerous in the treatment of dominance-related aggression.

Counterconditioning is training or conditioning an animal to respond to a stimulus in a manner that is incompatible with the response that was previously evoked by the stimulus. For treatment of fears and anxieties, a pleasant activity, such as eating or play, is often paired with the gradual introduction of the offending stimulus. The animal thus becomes conditioned to experience a different physiologic state with the stimulus rather than to associate it with fear or anxiety. Counterconditioning may also involve teaching the animal to assume a different motor response to specific stimuli. For example, the jumping dog could be taught to sit quietly while the owners gradually walk through the door.

Systematic desensitization is usually used in conjunction with specific counterconditioning procedures. The animal is gradually exposed to increasing intensities of a stimulus without evoking an undesirable response. A dog that is fearful of loud noises may be treated by exposing the dog to the fearful stimuli during meals, first at a volume so low so as not to evoke the fear, and then gradually increasing the volume.

Flooding is often used for the treatment of phobias in people but is used only occasionally in animals. During flooding, the patient is forced to experience the fear-evoking stimulus until the fear response is markedly reduced, or, ideally, ceases. Dogs that are mildly afraid of novel objects (plastic bags, garbage cans, umbrellas) may be treated using a program of gradual flooding. The dog is forced to experience the object at a distance. When it is obviously less afraid, the dog is moved closer and the flooding repeated. Eventually the dog should be able to experience the full-blown stimulus without displaying a fear response.

Habituation is the progressive decrease of a response with repeated application of a stimulus. It is often used in the treatment of separation anxiety in order to make a dog less anxious when exposed to pre-departure cues.

PATIENT MONITORING

Follow-up appointments are scheduled in order to monitor the progress of each patient at intervals dictated by the particular problem, severity, frequency, and the owners' motivation and time available to work on the problem. The intervals vary from weekly, as with litter box problems, to monthly, as with some fears. Many follow-ups are effectively done by telephone, while some require follow-up visits.

ADDITIONAL READING

Hart BL, Hart LA. Canine and feline behavioral therapy. Philadelphia: Lea and Febiger, 1985.

Voith VL. Behavioral disorders. In: Ettinger SJ, ed. Textbook of veterinary internal medicine. Philadelphia: WB Saunders, 1989: 227.

Voith VL, Borchelt PL, eds. Vet Clin North Am [Small Animal Practice] 1982; 12.

Voith VL, Borchelt PL. History taking and interviewing. Compendium of Continuing Education 1985; 7:432.

Voith Vl, Marder AM. Introduction. In: Morgan RV, ed. Handbook of small animal practice. New York: Churchill Livingstone, 1988: 1031.

66

AGGRESSION IN DOGS

Amy R. Marder

Aggression is the most common and potentially the most serious canine behavioral problem encountered by both dog owners and veterinarians. Annual estimates of dog bites in the United States are over 1 million, large numbers going unreported. Although most bites are minor, occasionally serious injuries and fatalities occur.

CAUSES

Aggression is a complex, multidimensional phenomenon that is influenced by numerous factors: genetic predisposition, early experience, maturation, sex, age, body size, learning, hormonal status, physiologic state, and external stimuli. The classification and causes have therefore often been the subject of controversy among behaviorists. A functional classification, based on an analysis of sequences and patterns of behaviors and the circumstances in which they occur, is the most useful. This type of classification is objective and allows the clinician to determine the motivation of the animal and the stimuli eliciting the behavior. As with most behavioral problems, most dogs exhibiting aggressive behavior are not abnormal. They are exhibiting normal species-typical behavioral patterns that are incompatible with human life style.

Dominance-related aggression is the most common type of canine aggression problem that is presented to animal behaviorists, probably because it is the most disturbing to the owners. The aggressive acts are directed toward one or several family members or other household pets. Dogs, like their highly social wolf ancestors, are pack animals; they maintain dominance-subordinate relationships through the use of aggressive displays. Dogs, when taken into human families, relate to humans as members of their own species and pack members. Most dogs respect the dominant status of family members. Some, however, attempt to or actually do achieve dominance over one or several family members and repeatedly exhibit aggressive behavior in order to affirm their position in the pack social hierarchy.

Possessive aggression is often associated with dominance-related aggression and consists of aggression directed to animals or humans when food or objects are approached.

Protective aggression is directed towards approaching animals or people outside of the pack in defense of a dog's area (home, room, or yard), the owners, or animal pack member. Territorial aggression is included within this category.

Predatory aggression is directed toward anything that the dog considers prey. It is usually directed toward animals but may be elicited by any quickly moving stimulus such as a child, bicycle, or car.

Fear-induced aggression occurs when people or animals approach or reach for a fearful dog. It is common when the dog cannot escape, such as in a cage or on the veterinary examination table. It is sometimes seen when the owners use severe punishment techniques. Active, unpredictable small children may also elicit fear-induced aggression.

Pain-induced aggression is elicited by a person or animal that causes the dog to feel pain. It often occurs when a person attempts to manipulate a painful area or when injections are administered.

Parental aggression is directed toward any person or animal who approaches a bitch with puppies or is in pseudocyesis.

Redirected aggression occurs when a dog that is aggressively motivated is interfered with. The aggression is then redirected from the person or animal that initially evoked the aggression onto another individual in the vicinity. For example, a dog that is barking at the door may redirect its aggression onto the person who is pulling it back by its collar. Dominant dogs often redirect onto subordinates, whether animal or human.

Play aggression refers to the normal growling, nipping, and biting directed toward people or other animals during play. Intermale aggression occurs between adult male dogs and often involves territorial or dominance disputes.

Interfemale aggression occurs between adult females usually in the same household. Competition over status within the pack hierarchy is usually involved.

Aggression caused by pathophysiologic disorders is rare; few well-documented cases exist. The signalment, history, and clinical signs of aggressive behavior are listed in Table 66-1.

Table 66–1 *Signalment, History, and Clinical Signs of Aggression in Dogs*

Classification	Presenting Complaints	Sex	Age	History
Dominance-related aggression	Unprovoked attacks on family members, moody Dr. Jekyl and Mr. Hyde personality	Either but usually males and purebreds	Usually adults	Aggressive when: Approached or attempt is made to take food or coveted objects; disturbed while resting or sleeping; restrained, pushed, pulled by collar or neck, stared at, disciplined, threatened, or hit; groomed, towel-dried, medicated; lifted Dog often assumes dominant postures over the people (paw, stand over) Often not aggressive to strangers
Possessive aggression	Aggressive to animals or people when dog is approached or threatened when in possession of food or objects.	Either	Any age	Often but not always related to dominance aggression
Protective and territorial aggression	Aggressive to strangers, either people or other animals	Either	Usually after 9 months	Occurs when person or animal approaches another person, animal, or area that dog is defending
Predatory aggression	Attack of animal or person, usually moving	Either	Any	Predation on small mammals, birds, etc., often accompanied by a chase, stalking, and other hunting behavior

(continued)

Table 66–1 (continued)

Classification	Presenting Complaints	Sex	Age	History
Fear-induced aggression	Aggressive to people or animals, sometimes small children	Either	Any age	Aggressive when approached or reached for, cornered, threatened, or punished; accompanied by fearful body and facial expressions (ears back, tail tucked); some fearful dogs do not bite when a person is facing them but do when the person turns away
Pain-induced aggression	Aggressive to people or animals; usually sudden onset	Either	Any age	Aggressive when person attempts to groom, medicate, touch, or approach painful area. Related to disease or injury.
Parental aggression	Aggressive to people or animals when bitch or puppies are approached	Usually female	Any age	Puppies present in house or bitch in pseudocyesis (6 to 8 weeks after estrus)
Redirected aggression	Aggressive to people or other animals when touched or restrained while fighting or threatening	Either	Any age	Occurs when dog is touched, restrained, or close to another individual; while the dog is threatening, fighting, or attempting to reach an eliciting stimulus
Play aggression	Growling, nipping, and biting other animals and people in play	Either	Usually young dogs	Usually directed toward moving body parts (hands, arms, legs); accompanied by play bows and other play gestures; bites usually do not break the skin.
Intermale aggression	Aggressive to other male dogs	Males	Usually 1 to 3 years	Body and facial expressions are usually indicative of dominance or offensive aggression
Interfemale aggression	Aggression to another female dog, usually in same household	Female	Usually 1 to 3 years	Usually involves dominance gestures; unlike males, females do not give extensive threats, and fights may result in serious injury or death
Aggression of pathophysiologic origin	Directed toward people or other animals; usually sudden onset	Either	Any age	Aggressive behavior does not fit any canine species-typical behavior patterns; is not adaptable

MANAGEMENT

Although most of the behaviors that aggressive dogs exhibit can be considered to be normal, they may still have severe consequences. The prognosis for the treatment of aggressive disorders must always be guarded. The owners must be made aware that they are responsible for the animal's behavior at all times. Although the frequency and severity of the aggression may be reduced, in most cases it cannot be eliminated completely. One cannot guarantee that the aggression will never occur again. The most that may be accomplished is to reduce the probability that the aggression will occur. The owners must weigh the risks of keeping an aggressive dog against the benefits. Most people who seek help are extremely emotionally attached to their dogs and do not want to give them up.

In general, the treatment for any type of aggressive behavior problem may consist of a combination of drug therapy, surgery (*e.g.*, castration), avoidance of eliciting stimuli, management (*e.g.*, leash), and behavior modification techniques (habituation, counterconditioning, and desensitization). Each case is different, and a treatment program varies not only according to diagnosis but also according to the owners' capability, motivation, and time.

Dominance Aggression

The primary goal is to get the dog to assume submissive or nonaggressive behaviors in situations that previously elicited aggression while avoiding personal injury to the owners. All situations known to elicit aggression should first be identified and initially avoided in order to prevent the dog from reinforcing its dominant position, as well as to prevent possible injury to the owners. The dog is then taught commands such as sit-stay and down-stay, preferably with food rewards. All affection and attention is withheld from the dog unless he obeys a command. For example, every time the dog is petted he must sit or lie down first. The owners are then taught to carefully countercondition the dog to assume nonaggressive behaviors while the owners engage in dominant gestures, such as touching, pushing, or staring.

Castration is effective in reducing dominance aggression in some male dogs. Spaying does not seem to affect the signs of dominance aggression in females. Progestins can be helpful adjuncts to behavior modification (*e.g.*, megestrol acetate [Ovaban] 2.2–4.4 mg/kg PO, daily for 2 weeks, then 1.1–2.2 mg/kg PO, daily for 2 weeks, then wean off, or medroxyprogesterone acetate [Depoprovera] 11 mg/kg IM or SC). Before using the progestins, however, be familiar with the side effects of these drugs (see Appendix II). The progestins often reduce the intensity and frequency of the aggression, thus enabling an owner to more safely implement a behavioral modification program. The aggressive behavior usually returns when the drug therapy is terminated if behavioral modification has not been successful. Physical punishment usually elicits severe aggression in dominant aggressive dogs and should be avoided. It should only be used if the the dog is highly likely to submit to the threat of punish-

ment. Treatment usually reduces the frequency and intensity of the aggression but rarely eliminates the problem entirely. It is therefore extremely important at all times that every family member understand the problem and does his or her best to avoid eliciting the aggression. As avoidance is sometimes impossible when small children, some elderly and handicapped persons are involved, families with these types of members should be particularly advised of the dangers involved in keeping such dogs. The prognosis is always guarded.

Protective and Territorial Aggression

Prohibiting access to the target by the use of fences and leashes is the most effective and safest way to prevent injury. It is often necessary to emphasize to the owners that their dog is dangerous and that they are liable if the dog bites someone, so that they understand the seriousness of the problem. Castration or spaying is unlikely to affect this type of aggression. The dog may be counterconditioned to assume a nonaggressive attitude while the eliciting stimuli are gradually introduced. Punishment is often used but should be combined with counterconditioning techniques. The owners should also understand that, although the dog may not be aggressive in his or her presence, it will probably still be aggressive when the owners are not around. The prognosis is guarded.

Fear-Induced Aggression

All of the fear eliciting stimuli must first be identified (*e.g.*, tall men) and initially avoided. A counterconditioning and desensitization program is then set up. The stimuli are first arranged on a continuum of intensities. Then, while the dog is in a nonfearful state (sitting and staying for food rewards and "happy" verbal praise or playing), the stimuli are gradually presented, the least threatening stimuli first, followed by the more threatening stimuli. The dog should never be allowed to become afraid or aggressive during treatment, and punishment should not be used unless absolutely necessary. Calming praise ("It's okay") should be avoided as it may actually act to reinforce the aggression. Comfortable basket muzzles that allow the dog to eat may be used for safety. If the dog is afraid of small children in the family, the children need to be taught to approach, touch, and pet the dog in a gentle manner. The children should never have unsupervised access to the dog. The owners should again be advised that they are responsible for the dog's behavior. The prognosis is guarded, due to the fact that the treatment program is difficult and lengthy.

Pain-Induced Aggression

The cause of the painful disorder must first be treated (see Chapter 12). The dog is then counterconditioned to engage in nonaggressive behavior when approached and touched. Punishment is contraindicated.

Parental Aggression

Eliciting the aggression should be avoided while the dog is gradually counterconditioned to assume a nonaggressive attitude (see Chapter 65).

Redirected Aggression

The owners must be strongly advised to avoid physically interfering in aggressive situations (*e.g.*, dog fights). If they must interfere, they should use inanimate objects such as pillows or blankets to protect themselves. Sometimes spraying the dog with water is helpful as punishment. The cause of the initial aggression should be treated as well as any existing dominance problem.

Predatory Aggression

Confinement is the only reliable method of preventing predatory aggression. Remote punishment, such as that delivered by a shock collar, may be effective. Counterconditioning the dog to assume a nonaggressive attitude in the presence of prey may also be effective but only in the presence of the owners.

Possessive Aggression

The dog is counterconditioned to assume a nonaggressive attitude when it is approached. Food rewards are often used. Punishment may be effective early on but may increase the intensity of the aggression and elicit fear-induced or defensive aggression.

Play Aggression

Inappropriate play should first be ignored so it is not reinforced, and then play is redirected onto appropriate toys. Punishment is often not effective, as many puppies respond to punishment as if it is cooperative play. If ignoring does not work, punishment may be tried with loud noises and scolding.

Intermale Aggression

Castration has a 62% chance of reducing fighting between male dogs (Hopkins, Additional Reading). It is more likely to be effective if both dogs are castrated. The synthetic progestins may also be helpful. The dog may also be counterconditioned to assume a nonaggressive or immobile stance when encountering other male dogs. If the aggression involves two dogs in the same family, the owners should support a stable dominance hierarchy, if it exists, by giving the dominant dog the first of everything (food, attention, greeting, etc.). If treatment is not successful, the owners should be advised to find one dog another home without other male dogs. Dogs that are aggressive to other dogs are not necessarily aggressive to people and may make very nice pets.

Interfemale Aggression

Spaying is unlikely to affect the aggression unless it is related to the estrus cycle. Often interfemale aggression worsens during estrus and pseudopregnancy. As with males, females may be conditioned to assume a nonaggressive attitude in circumstances that previously elicited aggression. Because the aggression is often severe, it may be necessary to either maintain the female dogs separately or find another home for one of them. Progestin therapy is unlikely to help the problem. The owners should support a stable dominance hierarchy, if it exists, like in males. Finding one dog a new home is often the best solution.

PATIENT MONITORING

All cases of aggression must be considered serious problems and given a guarded prognosis. Follow-up examinations are done initially by telephone on a weekly basis. The treatment program is altered as needed. Follow-up appointments are best done at least monthly. The length of treatment depends on the type of aggression, severity, and the owners' motivation, many lasting to some degree for the life of the dog. For all aggression cases, euthanasia must be fully discussed.

ADDITIONAL READING

Borchelt PL, Voith VL. Aggressive behavior in dogs and cats. Compendium of Continuing Education 1985; 7:949.

Borchelt PL. Aggressive behavior of dogs kept as companion animals: Classification and influences of sex, reproductive status, and breed. Applied Animal Ethology 1983; 10:45.

Hopkins SG, Schubert TA, Har BL. Castration of adult male dogs: Effects on roaming, aggression, urine marking and mounting. J Am Vet Med Assoc 1976; 168:1108.

Line S, Voith VL. Dominance aggression of dogs towards people: Behavior profile and response to treatment. Applied Animal Behavioral Science 1986; 16:77.

Voith VL, Borchelt PL. Vet Clin North Am [Small Animal Practice] 1982; 12.

Voith VL, Marder AR. Canine behavioral disorder. In: Morgan RV, ed. Handbook of small animal practice. New York: Churchill Livingstone, 1988: 1039.

67

AGGRESSION IN CATS

Amy R. Marder

Aggression directed toward people or other cats is the second most common behavioral problem reported by cat owners. Cat bites and scratches, although not usually severe, can lead to serious infections in both people and cats. Signs of aggression may consist of stalking, chasing, pouncing, scratching, biting, growling, and hissing.

CAUSES

As in dogs, feline aggression is a complex phenomenon affected by many factors. Also as discussed under canine aggression, a functional classification system is the most useful when making a diagnosis and setting up a treatment plan.

The majority of aggressive cats are exhibiting normal and appropriate species-typical behavior. Some diseases, however, cause signs of aggression but in patterns that are not consistent with normal species-typical aggressive behavior. A good knowledge of normal feline behavior is therefore essential in order to differentiate normal behavior from aggression, which has a pathophysiologic basis. In addition, organically caused be-havior changes are usually accompanied by other signs of the disease, which will be evident on a thorough physical examination.

Interfeline Aggression

Intermale Aggression

As males reach adulthood, they often start to threaten each other over territory and mates. Sometimes these encounters lead to fighting. The aggressive interaction usually begins with a threat ritual and is accompanied by growls and loud howls. If an attack occurs it often results in only one bite, but if infection ensues it may be serious.

Territorial Aggression

Aggression that occurs between two cats in defense of territory generally involves an aggressive pursuit accompanied by growling and hissing. One cat is usually the aggressor and relentlessly pursues the other cat, attempting to chase it away.

911

Fear-Induced or Defensive Aggression

A cat that is frightened often defends itself by being aggressive. A defensive cat will crouch, flatten its ears, hiss, spit, and exhibit piloerection. If approached, the cat is likely to attack. Sometimes two cats within the same household will suddenly begin fighting after a frightening incident occurs. For instance, two cats that were previously friendly may become aggressive toward each other after a lamp falls off a table.

Redirected Aggression

A very common cause of intercat aggression, redirected aggression often occurs when one cat interferes with another in an aggressive state. A typical example is the cat that becomes aggressively aroused on seeing an outdoor cat and attacks its housemate, which is walking by.

Aggression Toward People

Play Aggression

Although most often misinterpreted by owners, aggression as a part of play is probably the most common type of aggressive behavior that cats exhibit toward people. Young mammals in general spend a considerable portion of their day engaging in play. Normal play consists of behaviors that closely resemble components of predation and fighting (stalking, pouncing, scratching, and biting). During play they "practice" to help them prepare for hunting and intercat disputes later in life.

Redirected Aggression

Aggression is also sometimes directed toward people if a cat while aggressively motivated is interfered with. Redirected aggression often occurs unexpectedly in otherwise very friendly and affectionate cats. Many people are scratched or bitten by their cats while trying to calm them down. Aggressive cats should not be touched until they have clearly demonstrated that they are no longer in an aggressive mood by engaging in an activity such as grooming or eating.

Fear or Defensive Aggression

Cats that are frightened may also aggressively defend themselves from a person. A typical example is a cat that is disciplined for hissing at a house guest out of fear and responds aggressively.

Territorial Aggression

Although rare, some cats defend their homes from people. This sometimes occurs when the owners are away and cat-sitters enter the house to care for the cat.

Aggression Related to Being Petted

Some cats do not like to be held or petted excessively and may respond to these activities by biting or scratching. In most cases, these are just signals to tell people to stop. Often people, because of previous experience and expectations, have difficulty accepting the fact that they just do not own a huggable cat.

Idiopathic Aggressive Behavior

There have been occasional reports of cats that suddenly become aggressive with no warning and without any identifiable eliciting stimulus. Many of these cats probably have cases of redirected or defensive aggression, but many are euthanized before a good behavioral history can be taken.

CLINICAL SIGNS AND DIAGNOSTIC APPROACH

A detailed and thorough behavioral history is essential in order to make a diagnosis (see Chapter 65). The signalment, history, and clinical signs of aggressive behavior are listed in Tables 67-1 and 67-2.

MANAGEMENT

Intercat Aggression

Intermale Aggression

Castration has a 90% probability of stopping or reducing intermale aggression regardless of age or duration of the problem. It may also be reduced

Table 67–1 *Intercat Aggression Problems*

Diagnosis	Age	Sex	History	Behavioral Description
Intermale aggression	Onset 2 to 3 years	Male	May be sudden or gradual onset	Yelling, yowling, scratching, hissing, attacking other male cats; usually accompanied by ritualized threat displays
Territorial aggression	Onset 2 to 3 years	Either	May be sudden or gradual onset	Characterized by one cat pursuing the other, growling, chasing, attacking, scratching, and biting
Fear-induced aggression	Any age	Either	Sudden onset; may begin after frightening event or redirected aggression	Both cats assume defensive attitudes (ears back, body hunched, dilated pupils, paw blows, piloerection); cats usually do not seek each other; cats seem to misinterpret each others signals
Redirected	Any age	Either	Sudden onset; usually occurs after some type of aggressive event	Same as fear-induced

Table 67–2 *Feline Aggression Toward People*

Diagnosis	Age	Sex	History	Behavioral Description
Play aggression	Usually less than 3 years, but may be less than 1 year	Either	Usually occurs in single cat households or with young cat and older unplayful cat; directed toward one or several family members	Predatory-like behaviors (stalking, chasing, pouncing, biting and scratching); bites are not usually severe; cat attacks moving body parts such as hands and legs; pupils often dilate; does not growl.
Redirected aggression	Any	Either	Occurs suddenly; happens when person approaches or touches cat in aggressive mood; may be elicited by smell.	Usually involves hissing, growling, biting, and scratching; cat may even pursue person
Fear-induced aggression	Any	Either	Usually directed toward new person; problem is frequently made worse with punishment	Cat assumes fearful or defensive posture (crouch, flattened ears, piloerection), hisses, and growls; may bite and scratch if approached or touched
Territorial	Any	Either	Directed toward visitors; usually very friendly to family	Cat assumes offensive attack posture, ears forward, sometimes swiveled outward, body erect; often accompanied by a growl; cat follows person
Aggression while being petted or hugged	Any	Either	Directed toward anyone who pets or hugs the cat	Cat enjoys or tolerates petting up to a point, may even purr, but then bites and runs away; may also resist being held and petted; bites are inhibited
Idiopathic aggression	Any	Either	Sudden attack with no apparent eliciting stimulation	Severe and repeated attacks with biting, scratching, and sometimes chasing

by progestins at the same dosage used to treat spraying or marking (i.e., megestrol acetate or medroxyprogesterone acetate) (see Chapter 65 and Table 65-3). If the problem persists after castration, separating the male cats is the best prevention.

Territorial Aggression

This feline problem is one of the most difficult to treat, and the prognosis is poor. Recommending finding a new home for one of the cats, preferably the aggressor if in a multicat household, is often the best plan for both cats and owners. Drug therapy either with progestins or tranquilizers is rarely, if ever, curative. A program consisting of counterconditioning and habituation techniques may be attempted if the owners are motivated. A few reports have had successful treatment with these techniques. The cats are initially separated and then gradually introduced using a cage at first and then leashes. They are first exposed to each other at a long distance (20 feet, for instance) and only during feeding time. The intercat distance is gradually shortened and the time of exposure is then gradually lengthened. If at any time during the process there are signs of aggression, they are separated again or they are kept together with one in a cage until the aggression ceases. The owners should be advised to use a pillow or blanket when handling an aggressive cat, as many will redirect their aggression to the owners.

Fear-Induced Aggression

Unlike territorial aggression, fear-induced aggression has a very good prognosis. The two cats must first be separated so that they are unable to see each other. When the two cats are no longer in an obviously aggressive state (as when they start to play with each other under a closed door), a gradual introduction program should be initiated as described under territorial aggression. The program must be done slowly so as to avoid provoking aggression and may last anywhere between 1 week and several months. Occasionally, a tranquilizer such as diazepam (1–2 mg per cat, once or twice a day) is helpful and may shorten the length of treatment.

Redirected Aggression

Redirected aggression between cats is treated in the same manner as territorial aggression or fear-induced aggression. The prognosis is very good. The owners must be aware that the problem could recur and should work on eliminating the original stimulus of the aggression. Reducing or eliminating access to outdoor cats is often helpful, as they are common initiators. Examples are keeping shades closed, trapping strays, keeping cat indoors, spraying outdoor cats with water, or putting mothballs outside in cloth sacs.

Aggression Toward People

Play Aggression

As play aggression usually occurs in single cat households and in cats under 1 year of age, the easiest method of treatment for some people is just to get another cat of approximately the same age. If a feline playmate is present, the young playful patient usually prefers the cat over the human. If getting another cat is not convenient or possible, then a program consisting of daily vigorous and appropriate play combined with mild punishment should be initiated. String toys that can be pulled across the floor, Ping-Pong balls, and balls of crumpled paper or foil are effective ways to get a cat to play vigorously. Paper bags and boxes often stimulate exploration and play. Bird feeders placed on windows also keep bored cats occupied. If the cat's playful attacks can be predicted, as they often can, the attack can be redirected to a moving toy first. For example, the owners can dangle a string while stepping out of the shower, or throw a Ping-Pong ball before coming down the stairs. Punishment, when used, must be combined with active play, as the cat needs to play. Sometimes, a water sprayer or loud air horn is an effective method of punishment. Whatever is used, it must be used every time the cat begins the play attack. The owners should be warned not to hit or otherwise physically punish playfully aggressive cats, as they are likely to become defensive and injure the owners. The prognosis for play aggression is generally good.

Redirected Aggression

The best method of treating redirected aggression is preventing it from occurring in the first place. The owners often try to calm an aggressive cat by petting it. They should be advised that it is very dangerous to approach, touch, or pick up an aggressive cat. One should always wait until the cat is out of its aggressive mood before interacting with it. Physical punishment is contraindicated as it often makes the cat more aggressive. Occasionally, the cat's aggressive state lasts for days. In these cases, tranquilizers (diazepam 1–2 mg per cat, twice a day) are helpful. Separation from the cat, except during feeding time, also often helps to solve the problem. Petting the cat should be avoided until the cat has clearly demonstrated that it is no longer in an aggressive mood by engaging in an activity such as grooming or eating. The prognosis is very good, but the problem may recur.

Fear-Induced Aggression

A problem that occurs quite often when a cat living with a single person must accept a new person (such as a roommate, boyfriend, or girlfriend). The best method of treatment is to avoid all behaviors that frighten the cat (loud voices, forced petting, punishment) and encourage those that the cat enjoys. The easiest way to desensitize the cat's fear of a person is to associate that person with delicious food and play. The cat should at first eat its favorite food at a distance from the person. Gradually, the cat should eat closer and closer to the person until it will eat directly from the person's hand. Pulling string toys along the ground is a good method of initiating play in fearful cats. The prognosis is usually good.

Aggression Related to Being Petted

Probably the most important part of the treatment for this type of aggression is to get the owners to accept that their cat does not like excessive petting. They must understand that it is not that their cat doesn't like them, it is just that some cats like physical contact and others do not. Physical punishment should be avoided as it is likely to provoke a defensive response. Rather than punishing after the bite, the owners should carefully observe the cat for signs of discomfort before the actual bite and stop petting first. The owners should also interact with their cats in ways that the cat clearly enjoys, such as play. Most people find that when they stop trying to force physical affection on their cats, their cats start to become more affectionate in other ways. For example, many begin to sit next to the owners more often and sleep with them. In general, the prognosis is good.

Idiopathic Aggression

In many cases of seemingly unprovoked aggressive attacks, a thorough behavioral history reveals a cause, such as redirected or defensive aggression. But if no medical, environmental, or behavioral reason for the attacks can be determined, then they cannot be treated. Sudden, unprovoked feline attacks are extremely dangerous and euthanasia must be considered.

PATIENT MONITORING

All cases of feline aggression must be treated as serious problems. Follow-ups are generally done by telephone on a weekly basis to monitor both the progress of the cat and the owners. The treatment program is altered if necessary. The length of treatment varies according to the type of aggression, the severity of the aggression, and the motivation of the owners. When and if the problem is controlled, the owners are told to call if it recurs.

ADDITIONAL READING

Borchelt PL, Voith VL. Aggressive behavior in cats. Compendium of Continuing Education 1987; 9:49.

Borchelt PL, Voith VL. Aggfessive behavior in dogs and cats. Compendium of Continuing Education 1985; 7:949.

Hart BL, Barrett RE. Effects of castration on fighting, roaming, and uring spraying in adult male cats. J Am Vet Med Assoc 1973; 163:290.

Leyhausen P. Cat behavior: The predatory and social behavior of domestic and wild cats. New york: Garland Press, 1979:.

Voith VL, Borchelt PL. Social behavior of domestic cats. Compendium of Continuing Education 1986; 8:643.

Voith VL, Borchelt PL. Diagnosis and treatment of aggression problems in cats. In: Voith VL, Borchelt PL, ed. Vet clinics of North American animal behavior. Philadelphia: W.B. Saunders, 1982: 673.

Voith VL, Marder AR. Feline behavioral disorders. In: Morgan RV, ed. Handbook of small animal practice. New York: Churchill Livingstone, 1988: 1047.

Voith VL, Marder AR. Feline behavioral disorders. In: Morgan RV, ed. Handbook of small animal practice. New York: Churchill Livingstone, 1988: 1047–1049.

68

DESTRUCTIVE BEHAVIOR AND BARKING

Amy R. Marder

Destruction of household possessions and property by scratching, digging, or chewing is one of the most common behavioral complaints of pet owners. According to Voith (Voith, 1984, Additional Reading) in a survey of more than 700 dog owners, destructiveness was the third most common complaint. Out of 800 people with cats, destructive behaviors were the second most common.

CANINE DESTRUCTION

Causes

Separation anxiety is one of the most common reasons that a dog engages in destructive behavior. Dogs also commonly become destructive during play and when frightened as occurs in noise-phobic dogs.

Separation Anxiety

Attachment and attachment behaviors are essential for the survival of social animals like dogs. Distress responses, such as crying and active seeking, occur when many social animals are separated from their companions. Just as an infant cries and increases its activity level in order to be reunited with its mother, an adult dog may also exhibit similar separation distress responses when separated from its owners. The anxiety response may not only be manifested by crying and destructive attempts at reunion but also by elimination (i.e., inappropriate urination and defecation).

Play Behavior

Dogs are naturally playful animals. Many times destruction and digging are a part of normal play behavior, especially in young animals.

Fears and Phobias

Dogs that are afraid of loud noises, such as thunderstorms and firecrackers, often become destructive while attempting to get away from the fear-inducing stimulus.

Table 68-1 lists the clinical signs, history, and diagnostic approach to canine destruction.

917

Table 68–1 *Clinical Signs, History and Diagnostic Approach in Dogs*

Diagnosis	Sex	Age	History
Separation anxiety	Either	Any	Destruction occurs when dog is separated from its owner and is usually around exits (doors and windows); usually occurs within 30 minutes of separation and close to 100% of the time when left alone. Dog usually follows the owners from room to room, looks despondent, or is excited when the owners leave, and greets them very exuberantly upon return. Destruction is sometimes accompanied by barking and elimination. Dogs with separation problems share common histories: never or rarely left alone as puppies, spent a recent period of constant contact with the owners, were kennelled, given up to a shelter, or left to stray. The owners often interpret behavior as spiteful.
Play destruction	Either	Usually under 2 years	Destruction usually occurs both when the owners are there and when they are gone. Usually involves "fun" things such as pillows, clothing, shoes, and toys; occurs much less than 100% of the time when left alone; not accompanied by other signs of anxiety. Often occurs in playful dogs that are deprived of adequate exercise or confined to small areas for prolonged periods of time
Fear-induced	Either	Any	Destruction occurs during periods of loud noise, such as occurs during thunderstorms or fireworks. Often involves exit points (doors and windows) but may be directed at anything. Sometimes occurs only when dog is left alone and it experiences a loud noise. Unlike separation anxiety, occurs only occasionally, but sometimes leads to true separation anxiety.

Management

Separation Anxiety

The treatment for separation anxiety involves gradually getting the dogs used to being alone without becoming distressed. Habituation, desensitization, and counterconditioning techniques are first used to modify the dog's response to specific stimuli related to departure, for example, rattling the car keys, opening the door. A series of gradual departures is then performed by the owners. The dog is left alone for increasing amounts of time, while never allowing it to become afraid. Usually when the owners get up to two hours, the problem is cured. Although cage training is often helpful to control play destruction, cages and other types of confinement often worsen separation anxiety. Dogs with severe separation anxiety often injure themselves attempting to get out of cages. Anti-anxiety medication is often a helpful adjunct to behavioral modification therapy. Amitriptyline (Elavil) is the drug I prefer, given at a dose of 2.2 to 4.4 mg/kg PO once daily. It is usually administered 1 hour before departure and is continued for 2 to 3 months and then gradually withdrawn. Others have used megestrol acetate (Ovaban) at 2.2 to 4.4 mg/kg PO once daily decreasing the dose as the dog comes under control (see Table 65-3). The owners should always try the animal on the medication first when they are at home for the entire day in order to watch for side effects. Veterinarians should be thoroughly familiar with side effects of these drugs (Appendix II).

Play Destruction

The owners should provide the dog with an adequate amount of exercise and active play daily. Although each dog's requirement for play varies, young dogs should get at least 30 minutes of vigorous play or exercise daily. The owners should also make appropriate play items available for the dog and encourage the dog to chew on them and play with them. In addition to redirecting the play to appropriate objects, punishment may be helpful. Remote punishment in the form of booby traps, such as mouse traps (placed upside down), balloons, or bad-tasting substances are often effective in deterring dogs. If the dog is caught in the act of destruction, verbal discipline can be applied. Punishment alone usually does not correct a play behavioral problem, and delayed punishment is usually ineffective. Some dogs, especially puppies, need to be restricted to "puppy proof" areas or cages until they grow older and demonstrate their trustworthiness.

Fear-Induced Destruction

A program consisting of counterconditioning and desensitization to the fearful stimulus is often effective. Anti-anxiety drugs are very helpful (see Chapter 70).

Patient Monitoring

The prognosis for canine destructive behavioral problems is good in general. A separation anxiety program may last for months, but the outcome is usually successful. Most dogs outgrow playful destruction. Probably the most difficult to control is fear-induced destruction, because duplicating the fearful stimulus is sometimes not possible. For any of the problems, follow-ups should be done by telephone weekly or every 2 weeks.

FELINE DESTRUCTIVE BEHAVIORAL PROBLEMS

Causes

Scratching

Claw-sharpening is a normal feline species-typical behavior. It serves to remove old sheaths from the claws as well as a visual marking behavior.

Ingestive Behaviors

Ingestion of grass and plants is a normal behavior of cats. Chewing on other objects, such as electrical cords and leather, may be related to play, displacement activity, or a redirected behavior. Wool and cloth sucking, chewing, and eating are probably abnormal, hereditary behaviors. This behavior is primarily seen in Siamese and Siamese crosses.

Scratching and ingestive behavioral problems are easily diagnosed by the history. Neither behavior is age or sex related.

Management

Scratching

The cat should be provided with its own scratching post or materials and encouraged to use them. Wooden logs and rope covered posts are best. The owners should punish the cat immediately and consistently every time the cat scratches the inappropriate item with either a loud noise or a spray of water. Remote punishment should be used as well: commercial cat repellents or double-sided sticky cellophane tape on the inappropriate object works well for many people. As a last resort, the cat may be surgically declawed. There is no evidence that declawing is psychologically harmful to cats. Declawed cats are not more aggressive than cats with claws and continue to engage in scratching behavior.

Ingestive Behaviors

The owners should provide the cat with its own plants, grass, or as a last resort a wool blanket. Occasionally making a high bulk dry cat food (*e.g.,* Hill's r/d or w/d) available at all times is also helpful. At the same time, immediate and consistent punishment (loud noises and water spray) for chewing on inappropriate objects should be applied. Remote punishment, in the form of booby traps (upside down mousetraps, bad tasting substances), should also be tried. Prohibiting access to all tempting materials is the only sure way to prevent destruction, however.

Patient Monitoring

The prognosis for destructive behavioral problems in cats varies according to individual animal and owner compliance. Follow-ups should be done by telephone at weekly or 2-week intervals.

BARKING

Howling, whining, or barking in excess of what is acceptable to the owners and neighbors is another common canine behavioral problem. The owners of barking dogs are often threatened with eviction, and the dogs themselves with unusually cruel methods to silence them.

Causes and Diagnostic Approach

Separation Anxiety

Dogs that become anxious when separated from their owners often vocalize excessively and they also become destructive and eliminate in the home. The howling, whining, or barking usually begins at the time of the owners' departure or shortly thereafter and may be continuous or intermittent for several hours. The diagnosis is easily made by taking a thorough behavioral history (see Table 68-1).

Reaction to Specific Stimuli

Some dogs bark excessively in response to certain exciting stimuli, such as mail carriers, motorcycles, other dogs, and unusual noises. This type of vocalization may be merely an arousal response or a combination of alertive, protective, or fearful behaviors. Territorial aggression is often accompanied by threatening barking. Fearful dogs often assume a fearful body posture (crouched, tail tucked) and facial expression (ears back, eyes narrowed) and bark in order to keep certain stimuli (*e.g.*, children) away. Stimulus-induced barking may be self-reinforcing and is frequently facilitated by the vocalizations of other dogs. The behavioral history and direct observation of the dog easily lead to the diagnosis.

Play Behavior

Normal components of play behavior, play vocalizations are accompanied by play postures such as the "bow." Owners often unknowingly reward the vocalizations by continuing to engage in play with the dog. Again a diagnosis is easily made through the behavioral history and direct observation.

Reinforced Vocalizations

Many dogs bark because they have been reinforced for barking inadvertently by the owners by actions such as being paid attention to, let through a door, fed a treat, petted, or praised. History and observation of the owners' interaction with the dog usually reveal if the barking behavior is being reinforced.

Management

Separation Anxiety

See Management under the Canine Destruction section for actions to take.

Reaction to Specific Stimuli

The eliciting stimuli should be identified and a program consisting of counterconditioning, desensitization, and flooding instigated (see Chapter 65). Punishment is also indicated if fear is not a major component of the response. Common forms of punishment include a verbal reprimand, water, and loud noises (air horns, coin-filled "rattle" cans), a bark-stimulated electric shock collar (Tritronics, Bark Eliminator). In order to be effective, the punishment must be administered immediately at the onset of each episode of barking and every time the bark occurs. If shock collars are used, the owners should be supervised by an experienced individual. Care should be taken as painful punishment, such as shock, may elicit aggressive behavior.

Play Behavior

Play episodes should be terminated each time excessive barking begins, or play should be encouraged at other times of the day when the barking may be more acceptable.

Reinforced Barking

Vocalizations may be extinguished by discontinuing the reinforcement. Punishment may be applied if fear is not a component of the behavior and the punishment is properly done. The dog may also be counterconditioned to the stimuli that elicit the barking.

Patient Monitoring

The prognosis for excessive vocalization is generally good but varies widely based on cause and owner compliance. Follow-up re-evaluations are done by telephone or in person at weekly or 2-week intervals. The treatment program is modified as needed.

ADDITIONAL READING

Voith VL. Human/animal relationships. In: Anderson RS, ed. Nutrition and behaviour in dogs and cats. New York: Pergamon Press, l984: 147.

Voith VL, Marder AR. Canine behavioral disorders and feline behavioral disorders. In: Morgan RV, ed. Handbook of small animal practice. New York: Churchill Livingstone, 1988: 1033.

Voith VL, Borchelt PL. Separation anxiety of dogs. Compendium of Continuing Education 1985; 7:42.

69

ELIMINATION PROBLEMS IN DOGS AND CATS

Amy R. Marder

CANINE ELIMINATION PROBLEMS

Elimination problems are one of the most common complaints of dog owners. An elimination problem exists when a dog urinates or defecates in an objectionable location, usually in the house. The smell and presence of canine urine and feces in a family's living area are not only extremely unpleasant but also damage household items.

Causes

When a dog urinates or defecates in the house, he or she may be doing so because of a real need to eliminate (*e.g.*, empty the bladder) or as part of normal marking or communication.

A medical etiology for inappropriate elimination behavior must always be ruled out first before investigating a behavioral etiology. Except for neurogenic problems, if a dog is both urinating and defecating in the home, disease is rarely the cause. Numerous possible medical etiologies can be found, however, if a dog is only urinating or only defecating in inappropriate areas. For example, dogs with cystitis often have "accidents" in the house (see Chapter 46). Dogs with diarrhea problems also frequently defecate inside (see Chapter 37).

After ruling out medical causes, a behavioral etiology must then be investigated. Probably the most common behavioral cause of elimination problems is related to housebreaking. A dog that is not housebroken generally does not inhibit itself from urinating or defecating in the house.

Separation anxiety is another common reason for eliminating inside. Dogs with separation anxiety become distressed when separated from their owners and often urinate or defecate when left alone.

Animals also frequently urinate or defecate in response to fear-eliciting stimuli, so that dogs with noise phobias often have elimination problems as well.

Puppies and young adult dogs frequently urinate submissively on greeting. Urination is a normal component of the canine submissive behavior pattern.

Dogs, especially young ones, may also dribble urine when excited. Excitement urination often occurs during play. Urine marking is usually performed by sexually mature male dogs in the leg-lifting stance. A species-typical behavior, it may occur not only outdoors but indoors as well. Fecal marking has been observed in male dogs in outdoor situations and probably occurs in the home as well, but much less frequently. For the history and diagnostic approach to canine elimination problems, refer to Table 69-1.

Management

Punishment alone is generally not an effective method of treatment for elimination problems and can lead to other behavioral problems. When indicated, owners should be advised to apply punishment only when the dog is caught in the act of eliminating. It is ineffective when applied at other times. Punishment should be avoided in the treatment of submissive and fear-induced elimination problems. The owners' observation that their dog "looks guilty" only when they have misbehaved is probably a misinterpretation of their dog's expression. The guilty look is usually applied to a dog's submissive body posture, which is assumed in anticipation of punishment by the owners. The dog has learned that the stimuli of feces or urine in the presence of the owners is usually followed by some kind of punishment. Rather than the dog feeling guilty that it has done something wrong, the dog is displaying signs of submission to a dominant pack member.

Table 69–1 *History and Diagnostic Approach to Elimination Problems in Dogs*

Diagnosis	Sex	Age	History
BOTH URINE AND FECES			
Housebreaking	Either	Any	Often dog has eliminated in the house since puppyhood. Elimination is usually unrelated to the presence or absence of the owner; it is related in most cases to the length of time since the dog last had access to the appropriate area. Urine and/or feces may be found in one or more areas; large amounts are voided at one time.
Separation anxiety	Either	Any	Elimination occurs when dog is separated from the owner. It usually occurs within 30 minutes of separation and is usually unrelated to the length of time since the dog last eliminated (see Chapter 68).
Fear-induced	Either	Any	Dog eliminates in the house only when fear-eliciting stimuli occur (for example, punishment, thunderstorms).
URINATION ALONE			
Urine-marking	Usually male	Postpuberty	Usually unrelated to the owner's presence. May be initiated by specific stimuli (for example, another dog, mailperson); usually involves small amount of urine.
Submissive urination	Either	Usually puppies and young adults	Usually occurs during greeting or when person reaches toward dog; accompanied by submissive postures (lowered head, ears back, tail down, rolling over on side).
Excitement	Either	Usually young	Urinates in house only when excited (for example, greeting, play). Dog stands, squats, or dribbles urine while moving.
Housebreaking			See above
Separation anxiety			See above
Fear-induced			See above
DEFECATION ALONE			
Marking	Either	Any	Feces is often deposited on objects; may occur after major changes such as moving or new person in house.
Housebreaking			See above
Separation anxiety			See above
Fear-induced			See above

Housebreaking

The dog's natural instinct to avoid urinating and defecating in it's "den" (where it eats and sleeps) enables owners in most cases to easily housebreak their dogs. A housebreaking program should take advantage of this basic canine characteristic. To simulate the den, the dog should be restricted at first to a small area (cages are useful) except for times after it has just fully eliminated. When outside of this small area, the dog should be supervised at all times. The dog should be provided with frequent walks (every 2–3 hours) so there is ample opportunity to develop a preference for eliminating outside. The walks should be organized around the times that dogs usually demonstrate a need to eliminate (*e.g.*, after eating, waking, and during play.) Praise or food rewards should always follow elimination in the appropriate place. If the dog is seen eliminating in the house, immediate punishment, such as a loud verbal reprimand is indicated. Delayed punishment is counterproductive. If the elimination in the house occurs in only one location, the dog should be prevented access to the area or repelled from the area (*e.g.*, by using a citrus odor, like lemon-scented air fresheners), or the area's significance should be changed (*e.g.*, by putting food in the area). The dog should not be allowed full access to the house until it has had no "accidents" for 1 month.

Separation Anxiety

For an in-depth discussion of separation anxiety, see Chapter 68.

Fear-Induced Elimination

A program utilizing the techniques of counterconditioning and desensitization is prescribed (see Chapter 65). Anti-anxiety medication may be a helpful adjunct to behavior modification therapy. See Chapter 70 for detailed discussion of treatment of fears and phobias.

Urine-Marking

Castration has a 50% probability of decreasing urine-marking behavior in male dogs regardless of their age or length of time that the dogs have been marking (Hopkins, Additional Reading). Progestins may also suppress marking. Megestrol acetate (2.2–4.4 mg/kg, orally once a day) is given for 1 week followed by a weekly reduction to the lowest dose that still controls the problem. The dog should be carefully monitored for side effects and the drug discontinued if necessary (Appendix II).

Punishment, if applied consistently and at the time the dog begins to urine-mark, may prevent the behavior when the owners are present. The marking will probably still occur in the owners' absence, however. If the marking occurs in only one or a few locations, the dog can be prevented access to these locations, the locations made aversive (*e.g.*, by using citrus odors or commercial repellents, Boundary or Off), or the significance of the locations changed (*e.g.*, to a feeding area). If specific stimuli that elicit the urine-marking can be identified, a program consisting of counterconditioning and desensitization is sometimes useful.

Submissive Urination

Because a dog that is submissively urinating is usually greeting, friendly, and already submissive, punishment is contraindicated. It may just make the dog fearful and more submissive. Ignoring the behavior, thus avoiding either inadvertent reward or punishment, is a better method of treatment. If the eliciting stimuli can be identified, these should be avoided (*e.g.*, reaching for the dog, bending over the dog). Many dogs stop urinating submissively if the owners do not greet them at all on arriving home. If ignoring is not helpful, then redirecting the dog's greeting behavior to play (*e.g.*, throwing a ball) often is. If still not effective, then the dog can be counterconditioned to assume a standing nonurinating posture in situations that previously evoked the behavior. Most dogs naturally outgrow submissive urination.

Excitement Urination

Again the behavior should not be associated with either punishment or reward, as both may facilitate it. If the stimuli that elicit the behavior can be identified, they should be avoided if possible. If not, the dog's response to the eliciting stimuli can be habituated or counterconditioned (see Chapter 65).

Marking With Feces

As little is known about fecal marking by dogs in the home, no specific treatment techniques have been developed. There is no reason to believe that the behavior modification techniques that have been developed for urine marking should not be effective for fecal marking.

Patient Monitoring

Most canine elimination problems are controllable but require multiple and frequent rechecks. These are best done by telephone on a weekly basis.

FELINE ELIMINATION PROBLEMS

House soiling is the most common feline behavioral problem seen by veterinary animal behaviorists. Although more people with cats in general may be bothered by scratching and walking on countertops, these types of problems are usually tolerable and do not often cause the people to give up a pet. A daily greeting of fresh feces or urine in the corner of the living room, however, often ruins a previously good human-feline relationship and ends in pet relinquishment.

Causes

A cat that is urinating or defecating outside of the litter box may be doing so for either medical or behavioral reasons. If the cat is *either* urinating or defecating outside of the box, a medical etiology is a strong possibility. Lower urinary tract inflammation (see Chapter 48) and diseases that cause polyuria (diabetes mellitus) often lead to inappropriate urination. Diarrhea (see Chapter 37) often leads to litter box problems as well.

Although most cats with medical problems have other signs in addition to house soiling (*e.g.*, polydipsia, stranguria), some do not, or have not been observed by their owners. Therefore, in order to rule out disease, a complete urinalysis or fecal examination is necessary. If a cat is both urinating and defecating in inappropriate areas, the cause is most likely behavioral, although neurogenic incontinence should be considered (see Chapter 42).

After the possibility of disease has been ruled out, a behavioral diagnosis must be pursued. A cat that is urinating or defecating in objectionable locations may be marking or eliminating.

Urine marking is an innate, genetically based behavior that occurs in territorial, agonistic, sexual, or other highly arousing situations. It is most often performed in a spraying posture (standing, with tail upright and quivering while urine is sprayed onto vertical surfaces) but may also be done while squatting. The expression of marking behavior is influenced by many factors, hormones and environmental stimuli being the most important. Androgens and estrogens facilitate urine marking, while progestins inhibit it. Intact male cats mark more frequently than castrated males, and intact female cats more than spayed females (primarily during estrus). The sights, odors, and sounds of outdoor cats may cause a cat to mark, as does competition among indoor cats. Often, a male (intact or castrated) cat may start to mark if a female housemate goes into estrus.

Urination, defined as the emptying of the bladder for the purpose of eliminating waste products, is performed in a squatting posture. Defecation, or the voiding of feces, is also performed while squatting. The marking function of feces has not been clearly demonstrated in domestic cats. However, the fact that it serves a communication function in many other species makes a marking function in some situations likely. Still, in most cases, defecation is performed merely for the purpose of elimination.

Cats that are urinating or defecating outside of the litter box for the purpose of elimination usually are doing so due to the instinctive urge of cats to eliminate in a variety of substrates and locations (*e.g.*, loose dirt, leaves, sand), combined with learned aversions and preferences. Cats very often will faithfully use the box for one form of excrement but avoid the box for the other. A cat may avoid using the litter box if the litter or the box area is or has been associated with something aversive, for example, new litter, hood on box, dirty box, the use of a deodorizer, punishment, loud noises near the box, feeding near the box, or a bout of painful cystitis. Whether or not a cat clearly demonstrates a litter aversion, most cats with elimination problems also show either a location or surface preference. Cats with location preferences generally choose areas that are quiet and somewhat secluded (*e.g.*, the corner of the dining room). The most common surface preference is for carpeting, although some cats choose smooth surfaces such as bathtubs, sinks, and linoleum. Cats are probably not drawn back to an area because of the odor there; however, that hypothesis is controversial. In fact, a dirty litter box or a very soiled area is more likely to deter cats than attract them. Emotional causes of house soiling problems are rare—contrary to popular belief. Separation anxiety occasionally causes cats to mark or eliminate outside of the litter box, and the introduction of new household members (new baby, spouse) may precipitate territorial

marking. A thorough behavioral and medical history, physical examination, and appropriate laboratory tests (urinalysis and fecal examination) are necessary in order to make a diagnosis (Table 69-2).

Management

Before any behavioral therapy is initiated, physical disorders (*e.g.*, cystitis, diarrhea) must first be corrected.

Marking

Because marking behavior is influenced by a number of hormonal, environmental, and behavioral variables, a variety of treatment techniques may be effective. Surgical therapies include neutering and olfactory tractotomy. Castration has an 87% probability of reducing spraying in male cats, regardless of the age preformed or the duration of spraying (Hart and Barrett, Additional Reading). Spaying is likely to reduce marking by a female cat only if the incidence of marking is related to the estrus cycle. Olfactory tractotomy

Table 69–2 *Diagnosis of Feline Elimination Problems*

Diagnosis	Posture	Location	Amount	History
Urination	Squat	Horizontal surfaces	Usually large	Occurs when cat needs to empty bladder; cat usually scratches before and after. Cat often shows signs of litter or box aversion: doesn't dig or cover, stands on the sides of the box, runs from box. Obvious causes for aversion: dirty box, hood, food close to box, inaccessible, noisy area, perfumed litter. Cat shows location or substrate preference (carpet, sinks); usually urinates in only a few locations. Cat often uses box for feces.
Defecation	Squat	Horizontal surfaces	Normal bowel movement	Occurs when cat has urge to defecate; same as urination. Cat will often use box for urine.
Urine-marking	Spray	Vertical surfaces	Usually small	Often occurs in many locations. Occurs in context of territorial, sexual, or competitive interactions or other highly arousing circumstances; often seasonal. Often occurs at exit points, for example, doors and windows. May be initiated by introduction of new family member (baby, spouse) or animal.
	Squat or semisquat	Horizontal surfaces	Usually small	Occurs in same circumstances as spray; often occurs on objects, beds, and clothing.
Fecal-marking	Squat	Horizontal surfaces	Normal bowel movement	Very little is known; but may occur in same circumstances as urine marking.

is reported to reduce or stop spraying in about 50% of cats refractory to castration and progestin drug therapy (Hart, Additional Reading).

Manipulation of the environment is the least invasive of all techniques and is sometimes helpful. If a cat is marking in only a few locations, changing the significance of the areas by feeding or playing with the cat in them may at least stop the problem in those locations. Making the locations unpleasant by placing citrus-scented air fresheners or aluminum foil at the spots may also help. Preventing access to outdoor cats (closing a shade or door) or changing (increasing or decreasing) the amount of time a cat spends outdoors may reduce marking in the home.

Behavior modification in the form of reward or punishment is rarely, if ever, effective. Although some cats may no longer mark in the owners' presence, they continue to do so at other times.

The most effective treatment for marking in already neutered cats includes drug therapy. The progestins, diazepam, and other anti-anxiety drugs have been shown to be effective in reducing or eliminating marking behavior. When using drug therapy, the owners should be advised that no drugs are approved or marketed for treatment of behavioral problems in cats. Drug therapy of any kind should be gradually stopped every 1 to 2 months to determine if the cat is still motivated to mark, as many cats are seasonal sprayers. Because the range of minimum therapeutic doses is wide, the lowest effective dose should be utilized. Diazepam (Valium), at a dose of 1 to 2 mg, orally twice a day, significantly reduces spraying in more than 70% of cats (Marder and Voith, Additional Reading). Side effects include increased appetite and affection, sedation, and ataxia. In addition cats develop a tolerance to the drug and thus should be gradually withdrawn when discontinuing therapy. The progestins megestrol acetate (Ovaban), at a dose of 5 mg, orally once a day for 7 to 10 days, and then 5 mg, orally once weekly for 1 month, and medroxyprogesterone acetate (Depoprovera), at a dose of 10 to 20 mg/kg, SC or IM repeated as needed for a maximum of three injections per year, reduce or eliminate marking in about 30% of cats (Hart, Additional Reading). Potential side effects include increased appetite, lethargy, transient hyperglycemia, dia-

betes mellitus, aspermatogenesis, mammary gland hyperplasia, mammary adenocarcinoma, and pyometritis. If used, blood glucose, mammary gland development, and body weight should be carefully monitored during the course of therapy. Oral therapy is preferred because it is slightly more effective and can be rapidly withdrawn if side effects occur.

Urination or Defecation Problems

When a cat chooses a new area in which to eliminate, the new behavior becomes ingrained, somewhat like a bad habit. At this point, just changing the initiating cause (such as cleaning a once dirty litter box) is unlikely to correct the problem. The factors that are operating to maintain the problem at the present time as well as the initiating factors must be considered when designing a program for inappropriate elimination problems. (In many cases, the original cause is not even present at the time of treatment.)

Two treatment techniques, which are commonly prescribed but are rarely effective, are punishment and confinement. Punishment many hours after the fact, followed by putting the cat in the box, is more likely to cause a litter box aversion than cure an elimination problem. Confinement forces the cat to use the box but at the same time does not allow access to the inappropriate area. Once the cat is again permitted into the area, it usually resumes eliminating there.

A simple way to approach elimination problems is to make the litter box very desirable from the cat's point of view and make the inappropriate areas very unpleasant. If both are done at the same time, then in most cases both the initiating and maintaining factors are addressed.

Making boxes more desirable generally corrects the initiating factors. Ways to do this include: eliminating the hood if present, using plain clay litter rather than deodorized or perfumed types (the new sand-like clay litters are best); keeping the box clean by scooping both feces and urine-soaked litter daily and changing the entire box weekly; keeping 2 to 3 inches of litter in the box at all times; moving the box to a more accessible or quieter location; if the cat has a strong location preference, then moving it to the inappropriate area; providing at least two boxes and one box per cat (within limits); feeding the cat a distance from the box; or, if the cat does not seem to like clay at all, providing another type of substrate such as newspaper or wood shavings.

At the same time that the changes in the box are made, the inappropriate area must be made relatively intolerable. This action usually eliminates the maintaining factors. Ways to do this may include: covering a carpeted area with a thick plastic drop cloth in order to change the feeling of the substrate; putting a citrus-scented solid air freshener at the area; feeding the cat or playing with it at the problem location; leaving a few inches of water in the bathtub or sink.

Sometimes rewarding the cat with praise and a special treat every time it uses the box is also helpful.

Once the cat begins to use the box again, things should not be changed too quickly back to the way the owners might prefer them. If the owners progress too quickly, the cat usually goes back to its old habits. Things should be left in place for 1 month, then changes can be made. For instance, the owners might start to cut away the plastic, move the box a few inches each day back to a more desirable location, start mixing in clay litter with wood shavings, and so on, over a period of another month. Most households are back to normal within 3 months. Special care should be taken not to initiate the problem again or the process may start all over.

Patient Monitoring

The prognosis for control of house soiling in general is good. Although relapses are common, in the majority of elimination problem cases, cats can be converted back to using the litter box. Unless environmental factors radically change, marking behavior is rarely completely "cured." It can usually be well controlled, however, and kept to a tolerable minimum. Follow-ups are done by telephone on a weekly basis.

ADDITIONAL READING

Hart BL. Olfactory tractotomy for control of objectionable urine spraying and urine marking in cats. J Am Vet Med Assoc 1981; 179:231.

Hart BL, Barrett RE. Effects of castration on fighting, roaming, and urine spraying in adult male cats. J Am Vet Med Assoc 1973; 163:290.

Hopkins SG, Schuber TA, Hart BL. Castration of adult male dogs: Effects on roaming, aggression, urine marking and mounting. J Am Vet Med Assoc 1976; 168:1108.

Marder AR, Voith VL. Effectiveness of diazepam for the treatment of spraying in cats. Paper presented at the Animal Behavior Society Meeting, Raleigh, 1985.

Voith VL, Marder AR. Canine behavioral disorders, feline behavioral disorders. In: Morgan RV, ed. Handbook of small animal practice. New York: Churchill Livingstone, 1988: 1033.

Voith VL, Borchelt PL. Diagnosis and treatment of elimination behavior problems in dogs. Vet Clin North Am 1982; 12:637.

Borchelt PL, Voith VL. Elimination behavior problems in cats. Compendium of Continuing Education 1986; 8:197.

70

FEARS AND PHOBIAS IN DOGS

Amy R. Marder

Fearful and phobic responses are very common in dogs. Dogs are most often presented to veterinarians because of fears of loud noises, (thunder or fireworks), people, traffic, and stressful environments (dog shows).

The typical fear response of a dog may involve freezing, trembling, panting, urinating, defecating, increased heart rate, digging, hiding, or fleeing when possible. Very often animals become destructive, attempting to hide or escape. If an animal is cornered and cannot escape, however, aggressive or fighting responses, such as growling, barking, snapping, or biting may occur. A phobia is an excessive fear response that is out of proportion to the real threat of the stimulus. The behaviors exhibited are not adaptive and are often harmful to the animal.

CAUSES

Fears and phobias can develop at any age, and no sex predilection appears to exist. Numerous anecdotal reports of breed or strain predispositions exist, but, as of now, there are no good data to support these reports have been found. Sometimes, a fear or phobia can be traced to a specific frightening event; but in most cases the owners are unaware of any precipitating cause. Many studies have shown that early experience with humans and novel environments influence the development of fears in dogs. Dogs raised in restrictive environments (without exposure to people) at various ages are more likely to exhibit a fear of people. (This fear resulting from early restriction of experiences can be reduced by later experiences, however.) Fears and phobias often generalize to other similar stimuli. For example, a loud noise phobia may initially involve only thunder and fireworks but may eventually generalize to other loud noises, such as traffic sounds. Similarly, an initial fear of tall men may progress to a generalized phobia of all people.

CLINICAL SIGNS AND DIAGNOSTIC APPROACH

The fearful dog may freeze, pace, pant, dig, eliminate, try to escape, shiver, and bark when exposed to the fear-inducing stimulus. The history and direct observation of the dog most often leads to the diagnosis. Dogs with loud noise phobias display a fearful response whenever they are exposed to thunderstorms, firecrackers, gunfire, or similar noises. Very often a dog with a thunderstorm phobia can detect a storm long before the owners can. In many dogs, the fear generalizes to any type of rain whether or not it is accompanied by thunder. In addition, over time, the fear usually gets progressively worse. The diagnosis is sometimes confusing, as many dogs with loud noise phobias develop signs of separation anxiety as well.

Dogs that are afraid of people may not only display fearful behavior but may also exhibit aggression or submissive urination as well. A dog may be afraid of all strangers or only one type of individual, such as men or children. The fear often generalizes to all types of people over time.

MANAGEMENT

A program that allows the animal to experience the fear-eliciting stimulus without being afraid is prescribed. The techniques used may include counterconditioning, desensitization, or flooding. Anti-anxiety medication is often used but not during the actual treatment sessions.

For dogs that are afraid of noises, the noises are first identified and replicated by tape recording or if possible produced in a muted way, such as at a distance. The noises are then presented to the dog at a low volume while the dog is in a relaxed state, as when eating or playing. The volume is then gradually increased, taking care not to cause the dog to become fearful. Anti-anxiety medication, preferably the benzodiazepines (clorazepate dipotassium SD, 11.25–22.5 mg/dog, one or two times a day; Diazepam 0.5–2.2 mg/kg, orally as needed), are used between treatment sessions if the dog is exposed to the real noises of higher volume.

For dogs that are afraid of people, again, all the eliciting stimuli must first be identified and placed on a gradient. The least threatening stimulus is presented to dog first, followed by the more threatening stimuli while the dog is in a relaxed state. Again, the dog should never be allowed to become afraid. Flooding may be effective in some mild cases of fear of people but should be used only when signs of aggression are absent. If aggression is present, the use of a comfortable basket muzzle may make a behavioral modification program possible. The owners should be advised not to reinforce the fearful behaviors with petting, praise, or calming words. Exposure to the fear-eliciting stimuli should be prevented between treatment sessions. Extreme care should be taken if anti-anxiety medication is prescribed, as many dogs become more aggressive once the fear is decreased with medication. I prefer to stay away from drug therapy in the treatment of dogs that are afraid of people.

PATIENT MONITORING

The prognosis for phobic dogs is generally good. Desensitization is often difficult because many times dogs do not "believe" the artificial noises on tape. In these cases, drug therapy must be used every time the real noise (*e.g.*, thunderstorm) occurs. Extra care should be taken in dogs that are displaying fear-induced aggression. These dogs are often very dangerous to treat, as the treatment program must involve exposing a potentially aggressive dog to people. Follow-up evaluations are done on weekly or 2-week intervals, either by telephone or in person.

ADDITIONAL READING

Voith VL, Borchelt PL. Fears and phobias in companion animals. Compendium of Continuing Education 1985; 7:209.

Voith VL, Marder AR. Canine behavioral disorders. In: Morgan R, ed. Handbook of small animal practice. New York: Churchill Livingstone, 1988: 1033.

BLOOD-GAS, BIOCHEMICAL PROFILE, AND PERIPHERAL BLOOD

13

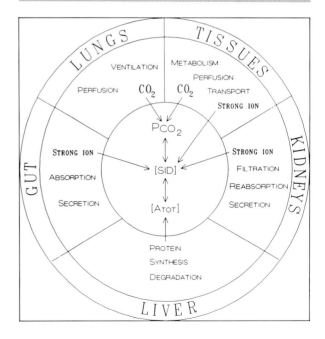

71

ACID-BASE AND BLOOD-GAS ABNORMALITIES

Peter J. Pascoe

In the past it has been customary to talk of acid-base and electrolyte abnormalities as separate entities. As we develop our understanding of the pathophysiology of these abnormalities, it becomes clear that the separation is artificial. The chemical reactions that alter the concentrations of substances within the body are interwoven, and it is almost impossible to change one thing without affecting many others. The neuroendocrine system controls various ion exchange mechanisms in the body, and the secretion of the hormones are in turn controlled by these ions. Also, feedback loops act directly on the ion exchanges across cell membranes and increase or decrease the exchange rate as the level of the ion alters. The purpose of this chapter is to present a cohesive approach to these alterations in a way that can be utilized in a modern practice.

Alterations in acid-base and electrolytes are usually not very important in and of themselves but are a reflection of the disease process affecting the animal. Despite the fact that homeostatic mechanisms maintain the levels of ions within very strict limits, animals tolerate marked derangements with apparent equanimity. Even under rigorous experimental conditions, it has been impossible to consistently demonstrate any major problems with a blood pH as low as 7.2 or as high as 7.6. In a study that reported on the acid-base values of 220 dogs suspected of having acid-base changes, only 9 animals had a pH less than 7.2, and none had a pH greater than 7.6.

Acidemia and alkalemia are the terms used to define a decrease or increase in the blood pH or hydrogen ion concentration from normal ranges. Acidosis and alkalosis are the terms used to denote the process that is tending to alter the pH. Alterations in acid-base balance produced by changes in the exchange of carbon dioxide are termed respiratory acidosis or respiratory alkalosis and all other changes are termed metabolic acidosis or metabolic alkalosis. These terms, then, are used to define the four simple derangements. Under normal circumstances, a metabolic derangement will stimulate an opposite respiratory compensation and vice versa. These compensatory mechanisms rarely achieve a full return to normal values. It is also possible that two or more derangements may occur at the same time, and these are generally termed mixed acid-base disturbances.

CAUSES

Any process that alters the normal balance of ionic intake, output, or internal regulation may lead to an acid-base disturbance. In addition, certain poisons may cause profound changes in acid-base balance. In the dog, the most common abnormality is a metabolic acidosis, with metabolic alkalosis next, and the respiratory changes being less common. Table 71-1 lists the common causes of acid-base disturbances in small animals.

Metabolic Acidosis

Diseases involving the gastrointestinal tract can produce an acidosis due to the loss of electrolytes. It was expected that an animal that was vomiting frequently would have an alkalosis due to the loss of acid from the stomach. Although this condition does occur with high intestinal obstruction, it is more common to see bile stained vomitus, which is likely to represent a loss of bicarbonate from the duodenum. In the study reported above, 12 dogs presented with vomiting had a metabolic acidosis, whereas only 7 had a metabolic alkalosis. Various circulatory disturbances (*e.g.*, dehydration and shock) can result in a metabolic acidosis due to a failure of the microcirculation and a build up of lactic acid. Other organic acids may accumulate in excess in renal disease, keto-

Table 71–1 Causes of Acid-Base Disturbances in Small Animals

METABOLIC ACIDOSIS

Vomiting (Is the vomitus bile stained?)
Diarrhea
Renal insufficiency (impaired excretion of H^+)
Diabetic ketoacidosis (Ketoacidosis may also occur in severe starvation.)
Shock (impaired circulation results in anaerobic metabolism and an accumulation of lactic acid)
Heart failure (lactic acidosis)
Hypoadrenocorticism
Ethylene glycol poisoning
Salicylate toxicity
Carbonic anhydrase inhibitors
Malignancies (lymphoma, leukemia, sarcoma)
Status epilepticus

METABOLIC ALKALOSIS

Vomiting (high intestinal obstruction with little reflux of duodenal secretion)
Sequestration of gastric acid (gastric dilation-volvulus complex)
Heartworm disease
Hyperadrenocorticism
Excess alkali (for example, sodium bicarbonate, citrate in blood transfusion)

RESPIRATORY ACIDOSIS

Impaired alveolar ventilation (for example, pleural effusion, diaphragmatic hernia, obstructive lung disease, pulmonary edema, pulmonary neoplasia)
CNS depression (mainly seen during anesthesia)
Neuromuscular disorders (for example, coonhound paralysis)

RESPIRATORY ALKALOSIS

Hypoxia (for example, pulmonary edema, pneumonia, anemia)
CNS stimulation (for example, anxiety, pain, fever, heatstroke, neoplasia)
Salicylate poisoning
Hepatic encephalopathy
Early septic shock

---

acidosis, and in certain poisonings (*e.g.*, ethylene glycol). Diseases that affect the renal control of electrolyte balance may also produce a metabolic acidosis. Examples include hypoaldosteronism (Addison's disease), the use of carbonic anhydrase inhibitors (*e.g.*, acetazolamide), and renal diseases that involve a decreased response to aldosterone.

Metabolic Alkalosis

Metabolic alkalosis is much less common because the kidneys are very efficient at excreting alkali. Therefore, a metabolic alkalosis is more likely in an animal with compromised renal function if it has an increased alkali load. Loss of hydrochloric acid from the stomach is still the most common primary cause for metabolic alkalosis, but it has also been reported to occur as a primary condition in dogs with heartworm disease. Metabolic alkalosis may also occur in hyperadrenocorticism where aldosterone stimulates the reabsorption of sodium and the secretion of hydrogen ions in the distal nephron. An iatrogenic alkalosis can occur with the excessive administration of sodium bicarbonate, during the administration of blood containing citrate, or by an overdose of antacids.

Respiratory Acidosis

Respiratory acidosis is most commonly seen as part of syndromes that impair alveolar ventilation. Under normal circumstances, control of CO_2 by the central nervous system (CNS) is such that the P_{CO_2} is maintained within very narrow limits. The presence of a respiratory acidosis in primary pulmonary disease indicates that the animal has begun to decompensate and that further increases in ventilation are either impossible or represent an excessive effort for the benefit gained. In severe respiratory acidosis, as the P_{CO_2} rises, the P_{O_2} falls, and the hypoxemia may provide an extra stimulus to ventilation. Depression of the CNS, in particular the respiratory center, may also result in a respiratory acidosis. This depression is most commonly seen during anesthesia when drugs producing CNS depression are administered. Opioids are well known for their effects as respiratory depressants, but in the dog it is uncommon to see a respiratory acidosis following the administration of an opioid on its own. Some opioids produce a lowering of the animal's thermoregulatory set point, and the stimulus to lose heat overrides the ventilatory depression, causing the dog to pant in order to lose heat. This effect prevents the development of a respiratory acidosis. However, when an opioid is combined with other respiratory depressants (*e.g.*, inhalants or barbiturates), a significant respiratory acidosis may result. Respiratory acidosis is also seen when interference with the muscles of ventilation occurs. This condition can occur in coonhound paralysis when the disease begins to affect the control of the diaphragm.

Respiratory Alkalosis

In dogs and cats, this disorder is most commonly associated with conditions that cause hypoxemia. Animals with pneumonia or pulmonary edema tend to become hypoxic on room air, and ventilation is driven by the low oxygen tension, thus lowering the tension of carbon dioxide. Ventilation may also be driven centrally by CNS excitation. This condition can occur because of anxiety or pain, fever or heatstroke, or CNS disease such as a tumor or meningitis. Salicylate intoxication produces an acute respiratory alkalosis due to a direct effect on the respiratory center. However, the uncoupling of oxidative phosphorylation in the peripheral tissues caused by the salicylate leads to a primary metabolic acidosis as well.

PATHOPHYSIOLOGY

According to Stewart's quantitative approach to acid-base changes, relationships exist for all the chemical reactions that concern the charged particles in an electrically neutral solution. This relationship exists because of the requirement for electrical neutrality in any particular solution. Hence, the sum of the positive charges must equal the sum of the negative charges.

For example

$$[Na^+] + [K^+] + [H^+] - [Cl^-] - [OH^-] = 0.$$

In biologic solutions, strong ions (*e.g.*, sodium, chloride, and potassium), which are completely dissociated, can be found, and also other ions, which are mostly dissociated (*e.g.*, lactate, aceto-acetate, β-hydroxybutyrate) and which can also be classed as strong ions, can be found. Other types of ions that are part of a reversible reaction where the concentrations of the ionic form are dependent on the conditions within the solution are also present. At body *p*H and temperature, these weaker ions are largely undissociated. Stewart has taken the strong ions as a group and, in a biologic solution, subtracts the anions from the cations and calls this result the strong ion difference [SID]. The above reaction becomes the following:

$$[SID] + [H^+] - [OH^-] = 0$$

Three other relationships exist in a biologic solution:

1. The dissociation of water to hydroxyl and hydrogen ions
2. The plasma protein and other weak acids and bases that are in a partially ionized form
3. The solution of carbon dioxide in water and the production of bicarbonate and carbonate ions from this reaction

These relationships can be expressed mathematically (see the Appendix at the end of this chapter) and produce an equation in which the variables are the [SID], the total amount of weak acids and bases (mainly accounted for by the plasma proteins), and the P_{CO_2}. This comprehensive theory leads to two interesting conclusions:

1. The behavior of $[H^+]$ and hence *p*H in a biologic system cannot be explained on the basis of a single variable. As a simple example, if CO_2 changes, it will produce HCO_3^- and H^+. Some of the hydrogen ions may be removed by the weak bases, altering the electrical neutrality, so a change in the [SID] must occur.
2. The independent variables or factors that will alter acid-base balance, are [SID], plasma proteins, and P_{CO_2}.

Understanding that these are the independent variables leads us to consider how they can be

altered in the body. While significant variations in plasma protein may affect acid-base balance, it is unusual for the variations to be the primary causes of an acid-base disturbance. Therefore, the most important components are [SID] and P_{CO_2}.

The organs involved in each of these variables are depicted in Figure 71-1.

Alterations in the [SID] produce changes in the dependent variables (*e.g.*, $[H^+]$, $[HCO_3^-]$). An increase in [SID] produces a fall in $[H^+]$ (alkalosis), and a decrease in [SID] results in a rise in $[H^+]$ (acidosis). These effects fit well with common changes such as a hypochloremic alkalosis caused by the loss of gastric acid. In this case, more chloride is lost than sodium, so the [SID] increases, and we have an increase in *p*H. In diabetic keto-acidosis, an accumulation of strong ions occurs (acetoacetate, β-hydroxybutyrate), which will narrow [SID], leading to a fall in *p*H. In the clinical setting, we do not measure all the components of [SID], a fact that makes it impossible to apply the computer models developed by Stewart. However, we do measure the main components of [SID] under normal circumstances (Na^+, K^+ and Cl^-), and we can use another approach to infer if other abnormal strong ions are present. This measurement is the anion gap, which is normally calculated by the following formula:

$$Anion\ gap = [Na^+ + K^+] - [Cl^- + HCO_3^-]$$

This measurement is obviously related to the [SID], but, by including the measurement of bicarbonate, it may give an indication of the unmeasured ions present that are causing the acid-base disturbance. To use the above examples in the hypochloremic alkalosis, an increase in [SID] occurs, but the anion gap is often normal because of the increase in bicarbonate. However, in the diabetic with ketoacidosis, the [SID] may be in the normal range, but the anion gap is increased because the presence of the other strong ions reduces the amount of bicarbonate.

As indicated in Figure 71-1, the main regulation of [SID] is by way of the tissues, the gut, and the kidneys. The responses in the tissues and the gut are relatively passive, so the regulation of the [SID] is mainly dependent on renal function. The ability of the kidney to alter ionic excretion is a very complicated and involved subject beyond the scope of this chapter. A few of the important

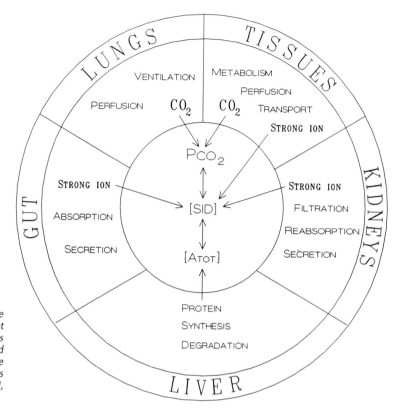

Figure 71–1. *The illustrated organs and tissues are responsible for the alterations in the independent variables P_{CO_2}, [SID], and $[A_{TOT}]$. ($[A_{TOT}]$ describes the total amount of weak acid present in the ionized $[A^-]$ and unionized [HA], forms.) Changes in these variables produce quantitatively defined alterations in the dependent variables, such as $[H^+]$, $[OH^-]$, $[HCO_3^-]$ and $[A^-]$.*

features include: the ability of the kidney to "buffer" urine, and the effect of potassium on renal function. The two main buffers in urine are ammonia and phosphate. Ammonia is produced from glutamine mainly in the proximal tubules. When ammonia is secreted into the tubule lumen, it will react with hydrogen ions to produce ammonium ions: $NH_3 + H^+ \rightleftharpoons NH_4^+$. At a neutral or low pH, this reaction proceeds largely to the right side, and hence it can remove significant amounts of hydrogen ion. Phosphate is also used to buffer urine, but its significance is much less than ammonia.

The role of potassium in acid-base regulation is not as clearly understood. In the plasma, a reduction of potassium from 5 mmol/L to 1 mmol/L (or 5 to 1 mEq/L) would only change [SID] by 4 mmol/L, producing minimal effects on pH (pH would drop by 0.05). However, although serum potassium levels are not a good indicator of whole body potassium, a reduction of this magnitude probably represents a significant fall in the intra-cellular levels of this cation. Under these circumstances, hydrogen ions and sodium ions shift into the cell in exchange for potassium, which tends to produce an alkalosis (loss of hydrogen ions from the extracellular fluid). In addition, potassium affects the rate of absorption of bicarbonate in the proximal renal tubules, and, in several species, a chronic potassium depletion leads to a severe metabolic alkalosis. This condition has been difficult to reproduce in the dog because potassium depletion reduces circulating aldosterone concentrations and also interferes with the tubular excretion of hydrogen ions. Such an opposing change reduces the degree of alkalosis. It is important to recognize potassium depletion since it may be difficult to correct an acid-base disturbance without first repairing the potassium deficit.

Carbon dioxide is produced during normal cellular metabolism and is transported to the lungs for excretion. The normal capacity of the ventilatory system for CO_2 removal is high, so it is rare for an increased production to result in an increased P_{CO_2}. Ventilation is controlled by the respiratory centers in the CNS. The peripheral nervous system and an effective mechanical system must be intact to provide ventilation. Interference at any of these levels can lead to an alteration and hence an effect on CO_2 removal. This interference may be caused by a primary injury to the system or it may be a compensatory alteration due to a change in the metabolic acid-base balance. The ability of the ventilatory system to compensate for metabolic changes is limited. When a metabolic acidosis stimulates an increase in ventilation, the concentration of carbon dioxide falls. Since the P_{CO_2} is inversely proportional to the alveolar ventilation, it follows that alveolar ventilation must be doubled in order to halve P_{CO_2}, or quadrupled to reach one quarter of the normal P_{CO_2}. In the awake animal it is hard to sustain such a significant increase in ventilation because of the energy required to do so. Conversely, a metabolic alkalosis will result in a retention of CO_2, but this retention is limited in that as the alveolar ventilation falls so does the level of oxygen in the alveolus. If alveolar ventilation is halved, then the P_{CO_2} will rise to about 80 mm Hg, resulting in a P_{O_2} of 50 mm Hg. As this fall in P_{O_2} is detected, it will begin to drive ventilation and prevent a further rise in P_{CO_2} (assuming that the animal is breathing room air at 760 mm Hg pressure—increasing the inspired oxygen concentration will allow a further decrease in ventilation. Decreasing the atmospheric pressure, for example, high altitude, will prevent even this much reduction in ventilation). Some drugs, notably the inhaled anesthetics, depress the ability of the animal to respond to hypoxia; this response can lead to a dangerous acidosis and hypoxia.

Compensation for primary respiratory acidosis or alkalosis occurs in two stages. With a respiratory acidosis, an initial change in the dependent variables occurs due to the alterations in the above reactions. If the condition has persisted for less than 6 hours, the following formula estimates the appropriate change in bicarbonate.

Change in $[HCO_3^-]$ = 0.1 × change in P_{CO_2}

That is, if the P_{CO_2} has risen by 20 mm Hg, the bicarbonate will increase by 2 mmol/L (mEq/L). As the condition persists, there is a shift of sodium out of the cells and a movement of chloride into the cells. The kidneys also begin to alter the rate of ionic excretion, and chloride excretion is increased. Both of these changes lead to an increased [SID] and hence to an increased bicarbonate and pH. In chronic respiratory failure, the rise in sodium leads to a retention of water, and the renin-angiotensin-aldosterone system is activated, leading to an increase in potassium excretion. The end result is that these animals may have marked sodium and water retention with a potassium and chloride deficiency. The expected change in bicarbonate in chronic respiratory acidosis follows:

Change in $[HCO_3^-]$ = 0.3–0.4 × change in P_{CO_2}

That is, for the same change in P_{CO_2} (20 mm Hg), the bicarbonate will increase by 6 to 8 mmol/L (mEq/L). Even in the chronic state, it is rare for this compensation to completely return the pH to a normal level. Therefore, in the dog and cat, bicarbonate is unlikely to exceed 40 mmol/L (mEq/L) in a pure respiratory acidosis.

In respiratory alkalosis, the same change in the dependent variables occurs in the acute stage:

Change in $[HCO_3^-]$ = 0.2 × change in P_{CO_2}

That is, for a fall in P_{CO_2} of 15 mm Hg, the bicarbonate will fall by 3 mmol/L (mEq/L). In the chronic state, a similar initial ionic shift across the cell membranes allows the chloride to move into the plasma and sodium to move into the cells. A rise in intracellular pH is associated with a stimulation of the glycolytic enzymes and an increase in the production of lactic acid, followed by a retention of chloride by the kidneys. These mechanisms tend to reduce [SID], thus, a decrease in bicarbonate and a fall in pH is evident. The full adaptive process can take several weeks, but it is the only compensatory mechanism that can return the pH to virtually normal levels. This mechanism is seen most commonly as an adaptive mechanism at high altitudes where the increased ventilation is produced by the relative hypoxia. In chronic hypocapnia the expected change in bicarbonate can be expressed by the following formula:

Change in $[HCO_3^-]$ = 0.3–0.5 × change in P_{CO_2}

That is, for a fall in P_{CO_2} of 15 mm Hg, the

bicarbonate will fall by 4.5 to 7.5 mmol/L (mEq/L), depending on the duration of the condition. Because of the limits to ventilatory capacity, the bicarbonate, will not fall below about 10 mmol/L (mEq/L) in a pure respiratory alkalosis.

When dealing with acid-base disturbances, it should also be remembered that the oxygen-hemoglobin dissociation curve is affected by alterations in *p*H. As the *p*H falls (acidosis), hemoglobin releases oxygen more easily, meaning that it will not be able to carry oxygen quite as well. The opposite occurs in alkalosis, and this effect becomes particularly important for the patient with a respiratory alkalosis caused by hypoxia. In this instance, less oxygen is picked up at the lung, and the alkalosis reduces the ability of the hemoglobin to release the oxygen to the tissues.

A metabolic alkalosis will also lead to an increase in lactate production because a rise in cellular *p*H forces glucose to be metabolized through the Embden-Meyerhof pathway to produce lactate. A rise in lactic acid will tend to counteract the alkalosis.

CLINICAL SIGNS

No specific signs associated with disorders of acid-base balance are seen; the manifestations are those of the primary disease. Severe alterations in *p*H affect neuronal conduction; hence, these patients may demonstrate muscle weakness, fatigue, and mental depression ranging from barely noticeable to a comatose state. These alterations in conduction may also affect the heart, and arrhythmias that develop may be refractory to normal therapy until the acid-base disturbance is corrected. In people with severe alkalosis (respiratory or metabolic), a reduction of ionized calcium is found, and signs of tetany may appear. This kind of response has not been documented in the dog and cat. In a metabolic acidosis or a respiratory alkalosis, one would expect an increase in ventilation, whereas in respiratory acidosis and metabolic alkalosis one would expect a decrease. However, this change may be difficult to detect, since the alteration in ventilation may be achieved by changing tidal volume rather than rate; and it is unusual to measure

minute or tidal ventilation in the awake veterinary patient. Because the dog and the cat may also alter ventilatory rate for the purposes of thermoregulation, it is difficult to assign such an alteration strictly to a change in acid-base balance.

DIAGNOSTIC APPROACH

Since the signs of acid-base and electrolyte disorders are often non-specific, the clinician must be alert to aspects of the patient's history that could lead to alterations in acid-base and electrolyte balance. An approach to diagnosis is presented in Figure 71-2. Some assessment of the severity of the change can also be obtained from the history. A cat that has had profuse diarrhea over several days is likely to have a severe metabolic acidosis, but almost no change may be apparent if the diarrhea has only been present for a few hours. A list of clinical signs and the associated disorders is presented in Table 71-2. The list also attempts to rank the changes, such that a vomiting animal is more likely to have a metabolic acidosis than a metabolic alkalosis. This list does not include the compensatory events that may result from the primary change.

Once the index of suspicion has been raised from the history, the physical examination is used to attempt to quantify and perhaps qualify the disturbance. This step is important in the situation where limited laboratory testing is available to assist in quantifying the change. The patient may have clinical signs of extracellular volume depletion (*e.g.*, increased skin turgor, tachycardia, prolonged capillary refill time). The more severe these signs appear, the more likely the presence of a metabolic acidosis. A depressed patient with "sweet" smelling breath and excessive ventilatory effort may have diabetic ketoacidosis with ventilatory compensation. In general, specific therapy for the acid-base disturbance is only necessary for the more severe disturbances. The clinician should, therefore, gauge the degree of dehydration, dyspnea, exercise intolerance, and so on, in order to arrive at a rationale for therapy.

In order to further define an acid-base disturbance, it is necessary to take a blood sample. Recently, dry chemistry machines have become

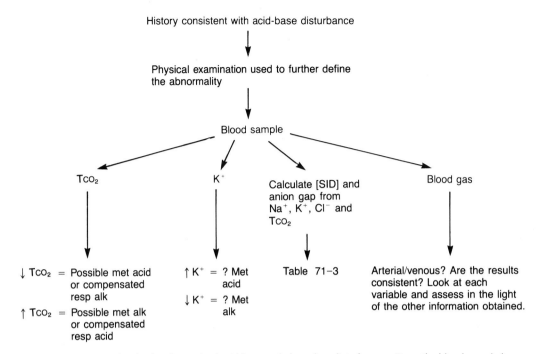

Figure 71–2. *Algorithm for the diagnosis of acid-base and electrolyte disturbances. Once the blood sample has been obtained, the approach can progress from left to right.*

Table 71–2 *Clinical Signs and Conditions Which May Produce Acid-Base Disturbances**

Sign/Condition	Possible Changes in Order of Likelihood
Vomiting	Met acid,† met alk‡ (resp acid,§ resp alk‖)
Diarrhea	Met acid
Bloat	Met alk, met acid, resp acid, resp alk
Anorexia	Met acid, met alk
Ingestion of toxin (ethylene glycol, salicylate)	Met acid, resp alk [salicylates]
Polyuria/Polydipsia	Met acid, (met alk)
Dehydration	Met acid, (met alk)
Shock	Met acid, resp alk, (met alk)
Exercise intolerance	Met acid, resp acid, resp alk
Dyspnea/Coughing	Met acid, resp acid, resp alk, met alk
Increased ventilation (chronic tachypnea or chronic increase in tidal volume)	Resp alk, met acid
Decreased ventilation (shallow breaths/slow respiratory rate)	Resp acid, met alk
Mental depression/Coma	Met acid, resp acid, met alk
Paresis/Paralysis	Met acid, resp acid

* *Changes in parentheses ( ) can occur but are rare.*
† *Metabolic acidosis*
‡ *Metabolic alkalosis*
§ *Respiratory acidosis*
‖ *Respiratory alkalosis*

available that can measure Na^+, K^+, Cl^-, and Tco_2 on blood, serum, or plasma. The Tco_2 is a measurement of the CO_2 when the blood is titrated with a strong acid and represents the carbon dioxide present in the sample as bicarbonate, dissolved CO_2, and CO_2 associated with organic ions (carbamino compounds). Since the majority of CO_2 is present as bicarbonate, it is a good indicator of the bicarbonate concentration in blood. An elevated Tco_2 is most likely to be associated with a metabolic alkalosis or a compensated respiratory acidosis; a decreased Tco_2 is normally associated with a metabolic acidosis or a compensated respiratory alkalosis. The potassium concentration should also be evaluated, since a decreased potassium is usually associated with a metabolic alkalemia, and an increased potassium is associated with an acidemia. The Tco_2, Na^+, K^+, and Cl^- can be used to calculate the [SID] and anion gap, which can then be interpreted as described in Table 71-3.

The most complete analysis would ideally include an arterial and a mixed venous (blood taken from the pulmonary artery) blood sample analyzed to measure pH, Pco_2, Po_2, Na^+, K^+, Cl^-, hematocrit, and total protein. From the first two values (pH, Pco_2), the $[HCO_3^-]$ and base excess (BE) can be calculated. The base excess may be reported as the actual base excess (ABE) or the standard base excess (SBE). These values represent the deviation from normal ($pH = 7.4$, $Pco_2 =$

40) of the buffers in the blood. The ABE is based on a correction factor measured in whole blood in vitro, whereas the SBE is based on in vivo measurements and includes the extracellular space. The SBE is, therefore, the more appropriate clinical measurement. An arterial sample assists in the interpretation of ventilatory abnormalities, and the differences between the arterial and mixed venous sample reflects the state of the circulation (*e.g.,* in low flow states, the difference between the arterial and the mixed venous values is increased).

The measurement of pH, Pco_2, and Po_2 requires a blood-gas machine, which is an expensive piece of equipment and, therefore, is not commonly available in practice. Despite the reliability of modern blood-gas machines, it is important to check that the results are consistent with the condition of the patient and that no sampling errors have been made.

For metabolic disturbances, a peripheral venous sample is usually adequate, but an arterial sample is essential for the interpretation of respiratory disorders. Venous samples can be taken from the jugular, cephalic, or saphenous vein in the dog and also from the femoral vein in the cat. Arterial samples can be obtained from the radial artery, the femoral artery, and the dorsal pedal artery in both species. When obtaining arterial samples, it is important not to struggle with the animal because this causes the dog or cat to

Table 71–3 *Interpretations of Anion Gap (AG) and Strong Ion Difference (SID)**

NORMAL [SID] ***NORMAL AG*** Normal or Respiratory acidosis or Respiratory alkalosis	***INCREASED [SID]*** ***NORMAL AG*** Metabolic acidosis Compensated respiratory alkalosis
DECREASED [SID] ***INCREASED AG*** Metabolic acidosis	***DECREASED [SID]*** ***NORMAL AG*** Metabolic Acidosis Compensated respiratory alkalosis
NORMAL [SID] ***INCREASED AG*** Metabolic acidosis	***INCREASED [SID]*** ***INCREASED AG*** Mixed metabolic alkalosis and acidosis

* *([SID] = [Na$^+$] + [K$^+$] − [Cl$^-$]). It should be emphasized that changes detected by these methods tend to be relatively severe since the range for normal values is wide. The definitive diagnosis of an acid-base disturbance requires the measurement of pH and Pco$_2$ as well as the electrolytes.*

hyperventilate, making it more difficult to obtain an accurate interpretation. In the anesthetized animal, a lingual artery can be used. It has also been shown that "arterial" samples can be obtained from the lingual veins and from a toe nail that has been clipped down to the vascular bed. The correlation between the results obtained from these sites and from arterial blood is good as long as circulation is not compromised. Hence, these latter sites should not be used in animals suffering from hypovolemia or peripheral vasoconstriction. When collecting the sample it is important that the blood be free flowing and that the vein or other vessel not be occluded for more than 5 to 10 seconds. No air should get into the syringe, since it will change the gas tensions toward those of room air (P_{CO_2} less than 5 mm Hg and P_{O_2} 150 mm Hg).

Heparin is normally used as the anticoagulant, and the powdered form is most appropriate since it does not dilute the sample. When liquid heparin is used, it is important to draw at least 20 times as much blood as heparin. Once the sample has been obtained, any air bubbles should be expelled and the sample capped. It should be analyzed immediately or placed in iced water if this is not possible. As long as the sample is kept in iced water, little deterioration occurs for about 2 hours (with the exception that samples with a P_{aO_2} of greater than 150 mm Hg may show rapid decline). Normal values for [SID] determined at the University of California are 44 ± 5 and 40 ± 2 mmol/L for the dog and cat respectively (the normal range is 34–54 mmol/L in the dog and 36–44 mmol/L in the cat). The normal range for anion gap quoted in the literature is 15 to 25 mmol/L for both the dog and cat.

Metabolic Acidosis

This condition is characterized by a rise in hydrogen ion concentration and, therefore, a fall in pH. In the uncompromised animal, ventilation will increase, and the decrease in P_{CO_2} will shift the equilibrium reaction to the left, thus removing hydrogen ions from the system. As the acidosis becomes more severe, the increasing energy cost of ventilation will limit the ability to compensate.

As a rough guide, in people, the expected P_{aCO_2} can be calculated from the following equation:
$$P_{aCO_2} = (1.5\ [HCO_3^-] + 8) \pm 2$$

For example, if the HCO_3^- is 16, then P_{aCO_2} = 30 to 34. This formula has not been tested in the dog and cat, but the expectation would be that it would underestimate the response, since the normal P_{aCO_2} values in the dog and cat are less than in people to begin with. Thus, if the P_{aCO_2} is greater than this value, then the animal is failing to compensate for the metabolic derangement. If the P_{aCO_2} is less, then a respiratory alkalosis is occurring at the same time. It is very unusual for the P_{CO_2} to be less than 10 mm Hg in a pure metabolic acidosis. Measured values less than 10 mm Hg usually indicate a concomitant respiratory alkalosis. In a pure metabolic acidosis, the bicarbonate concentration is reduced and the base excess is negative (base deficit).

With respect to the electrolyte and anion gap abnormalities, the alterations will depend on the cause of the acidosis:

1. Normal [SID] plus increased AG. When the anion gap is increased, it indicates the presence of unmeasured anions; the [SID] is unchanged because the anion has not affected the relative concentrations of sodium, potassium, or chloride. This condition is most commonly seen with lactic acidosis, ketoacidosis, hyperglycemic nonketotic coma, uremia, and in toxicities such as ethylene glycol poisoning.
2. Decreased [SID] plus normal AG. This condition is usually seen in what is classically referred to as a hyperchloremic acidosis. A hyperchloremic acidosis can be found following diarrhea with minimal dehydration. Once dehydration occurs, the anion gap usually increases as well. This process can also occur in some cases of diabetic ketoacidosis during the recovery phase. The keto acids have been removed, but a hyperchloremia persists and is slower to respond to therapy. It occurs in renal tubular acidosis and some other forms of renal failure. These cases can also be quite difficult to manage since the ultimate regulation of electrolytes in the body requires adequate renal function.
3. Decreased [SID] plus increased AG. The decreased [SID] indicates a hyperchloremic acidosis, and the increased anion gap suggests the accumulation of an unmeasured anion. This will be a metabolic acidosis and will generally be

rather severe since both factors contribute to the acidosis. It can occur occasionally in diabetic ketoacidosis and in renal insufficiency where a hypovolemia has been superimposed on the renal disease. In this instance, a hyperchloremic acidosis exists together with a lactic acidosis as a result of the poor circulation.

Metabolic Alkalosis

This condition is characterized by a fall in hydrogen ion concentration and, therefore, a rise in pH. Ventilation normally decreases, and $Paco_2$ will rise to compensate for the alkalosis. As indicated previously, the ability to increase Pco_2 is limited by the resulting hypoxemia. The expected change in $Paco_2$ can be calculated:

$Paco_2 = 0.9 [HCO_3^-] + 15$ mm Hg

For example, for a bicarbonate of 36, the $Paco_2$ should be 47.6 mm Hg. If the $Paco_2$ is much less than this amount, then it indicates a failure of compensation or a coexisting respiratory alkalosis. If the $Paco_2$ is much higher than this amount, then it indicates a coexisting respiratory acidosis. The normal limit for compensation is a $Paco_2$ of about 55 mm Hg. In metabolic alkalosis, the bicarbonate is increased and the base excess is positive. The most common electrolyte disturbance seen in a pure metabolic alkalosis is a hypochloremia with an increase in bicarbonate. This condition will produce a rise in inorganic [SID] with no change in the anion gap.

Mixed Metabolic Disturbances

It is quite feasible for two opposing changes to be occurring independently at the same time. These changes may lead to a relatively normal pH but abnormal electrolytes, characterized by an increased [SID] and an increased anion gap. The increased [SID] indicates a metabolic alkalosis, but the increased anion gap suggests that some unmeasured anions are present. This condition might be found in a dog with gastric dilation-volvulus, where the initial sequestration of acid in the stomach has produced the increased [SID], but the ensuing shock has caused an anaerobic increase in lactic acid production.

Respiratory Acidosis

An acute respiratory acidosis cannot be characterized on the basis of [SID] or anion gap and can only be defined on the basis of pH and $Paco_2$. The pH is decreased, the $Paco_2$ is increased, and the Pao_2 is below that expected for the amount of oxygen inspired (*e.g.*, a Pao_2 of 95 mm Hg is expected for a normal animal breathing room air but could indicate severe hypoventilation in the animal breathing 50% O_2). The formulae for the expected changes in bicarbonate have been given above. In a chronic respiratory acidosis, a loss of chloride occurs, which may lead to an increased [SID], but little change in the anion gap is found because of the increased bicarbonate concentrations.

Respiratory Alkalosis

This is the result of hyperventilation and is characterized by a rise in pH and a fall in $Paco_2$. In the acute condition, no changes occur in [SID] or anion gap, but if the ventilatory stimulus persists, an increase in chloride ions occurs, leading to a decreased [SID]. The anion gap is normal since bicarbonate decreases.

It is not possible for a respiratory acidosis to occur at the same time as a respiratory alkalosis, but it is possible to superimpose one of these alterations on one or both metabolic disturbances. For example, in gastric dilation-volvulus, the distended stomach limits the movement of the diaphragm and leads to a respiratory acidosis. The animal may already have a metabolic acidosis and metabolic alkalosis as indicated above. Iatrogenic disturbances have not been included in the above discussion, but they do occur and are normally diagnosed on the basis of the therapy and dose of drugs given.

MANAGEMENT

It is beyond the scope of this chapter to describe the management of individual disorders such as diabetic ketoacidosis, hypoadrenocorticism, or renal tubular acidosis. As with most clinical entities it is most important to treat the primary problem. However, the management of the four main types of disturbance is discussed here.

Metabolic acidosis

The aim of therapy in metabolic acidosis is to increase the [SID] and remove any unmeasured anions that are involved in the acidosis. In situations where there is a decreased [SID] with no alteration in anion gap, the normal approach is to provide sodium ions in excess of strong anions (usually chloride). Since the solutions administered have to be electrically neutral, this is normally achieved by adding a metabolizable anion with the sodium so that once the anion is removed the excess sodium will increase the [SID]. The sodium salts of lactate, gluconate, acetate, citrate, and bicarbonate are most commonly utilized. Sodium bicarbonate is the most effective because the bicarbonate can be rapidly excreted as carbon dioxide and can be given as a solution on its own. The other salts are usually used as part of a balanced electrolyte solution. Acetate is the next most effective because it is a relatively weak ion and therefore contributes little to the [SID]. It is also metabolized throughout the body and is removed rapidly. Lactate is a strong ion and is metabolized mainly in the liver. Gluconate is metabolized relatively slowly, and citrate is not used in any standard solutions except as an anticoagulant for blood.

In the case of the increased anion gap acidosis, the main aim should be to restore homeostasis so that the animal can metabolize or excrete the unmeasured anion. In the case of diabetic ketoacidosis the use of sodium bicarbonate has been largely curtailed because it was found that patients tended to become alkalotic if the acidosis was corrected with sodium bicarbonate before the ketoacids were metabolized or excreted. It should not be forgotten that severe acidosis interferes with myocardial and neuronal function and that the rapid restoration of acid-base balance significantly improves the patient's condition. Over the last few years there has been increasing debate over the use of sodium bicarbonate for metabolic acidosis, but in my opinion it is still a

valid treatment, particularly in patients with a TcO_2 less than 10 mmol/L or an SBE greater than 15 mmol/L. However, it should be given slowly and titrated to the animal's needs. Sodium bicarbonate usually comes as a hypertonic solution (8.4% or 2000 mOsmol/L) and this alone should dictate that it is given by slow intravenous injection. In the hypovolemic patient it can also cause cardiovascular collapse (myocardial depression and peripheral vasodilation), so it should be given only after an initial bolus of fluids. The normal calculation for its administration is based on its distribution into the whole extracellular space (0.3 × body weight in the adult, 0.5 × body weight in the neonate) and the correction of the base deficit (dose in mmol = 0.3 or 0.5 body weight in kg × base deficit). The calculation can also be based on TcO_2 (normal TcO_2 − measured TcO_2) although this is not as accurate because it does not allow for other buffers in the system. In most clinical cases it is unnecessary to administer the whole dose calculated above, and it is better to use smaller doses and recheck the patient's base deficit and TcO_2 after this therapy. In order to titrate the bicarbonate, the initial volume of distribution should be assumed to be the blood volume (0.1 × body weight in the dog, 0.05 × body weight in the cat), so the formula follows:

dose $NaHCO_3$ in mmol = 0.1 (dog) or 0.05 (cat) × body weight (kg) × (base deficit) or (normal TcO_2 − measured TcO_2)

This should be given over 15 to 20 minutes and the base deficit and TcO_2 reassessed after another 15 minutes. If the patient already has hypokalemia, the administration of sodium bicarbonate may cause a further decrease. Potassium supplementation should be started at the same time as alkali therapy.

The use of sodium lactate (Ringer's lactate) in animals with a lactic acidosis has often been questioned because it is expected to produce an increase in lactate levels. However, in most instances it is the restoration of the circulating volume that is most important in restoring normal acid-base status. Therefore, it is appropriate to use a balanced electrolyte solution because it increases circulating volume without altering the electrolyte balance. In clinical hypovolemic states with lactic acidosis, therapy with Ringer's lactate has resulted in a decrease in blood lactate because of the restoration of hepatic blood flow and metabolism.

Recently dichloroacetate has been advocated for the therapy of lactic acidosis. This drug stimulates the enzyme pyruvate dehydrogenase, which increases the conversion of pyruvate to acetyl CoA. The result is that less pyruvate is available for the production of lactate. This therapy has been beneficial to some people with marked-lactic acidosis, but it is not as effective in cases in which the basic cause of the lactic acidosis is tissue hypoxia. It has been used experimentally in the dog but there are no clinical reports of its use to date.

Metabolic Alkalosis

The aim of therapy is to reduce [SID], which is normally carried out by the use of a solution containing excess chloride (*e.g.*, 0.9% sodium chloride). Stronger acids are not usually used in clinical practice. The maintenance of a metabolic alkalosis may be dependent to some extent on a hypokalemia, so it is important to treat the potassium deficit at the same time by including up to 40 mmol/L of potassium chloride in the solution, depending on the severity of the deficit. Potassium chloride should not be infused at a rate greater than 0.5 mmol/kg/hr (mEq/kg/hr). Metabolic alkaloses produced by hyperadrenocorticoid states do not respond as well to this therapy until the hormonal imbalance is addressed.

Respiratory Acidosis

The aim of therapy is to reduce the level of carbon dioxide, which can only be achieved by increasing alveolar ventilation. It may be necessary to reverse agents that are causing respiratory depression (*e.g.*, naloxone to reverse the effects of an opioid). If this is not possible, the only other choice is to institute positive pressure ventilation. If the animal is not severely depressed and will not tolerate orotracheal intubation this may be achieved by heavily sedating the patient or by performing a tracheostomy and ventilating through the tracheostomy.

In patients with a chronic compensated respiratory acidosis, the patient tolerates the increased PCO_2 very well. It is normally best not to institute positive pressure ventilation in these patients. In this compensated state the increased PCO_2 is balanced by an increased bicarbonate such that the pH is nearly normal. If the PCO_2 is decreased rapidly, the patient may become severely alkalemic. This can produce coma and death because the loss of CO_2 across the blood–brain barrier occurs quickly, but the exchange of bicarbonate is slower, leading to a severe cerebral alkalosis. Reducing the PCO_2 may also make it difficult to wean the patient from the ventilator once the initial crisis is over. The animal is best controlled with limited oxygen administration; the aim is to improve the PaO_2 without further depressing ventilation. If IPPV is instituted to improve oxygenation, it is important not to lower the PCO_2, so the ventilator should be set to match the patient's ventilation.

Respiratory Alkalosis

The aim of therapy is to reduce alveolar ventilation by finding the cause and treating it. If the animal is hyperventilating because of hypoxemia, the provision of oxygen may be sufficient to treat the problem. It may be necessary to bronchodilate the animal and provide a humidified source of gas. An analgesic may provide sufficient pain relief to prevent hyperventilation caused by pain. In the case of some CNS lesions that are not amenable to therapy, one could reduce the alkalosis by increasing dead space breathing, but this is hard to maintain in a conscious patient.

PATIENT MONITORING

Once therapy has been initiated for acid-base disturbances, it is essential that the status of the animal be followed, using the same biochemistry tests described. These tests must be carried out in conjunction with corrections of the initiating disease and other abnormalities that do not necessarily play a large part in these measurements (*e.g.*, potassium).

The prognosis for dogs and cats suffering from acid-base disturbances is related to the initiating disease and the severity of the disturbance. In one study of 20 dogs with alkalemia (*p*H greater than 7.50), 7 died within 48 hours of the diagnosis of alkalemia, suggesting that an alkalemia carries a rather poor prognosis. However, no studies in the veterinary literature tie prognosis to the severity of acid-base disturbances in specific conditions in the dog and cat.

ADDITIONAL READING

Brobst D. Pathophysiology and adaptive changes in acid-base disorders. J Am Vet Med Assoc 1983; 183:773.

Cornelius LM, Rawlings CA. Arterial blood gas and acid-base values in dogs with various diseases and signs of disease. J Am Vet Med Assoc 1981; 178:992.

Hartsfield SM, Thurmon JC, Benson GJ. Sodium bicarbonate and bicarbonate precursors for the treatment of metabolic acidosis. J Am Vet Med Assoc 1981; 179:914.

Haskins SC. Blood gases and acid-base balance: Clinical interpretation and therapeutic implications. In: Kirk RW, ed. Current veterinary therapy VIII. Philadelphia: WB Saunders, 1983: 201.

Polzin DJ, Osborne CA. Anion gap: Diagnostic and therapeutic applications. In: Kirk RW, ed. Current veterinary therapy IX. Philadelphia: WB Saunders, 1986: 52.

Robinson EP, Hardy RM. Clinical signs, diagnosis, and treatment of alkalemia in dogs: 20 cases (1982–1984). J Am Vet Med Assoc 1988; 192:943.

Stewart PA. Modern quantitative acid-base chemistry. Can J Physiol Pharmacol 1983; 61:1444.

Wilson EA, Green RA. Clinical analysis of mixed acid-base disturbances. Compendium of Continuing Education 1985; 7:364.

APPENDIX

The relationships referred to in the text can be expressed in the following six equations:

(i) $[H^+] \times [OH^-] = K'w$. Dissociation of water

(ii) $[H^+] \times [A^-] = K_A [HA]$. Dissociation of weak acids

(iii) $[HA] + [A^-] = A_{TOT}$. Conservation of weak acids

(iv) $[H^+] \times [HCO_3^-] = K_C \cdot Pco_2$. Bicarbonate formation from CO_2

(v) $[H^+] \times [CO_3^{-2}] = K_3 [HCO_3^-]$. Carbonate formation from CO_2

(vi) $[SID] + [H^+] - [HCO_3^-] - [A^-] - [CO_3^{-2}] - [OH^-] = 0 -$ Electrical neutrality

Where $K'w$, K_A, K_C, and K_3 are constants, and A_{TOT} represents the total amount of weak acid present in either the ionic or nonionic form, these six equations can be simplified to an equation in the form $ax^4 + bx^3 + cx^2 + dx + e = 0$, containing the variables $[SID]$, A_{TOT}, and Pco_2 with the constants $K'w$, K_3, K_A, and Kc where $x = [H^+]$. This standard format can be solved using a computer, and the alterations in any one of the variables can be used to calculate the effects on the other variables.

72

ELECTROLYTE IMBALANCES

Dana G. Allen

Fluid and electrolyte changes commonly accompany and are associated with clinical manifestations of endocrine, renal, gastrointestinal, metabolic, biochemical, and drug-induced diseases in the dog and cat. Many of these changes are relatively benign and resolve spontaneously with resolution of the primary disease. Some electrolyte imbalances, however, are potentially life threatening and require immediate treatment.

CAUSES

The causes of specific electrolyte changes are listed in Tables 72-1 through 72-3.

PATHOPHYSIOLOGY AND CLINICAL SIGNS

Water accounts for approximately 60% of total body weight in the adult animal. In neonates, water may account for up to 80% of total body weight. Approximately two thirds of total body water is in the intracellular fluid (ICF) compartment and one third is in the extracellular (ECF) compartment. Most cells in the body are permeable to water, and an osmotic equilibrium is maintained between the ICF and the ECF compartments by the presence of dissolved solutes. The principle ICF solutes are potassium, magnesium, organic phosphates, and protein. The principle ECF solutes are sodium, chloride, and bicarbonate. Imbalances in the concentration of these solutes between the ICF and ECF accounts for many of the clinical signs associated with the primary disease initiating the imbalance.

Sodium Imbalances

Sodium is the principle extracellular cation and is responsible for maintaining extracellular osmolality. Sodium governs the distribution of water between the ECF and ICF. Clinical signs of sodium imbalance are primarily a reflection of changes in ECF status.

Hyponatremia

Hyponatremia is defined as serum sodium levels less than 136 mEq/L (mmol/L).

Table 72–1 Causes of Hyponatremia and Hypernatremia

HYPONATREMIA

NORMALLY HYDRATED ANIMAL
Pseudohyponatremia (hyperlipemia, hyperproteinemia, hyperglycemia)

DEHYDRATED ANIMAL
Salt-losing kidney disease
Hypoadrenocorticism
Gastrointestinal loss (vomiting, diarrhea)
Diuretic therapy (furosemide, ethacrynic acid, mannitol)
Hypertonic fluid loss (burns, large wounds, body cavity lavage)
Third space fluid and salt loss (pancreatitis, peritonitis, uroabdomen)

OVERHYDRATED ANIMAL
Congestive heart failure
Renal failure
Nephrotic syndrome
Hepatic cirrhosis
Psychogenic polydipsia
Iatrogenic water loading (5% dextrose)
Syndrome of inappropriate ADH secretion (CNS disease, canine heartworm disease, carcinoma, morphine, barbiturates, chlorpropamide, cyclophosphamide, vincristine, isoproterenol, neoplasia)

HYPERNATREMIA

EXCESS SODIUM GAIN
Iatrogenic salt containing infusion (saline, sodium bicarbonate, lactated Ringer's, hypertonic saline enemas)
Hyperadrenocorticism
Hyperaldosteronism

EXCESSIVE WATER LOSS
Pure water loss or lack of adequate intake
  Unable or unwilling to ingest water
  Diabetes insipidus
  Hyperventilation or heat prostration
  Fever
  Essential hypernatremia (defective thirst mechanism +/− impaired osmoregulation of ADH release)
Hypotonic water loss
  Excessive vomiting, diarrhea, diuretic therapy
  Acute and chronic renal failure
  Postobstructive diuresis (when water intake low)
  Diabetes mellitus

Clinical signs, however, are usually not apparent until serum sodium falls to values less than 120 mEq/L (mmol/L). Clinical signs vary depending on the severity of the deficit and are especially marked at levels below 110 mEq/L (mmol/L). Anorexia, apathy, weakness, muscle cramping, myoclonus, tachycardia, hypothermia, and cold extremities, shock, stupor, seizure, or coma may occur. Hyponatremia may be associated with hypo-osmolar states (vomiting, diarrhea, salt wasting renal disease, hypoadrenocorticism, diuretic therapy, burns), hyperosmolar states (hyperglycemia of diabetes mellitus, hyperproteinemia associated with multiple myeloma, the administration of glucose, mannitol or radiographic contrast material), and normal osmolar states (artifactual; due to the presence of excess lipid or protein causing a proportional displacement of the water phase of plasma in which sodium is dissolved and should be suspected in

Table 72–2 *Causes of Hypokalemia and Hyperkalemia*

HYPOKALEMIA

Chronic anorexia
Excessive gastrointestinal loss
   Vomiting, diarrhea
Excessive renal loss
   Chronic renal failure (cats especially)
   Increased sodium intake
   Excessive bicarbonate or lactate administration
   Nephrotoxic drugs (aminoglycosides, amphotericin B, outdated tetracyclines,
     cisplatinum)
   Renal tubular acidosis, Fanconi-like syndrome
   Postobstructive diuresis
   Chronic pyelonephritis
   Polyuria due to diabetes mellitus
   Diuretic therapy (furosemide, acetazolamide)
   Mineralocorticoid therapy
Chronic liver disease
Alkalosis
Excessive insulin therapy
Dilutional (fluid therapy low or devoid of potassium)
Other drugs (terbutaline, IV carbenicillin, theophylline, barium salts)

HYPERKALEMIA

Acidosis
Acute renal failure
Urinary tract obstruction (urolithiasis, neoplasia, trauma)
Urinary tract rupture
Hypoadrenocorticism
Hypovolemia
GIT disease (diarrhea)
Massive soft tissue trauma and possibly tumor lysis syndrome
Drug induced
   overdose of potassium containing solutions, digitalis, succinylcholine, spironolactone,
     heparin, captopril, β adrenergic blocking agents, potassium penicillin G, op'-DDD,
     lithium, nonsteroidal anti-inflammatory agents, verapamil, cyclosporine, progesterone
Exercise
Hypertonicity (hyperglycemia, hypernatremia)
Hyperthermia (body temperature > 42°C)
Pseudohyperkalemia
   Thrombocytosis (platelet counts > 600,000/mm³ or 600 × 10⁹/L)
   Leukocytosis (wbc counts > 100,000/mm³ or 100 × 10⁹/L)
   Red cell hemolysis (Akitas)

cases where measured osmolality is normal but an osmolal gap is present), in dehydrated animals (decreased ECF) and overhydrated animals (increased ECF). In the dehydrated patient, skin tenting is present. It is absent in the overhydrated hyponatremic animal. In these animals, peripheral edema and ascites may be present.

Hypernatremia

Hypernatremia in the dog is defined as a serum sodium in excess of 156 mEq/L (mmol/L) and in the cat as a serum sodium in excess of 161 mEq/L (mmol/L). It is most common in patients unable or unwilling to ingest water or who have a primary disease causing the loss of water in excess of sodium (*e.g.*, diabetes insipidus or mellitus, excessive vomiting, diarrhea, or diuretic therapy). Serum hyperosmolality commonly results from hypernatremia, hyperglycemia, or azotemia. In the nondiabetic, nonazotemic patient plasma osmolality can be calculated by the following formula:

Plasma osmolality (mOsm/kg) or (mmol/kg) = 2 × Sodium (mEq/L) or (mmol/L) + 10

Hyperosmolality causes neuronal intracellu-

Table 72–3 Causes of Hypocalcemia and Hypercalcemia

HYPOCALCEMIA

Hypoparathyroidism
Nutritional secondary hyperparathyroidism
Acute pancreatitis
Acute or chronic renal failure
Hypoproteinemia
  Malabsorption, protein losing enteropathy, protein losing nephropathy, liver disease
Intestinal malabsorption of calcium or vitamin D
Eclampsia (dogs)
Hyperphosphatemia (phosphate containing enemas)
Ethylene glycol toxicity
Sodium bicarbonate toxicity
Rapid volume expansion (dilutional cause)
Hypomagnesemia (humans only?)
Sampling error (calcium binding anticoagulant)

HYPERCALCEMIA

Hypercalcemia of malignancy (pseudohyperparathyroidism)
  Lymphoma, perianal adenocarcinoma, mammary gland adenocarcionoma, leukemia, gastric
    adenocarcinoma, multiple myeloma
Primary hyperparathyroidism
  Parathyroid adenoma, carcinoma, or hyperplasia
Hypoadrenocorticism
Acute or chronic renal failure
Hyperproteinemia
Hemoconcentration
Hypervitaminosis D
  Dietary oversupplementation
  Ingestion of toxic plants
  Cestrus diurnum (day blooming jessamine)
  Solanum malacoxylon
  Trisetum flavescens
  Ingestion of cholecalciferol rodenticides
    Quintox, Rampage, Rat-Be-Gone, Mouse-Be-Gone
  Blastomycosis
Osteolytic disease
  Primary bone neoplasia (osteosarcoma, multiple myeloma)
  Metastatic bone disease
Immobilization
Severe hypothermia
Nonpathologic hypercalcemia
  Lipemia
  Young growing animals (usually in association with increased serum phosphorus and alkaline
    phosphatase and normal serum urea)

---

lar dehydration. Initial clinical signs include irritability, lethargy, weakness, and ataxia. As the hypernatremia worsens, stupor progresses to coma and seizure. Clinical signs are more prominent when serum sodium changes are acute. Central nervous system depression or coma are more likely seen when serum osmolality exceeds 375 mmol/kg (normal 295–315). With chronic hypernatremia these signs are less pronounced because of the formation of intracellular neuronal idiogenic osmoles that help protect the brain from dehydration by increasing intracellular tonicity. Patients with pure water loss, that is, diabetes insipidus, may not appear clinically dehydrated even though total body water is severely depleted. Water leaves the intracellular compartment and enters the extracellular compartment to reestablish osmotic equilibrium and maintain blood pressure. Other clinical signs depend on the primary disorder present.

Potassium Imbalances

Potassium is a principle intracellular cation. It plays an active role in acid-base balance, cell volume, electrophysiologic properties of cells, and synthesis of protein and glycogen. Total body potassium concentration is governed by the balance between oral intake and renal excretion. Renal potassium excretion is the principle factor affecting serum levels. Losses through the gastrointestinal tract and in sweat are small. Almost all the potassium filtered by the glomeruli is reabsorbed by the proximal tubules. Movement of potassium from the renal tubular cells is passive and occurs in exchange for sodium and chloride ions. Potassium excretion increases when sodium and urine flow is increased; conversely, hypovolemia and decreased urine flow lead to an increase in serum potassium. Greater than 95% of body potassium is intracellular. Only 2% to 5% is present in the ECF. Therefore, measurement of serum values are not necessarily indicative of total body potassium concentrations. Serum potassium is significantly higher (mean difference 0.63 ± 0.17 mEq/L) than plasma potassium in normal dogs due to the leakage of potassium from cells during the clotting process. It has, therefore, been recommended that potassium in blood is more accurately measured by using plasma. If serum potassium exceeds plasma concentrations by greater than 0.2 to 0.3 mEq/L (mmol/L), pseudohyperkalemia should be suspected. Pseudohyperkalemia is an in vitro artifactual elevation in measured potassium levels related to the escape of potassium from cells and may be seen with thrombocytosis, leukocytosis, or hemolysis of red blood cells in the Akita.

Hypokalemia

Hypokalemia is defined as a serum potassium of less than 3.5 mEq/L (mmol/L). Clinical signs seldom occur if serum levels are maintained above 2.5 mEq/L (mmol/L). Hypokalemia impairs electrical conduction at the cell membrane. In early potassium deficiency, ECF potassium falls more rapidly than ICF potassium, causing the resting membrane potential difference to increase (hyperpolarization). A greater than normal stimulus is required for depolarization and impulse conduction, and muscle contraction is impaired. With severe hypokalemia, the resting membrane potential difference decreases (hypopolarization), and muscular weakness progressing to paralysis results. The extent of clinical signs is related to the severity of the deficit. Hypokalemia may be characterized by muscle weakness, muscular cramping, anorexia, dysphagia, vomiting, constipation, lethargy, or paralysis. A condition of hypokalemic polymyopathy has been described in cats. It is characterized by an acute onset of weakness, apparent muscle pain, and ventroflexion of the neck. Decreased potassium intake and increased urinary loss are believed to be contributive factors. Hypokalemia can contribute to a metabolic alkalosis, which may serve to maintain the hypokalemia. In the absence of a history or clinical signs suggestive of renal or gastrointestinal disease, hypokalemia is likely due to alkalosis or insulin excess. Pseudohypokalemia, although uncommon, may occur secondary to hyperlipemia or severe hyperproteinemia.

Hyperkalemia

Hyperkalemia is present when serum potassium levels are in excess of 5.6 mEq/l (mmol/L). Values above 7 mEq/L (mmol/L) are potentially life threatening (cardiotoxic). Hyperkalemia causes a sustained depolarization of muscle cell membranes characterized by muscular weakness. Paralysis may also occur. Affected animals may have bradycardia, weak femoral pulses, vomiting, or diarrhea depending on the etiology of the electrolyte imbalance. Hyperkalemia may be due to increased intake, decreased excretion, or a redistribution from the ICF to the ECF. The most common cause is decreased renal excretion. A case of hyperkalemic periodic paralysis has been documented in the dog. The dog exhibited frequent, short bouts of weakness and paralysis precipitated by exercise or excitement. Pseudohyperkalemia is a test tube phenomenon that is of no direct clinical consequence to the patient.

Calcium Imbalances

Calcium is an important component of bone and plays an essential role in neuromuscular transmission, muscle contraction, membrane stability, and hemostasis. Most body calcium (99%) is stored in bone. Half of total serum calcium is bound to protein, 40% is ionized, and 10% is complexed (*e.g.*, with citrate). Most laboratories report calcium as total serum calcium, although it is the ionized fraction that is the biologically active portion, and changes in it are responsible for the clinical signs of calcium imbalance. The ionized fraction is affected by changes in blood *p*H and protein content. Acidosis increases the ionized fraction, and alkalosis decreases it. Consequently, clinical signs of hypocalcemia may become apparent in patients with alkalosis at total serum calcium concentrations not generally considered significant. Total serum calcium varies with changes in serum protein. With hypoalbuminemia, the ionized fraction is increased, and clinical signs of hypocalcemia may not be apparent in spite of an abnormally low total serum calcium. To account for the influence protein has on serum calcium concentration, correction formulae have been devised for use in the dog. In the cat, marked variability among calcium and albumin concentrations invalidates the use of these formulae in this species: Corrected calcium (mg/dl) = calcium (mg/dl) − albumin (g/dl) + 3.5; or corrected calcium (mg/dl) = calcium (mg/dl) − [0.4 × total serum protein (g/dl)] + 3.3.

Hypocalcemia

Clinical signs associated with hypocalcemia generally become apparent when serum calcium falls to values less than 6 to 7 mg/dl (1.5 to 1.75 mmol/L) or when the ionized fraction is less than 2.5 mg/dl (0.625 mmol/L). Clinical signs are due to neuromuscular excitation and may include anxiety, irritability, weakness, muscle tremors, or fasciculations, tetany, stiff gait, hypersensitivity to light and sound, and seizures. Signs may be intermittent. Cataracts may also be observed in cases of chronic hypocalcemia. Hyperkalemia and hypomagnesemia potentiate the toxic effects of hypocalcemia. Hypoparathyroidism, ethylene glycol toxicity, and eclampsia may be associated with clinical signs of hypocalcemia. Although acute pancreatitis, renal failure, hypoproteinemia, and nutritional secondary hyperparathyroidism may also cause hypocalcemia, clinical signs of hypocalcemia are less common.

Hypercalcemia

Hypercalcemia is defined as a total serum calcium in excess of 12 mg/dl (3.0 mmol/L) in the dog and 11 mg/dl (2.75 mmol/L) in the cat. The most common cause of hypercalcemia in dogs and cats is neoplasia, especially lymphoma. Clinical signs associated with hypercalcemia are due to the suppression of lower motor neuron activity and neuromuscular excitability. Hypercalcemia may be characterized by anorexia, nausea, vomiting, constipation, abdominal pain, polyuria, polydipsia, dehydration, and depression. Cardiac arrhythmias, including ventricular fibrillation, muscle twitching, and seizure activity are uncommon manifestations of hypercalcemia. Serum concentrations greater than 16 mg/dl (4.0 mmol/L) may precipitate acute renal failure and death.

DIAGNOSTIC APPROACH

The minimum data base for animals with suspected electrolyte abnormalities includes a complete blood cell count, serum biochemistry profile, including electrolytes, blood-gas analysis, urinalysis, and an electrocardiogram (Table 72-4). The extended data base is directed at the underlying primary cause.

MANAGEMENT

The goal of fluid therapy is to restore and maintain normovolemia and electrolyte balance. In the dehydrated patient, fluid requirements are met by calculating replacement deficits (including ongoing losses, as with vomiting) and daily maintenance requirements. Half of the total calculated volume (replacement + maintenance requirements) is given over a 4-hour period and the

Table 72–4 Common Electrocardiographic Changes Associated With Electrolyte Abnormalities*

Electrolyte	Associated Electrocardiographic Change(s)
Hypokalemia	Prolonged QT interval, ST segment depression, flattening of T wave
Hyperkalemia†	Increased amplitude of T wave with tenting of the wave, decreased amplitude of R wave, prolonged QRS complex and PR interval, ST segment depression, decreased amplitude of P wave, prolonged QT interval, disappearance of P wave, bradycardia, ventricular flutter, fibrillation, or asystole
Hypocalcemia	Prolonged QT interval, ventricular flutter or fibrillation
Hypercalcemia	Prolonged PR interval, shortened QT interval, ST segment coving +/− ventricular fibrillation

* The electrocardiographic changes are not specific for electrolyte abnormalities, nor are they a reliable indicator of the severity of the electrolyte change.
† Listed in order of occurrence as serum potassium levels increase.

remainder over 20 hours. If the clinical situation continues to warrant it (*e.g.*, azotemia), maintenance fluids are continued at one and a half to two times basal rate (90–120 ml/kg/day) until normal hydration, electrolyte, and acid-base balance are reestablished. Monitoring central venous pressure (see Chapter 80) helps gaurd against overhydration.

Replacement fluids closely match the composition of the ECF, the volume of which can be calculated by the following formula:

percent dehydration (%) × body weight (kg) × 1000 = ml of fluid required

Examples of replacement fluids are listed in Table 72-5. Maintenance fluids are lower in sodium

Table 72–5 Parenteral Fluid Solutions for Use in Small Animals

REPLACEMENT FLUIDS
Lactated Ringer's solution
Normal saline
Normosol R
Plasmalyte 148
Ringer's solution

MAINTENANCE FLUIDS
2½% dextrose/0.45% saline
2½% dextrose/½ strength lactated Ringer's solution
Normosol M
Normosol M in 5% dextrose in water
Plasmalyte 56 with 5% dextrose

and higher in potassium than replacement fluids because normal losses in the urine and stool are low in sodium and insensible losses through the skin and respiratory tract are essentially sodium-free. Normal daily maintenance fluid requirements in the adult dog and cat are approximately 60 ml/kg. (Smaller patients warrant larger volumes—up to 100 ml/kg). Examples of maintenance fluids are listed in Table 72-5. A discussion of the management of specific electrolyte abnormalities follows.

When metabolic acidosis contributes to acid-base and electrolyte imbalance after fluid deficit replacement has occurred, administer 2 mEq/kg of bicarbonate over 15 minutes to 1 hour. In cases of moderate to severe acidosis, larger amounts of bicarbonate may be required (Table 72-6). If the patient's plasma bicarbonate concentration is known, the approximate quantity of bicarbonate required to correct the deficit can be estimated by the following formula:

Bicarbonate Required (mEq) = 0.3 × body weight (kg) × plasma bicarbonate deficit where bicarbonate deficit is calculated as normal bicarbonate [24 mEq/L] − patient's bicarbonate

Half the calculated bicarbonate needs can be given over the first 4 to 6 hours. Further correction may be accomplished (generally over a 24-hour period) with the use of maintenance fluid therapy (*e.g.*, Plasmalyte 56, Normosol M). The acid-base status is then reevaluated.

Table 72–6 *Estimated Bicarbonate Requirements in Animals With Metabolic Acidosis*

Severity of Clinical Signs	Bicarbonate Required (mEq/kg)
Mild	1.5
Moderate	3.0
Severe	4.5

Hyponatremia

Hyponatremia occurring in animals with a normal hydration and osmolal status is artifactual and simply requires correction of the underlying problem (*e.g.*, hyperproteinemia due to multiple myeloma, hyperglycemia associated with diabetes mellitus, or hyperlipidemia caused by hypothyroidism, familial hyperlipidemia, or diabetes mellitus). Serum sodium levels should be measured after a 12 hour fast because hyperlipemia from the ingestion of a fatty meal may cause pseudohyponatremia.

Treatment of hyponatremia in dehydrated animals requires treatment of the underlying primary problem and the administration of isotonic (0.9%) sodium chloride or lactated Ringer's to correct the dehydration and expand ECF. The following equation can be used to calculate the required sodium replacement:

$$\text{mEq of sodium required} = 0.6 \times \text{body weight (kg)} \times \text{normal serum sodium} - \text{patient's serum sodium}$$

Animals with hyponatremia in the face of overhydration are treated by addressing the causative disorder, restricting access to water, and administering diuretics and isotonic fluids to expand ECF. Restriction of sodium is indicated in disorders characterized by sodium retention, for example, congestive heart failure, cirrhosis, and nephrotic syndrome. The syndrome of inappropriate antidiuretic hormone secretion is characterized by renal sodium excretion and relative water excess. In this case, sodium chloride is added to the diet, and water intake is restricted. In those cases associated with protein loss, attempts are made to increase protein intake (*e.g.*, high protein diet). Severe, symptomatic, hyponatremia of rapid onset may be treated with a slow infusion of (3%) hypertonic saline (3% sodium chloride contains 520 mEq/L of sodium).

Hypernatremia

Hypernatremia is treated by eliminating the cause and lowering serum sodium levels in accordance with the animal's volume status. If significant dehydration is present, initial treatment is directed at expanding the ECF by the intravenous administration of isotonic (0.9%) saline or lactated Ringer's solution at a rate of 90 ml/kg per hour IV, until capillary refill time and pulse pressure improve. Ringer's solution is preferred if electrolytes are lost along with water, as with some renal and gastrointestinal problems. In the hypernatremic patient, isotonic fluids are hypotonic relative to the patient's plasma, and a dilutional effect occurs, lowering serum sodium. Once the hypovolemia is corrected, 5% dextrose in water can be used to replace the remaining water deficit and correct the hypernatremia.

Pure Water Loss

Animals with pure water loss (see Table 72-1) require solute free water, that is, 5% dextrose in water. Alternatively, the hypertonicity can be corrected using half-strength lactated Ringer's and 2.5% dextrose solution or half-strength (0.45%) saline. The volume of fluid required to correct the water deficit is calculated by the following formula:

$$\text{Water deficit (L)} = 0.6 \times \text{body weight (kg)} \times 1 - \frac{\text{normal serum Na}}{\text{patient's serum sodium}}$$

If the hypernatremia is severe (greater than 180 mEq/L or mmol/L and plasma osmolality greater than 375 mmol/kg), the imbalance should be corrected over a 48- and preferably a 72-hour period. Serum sodium concentration and neurologic status should be monitored every 4 to 6 hours during therapy. Generally, no greater than 50% of the calculated volume of fluid should be given over the first 24 hours. Serum sodium should not fall more rapidly than 0.5 to 1.0 mEq/L per hour. Lowering serum sodium too quickly can induce cerebral edema by allowing the idiogenic osmoles to draw water into neurons. Worsening of neurologic status or the sudden onset of seizure activity may be indicative of cerebral edema. Lowering serum sodium too slowly may permit the existing neuronal dehydration to be fatal.

Dietary sodium restriction for the long-term management of chronic hypernatremia can be accomplished with the use of Hill's Prescription diet h/d. Other less restricted sodium diets from Hill's include k/d, u/d, and w/d.

Hypotonic Water Loss

Animals suffering from hypernatremia secondary to hypotonic fluid loss (see Table 72-1) can be treated initially by correcting the hypovolemia with isotonic (0.9%) saline. Following rehydration, the hypernatremia may be addressed by the administration of half-strength (0.45%) saline.

Sodium Gain

The first course of action in the hypernatremic patient with volume expansion is to discontinue the administration of any fluids containing excess sodium (see Table 72-1). If renal function is normal, the increased serum sodium will initiate a diuresis and return the sodium load and the increased extracellular volume to normal over time. Furosemide may be given to increase the renal elimination of sodium and 5% dextrose in water may also be given to help lower it.

Hypokalemia

Hypokalemia is managed by treating the underlying disease process and replacing the potassium deficit. If the deficit is mild (not less than 3 mEq/L or mmol/L), oral administration of foods high in potassium content (*e.g.*, bananas, nuts, grapes, oranges) or the addition of potassium gluconate elixir (Kaon) to the diet at a dose of 5 to 10 mEq per day for cats and a dose of 5 ml of a 20 mEq/ml solution every 8 to 12 hours for dogs is

indicated. If the deficit is moderate to severe (2.5–3 mEq/L or mmol/L), parenteral administration of potassium is recommended. Because potassium is an intracellular cation, and laboratories only assay ECF potassium, exact requirements can not be given. The following guidelines, however, are useful: for mild deficits (3.0–3.5 mEq/L or mmol/L), daily potassium requirements are in the order of 1 to 3 mEq/kg; for moderate potassium deficits (2.5–3 mEq/L or mmol/L), daily potassium requirements are in the order of 4 to 6 mEq/kg; for severe potassium deficits (less than 2.5 mEq/L or mmol/L), 7 to 9 mEq/kg per day of potassium is recommended. Infusion rates should not exceed 0.5 mEq/kg per hour and may need to be decreased further in animals with renal failure. Treatment must be more conservative if blood potassium is measured in the face of alkalosis. Conversely, acidosis may mask a severe hypokalemia and must be treated accordingly. A change in blood *p*H of 0.1 is reflected by a corresponding change in potassium of 1.6 mEq/L or mmol/L.

Hyperkalemia

Hyperkalemia is treated by correcting the underlying disease process, antagonizing the cardiotoxic effects of potassium with calcium gluconate, increasing potassium urinary excretion with sodium chloride, and directing the intracellular redistribution of the cation with sodium bicarbonate, lactated Ringer's, or glucose and insulin therapy.

If hyperkalemia is not severe (less than 8.0 mEq/L) and no evidence of cardiotoxicity is found, the administration of sodium chloride will generally suffice to lower blood potassium levels as long as urine output is adequate. The mineralocorticoids, desoxycorticosterone acetate (1–5 mg/dog every 24–72 hours) or fludrocortisone (0.1–1.0 mg/dog per day) offer another approach to effectively lower blood potassium. Cation exchange resins (*e.g.*, Kayexalate, 2 g/kg; each gram suspended in 4 ml water) may be given orally or rectally. If the resin is given orally, it should be given with a laxative to prevent constipation. These products should be used with caution in animals with heart failure, edema, or oliguric renal failure, as potassium is exchanged for sodium, and excessive sodium loading and hypervolemia may occur in these patients.

If hyperkalemia is acute or severe (greater than 8.0 mEq/L or mmol/L), immediate therapy with calcium gluconate, sodium bicarbonate, or regular insulin and dextrose is indicated. Intravenous 10% calcium gluconate (0.5–1.5 ml/kg) is administered over a 10 to 15 minute period. This regimen successfully antagonizes the effects of potassium on the heart for about 5 to 15 minutes; it does not lower measured blood potassium levels. It should, therefore, be repeated as indicated by changes in the electrocardiogram. The infusion should be stopped when the heart rate becomes normal or if it increases significantly.

Intravenous sodium bicarbonate may be used to help redirect potassium back into cells. It is especially advantageous in countering the acidosis that commonly accompanies hyperkalemia. If serum bicarbonate or total carbon dioxide levels can not be established, 2 to 3 mEq of $NaHCO_3$/kg can be safely administered over a 30-minute period if renal failure, diabetic ketoacidosis, or severe decreased tissue perfusion does not exist. Animals with heart failure are at greater risk to the consequences of hypervolemia and hyperosmolality, which may accompany this treatment. The potassium lowering effect of sodium bicarbonate lasts a few hours.

Dextrose given with insulin has also been used to lower blood potassium levels. A dose of 0.5 unit regular insulin/kg given with 2 g dextrose per unit of insulin administered intravenously has been recommended in the cat. Dogs generally require more insulin than cats (that is, 5 units/kg per hour). Except in animals with diabetes mellitus, insulin should not be given without concurrent administration of glucose, glucagon, or both, or severe hypoglycemia may occur.

These measures only temporarily decrease blood potassium levels or antagonize its effects. The primary causative disease must be effectively managed to maintain a normal potassium balance. In cases resistant to these forms of therapy, peritoneal dialysis (see Peritoneal and Pleural Dialysis in Chapter 80) may be considered as a last resort to normalize blood potassium concentrations.

Hypocalcemia

Hypocalcemia is potentially life threatening and should be treated as an emergency. Calcium gluconate (10%) is administered by slow intravenous infusion (0.5–1.5 ml/kg) over a 20 to 30 minute period. If the heart rate increases significantly or if an arrhythmia develops during therapy, the infusion should be stopped. Calcium gluconate should not be added to solutions containing bicarbonate, or precipitation of calcium bicarbonate may ensue.

In cases of hypocalcemia due to hypoparathyroidism, long-term management with vitamin D supplementation is required. Dihydrotachysterol (Hytakerol; 0.02–0.03 mg/kg per day initially, and 0.01–0.02 mg/kg every 24–48 hours for maintenance) and 1,25-dihydroxyvitamin D_3 (Rocaltrol; 0.03–0.06 ug/kg per day) are suggested therapeutic agents. The time required for maximal effect of these drugs is 1 to 7 days (dihydrotachysterol) and 1 to 4 days (1,25-dihydroxyvitamin D_3). Iatrogenic hypercalcemia may occur with the use of these agents. In this case, the time to normocalcemia following excessive dosage of these agents may be 1 to 3 weeks with dihydrotachysterol and 1 day to 2 weeks with dihydroxyvitamin D_3. Dihydrotacysterol has a more rapid onset of action and a shorter duration of action should hypercalcemia be encountered and may be the preferred agent. Early in the course of therapy, oral calcium supplementation may be required. Calcium carbonate (cat: 0.5–1 g per day divided; dog: 1.0–4.0 g per day divided) is recommended. As the vitamin D dose reaches a steady state, the dose of calcium can be gradually reduced over a period of 2 to 4 months. For the management of cats with hypocalcemia occurring after surgical thyroidectomy (causing concurrent loss or trauma to the parathyroid glands), the reader is referred to Chapter 61.

Hypercalcemia

Hypercalcemia, if severe, may also be life threatening and should be treated accordingly. The most effective approach to treating hypercalcemia is to rehydrate the animal and promote diuresis with 0.9% saline (80 ml/kg per day). Urinary calcium excretion is enhanced by the saline infusion, and sodium competitively inhibits renal tubular reabsorption of calcium.

In cases with moderate hypercalcemia (14–16 mg/dl or 3.7–4.0 mmol/L), furosemide may be given to enhance calciuresis after hydration status has been corrected. An initial intravenous dose of 5 mg/kg followed by a maintenance dose of 5 mg/kg per hour has been shown to effectively decrease serum calcium levels by a mean value of 2.7 mg/dl (0.675 mmol/L). Alternatively, an oral dose of 2.5 to 4.5 mg/kg three to four times a day has been suggested. It is imperative that hydration status be corrected before furosemide is given and maintained throughout the treatment protocol. Glucocorticoids are often effective in lowering serum calcium levels in the treatment of hypercalcemia due to lymphoma and vitamin D intoxication (*e.g.*, cholecalciferol) and may be given in addition to saline diuresis and furosemide in patients with moderate hypercalcemia. Glucocorticoids do not, however, decrease serum calcium levels in patients with hyperparathyroidism. These drugs limit bone resorption, increase urinary calcium excretion, inhibit absorption from the intestinal tract, and have a direct toxic effect on some tumor cells. Prednisone (4 mg/kg divided, orally twice day) has been recommended for this purpose. These drugs are lymphocytolytic and should be avoided before a biopsy of a suspect neoplastic lesion is secured.

In addition to fluid therapy, diuretics, and corticosteroids, salmon calcitonin (Calcimar) has been used to lower serum calcium concentrations in dogs with vitamin D toxicosis. The drug was given at a dose of 4 to 7 units per kilogram subcutanously every 6 to 8 hours. Anorexia was the principle adverse effect of the drug.

Recently, diphosphonates have been used to treat refractory hypercalcemia. These drugs decrease serum calcium by blocking osteoclast-mediated bone resorption. Dichloromethylene diphosphonate, as yet an investigational drug (10–30 mg/kg, orally two to three times a day), has resulted in a lowering of serum calcium concentrations in dogs with parathyroid adenomas and perianal gland adenocarcinoma. Etidronate disodium (Didronel) is commercially available, and, although a dose has not been established in small

animals, an initial dose of 5 mg/kg per day per os is recommended in humans.

In cases with severe hypercalcemia (greater than 16 mg/dl or 4 mmol/L), immediate reduction of ionized calcium may be accomplished with the intravenous infusion of sodium EDTA (25–75 mg/kg per hour). This agent is potentially nephrotoxic, and acute renal failure may occur with its use; therefore, it is only recommended in animals with severe hypercalcemia unresponsive to other therapeutic modalities. Sodium bicarbonate (1–3 mEq/kg) can also be used to decrease the ionized portion of total serum calcium. Mithramycin, a potent inhibitor of osteoclastic bone resorption, is cytotoxic and can cause severe hepatotoxicity and is not recommended. The efficacy of these forms of treatment is transient, and the primary cause of the electrolyte imbalance must be corrected if long-term control of the hypercalcemia is to be expected. In all cases of hypercalcemia, a low calcium diet (*e.g.*, Hill's Prescription diets s/d, u/d, and k/d) and free access to water is recommended.

PATIENT MONITORING

Serum electrolytes and acid-base balance should be monitored frequently (every 4–6 hours) during initial therapy. It is also prudent to monitor electrocardiographic changes throughout the treatment regimen (see Table 72–4). Other recommendations pertaining to patient monitoring are dependent on the underlying disease process. Because the causes of electrolyte imbalances are so diverse, the prognosis of these disorders depends on the causative disease, and the reader is directed to the appropriate chapter.

ADDITIONAL READING

Abrams KL. Hypocalcemia associated with administration of sodium bicarbonate for salicylate intoxication in a cat. J Am Vet Med Assoc 1987; 191:235.

Berger B, Feldman EC. Primary hypoparathyroidism in dogs: 21 cases (1976–1986). J Am Vet Med Assoc 1987; 191:350.

Brobst D. Review of the pathophysiology of alterations in potassium homeostasis. J Am Vet Med Assoc 1986; 188:1019.

Bruyette DS, Feldman EC. Primary hypoparathyroidism in the dog. Journal of the American College of Veterinary Internal Medicine 1988; 2:7.

Cornelius LM. Abnormalities of the standard biochemical profile. In: Lorenz MD, Cornelius LM, eds. Small animal medical diagnosis. Philadelphia: JB Lippincott, 1987: 539.

Crawford MA, Kittleson MD, Fink GD. Hypernatremia and adipsia in a dog. J Am Vet Med Assoc 1984; 184:818.

Crow SE, Stockham SL. Profound hyponatremia associated with glucocorticoid deficiency in a dog. Journal of the American Animal Hospital Association 1985; 21:393.

Degen M. Pseudohyperkalemia in Akitas. J Am Vet Med Assoc 1987; 190:541.

DiBartola SP. Hyponatremia. In: Schaer M, ed. Fluid and electrolyte disorders. Vet Clin North Am 1989; 19:215.

Dow SW, Fettman MJ, Curtis CR, LeCouteur RA. Hypokalemia in cats: 186 cases (1984–1987). J Am Vet Med Assoc 1989; 194:1604.

Dow SW, Fettman MJ, LeCouteur RA, Hamar DW. Potassium depletion in cats: Renal and dietary influences. J Am Vet Med Assoc 1987; 191:1569.

Dow SW, LeCouteur RA, Fettman MJ, Spurgeon TL. Potassium depletion in cats: Hypokalemic polymyopathy. J Am Vet Med Assoc 1987; 191:1563.

Drazner FH. Hypercalcemia in the dog and cat. J Am Vet Med Assoc 1981; 178:1252.

Edwards DF, Richardson DC, Russell RG. Hyper-natremic, hypertonic dehydration in a dog with diabetes insipidus and gastric dilatation-volvulus. J Am Vet Med Assoc 1983; 182:973.

Feldman EC, Krutzik S. Case reports of parathyroid levels in spontaneous canine parathyroid disorders. Journal of the American Animal Hospital Association 1981; 17:393.

Finco DR. Interpretations of serum calcium concentration in the dog. Compend Contin Educ 1983; 5:778.

Flanders JA, Scarlett JM, Blue JT, Neth S. Adjustment of total serum calcium concentration for binding to albumin and protein in cats: 291 cases (1986–1987). J Am Vet Med Assoc 1989; 194:1609.

Haskins SC. Fluid and electrolyte therapy. Compendium of Continuing Education 1984; 6:244.

Jezyk PF. Hyperkalemic periodic paralysis in a dog. Journal of the American Animal Hospital Association 1982; 18:977.

Kornegay JN. Hypocalcemia in dogs. Compendium of Continuing Education 1982; 4:103.

Kornegay JN, Greene CE, Martin C et al. Idiopathic hypocalcemia in four dogs. Journal of the American Animal Hospital Association 1980; 16:723.

Peterson ME, Feinman JM. Hypercalcemia associated with hypoadrenocorticism in sixteen dogs. J Am Vet Med Assoc 1982; 181:802.

Reimann KA, Knowlen GG, Tvedten HW. Factitious hyperkalemia in dogs with thrombocytosis. Journal of the American College of Veterinary Internal Medicine 1989; 3:47.

Scott RC. Disorders of sodium metabolism. In: Schaer M, ed. Vet Clin North Am 1982; 12:375.

73

ANEMIA
Robert M. Jacobs

Anemia is present when the red blood cell (RBC) count, packed-cell volume (PCV), or the hemoglobin (Hb) concentration are below the lower reference limit. Reference intervals are appropriate only for the methodology by which they were determined and for the laboratory in which the work was done. Differences in measurements between breeds, age, sex, and pregnant and nonpregnant animals likely exist but are largely ignored in veterinary medicine. Results will vary between manual techniques and different automated instruments.

Anemia is considered a secondary phenomenon—a symptom of an underlying disease. Generally, effective treatment of the primary disease results in resolution of the anemia.

CAUSES AND PATHOPHYSIOLOGY

Anemia can be characterized by changes in RBC indices (mean corpuscular volume [MCV], mean corpuscular hemoglobin [MCH], mean corpuscular hemoglobin concentration [MCHC]) or pathogenesis. The advantage of categorizing anemias by pathogenesis is that the cause of the anemia is often denoted by the classification into which the anemia is placed (Fig. 73-1). A few simple and widely available tests will allow classification of

the anemia by pathogenesis and indicate the route to be taken to further characterize the lesion or determine its cause. Basically, anemia is due to either inadequate numbers of RBCs reaching the peripheral blood or, once in the peripheral blood, decreased life span.

Regenerative Anemias

Anemias due to decreased RBC life span in peripheral blood are generally regenerative. Hemorrhage or hemolysis account for the loss of RBCs; hemorrhagic anemias are generally less regenerative than hemolytic anemias. Acute hemorrhagic or hemolytic episodes may appear initially as nonregenerative anemias since the appropriate bone marrow response has not had time to develop. It may take 5 to 7 days to develop a marked reticulocytosis. Anemia from acute hemorrhage is not evident until fluid shifts from extravascular to intravascular sites, which takes about 24 hours. The nature of the hemorrhage is usually blood loss from the body, most often from the gastrointestinal tract. Urogenital and pulmonary hemorrhage and hemorrhage into a body cavity may also result in anemia. External blood loss results in a regenerative anemia, until iron stores are depleted. Hemorrhage into body cavi-

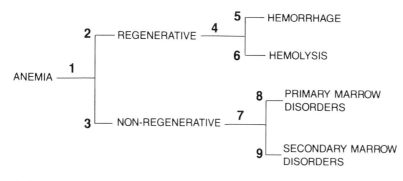

1. Determine absolute reticulocyte count
2. Absolute reticulocyte count greater than 80,000/μL (80 × 10⁹/L)
3. Absolute reticulocyte count less than 50,000/μL (50 × 10⁹/L)
4. Determine serum protein concentration
5. Protein concentration less than 60 g/L (6 g/dl) (adult)
6. Protein concentration greater than 60 g/L (6 g/dl) (adult)
7. Complete blood cell count and platelet count
8. Single or multiple (usually) cytopenias
9. Normal or increased leukocyte and platelet counts

Figure 73–1. *Flow diagram showing the initial steps in determining the cause of anemia.*

ties may result in transient but potentially severe anemia. A large fraction of blood lost into a body cavity is returned to the circulation, essentially as an autotransfusion. Where continuous hemorrhage into a body cavity or chronic low grade hemolysis occurs, the anemia may be persistently regenerative.

Hemolysis is divided into intravascular and extravascular types. Intravascular hemolysis is unusual in animals. Immune intravascular hemolysis is seen when certain immunoglobulin classes that fix complement efficiently are involved and the complement cascade goes to completion. Some of the other causes of intravascular hemolysis are bacterial toxins (lecithinases), hypophosphatemia, parasitism (partially mediated through immune mechanisms), RBC oxidants (copper and iron toxicity), and water intoxication.

Classic immune hemolytic anemia is due to extravascular hemolysis resulting from opsonization of the RBC with antibody. Red blood cell parasitism may also cause RBCs to be removed at extravascular sites for immune and nonimmune reasons. In particular, those parasites that are membrane associated decrease the fluidity and flexibility of the RBC membrane so that the RBC can no longer change shape and traverse the splenic vasculature. Spherocytes (resulting from

the attachment of antibody to the RBC), RBCs with Heinz bodies (resulting from the oxidative denaturation of hemoglobin), and fragmented RBCs (resulting from intravascular deposition of fibrin seen with localized or disseminated intravascular coagulation) are removed from circulation for similar reasons. Liver disease is also associated with decreased RBC life span, possibly because of acquired shape changes and decreased flexibility resulting from cholesterol loading of RBC membranes. Opsonized or inflexible RBCs are phagocytized by cells of the mononuclear phagocyte system located in the spleen, liver, bone marrow, and lymph nodes.

Nonregenerative Anemias

Either decreased (lack of erythroid marrow) or, less commonly, increased ineffective production (increased rate of intramarrow death) of RBCs can result in lack of delivery of mature red cells to the peripheral blood. These anemias are nonregenerative. Primary bone marrow diseases causing a relative (erythroid hypoplasia) or absolute (erythroid or pure red cell aplasia) lack of erythroid marrow can be neoplastic or associated with metabolic, infectious, toxic, drug, or immune-mediated insults directed at erythroid precursor cells. Tumors in the marrow-causing anemia can be myeloproliferative (granulocytic, monocytic, myelomonocytic, megakaryocytic, myelofibrotic, osteosclerotic, erythroid), lymphoproliferative, or rarely metastatic. Marrow neoplasia causes anemia by occupying marrow space, competing with normal cells for essential nutrients, producing inhibitors of normal hematopoiesis, and indirectly by causing anemia of chronic disease mediated through immunosuppression and leukopenia. Myelofibrosis may be seen in association with pyruvate kinase deficiency in Basenjis and beagles and other diseases affecting the marrow. Osteosclerosis has been reported to occur in people with a particular carbonic anhydrase deficiency. Erythrosuppression has been associated with storage diseases, tuberculosis, infection with *Ehrlichia* organisms, infections with parvoviruses, and feline leukemia virus (FeLV). Although parvoviruses kill rapidly dividing cells, including early erythroid cells, anemia resulting from this infection in dogs is due to hemorrhage. In cats, an anemia is generally not seen with panleukopenia virus infection since the animals die or recover in a relatively short time period compared with the RBC life span. Treatment with estradiol, phenylbutazone, mitotane, phenobarbital, numerous chemotherapeutic agents used for tumor therapy, and, possibly, chloramphenicol may be associated with marrow stem cell injury. There are anecdotal reports of numerous other drugs causing marrow stem cell injury in animals. The list of proven agents in people is extensive and includes all classes of drugs. Whole body irradiation will also destroy the marrow. Immune-mediated mechanisms are thought to be involved in those patients where the aplasia or hypoplasia apparently responds to corticosteroid treatment. Direct evidence for an immune mechanism in these patients is rarely proved.

Patients with primary bone marrow diseases causing nonregenerative anemia with erythroid hyperplasia are anemic due to ineffective erythropoiesis. Here the more mature cells of the marrow erythroid series are more severely affected by offending stimuli and never leave the marrow compartment. Ineffective erythropoiesis is also seen in the myelodysplasia syndrome along with additional peripheral blood cytopenias, megaloblastic changes, and other morphologic abnormalities. Although the biology of myelodysplasia is not well characterized in animals, it appears that some affected animals become frankly leukemic after a variable period of time.

Almost three quarters of anemic cats are FeLV-infected. Anemia associated with FeLV infection is most often nonregenerative due to interference with erythroid stem cells. Erythroid hypoplasia or pure red cell aplasia associated with FeLV infection is almost always due to infection with the subgroup C variant of FeLV, either alone or in combination with other variants. A structural antigen of the subgroup C variant has been shown to suppress erythropoiesis at the committed stem cell level. Other expressions of FeLV infection can also be associated with anemia. The anemia of FeLV-related myelodysplasia is often seen with leukopenia or thrombocytopenia. The FeLV-related panleukopenia-like or pancytopenia syndrome occurs when the three cell lines of the peripheral blood are suppressed simultaneously. Pancytopenia is more often associated with marrow hypocellularity rather than hypercellularity; one assumes the hypocellularity is due to damage to the multipotential stem cell. With marrow neoplasia, it is not unusual to find a marrow filled with neoplastic cells, almost to the exclusion of normal cells, a lack of circulating neoplastic cells (aleukemic leukemia), and pancytopenia.

Secondary bone marrow diseases causing anemias are much more common than primary problems. The anemia of chronic disease is a common secondary cause. It is apparently mediated through failure of efficient transfer of storage iron to developing erythroid cells, shortened RBC survival, and inappropriately poor marrow response to the anemia. Other causes of secondary bone marrow problems include renal disease and diseases of the pituitary-thyroid and pituitary-adrenal axes. Decreased erythropoiesis associated with chronic renal disease is due to decreased erythropoietin production, shortened RBC survival (possibly mediated through parathyroid hormone excess), and relative marrow refractoriness to erythropoietin stimulation. Hypothyroidism is also associated with mild to moderate anemia, which may be related to decreased oxygen demand. Anemia is seen with hypoadrenocorticism but is sometimes masked by dehydration.

Traditionally, iron deficiency in people has been categorized as a poorly or nonregenerative anemia, but this categorization is relatively uncommon in animals. Differences in the common causes for the iron lack between animals and people may account for this discrepancy. Iron deficiency in animals is almost always due to blood loss, and this loss is most often gastrointestinal in origin. Depending on the site of the gastrointestinal lesion, an opportunity may arise for reabsorption of iron from digested blood. In this situation, iron will not be rate limiting and regenerative anemia results. It is also likely that with continued hemorrhage over a longer period of time a previously regenerative anemia would become poorly regenerative then nonregenerative as iron stores become progressively depleted. This progression represents a change from iron deficient erythropoiesis to iron deficient anemia. Dietary iron deficiency is seen only in suckling animals resulting in a phase of physiologic iron deficiency. This deficiency resolves spontaneously once adult foods are fed. Heavy infestations of fleas, tick, and hookworms are common causes of hemorrhage and iron deficiency anemia in young animals.

Other trace minerals, such as copper and cobalt, and vitamins, such as pyridoxine, vitamin B_{12}, and folic acid, are required for normal erythropoiesis. Deficiencies of these materials may rarely cause poorly or nonregenerative anemias in animals, most often without the characteristic morphologic changes (megaloblastosis, macrocytic, normochromic anemia with vitamin B_{12} and folate deficiency; microcytic, hypochromic anemia in copper deficiency) seen in some other animal species and people.

CLINICAL SIGNS

Clinical signs, as they relate to specific organ systems are listed in Table 73-1. Many of the clinical signs are directly related to attempts at compensation for decreased delivery of oxygen to tissues. Other clinical signs relate more directly to the cause of the anemia. The severity of symptoms are

Table 73–1 *Clinical Signs of Anemia*

CARDIPULMONARY

Amplified arterial pulse
Cardiomegaly
Dyspnea with or without exercise
Increased rate and depth of respirations
Pale mucous membranes
Shock
Tachycardia
Systolic (anemic) murmur

DIGESTIVE

Anorexia
Constipation
Diarrhea

INTEGUMENTARY

Icterus
Poor quality hair coat

NEUROMUSCULAR

Cold sensitivity
Depression
Exercise intolerance
Fainting, collapse, seizures
Lack of endurance
Listlessness
Muscle atrophy
Ocular fundus pathology
Weakness

URINARY

Hemoglobinuria

directly related to the degree of anemia and the rapidity of onset. Anemias that develop quickly are less well tolerated than those developing over a longer period, since less time is allowed for effective compensation. Signs tend to be more severe in aged animals and animals with preexisting diseases, particularly of the cardiopulmonary system. Cats and sedate animals show less severe signs than active animals with comparable degrees of anemia.

DIAGNOSTIC APPROACH

The basic laboratory tests required to initially categorize an anemia according to Figure 73-1 are: complete blood cell count (CBC) (includes PCV, Hb, RBC count, MCV, MCH, MCHC, total nucleated cell count, differential nucleated cell count including nucleated RBCs), total plasma or serum protein concentration, and the absolute reticulocyte count. Sequential CBC counts and reticulocyte counts are usually required for diagnosis and monitoring. Once anemia is established, it is then divided into regenerative and nonregenerative forms by use of the absolute reticulocyte count. Normally, dogs and cats have between 50,000 and 80,000 reticulocytes/μL blood (50 and 80 × 10^9/L respectively), which corresponds to reticulocyte percentages of about 1% in the dog and 0.4% in the cat. Reticulocyte percentages can be corrected by the following formula:

% Reticulocytes (corrected) = % Reticulocytes × PCV patient/PCV normal

A further correction can be made for reticulocyte maturation time. Anemias in animals with reticulocyte counts below this range are considered nonregenerative. Acute hemorrhagic (*e.g.*, trauma, laceration, surgery) or hemolytic episodes may not have absolute reticulocyte counts above normal if there has been insufficient time (less than 2 or 3 days after the episode) for the development of a bone marrow response. Subsequent CBCs will reveal the regenerative nature of these anemias. Normally, the more severe the regenerative anemia, the greater the reticulocyte response. Blood loss anemias tend to have lower absolute reticulocyte counts than hemolytic anemias. Regenerative anemias most often are macrocytic hypochromic but can be normocytic normochromic or microcytic hypochromic, as in iron deficiency. As discussed previously, most chronic blood loss anemias complicated by iron deficiency have increased absolute reticulocyte counts; only rarely does iron deficiency present as a nonregenerative anemia.

Regenerative Anemias

Animals with regenerative anemias are subsequently divided into the hemorrhagic or blood loss and hemolytic categories on the basis of plasma or serum protein concentrations. Causes of blood loss anemia are listed in Table 73-2. A decreased plasma or serum protein concentration is generally present with a single hemor-

Table 73–2 *Causes of Hemorrhagic or Blood Loss Anemia*

CLOTTING DISORDERS

Congenital deficiencies of coagulation factors
Disseminated or localized intravascular coagulation
Hyperviscosity syndrome
Thrombasthenia or thrombopathia (acquired or congenital)
Thrombocytopenia (immune, systemic lupus erythematosus, rickettsial, intravascular coagulation, hypersplenism)
Vitamin K antagonists (warfarin and related compounds)

GASTROINTESTINAL ULCERATION

Drug associated
Neoplasia associated

NEOPLASIA

Adenocarcinoma
Hemangiosarcoma
Leiomyoma
Lymphoma

PARASITISM

Coccidiosis
Fleas
Hookworms
Lice
Ticks

PARVOVIRAL INFECTION

SURGICAL PROCEDURES

TRAUMA AND LACERATIONS

rhagic episode that is of more than 24 hours duration. Until fluid shifts have taken place to increase intravascular volume, these patients will have normal PCVs and protein concentrations. Most often the site of blood loss is obvious from the history or the physical examination. Sometimes a more thorough search is required. The gastrointestinal tract should be the first organ system examined. Feces should be examined for hookworm eggs. If the feces are not melenic, then a test for occult blood should be done and repeated several times over several days. If gastrointestinal hemorrhage is present, then a platelet count should be done. Plain and contrast radiography, endoscopy, and biopsy at laparotomy may be required to discover an ulcer or a tumor causing the hemorrhage. Finding decreased serum iron and total iron binding concentrations is useful in confirming an already suspected (on the basis of microcytosis and hypochromia) iron deficiency. Serum iron and total iron binding concentrations should always be interpreted carefully since they may be influenced by inflammatory disease. With inflammation, the serum iron concentrations tend to decrease, while the total iron binding concentrations remain unchanged or decrease slightly.

Hemolytic anemias have normal or increased serum or plasma protein concentrations. Causes of hemolytic anemias are listed in Table 73-3. Intravascular hemolysis is unusual in animals, and, if severe, is typified by hemoglobinemia and hemoglobinuria. Milder intravascular hemolysis can be detected by measuring plasma concentrations of hemoglobin, haptoglobin, or hemopexin. Concentrations of the latter two analytes increase with inflammatory disease, which may mask a decrease caused by hemolysis. Once hemolysis is thought to be occurring, a careful search of the blood smear may reveal the etiology. Parasitic agents may be found. Spherocytes or agglutination indicate immune hemolysis. A positive Coombs' test result will confirm a preliminary diagnosis of immune hemolytic anemia, but a negative test will not eliminate the diagnosis. The presence of spherocytes, which are difficult to recognize in the cat, can be confirmed by lysis of red cells in hypotonic saline (osmotic or saline fragility test). The immune complex disease, systemic lupus erythematosus (SLE), is expressed as some combination of immune hemolytic anemia, immune thrombocytopenia, proteinuria, arthritis, and skin disease. The antinuclear antibody test (ANA) has the greatest sensitivity for SLE. Red blood cell fragmentation with or without thrombocytopenia suggests disseminated or localized intravascular coagulation (see Chapter 16). Increased concentrations of fibrin degradation products in blood or urine support a diagnosis of intravascular coagulation. The presence of increased numbers of Heinz bodies suggests exposure to drugs and chemicals capable of inducing hemoglobin denaturation. Other RBC shape changes, such as acanthocytes and target cells indicate chronic inflammatory disease or liver disease. In a large breed of dog, the presence of acanthocytes, fragmented RBCs, and inappropriate numbers of nucleated RBCs for the degree of anemia are highly suggestive of hemangiosarcoma (see Chapter 15).

Table 73-3 *Causes of Hemolytic Anemia*

BACTERIAL

Clostridiosis
Leptospirosis
Other bacteremias

**CHEMICAL TOXICITIES
(MOST CAUSE HEINZ BODY FORMATION)**

Acetaminophen
Acetohydroxamic acid
Aspirin
Benzocaine
Copper (Bedlington terrier)
Iron
Lead
Methylene blue
Napthalene in moth balls
Propylene glycol
Soap
Toilet bowl cleaners

FeLV INFECTION

IMMUNE-MEDIATED HEMOLYTIC ANEMIAS

Altered RBC antigen, cross-reactive antigen, or hapten (bacterial, chemical, drug [for example, propylthiouracil], viral) (common)
Autoimmune (uncommon)
Systemic lupus erythematosus
Transfusion reaction

MISCELLANEOUS

Heat stroke
Hypersplenism
Hypophosphatemia (associated with hyperalimentation)
Liver disease
Malignant hyperthermia
Water intoxication

PARASITISM

Babesiosis
Cytauxzoonosis
Ehrlichiosis
Hemobartonellosis

POISONOUS PLANTS AND VENOM

Onions, fava beans, jasmine, and others
Tiger snakes and others

RBC METABOLIC DISEASES

Feline porphyria
Methemoglobinemia (acquired)
Methemoglobin reductase deficiency
Phosphofructokinase deficiency (English springer spaniel)
Pyruvate kinase deficiency (Basenji, beagle)

Nonregenerative Anemias

Anemias in patients with absolute reticulocyte counts less than normal are considered nonregenerative. These anemias are most often due to secondary effects on the marrow, caused by abnormalities in tissues outside of the bone marrow. Primary bone marrow disorders are seen less frequently. Primary and secondary marrow changes can often be separated simply by examination of the CBC results. With primary marrow problems, multiple, unexplained cytopenias are often found so that thrombocytopenia and anemia, leukopenia and anemia, or pancytopenia are seen. Alternatively, unexplained increases in leukocytes or platelets may be seen. With secondary marrow problems, platelets and leukocytes are usually present in normal or increased numbers, depending on the underlying disease process.

Causes of primary bone marrow diseases are listed in Table 73-4. Lymphoid or myeloid leuke-

Table 73–4 *Primary Marrow Disorders Resulting in Anemia*

Estrogen toxicity (exogenous or Sertoli's cell tumor)
Immune stem cell disease
Infectious diseases
  Ehrlichiosis
  Feline leukemia virus infection
  Feline immunodeficiency virus infection
  Tuberculosis
Metabolic diseases
  Pyruvate kinase deficiency leading to myelofibrosis
  Storage diseases
Mineral deficiencies
  cobalt (?), copper, iron, selenium (?)
Miscellaneous
  Chloramphenicol
  Other drugs (trimethoprim-sulfa, fenbendazole)
  Phenylbutazone
  Uncharacterized environmental chemicals
Myelodysplasia
Myelofibrosis (separate from myeloproliferative disease)
Neoplastic disorders
  Cancers metastatic to marrow
  Lymphoproliferative disorders
    Lymphoid leukemia
    Lymphosarcoma metastatic to marrow
  Myeloproliferative disorders
    Erythremic myelosis
    Granulocytic leukemia
    Megarkaryocytic or blastic leukemia
    Monocytic leukemia
    Myelofibrosis
    Myelomonocytic leukemia
    Osteosclerosis
Protein deficiency (?)
Vitamin deficiencies (?)
  B_{12}, folate, niacin, pyridoxine, pantothenic acid, riboflavin, thiamine, vitamins A, C, and E
Whole body radiation

mias, if detected on a CBC, are often associated with suppression of the normal erythroid and megakaryocytic cell lines. In fact, atrophy of the normal components of the marrow is an important observation to make before leukemia is diagnosed. If the diagnosis of leukemia is unequivocal on the basis of examination of peripheral blood, then a bone marrow aspirate generally does not add further information. Sometimes, there may be only small numbers (subleukemic leukemia) or an absence (aleukemic leukemia) of leukemic cells in circulation. In these situations, making a diagnosis on the peripheral blood is difficult or impossible. With the aleukemic and subleukemic varieties of leukemia, nucleated RBCs and immature leukocytes often appear in the peripheral blood (leukoerythroblastic reaction) because of interference with the normal age-related release of cells and extramedullary hematopoiesis. The presence of nucleated RBCs in peripheral blood with little polychromasia does not indicate a regenerative erythroid response. In these situations, and in all other situations where primary marrow disease is suspected, a bone marrow aspirate or core biopsy must be done to arrive at a final diagnosis (see Bone Marrow Aspiration and Biopsy in Chapter 80).

Macrocytosis is commonly observed in cats with FeLV-related anemias. This finding should not be interpreted as a sign of regeneration since reticulocytopenia is usually present. A prior hemolytic episode is seen in about 20% of cats destined to develop FeLV-related erythroid hypoplasia. It is thought that macrocytes produced at the time of the hemolytic episode persist in the circulation, possibly accounting for the macrocytosis.

Myelofibrosis can be seen as a myeloproliferative disorder or as a consequence of other diseases impacting on the marrow. Occasionally, excess fibroblasts can be detected on marrow aspirates, but core biopsies are preferred. In addition to a lack of production of cells, the RBCs exiting the marrow often undergo shape changes to form teardrop (apple stem) cells or, less commonly, stomatocytes.

Deficiencies of minerals and vitamins rarely cause anemia except for iron deficiency, and even then iron deficiency anemias as experienced in animals are most often regenerative. Although iron deficiency is indicated by the presence of microcytosis and hypochromia, copper deficiency in some species is expressed as a normocytic normochromic anemia. The changes in the marrow with iron deficiency are characteristic. With iron deficiency anemia, no stainable marrow iron will be found, but this result is unreliable in young animals since they do not have any normally.

Myelodysplasia may be a cause of ineffective erythropoiesis. It is sometimes difficult to differentiate myelodysplasia from acute leukemia. Essentially, the differentiation depends on determining the fraction of marrow cells that are blasts. Above a certain threshold (about 30% in people), leukemia is diagnosed. A similar threshold has been adopted in animals, but more study is required to assess the situation. If diagnoses of myelodysplasia or equivocal leukemia are given, then sequential CBCs should be done to further characterize the abnormality.

Single or multiple peripheral blood cytopenias can be seen in infection with *Ehrlichia* organisms. Marrow failure is more often seen in the German shepherd, while myeloid hyperplasia is more common in other breeds. Since the organism is rarely seen in biopsy specimens, a presumptive diagnosis is made using serology (see Chapter 79).

Immune hemolysis can also be seen as a nonregenerative or reticulocytopenic form if the immune response is directed against a red cell precursor. Depending on the particular stage of development affected, hyperplasia of the more immature stages may be present; if the earliest forms are involved, pure red cell aplasia will be found. A serum IgG inhibitor of *in vitro* erythropoiesis has been demonstrated in some people and dogs with pure red cell aplasia. In people T lymphocyte mediated suppression of erythroid precursors has also been shown. However, due to the complexity of the assays, direct proof of an immune pathogenesis in these cases is rarely provided. Recognition of erythrophagy in the marrow and response to immunosuppressive therapy provide supportive but indirect evidence.

Estrogen toxicity, whether present as a paraneoplastic syndrome (Sertoli's cell tumor) or caused by the administration of estrogen-containing drugs, begins as myeloid hyperplasia with marked leukocytosis. The leukocytosis wanes and is followed by leukopenia, thrombocytopenia, and anemia. Other drugs and environmental chemicals are often thought to be involved in marrow disease, but it is either difficult or impractical to prove cause and effect.

Of the disorders causing secondary marrow failure and anemia (Table 73-5), chronic inflammatory disease is the most common. Often the sites of inflammation are obvious at physical examination. Any organ system can be involved. Generally the anemia is mild or moderate, normocytic normochromic, and roughly proportional to the extent and duration of the lesion. Despite poor turnover of iron, anemias of chronic disease in animals are normocytic normochromic and not microcytic hypochromic, although in people microcytosis and hypochromia are reported occasionally. Other causes of secondary marrow disorders will become evident with the physical examination, radiography, serum biochemistry profile, and tests of endocrine function.

MANAGEMENT

Since anemia is always secondary to other problems, the underlying abnormality must be identified. If the primary disease is successfully treated then, as long as adequate materials for erythropoiesis are present, the anemia will resolve spontaneously.

Treatment of patients with acute anemias, where there is inadequate time for physiologic adaptations, should be directed at preventing shock and decreasing hypoxia (see Chapter 4). The patient should be maintained in a quiet environment and not stressed. An oxygen cage or pro-

Table 73–5 *Secondary Marrow Disorders Resulting in Anemia*

Chronic inflammatory diseases
Endocrine disease
  Hypothyroidism
  Hypoadrenocorticism
Neoplasia
Renal disease

vision of oxygen through a nasal tube is sometimes appropriate. Fluid therapy is given to enhance perfusion but may further decrease the PCV. Transfusions should be given to alleviate acute hypoxic episodes. It has been recommended that whole blood be given at a dose of 10 to 20 ml/kg body weight. It is preferable to estimate the patient's total blood hemoglobin deficit (based on 8%–9% blood volume in the dog and 6%–7% blood volume in the cat), and then transfuse adequate blood to bring the hemoglobin concentration into the normal range (see Chapter 16). There are no thresholds below which a transfusion must be given; the decision to transfuse should be made solely on the basis of the severity of clinical signs. Although cross-matching and blood typing should be done, often the time is not adequate. To deal with this problem, many busy hospitals maintain blood-typed, splenectomized, iron-replete, and tetracycline-treated universal donor dogs. Spontaneous transfusion reactions have been reported in both dogs and cats. Transfusing blood into patients that are actively hemolyzing may cause or augment an existing hemoglobinemia, precipitate disseminated intravascular coagulation, and potentially cause nephrosis. If mild or moderate signs of hypoxia are present and evidence of increased erythropoiesis is already found, it is likely the hemolytic or hemorrhagic event occurred at least several days prior. In these situations, transfusion is unnecessary and, if given in large enough amounts, will effectively slow down or turn off the endogenous response.

Specific treatment of immune hemolytic anemia is directed at decreasing the rate of immune-mediated destruction of red cells. Corticosteroids, with or without other immunosuppressive drugs, such as cyclophosphamide and azathioprine, are given at immunosuppressive dose rates (Table 73-6). As the hemolysis comes under control, the dose is decreased slowly and finally stopped. Some animals may be resistant to or poorly tolerate one or more drugs. In recurrent immune hemolytic anemia, which may be seen as an annual phenomenon, apparent drug resistance may develop.

Splenectomy has, from time to time, been advocated in the treatment of immune hemolytic anemias that are refractory to medical treatment. Splenomegaly, which is often seen in patients with immune hemolytic anemia, is due to reticuloendothelial hyperplasia and extramedullary hematopoiesis. The mononuclear phagocyte system is found in several organs, so splenectomy, at best, removes only part of the problem and, at worst, may compromise a developing response by eliminating a site of RBC production. Splenectomy may be used to prolong the RBC life span when intrinsic red cell defects are present, such as with pyruvate kinase deficiency and inherited disorders of RBC shape. Splenectomy is indicated in hypersplenism, where the splenic transit time is increased due to neoplasia or inflammation (see Chapter 15).

Clinical signs in animals with chronic anemia are less severe than those associated with acute anemia. Some of these patients, particularly cats,

Table 73–6 *Drugs Commonly Used in the Treatment of Anemia*

Drug	Dose*	Route
Azathioprine	2 mg/kg, s.i.d.	PO
Cyclophosphamide	6.6 mg/kg for 3 days then 2.2 mg/kg, s.i.d.	PO
Ferrous sulfate	100 to 300 mg/kg/day (dog)	PO
	50 to 100 mg/kg/day (cat)	PO
Iron dextran	10 mg/kg/day (in divided doses)	IM
Nandrolone decanoate	1 mg/kg/wk	IM
Oxymetholone	1 mg/kg, s.i.d.–t.i.d.	PO
Prednisone	2 to 4 mg/kg/day	PO

* All doses are for dogs and cats unless indicated otherwise.

can have remarkably low PCVs, yet the only sign is paleness of mucous membranes. Generally, chronic anemias do not need transfusions. With those chronic anemias that are regenerative, the prognosis is good. If microcytosis and hypochromia are present, the site of blood loss identified, and the cause (thrombocytopenia, neoplasia, hookworms, fleas) rectified, then iron replacement therapy is indicated. Young animals that are iron deficient should be dewormed even if the results of a fecal examination are negative. Iron can be given parenterally as iron dextran. Oral administration is preferred; iron sulfate is the usual choice. With nonregenerative chronic anemias, the prognosis is much worse because of the association with primary bone marrow disorders, such as leukemia and myelofibrosis. Anabolic androgenic steroids (oxymetholone, nandrolone decanoate) have been recommended for use in erythroid hypoplasia or pure red cell aplasia resulting from either a primary or secondary (*e.g.*, renal) bone marrow disorder. Where an immune mechanism is thought to be involved, corticosteroids and other drugs (*e.g.*, cyclophosphamide, azathioprine) are given at immunosuppressive doses.

If an association is found between drug therapy and the development of anemia, then therapy should be suspended or changed. A change in the animal's environment should be made if chemical exposure is suspected.

PATIENT MONITORING

Sequential CBCs and absolute reticulocyte counts should be done to confirm a diagnosis and monitor therapy. Other tests should be requested depending on the underlying disease.

ADDITIONAL READING

Badylak SF. A pathophysiologic approach to the diagnosis of hemolytic anemia in the dog. Compendium of Continuing Education 1981; 3:827.

Christopher MM. Relation of endogenous Heinz bodies to disease and anemia in cats: 120 cases (1978–1987). J Am Vet Med Assoc 1989; 194:1089.

Christopher MM, Perman V, Eaton JW. Contribution of propylene glycol-induced Heinz body formation to anemia in cats. J Am Vet Med Assoc 1989; 194:1045.

Feldman BF, Handagama P. Splenectomy as adjunctive therapy for immune mediated thrombocytopenia and hemolytic anemia in the dog. J Am Vet Med Assoc 1985; 187:617.

Feldman BF, Kaneko JJ. Anemia of inflammatory disease in the dog: Clinical characterization. Am J Vet Res 1981; 42:1109.

Feldman BF, Kaneko JJ, Farver TB. Anemia of inflammatory disease in the dog: Availability of storage iron in inflammatory disease. Am J Vet Res 1981; 42:586.

Sherding RG, Wilson GP, Kociba GJ. Bone marrow hypoplasia in eight dogs with Sertoli cell tumor. J Am Vet Med Assoc 1981; 178:497.

Weiser MG. Correlative approach to anemia in dogs and cats. Journal of the American Animal Hospital Association 1981; 17:286.

74

POLYCYTHEMIA

Robert M. Jacobs

An increase in red blood cell (RBC) count, packed-cell volume (PCV), or hemoglobin concentration above the upper reference limit is considered polycythemia. The upper reference limit depends on such factors as age, breed, sex, and altitude. Reference intervals represent about 95% of a population so that 2.5% of normal individuals may have values above the upper limit.

CAUSES AND PATHOPHYSIOLOGY

The types and causes of polycythemia are summarized in Table 74-1. Polycythemia most often results from dehydration. This type is referred to as relative polycythemia since a decrease in plasma volume occurs. A PCV of 70% (0.70 L/L) or greater may be noted. Physiologic polycythemia occurs as a result of splenic contraction mediated through epinephrine release. Plasma volume does not change with splenic contraction, but the total blood volume and PCV may increase 10% to 15% due to an increase in red cell mass. The primary and secondary forms of absolute polycythemia are generally associated with normal or increased plasma volumes. Relative and absolute forms of polycythemia may coexist.

Primary polycythemia, or *polycythemia vera*, occurs rarely and is due to the autonomous prolif-eration of erythroid cells. Erythroid precursor cells are not dependent on erythropoietin for differentiation. Polycythemia vera is one variety of myeloproliferative disease. A range in PCV of 70% to 88% (0.70–0.88 L/L) has been found in dogs and cats with primary polycythemia.

Secondary polycythemia is seen occasionally and results most often from erythropoietin-stimulated erythropoiesis. Cardiopulmonary disease, right-to-left arteriovenous shunts, and acquired hemoglobinopathies (methemoglobin, sulfhemoglobin, and carboxyhemoglobins) can be involved. Congenital hemoglobinopathies (hemoglobins with an unusually high oxygen affinity) have not been identified in animals.

Although rarely reported, inappropriate erythropoietin synthesis and secretion causing secondary polycythemia can occur as a paraneoplastic syndrome or in association with space occupying renal lesions. The paraneoplastic form is almost exclusively associated with renal carcinomas and lymphomas. There are single reports of a renal pheochromocytoma and an apparent erythropoietin-producing nasal fibrosarcoma causing polycythemia in dogs. In addition to renal neoplasms, uterine leiomyomas, cerebellar hemangioblastomas, hepatomas, adrenal tumors, and several other tumors in people are also associated with the paraneoplastic syndrome. Non-neoplas-

Table 74–1 *Types and Causes of Polycythemia*

Absolute primary
  Myeloproliferative disease
    Polycythemia vera
Absolute secondary
  Cardiopulmonary disease (hypoxemia)
  Familial*
  Hemoglobinopathy (hypoxemia)*
  Hormonal excess
    Adrenal
    Thyroid
  Paraneoplastic syndrome
Physiologic
  Splenic contraction
Relative
  Dehydration

* *Not reported in dogs and cats.*

tic space occupying renal lesions, such as hydronephrosis, renal cysts, and polycystic disease, possibly causing renal ischemia and increased erythropoietin release, are also associated with polycythemia in animals and people.

Adrenocortical and thyroidal hormonal excess, from either endogenous or exogenous sources, can result in mild polycythemia (10% increase in PCV). These hormones may act directly on the erythroid marrow or indirectly by creating increased oxygen demand. Relative polycythemia may also be involved.

Familial polycythemia, although characterized in people and in large animals, has not yet been reported in dogs and cats.

CLINICAL SIGNS

Most clinical signs are related to hyperviscosity. Blood viscosity increases exponentially with increasing PCV; the greater the viscosity the more severe the clinical signs. Mucous membranes are often congested and blood vessels dilated as a result of increased blood volume and sludging of blood particularly in small bore vessels. Frequently, a bleeding diathesis is found related to decreased platelet function. Sludging of blood may also lead to thrombosis and loss of integrity of blood vessel walls. Depending on the site of

hemorrhage, epistaxis, hematemesis, melena, or hematuria may occur. Polydipsia and polyuria are noted frequently. Lameness may be present. Neurologic disturbances, resulting from sludging of blood and leading to anoxia and central nervous system hemorrhage, include lethargy, disorientation, tremors, ataxia, weakness, dementia, seizures, and blindness.

DIAGNOSTIC APPROACH

Clinical signs of dehydration, increased serum or plasma protein concentration (and other biochemical analytes), and urinary specific gravity are often adequate to confirm a suspicion of relative polycythemia. If the increase in PCV is mild (PCV of 55%–65% or 0.55–0.65 L/L in the dog) and no fluid loss is obvious, then direct measurement of the total blood volume and calculation of the red cell mass and plasma volume are required. Although not done frequently in veterinary medicine, clinically useful radioisotopic and nonradioisotopic procedures are available to measure total blood volume, red cell mass, and plasma volume. Animals with relative polycythemia have decreased blood volumes.

If absolute polycythemia is established, then the primary and secondary forms must be differentiated. Primary polycythemia is sometimes diagnosed once the causes of secondary polycythemia have been eliminated. People with primary polycythemia sometimes have microcytic hypochromic red cells due to the RBC production rate exceeding the rate at which iron is supplied to erythroid marrow. This phenomenon has not been reported in dogs or cats with primary polycythemia. Measurement of arterial blood oxygen tension and serum, plasma, or, less commonly, urinary erythropoietin concentrations can be quite helpful. Better assays for measuring erythropoietin concentrations are becoming available, but few have been evaluated in animals. The exhypoxic polycythemic mouse assay is available through some research laboratories. A patient with polycythemia with undetectable or low concentrations of erythropoietin and normal arterial oxygen tension (depending on the laboratory, about 80 mm Hg and 92% saturation) proves primary polycythemia or polycythemia vera.

Most of the semi- or fully-automated blood-gas analyzers used in clinical laboratories are highly flow rate dependent; excessively viscous samples result in an instrument error. It is often not possible to measure blood gases by conventional means in patients severely affected with polycythemia because of the high blood viscosity.

The leukocytosis, thrombocytosis, and hepatosplenomegaly commonly associated with polycythemia vera in people are rarely seen in animals; hence, the trend in calling the animal disease *erythrocytosis* is justified. In people, a progression from polycythemia vera to other myeloproliferative disorders (*e.g.*, lineage infidelity) may occur, but this progression is unreported in animals. Bone marrow examination is often not helpful since, even if the marrow is hyperplastic, the myeloid to erythroid ratios may be within the normal range. Decreased myeloid to erythroid ratios have been reported in some cases.

Electrocardiography, ultrasonography, and plain and contrast radiography usually identify cardiac or pulmonary problems causing secondary polycythemia. These patients will have decreased arterial oxygen tensions and increased erythropoietin concentrations. Hemoglobin changes associated with chronic exposure to toxic drugs and chemicals are best characterized by measuring the concentrations of methemoglobins, sulfhemoglobins, and carboxyhemoglobins. Hemoglobins with increased oxygen affinity have been described in people; these can be characterized by measuring the oxygen tension at which the hemoglobin is 50% saturated.

Once the hypoxic causes of secondary polycythemia are eliminated, then inappropriate release of erythropoietin is considered. Plain radiography, renal ultrasonography, and intravenous pyelography should be done since the lesions in animals are almost always renal. Rarely, a search for an extrarenal mass may be required. Sophisticated techniques, such as molecular hybridization, are done in a few research laboratories to prove that the neoplasm is actually synthesizing erythropoietin.

Mild polycythemia may be seen with an excess of adrenocortical and thyroidal hormones. Standardized protocols have been established for the assessment of the pituitary-adrenal and pituitary-thyroid axes (see Chapters 59 and 62).

MANAGEMENT

Appropriate fluid therapy resolves relative polycythemia. Treatment of absolute polycythemia usually begins with phlebotomy and fluid replacement to arrest the immediate complications of hyperviscosity. Further therapies for absolute polycythemia depend on the underlying cause. In polycythemia vera, phlebotomy at frequent intervals, aimed at maintaining the PCV in the high normal range, has been used successfully. Approximate guidelines for blood volume taken at phlebotomy in cats and dogs are 10 ml/kg body weight per day and 20 to 30 ml/kg body weight at 2 to 4 day intervals, respectively. At least in dogs, this regime often needs to be repeated at 2- to 3-month intervals.

Iron deficiency may occur because of the high rate of erythropoiesis and chronic phlebotomy treatments. Polycythemic people with iron deficiency are not treated with iron since the iron lack helps to reduce the PCV. Smaller red cells, however, may tend to increase blood viscosity. The problem of increased production of red cells can be attacked directly by using radiophosphorus and chemotherapeutic agents, such as chlorambucil, nitrogen mustard, busulfan, melphalan, or hydroxyurea. Prior to starting cytoreductive treatment, the PCV should be reduced to within the normal range by phlebotomy and fluid or plasma replacement. Hydroxyurea specifically inhibits DNA synthesis and is given at an initial oral rate of 30 mg/kg for 7 to 10 days and is then decreased to 15 mg/kg or lower as a maintenance dosage. Carefully monitored animals with primary polycythemia can survive for at least several years.

With the secondary polycythemias, the lesions (usually cardiac or pulmonary) responsible for the hypoxia may or may not be amenable to treatment. Since the increased PCV is an adaptive mechanism in these cases, phlebotomy is not indicated unless the consequences of hyperviscosity are life threatening. The paraneoplastic syndrome of inappropriate erythropoietin secretion is treated initially by phlebotomy and fluid or plasma replacement, followed by chemotherapy or surgical excision of the tumor. The survival of the animal with secondary polycythemia is dependent on the nature of the underlying cause.

PATIENT MONITORING

The simplest way to monitor patients with polycythemia undergoing phlebotomy or chemotherapeutic treatments is to perform sequential PCV determinations. A trend to increasing PCVs indicates decreasing effectiveness of the therapy or regrowth of a surgically excised tumor. Adjustment of the rate of phlebotomy, chemotherapeutic dosage, or surgery is indicated. When using cytoreductive therapy, CBCs should be done at regular intervals (minimum of once per month) to prevent life threatening thrombocytopenia, leukopenia, or anemia. It is often helpful to have the owners monitor the animal's temperature on a daily basis; an increase in body temperature may signify sepsis as a result of leukopenia.

ADDITIONAL READING

Carothers MA, Couto CG. Erythrocytosis in 7 dogs. In: Proceedings of the Veterinary Cancer Society, Eighth Annual Conference. Estes Park, CO, 1988: 27.

Legendre A, Appleford M. Secondary polycythemia and seizures due to right to left shunting patent ductus arteriosus in a dog. J Am Vet Med Assoc 1974; 164:1198.

McGrath CJ. Polycythemia vera in dogs. J Am Vet Med Assoc 1974; 164:1117.

Peterson ME, Randolph JF. Diagnosis of canine primary polycythemia and management with hydroxyurea. J Am Vet Med Assoc 1982; 180:415.

Peterson ME, Zanjani ED. Inappropriate erythropoietin production from a renal carcinoma in a dog with polycythemia. J Am Vet Med Assoc 1981; 179:995.

Smith M, Turrel JM. Radiophosphorus treatment of bone marrow disorders in dogs: 11 cases (1970–1987). J Am Vet Med Assoc 1989; 194:98.

75

LEUKOCYTOSIS

John H. Lumsden

Leukocytosis is an increase in peripheral blood leukocytes when compared to reference limits established for the species. Leukocytes include granulocytes (neutrophils, eosinophils, and basophils), monocytes, and lymphocytes. All leukocytes participate in body defense with some degree of interaction but, for clinical interpretation, are considered to be kinetically and functionally independent. Leukocytosis may involve an increase in one or more cell types concurrent with a decrease in other cell types. The type and morphology of the predominant cells and the patterns of change often provide significant clinical information.

Leukocytosis is most frequently a benign process secondary to inflammation or physiologic stimuli (*e.g.*, fever, excitement, pain), but it may be primary due to neoplasia of leukocyte cell lines (leukemia). Serial blood samples or bone marrow evaluation may be required to differentiate the primary abnormality.

Hematologic examination contributes to the routine data base for most sick dogs and cats. Changes in numbers and distribution of cell types and their morphology may be used to support or rule out differential diagnoses.

CAUSES

Leukocytosis may occur for many reasons. The predominant cell type contributing to the leukocytosis or the distribution of leukocyte types is correlated with the patient history and clinical signs to indicate the more likely cause. Leukemia of any cell line may produce leukocytosis. Most frequently, leukocytosis is a response to physiologic, corticosteroid, or inflammatory stimuli affecting neutrophils and monocytes.

Neutrophilia may occur due to physiologic influences or the use of drugs, or it may indicate inflammation, infection, tissue damage, or marrow stimuli, such as due to tumor metastasis. Major causes for neutrophilia are listed in Table 75-1.

Eosinophilia is generally associated with parasitic infection or hypersensitivity (Table 75-2). Some of the more common parasites associated with eosinophilia in dogs and cats are Dirofilaria immitis (not Dipetalonema reconditum), paragonimiasis, Strongyloides stercoralis, aelurostrongylosis, ancylostomiasis, Filaroides osleri and Spirocerca lupi. Less frequently, eosinophilia may be expected from infection with de-

Table 75–1 Causes of Neutrophilia

ACUTE NEUTROPHILIA

Physical stimuli
    Exercise, convulsions, heat, cold, surgery, anesthesia, stress
Inflammation or tissue necrosis
    Trauma, burns, infarction, anoxia, acute vasculitis, antigen-antibody reactions, complement
        activation
Infection
    Many localized and systemic bacterial, mycotic, rickettsial, spirochetal and some viral
        infections
Toxins, hormones and drugs
    Endotoxin, venoms, corticosteroids, epinephrine

CHRONIC NEUTROPHILIA

Infections
    Persistence of infections that cause acute neutrophilia
Inflammation
    Continuation of acute inflammatory reactions such as myositis, pancreatitis, dermatitis,
        rheumatoid arthritis
Toxins, hormones and drugs
    Chronic exposure to substances which cause acute neutrophilia, such as endotoxins or
        glucocorticoids. The effects tend to become modulated with time (e.g., acetaminophen
        toxicity, corticosteroids)
Tumors
    Various tumors especially carcinomas, less likely diseases; in some, tissue necrosis may be a
        factor
Hematologic disorders
    Response to hemolysis and hemorrhage, myeloproliferative disorders, idiopathic leukemoid
        response

---

modecosis, fleas, ascariasis, and coccidiosis. Hypersensitivity-induced eosinophilia may be expected with flea allergy and eosinophilic pneumonitis but is unpredictable with canine eosinophilic gastroenteritis, pneumonitis, panosteitis, and canine and feline granuloma complex. Eosinophilia, and possibly lymphocytosis, may accompany hypoadrenocorticism and is frequently observed with mast cell tumor in dogs.

Basophilia occurs with many allergic and inflammatory diseases, including parasites (*e.g.*, *Dirofilaria immitis*), and with food or drug related hypersensitivities and may occur with alterations in lipid metabolism (*e.g.*, hypothyroidism, hyperadrenocorticism, nephrotic syndrome; Table 75-3). Basophilia is usually present in association with eosinophilia. Basophilia has been noted with megakaryocytic leukemia.

Monocytosis is primarily associated with chronic inflammation but does occur with acute and chronic diseases (*e.g.*, bacteremia, bacterial endocarditis, nocardiosis, hepatozoonosis). Table 75-4 lists causes of monocytosis. In the dog, exogenous and endogenous corticosteroids will in-crease the numbers of circulating monocytes, at least for a few days, but this response is variable in the cat. Monocytosis occurs in cats with hemobartonellosis. Absolute numbers of circulating monocytes, as with most leukocyte types, appear to have better correlation with clinical syndromes than percentage.

Lymphocyte counts are higher in young ani-

Table 75–2 Causes of Eosinophilia

HYPERSENSITIVITIES

Eosinophilic pneumonitis, flea allergy
Variable: canine eosinophilic gastroenteritis, myositis and panosteitis, canine and feline granuloma complex, atopy

PARASITISMS

Anclyostomiasis, dirofilariasis, paragonimiasis, strongyloidosis, *Spirocerca lupi, Filaroides osleri*
Variable: coccidiosis, demodicosis, ascariasis, fleas, trichuriasis

OTHER

Estrus, neoplasia including mast cell tumor and eosinophilic leukemia

---

Table 75–3 *Causes of Basophilia*

HYPERSENSITIVITIES
IgE mediated, immediate and delayed type parasitemia, food and drugs in association with eosinophilia

CHRONIC INFLAMMATION
Variable

HEMATOLOGIC DISORDERS
In association with eosinophilia

LIPEMIA
Altered lipid metabolism
Hyperadrenocorticism
Hyperthyroidism

NEOPLASIA
Mast cell tumor
Basophilic leukemia

Table 75–5 *Causes of Lymphocytosis*

PHYSIOLOGIC
Higher in young animals
Excitement, stress especially in cats

CHRONIC INFLAMMATION
After vaccination
Rocky Mountain spotted fever in the dog

NEOPLASIA
Lymphocytic leukemia

---

mals. Counts may increase during acute stress due to the effects of epinephrine, particularly in the cat. Chronic stress induces an increase in endogenous corticosteroid production, which reduces lymphocyte counts owing in part to lympholysis. Persistent lymphocytosis has been reported with certain chronic infections, such as Rocky Mountain spotted fever. Chronic antigenic stimulation frequently induces lymphadenopathy but infrequently lymphocytosis. Post-vaccinal lymphocytosis is often accompanied by increased cytoplasmic basophilia in circulating lymphocytes, indicating increased immunoglobulin production or preparation for cell division (Table 75-5).

Table 75–4 *Causes of Monocytosis*

PHYSICAL STIMULI
Pain, stress

INFLAMMATION OR TISSUE NECROSIS
Including immune-mediated diseases

CHRONIC INFECTION
Persistence of many infections that cause neutrophilia

HORMONES AND DRUGS
ACTH, corticosteroids

HEMOLYTIC DISORDERS
Response to hemolysis and hemorrhage, monocytic and myelomonocytic leukemia, persistent neutropenia

PATHOPHYSIOLOGY

Leukocytes, except for lymphocytes, are produced by hematopoietic stem cell division within the special microenvironment of bone marrow. Lymphocytes are produced in lymphoid tissue, although B lymphocytes are originally of bone marrow derivation. Colony stimulating factors initiate division and differentiation of pluripotential stem cells into committed myeloid or lymphoid stem cells (Fig. 75-1). Further differentiation and division of committed stem cells (mitotic pool) leads to a maturing population of leukocytes (maturation pool). Segmented and band neutrophils (storage pool) are released into the peripheral circulation on demand. The storage pool is considered to contain about three times as many neutrophils as the peripheral circulation contains, or about a 5-day supply. Neutrophils have a half-life of 6 to 10 hours in the circulation. The tissue half-life is unknown but is considered to be about 3 days.

The degree of leukocytosis must be considered when clinical significance is being evaluated. For practical reasons, the reference values provided in *Schalm's Veterinary Hematology* will be referred to in this section (Table 75-6). The range of leukocytes observed in most healthy adult dogs and cats is 6 to 17 $\times$ 10^9/L ($\times$ 10^3/μL) and 5.5 to 19.5 $\times$ 10^9/L ($\times$ 10^3/μL), respectively.

The pathophysiology associated with increases in individual leukocyte types is reviewed briefly, and some of the more common patterns of change are described. Qualitative abnormalities are presented for neutrophils. The major types of leukemia are outlined.

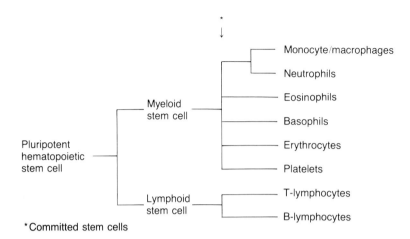

Figure 75–1. Simplified schematic diagram of relationship between differentiating hematopoietic, myeloid, and lymphoid cells.

Neutrophilia

Neutrophils are the predominate leukocyte in the peripheral blood of healthy dogs and cats. Leukocytosis usually implies neutrophilia. Neutrophilia is defined as a blood neutrophil count greater than 11.5 or 12.5 × 10⁹/L (× 10³/μL) for adult dogs and cats, respectively (see Table 75-6). Neutrophilic leukocytosis and polymorphonuclear leukocytosis are used interchangeably with neutrophilia. Granulocytosis refers to an increase in neutrophils, eosinophils, or basophils, although it has been used synonymously with neutrophilia.

Leukemoid reactions refer to a marked increase in leukocytes, for example three to four times the upper reference limit. The leukocytes are primarily neutrophils and monocytes, but the initial appearance can resemble leukemia, which may accompany hemolytic anemia in the dog. Careful peripheral blood and bone marrow examination may be required in context of the clinical picture to differentiate the leukocyte reaction.

Three major mechanisms are responsible, alone or in combination, for most neutrophilic reactions: (1) Increased numbers of mature neutrophils may be mobilized from the marginal pool or released from the bone marrow stores into the circulating pool; (2) Increased blood neutrophil survival may occur owing to release of increased numbers of immature neutrophils or decreased outflow into the tissues; and (3) In-

Table 75–6 Blood Leukocyte Reference Values for the Dog and Cat

	Dog		Cat	
	Limits	Average	Limits	Average
	×10⁹/L		×10⁹/L	
Leukocytes	6 to 17	11.5	5.5 to 19.5	12.5
Neutrophils (band)	0 to 3	0.07	0 to 3	0.1
Neutrophils (mature)	3 to 11.5	7	2.5 to 12.5	7.5
Lymphocyte	1 to 4.8	2.8	1.5 to 7	4
Monocyte	0.15 to 1.35	0.75	0 to 0.85	0.35
Eosinophil	0 to 1.25	0.55	0 to 1.5	0.65
Basophil	Rare	0	Rare	0

Modified from Jain NC. ed. Schalm's veterinary hematology, 4th ed. Philadelphia: Lea and Febiger, 1986.

creased production of neutrophils in the marrow may occur owing to increased differentiation of precursor cells into the neutrophil series, increased stimulation of precursor cells in the mitotic pool, or shortening of the cell mitotic cycle of the proliferating cells. Various causes of acute and chronic forms of neutrophilia are listed in Table 75-1. The marginal pool, that is, the neutrophils that are marginated against the walls of the peripheral blood vessels and not sampled during venipuncture, contain approximately an equal number of neutrophils as the circulating pool.

Acute neutrophilia can develop within minutes and last for minutes to hours or may develop more slowly and last for hours to days, depending on the cause. The increase is almost always due to mobilization of neutrophils from the marginal pool or the marrow storage pool. Acute neutrophilia is usually associated with sudden excitement, pain, exercise, temperature change, or the administration of drugs or biologicals. It is usually due to the mobilization of the marginal neutrophil pool in association with increased blood flow or stimulation of β receptors regulating small vessel blood flow. The exact mechanism is still controversial. When exercise or epinephrine induce neutrophilia, the response is usually of short duration (20–30 minutes).

A more delayed type of acute neutrophilia developing over 4 to 24 hours is recognized. This type of response can be elicited by glucocorticoids, acute anoxia, inflammation, bacterial, and parasitic infections, antigen-antibody complexes, and complement activation. The neutrophils are released from the marrow storage into the circulating pool in response to neutrophil releasing factors, such as interleukin-1, and tissue necrosis factor. The delay in neutrophilia has been suggested to be due to margination of many of the initially released neutrophils. Administration of glucocorticoids will increase the neutrophil half-life in the circulating pool by slowing the random emigration of circulating neutrophils into the tissues. Glucocorticoids also increase the rate of release of neutrophils from the marrow storage pool. A left shift (the release of immature neutrophils into the peripheral circulation) is not expected following glucocorticoid administration as long as adequate stores of segmented neu-

trophils are available. In contrast, when a hemolytic or inflammatory process accompanies corticosteroid administration, a left shift may follow.

Acute anoxia, inflammation, and bacterial or parasitic infection may initiate prompt release of immature neutrophils into the circulation. When marked immaturity of neutrophils, that is, circulating band, metamyelocyte, and earlier forms, is found without an increase in total neutrophil count, the term *degenerative left shift* has been used. This observation may suggest the presence of an overwhelming septicemia or toxemia. Interpretation should be made in association with the clinical information and following sequential blood examinations, as the marked immaturity and decreased total neutrophil count may be transient. Anesthetic agents and surgery may precede the development of neutrophilia that lasts several days. Complement activation and immunologic hypersensitivity may be factors initiating neutrophilia.

Chronic neutrophilia is usually the consequence of continued stimulation of neutrophil release, resulting in greater feedback to the marrow, which increases colony stimulating factor and neutrophil production. Continued stimulation over days to weeks will result in a marked increase in neutrophil availability. The degree of left shift depends on the strength of the stimulus and the availability of mature neutrophils in the marrow storage pool.

Bacterial infection is a very common cause of chronic neutrophilia. Endotoxemia, complement activation, or other products of inflammation may induce a temporary neutropenia, followed by a neutrophilia with or without an initial left shift. The leukocyte response to chronic infection is extremely variable. The type and virulence of the organism, location of the infection, resistance of the animal to infection, and the capacity of the host to respond influence the degree of leukocyte response. For example, moderate to marked leukocytosis occurs in response to pneumonia, endocarditis, cellulitis, and closed pyometra. In contrast, minimal leukocytosis or even leukopenia may occur with open pyometra, and enteritis due to neutrophil loss concomitant with endotoxin absorption, depending on bacteria involved.

Mild to moderate leukocytosis may occur in some systemic mycotic and protozoal infections and in the early phase of some viral infections.

Chronic stimulation of the marrow in response to hemolysis or hemorrhage may result in leukocytosis, which is primarily neutrophilic and may be accompanied by release of immature neutrophils (a left shift). Following induced neutropenia due to endotoxemia (which may be associated with leukopenia or agranulocytosis), a rebound period may occur when the leukocyte count significantly increases. The leukocytosis may last 1 to 3 weeks before feedback mechanisms allow complete recovery to normal homeostasis.

Nonbacterial chronic inflammation can be responsible for persistent neutrophilic leukocytosis. Disorders that induce tissue damage, such as hepatic necrosis and cutaneous inflammation, and reactions due to certain drugs or chemicals may be associated with neutrophilic leukocytosis.

Leukocytosis frequently occurs when tumors are widespread and necrotic. When anemia and thrombocytopenia are present and release of early erythroid and myeloid cells from the marrow occurs, differentiation from leukemia may be difficult. This condition has been called a *leukoerythroblastic reaction.*

Continued administration of low to medium dosages of glucocorticoids (1–2 mg/kg per day of prednisone) results in neutrophilic leukocytosis peaking in many dogs at about 2 weeks. In many of these animals, with continued administration, the cell numbers gradually return to premedication counts. Lithium salt administration in humans will produce an increase in the neutrophil count of 3 to 5 $\times$ 10^9/L ($\times$ 10^3/μL). The increased granulocytopoiesis is associated with an increased colony-stimulating activity that persists while the drug is administered. A similar response appears to occur in some dogs.

Qualitative Abnormalities of Neutrophils

Qualitative abnormalities of neutrophils have been extensively studied in humans. Although they have been observed in dogs and cats, only a few have been studied in detail. Chemotaxis and phagocytosis are functions required by neutrophils to perform their key role of protecting the host against infection. With structural or biochemical deficiency of any aspect of these functions comes increased risk for infection. Neutrophil function relies on plasma factors, such as complement, to provide stimuli for adherence, chemotaxis and degranulation, and antibodies to opsonize microorganisms.

The Chédiak-Higashi syndrome is a lethal autosomal recessive disease in humans, which has been discovered in cats, mink, cattle, mice, and killer whales. A defective degranulation of abnormal neutrophil granules results in increased susceptibility to infection. The cellular dysfunction is generalized and not restricted to leukocytes. Giant cytoplasmic granules can be seen in the cytoplasm of neutrophils, monocytes, and eosinophils of affected individuals, and in cats the eosinophil granules may be round instead of elongated. Albinism occurs in this defect due to pathologic aggregation of melanosomes. Neutropenia, thrombocytopenia, deficiency of lymphocyte natural-killer cells, recurrent unexplained fever, and peripheral neuropathy are other features of the disease in humans. Three Persian cats with the combination of yellow eye color and "blue smoke" hair color in a single line of Persian cats have been studied. Enlarged granules were found in neutrophils, eosinophils, basophils, and melanocytes. A bleeding tendency was observed, but no increased susceptibility to infection was seen.

Mucopolysaccharidosis (Alder-Reilly anomaly) is an autosomal recessive trait in which coarse intensely stained azurophilic granules may be seen in mature neutrophils, other leukocytes, and marrow reticulum cells. Due to an enzyme deficiency, an abnormal mucopolysaccharide catabolism affects the function of many cells. Six genetic forms of mucopolysaccharidosis (MPS) have been described in humans. Two genetic forms have been described in domestic cats with central nervous system abnormalities, corneal clouding, or skeletal deformities. Mucopolysaccharidosis I (MPS I), due to a deficiency of α-L-iduronidase, is described in domestic short haired cats, while MPS VI, associated with a deficiency of arylsulfatase B activity, is observed in

Siamese cats. Ultrastructural study is required to demonstrate the granules for MPS I deficiency. With MPS VI, the granules may be seen in neutrophils with Wright's stain and differentiated from primary granules with toluidine stain. A toluidine blue (Berry) spot test can be used to detect excessive urine glycosaminoglycans. Three dachshund puppies have been reported with abnormal granulation in leukocytes.

Pelger-Huët anomaly is a benign, hereditary trait characterized by a decreased number of nuclear segments of granulocytes and cells of the bone marrow (megakaryocytes) and a coarseness of nuclear chromatin of monocytes and lymphocytes. In humans, the cells have only minor alterations in function. The anomaly has been reported in dogs as a hereditary or acquired defect. Impaired neutrophil mobilization into skin and antibody response has been reported in foxhounds. The anomaly has been reported in cats where it may be a lethal trait. A pseudo–Pelger-Huët anomaly has been reported to occur in myeloproliferative disorders and with severe infections and malignancies in humans and dogs. Differentiation of this anomaly from a true left shift should be recognized.

Cyclic hematopoiesis is an autosomal recessive semi-lethal disorder, which has been well characterized in silver-gray collie dogs and compared to a similar condition in humans. Many pups are born weak and succumb to infections associated with neutropenia early in life. A cyclic maturation arrest occurs at the pluripotential stem cell level that affects all blood cell lines but is more apparent in the neutrophil series, presumably because of the shorter neutrophil half-life. Bone marrow transplantation following whole body irradiation has been successful in correcting the cyclic defect. Cyclic changes in the formation of neutrophils, platelets, and reticulocytes have been eliminated by daily administration of endotoxin over several weeks and by treatment with lithium carbonate (20–25 mg/kg per day, orally). Cyclic hematopoiesis has been reported in association with feline leukemia virus infection.

A granulocytopathy syndrome has been described in Irish setters and defective neutrophil function reported in eight closely related Doberman pinscher dogs.

Eosinophilia

Eosinophils appear to be important in controlling infection with parasites that have prolonged host-tissue interaction, and in playing an active role in regulating allergic and inflammatory reactions. Eosinophils are attracted chemotactically to sites of excess histamine release from activated mast cells. However, experimental data have suggested that eosinophils may initiate inflammation by contributing to histamine release and the degradation of platelet lytic factor.

An increase in blood eosinophils in conjunction with a neutrophilic left shift is often an unfavorable sign. These changes may be an indication that the marrow is severely stressed and unable to meet demands in a normal fashion.

The eosinophil is produced in the bone marrow from a precursor cell, which appears to antedate the myeloblast. A low molecular weight protein has been identified with eosinophilopoietin properties. Studies suggest this protein may be of T lymphocyte or of monocyte origin. Less than 1% of the total body eosinophils are present in the blood. Most are in the bone marrow and tissues of the skin, lung, and gastrointestinal tract. In the dog, the circulating half-life of the eosinophil is approximately 30 minutes compared to 4 to 10 hours for the neutrophil. Eosinophil granules vary in size in the dog. In the adult greyhound, more vacuoles than granules may be visible.

Eosinophils have four types of granules, which contain several enzymes and proteins. The major basic protein present in the specific granules neutralizes heparin, induces noncytotoxic mast cell and basophil degranulation, and is cytotoxic for helminths. Eosinophil-derived histaminase inactivates histamine from mast cells. The reappearance of eosinophils into the blood of a sick dog or cat is often a favorable sign, especially when supported by improvements in the clinical appearance of the patient.

Basophilia

The presence of more than a few basophils on a blood smear warrants consideration for possible cause. Basophilia occurs most frequently in association with eosinophilia when due to an IgE related hypersensitivity response.

The cytoplasmic granules of canine basophils contain glycosaminoglycans, which stain metachromatically with basic dyes, such as Wright's stain, and are readily visible as reddish purple granules. The granules may be difficult to detect in feline basophils. Basophil granules do not stain well with water soluble stains, such as new methylene blue.

The role of the basophil is not well defined but is considered to perform functions similar to mast cells. The basophil cytoplasmic granules contain histamine, heparin, chondroitin sulfates, and several other substances that are important mediators of inflammation. Basophils degranulate within minutes in immediate hypersensitivity reactions. They enter the tissues and make a significant contribution to delayed hypersensitivity reactions in some species. The role of the mast cell is increasingly associated with the nervous system in the functional response of many organ systems, especially the intestinal mucosa. The response of the basophil to nervous system stimulation has not been defined.

Heparin from basophil granules may activate lipoprotein lipase of endothelial cell origin. The lipoprotein lipase cleaves circulating lipids, contributing to their removal from the plasma. Corticosteroid administration results in a marked decrease in basophils within hours, but unexplainable basophilia has been reported in some dogs with adrenocortical hyperfunction. Hormones, such as estrogen, produce basophilia, while progesterone and thyrotropin produce a basopenia experimentally.

Both basophils and mast cells originate from bone marrow precursor cells. Basophils differentiate in the marrow prior to release, whereas mast cells multiply in tissues.

Monocytosis

Monocytes are large leukocytes with a blue-gray cytoplasm that may contain a few small vacuoles and even dust-like azurophilic granules. The nucleus is variable in shape and can resemble the nucleus of immature granulocytes, especially band neutrophils in the dog. Cytoplasmic basophilia and vacuolation usually allows ready differentiation unless a severe immaturity of the neutrophils with basophilia and toxic vacuolation is present. Monocytes may be confused with some large lymphocytes, especially when lymphoid leukemia is present.

Monocytes are produced in the bone marrow from monoblasts and differentiate into promonocytes, which divide once or twice varying with the species. Monocytes are released within several hours of stimulation and circulate to enter tissues and cavities to supply free and fixed tissue macrophages. The marrow storage pool is not significant in most species studied. Some species appear to have a marginal pool, but it has not been reported for the dog and cat. The circulating time in the peripheral circulation varies with the species and ranges from a half-life of 8.5 hours in humans to 2 days in the rat. The monocyte and macrophage are closely related in function. The mononuclear phagocyte system includes both monocytes and macrophages. This system has many important functions. One of the earlier functions recognized was phagocytosis and microbicidal action against intracellular bacteria, viruses, protozoa, and fungi. The system interacts closely with both the afferent and efferent limbs of the immune response, is closely involved with regulation of hematopoiesis and inflammation, is the source of several factors or activators required for coagulation, is a scavenger system for cells and debris, and contributes to a cytotoxic effect against tumor cells.

Lymphocytosis

The reference values for young healthy animals is higher than for adults. The number of circulating lymphocytes is not a good indication of total body lymphocytes or the rate of production, as lymphocytes recirculate from lymphatic vessels and lymphoid tissues into the peripheral blood. The lymphocytosis observed in physiologic leukocytosis is considered to be epinephrine related. Lymphocytosis may be present with certain infections, especially viral, but the number present has limited clinical significance. An increase in lymphocyte cytoplasmic basophilia suggests increased antigenic stimulation with immunologic response, as is observed with post-vaccinal lymphocytosis.

Lymphocytes are produced in bone marrow and populate the lymphoid tissue throughout the body. Three major types with several subtypes are currently recognized using special techniques: bone marrow derived (B lymphocytes), thymus-dependent (T lymphocytes) and non-T, non-B, or *null* lymphocytes. In most species, T lymphocytes predominate in the peripheral blood (up to 80% of the circulating lymphocytes), thymus, lymph nodes, and thoracic lymphatics. B lymphocytes predominate in the bone marrow and spleen and make up as high as 20% of the circulating lymphocyte population. A small number of lymphocytes are identified as null cells. The relative numbers of lymphocytes change during disease, but the techniques used for identification usually are available only in research laboratories. Surface membrane antigens, surface receptors, surface or cytoplasmic immunoglobulins, and cytochemistry staining reactions are used for classification.

T cell function is complex and involves cellular immunity and immunoregulation, whereas B cell function is most closely associated with antibody production.

Leukemia

Leukemia is a malignant disease of a hematopoietic cell line in which leukocytosis is frequently, but not always, present. Diagnosis is made by observing abnormal cells in the blood or bone marrow. Leukemia is divided into myeloproliferative and lymphoproliferative disorders. Leukemia of nonlymphoid hematopoietic origin cells is called myeloproliferative disease. Leukemia of the lymphoid cell line is lymphoproliferative disease. The adjusted annual incidence rate for all leukemias per 100,000 dogs and cats has been reported as 30.5 and 224.3, respectively, with cats having 6.1 times more lymphoma and 15.7 times more myeloproliferative disorders than dogs.

Leukemias are classified in many ways; each approach has been used in an attempt to find a relationship between clinical progression and prognosis or response to therapy. One of the more useful classifications is based on maturity of the cells. If all the cells are well differentiated, such as mature neutrophils or eosinophils, the leukemia is classified as chronic. If immature or poorly differentiated (blast) cells are present in peripheral blood or increased numbers present in marrow, the leukemia is acute. Acute leukemia tends to present with sudden onset and has a shorter clinical course. This presentation is the more common one in dogs and cats. In chronic leukemia, the affected cells are well differentiated and usually markedly increased in number. The criteria used to categorize acute and chronic leukemias in human medicine can be applied to typical cases of leukemia in dogs and cats; however, for many cases, the classification is rather arbitrary because precise criteria have not been established for each species. Cytochemistry stains and electron microscopy studies are used to classify some poorly differentiated leukemias. Classification of poorly differentiated (acute) leukemia is warranted when specific guidance for therapy and prognosis are available.

The presenting clinical signs for dogs and cats with leukemia vary considerably. Weight loss and progressive weakness are common complaints, but many animals may present with sudden onset of anorexia, vomiting, diarrhea, polyuria, and anemia. Lymphadenopathy, splenomegaly, and hepatomegaly may be present. The predominant clinical signs vary with the species and the organ system affected. Initial hematologic examination may reveal the nature of the disease, but, in many cases, serial blood examinations with bone marrow and lymph node aspiration or core biopsy are required. Cytologic and histologic examination, including cytochemistry, immunochemistry, and electron microscopy studies of bone marrow, lymph node, and sometimes spleen and liver, are used to define the extent of the disease process for evaluation of therapeutic trials.

Animals may present with various hematologic changes that may not be readily diagnosed. With the development of recognizable leukemia, the changes can be classified retrospectively as due to preleukemia. Further details regarding diagnosis, prognosis, and therapy of leukemia in the dog and cat are available (Jain; Latimer and Meyer; Theilen and Madewell, Additional Reading).

Myeloproliferative Disorders

Myeloproliferative disorders can involve any of the nonlymphoid hematopoietic cell lines and may be acute or chronic. Chronic myeloproliferative disorders can revert to acute leukemia. A greater variety of myeloproliferative disorders are observed in the cat than the dog. Until proven otherwise, most myeloproliferative and lymphoproliferative disorders in the cat are considered to be feline leukemia related. The role of feline immunodeficiency virus is unproven at this time.

Granulocytic leukemia usually refers to the neutrophil cell line as distinct from the eosinophil and basophil, which are also granulocytes. Peripheral blood neutrophil counts are often very high. Granulocytic leukemia may not be readily diagnosed if the neutrophilia is not accompanied by early stages such as promyelocytes or myeloblasts. Even with a count of 50 × 10⁹/L (× 10³/μL), if all the neutrophils are of the band or segmented forms, differentiation from the leukemoid response may be difficult. Close examination of the patient should be made for a source of inflammation. Serial blood samples should be examined. Careful examination of more than one blood smear or even a buffy coat preparation should be made for the presence of precursor cells to confirm that leukemia rather than a chronic inflammatory response is responsible for the neutrophilia. If precursor cells predominate without distinct differentiation, special stains may or may not be helpful in differentiating monocytic, lymphocytic, and neutrophilic blast cells. In some cases, normal appearing mature neutrophils are accompanied by an asynchronous population of less differentiated neoplastic cells (leukemic hiatus). Bone marrow aspiration and core samples may assist in differentiation (see Bone Marrow Aspiration and Biopsy in Chapter 80).

In the cat, differentiation of granulocytic leukemia from the leukemoid response must also be considered. Granulocytic leukemia may occur after erythremic myelosis and erythroleukemia

(lineage infidelity). The leukemic neutrophils are generally adequately differentiated for classification into the granulocytic series. A form of preleukemia, which may progress to granulocytic leukemia, is recognized in the cat and also has been reported in the dog. Initially, persistent neutropenia is present. Only a few immature neutrophils may be present in the peripheral blood but usually a greater number is found in the bone marrow, along with evidence of marrow granulocytic hyperplasia and nonregenerative anemia. Subleukemic granulocytic leukemia (low to normal leukocyte count but circulating precursor cells) can be confused with systemic toxemia when leukopenia and marked immaturity are present. Careful examination of the bone marrow may be required for differentiation.

Marked nonregenerative anemia along with thrombocytopenia are common presenting observations in both dogs and cats with granulocytic leukemia. The bone marrow has marked granulocytic hyperplasia with immaturity and often decreased megakaryocytes and erythroid precursors.

Eosinophilic leukemia has been reported for several cats but is rare in the dog. All cats tested have been feline leukemia virus negative.

Basophil leukemia is rare in the dog and cat. Increased numbers of basophils in bone marrow smears support the diagnosis. Mast cell leukemia can be confused with basophilic leukemia. Basophils have segmented nuclei. Mast cells have round nuclei and larger basophilic intracytoplasmic granules that can obscure the nucleus. Mast cell leukemia is a frequent manifestation of mastocytoma. Examination of buffy coat smears is warranted if mastocytoma is suspected.

Monocytic leukemia has been documented for dogs and cats. Increased numbers of mature and immature monocytes in peripheral blood and bone marrow should initiate consideration of monocytic leukemia when no other apparent cause for chronic inflammation is found. Cytochemistry stains are frequently required to differentiate monocyte, neutrophil, and lymphocyte precursors. Monocytic leukemia may progress to myelomonocytic leukemia in which both immature monocytes and neutrophils are present. Anemia may be mild to severe, and thrombocytopenia may be present. Erythremic myelosis is a myeloproliferative disorder reported in feline leukemia positive cats. The disease is characterized by a severe anemia without polychromasia in the presence of either a few erythrocytes with asynchronous nuclear and cytoplasmic maturation or a marked increase in late and early stage erythroid precursor cells in peripheral blood and marrow smears without the normal maturation sequence. Megaloblastoid erythrocytes may be present. When only blast forms of the cells appear, the disorder has been called *reticuloendotheliosis*. Serial examination of several cats has demonstrated the progression of erythremic myelosis to erythroleukemia and granulocytic leukemia. Erythroleukemia is considered to be a transitory stage between erythremic myelosis and granulocytic leukemia when precursor cells of both erythroid and myeloblast morphology are present in the blood.

Megakaryocytic leukemia is rare but has been reported in dogs and cats. In dogs, anemia, thrombocytopenia, and blasts cells were observed in blood smears, and blast cells and increased numbers of megakaryocytes were found in bone marrow and various organs. Basophilia has been observed in dogs. In cats, severe nonregenerative anemia with bizarre appearing platelets in peripheral blood and increased numbers of megakaryocytes in the bone marrow, spleen, and liver has been observed.

Lymphoproliferative Disorders

Lymphoproliferative disorders include all the neoplastic diseases of lymphocytes and plasma cells. Leukocytosis may be a feature of this disorder. Many schemes are used for classification based on either anatomic distribution, histologic architecture of affected lymph nodes, or cytology of neoplastic cells. Classification schemes are useful if they assist diagnosis or if they can be related to the expected clinical course, likely prognosis, or response to therapy. Classification schemes adopted in human medicine have been applied to animals with some success. Staging of the disease is used in dogs to direct therapy and to estimate prognosis. Lymphosarcoma is a commonly applied general term that can be used to include those cases where sarcomatous masses are present in lymphoid tissue (also called lymphoma), or where neoplastic lymphocytes are present in the peripheral blood and bone marrow (lymphocytic leukemia). Either form may develop independently or a progression from one to both disorders in the same animal may appear (see Chapter 15).

Lymphosarcoma is the most common form of the leukemia complex in the dog (24 of 100,000 dogs annually in one study, or 5%–7% of all dogs with cancer) with lymphocytic leukemia occurring less frequently. Multicentric, alimentary, thymic, skin, and leukemic forms are found in dogs. Clinical signs often relate to the anatomic involvement. Dysproteinemias (abnormal protein production as determined using electrophoresis or immunoelectrophoresis of serum or urine) occur when B lymphocytes and plasma cells are the primary neoplastic population of cells. Leukemia is present in about 50% of dogs on initial examination with an increased incidence in advanced disease. There may be leukocytosis with a high percentage of lymphocytes (well or poorly differentiated), or there may be normal to low leukocyte counts where leukemia is identified by the presence of a population of less differentiated or abnormal appearing lymphocytes in blood or bone marrow. Lymphadenopathy occurs more frequently in dogs than in cats with lymphosarcoma. Mild nonregenerative anemia and thrombocytopenia are common, especially when bone marrow is involved. A leukemoid blood picture due to granulocytosis may confuse interpretation in some cases. Hypercalcemia of malignancy has been reported to occur in one third of dogs with mediastinal lymphosarcoma.

In cats, lymphosarcoma and lymphocytic leukemia together account for 80% to 90% of all hematopoietic neoplasms. About 70% of cats with lymphosarcoma are feline leukemia test result positive. Those that are negative frequently are over 7 years of age and have the alimentary or unclassified type. Leukemia, usually involving B lymphocytes, is present in about 30% of cats with lymphosarcoma. More cats with lymphoproliferative disorders have leukopenia or normal leukocyte counts than have leukocytosis. Nonregenerative anemia is often present and is associated with feline leukemia virus infection or bone marrow myelophthisis. Bone marrow examination is warranted to confirm leukemia in some cases and to assist identification of the primary cell line, to determine the extent of marrow involvement, or to investigate leukopenia, anemia, or thrombocytopenia.

DIAGNOSTIC APPROACH

Leukocytosis is an indication of altered homeostasis and possibly a disease process that requires identification. The pattern of response can often be used with other clinical information pertaining to a case to rule-in or rule-out differential diagnoses. Some leukemias may be readily identified by blood examination alone but many require further evaluation before a diagnosis can be confirmed.

Initial or complete hematologic examination can be done in-clinic or at a referral laboratory. Peripheral blood is collected in EDTA anticoagulant. For optimum cell morphology, blood smears should be made when blood is collected from the animal. Each hour that blood cells are in anticoagulant prior to preparation of blood smears increases the degree of in vitro changes in morphology. Since many of these in vitro changes are similar to those used by hematologists to estimate the likely in vivo influences, interpretation may be misleading. The stained blood smear is examined for platelet numbers and morphology, red cell morphology, and leukocyte types and morphology. The percentage times the total count is used to calculate the absolute numbers of each major leukocyte type. Extra unstained labelled slides should be prepared if consultation is anticipated for difficult cases. The clinician should determine that the techniques used are appropriate for the species, quality control is maintained, and that appropriate reference values are available for the techniques used.

Interpretation of leukocytosis requires correlation with history, clinical signs, and problems identified by the clinician. If neutrophilia is present, one should relate a left shift and degenerative changes, such as increased cytoplasmic basophilia, granulation, vacuolation, or Döhle's bodies, to possible systemic toxicity. Marked degenerative changes in neutrophils of a blood slide prepared immediately after collection are often due to bacterial infection. The patient should be reexamined, if not originally noted, for supporting clinical information, such as pyrexia and localizing signs, for a particular organ system or location. If the patient was excited, chronically stressed, or had been given steroids, leukocytosis due primarily to neutrophilia can be expected. The pattern of neutrophilia, monocytosis, eosinopenia, and lymphopenia typical of steroid administration is frequently present but can be variable.

Eosinophilia requires consideration of parasitemia or a hyperimmune response. Heartworm disease tests should be done and the animal evaluated for flea allergy and insect bites. Reference values must be adjusted for the geographic area and season. Because of the decreased steroid effect, eosinophilia is often present in adrenocortical insufficiency. The return of eosinophils and increasing numbers of segmented neutrophils to the peripheral blood of a seriously ill patient has been considered to be a favorable prognostic sign. Basophilia in the dog and cat is unusual and should initiate consideration of a hyperimmune response. If eosinophilia does not accompany the basophilia, consider disorders associated with altered lipoprotein metabolism, such as endocrine disease, nephrotic syndrome, and chronic liver disease.

Monocytosis is usually associated with some degree of neutrophilia. Monocytosis can occur with both acute and chronic disorders. If endogenous or exogenous steroid effects are ruled out, inflammatory response associated with tissue necrosis, suppuration, hemolysis, hemorrhage, malignancy, and some pyogranulomatous diseases must be considered.

Lymphocytosis is more often due to changes in lymphocyte circulation rather than production rate. Reactive lymphocytosis or plasmacytosis is associated with some viral infections or vaccinations (*e.g.*, canine distemper and hepatitis vaccine). The primary challenge to the hematologist or clinician is differentiation of benign from neoplastic lymphocytosis. Morphology is frequently more important than numbers in the peripheral blood. Bone marrow and lymph node aspiration or core biopsy are required for confirmation of many cases with suspect lymphoproliferative disease. The approach to classification of lymphocytic leukemia or lymphosarcoma should be determined by the clinician or oncologist in association with the pathologist or hematologist. The reader is referred to the Additional Reading section for more details regarding diagnosis, classification, therapy, and prognosis.

Leukemia is readily apparent from peripheral blood examination in a minority of cases. These are more often chronic leukemia in which well-differentiated cells, more often neutrophils, lymphocytes, or eosinophils, are present in excessive numbers or acute leukemia in which significant numbers of less differentiated cells are present. In acute leukemia, cell numbers may or may not be increased. Careful examination of blood smears may be required to detect abnormal, immature, or an asynchronous population of cells. Bone marrow aspiration and core biopsy examination will more frequently confirm the presence of acute leukemia. Lymph node, liver (see Liver Biopsy in Chapter 80) and spleen biopsies contribute to the diagnosis of lymphosarcoma associated with lymphocytic leukemia. Cytochemistry and immunocytochemistry stains and ultrastructural study are used in an attempt to identify poorly differentiated myeloproliferative and lymphoproliferative leukemias.

MANAGEMENT

Leukocytosis is an indicator of altered homeostasis and not a disease requiring treatment unless due to leukemia. Correlating the degree and pattern of leukocytosis with the history, clinical signs, and drug administration leads to interpretation of the cause of leukocytosis for most cases. Medication history should be reviewed. If physiologic reasons are suspect, leukocyte counts decrease to within reference limits in a few hours to days. Physical examination of the patient for localizing signs of inflammation, especially monitoring temperature, urine sediment, and cavity fluids, assists detection of many inflammatory or infectious causes. Examination of plasma, serum, and urine for hemoglobin or bilirubin pigment and peripheral blood smears

for evidence of increased erythroid response or erythrocyte agglutination may indicate a hemolytic or hemorrhagic etiology. Many metabolic diseases can be detected with routine serum and urine clinical chemistry tests. Testing for aberrant antibodies may indicate systemic immune-mediated disease.

If the cause of the leukocytosis is not readily apparent, further evaluation of the patient is warranted, especially when differentiating a leukemoid reaction from leukemia. Serial blood sampling and bone marrow biopsy may be required. Bone marrow biopsy is indicated if leukemia is suspected.

For therapy of individual diseases, the reader is directed to appropriate chapters in this text or elsewhere. Unless leukemia is present, specific treatment is indicated for the underlying disease but not for the leukocytosis.

ADDITIONAL READING

Breitschwerdt EB, Brown TT, DeBuysscher EV et al. Rhinitis, pneumonia, and defective neutrophil function in the Doberman pinscher. Am J Vet Res 1987; 48:1054.

Carter RF, Valli VEO, Lumsden JH. The cytology, histology and prevalence of cell types in canine lymphoma classified according to the National Cancer Institute Working Formulation. Can J Vet Res 1986; 50:154.

Duncan JR, Prasse KW. Veterinary laboratory medicine: Clinical pathology, 2nd ed. Ames, Iowa: Iowa State Press, 1986.

Jain NC. Schalm's veterinary hematology, 4th ed. Philadelphia: Lea and Febiger, 1986.

Latimer KS, Meyer DJ. Leukocytes in health and disease. In: Ettinger SJ, ed. Textbook of veterinary internal medicine. Philadelphia: WB Saunders. 1989: 2181.

Prasse KW. White cell disorders. In: Ettinger SJ, ed. Textbook of veterinary internal medicine: Diseases of the dog and cat, 2nd ed. Philadelphia: WB Saunders, 1982.

Renshaw HW, Chatburn C, Bryan GM et al. Canine granulocytopathy syndrome: Neutrophil dysfunction in a dog with recurrent infections. J Am Vet Med Assoc 1975; 166:443.

Searcy GP. Hematopoietic System. In: Thomson RG, ed. Special veterinary pathology. Toronto: BC Decker, 1988: 269.

Theilen GH, Madewell BR. Veterinary cancer medicine. Philadelphia: Lea and Febiger, 1979.

Zinkl JG. The leukocytes. In: Jain NC, ed. Symposium on clinical hematology. Vet Clin North Am 1981; 11:237.

76

LEUKOPENIA

John H. Lumsden

Leukopenia is a decrease in total circulating leukocytes involving one or more types of cells. Leukopenia may be temporary and last for a few hours to days or it may last for weeks to years. If persistent, leukopenia may be associated with recurrent infections and is indicative of a grave clinical prognosis. When persistent leukopenia has been confirmed by repeat hematologic examinations, further diagnostic procedures are usually required for differentiation of the cause. The underlying etiology may not be readily apparent. Drug-induced and immune-mediated mechanisms are increasingly recognized as likely causes for neutropenia, but convenient methods for confirmation are not readily available.

Neutropenia is the most common cause of leukopenia and may be accompanied by a decrease in any or all of the major types of leukocytes. Because the numbers of circulating monocytes, eosinophils, and basophils are low in healthy dogs and cats, an absolute decrease in any of these cell populations is not readily detected from examination of total white cell counts.

CAUSES

Leukopenia may occur due to decreased production and increased destruction or sequestration. One or more cell types may be involved, depending on the cause. Although leukocytes interact closely, for clinical interpretation they are often considered to be kinetically and functionally independent.

The major causes of leukopenia are presented for each type of leukocyte followed by the more frequently encountered clinical syndromes.

Neutropenia

Neutropenia is of immediate concern to the clinician. Classification of neutropenia according to kinetic mechanisms provides a useful conceptual approach (Table 76-1). Non-drug causes of neutropenia are listed in Table 76-2. A simple classification of neutropenia follows: It can be classified as due to a decrease in production, increased ineffective granulopoiesis, reduced survival, or unknown mechanisms. Decreased neutrophil production is found in dogs with canine cyclic hematopoiesis, parvovirus, infectious canine hepatitis, infection with *Ehrlichia* organisms, and late stage estrogen therapy; in cats, with feline infectious panleukopenia and feline leukemia virus (FeLV) infection; and in dogs and cats, with myelophthisis, irradiation, and cancer chemotherapy. Decreased granulopoiesis occurs with FeLV, myelophthisis, chemotherapy, and diphenylhydantoin administration. Common causes of decreased neutrophil

Table 76–1 *Kinetic Classification of Neutropenias*

Type I	Reduced granulocytopoiesis
	Marrow granulocyte hypoplasia, both total and effective neutrophilic granulocytopoiesis
	Ia Predictable (chemotherapy) drug-induced
	Slow onset, dose-dependent damage to stem cells and progenitor cells by alkylating agents (e.g., cyclophosphamide, doxorubicin)
	Ib Idiosyncratic (chemotherapy) drug-induced
	Slow onset, dose-dependent with wide variation in susceptibility (e.g., chloramphenicol, estrogens, sufladiazine, phenylbutazone, methotrexate)
	Ic Idiosyncratic (hypersensitivity) drug-induced
	Variable onset, usually dose-dependent. Reactions may be acute, lasting from days to weeks, or chronic, lasting from months to years (e.g., chloramphenicol)
Type II	Increased ineffective neutrophilic granulocytopoiesis
	Increased intramedullary destruction with variable marrow granulocyte cellularity
	IIa Predictable ineffective drug-induced
	Slow onset, dose-dependent with wide individual susceptibility. (e.g., estrogen toxicity in the dog)
Type III	Reduced neutrophil survival
	Increased destruction or utilization (e.g., sepsis, hypersplenism, antibody)
	IIIa Idiosyncratic (drug-hapten-antibody) neutropenia
	Rapid onset, dose-independent in sensitized animal
Type IV	Combination (type I or II and type III) neutropenia
	Decreased effective granulocytopoiesis combined with increased peripheral destruction or utilization
	IVa Drug-induced (combination) neutropenia
	Drug-activated antibody may decrease peripheral survival and lead to marrow myeloid damage
Type V	Pseudoneutropenia
	Due to decreased release from marrow granulocyte reserve or shift from circulating to marginated pool
	Va Drug-induced pseudoneutropenia
	Usually secondary to vasomotor changes (e.g., histamine)

Note: Many drug effects have not been adequately characterized for dogs and cats.
(Modified from Finch SC. Neutrophil disorders: Benign, quantitative abnormalities of neutrophils. In: Williams WJ, Beutler E, Erslev AJ. et al, eds. Hematology, 3rd ed. New York: McGraw-Hill, 1983.)

survival are overwhelming sepsis, endotoxemia, and immune-mediated mechanisms. The exact mechanism leading to neutropenia is uncertain for canine distemper and Rocky Mountain spotted fever. The most common cause of neutropenia is increased utilization (decreased survival) of neutrophils, which occurs early in infectious diseases.

Eosinopenia

Eosinopenia is difficult to differentiate from a normal low eosinophil count. Eosinophil counts will decrease in association with stress, acute infection, exogenous corticosteroid administration, or hyperadrenocorticism. Eosinopenia associated with increased systemic glucocorticoids persists for about 24 hours.

Basopenia

Basophils are rare in the peripheral blood of dogs and cats. No clinical significance can be attached to a hematology report indicating lack of basophils.

Monocytopenia

Lack of monocytes is of limited clinical significance unless it is persistent and accompanied by neutropenia.

Lymphopenia

Lymphopenia is commonly observed in the leukogram of sick animals. Causes of lymphopenia are listed in Table 76-3 according to mechanisms as

Table 76–2 *Non–Drug-Induced Neutropenic Disorders**

Type	Possible Kinetic Mechanism(s)†
STEM CELL DISORDERS	
Cyclic neutropenia	I
Preleukemia	I, II
Myelophthisis (tumor, fibrosis)	I, II
T AND B CELL DISORDERS	
Dysgammaglobulinemias	I
T cell lymphocyte disorders	I, II
Chronic hypoplastic neutropenia	I, II
PROGENITOR CELL DISORDERS	
Chédiak-Higashi syndrome	II
Chronic idiopathic neutropenia	I, II, V
Severe bacterial sepsis	I–IV
Mycobacterial infections	I, III
Starvation (copper) deficiency	I, IV, V
ANTIBODY-RELATED DISORDERS	
Isoimmune neonatal neutropenia	III, IV
Autoimmune neutropenia	III, IV
Systemic lupus erythematosus	III, IV
COMPLEX MECHANISMS	
Splenic neutropenia (hypersplenism)	III, IV
Viral and rickettsial infections	I, IV, V
Bacterial and protozoal infections	I, IV, V
PSEUDONEUTROPENIA	
Acute: endotoxin, dialysis, etc.	III, IV
Chronic: starvation, cold, etc.	V

* *Partial list of documented and potential types of neutropenia, observed in humans which may occur in dogs and cats.*
† *Refers to kinetic classification in Table 76–1.*

discussed in the section on pathophysiology. The lymphopenia associated with increased systemic levels of glucocorticoids persists for about 24 hours.

PATHOPHYSIOLOGY

Because neutrophils and lymphocytes are the most numerous leukocytes in the peripheral blood of normal dogs and cats, leukopenia usually implies neutropenia and frequently lymphopenia. There are significant differences in the kinetics of each leukocyte type. Different stimuli activating the mechanisms leading to a decrease in each leukocyte type can be initiated within the same disease process. The pathophysiology involved is discussed for each major leukocyte type.

Neutropenia

Neutrophils are produced in the special microenvironment of bone marrow from progenitor stem cells. Alterations in this microenvironment because of decreased blood supply, inflammation, or tumor invasion may interfere with stem cell differentiation and neutrophil production. Chemicals, drugs, toxins, and antibodies may interfere with cell division and maturation, leading to ineffective or inadequate neutrophil production.

Table 76–3 *Causes of Lymphopenia*

Acute infection
    Septicemia, endotoxemia, canine parvovirus, distemper, hepatitis or corona virus, feline
      infectious panleukopenia
Corticosteroid-induced
    Hyperadrenocorticism, ACTH, or exogenous corticosteroid administration, pain, severe heat
      or cold exposure
Irradiation or immunosuppression therapy
Loss of lymphocyte-rich afferent lymph
    Granulomatous enteritis, protein-losing enteropathy, enteric neoplasms, alimentary
      lymphosarcoma
Loss of lymphocyte-rich efferent lymph
    Ruptured thoracic duct, feline cardiovascular disease
Acquired T lymphocyte deficiency (neonatal infections)
    Canine distemper, feline infectious panleukopenia, feline leukemia virus (fading kitten
      syndrome), feline immunodeficiency virus
Altered lymph node architecture
    Lymphosarcoma, generalized granulomatous diseases

(Modified from Duncan JR, Prasse KW. Veterinary laboratory medicine: Clinical pathology, 2nd ed. Ames, Iowa: Iowa State University Press, 1986.)

The classification of kinetic causes for neutropenia, listed in Table 76-1, is modified from one developed for use in people and appears to be applicable for use in dogs and cats. Differentiation of the cause of neutropenia is often difficult, but integration of the kinetic relationships and pertinent clinical information leads to identification of probable etiology in many cases.

A simplified list of non–drug-induced causes of neutropenia is presented in Table 76-2. In most bacterial infections, chemoattractants are produced that result in neutrophil margination against blood vessel endothelium. This process may create a temporary pseudoneutropenia. Other stimuli, such as leukotrienes and neutrophil-releasing factors, release neutrophils at an increased rate from the marrow storage pool reserve. When demand exceeds supply, less mature cells (band neutrophils, metamyelocytes) are released (left shift). In normal health, the storage pool is considered to contain about a 5-day supply of mature neutrophils. In severe infections, the increased demand may exhaust reserves quickly. Endotoxins may initiate temporary sequestration of leukocytes in blood vessels, particularly in the lungs and intestines of the dog and cat. With severe endotoxemia, destruction of neutrophils in blood vessels and marrow storage pools may limit neutrophil availability until mitotic and maturation pools are replenished.

Neutropenia occurs every 11 to 12 days in collie dogs with cyclic hematopoiesis due to altered stem cell kinetics. Other cell lines are affected also, but the lack of production is less apparent because of the longer cell half-lives. In FeLV infection, neutropenia is one of the several non-neoplastic hematopoietic disorders that may occur. Others include pancytopenia, panleukopenia, thrombocytopenia, and regenerative and nonregenerative anemias. In anaphylaxis, leukopenia and neutropenia usually last several minutes to a few hours.

Many drugs have been demonstrated to cause neutropenia in humans. The frequency of neutropenia induction and the relative risk is high for phenothiazines, phenylbutazones, sulfonamides, semisynthetic penicillins, antithyroid drugs, and chloramphenicol. The list of documented drugs is short for dogs and cats, but the potential must be considered in all cases with neutropenia.

Eosinopenia

Because eosinophils are present in low numbers in the blood of healthy dogs and cats, a decrease is not readily recognized. Stress and endogenous corticosteroid release or exogenous corticosteroid administration will decrease the number of circulating eosinophils. The eosinopenia induced by catecholamines is considered to be due to affects on the β-adrenergic receptors. The mechanism of corticosteroid-induced eosinopenia is complex. Histamine is chemotactic for eosinophils but is neutralized by corticosteroids, resulting in decreased eosinophil release from the bone marrow. Corticosteroids also inhibit degranulation of basophils and mast cells, reducing the histamine eosinotactic effect. Corticosteroids diminish eosinophil adherence and chemotaxis and are considered to be able to lyse intravascular eosinophils. Corticosteroids are associated with increased emigration of eosinophils into lymphoid organs possibly due to release of eosinophilotactic lymphokines following corticosteroid-induced lympholysis. Prolonged corticosteroid administration may cause decreased eosinophil production.

Eosinopenia is characteristic of acute infection and inflammation. The release of catecholamines and corticosteroids is usually considered to be the cause, but other factors may be involved. The rate of eosinophil emigration into areas of inflammation may be increased in response to locally produced eosinophil chemotactic factors. Complement activation may be involved. There may be a decreased rate of release of cells from the bone marrow during acute inflammation and decreased production during chronic inflammation, the latter due to decreased lymphokine stimulation.

Basopenia

No clinical significance is attached to basopenia because of the low numbers normally present in canine and feline blood. The functions of basophils are not as well characterized but are considered to be similar to mast cells. Basophils participate in allergic reactions, primarily due to the release of vasoactive and other potent mediators contributing to the immediate hypersensitivity reaction, in inflammation, and in triglyceride metabolism. Corticosteroid injection will result in a decrease in basophils. Basophil numbers decrease in some species with urticaria and anaphylactic shock.

Monocytopenia

Monocytes are the circulating component of the mononuclear phagocyte system. Marked stress may induce a temporary monocytopenia in the cat, which can be followed by monocytosis. Endotoxins can also induce monocytopenia. Corticosteroid effects differ with the species. Monocytosis develops in the dog, while the response is variable in the cat. Monocyte production in the bone marrow may decrease when an increase in circulating corticosteroids occurs.

Lymphopenia

Although lymphopenia is a common abnormality in the blood of sick animals, often the cause can be identified only in retrospect. The number of lymphocytes in the blood is a balance between the cells entering and leaving the circulation and does not necessarily reflect the total numbers of lymphocytes, the rate of lymphopoiesis, or lympholysis. There may be no correlation between the size of the lymphoid organs and the lymphocyte count, although a decrease in lymphopoiesis and lymph node size due to thymectomy, corticosteroid administration, and irradiation is usually associated with lymphopenia. Lymphocyte subpopulations, such as T and B lymphocyte subsets, have different surface characteristics that probably affect adherence to endothelial cells, locomotion, and trapping within lymph follicles.

Common causes of lymphopenia are listed in Table 76-3. In acute septicemias, antigen production can result in entrapment of recirculating lymphocytes and increased antibody production. The lymphopenia and lymphadenopathy tend to disappear with time. Endotoxemia may induce lymphopenia through similar mechanisms, although the immediate lymphopenia following endotoxin administration is more likely due to sequestration and the lympholytic effect of the corticosteroids that are released. In localized infections, entrapment of lymphocytes within the draining lymph nodes occurs, but lymphopenia is rare. Irradiation and immunosuppressive therapy suppress lymphopoiesis, resulting in a slow decrease in circulating lymphocytes. Lymphopenia develops when lymphocyte-rich plasma is lost through damaged intestinal mucosa, as occurs with lymphangiectasis, granulomatous enteritis, and intestinal neoplasms. Rupture of the thoracic duct and feline cardiovascular disease result in the pooling of large numbers of lymphocytes within the pleural cavity. With chronic drainage, lymphopenia frequently develops. Lymphopenia is seen in early viral infections due to lympholysis or due to altered circulation of lymphocytes through lymphoid tissues. An acquired T lymphocyte deficiency can be produced by certain viral infections in the neonatal dog and cat. Other T and B lymphocyte deficiencies described in humans have not been adequately characterized for the dog and cat. Lymphopenia may be observed in generalized granulomatous diseases (e.g., systemic mycosis) and is probably due in part to altered lymphocyte recirculation. Lymphopenia, without other changes in leukocyte numbers, is observed in some dogs with uremia. The mechanism has not been defined.

DIAGNOSTIC APPROACH

When leukopenia is present, the leukocytes that are decreased, or in some situations increased, should be noted. History of the patient and clinical signs should be reviewed for indications of infection, inflammation, or neoplasia. Hepatosplenomegaly, lymphadenopathy, superficial or deep bacterial infections, and signs of chronic illness should be evaluated. All drug therapy used during the previous months should be noted. Red blood cell and platelet numbers should be noted for indications of disease processes or general marrow failure. Sequential blood samples are very important in differentiating causes of leukopenia, especially persisting neutropenia.

Neutropenia may occur in the early stages of severe septicemia or endotoxemia or if the infection becomes overwhelming. Depletion of neutrophil storage pools is indicated by the release of immature neutrophils, band neutrophils, metamyelocytes, and occasionally myelocytes. A degenerative left shift is characterized by the presence of a greater number of circulating immature than mature (segmented) neutrophils. The total leukocyte count may be normal or decreased. Septicemia or endotoxemia are often accompanied by changes in the neutrophil cytoplasm, including "toxic granulation" and "vacuolation" (which should be evaluated only on blood smears made following blood collection), increased cytoplasmic basophilia, and Döhle's bodies. The history and clinical examination will usually provide additional support for infection or toxemia.

Pseudoneutropenia may develop during hypersensitivity and antigen-antibody reactions but are less likely to be associated with a left shift and toxic changes in the neutrophil cytoplasm. Sequential blood samples usually reveal a return to normal neutrophil counts within hours to days.

Dogs with estrogen toxicity are usually presented because of petechial and ecchymotic hemorrhages typical of thrombocytopenia. At this time, neutrophilia is often present. If the dose of estrogen was high, pancytopenia with neutropenia may develop. The prognosis is guarded if bone marrow damage has progressed to pancytopenia. Estradiol is considered to be about ten times more potent than diethylstilbestrol.

The degree and duration of the neutropenia will guide the extent of laboratory evaluation required. If the etiology is not apparent and no clinical signs of infection are evident in a closely monitored patient, serial neutrophil counts should be examined over several days to weeks to document that the neutropenia is persistent. Bone marrow aspiration and biopsy are indicated in unexplained acute or persistent neutropenia to allow evaluation of the marrow cellularity, granulocyte reserves, myeloid:erythroid ratios, ineffective granulopoiesis, myelophthisis, and myelofibrosis. Tests for FeLV and feline immunodeficiency virus should be included for all cats with persistent neutropenia. Neutrophil-specific antibodies and other tests indicative of immune-mediated or drug-related causes of neutropenia are only available in a few research laboratories. Colony forming unit, colony-stimulating activity, excess suppressor or cytotoxic T cell, and serum inhibitory factor measurements are useful if available.

Eosinopenia, basopenia, and monocytopenia are not readily diagnosed. They are usually detected during sequential leukogram evaluations for persistent neutropenia. Direct counts (utilizing specialized staining techniques) are a more accurate method of documenting eosinopenia and basopenia than routine leukocyte counts.

Lymphopenia often occurs due to altered circulation, which develops during acute infections and in early viremias or generalized granulomatous disease. Corticosteroid, immunosuppressive, or irradiation therapy should be differentiated by the history. Unexplained lymphopenia warrants the use of additional tests to rule out hyperadrenocorticism (see Chapter 59) and possibly chronic renal disease (see Chapter 44). Thoracic fluid should be examined to rule out thoracic duct leakage (see Chapter 32). Tests of cardiac function are used to differentiate feline cardiovascular disorders. Loss of lymphocytes due to diseases affecting the intestinal mucosal, such as lymphosarcoma, lymphangiectasis and granulomatous enteritis, is usually accompanied by loss of serum proteins (see Chapter 78). In a series of cats with intestinal lymphosarcoma, 48% had lymphopenia.

MANAGEMENT AND PATIENT MONITORING

The presenting history and clinical information should direct the approach to management of leukopenia, especially neutropenia. In patients where leukopenia and neutropenia are associated with severe bacterial infection, appropriate samples should be submitted for culture. Antibiotic (bactericidal) therapy should be started immediately. Clinical improvement should be accompanied by recovery of the neutrophil count and maturity. The return of eosinophils to peripheral circulation is considered to be favorable when associated with improving clinical signs but an ominous change in the face of continuing severe infection.

Neutropenia that develops quickly (acute neutropenia) requires immediate attention because of the increased susceptibility to infection. A neutrophil count less than $0.5 \times 10^9/L$, ($\times 10^3/\mu L$), should be rechecked on the original sample with careful examination for evidence of *in vitro* clotting. Sequential blood samples should be used to confirm the neutropenia. Bone marrow aspiration and biopsy should be examined. All medication should be discontinued immediately to eliminate possible drug-induced mechanisms. Body temperature should be monitored several times a day. If a fever develops, the patient should be examined and all suspicious sites investigated as required to confirm or rule them out as a source of infection (Chapter 6). Urine samples should be examined for pyuria and bacteriuria and submitted for culture and sensitivity testing (Chapter 46). Repeat blood cultures should be made. If neutropenia is caused by drugs or chemicals, days to weeks or longer may be required for granulocytopoiesis to return to normal,

if it does. Neutrophil-rich transfusions may assist in treating serious infections unresponsive to antibiotic therapy. The effect of neutrophil transfusions is temporary due to the short half-life of neutrophils in circulation. Some effort is required to transfer adequate numbers from the donor to the patient.

Chronic neutropenia, that is, neutropenia present for several days to months in a patient without apparent signs of infection, may not require treatment. The threat of bacterial infection is much lower, but the patient should be kept away from likely exposure to infectious agents. All drugs, chemicals, or physical agents (such as radiographs) that may harm the bone marrow should be avoided. The patient should be observed closely. Body temperature should be monitored regularly. If suspicious clinical signs of infection develop, the patient should be treated as for acute neutropenia. Tests for drug- or chemical-induction, immune-mediated etiology, inhibitory stimuli, and so forth can be pursued as available. Splenectomy may be beneficial if the spleen is enlarged and considered to be the source of neutrophil removal.

Neutropenia develops on an 11- to 12-day cycle in dogs with cyclic hematopoiesis. During the periods of neutropenia, close attention is required to detect early signs of infection so that appropriate antibiotic therapy can be initiated. Endotoxin has been used on an experimental basis to increase granulocytopoiesis and reduce the degree of cyclic change. Bone marrow transfusion from a normal donor after patient irradiation has been successful.

Lithium therapy (20–25 mg/kg per day orally) has been used to increase the release of neutrophils from the storage pool. Corticosteroids have no proven value in increasing granulopoiesis. In high doses, they may mask as well as increase susceptibility to infection. Corticosteroids may reduce immune-mediated destruction of neutrophils in circulation and interference with granulopoiesis. Prednisone (2–4 mg/kg per day orally) is suggested for these cases. Globulin administration may be considered in patients with hypogammaglobulinemia.

Primary disorders leading to eosinopenia and basopenia may respond to treatment.

Treatment for lymphopenia, if required, is directed at the primary disorder.

ADDITIONAL READING

Campbell KL. Canine cyclic hematopoiesis. Compendium of Continuing Education 1985; 7:57.

Duncan JR, Prasse KW. Veterinary laboratory medicine: Clinical pathology, 2nd ed. Ames, Iowa: Iowa State Press, 1986: 31.

Gabbert NH. Cyclic neutropenia in a feline leukemia positive cat: A case report. Journal of the American Animal Hospital Association 1984; 20:343.

Jain NC. Schalm's veterinary hematology, 4th ed. Philadelphia: Lea and Febiger, 1986.

Maddison JE, Hoff B, Johnson RP. Steroid responsive neutropenia in a dog. Journal of the American Animal Hospital Association 1983; 19:881.

Theilen GH, Madewell BR. Veterinary cancer medicine. Philadelphia: Lea and Febiger, 1979.

Zinkl JG. The leukocytes. In: Jain NC, ed. Symposium on clinical hematology. Vet Clin North Am 1981; 11:237.

77

HYPOGLYCEMIA

Robert M. Jacobs

Hypoglycemia can be a life-threatening problem; therefore, hypoglycemia must be recognized and treated promptly. Strictly speaking, hypoglycemia is present when the serum glucose concentration is below the lower reference limit. However, the onset of clinical signs associated with hypoglycemia is variable and cannot be predicted simply by measurement of the serum glucose concentration. Clinical signs of hypoglycemia are often attributable to central nervous system (CNS) dysfunction.

CAUSES AND PATHOPHYSIOLOGY

The serum glucose concentration is maintained within the reference limits by the correct hormonal balance, availability of precursors for hepatic gluconeogenesis, and hepatic adequacy for glycogenesis, glycogenolysis, and gluconeogenesis. Hormones that influence glucose metabolism are catecholamines, cortisol, growth hormone (somatotropin), insulin, and insulinlike growth factors (somatomedins), somatostatin, and thyroxine.

Compensatory mechanisms to adjust for hypoglycemia include the release of catecholamines, cortisol, glucagon, and growth hormone. Effective compensation results in an increase in the serum glucose concentration derived from hepatic glycogenolysis and gluconeogenesis. Insulin release is inhibited and peripheral glucose utilization decreased. With prolonged and severe hypoglycemia or repeated episodes of hypoglycemia, these compensatory mechanisms may become exhausted.

Causes of hypoglycemia that have been reported in small animals are listed in Table 77-1. Laboratory error should always be considered if the clinical signs are inconsistent with the laboratory abnormality. Inappropriate sample handling is perhaps the most common error to cause decreased serum glucose concentrations. Failure to quickly separate serum from clotted blood allows for the metabolism of glucose by erythrocytes and leukocytes. Serum or plasma allowed to sit on the clot for 1 hour after taking the specimen have about a 7% decrease in glucose concentration. Some sources recommend that samples to be analyzed for glucose concentration be taken in an anticoagulant with sodium fluoride added. The fluoride inhibits glycolysis by blood cells. Fluoride, however, interferes with methodologies on some instruments. Bacterial contamination will rapidly deplete the glucose in a sample. A marked leukocytosis, as seen with chronic leukemia, may cause the glucose concentration to decrease *in vitro* faster than anticipated. The para-

Table 77–1 *Causes of Hypoglycemia in Dogs*

Artifact of sample handling
Bacterial
Chemicals
  Acetylcholinesterase inhibitors
    Edrophonium
    Neostigmine
    Organophosphates
    Physostigmine
  Ethanol
  Disopyramide
  Plant toxins
  Propanolol
  Salicylate
  Sulfonylurea compounds
    Chlorpropamide
    Acetohexamide
    Tolbutamide
Functional
  "Hunting dog" hypoglycemia
  Neonatal hypoglycemia
  Pregnancy-associated hypoglycemia
  Starvation
  "Toy breed" hypoglycemia
Glycogen storage diseases
  Type I (von Gierke's disease)
  Type II (Pompe's disease)
  Type III (Cori's disease)
Insulin or insulin-like hormones
  Extrapancreatic tumor
  Iatrogenic
  Pancreatic islet β-cell tumor (dog and cat)
Organ disease
  Cardiac-induced hypoglycemia
  Hepatic-associated
    Cirrhosis
    Fibrosis
    Neoplasia
    Vascular shunts
  Hypoadrenocorticism
  Malassimilation
  Pituitary dwarfism
  Renal-associated
    Tubular acidosis
    Fanconi-like syndrome
    Chronic renal failure (cat)

sitemic phase of hemoparasitic infection may also be associated with hypoglycemia *in vitro* or *in vivo*. Most automated glucose methodologies are now highly specific for glucose, but some older methods still in use are susceptible to interference by other sugars and chemicals leading to falsely increased test results.

Bacterial infections may result in hyperglycemia possibly mediated by catecholamine inhibition of insulin secretion and glycogenolysis.

In some severe bacterial infections, there may be depleted glycogen stores, increased tissue glucose utilization, and decreased gluconeogenesis leading to hypoglycemia. Tissue hypoxia causes a shift to anaerobic metabolism and acidosis. Anaerobic metabolism is much less efficient in using glucose to produce energy, and the acidosis decreases hepatic gluconeogenesis. Insulin release may be augmented in endotoxemia.

The functional causes of hypoglycemia are related to unique circumstances (*e.g.,* overexertion, starvation, young age) or breed. Hypoglycemia can occur in lean, high-strung hunting dogs for unknown reasons. Marathon runners or people who exercise to exhaustion also may develop hypoglycemia. Depletion of hepatic glycogen stores may be involved.

Neonates are susceptible to the development of clinical signs associated with hypoglycemia, since, when starved, they deplete glycogen stores rapidly, their brain to body weight ratios are 2 to 4 times greater than in adult animals, and they have relatively little muscle and fat for gluconeogenic activity. Gluconeogenic activity may be further compromised by immaturity of gluconeogenic enzyme systems. Neonates are not efficient in using free fatty acids as an energy source. Despite good reasons for the development of severe complications of hypoglycemia, neonates are relatively resistant to the development of irreversible lesions since lactate is used as an alternative energy source. Hypoglycemia in neonates has been associated with dehydration, diarrhea, dystocia, hypothermia, hypoxia, maternal rejection, poor maternal nutrition, prematurity, septicemia, toxic milk syndrome, and trauma.

A case of hypoglycemia-ketonemia in a pregnant bitch has been described, but the pathogenesis was not determined. The hypoglycemia-ketonemia resolved after parturition.

Despite weeks of starvation, the serum glucose concentration in dogs remains normal. Hypoglycemia may ensue once glycogen stores are completely depleted and substrates for gluconeogenesis are limited.

Hypoglycemia is sometimes seen in young (6–12 weeks old) toy or miniature breeds of dogs. The hypoglycemic crisis is often associated with anorexia, diarrhea, hypothermia, infectious disease, parasitism, starvation, and stress associated with environmental changes. Inadequate substrates for gluconeogenesis and immaturity of gluconeogenic and glycogenolytic enzyme systems may be involved in the pathogenesis.

Glycogen storage diseases are inherited defects such that glycogenolytic enzymes are either lacking or defective. Three types have been reported (although some have not been proven by enzymatic analysis) in dogs; Types I, II, and III are due to lack of activities of glucose-6-phosphatase, 1,4-glucosidase, and amylo-1,6-glucosidase, respectively.

Hyperinsulinism can be iatrogenic or is seen as a paraneoplastic syndrome in association with a pancreatic islet β-cell tumor or some extrapancreatic tumors. Any animal receiving insulin can suffer hypoglycemic episodes. Precipitating events include anorexia, starvation, unusual level of exercise, and inadvertent insulin overdose. Failure to monitor serum glucose concentrations and adjust the insulin dose accordingly can lead to an insulin overdose.

The paraneoplastic syndrome of hyperinsulinism is most often associated with a functional pancreatic β-cell tumor (insulinoma). Most reports are in dogs, but a feline case has been documented. Decreased glucose production, rather than increased utilization, may be more important in the pathogenesis of hypoglycemia associated with insulin-secreting tumors. These tumors have a high rate of metastasis to liver and regional lymph nodes. Insulinomas tend to respond to normal and provocative stimuli by an exaggerated insulin release. Hence, affected dogs may show hypoglycemic clinical signs 1 to 4 hours after eating. If fed once per day, clinical signs may occur close to feeding time or may be associated with excitement at feeding.

Extrapancreatic tumors may produce insulin or insulinlike growth factors (somatomedins). A large tumor in a cachectic, glycogen depleted animal may consume glucose at a rate exceeding the gluconeogenic rate. Replacement of normal hepatic parenchyma with tumor or hormonal alteration of the gluconeogenic and glycogenolytic enzyme systems has also been suggested to play a role in the hypoglycemia of malignancy. In people, adrenocortical carcinoma, hemangiosarcoma, hepatocellular carcinoma, hepatoma, hypernephroma, leiomyosarcoma, liposarcoma, mesothelioma, and rhabdomyosarcoma can produce insulinlike growth factors and have been associated with hypoglycemia. Hypoglycemia with normal or low serum insulin concentrations have been noted in dogs with hemangiosarcoma, heptocellular carcinoma, hepatoma, leiomyosarcoma, lymphoplasmacytoid splenic tumor, melanoma, and salivary gland adenocarcinoma.

Individuals with adrenal, cardiac, hepatic, pituitary, and renal disease may show clinical signs associated with hypoglycemia. The pathogenesis varies with the organ involvement. With hypoadrenocorticism, a relative or absolute lack of counter-regulatory hormones (catecholamines, cortisol) may cause decreased hepatic gluconeogenesis and increased peripheral glucose utilization. The role of counter-regulatory hormones in diabetic individuals is receiving more attention, since lack of or poor regulation of these hormones may precipitate hypoglycemic episodes. Hypoglycemia in malabsorption is uncommon, since in most cases residual absorption of gluconeogenic substrates (fats and amino acids) is not limiting. Hepatic diseases associated with hypoglycemia may be acquired (inflammation, fibrosis, neoplasia) or congenital (glycogen storage, vascular shunts). The loss in functional hepatic mass must be greater than 70% before hypoglycemia is seen. Pituitary dwarfism could result in hypoglycemia due to decreased growth hormone secretion but is so far unreported. Proximal and distal renal tubular acidosis and congenital or acquired Fanconilike syndrome are potential causes of hypoglycemia.

CLINICAL SIGNS

The lower reference limit for serum glucose concentration in dogs and cats is between 60 and 70 mg/dl (3.3–3.9 mmol/L). Clinical signs associated with hypoglycemia generally do not occur until the serum glucose concentration falls below 45 mg/dl (2.5 mmol/L). However, the onset of clinical signs is variable and is influenced by such factors as the underlying disease process, individual susceptibility, and rate of onset, degree, and duration of hypoglycemia. Neurologic abnormalities are most often seen because of the high metabolic activity of the CNS, CNS-dependency on carrier-facilitated diffusion of glucose across the blood–brain barrier for metabolism, and accumulation of excitatory amino acids and anaerobic glycolytic metabolites. Hypoglycemia differentially affects the CNS, the more primitive, less metabolically active parts of the brain (mesencephalon and myelencephalon) being more resistant.

Adrenergic stimulation and the direct effect of neuronal glucose deprivation cause most of the clinical signs of hypoglycemia if the decrease in blood glucose concentration is rapid. With hypoglycemia, sympathetic tone is increased following stimulation of glucoreceptor-containing hypothalamic cells. Pupillary dilatation, increased heart rate, nervousness, vocalization, muscle twitching, and irritability may occur. The CNS signs associated with hypoglycemia are usually multifocal (diffuse) or less often focal and include visual disturbances, blindness, mental dullness, confusion, behavioral changes (*e.g.*, aggression, anxiety, hysteria, obsessive running, loss of bladder and bowel control), weakness, ataxia, hypothermia, generalized seizures, bradycardia, decerebrate rigidity, miotic pupils, and absence of deep tendon reflexes; eventually, coma can occur. If the hypoglycemia is severe and prolonged, the CNS lesions may be irreversible. Peripheral nervous system abnormalities (*e.g.*, posterior paresis) may occur.

DIAGNOSTIC APPROACH

Hypoglycemia must be established using laboratory methods. The association of the hypoglycemia with clinical signs is proven if resolution of the clinical signs occurs after glucose administration. Once this resolution is accomplished, the cause is determined.

Most of the causes will be evident once an accurate history is obtained and the physical examination, complete blood cell count, urinalysis, and serum biochemistry profile are completed. If a temporal association between drug treatment and the development of hypoglycemia is established, alternative therapy should be instituted. The glycogen storage diseases are diagnosed by enzyme quantitation and histopathology of a liver biopsy.

Iatrogenic hyperinsulinism and hyperinsulinism as part of a paraneoplastic syndrome are the most common causes of hypoglycemia in companion animals. Functional pancreatic and extrapancreatic tumors secrete insulin, in which case the serum immunoreactive insulin concentrations are inappropriately (relative to the glucose concentration) or absolutely increased. Extrapancreatic tumors can also secrete insulinlike growth factors; in these instances, the serum immunoreactive insulin concentrations will be low-normal or decreased. Often the extrapancreatic tumors causing hypoglycemia are located in the liver. Hepatomegaly may be detected by palpation, radiographs, or ultrasound. Liver-dependent serum chemistry analytes are often increased. Assays for various human insulinlike growth factors are available, but cross-reactivity in animal species is unknown.

Islet cell tumors in animals are generally not associated with organomegaly or serum biochemistry abnormalities apart from episodic hypoglycemia, although hepatic and regional lymph node metastasis is often present at the time of diagnosis. In dogs with functional islet cell tumors, random serum glucose concentrations are often below the reference interval. Measurement of serum glucose and immunoreactive insulin concentrations after withholding food overnight is diagnostic in most dogs with insulinoma. Alternatively, food can be withheld from dogs until the serum glucose concentration is below 60 mg/dl (3.3 mmol/L). Most dogs with insulinoma develop hypoglycemia within 8 hours, but in some dogs it may take 24 to 72 hours. Once hypoglycemia is apparent, a sample is taken for insulin determination. If the immunoreactive insulin concentration remains within the reference interval (8–20 μU/ml), then the glucose:insulin ratio (normal range equals 3.31–12.67, where glucose is mg/dl and insulin is μU/ml), insulin:glucose ratio (normal range equals 0.042–0.234, where insulin is μU/ml and glucose is mg/dl), or amended insulin:glucose ratio (AIGR equals serum insulin [μU/ml] × 100 divided by serum glucose [mg/dl] minus 30) are calculated to demonstrate inappropriately (relative to the glucose concentration) increased insulin secretion. In the formula for the AIGR, it is assumed that when the serum glucose concentration is 30 mg/dl (1.7 mmol/L), the serum insulin concentration is zero. An AIGR greater than 30 μU insulin/ mg glucose is considered diagnostic for insulinoma. In a series of 23 dogs with insulinomas, the AIGR ranged from 16 to 7,000 μU insulin/mg glucose. Compared with serum insulin concentration alone, the AIGR provides fewer false-negative test results among dogs with insulinoma, but increased false-positives are seen in cases where marked hypoglycemia (40 mg/dl [2.2 mmol/L] or less) occurs for reasons other than hyperinsulinism (*e.g.*, bacterial infection, hypoglycemia associated with extrapancreatic tumors). Therefore, other causes of hypoglycemia should be eliminated before the AIGR is applied.

If prolonged fasting (24–48 hours) does not precipitate hypoglycemia, the administration of calcium, glucagon, glucose, leucine, or tolbutamide may be used as provocative tests for the diagnosis of insulinomas. The glucagon tolerance test is used most often, but insulinomas vary in their sensitivity to different provocative agents. Glucagon causes rapid glycogenolysis and subsequent hyperglycemia. Dogs with insulinomas demonstrate an exaggerated glucagon effect on insulin release. After withholding food overnight, 0.03 mg glucagon/kg body weight is given intravenously. Serum glucose concentrations are determined when the glucagon is given and at 15, 30, 60, and 120 minutes after administration. Additional samples for serum glucose concentration at 1 minute and immunoreactive insulin concentrations at zero time and at 1 minute after giving glucagon are also useful. In dogs with insulinoma, the serum glucose concentration does not exceed 135 mg/dl (7.5 mmol/L) and decreases to 50 mg/dl (2.8 mmol/L) or less by 120 minutes. In the 1 minute sample, dogs with insulinoma usually have an insulin concentration above 50 μU/ ml, an insulin concentration increment between zero time and 1 minute greater than 18 μU/ml, decreased glucose concentration (due to rapid release of insulin from the tumor), and an insulin:glucose ratio greater than 0.75 (where insulin is μU/ml and glucose is mg/dl). If hypoglycemic signs develop, glucose should be given immediately.

The diagnosis of insulinoma can be confirmed at biopsy. Most of the pancreatic tumors are visible to the surgeon, but careful palpation of the pancreas may be necessary to detect multiple small masses. Intravenous methylene blue prior to surgery appears to be helpful in the gross identification of insulinomas. At presentation, most insulinomas have metastasized. From 70% to 95% of insulinomas are considered malignant.

MANAGEMENT

If the patient is conscious, 50% dextrose, Karo syrup, or honey can be given orally. When the intravenous route is chosen, 50% dextrose (1–2 ml/kg body weight) should be diluted 1:1 with sterile water and infused slowly. In neonates, warmed half-strength lactated Ringer's solution in 2.5% dextrose (0.04 ml/gm body weight) is given subcutaneously. Neonates should be kept warm and nursing resumed as soon as possible. Any underlying problems must be identified and effectively treated to prevent further occurrences. Some conditions, such as neonatal and "toy breed" hypoglycemia, resolve as the animals mature. More frequent high carbohydrate, high protein feedings (*e.g.*, Hill's Prescription Diet, canine p/d) in the interim may be useful. Where dehydration is present, fluid replacement is necessary. With "hunting dog" hypoglycemia, feeding prior to exercise may prevent a hypoglycemic episode. Alternatively, carbohydrate-rich treats during periods of strenuous exercise are useful. Hypoglycemia associated with sepsis is best treated with dextrose, insulin, potassium, and glucocorticoids in addition to appropriate antibiotic therapy. Fluid therapy is important to maintain tissue perfusion.

Extrapancreatic tumors are treated with chemotherapy, radiation, surgery, or a combination of two or more modalities, if an efficacious protocol is available.

The preferred treatment for insulinomas is surgical resection. Frequent feedings may prevent acute episodes of hypoglycemia, but as the disease progresses, maintaining the individual in a euglycemic state becomes increasingly difficult. Glucocorticoids (prednisone, 0.25–0.5 mg/kg body weight) enhance hepatic gluconeogenesis and decrease peripheral glucose utilization and have been beneficial when used in conjunction with frequent feedings. If frequent feedings and glucocorticoids fail to maintain adequate blood glucose concentration, diazoxide, initially given at 10 mg/kg per day, increasing to 40 mg/kg per day, and used along with frequent feedings, controls hypoglycemia, at least temporarily, in about 70% of dogs with insulinomas. Propanolol and diphenylhydantoin have also been used as hyperglycemic agents in people with insulinomas, but only 30% of affected people appear to benefit from the use of diphenylhydantoin, and propanolol may sometimes induce hypoglycemia. The only antineoplastic drug to be tried is streptozotocin (Zanosar), and, although it temporarily controls clinical signs, it does so at the expense of hepatic and renal toxicity.

At surgery, tumors should be widely excised. Palpation of tumors may cause the release of large amounts of insulin, so 5% dextrose should be added to the fluids (given at twice the maintenance rate) administered during surgery. Postsurgical care should be directed at maintaining the serum glucose concentration within the reference interval and monitoring serum amylase activity for possible pancreatitis. Dogs should not be fed or fed small amounts until stabilized (36–48 hours after surgery). A transient (most often 2–4 day duration, but up to 6 months) diabetic state may occur in about 25% of dogs postoperatively, since normal β-cells will have become atrophic. When most of the pancreas is removed or normal β-cells fail to hypertrophy, a permanent diabetic state requiring insulin supplementation is seen (see Chapter 58). It is assumed that most dogs with insulinoma have metastases when presented. Surgery is therefore palliative, but clinical signs may be controlled for months to years (mean survival time is 19.4 months). Subsequent surgery is often as helpful as the initial surgery in controlling the hypoglycemia. Glucocorticoids or diazoxide can be used postoperatively to control hypoglycemia if the tumor cannot be adequately removed.

PATIENT MONITORING

Close observation of the animal for signs attributable to hypoglycemia and prompt treatment will prevent any permanent effects. Monitoring of serum glucose concentrations is most useful in heralding further tumor growth.

ADDITIONAL READING

Allen TA. Canine hypoglycemia. In: Kirk RW, ed. Current veterinary therapy VIII. Philadelphia: WB Saunders, 1983: 845.

Atkins CE. Disorders of glucose homeostasis in neonatal and juvenile dogs: Hypoglycemia. Part II. Compendium of Continuing Education 1984; 6:353.

Caywood DD, Wilson JW, Hardy RM, Shull RM. Pancreatic islet cell adenocarcinoma: Clinical and diagnostic features of six cases. J Am Vet Med Assoc 1979; 174:714.

Chrisman CL. Postoperative results and complications of insulinomas in dogs. Journal of the American Animal Hospital Association 1980; 16:677.

Feldman EC. Diseases of the endocrine pancreas. In: Ettinger SJ, ed. Textbook of veterinary internal medicine: Diseases of the dog and cat, 2d ed. Philadelphia: WB Saunders, 1983: 1640.

Fingeroth JM, Smeak DD, Jacobs RM. Intravenous methylene blue infusion for intraoperative identification of parathyroid gland and pancreatic islet cell tumors in dogs. Part I: Experimental determination of dose-related staining efficacy and toxicity. Journal of the American Animal Hospital Association 1988; 24:165.

Hawkins KL, Summers BA, Kuhajda FP, Smith CA. Immunocytochemistry of normal pancreatic islets and spontaneous islet cell tumors in dogs. Vet Pathol 1987; 24:170.

Knowlen GG, Schall WD. The amended insulin-glucose ratio: Is it really better? J Am Vet Med Assoc 1984; 185:397.

Kruth SA, Feldman EC, Kennedy PC. Insulin-secreting islet cell tumors: Establishing a diagnosis and the clinical course for 25 dogs. J Am Vet Med Assoc 1982; 181:54.

Leifer CE. Hypoglycemia. In: Kirk RW, ed. Current veterinary therapy IX. Philadelphia: WB Saunders, 1986: 982.

Leifer CE, Peterson ME, Matus RE, Patnaik AK. Hypoglycemia associated with nonislet cell tumor in 13 dogs. J Am Vet Med Assoc 1985; 186:53.

McMillan FD, Barr B, Feldman EC. Functional pancreatic islet cell tumor in a cat. Journal of the American Animal Hospital Association 1985; 21:741.

Mehlhaff CJ, Peterson ME, Patnaik AK, Carrillo JM. Insulin-producing islet cell neoplasms: Surgical considerations and general management in 35 dogs. Journal of the American Animal Hospital Association 1985; 21:607.

Meyer DJ. Temporary remission of hypoglycemia in a dog with an insulinoma after treatment with streptozotocin. Am J Vet Res 1977; 38:1201.

Nelson RW, Foodman MS. Medical management of canine hyperinsulinism. J Am Vet Med Assoc 1985; 187:78.

O'Brien TD, Hayden DW, O'Leary TP et al. Canine pancreatic endocrine tumors: Immunohistochemical analysis of hormone content and amyloid. Vet Pathol 1987; 24:308.

Rogers KS, Luttgen PJ. Hyperinsulinism. Compendium of Continuing Education 1985; 7:829.

Steinberg HS. Insulin secreting pancreatic tumors in the dog. Journal of the American Animal Hospital Association 1980; 16:695.

Turnwald GH, Troy GC. Hypoglycemia. Part I: Carbohydrate metabolism and laboratory evaluation. Compendium of Continuing Education 1983; 5:932.

Turnwald GH, Troy GC. Hypoglycemia. Part II: Clinical Aspects. Compendium of Continuing Education 1984; 6:115.

78

INTERPRETATION OF CHANGES IN SERUM PROTEIN

Rebecca Baker

Plasma contains many different proteins, each with specific functions. The proteins function as proteinase inhibitors, enzymes, clotting factors, antibodies, complement, and as transport substances for hormones, vitamins, bilirubin, metals, and lipids. Each protein is subject to variation in health and disease.

Plasma proteins are arbitrarily divided into α-, β-, and τ-globulins based on their zonal migration in an electric field. Since the individual proteins contributing to each zone are not separated, finding a normal concentration within each electrophoretic zone does not exclude an abnormal concentration of any individual protein.

Most plasma proteins are synthesized within the liver, excluding the immunoglobulins, which are synthesized by the reticuloendothelial system. Protein electrophoresis is generally performed on serum, as plasma contains fibrinogen, which exists as a broad dense band in the β region, obscuring other proteins of interest. Coagulation factors V and VIII are also present in plasma but not in serum.

Basic plasma protein analysis begins with measurement of total serum protein, serum albumin, and globulin concentrations. For further analysis, serum protein fractionation is done by electrophoresis. Quantitation of specific proteins may be assayed with biochemical or immunochemical techniques.

MEASUREMENT OF SERUM PROTEIN

Total Serum Protein

Biuret Reaction

Total serum protein can be measured on most automatic analyzers using the biuret reaction. This test depends on the presence of peptide bonds in proteins. A reaction between the cupric ion, the organic compound biuret, and the peptide bond results in a color change measured spectrophotometrically. This method is very accurate for the protein concentrations normally found in serum (1–100 g/L or 0.1–10 g/dl), but is not sensitive enough for fluids with normally low protein concentrations (*e.g.*, cerebral spinal fluid). Hemolyzed samples may falsely elevate the total protein and should be avoided.

Refractometer

The refractometer is widely used for the determination of serum protein concentration (total solids). If used properly, it is accurate and correlates closely with total protein concentration assayed by the biuret reaction. Proteins in solution cause a change in refractive index proportional to their concentration. Other plasma solids (glucose, urea, sodium, chloride, cholesterol) also contribute to the refractive index, hence the term *total solids*. Serum refractometry assumes that the concentration of inorganic electrolytes and nonprotein compounds do not vary markedly; therefore, differences in serum refractive index reflect changes in protein concentration (proteins form 85% of the plasma solutes). However, estimated total protein concentration can be falsely increased in conditions where these parameters are increased. Hemolysis causes a mild increase in the measurement of total solids. When lipemia is visible, the refractive index should not be used to estimate protein concentration.

Hand held temperature controlled refractometers are the best for clinical practice and are scaled to read total serum protein concentration and urine specific gravity. At protein concentrations less than 35 g/L (3.5 g/dl), the refractometer is inaccurate.

Plasma Albumin

Plasma albumin is measured using protein binding dyes such as bromocresol green. Bromocresol green and albumin form a colored complex that is measured spectrophotometrically. Hemolysis and lipemia do not interfere with the assay. At very low albumin concentrations (less than 10 g/L or 1 g/dl), nonspecific binding of other serum proteins to the dye occurs and causes an artifactual increase in the protein value. Anticonvulsants and some antibiotics can compete with albumin and give a false low value. Serum albumin concentrations are accurately determined using serum protein electrophoresis, which is the method of choice when monitoring low albumin concentrations.

Globulins

On automated chemical analyzers, the total globulin concentration is calculated as the difference between the total protein and albumin concentrations (globulin equals total protein minus albumin). Therefore, α-, β-, and τ-globulins are included in this result. The globulin concentration can be determined from the electrophoretic strip by measuring the area under the curve (using a densitometer).

ELECTROPHORESIS

Total protein is separated electrophoretically into its component parts. Although only a few changes in pattern are diagnostically specific, it is still a valuable clinical tool. The electrophoretic principle is based on the migration of charged particles in an electric field. The distances protein migrate depend on the charge on the protein, the size of the protein, the intensity of the electric field, and the support medium.

Electrophoretic techniques between laboratories vary mainly in the support medium utilized. Cellulose acetate and agarose are the most common. On either medium, a serum sample is applied to a designated area, and a given voltage is applied for a specified time. Most serum proteins are negatively charged and under the designated electrophoretic conditions migrate towards the anode. Albumin being the most negatively charged migrates the furthest, followed by the α- and β-globulins. Feline albumin has the fastest migrating albumin of the domestic species. Some τ-globulins migrate slightly anodally and others move towards the cathode. Protein bands are then visualized by staining with Amido black B or Coumassie brilliant blue dyes. Electrophoretic profiles can be evaluated qualitatively by looking at the bands on the electrophoretogram, and quantitatively by scanning the staining intensity of the bands with a densitometer. Since overlap of protein bands occurs, albumin is the only protein that can be clearly quantitated. The interlaboratory variability in methods requires that normal species reference values be developed in each laboratory. Depending on the species and support medium, there may be one or two α, one or two β and one or two γ fractions.

Cellulose acetate electrophoresis in the dog and cat normally yields albumin, α_1, α_2, β_1, β_2, τ_1, and τ_2 zones. Agarose electrophoresis in the dog yields albumin, α_1, α_2, β_1, β_2, and τ, and in the cat yields albumin, α_{1a} α_{1b}, α_{2a}, α_{2b}, β_{1a}, β_{1b}, β_2, and τ zones (Figs. 78-1 through 78-2).

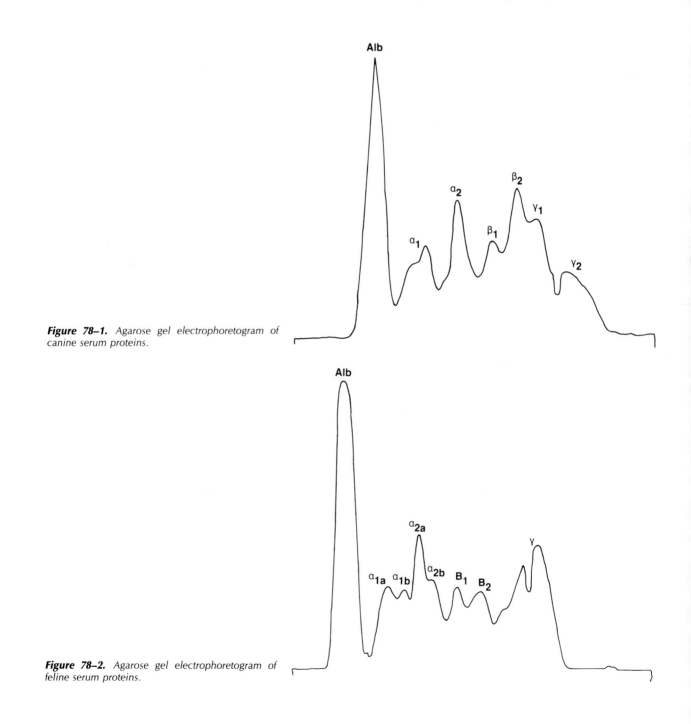

Figure 78–1. *Agarose gel electrophoretogram of canine serum proteins.*

Figure 78–2. *Agarose gel electrophoretogram of feline serum proteins.*

Quantitative values for these zones using agarose electrophoresis are listed in Table 78-1.

ALBUMIN

Albumin is a water soluble globular protein with a molecular weight of 66,000 daltons. Albumin is synthesized and released by the liver but is not stored in the body in significant quantities. Albumin is catabolized in many tissues, where it is taken up by pinocytosis, releasing the constituent amino acids by intracellular proteolysis. The half-life of albumin varies between species and is inversely proportional to body size (dogs: approximately 10–16 days; cats: approximately 20 days). In conditions of decreased albumin synthesis or increased albumin loss, the albumin half-life increases, presumably as a compensatory phenomenon. With albumin loss, the liver increases its synthetic capacity to maintain normal serum levels. The exact mechanisms that control the rate of hepatic albumin synthesis are unknown, although plasma oncotic pressure and serum viscosity may be important. Eventually this capacity is exceeded and a decreased serum albumin results. Albumin has three important physiologic functions.

1. Transport and storage of ligands. By binding to nonpolar compounds, albumin solubilizes substances, allowing for their effective transport in serum. The large number of albumin molecules, as well as the large number of negative charges available on the albumin molecule, make it efficient at this function. It transports many ligands such as unconjugated bilirubin, free fatty acids, hormones, calcium, phenylbutazone, warfarin, and salicylates. Binding to albumin prevents loss of many compounds in the glomerular filtrate and also acts as a reservoir by storing these compounds in an inactive form until needed. Approximately 40% of serum calcium is bound to albumin, 10% is complexed with anions (citrate, phosphate, and sulfate) and 50% is ionized. Only the ionized fraction is biologically active. In hypoalbuminemia, the protein bound fraction and total serum calcium decrease, but ionized calcium remains normal (see Chapter 72).

2. Maintenance of plasma oncotic pressure. Albumin is the most osmotically active plasma protein due to its abundance and small size, accounting for 75% of the osmotic activity of plasma. The oncotic pressure of the plasma protein counterbalances the hydrostatic blood pressure and thereby maintains an effective circulatory blood volume. The partitioning of water between intravascular and extravascular compartments is, therefore, regulated by the serum albumin concentration. Logically, low serum albumin concentrations (less than 10–15 g/L or 1–1.5 g/dl) allow water to move out of the vascular bed and into tissue, causing edema (see Chapter 10).

3. Provides a source of endogenous amino acids. Albumin provides a source of immediately available amino acids at times of nutritional need.

Increased or decreased serum albumin concentration is a frequent observation. Interpretation depends on an adequate understanding of the variability involved in albumin synthesis, degradation, and loss (Fig. 78-3).

Hyperalbuminemia

The only known cause of hyperalbuminemia in animals is dehydration. In dehydration, both albumin and the globulins will be increased and, therefore, the albumin:globulin (A:G) ratio will remain the same. An accompanying increase in packed-cell volume (PCV) supports dehydration. An increase in PCV with normal protein levels suggests splenic contraction.

Hypoalbuminemia

Causes of hypoalbuminemia can be divided into two groups pathophysiologically: increased albumin loss and decreased albumin synthesis.

Table 78–1 *Reference Values for Agarose Electrophoresis*

Electrophoretic Zones	Canine	Feline
Albumin g/dl	2.2 to 3.5	2.5 to 3.9
α_1 g/dl	0.5 to 0.8	0.2 to 0.5
α_2 g/dl	0.5 to 0.8	0.8 to 1.1
β_1 g/dl	0.5 to 1.1	0.3 to 0.5
β_2 g/dl	0.3 to 0.7	0.3 to 0.6
γ g/dl	0.5 to 1.8	1.2 to 3.2

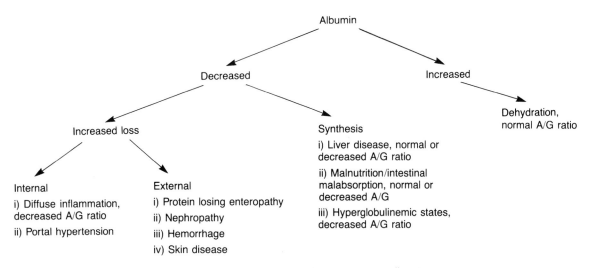

Figure 78–3. *Interpretation of changes in serum albumin.*

Increased Albumin Loss

Serum albumin loss can be internal (lost from the circulation while remaining in the body) or external (*e.g.,* nephropathy, enteropathy, skin diseases).

INTERNAL LOSS. In areas of diffuse inflammation, leakage of serum proteins into the affected area results in decreased serum albumin. The τ-globulin concentration remains normal or increases from antigenic stimulation. Hypoalbuminemia may be seen in pleuritis, peritonitis, or hemorrhagic pancreatitis. Severe trauma or inflammation increases catabolism and shortens albumin half-life, contributing to the hypoalbuminemia. A similar increased catabolism of protein occurs in the febrile stages of inflammation and in gastrointestinal malabsorption.

Portal hypertension results from intrahepatic or posthepatic obstruction of portal venous flow. Hepatic lymph production increases, and, when the capacity of the thoracic duct is exceeded, the hepatic lymph escapes from the space of Disse, percolates through the liver capsule, and accumulates in the peritoneal cavity leading to hypoalbuminemia (see Chapter 11).

EXTERNAL LOSS. The plasma albumin concentration decreases after severe hemorrhage, as the plasma volume is restored faster than the plasma protein. Peak depression occurs by 24 hours and is normal within a week (sooner than the red blood cell parameters). Therefore, an anemia with a normal plasma protein suggests the anemia is not likely hemorrhagic in origin.

Gastrointestinal disease also alters serum protein concentrations in a number of ways. Malabsorption of nutrients, loss of appetite, and enteric protein loss all contribute to decreased serum protein concentration. The digestion and assimilation of nutrients is mediated intraluminally by pancreatic and biliary secretions and by enzymes on the surface of the enterocytes. Pancreatic exocrine insufficiency due to pancreatic hypoplasia or repeated episodes of pancreatic necrosis can, therefore, lead to maldigestion and a decrease in serum protein concentration. In erosive lesions, loss of red blood cells and plasma proteins can be extensive. If hypoproteinemia coexists with anemia, blood loss due to intestinal neoplasia, bleeding ulcers, or parasitism should be ruled out. With increased vascular permeability due to inflammation, increased intrapropial hydrostatic pressure (*e.g.,* congestive heart failure), or lymphatic obstruction, the permeability of tight junctions between epithelial cells can be damaged, permitting transport of plasma protein and nonselective protein loss.

In dogs, several gastrointestinal disorders are commonly associated with protein loss. Lymphangiectasia results in chronic diarrhea, lymphopenia, decreased serum protein, and decreased cholesterol concentrations. Histologically, dilation of lacteals and lymphatics of the submucosa, intestinal wall, serosa, and mesentery are present. Eosinophilic gastroenteritis affects all breeds, but the German shepherd appears at increased risk. The disease is usually segmental, affecting any one area of the gastrointestinal tract. In cats, a hypereosinophilic syndrome can involve many organs, including the gastrointestinal tract. Both disorders are associated with hypoproteinemia (see Chapter 37).

Lymphocytes and plasma cells infiltrate the lamina propria of the villi and crypts in the syndrome lymphocytic plasmacytic enteritis. The Lundehund and Basenji are at increased risk, but the disease may occur in any dog or cat. Chronic diarrhea and wasting are accompanied by a decreased serum albumin and increased α_2- and τ-globulins, resulting in a low A:G ratio (0.21–0.5). Other causes of hypoproteinemia associated with gastrointestinal disease include granulomatous enteritis and colitis (histoplasmosis), amyloidosis, ulcerative colitis, intestinal tumors (lymphoma), congestive heart failure, and intestinal parasites.

Decreased serum protein concentrations are associated with lesions involving large areas of the skin. In patients with extensive burns or superficial trauma, exudation of albumin and globulin can be marked.

In healthy kidneys, only small quantities of albumin are filtered, and 90% of it is reabsorbed by the renal tubules. With glomerular disease, albumin leaks into the filtrate. As the glomerular lesions progress, larger proteins pass into the filtrate, including τ-globulins. The glomerular protein loss eventually results in hypoproteinemia. With the decrease in albumin concentration, the accompanying decrease in plasma oncotic pressure results in a decrease in intravascular volume. The renin-angiotensin system is then activated, with accompanying increases in antidiuretic hormone and aldosterone secretion. As a result, the kidneys retain sodium and water. The decreased oncotic pressure of plasma also reduces fluid removal from the interstitial tissues. These factors all contribute to the edema associated with hypoproteinemia levels frequently seen in the nephrotic syndrome. Generally, serum albumin levels less than 10–15 g/L (1–1.5 g/dl) may be associated with edema. In the early stages of glomerular disease, albumin decreases while globulins remain normal, resulting in a decreased A:G ratio. Eventually this ratio normalizes as globulins are also lost (see Chapter 45).

Normal dog urine contains less than 20 mg of protein/kg per 24 hours. Determination of the protein:creatinine ratio in a single sample is more practical and correlates closely with a 24-hour sample. In dogs with primary glomerulonephropathy, the ratio is generally greater than 1.0.

Decreased Albumin Synthesis

MALNUTRITION AND INTESTINAL MALABSORPTION. In cases of prolonged malnutrition due to starvation or severe intestinal malabsorption, plasma albumin concentrations eventually decrease. However, this decrease requires prolonged starvation as extravascular albumin is redistributed to the intravascular pool. When animals are deprived of food or are on protein-deficient diets, albumin synthesis decreases by 50% within 24 hours. To compensate, the fractional and absolute degradation rates decrease, thereby conserving the available albumin pool. The plasma protein concentration thus regulates the metabolic rate of production or degradation.

LIVER DISEASE. Hepatocytes synthesize proteins and secrete them into the space of Disse where they enter the sinusoidal blood. Most proteins are catabolized by the reticuloendothelial system of the liver. In chronic liver disease, decreased functional hepatic mass leads to decreased synthesis of albumin, resulting in a decreased A:G ratio. However, 60% to 80% of the hepatic mass must be lost before this process occurs. Increased synthesis of IgA and IgG in chronic liver disease explains the electrophoretic phenomenon of β-τ bridging seen in chronic active hepatitis.

Hypoalbuminemia can be seen in liver disease even when synthetic capacity is normal. Obstruction of the intrahepatic portal venous system inhibits return of interstitial fluid from the viscera to the portal circulation. In portal hypertension, newly synthesized albumin also leaks into the abdominal cavity through the liver capsule. Extravascular albumin pooling, edema, and ascites result.

The decrease in plasma oncotic pressure and plasma volume due to hypoalbuminemia causes renal sodium and water retention. This retention further dilutes the serum albumin levels and exacerbates the hypoalbuminemia and edema.

In liver disease, there is decreased synthesis of the coagulation factors and a potential for hemorrhage, with further loss of protein.

INHIBITED SYNTHESIS. When globulins increase, a concomitant decrease in albumin occurs. This inverse relationship exists regardless of the cause for increased τ-globulin concentration. This relationship is due to a decrease in hepatic synthesis of albumin likely in response to increased oncotic pressure or viscosity of the blood perfusing the liver.

The mechanism for decreasing albumin is most sensitive with small increases in τ-globulin and becomes less efficient at higher concentrations. In animals, decreased albumin levels are commonly seen in hyperglobulinemic states (*e.g.*, severe chronic inflammation and myeloma).

α- AND β-GLOBULINS

The α- and β-globulins represent a diverse group of serum proteins. Included in this group are α_1-antitrypsin, orosomucoid, haptoglobin, α_2-macroglobulin, ceruloplasmin, transferrin, complement (C3), and hemopexin. α_1-Antitrypsin, orosomucoid, haptoglobin, and C-reactive protein (which migrates in the τ region) are the principle members of the group of acute reacting proteins. The acute phase proteins are a component of the overall systemic response to infection, inflammation, or tissue damage. The acute reacting proteins in humans are well documented and are routinely assayed in any patient with a potential inflammatory disorder. Acute reacting proteins are especially useful when the leukocyte count is either normal or elevated due to leukemia and, therefore, not indicative of inflammation. Concomitant decreases in concentrations of albumin, transferrin, α- and β-lipoproteins are also seen. α_2-Macroglobulin does not participate in the acute phase response.

Most of the acute phase proteins are synthesized by hepatocytes. Stimulus for their production is mediated by macrophage products (interleukin-1) released as a result of trauma, bacteria, viruses, fungal infection, ischemic necrosis, allergic inflammation, or neoplasia. Increased circulating levels of acute phase proteins are due to de novo hepatic synthesis. Even with massive utilization of amino acids for repair of damaged tissue, the acute phase response goes on unabated, indicating its importance to survival. Their exact role is still poorly understood but likely involves restricting injury and promoting resolution and repair of damaged tissue.

The acute phase response in the dog and cat has not been adequately studied; however, routine analysis of the acute phase proteins in dogs and cats would be useful in assessing response to treatment or postoperative recovery. Several studies have suggested that C-reactive protein in the dog rises quickly after induction of inflammation, peaking on days 1 to 3 at values approximately 1000 times the normal serum level.

α₁-Protease Inhibitor/Formerly Antitrypsin

α_1-Protease inhibitor is a glycoprotein found in the α_1 electrophoretic region with a molecular weight of 54,000 daltons. It has a half-life of 5 to 7 days. It is involved in the inactivation or neutralization of many proteolytic enzymes including chymotrypsin, elastase, collagenase, thrombin, and trypsin. In humans, a deficiency of α_1-AT leads to loss of lung elasticity and emphysema. In dogs with induced inflammation, serum α_1-AT increased approximately 50%.

Orosomucoid

Orosomucoid is a glycoprotein also found in the α_1 region with a molecular weight of 40,000 daltons and a half-life of 5 days. Its high lipid content prevents it from staining clearly on the electrophoretic strip. In dogs, orosomucoid increased to 17 times its normal value after turpentine-induced abscesses. It may, therefore, prove one of the most useful acute reacting proteins in dogs, indicative of inflammation.

α_2-Macroglobulin (α_2-M)

α_2-Macroglobulin is an α_2-glycoprotein with a molecular weight of 900,000 daltons. It inhibits trypsin, chymotrypsin, plasmin, kallikrein, thrombin, and elastase and as such is very important in coagulation and fibrinolysis. It does not participate in the acute phase response. A significant increase in α_2-M is seen in the nephrotic syndrome. The increased serum levels may be due to loss of plasma volume with selective retention of high molecular weight proteins. Some evidence for increased half-life or increased rate of synthesis also exists.

Haptoglobin (Hp)

Haptoglobin is an α_2-globulin, molecular weight 100,000 daltons, with a half-life of 5 days. It binds α and β dimers of hemoglobin through globin chain attachment. This irreversible complex is rapidly cleared via specific hepatic receptor sites and degraded to bilirubin and iron. These complexes, therefore, prevent renal excretion of heme, serving as an iron trap (Fig. 78-4). Unbound Hp is measured spectrophotometrically by estimating the total hemoglobin-binding capacity. It is reported as milligrams of cyanmethemoglobin-binding capacity per deciliter. Normal serum Hp levels in the dog and cat are 20 to 190 mg/dl.

Haptoglobin is an important component of the acute phase response. Hepatic Hp synthesis in-

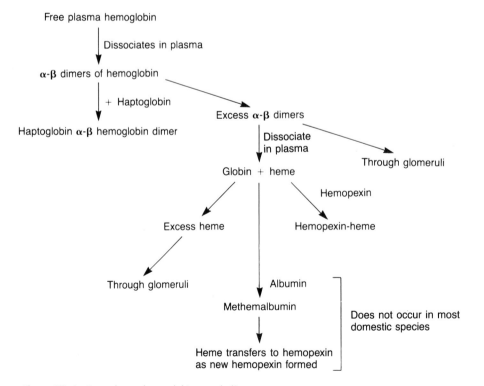

Figure 78–4. *Free plasma hemoglobin metabolism.*

creases in response to inflammation. With experimentally induced inflammation in the dog, plasma Hp concentration peaked on day four at four to 10 times normal levels. In two cats with experimental abscesses, one cat after splenectomy, and cats with feline infectious peritonitis, plasma Hp levels were increased two to four times normal serum levels.

Ceruloplasmin

Ceruloplasmin is an α_2-glycoprotein, molecular weight 160,000 daltons, with a half-life of 4 to 7 days. Normal serum concentrations are too low to be detected on an electrophoretic strip stained for protein. Ceruloplasmin is important in the transport of copper, in the mobilization of iron from tissue storage sites, and in protecting lipids from auto-oxidation. Ceruloplasmin is a participant in the acute phase response. In the dog, serum levels increase slowly (over 1–2 weeks) and slowly return to normal. Decreased concentrations of ceruloplasmin in humans are associated with the genetic defect Wilson's disease. Inherited copper toxicosis in Bedlington terriers is similar to Wilson's disease. Massive accumulation of copper in the liver, kidney, and brain with progressive hepatic cirrhotic change is a feature of the disease in humans and Bedlingtons. A defect in biliary excretion of copper in common to both, as is increased excretion of urinary copper. However, although serum ceruloplasmin is decreased in 90% to 95% of affected people, it is normal in Bedlingtons.

Hemopexin

Hemopexin is a β-globulin with a molecular weight of 70,000 daltons. When hemoglobin is released in excess of the haptoglobin-binding capacity, the unbound hemoglobin dissociates into its heme and globin components. The ferrous heme iron (Fe^{+2}) is oxidized to ferric iron (Fe^{+3}) on exposure to plasma and then binds to hemopexin in an equimolar ratio. This heme-hemopexin complex is carried to the liver where heme oxygenase begins the conversion of heme to bilirubin.

In humans, if the hemopexin capacity becomes saturated, the heme binds to albumin, forming methemalbumin until newly synthesized hemopexin becomes available for binding. Apparently, dog albumin does not bind heme in this way (see Fig. 78-4). As plasma haptoglobin is rapidly depleted with intravascular hemolysis, hemopexin may more accurately reflect the degree of hemolysis.

Transferrin

Transferrin is one of the main components of the β-globulins (approximately 50%) and has a molecular weight of 74,000 daltons. It is synthesized primarily in the liver, but some synthesis occurs in lymphoid tissue and peripheral blood lymphocytes. Transferrin binds two moles of free iron in the ferric form (Fe^{+3}). Ceruloplasmin oxidizes the Fe^{+2} to Fe^{+3} as a preliminary step for binding of Fe^{+3} to transferrin.

Plasma transferrin concentration is estimated indirectly by measuring plasma total iron-binding capacity (TIBC). The transferrin-iron complex appears red. As iron is added to serum, an increase in this red color develops and gives a measure of the unsaturated iron-binding capacity of the serum (UIBC). The sum of this measurement and the serum iron (SI), measured spectrophotometrically, gives the TIBC. The percent saturation of transferrin is frequently used as an index of Fe deficiency and is calculated as follows: SI $\div$ TIBC $\times$ 100 = % saturation.

Levels in the dog and cat are given in Table 78-2.

Transferrin functions in the transport of iron from the intestine to iron storage sites (especially the liver, spleen, and bone marrow) where iron is

Table 78–2 *Reference Value for Serum Iron and Iron-Binding Capacities in Dogs and Cats*

	Dog	**Cat**
SI (μg/dl)	72.6 to 189.8	68 to 215
TIBC (μg/dl)	362.9 to 474.6	173 to 420
% Saturation	16 to 40	16 to 40

stored as ferritin or hemosiderin and to cells that synthesize iron containing compounds (hemoglobin, myoglobin, cytochromes). Bone marrow cells of the erythroid series have specific surface receptors for transferrin iron. The transferrin iron complex is internalized, and the iron is used for hemoglobin production. The transferrin is then re-released to plasma.

Plasma concentrations of transferrin are altered in disorders of iron metabolism. With chronic inflammation, infection, trauma, or neoplasia, there are disturbances of iron utilization, characterized by a mild normochromic, normocytic, nonresponsive anemia. In these conditions, the unifying mediator is interleukin-1 released from inflammatory cells. Interleukin release results in decreased release of iron to the bone marrow for red blood cell production, decreased intestinal iron absorption, and decreased hepatic release of iron stores. This process can be assessed clinically as a decrease in serum iron concentration and a decreased transferrin percent saturation. It is associated with normal or increased iron stores in the bone marrow. Transferrin concentration may decrease as well. Similar changes are seen in cats. Cats also show a marked decrease in erythrocyte survival time.

In true iron deficiency anemia in dogs, the serum iron and percent saturation decrease, although the TIBC remains normal (Table 78-3). Accompanying decreases in the hematocrit, mean corpuscular volume (MCV) and mean corpuscular hemoglobin concentration (MCHC) are also present. The presence or absence of stainable bone marrow iron is useful in differentiating the anemia of chronic disease from true iron deficiency anemia (being absent in this disorder in adult animals).

C-Reactive Protein (CRP)

C-reactive protein is a unique protein found in the τ-globulin region but at serum concentrations far too low to affect the normal electrophoretic strip. It has a half-life of 4 to 6 hours. It is named for its reaction with the C polysaccharide of pneumococcus. It increases nonspecifically in most inflammatory states. Peak concentrations of CRP correlate well with the degree of tissue damage in humans. C-reactive protein has the most dramatic increase of all acute reacting proteins, rising and returning to normal the fastest. It fulfills most of the criteria for an ideal acute reacting protein, as it is undetectable in normal sera and has a large and rapid increase as well as rapid decrease, making secondary responses detectable. C-reactive protein in dogs under experimental conditions responds rapidly to inflammation and may be a useful screening technique when canine specific assays become available.

Fibrinogen

Fibrinogen is a large (molecular weight 340,000 daltons) fibrous protein consumed in the clotting process. It is, therefore, found only in plasma. It migrates as a broad band in the β region. Fibrinogen is a dimer, each half of which is formed of three polypeptide chains (α, β, τ) connected by disulfide bonds. Fibrinogen is essential to coagulation. Factor Xa, once activated by the intrinsic or extrinsic pathway in combination with factor V, converts prothrombin to thrombin, which then converts fibrinogen to fibrin monomers. These monomers polymerize and in the presence of factor XIIIa form a stable clot.

Fibrinogen can be measured clinically by measuring the plasma protein (on the refractometer) before and after precipitating fibrinogen by heating. Two microhematocrit tubes are filled with plasma, and the plasma protein content of one tube is measured with a refractometer. The other tube is placed in a 56°C water bath for 3 minutes

Table 78–3 *Serum Iron and Iron-Binding Capacities in Iron-Deficient and Normal Dogs*

Iron Capacities	Iron Deficient		Reference Values	
	Mean	Range	Mean	Range
SI (μg/dl)	30	(8–60)	149	(84–233)
UIBC (μg/dl)	357	(216–633)	243	(142–393)
TIBC (μg/dl)	387	(234–659)	391	(284–572)
% Saturation	8	(2–19)	39	(19.0–59.3)

(Harvey JW, French TW, Meyer DJ. Chronic iron deficiency in dogs. J. American Animal Hospital Association. 1982:18. 946.)

to precipitate the fibrinogen, then recentrifuged, and the protein remeasured. The difference in the refractometer readings represents the fibrinogen concentration. Alternatively, after heating and recentrifugation, the length of the fibrinogen column and total plasma column are measured under the microscope. The ratio of the length of the fibrinogen column to the total plasma is multiplied by 100. The resulting figure is equal to the fibrinogen concentration in g/L. Both measurements are slightly inaccurate and give lower concentrations than reference methods. Diagnostic laboratories obtain fibrinogen concentrations by using a fibrometer and measuring the thrombin time. When thrombin is added to diluted plasma, the time of clotting is linearly related to the fibrinogen concentration.

Fibrinogen is considered an acute reacting protein. It does not appear to be as useful an indicator of inflammation in the dog and cat as in the cow and horse. Fibrinogen can increase in any inflammatory, traumatic, or neoplastic condition. The increases in fibrinogen are not always proportional to the severity of the disease. Fibrinogen concentrations decrease in disseminated intravascular coagulation (DIC) and fibrinolysis due to consumption. However, conditions associated with DIC are often associated with extensive inflammation (tending to increase plasma fibrinogen levels). Thus, a normal or increased plasma fibrinogen level is difficult to interpret in these situations. As fibrinogen is produced by the liver, severe hepatic insufficiency can lead to decreased plasma levels.

The erythrocyte sedimentation rate (ESR) is now an infrequently used diagnostic test in animals. The ESR is positively influenced by rouleaux formation (high molecular weight proteins) and, therefore, plasma concentrations of fibrinogen, $_2$-globulin, and globulin. The ESR is negatively affected by reticulocytes, plasma albumin, and the number of red blood cells. Previously, it was used as an indication of acute inflammation (increased plasma fibrinogen). Direct measurement of plasma fibrinogen has replaced the ESR in most laboratories, although the two do not always correlate. In myelomas associated with elevated levels of IgM paraproteins (macroglobulinemia), a point may be reached where the

increased plasma viscosity inhibits sedimentation of the red blood cells, and, therefore, a high plasma protein is associated with a normal or decreased ESR.

IMMUNOGLOBULINS

Immunoglobulins in serum are found in the β and τ zones of the electrophoretic strip. IgA, IgG, and IgM are present at concentrations in normal serum to influence the electrophoretic pattern. Measurement of serum immunoglobulin concentrations is a common diagnostic procedure. Levels of β- and τ-globulin can be estimated from the electrophoretic strip after densitometer scanning. However, quantitation of individual immunoglobulin classes requires immunologic techniques. Radial immunodiffusion is the most frequently used method but is quickly being replaced by the more sensitive and reproducible enzyme-linked immunosorbent assay (ELISA). These tests are available at most diagnostic laboratories. Values for normal immunoglobulin concentrations in dogs and cats vary due to different laboratory techniques and the absence of reference laboratory standards. Normal reference values from my laboratory for dogs and cats are listed in Table 78-4.

In veterinary medicine, the measurement of serum immunoglobulins is important in three clinical situations: hypoglobulinemia, polyclonal hyperglobulinemia, and monoclonal hyperglobulinemia.

Hypoglobulinemia

Hypoglobulinemia is an important clinical entity in calves, foals, lambs, and kids, where failure of passive transfer leads to increased susceptibility

Table 78–4 *Normal Serum Immunoglobulin Concentrations*

Immunoglobulin	Canine	Feline
IgA (mg/dl)	100 ± 60	102−582
IgM (mg/dl)	150 ± 50	60−390
IgG (mg/dl)	1500 ± 500	1171−2258

to bacterial and viral infections. In dogs, similar decreases in immunoglobulins of colostrum-deprived pups are seen; however, associated illness is not as well documented.

Hypoglobulinemia is also seen in severe cases of protein-losing enteropathy and nephropathy where enterocyte and glomerular damage is severe and protein loss is nonselective. With hemorrhage, both albumin and globulins are lost and both are further diluted as tissue fluids enter the circulation to maintain blood volume.

Polyclonal Hyperglobulinemia

An increase in plasma immunoglobulin concentrations can be seen with a number of diseases (Table 78-5). A nonimmunologic mechanism is seen in dehydration.

Polyclonal gammopathies are caused by a large number of different B cell clones producing increased amounts of immunoglobulin. Electrophoresis detects an increase in the β- and τ-globulin region. No one specific immunoglobulin class is involved, and the magnitude of increase is less than in monoclonal gammopathy. An increase in acute reacting proteins is often associated with it. Polyclonal increases are associated with any chronic inflammatory condition or immune mediated disorder. Thus, they are seen with systemic lupus erythematosus, rheumatoid arthritis, feline infectious peritonitis, infectious canine hepatitis, pyometra, feline cho-langiohepatitis, infection with *leishmania*, *ehrlichia*, or neoplasia.

The terminal stages of tropical canine pancytopenia are associated with a doubling of the τ-globulin concentration. Leishmaniasis is frequently associated with a marked hypergammaglobulinemia (total serum protein 12–14 g/L [1.2–1.4 g/dl], globulin 50–90 g/L [5–9 g/dl]) and increased numbers of benign plasma cells in the bone marrow.

Increases in serum α_2-, β-, and τ-globulin are seen in feline infectious peritonitis. Total serum protein greater than 78 g/L (7.8 g/dl) is seen in 55% of effusive and in more than 70% of noneffusive cases of feline infectious peritonitis. Polyclonal increases in IgG account for most of the protein concentration increase, but increased β-globulin (likely due to complement) and increased α_2-globulin (likely haptoglobin) are also seen.

Monoclonal Gammopathy

Monoclonal gammopathies appear as a narrow based sharply defined peak, usually in the β or τ region (Fig. 78-5). The peak should be as narrow and as clearly defined as the albumin peak, as it represents a band of homogeneous immunoglobulin. Monoclonal gammopathies are associated with lymphoproliferative neoplasms and should be regarded as evidence for a functional B cell neoplasm. In humans "benign" monoclonal

---

Table 78–5 *Common Causes of Hyperglobulinemia*

Polyclonal	Monoclonal
Systemic lupus erythematosus	Myeloma
Rheumatoid arthritis	B cell leukemia
Feline infectious peritonitis	B cell lymphoma
Infectious canine hepatitis	"Benign" idiopathic
Pyometra	
Feline cholangiohepatitis	
Neoplasia	
Immune hemolytic anemia	
Any chronic inflammatory condition	
Leishmania	
Ehrlichia	

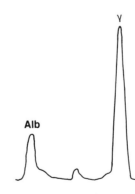

Figure 78–5. *Agarose gel electrophoretogram of a monoclonal gammopathy in the dog.*

gammopathies are occasionally found on routine electrophoretograms. A high incidence of developing myeloma and lymphoma occurs within this group.

Monoclonal gammopathies are associated with myeloma, B cell leukemia (chronic), and B cell lymphoma.

Myelomas

Myelomas represent 1% of hematopoietic canine tumors and are rare in the cat. The main clinical features of myeloma include monoclonal spike (IgG, IgM or IgA); lytic bone lesions of the long bones or flat bones; Bence Jones proteinuria; and plasma cell infiltration of bone marrow.

At the same time that the excess monoclonal protein is produced, development of normal clones of plasma cells are inhibited. Decreased T cell and complement function have also been associated with myeloma. Therefore, an increased incidence of recurrent infections, especially of the urinary and respiratory tract, are seen.

Hyperglobulinemia is seen in approximately 80% of myelomas in the dog. Several cases of nonsecretory myelomas in the dog, associated with plasmacytosis and lytic bone lesions, are reported. As well, solitary plasmacytomas have been reported in the gastrointestinal tract of the dog, unassociated with monoclonal spikes.

Diagnosis of multiple myeloma depends on clinical signs, radiographs, and laboratory assessment. The clinical signs are a manifestation of the excess immunoglobulin. Lethargy, depression, generalized pain, bone pain, and fractures are common presenting signs. Increased bleeding tendencies, especially into the gastrointestinal tract, occurs as a result of immunoglobulins complexing with platelets, causing a thrombocytopathia or immunoglobulin-binding coagulation proteins inhibiting their function. The large molecular weight of IgM (approximately 900,000 daltons) causes hyperviscosity of the blood when serum levels are increased, as in monoclonal gammopathy. IgA in canine serum is a dimer and may form a high molecular weight polymer, thus also increasing serum viscosity. The syndrome is rare in IgG myelomas. Hyperviscosity syndrome is associated with lethargy, weakness, depression, congestive heart failure, distended retinal veins, and a bleeding diathesis. The dogs often present with vague central nervous system deficits difficult to localize on neurologic examination.

The viscosity of serum is influenced by the concentration, degree of aggregation, molecular weight, and shape of the serum proteins, as well as by red blood cell numbers and the circulatory system status. Serum viscosity is measured using a viscosimeter. The time required for the test serum vs. water to flow through the viscosimeter column is measured. Normal viscosity is between 1 and 2. Hyperviscosity signs can appear at values of 4. Increases in serum immunoglobulins can also be seen on the peripheral smear, as an increased blue background and rouleaux formation. To qualify and quantify the offending immunoglobulins, immunoelectrophoresis, immunofixation and radial immunodiffusion are routinely performed.

Lytic bone lesions are present in approximately 60% of cases of multiple myeloma. Animals present with acute lameness due to pathologic fractures or neurologic signs associated with fractured vertebra. Increased serum calcium is frequently associated with multiple myeloma in dogs, especially in cases of severe osteolysis. These dogs are frequently hypercalciuric, and a normal calcium balance is maintained if adequate hydration and normal kidney formation are present. Prolonged hypercalcemia leads to renal tubular impairment and azotemia, frequently with resulting hypercalcemia (see Chapter 72). Some paraproteins actively bind calcium, and, although the total serum calcium is increased, no increase in free ionized calcium occurs.

Renal amyloidosis is a frequent complication of myelomas, leading to renal failure in humans, but seems less common in dogs.

Occasionally associated with the monoclonal protein is the presence of light chains in the urine Bence Jones proteins. These light chains have a molecular weight of approximately 16,000 daltons and pass easily through the glomeruli. They are found in 25% to 35% of canine myelomas. This persistent proteinuria eventually leads to renal tubular failure.

The detection of Bence Jones proteinuria can

be difficult. The routine protein dipstick does not detect Bence Jones proteins. Bence Jones proteins have the unique capacity to precipitate at 56°C and then redissolve as the sample is reheated to 100°C. This method is the most frequently utilized mode of detection, although the preferred technique involves concentration of the urine followed by immunoelectrophoresis or immunofixation.

Plasma cell infiltration of the bone marrow is the definitive technique for diagnosis of multiple myeloma. Normal dogs have low numbers of plasma cells in the marrow. With severe chronic inflammatory conditions, this percent can increase to 5% to 10%. In myeloma, the percent of plasma cells present is often markedly increased. The presence of large clusters of abnormally proliferating plasma cells is the key to diagnosis. Malignant plasma cells frequently demonstrate increased nuclear to cytoplasmic ratio, multiple prominent irregular nucleoli, binucleation, and a shaggy irregular nuclear contour. While aspiration bone marrow biopsy is frequently adequate, core biopsy is the approach of choice (see Bone Marrow Aspiration and Biopsy in Chapter 80). The malignant plasma cells often cluster in focal aggregates and thus can be missed if several core biopsy tissue sections are not obtained.

Infiltration of the bone marrow with plasma cells may inhibit myelopoiesis and erythropoiesis. Animals can, therefore, present with a combination of nonresponsive anemia or leukopenia. Occasionally, the anemia is immune mediated and, therefore, responsive in origin, owing to nonspecific adsorption of the elevated immunoglobulin onto the red blood cell membrane.

Thrombocytopenia can be due to marrow failure or consumption of platelets associated with chronic hemorrhage.

Chronic B Cell Leukemia and B Cell Lymphoma

Hyperviscosity syndrome associated with increased plasma monoclonal IgA or IgM was reported in three dogs with lymphoid leukemia. The dogs had increased blood and bone marrow lymphocytes. Lymphoma in the dog is also associated with monoclonal gammopathies. The frequency is unknown. These tumors are assumed to be functioning B cell clones.

ADDITIONAL READING

Degen MA, Breitschwerdt EB. Canine and feline immunodeficiency. Part II. Compendium of Continuing Education 1986; 8:379.

Duncan JR, Prasse KW. Veterinary laboratory medicine. Iowa: Iowa State University Press, 1986: 229.

Feldman BF, Kaneko JJ, Farver TB. Anemia of inflammatory disease in the dog: Ferrokinetics of adjuvant-induced anemia. Am J Vet Res 1981; 42:583.

Guilford WG. Primary immunodeficiency diseases of dogs and cats. Compendium of Continuing Education 1987; 9:641.

Harvey JW, French TW, Meyer DJ. Chronic iron deficiency anemia in dogs. Journal of the American Animal Hospital Association 1982; 18:946.

Shelly SM, Scarlett-Kranz J, Blue JT. Protein electrophoresis on effusions from cats as a diagnostic test for feline infectious peritonitis. Journal of the American Animal Hospital Association 1988; 24:495.

Williams DA. Gammopathies. Compendium of Continuing Education 1981; 3:815.

79

INTERPRETATION OF SERUM TITERS

Robert M. Jacobs

The use of serologic tests in veterinary medicine is widespread. Most commonly, the tests are used to detect individuals and groups affected by infectious diseases. In certain instances, serologic test results can be used to monitor response to treatment and to give a prognosis. Serologic tests are also used to detect autoimmune diseases and diseases with an immune pathogenesis.

Test kits for the detection of the most common infectious diseases are now available. These kits are designed for in-hospital use; however, they are usually available in commercial veterinary laboratories as well. Some commercial veterinary laboratories will also do testing for the less common diseases of veterinary importance. Generally, tests for zoonotic diseases are available through human and public health laboratories.

Many of the test systems marketed recently are based on monoclonal antibody technology. Consequently, the specificity and sensitivity of these tests are much improved. Despite this advance and advances in ease of performance, the tests should not be performed by untrained personnel. Appropriate positive and negative controls must be run at regular intervals to ensure the integrity of the test system.

The interpretation of serologic test results for common infectious agents is usually straightforward. Many test systems give a simple positive or negative test result, having been standardized by the manufacturer. When some test kits were introduced there were problems with manufacturer quality control, but most of the kits now appear to be highly reliable. Nevertheless, veterinarians and technical personnel should not ignore the fact that manufacturing errors do occur under the best of circumstances. If one is suspicious, the manufacturer should be contacted immediately. The burden of proof lies with the manufacturer. When referring sera for analysis to a commercial veterinary, human, or public health laboratory, it is up to the laboratory to provide guidelines for the interpretation of the test result. If the serologic test result and the physical abnormalities of the patient cannot be reconciled, the laboratory should be contacted and the test result confirmed.

The dilution of serum constituting a positive test result will vary between laboratories because of differences in technique, instrumentation, and source of antigen. Standardization of antigen sources is slowly occurring. Since titers are only approximate and interlaboratory variation is significant, laboratory personnel may be asked to assist in interpretation. Titers discussed in the following text are only general guidelines. For an animal sample sent to a human laboratory, the laboratory must be informed that it is an animal sample because in some tests, species-specific antisera must be used.

When interpreting serum titers, the patient should be considered in terms of state of the immune system (immunosuppression), vaccination history, and interference from maternal transfer of antibody. A single titer is often of no use for detecting infection with an agent that animals are commonly vaccinated against. In vaccinated animals, acute and convalescent serum samples are preferable. A positive test result indicates exposure, not necessarily active disease. The definitive diagnosis is by morphologic identification or culture. Without positive identification of an agent by cytology, biopsy, or culture, a positive serologic test result will give a presumptive diagnosis.

Where antigenic cross-reactivity is a problem, serologic tests should be requested for both (or multiple) agents involved; in this case, the one with the highest titer is assumed to be the primary agent. Acute and convalescent titers can help sort out cross-reactivity. When sending sera for indirect fluorescent antibody (IFA) or complement fixation (CF) tests or other assays in which the substrate or antigen is a cell culture or is not well-defined or standardized, it is best to send the acute (maintained by refrigeration) and convalescent serum samples at the same time, so that their reactivity is measured on the same quality of substrate simultaneously. This limits variation in titer due to changes in antigen expression in the substrate.

Tests that are positive early (within 2 weeks of exposure) are generally those designed to detect immunoglobin M (IgM), while those that become positive later (after 3 weeks) react with IgG. With those infectious agents that have a parasitemic phase, the antibody response peaks following parasitemia. Complement fixation tests are sometimes not useful in dogs because of the anticomplementary effect of some canine sera. In the future, molecular probes may replace serologic tools in the detection of infectious agents.

MYCOTIC DISEASES

Due to antigenic cross-reactivity between fungal agents it is difficult to interpret a single test result. It is often necessary to examine the reactivity of a serum sample to the group of systemic mycotic agents. The one eliciting the highest titer is assumed to be the pathogen. A fourfold increase in titer between acute and convalescent samples to one antigen is also helpful in making a presumptive diagnosis. With most mycotic infections, the antibody titer is often unrelated to the extent, duration, and outcome of infection, irrespective of treatment.

Aspergillosis

Agar gel immunodiffusion and counterimmunoelectrophoresis tests are used. A positive test result indicates exposure to *Aspergillus* or *Penicillium* organisms, since there is some antigenic cross-reactivity between the two agents. In dogs with chronic nasal discharge there is a high correlation of positive serologic test results and the presence of nasal aspergillosis. False-positive reactions generally do not occur, but false-negatives are seen.

Blastomycosis

Immunodiffusion, CF, counterimmunoelectrophoresis, and agar gel precipitin tests are used. A positive test result indicates at the least exposure to antigen, and possibly active infection. The immunodiffusion test in dogs has greater than 90% sensitivity and specificity in advanced cases. In acute cases the test is less reliable, since the antibody response may not have had time to develop sufficiently. With the immunodiffusion test there are no problems with antigenic cross-reactivity between *Blastomyces dermatitidis* and *Histoplasma capsulatum*. Other available tests are less commonly used because of cross-reactivity and unnecessary complexity. In addition to cross-reactivity problems, anticomplementary activity of canine serum limits the usefulness of the CF test. A CF titer greater than or equal to 1 : 8 has been considered positive. Antibody titers may decrease with the progression of disease, hence it is possible for an actively infected individual to be seronegative.

Candidiasis

Tests available are counterimmunoelectrophoresis, slide latex agglutination, and immunodiffusion. In humans, seroconversion, increase in the number of precipitin lines, or a fourfold or greater increase in titer are associated with systemic infection with *Candida* organisms. Interestingly, a fourfold decrease in titer is associated with successful antifungal therapy. Serologic tests for candidiasis in animals are considered unreliable.

Coccidioidomycosis

Complement fixation, immunodiffusion, counterimmunoelectrophoresis, and tube precipitin tests are used. The two tests used for detection of the canine disease are CF (despite the anticomplementary effect of canine serum) and tube precipitation. Suspect dogs are screened using immunodiffusion and then tested by CF. The interpretation of CF titers is as follows: less than 1:8 is negative, 1:8 is suspicious or represents early infection, and greater than or equal to 1:16 is positive. Titers usually parallel the extent and severity of disease, although antibody is not protective. Antibody titers decrease with treatment and increase upon relapse. Dogs with active infection can be negative on both tests if there is immunosuppression or if they are tested prior to the development of a sufficient immune response. If the physical findings continue to be suggestive, the patient should be retested in 2 weeks. Up to 40% of humans with chronic pulmonary infections are seronegative. A positive tube precipitin test and negative CF test indicates early infection in which the predominant immunoglobulin response is IgM (occurring 2–6 weeks after infection), to which the tube precipitin test is most sensitive. The CF test is more dependent on IgG concentration, and the CF titer peaks 8 to 10 weeks after infection or the increase in the IgM concentration. This temporal difference in immunoglobulin concentrations accounts for negative tube precipitin test and positive CF test results where there has been past exposure or a quiescent phase 4 to 5 weeks after active infection. In the few feline cases reported most CF test results were negative.

Cryptococcosis

Tests for the detection of antibody are of some use early in infection when there is little antigenemia. There is an inverse relationship between circulating cryptococcal antigen and antibody. Once the infection is well-established, individuals are often seronegative. With successful treatment antibody titers reappear, and therefore may be of prognostic value. Serologic responses are monitored using slide latex agglutination, tube agglutination, and IFA tests. Dogs and cats with active disease are generally seronegative.

A latex particle cryptococcal antigen test for detection of capsular antigen in cerebrospinal fluid, blood, urine, and other body cavity fluids has been developed. Since these latex particles are coated with antibody, sera from patients containing rheumatoid factor will cause false-positive test results. *Toxoplasma gondii* in cats has been reported to cross-react with cryptococcal antigens; this is another possible cause for false-positive reactions. False-negative reactions occur when there is nondisseminated disease and the cryptococcal burden is relatively low. Titers parallel the severity of disease and become negative with successful treatment. Titers as low as 1:16 have been reported in confirmed cases. The latex particle cryptococcal antigen test was used successfully in a small number of infected cats and should be widely used in dogs.

Histoplasmosis

The CF test is most widely used, but immunodiffusion, counterimmunoelectrophoresis, and latex agglutination tests may also be available. Generally, serologic tests for histoplasma are considered unreliable because of false-negative reactions and the anticomplementary activity of canine serum, making CF test results difficult or impossible to interpret. Some data indicate that in early infection the CF titer to the yeast phase antigens is strongest, while chronic disease is associated with high titers to the mycelial antigens. Infected dogs without active disease may have persistently increased titers.

Sporotrichosis

Slide latex, tube, and yeast cell agglutination tests are available, but have not been evaluated in animals.

RICKETTSIAL DISEASES

Ehrlichiosis

A highly sensitive and specific immunofluorescence test is widely used for the detection of antibody to *Ehrlichia canis*. A 1:10 titer (the lowest measured) is considered a positive test result. Positive titers can be detected as early as 7 days after exposure, but some dogs do not seroconvert for up to 30 days after exposure. Titers increase steadily with progression of the disease, but occasionally decrease quickly just before death. In successfully treated dogs the titers decrease steadily over several months, while in chronically infected dogs the titers remain increased. Dogs that are successfully treated can be reinfected. There is no relationship between the degree of hyperglobulinemia, which is commonly observed, and the titer. There is little or no antigenic cross-reactivity with *E. platys* (the agent of infectious canine cyclic thrombocytopenia) or *Rickettsia rickettsii* (the agent of Rocky Mountain spotted fever). There is no antigenic cross-reactivity between *E. canis* and one of the causative agents of salmon poisoning disease, *Neorickettsia helminthoeca*. The physical signs of acute ehrlichiosis and Rocky Mountain spotted fever are similar; therefore, acute and convalescent titers to both agents should be determined.

A fluorescent antibody test has been described to detect serum antibody in dogs infected with *E. platys*. In Florida about 5% of dogs in pounds, 35%

of thrombocytopenic dogs, and 54% of thrombocytopenic dogs with *E. canis* infection were seropositive for *E. platys*. The infection is widespread, and a common route of transmission is likely.

Dogs and cats are susceptible to infection with *E. risticii*, the agent of equine monocytic ehrlichiosis, and *E. equi*. With *E. risticii* there is serologic evidence for widespread infection of dogs and cats in endemic areas, but only infected cats show illness. Experimental *E. equi* infection in dogs and cats does not cause disease. Dogs infected with *E. equii* are not protected from infection with *E. canis*. There is little or no antigenic cross-reactivity between these two agents and *E. canis*.

Rocky Mountain Spotted Fever

Complement fixation, microagglutination, and microscopic immunofluorescence tests have been used to detect Rocky Mountain spotted fever infection in dogs. Generally, titers are not significantly increased for 2 or 3 weeks after exposure, which makes them of limited usefulness in the acute stages. Acute and convalescent sera should be submitted so that a presumptive diagnosis can be made. Antibody titers remain increased for prolonged periods (3–5 months) despite effective therapy, and will often remain above levels seen in unexposed individuals for up to 1 year. The CF test for Rocky Mountain spotted fever may show cross-reactivity with typhus antigens, and for a presumptive diagnosis one must demonstrate a fourfold increase in titer. The CF test is least sensitive, the microagglutination test is of intermediate sensitivity, and the microimmunofluorescence test is the most sensitive. The latter test is now the most widely used test for the serologic diagnosis of Rocky Mountain spotted fever, not only because of its high sensitivity but also because IgG and IgM antibodies can be detected. Because an IgM titer can be determined, the test is useful in identifying recent infection from a single serum sample. Using the microimmunofluorescence test, unexposed dogs and dogs with ehrlichiosis have titers less than 1:64. Actively infected dogs have titers greater than or equal to 1 : 128 and show a fourfold increase between acute and convalescent titers.

Salmon Poisoning Disease

There are no serologic tests available to detect infections with the two agents associated with this disease, *Neorickettsia helminthoeca* and Elokomin Fluke Fever Agent. Although ultrastructurally identical, these two agents do not show antigenic cross-reactivity.

PROTOZOAL DISEASES

Babesiasis

An immunofluorescence test is used to detect occult infections in dogs. A titer greater than 1 : 40 is considered positive, representing active infection. The test has been criticized for its lack of discrimination between *Babesia canis* and *B. gibsoni*. This differentiation is important, since infections with the two organisms are treated differently. Apparently, young dogs infected with *B. canis* do not mount an antibody response, as measured by immunofluorescence. Following exposure, dogs generally seroconvert by 3 weeks.

Cytauxzoonosis

Tests for the serologic detection of the organism and serum antibody titers have been reported, but are only available in some research laboratories.

Encephalitozoonosis

Although several tests have been used experimentally in monitoring antibody titers, only the IFA test has been used in spontaneous cases. Using the IFA test, dogs seroconvert as early as 3 days following inoculation; cats show low titers at 2 weeks and significant titers at 4 to 5 weeks after inoculation. Antigenic cross-reactivity with other agents has not been determined, but random source dogs do not have titers. Active infection has been associated with a titer greater than or equal to 1 : 40.

Giardiasis

An IFA test to detect anti-*Giardia* antibodies is used in humans. Anti-*Giardia* antibodies were not identified consistently in infected dogs using an enzyme-linked immunosorbent assay (ELISA). A counterimmunoelectrophoresis test to detect *Giardia* antigen in human feces has been reported.

Hepatozoonosis

A serologic test has not been designed due to difficulties in antigen preparation.

Leishmaniasis

Complement fixation, ELISA, IFA, direct agglutination, and indirect hemagglutination tests are available. Complement fixation titers are detectable 7 to 12 weeks after infection. From 30% to 60% of dogs with positive titers have clinical signs, while an additional 40% of seropositive dogs develop clinical signs within 1 year. Antigenic cross-reactivity with the agent of Chagas' disease (*Trypanosoma cruzi*) is a problem in all tests except for CF.

Toxoplasmosis

Indirect hemagglutination, IFA, CF, and ELISA tests are available. The Sabin-Feldman dye test (which uses methylene blue dye), although highly specific and sensitive, is no longer widely used because it requires live organisms and is complex and not easily automated compared with most of the newer tests. The IFA test gives similar results to the Sabin-Feldman dye test; the Sabin-Feldman dye test is sensitive to both IgG and IgM antibodies, while the IFA test can be used to detect either antibody class.

The indirect hemagglutination test is simpler to perform and of equal specificity, but is less sensitive than the IFA test. The indirect hemagglutination test, since it detects only IgG antibody, does not show seroconversion for 22 to 30 days after infection, in contrast to 10 to 15 days with the more sensitive tests. Antibody titers are absent or low in the acute phases of infection. The ELISA is easily automated and can be used to measure both IgM and IgG antibodies. False-positive reactions may occur with the IFA and ELISA tests in association with immune complex diseases, such as systemic lupus erythematosus and rheumatoid disease.

Tests detecting IgM antibody or the CF test can be used on a single sample basis to assist in identifying acutely infected individuals. Specific IgM and CF titers rise quickly and generally do not persist for longer than 3 or 6 months, respectively. An IgM titer equal to or greater than 1 : 20 is associated with recent infection, while 1 : 80 is associated with active infection. With other test systems, paired serum samples showing a fourfold increase in titer over a 2- or 3-week period are required for a presumptive diagnosis of acute infection. In these systems, titers of 1 : 64 and 1 : 2 indicate past infection in dogs and cats, respectively; 1 : 256 and 1 : 64 to 1 : 256 indicate recent infection; and 1 : 1024 to 1 : 4096 and greater than or equal to 1 : 1024 suggest active infection. Titers in these tests generally persist for long periods of time; oocysts are generally not shed from cats that have measurable antibody titers, unless immunosuppressed.

Trypanosomiasis (American)

Complement fixation, IFA, ELISA, direct agglutination, and hemagglutination tests are commonly used. In humans, a titer equal to or greater than 1 : 512 in the direct agglutination test is specific for Chagas' disease. Antigenic cross-reactivity with leishmanial antigens is small with the direct agglutination and CF tests, but may limit the usefulness of other tests for differentiating the two diseases. Serum antibodies to *Trypanosoma cruzi* indicate present or past exposure. Most infected individuals with positive titers are sub-

clinical carriers. A positive titer may or may not be associated with active infection. Although this disease is difficult to treat, if successful, the antibody titers will decrease over time.

VIRAL DISEASES

Canine Adenovirus Type 2

This agent causes infectious laryngotracheitis. Virus neutralization and hemagglutination inhibition tests are available. A fourfold increase in titer between acute and convalescent sera indicates an active infection. The type 1 adenovirus is antigenically distinct.

Canine Coronavirus

Antibodies to this agent cross-react with antibodies to feline infectious peritonitis virus, transmissible gastroenteritis virus of swine, and mouse hepatitis virus. Serum titers are generally low, since there is no systemic spread of virus. A fourfold increase in IFA or virus neutralization titer indicates active infection.

Canine Distemper

Virus neutralization and ELISA tests are available. Both tests can be designed to measure either IgG or IgM antibodies. A virus neutralization titer equal to or greater than 1 : 100 is considered protective. A fourfold increase between acute and convalescent titers is presumptive evidence for active infection. A cerebrospinal fluid sample obtained atraumatically with a titer greater than the titer of a paired serum sample is supportive of chronic distemper encephalitis.

Canine Herpesvirus

Virus neutralization and IFA techniques are used to determine the serologic response to this agent. A fourfold increase between acute and convalescent titers supports the diagnosis. Antibody responses are persistent, thus it is difficult to differentiate recent and past exposure unless the virus-specific IgM and IgG concentrations are measured.

Canine Infectious Hepatitis

The etiologic agent is canine adenovirus type 1. Tests that are available for the detection of this rare disease include indirect hemagglutination, charcoal agglutination, CF, immunodiffusion, ELISA, and virus neutralization. A fourfold increase in titer between acute and convalescent sera is presumptive evidence for active infection.

Canine Parainfluenza

Virus neutralization and IFA tests are available. A fourfold increase in titer between acute and convalescent sera indicates active infection. In experimentally infected dogs, the cerebrospinal fluid antibody titers remain persistently increased.

Canine Parvovirus

The immune response to this agent is rapid. The viremic phase is terminated once serum-neutralizing antibody increases; this is often at the time clinical signs become apparent. Since the immune response is rapid and prolonged, acute and convalescent titers may be uniformly high, making it difficult to differentiate recent from previous exposure unless IgM antibodies are measured. Hemagglutination inhibition, virus neutralization, and IFA tests are used to detect serum antibody. The hemagglutination inhibition test is less sensitive than the virus neutralization test; generally the titers are three to five times greater with the virus neutralization test. Some investigators consider a hemagglutination inhibition titer equal to or greater than 1 : 80 to be protective. Antigenic cross-reactivity with other parvoviruses may make the interpretation of a titer difficult. The IgM component of the antibody response can be estimated by measuring the hemagglutination inhibition titer with and without mercaptoethanol.

Serologic tests for the presence of fecal antigen are hemagglutination, direct immunofluorescence, and ELISA tests. The hemagglutination test is most widely used, but is not as sensitive as other serologic tests or direct visualization by electron microscopy. Maximal fecal hemagglutination titers of 1 : 320 to 1 : 10,240 are seen at the commencement of clinical signs. Nonspecific fecal hemagglutinating activity can be controlled for using antiparvoviral antibody.

Canine Rotavirus

A group-specific antigen is shared among all rotavirus isolates. An ELISA test is available. The virus is widespread and generally causes mild disease.

Feline Calicivirus

Virus neutralization, IFA, and CF tests are available. A fourfold increase in serum titer between acute and convalescent sera indicates active infection. Viral antigen can be demonstrated in tissue sections using an IFA test.

Feline Enteric Coronaviruses

There are at least two distinct feline enteric coronaviruses, designated types 1 and 2. The type 1 virus is not associated with clinical disease, but it is infectious and is shed in feces. Antibodies to the type 1 virus do not cross-react in tests to detect antibody to the feline infectious peritonitis virus. The type 2 virus is morphologically and antigenically indistinguishable from the feline infectious peritonitis virus. The type 2 virus causes a mild transient diarrheal disease of neonates and kittens. Infected individuals show coronaviral titers as high as 1 : 1024 six weeks after infection. Antibodies to this agent cross-react with feline infectious peritonitis virus, transmissible gastroenteritis virus of swine, and canine coronavirus in IFA, ELISA, and virus neutralization tests. Reactivity to the type 2 virus probably accounts for a large percentage of cases formerly attributed to feline infectious peritonitis virus. Type 2-infected kittens are more susceptible to infection with feline infectious peritonitis virus and development of disease compared with seronegative kittens. Currently there are no monoclonal antibodies that differentiate the coronaviral enteritis agent and the coronavirus associated with feline infectious peritonitis virus.

Feline Immunodeficiency Virus

This virus was previously termed the *feline T-lymphotropic lentivirus*. An ELISA (CITE) to detect antifeline immunodeficiency virus antibody is widely available. In one unique test system (CITE Combo) both feline leukemia virus antigen and antifeline immunodeficiency virus antibody can be detected simultaneously. Cats seroconvert about 2 weeks after exposure. Since this disease is associated with potent immunosuppression, chronically infected cats that were previously seropositive may appear negative serologically. When test kits were initially available, some weak reactions were due to cross-reactivity with the feline syncytium-forming virus. It is important to check with the laboratory performing the test or the manufacturer about the potential for false-positive test results from antigenic cross-reactivity.

An ELISA test (Petcheck-FIV-Ag) used to detect feline immunodeficiency virus core antigen has recently become available. The test requires cultivation of cells *in vitro* and may be useful in a research setting. Further work is needed to establish a role for this test in clinical diagnosis.

Feline Infectious Peritonitis

Currently, antibody titers to the feline infectious peritonitis virus and other feline coronaviruses cannot be differentiated. Antibody responses are not protective and may be associated with increased morbidity. Tests used to detect serologic responses to the coronavirus family are the IFA, enzyme-linked immunofluorescence assay (including the kinetic form), and virus neutralization tests. Titers greater than 1 : 3200 are associated with active infections, most commonly of the noneffusive form. False-positive nonspecific reactions may occur in recently vaccinated cats. Apparently, this nonspecific reactivity decreases to low levels over 3 to 4 months after vaccination. Cats with the effusive form and cats infected with coronaviruses other than feline infectious peritonitis virus have titers between 1 : 100 and 1 : 3200. A fourfold increase between acute and convalescent titers is supportive of a diagnosis of feline infectious peritonitis virus if the clinical signs are appropriate.

Not only is there lack of specificity with these serologic tests, but low or negative titers are sometimes seen in actively infected cats, particularly kittens with the effusive form and aged cats with the noneffusive form. Some cats with active infections that are seronegative using the immunofluorescence test will produce antibody detectable by virus neutralization. The serologic test results must be interpreted in conjunction with the physical findings and the results of other laboratory tests. In those rare cases in which the treatment of feline infectious peritonitis is successful, there may be a decrease in feline infectious peritonitis virus antibody titer. Conversely, unsuccessful therapy is associated with gradually increasing or unchanging titers.

Feline Leukemia Virus

Viral antigen or viremia can be detected by virus isolation, IFA, and ELISA (CITE, ClinEase, DiaSystems Flex II, Leukassay FII, Leukotest, Virachek) tests. Virus isolation is a research tool and is not widely available. The IFA test detects viral antigen within nucleated cells and platelets. Eosinophils autofluoresce, and this may be a cause for a false-positive reaction. If there is peripheral pancytopenia, then a smear of bone marrow should be used in the IFA test (leukopenia may cause a false negative result with IFA testing). About 98% of cats that are positive and negative by the IFA test are correspondingly virus isolation positive and negative.

The ELISA detects viral antigen circulating in blood, plasma, or serum. The results of this test are less well correlated with virus excretion and contagious transmission. Hence, the results by

IFA and ELISA sometimes are discrepant. About 10% of ELISA-negative cats are IFA positive. These cats may have been recently exposed, or a latent infection (unexpressed feline leukemia virus compartmentalized to the bone marrow) may be in the process of reactivation. Corticosteroid therapy and stress at surgery are examples of events associated with reactivation of latent feline leukemia virus infections. If laboratory error is suspected, the ELISA and IFA tests should be repeated on the same sample, and if consistent, new samples should be analyzed in 6 to 8 weeks. Most cats that are positive initially remain positive and are considered persistently viremic; viremia regresses in only 3% of feline leukemia virus-positive cats.

Studies show that anywhere from 31% to 88% of ELISA-positive cats are IFA-positive. The percentages at the lower end of this range come from studies that were done shortly after test kits became widely available. There are generally three explanations for this excess of ELISA-positive cats. From 1% to 3% of cats have naturally occurring antimouse antibody. Since the test kits contain a mouse monoclonal antibody, cats with such antimouse activity show a false-positive reaction. Some ELISA test kits control for this activity; if the intensity of color development in the control sample is less than that for the test sample, then the cat can be considered infected. If the result is ambiguous, then an alternative testing system must be used. False-positive reactions may also occur with poor laboratory technique. The problems most often encountered are inadequate attention to washing and incubation times, careless splashing of reagents, and poor sample quality (partially clotted or hemolyzed blood). In the third instance, the reaction is not a false-positive reaction, but occurs because of compartmentalization of the feline leukemia virus in non-myeloid tissues.

The ELISA tests can also be done on saliva, urine, and tears (CITE, DiaSystems Flex II, Virastat). This may be useful if it is particularly difficult to obtain a blood sample or perhaps for screening a cattery. Tests done on these fluids tend to have more frequent false-negative test results, but false positive test results have also been reported.

Tests for measuring virus neutralization antibody and antibody response to feline leukemia virus glycoprotein antigen have been described, but are only available through research laboratories. Since titers in individual cats are difficult to interpret, the general feeling is that these tests have little significance for the practicing veterinarian.

An indirect membrane immunofluorescence test is used to determine the antibody titer to the feline oncornavirus-associated cell membrane antigen (FOCMA). Although the threshold antibody titer varies between laboratories from 1 : 4 to 1 : 32, a titer of 1 : 8 or greater is often quoted as being protective against the neoplastic consequences of feline leukemia virus infection. Before interpreting the result, the laboratory's recommended threshold protective FOCMA titer should be checked. A cat with a protective FOCMA titer has been exposed to feline leukemia virus and is protected against feline leukemia virus-related neoplasia, but may remain susceptible to all of the non-neoplastic consequences of infection if viremic. Generally, cats with a high FOCMA titer also have good virus neutralization activity, and are not often viremic. A cat with a negative FOCMA titer may be unexposed, latently infected, or viremic.

Latent feline leukemia virus infection is often difficult to diagnose. Stress and drug treatments may cause a recrudescence that can be detected by sequential tests for viremia or antigenemia. Some latently infected cats will have FOCMA antibody. Some practitioners submit bone marrow aspiration smears for the IFA test in the hopes of proving latent feline leukemia virus infection. Bone marrow aspiration smears are no better than peripheral blood smears as long as there is no peripheral pancytopenia. Feline leukemia virus may reside in bone marrow cells, and if cultured *in vitro* may be expressed. This test is only available in a small number of research laboratories.

Feline Panleukopenia

Virus neutralization, IFA, and hemagglutination inhibition tests are available. The virus neutralization test is the most commonly used. A fourfold increase in serum titer between acute and convalescent sera indicates active infection.

Feline Rhinotracheitis Virus

Virus neutralization, IFA, and CF tests are available. A fourfold increase in serum titer between acute and convalescent sera indicates active infection.

Feline Syncytium-Forming Virus

Hemagglutination, IFA, and immunodiffusion tests are performed in some research laboratories. Dual infections of this virus and feline leukemia virus occur frequently. It is not clear if this virus causes disease, but it has been associated with chronic progressive polyarthritis, lymphoma, and myeloproliferative disease. The presence of antibody indicates persistent viral infection.

Pseudorabies

Virus neutralization, immunodiffusion, and ELISA tests are very useful in detecting this infection in pigs. Virus neutralization testing was unsuccessful in identifying infected dogs during an outbreak. Titers in acute and convalescent serum samples may be useful, but most often the disease runs a peracute course, so serologic testing is not practical. Viral antigen can be detected by IFA on tissue sections.

Rabies

Tests to detect specific antibody are virus neutralization, neutralization in mice, rapid fluorescent-focus inhibition, gel diffusion, and CF tests. Viral antigen can be demonstrated using IFA and hemagglutination tests. Recent exposure to rabies virus can be determined in serum if IgM titers are measured. At 3 to 4 days after exposure the IgM titer begins to increase, and at about 40 days it starts to decrease. Immunoglobulin G titers begin rising at about 10 days after exposure, and are decreased at 1 year. In rabies encephalomyelitis, caused by either virulent or vaccine virus, the cerebrospinal fluid titer is higher than in a paired serum sample. The measurement of antibody titer in aqueous humor is unreliable. Monoclonal antibody technology can differentiate between vaccine and virulent strains of rabies virus.

BACTERIAL DISEASES

Bordatellosis

Serum agglutination and ELISA tests are available. The latter is the more rapid and sensitive test. Experimentally infected dogs developed low agglutination titers that persisted for only 2 months; protection against reinfection persisted for a slightly longer period. Generally, serum agglutination titers do not correlate with protection, whereas there is a close association of protection with local mucosal humoral immunity. Vaccination results in titers up to 1 : 512.

Borreliosis

The agent *Borrelia burgdorferi* can be identified in tissue samples by fluorescent antibody and immunoperoxidase techniques. Serum titers are measured by IFA and ELISA tests. There is some antigenic cross-reactivity with leptospira, but vaccination for leptospirosis is not believed to interfere with interpretation of serologic test results. Dogs with clinical symptoms generally have high titers (1 : 512–1 : 16,384), but some dogs in endemic areas have overlapping titers (less than 1 : 32–1 : 8912). In nonendemic areas the titers range from less than 1 : 32 to 1 : 256. Some laboratories suggest that titers equal to or greater that 1 : 64 and 1 : 150 in the IFA and ELISA tests, respectively, signify past infection. Serologic data suggest that exposure is common in cats in endemic areas.

Brucellosis

Several tests are available; these are the rapid slide agglutination, rapid slide agglutination with mercaptoethanol, tube agglutination, tube agglutination with mercaptoethanol, counterimmunoelectrophoresis, IFA, CF, and immunodiffusion tests. Sera should be nonhemolyzed, since free hemoglobin causes false-positive test results in the tube agglutination test. Sera for analysis should be obtained no sooner than 1 month after exposure, since the interval between bacteremia and seroconversion is at least this long. If the time from exposure is not known, the individuals should be tested once monthly for several months. While a single high titer likely indicates active infection, intermediate or low titers are consistent with recent infection, prior disease, or antibiotic therapy. Asymptomatic individuals that are seropositive should be further studied using more sensitive and specific tests, such as the immunodiffusion test and blood culture.

The rapid slide agglutination test is often done as an in-office procedure. It has a high sensitivity and low specificity. If the result is negative there is very little chance (99% probability) that the dog is infected with *Brucella canis*. Up to 65% of the positive test results are false-positive results, since there is great antigenic cross-reactivity with other bacteria. Adding mercaptoethanol to this test eliminates reactivity due to IgM, which accounts for some of the false-positive reactions due to other bacteria.

Most veterinary diagnostic laboratories use the tube agglutination test to confirm infection in dogs that test positive using the rapid slide agglutination test with mercaptoethanol. False-positive test results from cross-reactivity with other agents occur. Addition of mercaptoethanol decreases the frequency of false-positive reactions. A titer of 1:50 is associated with early or recovering infections, while a titer equal to or greater than 1:200 indicates active or bacteremic infection. Titers between 1:50 and 1:200 are considered suspicious and should be repeated.

The immunodiffusion test is highly specific for *Brucella canis* infection and is used to confirm positive agglutination test results. Positive reactions are present 5 to 10 weeks after infection. Dogs with genitally restricted infections may remain seronegative. Infected dogs should have precipitin lines to both the somatic and cytoplasmic antigens, although male dogs with genitally restricted infections may not show a precipitin line with somatic antigen. Dogs generally show a precipitin line with the cytoplasmic antigen about 1 week prior to a precipitin reaction with the somatic antigen.

Campylobacteriosis

Agglutination and immunofluorescence techniques are available, but have not been used widely in animals. In humans, a fourfold or greater increase in IgG titer between acute and convalescent sera or a significant IgM titer is considered diagnostic.

Chlamydiosis (Feline)

Virus neutralization and CF tests are available. A fourfold increase in serum titer between acute and convalescent sera indicates active infection. A significant CF titer does not indicate protection; this is likely due to the agent being an obligate intracellular parasite.

Leptospirosis

The standard test is the microscopic agglutination test. An ELISA test has been developed. A fourfold or greater increase in titer between acute and convalescent sera (separated by 3–4 weeks) gives a presumptive diagnosis. Due to the nature of the test and variability in preparation of the antigen it is best to submit paired serum samples at the same time and same laboratory. The use of multiple leptospiral antigens may be required to identify the particular serovariety involved. Active infections are associated with titers greater than 1:300 in nonvaccinated individuals, while titers resulting from immunization are generally less than 1:300. A single titer equal to or greater than 1 : 1600 is presumptively due to active infection. The ELISA test may be better in identifying chronically infected dogs. Leptospiral-vaccinated dogs with borreliosis may have unusually high antileptospiral antibody titers due to antigenic cross-reactivity.

Yersiniosis

A fluorescent antibody test is available for the demonstration of *Yersinia pestis* in tissue samples. Demonstration of the organism confirms the diagnosis. A passive hemagglutination test is used in humans to determine serum titers to the agent. Serum agglutination tests are available for other species, but are generally unreliable for serologic diagnosis.

AUTOIMMUNE DISEASES

Antinuclear Antibody

The test is not species-specific in that several different cell types from various species can be used as substrate, but a species-specific fluorescinated anti-IgG must be used. Cultures of human epithelial cells and numerous other mammalian cell cultures have been used as substrate; these are generally more sensitive than frozen sections of mouse liver. Some human laboratories use *Crithidia luciliae*, which contains a kinetoplast composed of double-stranded DNA as substrate. This is a highly specific substrate for systemic lupus erythematosus in humans; unfortunately, affected dogs rarely react in this assay since antibody to double-stranded DNA is uncommon in dogs.

Low titers using mammalian cells are found in normal individuals. In one laboratory titers greater than 1 : 40 using human epithelial cells as substrate are considered positive, while in other laboratories using different substrates the threshold titer may be as high as 1 : 100. Some normal animals may have high titers; this possibly can be due to the effects of subclinical infectious agents. The pattern of fluorescence is reported as diffuse, granular, ring, or nucleolar. The nucleolar pattern is less often associated with systemic lupus erythematosus. Radioimmunoassays and slide latex agglutination tests for antinuclear antibody are unreliable in dogs, since canine serum contains a nonantibody DNA-binding protein.

Systemic lupus erythematosus is a rare disease in cats. Positive, but transient, antinuclear antibody titers (greater than 1 : 20 using the mouse hepatocyte as substrate) have been reported in association with methimazole or propylthiouracil treatments, feline leukemia virus and feline infectious peritonitis virus infections, and cholangiohepatitis.

Anti-Red Cell Antibody

The direct antiglobulin or Coombs' test is the standard test to detect anti-red cell antibody potentially causing immune hemolytic anemia. The test can be read as a hemagglutination test if adapted to round-bottomed 96-well plates. Doubling dilutions of a multispecific antiglobulin serum (anti-IgG, anti-IgM, anti-C3) are added to the wells. Although slightly more expensive and complex than traditional methods, fewer false-negatives occur when the test is performed in this fashion. An ELISA technique has also been described in dogs. Using the microtiter plate test, dogs with active hemolysis generally have titers equal to or greater than 1 : 64, while in cats a titer equal to or greater than 1 : 8 suggests immune hemolysis. Some individuals may be hemolyzing below these titers, but any chronic disease (mostly infectious, but also some noninfectious) seems to result in titers up to these thresholds. The titers will vary with the source of antiglobulin, and prozones (lack of a positive test result due to antigen or antibody excess) may occur because of the multispecific nature of the antiglobulin serum. Coombs' titers often remain increased for a prolonged period despite successful treatment. Positive Coombs' test may be seen in babesiosis. Infection with *Haemobartonella* organisms and feline leukemia virus infection should always be suspected of playing some role in immune hemolysis in the cat.

Rheumatoid Factor

Tests used are the slide latex agglutination and Rose–Waaler tests. Latex particles and red cells can be coated with canine, rabbit, or human immunoglobulin. For use in the dog, rabbit immunoglobulin appears to give the best sensitivity. Other tests are available but are not widely used. With the Rose–Waaler test, the result is considered positive at a titer equal to or greater than 1 : 16. About 70% of dogs with rheumatoid arthritis are positive with this test. Rheumatoid factor titers do not correlate with severity of disease. Titers tend to decrease in chronic cases. About 6% of normal dogs have positive titers. Rheumatoid factors may be seen in individuals with chronic infectious and lymphoproliferative diseases and keratoconjunctivitis sicca. Titers in affected dogs are generally much lower than those seen in affected humans. This difference is probably accounted for by the preponderance of IgG rheumatoid factor in the dog, whereas most human rheumatoid factors are IgM, which agglutinates particles more efficiently. In addition, canine rheumatoid factor tends to be complexed, and therefore sites are not available to bind sensitized particles. Some believe that latex particle agglutination tests are not useful in the detection of canine rheumatoid factor or that different autoantibodies are detected.

Acetylcholine Receptor Antibody

Antibodies to this receptor are found in the majority of canine and feline patients with acquired myasthenia gravis. Dogs with the congenital form do not have the autoantibody. The upper limit of normal for the dog is 0.03 nmol/L.

Anti-Platelet Antibody

The traditional test to detect these antibodies is the platelet factor 3 release assay. There is some controversy as to whether the test should be performed on serum or plasma; the clinician should check with the laboratory for particular sample requirements. The test is relatively complex, since donor platelets must be prepared fresh or stored frozen and species-specific contact product must be made. The patient sample is considered positive if it clots in a time two standard deviations less than the control. The time to clot in a positive sample is generally about 10 seconds shorter than the control. Drugs suspected of being involved can be incorporated into the test. Occasionally, the time to clot in the patient sample may be significantly prolonged; in these cases circulating inhibitors of coagulation may be present. Immunofluorescence to detect antibody on patient megakaryocytes or an indirect method designed to detect serum antibody reacting with normal donor megakaryocytes have been used with some success. An ELISA has also been described in dogs. This was much more sensitive than the platelet factor 3 release assay and had few false-positive reactions. The large number of tests used to detect anti-platelet antibody in humans suggests that there is still more to learn about detecting these antibodies and their clinical significance.

OTHER

Occult Heartworm Disease

From 10% to 67% (mean is 35%) of dogs with adult heartworms have no circulating microfilaria. Tests to detect these occult infections are ELISAs for anti-adult heartworm antibody (Dirocult, Dirotect) and adult heartworm antigen (CITE, ClinEase, DiaSystems, Dirochek, Equate, Filarochek) and IFA tests for anti-adult heartworm antibody and antimicrofilaria antibody. The sensitivity of these assays ranges from 70% for the test measuring antimicrofilaria antibody to 95% for the test measuring anti-adult heartworm antibody by IFA. A test for anti-adult heartworm antibody had a sensitivity of 77%, while a test for circulating adult heartworm antigen had a sensitivity of 99% (very few false-positives). The highest correlation between serologic test results and necropsy findings was 97% for the test detecting circulating adult heartworm antigen. Although 100% of the dogs with heartworm were detected by the IFA test for anti-adult heartworm antibody, this test had significant interference with intestinal parasitism (most commonly ascarid). This test and the other tests for antibody tend to suffer from relatively frequent false-positive results (where there are no adult worms found in the heart at necropsy). Intestinal parasitism, prepatent infections, infections with *Dipetalonema reconditum*, abortive heartworm infections, and cured infections can also cause false-positive test results. The presence of antimicrofilaria antibody does not preclude microfilaremia. Several test kits now available to detect circulating antigen use monoclonal antibody, which essentially eliminates cross-reactivity with intestinal parasites and *Dipetalonema reconditum*.

If microfilaria cannot be found using one of the concentration methods and the dog has clinical signs and radiographic changes consistent with occult heartworm infection, then one of the serologic tests should be done. The test with the least chances of a false-positive reaction should be chosen; with our current knowledge this would be a test for circulating adult heartworm antigen. Any of the ELISA kits used to detect antigen will identify all dogs with occult heartworm infection with clinical signs, since these dogs generally have burdens of 20 or more worms. With worm burdens between 5 and 20 the sensitivity drops to about 95%, and with less than 5 worms the sensitivity is around 50%. By diluting the patient's serum with saline one can estimate the worm burden; a titer of 1 : 128 to 1 : 256 suggests a heavy worm burden. Knowing the worm burden can alert the clinician to anticipate therapeutic complications.

ADDITIONAL READING

Fox JC, Jordan HE, Kocan KM, George TJ et al. An overview of serological tests currently available for laboratory diagnosis of parasitic infection. Journal of Veterinary Parasitology 1986; 20:13.

Green CE, ed. Clinical microbiology and infectious diseases of the dog and cat. Philadelphia: WB Saunders, 1984.

Halliwell REW, Gorman NT. Veterinary clinical immunology. Philadelphia: WB Saunders, 1989.

Rose NR, Friedman H, Fahey JL, eds. Manual of clinical immunology, 3rd ed. Washington, DC: American Society for Microbiology, 1986.

Timoney JF, Gillespie JH, Scott FW, Barlough JE. Hagan and Bruner's microbiology and infectious diseases of domestic animals, 8th ed. Ithaca, NY: Comstock Publishing Associates, 1988.

Tyler JW, Cullor JS. Titers, tests and truisms: Rational interpretation of diagnostic serologic testing. J Am Vet Med Assoc 1989; 194:1550.

SPECIAL
TECHNIQUES

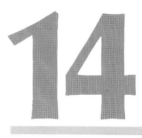

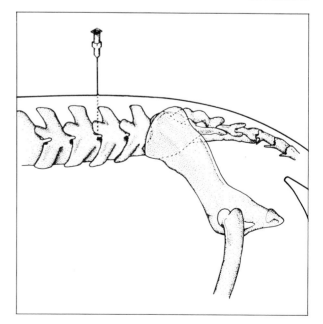

SPECIAL
TECHNIQUES

Dana G. Allen

CENTRAL VENOUS PRESSURE

The serial measurement of central venous pressure (CVP) is a simple and effective technique for monitoring fluid volume replacement and right heart function. The interaction of venous blood volume, the contractility and distention of the right atrium, intrathoracic pressure, and venous vascular tone contribute to right atrial pressure or CVP.

Right atrial pressure is determined by a balance between venous return and the ability of the right heart to pump this volume of blood to the pulmonary arteries. An increase in central venous pressure can be associated with an increase in venous return due to increased venous vascular tone or increased circulating blood volume. Significant elevations may occur with factors that impair right atrial or right ventricular function or conditions that limit the filling of the heart, such as pericardial effusion. Central venous pressure is not a direct measure of blood volume. Significant increases in central venous pressure may be recognized clinically by jugular venous distention and, sometimes, pleural effusion or ascites.

Indications

Central venous pressure monitoring is indicated in patients with ascites or jugular venous distention and in cases in which heart failure is present or appears imminent, and fluid therapy is required. In patients requiring fluid therapy in whom production of urine is low or unknown, it is wise to monitor CVP to avoid overhydration. In addition, body weight, hematocrit (packed-cell volume), and total protein should be monitored prior to and during fluid therapy. The gain or loss of 1 kg of body weight is equivalent to the gain or loss of 1 L of fluid.

An elevated CVP (greater than 5 cm H_2O) does not preclude the administration of fluids in patients whose clinical signs appear to warrant it. In some of these cases the CVP will actually fall with the restoration of normal hydration status. Fluid therapy is initially instituted slowly, and the CVP is monitored closely for further increases. Generally, the CVP should not be allowed to rise more than 5 cm H_2O in any 10-minute period in the dog or more than 2 cm H_2O in any 30-minute period in the cat. If the CVP does exceed these values, fluid administration should be slowed or stopped. Once the CVP line is in place it can also serve as an access for long-term intravenous fluid administration or parenteral alimentation.

Limitations

Central venous pressure does not accurately assess left heart function. Although many animals in heart failure have a component of left and right heart failure, a more accurate assessment of left heart function can be made from the measurement of pulmonary capillary wedge pressure. Pulmonary capillary wedge pressure is an estimate of mean left atrial, pulmonary venous, and left ventricular end-diastolic pressure and is an indication of the tendency for pulmonary edema (as with congestive heart failure). It may be elevated (greater than 20 mmHg) in cases of left heart failure and pulmonary edema, whereas CVP may be normal. Pulmonary capillary wedge pressure may be normal (14–18 mmHg) in cor pulmonale, while CVP is elevated. Consequently, animals with clinical signs of heart failure should have a complete cardiovascular examination, including a thorough physical examination, an electrocardiogram, chest radiographs, and an echocardiogram.

Patient Preparation and Technique

Most animals require only manual restraint. The area over the jugular vein is shaved and the skin is surgically prepared for intravenous catheterization. An intravenous catheter (Intracath [Deseret Medical], L-CATH [Luther Medical Products]) is inserted in the jugular vein and advanced to the level of the right atrium, about the level of the third intercostal space (Fig. 80-1). The largest possible gauge catheter should be used. The catheter is secured to the neck, bandaged, and then connected to a three-way stopcock. The stopcock is connected to a fluid administration set at one port and to a manometer at the other. Commercial manometers can be used (Manometer Tray [Pharmaseal Laboratories]) or extension tubing can be vertically aligned against a ruler with centimeter gradations. The zero point of the manometer is aligned at the level of the right atrium and the midpoint of the trachea near the thoracic inlet (see Fig. 80-1).

Fluid is allowed to flow from the delivery set to the patient to clear the catheter of blood. The access to the patient is closed and the manometer is allowed to fill with fluid from the delivery system. Once filled, the stopcock is turned to permit the fluid column to fall in the direction of the patient. Once the column of fluid in the manome-

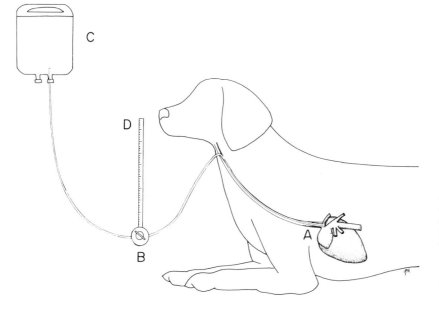

Figure 80–1. *Measurement of central venous pressure. With the patient in sternal recumbency, a jugular venous catheter is advanced to the level of the right atrium (A) and connected to a stopcock (B). The stopcock is connected to an intravenous delivery system (C) and a manometer (D). (Allen DG. Ancillary aids to cardiopulmonary medicine. In: Allen DG, Kruth SA, eds. Small animal cardiopulmonary medicine. Philadelphia: BC Decker, 1988: 142.)*

ter is stable, a reading is taken. Three readings should be taken each time and the average value recorded. Trends in the rise or fall of CVP are noted.

Normal CVP ranges from −1 to 5 cm H_2O. Slight changes in CVP (3 cm H_2O or less in the dog) are not considered clinically significant. Values consistently greater than 10 cm H_2O are associated with increased circulating blood volume. Values greater than 15 cm H_2O are associated with right heart failure or significant pericardial disease. Values less than normal may be associated with hypovolemia and severe hemorrhage (Table 80-1).

Central venous pressure normally changes in phase with the respiratory cycle. It falls during inspiration and rises during expiration. Falsely elevated readings may occur with tension pneumothorax, hemothorax, and positive pressure ventilation. Falsely low values may be caused by catheter occlusion, malposition, or kinking. When recordings are complete, the manometer is closed and fluids are permitted to run in the direction of the patient. If continual fluid administration is not indicated, periodic flushing of the catheter with heparinized saline is advised.

Complications and Contraindications

Although complications are rare, it is possible to traumatize the heart and initiate hemorrhagic pericardial effusion. Arrhythmias and sepsis are rare. Aseptic technique and careful catheter placement should obviate these complications. Bleeding tendencies or severe respiratory embarassment are the only contraindications.

THORACIC RADIOGRAPHY

Thoracic radiography permits the simultaneous evaluation of the cardiovascular and respiratory systems. It remains one of the most informative diagnostic tools available to the practitioner.

Indications

Animals with historical or physical findings suggestive of cardiopulmonary disease are candidates for chest radiography, as are those with suspected metastatic disease.

Limitations

The great variation in conformation and size of dogs makes cardiac mensuration difficult. The feline heart can be especially difficult to objectively evaluate radiographically. Echocardiography is a more sensitive tool for evaluation of cardiac structures.

Small volumes of pleural effusion (less than 100 ml in larger dogs) or intrapulmonary edema may be present without being obvious radiographically, especially in the early stages of disease. The historical and physical findings must be

---

Table 80–1 *Conditions Associated With Changes in Central Venous Pressure*

CONDITIONS ASSOCIATED WITH A SIGNIFICANT RISE IN CENTRAL VENOUS PRESSURE

Fluid overload
Pericardial effusion, cardiac tamponade, or restrictive pericarditis
Intracardiac neoplasia
Pulmonic stenosis
Tricuspid insufficiency
Tetralogy of Fallot
Eisenmenger's syndrome (which includes pulmonary hypertension, ventricular septal defect, atrial septal defect, or patent ductus arteriosus and right-to-left shunting of blood)
Rarely, cor pulmonale (severe heartworm, pulmonary thromboembolism)

CONDITIONS ASSOCIATED WITH A SIGNIFICANT FALL IN CENTRAL VENOUS PRESSURE

Hypovolemia (severe hemorrhage and shock)
Adverse reaction to venous vasodilators

considered with other laboratory data before an effective clinical evaluation can be made.

Patient Preparation and Technique

Radiographs are taken at peak inspiration in the right lateral and dorsoventral projections. If suspicious lesions are seen, a left lateral view should be taken as well. The dorsoventral view is better for the evaluation of the pulmonary arteries and the detection of pleural effusion. Consistency between radiographs is most important. The same body position and radiographic technique must be followed if subsequent radiographs are to be compared.

The normal features of the cardiac silhouette of the dog and cat are illustrated in Figures 80-2 and 80-3. These figures are only a guide for the evaluation of the heart and great vessels. The radiographs must be evaluated in conjunction with the history, physical presentation, and other laboratory tests before a clinical judgment can be given. Cardiac abnormalites and expected radiographic changes are listed in Table 80-2.

Three pulmonary radiographic patterns (bronchovascular, interstitial, and alveolar) are recognized in small animal medicine. A bronchovascular pattern is described as an increased prominence of the bronchi or an increase in pulmonary vessel number, size, or diameter. Bronchial patterns may become apparent in cases of chronic bronchitis, bronchiectasis, and asthma. Increased pulmonary arterial markings may be associated with heartworm disease as well as pulmonary venous congestion with left heart failure. Interstitial patterns obscure vascular markings and appear as fine, linear, honeycomb, or nodular densities. This pattern is associated with metastatic lung disease, mycotic or allergic pneumonitis, pulmonary hemorrhage, or pulmonary edema. Fluffy or patchy pulmonary densities that have a tendency to coalese plus air bronchograms (air-filled bronchioles surrounded by fluid-filled alveoli) are hallmarks of alveolar lung pathology. Alveolar patterns are seen with pneumonia, pulmonary infiltrate with eosinophils, advanced stages of left heart failure with pulmonary edema, pulmonary contusion or hemorrhage, and electric shock. In many diseases causing lung pa-

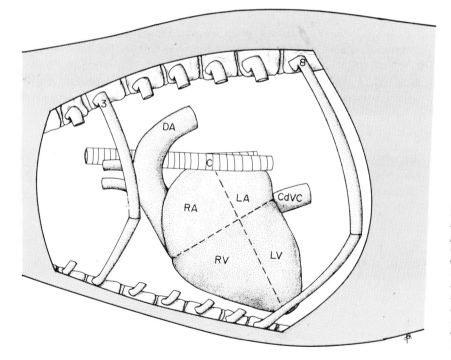

Figure 80–2. Cardiac silhouette and its associated structures in the lateral projection. (C = carina or tracheal bifurcation; CdVC = caudal vena cava; DA = descending aorta; LA = left atrium; LV = left ventricle; RA = right atrium; RV = right ventricle; 3 and 8 = 3rd and 8th ribs) (Modified from Allen DG. Ancillary aids to cardiovascular medicine. In: Allen DG, Kruth SA, eds. Small animal cardiopulmonary medicine. Philadelphia: BC Decker, 1988: 143.)

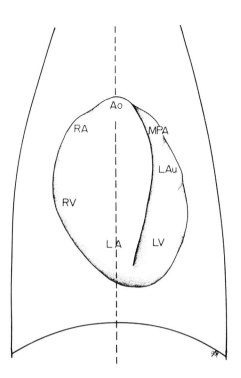

Figure 80–3. *Cardiac silhouette and its associated structures in the dorsoventral projection. (Ao = aorta; MPA = main pulmonary artery; LAu = left auricle; LV = left ventricle; LA = left atrium, RV = right ventricle; RA = right atrium) (Modified from Allen DG. Ancillary aids to cardiovascular medicine. In: Allen DG, Kruth SA, eds. Small animal cardiopulmonary medicine. Philadelphia: BC Decker, 1988: 144.)*

thology, a combination of the above lung patterns (mixed) is seen.

Lateral View

Generally, the cardiac silhouette in the dog should not occupy more than three intercostal spaces in the lateral projection. Extension beyond this is indicative of right ventricular enlargement. Left ventricular enlargement is indicated by a left ventricular caudal border that assumes a more vertical position relative to the sternum. It is usually accompanied by left atrial enlargement, which may be seen as an obvious bulging of that structure or as a separation of the left and right principle bronchi with compression of the left principle bronchus.

Loss of the cranial cardiac waist is associated with enlargement of the aorta, main pulmonary artery, or right atrium. Right atrial enlargement may also be seen with dorsal displacement of the trachea at a point just cranial to the carina of the trachea.

Dorsoventral View

At its widest point, the cardiac silhouette does not normally occupy more than two thirds of the chest cavity in the dorsoventral projection. Right ventricular enlargment is indicated by a rounding or bulging of the right ventricular border, creating an inverted "D" shape. The cardiac apex also appears rounder and is shifted to the left of the midline. A prominent buldge at the 1 to 2 o'clock position may be indicative of pulmonic stenosis, heartworm disease, pulmonary hypertension, or pulmonary thromboembolism.

With left ventricular enlargement, the left heart border appears closer to the left chest wall. The cardiac apex is more pointed, and it may be shifted to the right of the midline. It may also be accompanied by left auricular and left atrial enlargement. See the Additional Reading section for more detail about radiographic interpretation.

Complications and Contraindications

Animals in respiratory distress should be stablized prior to restraint for chest radiography. In many of these patients a standing lateral radiograph may be preferred.

NONSELECTIVE ANGIOCARDIOGRAPHY

Nonselective angiocardiography is the injection of contrast material into a peripheral vein with continuous or sequential radiographic recording. Selective angiocardiography is the injection of contrast material directly into a specified cardiac chamber or blood vessel. Nonselective angiocardiography is a safe and simple technique permitting the evaluation of ventricular size, wall thickness, intracardiac masses (thrombi, tumors),

Table 80–2 *Common Cardiac Abnormalities and Expected Radiographic Changes*

Cardiac Abnormality	Expected Radiographic Changes
Mitral valvular insufficiency	Depends on stage of disease: Left atrial or left ventricular enlargement Compression of left principle bronchus Pulmonary congestion or edema
Dilated cardiomyopathy	Generalized cardiomegaly Possibly pleural effusion Possibly pulmonary edema
Hypertrophic cardiomyopathy (cat)	Biatrial enlargement Valentine shape on dorsoventral view Possibly pulmonary edema
Patent ductus arteriosus	Left ventricular enlargement Left atrial enlargement Enlargement of aortic root Enlargement of main pulmonary artery and left auricular appendage Increased pulmonary circulation (arteries and veins) Pulmonary edema (if in left heart failure)
Pulmonic stenosis	Right ventricular enlargement Poststenotic dilation of pulmonary artery segment Normal or decreased pulmonary circulation
Aortic stenosis	Often normal Left atrial and ventricular enlargement Enlargement of ascending aorta
Tetralogy of Fallot	Right ventricular enlargement Coving of pulmonary artery segment Decreased pulmonary circulation
Ventricular septal defect	Often normal Left or biventricular enlargement Possibly increased pulmonary circulation
Pericardial effusion	Rounding of cardiac silhouette (with large amounts of effusion)

intracardiac congenital or acquired defects, pericardial effusion, and vascular patency (Figs. 80-4, 80-5, and 80-6).

Indications

Nonselective angiocardiography is a useful technique in cats and small dogs (less than 15 kg) for the demonstration of tetralogy of Fallot, right-to-left shunting lesions, pulmonic stenosis, and aortic stenosis and for the differentiation of pericardial effusion from generalized cardiomegaly and hypertrophic from dilated cardiomyopathy in cats. It is less useful in large dogs because of the

difficulty of injecting by hand in a limited time a sufficient volume of contrast agent to opacify cardiac structures.

Limitations

The basic limitation to angiocardiography in private practice is technique. Without intracardiac catheterization, rapid film changers, and power-assisted injection of contrast media, the study is limited to the evaluation of cats and small dogs. Other technical considerations include difficulties in timing radiographic exposures, patient postitioning, opacification with recirculation and

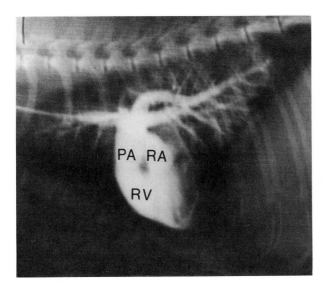

Figure 80–4. *Nonselective angiocardiogram of the right side of the heart in a mature cat. (RV = right ventricle; RA = right atrium; PA = pulmonary artery) (Courtesy of Drs. R. Downey and P. Pennock, Ontario Veterinary College.)*

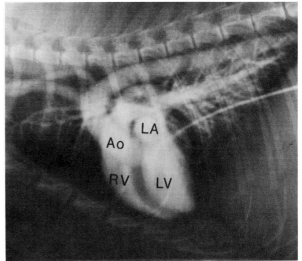

Figure 80–6. *Nonselective angiocardiogram outlining the right and left sides of the heart in a mature cat. (LV = left ventricle; RV = right ventricle; LA = left atrium; Ao = aorta) (Courtesy of Drs. R. Downey and P. Pennock, Ontario Veterinary College.)*

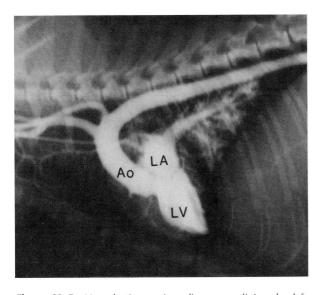

Figure 80–5. *Nonselective angiocardiogram outlining the left-sided cardiac structures in a mature cat. (LV = left ventricle; LA = left atrium; Ao = aorta) (Courtesy of Drs. R. Downey and P. Pennock, Ontario Veterinary College.)*

Patient Preparation and Technique

Sedation and manual restraint are required. Suggested chemical restraint is a ketamine hydrochloride and diazepam combination (100 mg/ml ketamine hydrochloride and 5 mg/ml diazepam mixed 1 : 1 and given at a dose of 0.1–0.15 ml/kg IV). Alternatively, dogs can be sedated with oxymorphone (0.05 mg/kg IM or IV, not to exceed a total dose of 4.5 mg).

Animals are positioned in right lateral recumbency, and an area over the jugular vein or cephalic vein is shaved and aseptically prepared. The needle tip is directed down toward the heart in the jugular vein. The jugular vein is preferred beause of its larger diameter and closer proximity to the heart. To facilitate rapid intravenous injection of the viscous contrast material, the largest possible diameter intravenous catheter should be used (Intracath [Deseret Medical]). The dose of contrast required for adequate opacification in the cat is 0.8 to 1.8 ml/kg, and in the dog is 1 to 2 ml/kg. A total dose of 6.6 ml/kg of contrast material should not be exceeded. A number of radiocontrast agents are available (Renografin 76 and Conray 400 [ER Squibb and Sons], Hypaque 75 [Winthrop Laboratories]). The dye should be

the superimposition of opacified structures. Abnormalities of left heart structures are more difficult to outline because of dilution of the dye during the course of its travel from the right heart and the lungs.

warmed to body temperature before injection to decrease adverse effects and viscosity.

Approximately four radiographic exposures are required. The approximate time at which various structures will be opacified is identified in Table 80-3. Generally, exposure should immediately follow the rapid intravenous injection of contrast and be repeated every 2 seconds thereafter for up to 10 or 15 seconds. Review of the films and adjustments in timing to suit the individual's situation are often required. For example, cats with hypertrophic cardiomyopathy or hyperthryoidism tend to have rapid passage of the dye through the heart and great vessels. Those with dilated cardiomyopathy will have much longer transit times.

Complications and Contraindications

Severely debilitated and weak animals and those with bleeding tendencies are poor candidates for angiocardiography. Complications of the procedure include vomiting, which may occur 1 to 3 minutes following injection of the contrast media. Anxiety, urination, defecation, coughing, sneezing, erythema, and urticaria have also been documented. Vascular trauma, sepsis, arrhythmias, congestive heart failure, hypotension, bradycardia, and oliguria are the most serious potential complications, and may result in death. The incidence of complications is increased in animals with hypovolemia and pre-existing renal or vascular disease. Most side effects are attributed to the hypertonicity of the contrast agent. They are usually transient and relatively benign. Contrast material can also adversely affect the interpretation of various laboratory tests. See Walter and associates (Additional Reading) for more detail on this subject.

ECHOCARDIOGRAPHY

The use of echocardiography as a diagnostic tool is no longer limited to academic institutions. Many private practices are utilizing this technique to enhance the investigation of the cardiac patient.

Indications

All patients with suspected cardiac pathology are potential candidates for study. Left ventricular function can be assessed prior to and following the institution of medical or surgical therapy. Echocardiography provides quantitative information on wall thickness, intraventricular dimensions, valvular and left ventricular function, and the presence of certain acquired or congenital defects. Pleural and pericardial effusion and intracardiac masses (tumors, heartworms, vegetations) may be identified (Table 80-4).

The two most commonly used forms of ultrasonography employed for cardiac examination are real time (two-dimensional) and M mode (motion mode) echocardiogaphy. Real time displays the beating heart in a longitudinal (long axis) or cross-sectional (short axis) plane. It is a moving picture image providing accurate spatial orientation. Appropriate areas for M mode echocardiography are selected and specific measurements of wall thickness and intraventricular, intra-atrial and aortic root dimension are taken (Fig. 80-7). Fractional shortening, a measure of left ventricular function, is calculated from measurement of the left ventricular diastolic and systolic dimensions.

New echocardiographic techniques include pulsed wave Doppler, continuous wave Doppler, and Color-Flow Doppler echocardiography. These techniques have the potential to obviate selective cardiac catheterization in many settings, as they have the capacity to measure cardiac output and document the presence and estimate the severity

Table 80-3 *Time Course of Opacification of the Heart and Vessels After Dye Injection*

Time*	Structures Opacified
1 to 3 seconds	Cranial vena cava, right atrium, right ventricle, pulmonary artery
4 to 8 seconds	Pulmonary veins, left atrium, left ventricle, aorta

* *May be markedly prolonged in states of low cardiac output*

Table 80–4 *Common Echocardiographic Findings in Selected Cardiac Diseases*

Cardiac Disease	Expected Echocardiographic Findings
Mitral valvular insufficiency	Left ventricular and atrial enlargement Normal or falsely increased fractional shortening (ventricular contractility) Thickened mitral valve leaflets Abnormal valvular motion with ruptured chordae
Dilated cardiomyopathy	Left ventricular and atrial enlargement Decreased fractional shortening Thin left ventricular wall and interventricular septum Possibly pericardial or pleural effusion
Hypertrophic cardiomyopathy (cat)	Decreased left ventricular cavity dimensions Left atrial enlargement Normal or increased fractional shortening Thickened left ventricular wall and interventricular septum
Patent ductus arteriosus	Left ventricular and atrial enlargement Increased amplitude of motion of aortic root
Pulmonic stenosis	Thickened right ventricular wall and interventricular septum Poststenotic dilation of pulmonary artery Abnormal pulmonic valve or subvalvular region Possibly paradoxical septal motion
Aortic stenosis	Thickened left ventricular wall and interventricular septum Possibly left atrial enlargement Narrowing of left ventricular outflow tract just below the level of the aortic valve Premature closure of aortic valve Systolic anterior motion of mitral valve
Tetralogy of Fallot	Aorta overrides the interventricular septum Ventricular septal defect Narrowed pulmonary outflow tract Thickened right ventricular wall
Ventricular septal defect	Possibly "drop out" of interventricular echo high in septum Left ventricular and atrial enlargement
Pericardial effusion	Echo-free epicardial–pericardial space Diminished motion of pericardium Parodoxical septal motion Collapse of right atrium and ventricle in diastole (tamponade)
Valvular vegetations (bacterial endocarditis)	Shaggy echoes at level of aortic or mitral valve Diastolic flutter of mitral valve with aortic valve lesions Left atrial and ventricular enlargement

of valvular insufficiencies noninvasively. In addition, estimation of the pressure gradient across a stenotic valve is possible. Due to the expense of these machines, the availability of these techniques will likely remain limited to veterinary schools or referral institutions for many years.

Limitations

Air prevents transmission of the ultrasound beam; therefore, pneumothorax, in addition to diaphragmatic hernia, or peritoneopericardio-diaphragmatic hernia may interfere with the

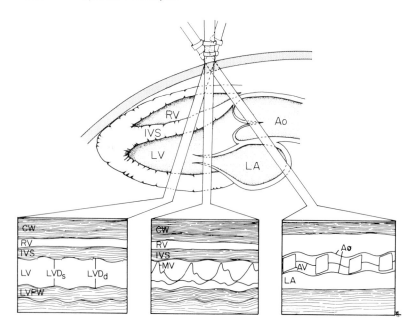

Figure 80–7. *Normal M mode echocardiogram of the dog and cat. Three areas are routinely examined: the left ventricle, the mitral valve, and the aorta and left atrium. (CW = chest wall; RV = right ventricle; IVS = interventricular septum; LV = left ventricle; MV = mitral valve; LVPW = left ventricular posterior wall; LVD$_d$ and LVD$_s$ = left ventricular diastolic and systolic dimensions; Ao = aortic root; AV = aortic valve; LA = left atrium)*

study. Abnormalities of thoracic conformation or intrathoracic masses may displace the heart or obstruct the ultrasound beam, making echocardiography difficult.

Structures smaller than 3 mm in diameter are not visualized. Small vegetative lesions in bacterial endocarditis, extracardiac lesions, and some cardiac lesions may not be obvious. Like most indicators of cardiac performance, echocardiographic measurements are dependent on factors other than cardiac contractility (preload, afterload, heart rate). Altered loading conditions present in mitral insufficiency make determination of myocardial function questionable. Mitral regurgitation can be documented and, at a minimum, semiquantitated with the use of Doppler echocardiography.

Patient Preparation and Technique

Routine cardiac ultrasonography is performed with the patient in left or right lateral recumbency. If necessary, the area over the second to fourth intercostal space near the sternum is shaved to facilitate a better air-free contact between the transducer and the skin. Most animals require only manual restraint. Cats requiring chemical restraint may be sedated with a ketamine hydrochloride and diazepam combination (100 mg/ml ketamine hydrochloride and 5 mg/ml diazepam mixed 1 : 1 and given at a dose of 0.1–0.15 ml/kg IV). Dogs may be sedated with oxymorphone (0.05 mg/kg IM or IV, not to exceed a total dose of 4.5 mg). These regimens are safe in most patients with cardiovascular disease, and although functional studies may be altered, they do not adversely affect anatomic evaluation.

Complications and Contraindications

Patients in severe cardiac or respiratory distress might be further comprimised if placed in lateral recumbency. In these patients a standing examination may be attempted. The study in these cases is generally limited to a cursory examination of gross cardiac structures, contractility, and the presence of pleural or pericardial effusion.

There are no known short- or long-term adverse biologic effects of ultrasound in the frequency range used for cardiac or abdominal investigation.

ELECTROCARDIOGRAPHY

Most practices use electrocardiography on a daily basis. Commercial electrocardiographic units, transtelephonic electrocardiography, and computerized interpretive electrocardiography are available to the practitioner. The electrocardiogram (ECG) is only one part of the cardiovascular examination, and it must be interpreted in light of the historical and physical findings as well as other laboratory data (see Chapter 18).

Indications

The ECG may indicate cardiac chamber enlargment, heart rate and rhythm abnormalities, and the response of these paramenters to anesthesia and medical therapy. Abnormalities in serum electrolytes, pericardial disease, myocardial hypoxia, and inflammation may be indicated by changes in the ECG.

Limitations

The ECG provides details on only one aspect of cardiac function, namely heart rate and rhythm. It does not provide information on other factors governing stroke volume (preload, afterload, and contractility). Therefore, the ECG must be interpreted in light of the patient's history, findings on the physical examination, and other ancillary data. Cardiac pathology may be present in the absence of changes in the ECG. For example, animals may have a normal ECG in the presence of gross cardiomegaly or changes in serum electrolytes.

Table 80-5 gives the normal maximum electrocardiographic values for the dog and cat. "Normal" reported values cover a wide range of conformations and size in the dog. Care must be taken not to overinterpret slight changes in the electrocardiogram.

Patient Preparation and Technique

Most animals require only manual restraint for an ECG. If chemical restraint is employed, care must be taken to use drugs that do not adversely affect the interpretation of the ECG. Drugs with minimal electrocardiographic effects include acepromazine (0.03 mg/kg IM), diazepam (0.2 mg/kg IV), and ketamine hydrochloride with diazepam (100 mg/ml ketamine hydrochloride and 5 mg/ml diazepam mixed 1 : 1 and given at a dose

Table 80–5 *Normal Maximum Electrocardiographic Values in Lead II*

Parameter	Dog	Cat
Heart rate (beats per minute)	70 to 160 (adults) to 180 (toy breeds) to 220 (puppies)	140 to 240
Rhythm	Sinus rhythm Sinus arrthythmia Wandering pacemaker	Sinus rhythm
P wave	0.4 mV, 0.04 sec	0.2 mV, 0.04 sec
PR interval	0.06 to 0.13 sec	0.05 to 0.09 sec
QRS complex	2.5 mV, 0.05 sec (small breeds) 3 mV, 0.06 sec (large breeds)	0.9 mV, 0.04 sec
QT interval	0.25 sec	0.18 sec
ST segment	No significant depression (<0.2 mV), or Elevation (>0.15 mV) or coving	No significant depression, elevation or coving
T wave	Not greater than ¼ R wave height	0.3 mV
Electrical axis	40 to 100 degrees	0 to 160 degrees

of 0.1–0.15 ml/kg IV). Agents to avoid include halothane, thiamylal sodium, atropine, and xylazine.

Dogs are positioned in right lateral recumbency. Cats may be positioned similarly or may remain in sternal recumbency.

The ECG is evaluated for heart rate, rhythm, enlargement patterns, mean electrical axis, and conduction abnormalities (Fig. 80-8). Serial changes are often more important than single electrocardiographic changes. See Table 80-6 for common electrocardiographic abnormalities in the dog.

Complications and Contraindications

Dyspneic animals may be stressed by positioning for electrocardiography.

PERICARDIOCENTESIS

Indications

Pericardiocentesis is a useful aid in confirming the diagnosis and possibly the etiology of pericardial effusion. It is also of therapeutic benefit to patients with clinical signs secondary to pericar-

dial effusion or tamponade (see Chapter 23). A suspicion of pericardial effusion should be substantiated with electrocardiography and chest radiography, and, where available, confirmed with echocardiography prior to pericardiocentesis. Echocardiography is the most sensitive tool for confirming a diagnosis of pericardial effusion.

Limitations

Cytologic and bacteriologic analysis of the pericardial fluid aspirate does not accurately differentiate between neoplastic and non-neoplastic disease. This does not, however, preclude the need for analysis (see Chapter 23). Pneumopericardiography, angiocardiography, echocardiography, or exploratory thoracotomy are usually required to establish the cause of the effusion.

Patient Preparation and Technique

In most cases, pericardiocentesis can be performed without sedation. If sedation is required a ketamine hydrochloride and diazepam combination may be used (100 mg/ml ketamine hydrochloride and 5 mg/ml diazepam mixed 1 : 1 and given at a dose of 0.1–0.15 ml/kg IV). Other alter-

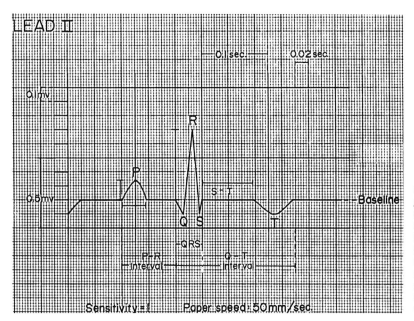

Figure 80–8. *Evaluation of the electrocardiogram. To calculate heart rate in beats per minute (at a paper speed of 50 mm/sec), divide the number of small boxes (0.02 sec) in one R-R interval into 3,000, or the number of large boxes (0.1 sec) in one R-R interval into 600. Note: the PR interval is actually calculated from the onset of the P wave to the onset of the Q wave (not the R wave). The height of the R wave is calculated from the top of the baseline to the peak of the R wave.*

Table 80–6 *Common Electrocardiographic Abnormalities in the Dog and Cat*

Parameter	Abnormality	Association
Heart rate	Bradycardia	Increased vagal tone, hyperkalemia, elevated central nervous system pressure, hypothermia, hypothyroidism, chronic obstructive pulmonary disease
	Tachycardia	Increased sympathetic tone, hypotension, fear, excitement, pain, anemia, hypovolemia, supraventricular and ventricular arrhythmias, atrial fibrillation, atrial or junctional tachycardia, ventricular tachycardia
P wave	Varying height	Vagal influences, "wandering pacemaker"
	Prolonged duration	Left atrial enlargement
	Increased amplitude	Right atrial enlargement
	Replaced by "f" waves	Atrial fibrillation or flutter
PR interval	Prolonged	First-degree heart block, digitalis intoxication, excessive vagal tone
QRS complex	Prolonged duration	Ventricular enlargement or bundle branch block
	Increased amplitude	Ventricular enlargement
	Decreased amplitude (<0.5 to 1 mV)	Obesity, pericardial or pleural effusion, hypothyroidism, hypoadrenocorticism, normal variant
	Abnormal configuration	Ventricular ectopia
	Varying R wave height	Pericardial effusion, supraventricular tachycardia
ST segment	Elevation or depression	Ventricular enlargement, myocardial hypoxia, electrolyte abnormalities
T wave	Change in shape or polarity	Myocardial hypoxia, electrolyte abnormalities
Axis deviation		Left or right ventricular enlargement, normal variant in the absence of other electrocardiographic changes

(Allen DG. Cardiac arrhythmias. In: Allen DG, Kruth SA, eds. Small animal cardiopulmonary medicine. Philadelphia: BC Decker, 1988: 98.)

natives include morphine sulfate (0.5 mg/kg IM in the dog) or oxymorphone (0.05–0.2 mg/kg IM or IV).

The area over the right thorax from the third to sixth intercostal space at the level of the costochondral junction is shaved and surgically prepared. The right side is preferred because the cardiac notch between lung lobes provides an area free of lung overlap and because there is less liklihood of traumatizing coronary arteries on the right side of the heart. In most patients local anesthesia is unnecessary. In cases in which it is required, lidocaine is infiltrated into the intercostal muscles down to the level of the parietal pleura. Animals are placed in left lateral recumbency or sternal recumbency or can remain standing.

An electrocardiogram is monitored for arrhythmias throughout the procedure (Table 80-7). Ectopic beats signal irritation of the epicardium by the catheter tip. A 14- to 16-gauge over-the-needle intravascular catheter attached to a 3-ml syringe is slowly advanced through the skin in the area of the fourth to sixth intercostal space near the costochondral junction. Additional side holes are cut near the tip of the catheter to facilitate fluid aspiration. Radiographs help determine the best site for needle insertion. The needle is inserted at the cranial border of the ribs to avoid the intercostal vessels. When fluid enters the syringe, the plastic catheter is advanced and the needle and 3-ml syringe are withdrawn. The catheter is connected to a 30- to 60-ml syringe

Table 80–7 Arrhythmias: Appearance and Treatment

Arrhythmia	Appearance	Treatment (if indicated)
Sinus bradycardia	Sinus rate <70 beats per minute (dog), <160 beats per minute (cat)	Atropine, glycopyrrolate, isoproterenol, isopropamide, pacemaker
Sinus tachycardia	Sinus rate >160 beats per minute (dog), >240 beats per minute (cat)	Carotid massage, digitalis, propranolol
Sinus arrest and block	Pauses in sinus rhythm more than twice the normal R-R interval (arrest), pauses in rhythm equal to twice the normal R-R interval (block)	Atropine, glycopyrrolate, isoproterenol, isopropamide, pacemaker
Sinoatrial standstill	Ventricular rate slow, no P waves	Treat primary cause, atropine, isoproterenol, isopropamide, pacemaker
Atrial fibrillation	Rapid, irregular ventricular rate, absence of P waves	Digitalis, propranolol, verapamil, diltiazem
First-degree heart block	Prolonged PR interval	Treat primary cause
Second-degree heart block	More P waves than QRS complexes	Treat primary cause, atropine, glycopyrrolate, isoproterenol, isopropamide, pacemaker
Third-degree or complete heart block	P waves and QRS complexes unrelated, ventricular rate usually <40 beats per minute	Atropine, glycopyrrolate, propantheline, isoproterenol, isopropamide, pacemaker
Ventricular ectopia	Ventricular complexes wide, aberrant in shape, and unrelated to P waves	Lidocaine, procainamide, propranolol, phenytoin

(Allen DG. Cardiac arrhythmias. In: Allen DG, Kruth SA, eds. Small animal cardiopulmonary medicine. Philadelphia: BC Decker, 1988: 99.)

using extension tubing and a three-way stopcock. Pericardial fluid is withdrawn and observed for clotting. Benign pericardial effusion does not clot. Clotting suggests vascular trauma, ventricular puncture, atrial tear, or an actively bleeding neoplasm. The catheter should be withdrawn and a new over-the-needle catheter redirected for a second attempt. The hematocrit (packed-cell volume) of the aspirate and peripheral blood can also be compared. Pericardial effusate usually has a lower packed-cell volume than that of peripheral blood. Collected fluid is saved for cytologic and bacteriologic analysis.

If the tap is unsuccessful, the needle can be redirected into a different intercostal space, or the body position can be changed and another attempt made. If the tap is still unsuccessful, the procedure should be repeated on the left side of the chest.

Complications and Contraindications

Relative contraindications include coagulopathies (except as a therapeutic measure in anticoagulant toxicity), severe uncontrolled ventricular arrhythmias, or septic thoracic disease. Inadequate restraint may lead to patient trauma. Complications of the procedure, although uncommon, may include pulmonary edema, pneumothorax, myocardial or coronary artery laceration, and hemorrhage.

NASAL BIOPSY

Indications

Nasal biopsy should be considered in any animal with a history of chronic unresponsive nasal discharge of unknown etiology. Nasal biospy is superior to nasal flush for cytologic diagnosis of suspect lesions.

Limitations

Lesions may not be evident radiographically, and the clinician may be visually hampered by the presence of blood or mucus. Most tumors are in the area of the ethmoturbinates, making biopsy samples difficult to obtain. Similarly, pathology may involve the paranasal sinuses. If a nasal biopsy does not render a definitive diagnosis and the problem persists, exploratory rhinotomy should be performed.

Patient Preparation and Technique

General anesthesia is required. Radiographs are taken, followed by rhinoscopy, to locate the lesion for biopsy. Animals are then placed in sternal recumbency. Four techniques for nasal biopsy are described. Personal preference dictates the technique of choice.

1. A 10F polypropylene urinary catheter cut at a 45-degree angle is connected to a 12-ml syringe for suction biopsy (Fig. 80-9). The length of the catheter required is determined by the location of the lesion, as identified radiographically. To avoid possible penetration of the cribiform plate the catheter must not extend beyond a distance measured from the external nares to the medial canthus of the eye. Nicks can be made along the length of the catheter and bent outward to create spurs. The catheter is advanced into the lesion and thrust back and forth over a short distance (0.5–1 cm) several times to obtain biopsy specimens. Saline may be flushed and aspirated at this time or the catheter withdrawn and flushed through with air and the biopsy specimens deposited on a gauze sponge to allow for the drainage of blood and fluid. The catheter is redirected and the procedure is repeated several times. Biopsy samples are fixed in 10% buffered formalin and examined histologically. Some tissue may also be saved for bacterial (aerobic and anaerobic) and fungal culture. Epistaxis is to be expected. It should stop within 5 minutes.
2. Punch biopsy can be performed with a Tru-Cut biopsy needle (Travenol Laboratories). The biopsy needle is advanced into the nares in a closed position and directed into the lesion. Several samples are obtained.
3. Aspiration biopsy using a large bore (3–5 mm) plastic cannula (see Fig. 80-9) is an alternative method described by Withrow and associates (Additional Reading). The technique is similar to that described for suction biopsy with the urinary catheter.

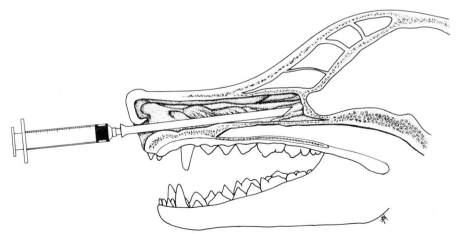

Figure 80–9. Nasal biopsy. The cannula is advanced to the level of the lesion.

4. Alligator forceps are advanced into the nares to the level of the lesion, and samples are grasped and pulled away for analysis. Alternatively, selected areas may be currettaged and the tissue samples evaluated histologically.

Complications and Contraindications

Coagulopathies predispose to profuse hemorrhage. If there is concern that the patient has a bleeding tendency, a full coagulation screen should be completed before a nasal biopsy is attempted.

TRANSTRACHEAL WASH

Indications

Transtracheal wash is indicated in dogs with a history of chronic cough, a productive cough, or radiographic evidence of bronchial or peribronchial disease. It provides cytologic and bacterial samples from the trachea and larger lower airways free of contamination from the oral cavity or upper airway.

Limitations

Transtracheal wash is of limited diagnostic value in patients with pulmonary parenchymal disease. In these cases, fine needle pulmonary biopsy is of greater diagnostic benefit (see Lung Biopsy). In some cases, thick tenacious material is impossible to aspirate through the catheter. In these animals general anesthesia and tracheobronchoscopy with bronchial brushing may be more rewarding (see Tracheobronchoscopy).

Patient Preparation and Technique

Manual restraint is preferred. Heavy sedation and general anesthesia tend to abolish the cough reflex. Fractious or uncooperative patients may be sedated with acepromazine (0.05 mg/kg IM or IV). Morphine sulfate and butorphanol suppress the cough reflex and should not used for this procedure.

The area over the cricothyroid membrane or the trachea near the thoracic inlet is shaved and surgically prepared. Lidocaine is infiltrated into the area over the puncture site. Animals are positioned in sternal recumbency and the neck is extended. A 12- to 18-inch, 14- to 16-gauge intravenous catheter (Intracath [Deseret Medical], or L-CATH [Luther Medical Products]) is preferred. Catheters of smaller gauge tend to become plugged with tenacious material. The trachea is stablized and the site for puncture is palpated. The needle is introduced into the trachea at a 45-degree angle (with the bevel of the needle facing away from the patient). The catheter is fully advanced into the trachea. Coughing is often elicited with this maneuver. Once the catheter is in place, the metal stylet and needle are removed from the trachea, leaving the catheter in place. A plastic guard covers the needle and prevents it from severing the catheter (Fig. 80-10).

Nonbacteriostatic saline (3–10 ml) is rapidly infused through the catheter. Larger volumes do not increase diagnostic yield. Aspiration should be performed as soon as a cough is elicited. Generally, less than 20% of the infused volume is recovered. The procedure should be repeated two to three times until a visibly productive sample is obtained. Representative samples contain respiratory epithelial cells on cytologic examination. Neutrophils are the predominant cell type collected in bronchopneumonia (see Chapter 29). Eosinophils are recovered in large numbers in animals with eosinophilic bronchitis, allergic lung disease (pulmonary infilitrate with eosinophils), feline asthma, or occult dirofilariasis (see Chapter 30). Bacteria, parasite larvae or eggs (see Chapter 33), microfilaria, or neoplastic cells may also be recovered from transtracheal aspirates.

The catheter should be removed while maintaining digital pressure over the puncture site. Gauze with povidone-iodine ointment is then placed over the area and the neck covered with a pressure bandage for a few hours. The patient

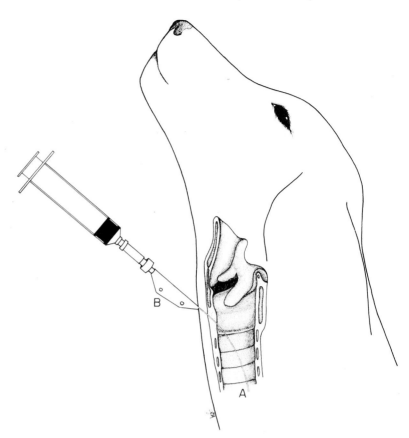

Figure 80–10. Transtracheal aspiration. The patient is positioned in sternal recumbency with the neck extended. An intravenous catheter (Intracath) is inserted through the cricothyroid membrane (A) or the interannular membrane at a 45-degree angle. The needle and metal stylet are removed, leaving the catheter in place. A plastic guard (B) prevents the needle from cutting the catheter.

must be observed closely for dyspnea for a minimum of 2 hours following the wash.

Complications and Contraindications

Although uncommon, tracheal or lower airway laceration leading to hemorrhage, hemoptysis, pneumomediastinum, pneumothorax, or dyspnea are possible sequelae. Other complications include subcutaneous emphysema and iatrogenic infection. The risk of inducing trauma is greater in cats, small dogs (less than 15 kg), puppies, and fractious or uncooperative animals. In these patients I prefer to use general anesthesia and wash the lower trachea and principle bronchi through the endotracheal tube or bronchoscope. Animals with bleeding tendencies should not undergo a transtracheal wash. If a cytologic sample is required, a tracheal wash can be obtained under general anesthesia through the endotracheal tube or bronchoscope.

TRACHEOBRONCHOSCOPY

Indications

Tracheobronchoscopy has diagnostic and therapeutic benefits. It allows direct visualization and biopsy of lesions of the trachea and bronchi and facilitates the removal of foreign bodies, mucus plugs, and blood. It is indicated in patients with a chronic cough of unknown etiology, hemoptysis, airway obstruction, parasitism of the respiratory system, or pulmonary bronchial disease. Cytologic preparations are superior to those obtained through transtracheal wash and aspiration.

Limitations

Tracheobronchoscopy is limited by the size of the patient and the diameter of the scope. In smaller animals the procedure is limited to the examination of the larynx, trachea, and principle bronchi. Lesions involving parenchymal tissue will not provide adequate cytologic samples unless there is concurrent involvement of bronchial tissue. The major limitation is the cost of the endoscope. Many endoscopes may also be used for esophagoscopy, gastroscopy, or proctoscopy. Smaller-diameter bronchoscopes can also be used for rhinoscopy.

Patient Preparation and Technique

General anesthesia is required. Tracheobronchoscopy is preceded by a thorough examination of the oral cavity; posterior pharyngeal and tonsillar areas, including the tonsillar crypts, soft palate, and caudal aspect of the nasal cavity; epiglottis; arytenoid cartilages; and glottis. Several rigid or flexible endoscopes are available.

Tracheobronchoscopy proceeds in a systematic fashion from the trachea to the carina, principle bronchi, and major lobar bronchi in the dog (Fig. 80-11). The right main stem bronchus is larger than the left. The normal trachea appears moist and pink. White cartilaginous tracheal rings and a fine network of submucosal blood vessels are evident. Changes in color and structure and the presence of abnormal secretions are noted. If an endotracheal tube is inserted, a "Y" adapter will permit the passage of the endoscope and the concurrent administration of anesthetic gases. Brush catheters, lavage and suction, and biospy may be completed through ports in the endoscope.

Complications and Contraindications

Although rare, trauma causing pneumothorax and hemoptysis can occur. In the cat, bronchospasm and hypoxemia are possible. Bronchospasm may be prevented by spraying the larynx with lidocaine prior to the procedure.

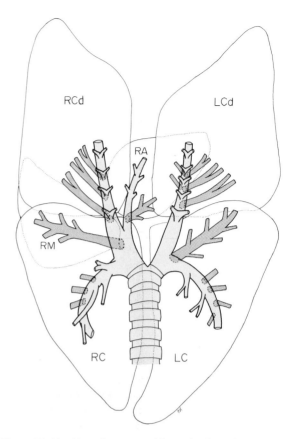

Figure 80–11. *Normal anatomy of the tracheobronchial tree in the dog. (RC = right cranial; RM = right middle; RCd = right caudal; RA = right accessory; LC = left cranial; LCd = left caudal lung lobes. Ventral structures are stippled) (Modified from Amis TC, McKiernan BC. Systematic identification of endobronchial anatomy during bronchoscopy in the dog. Am J Vet Res 1986; 47:2649.)*

Hypoxemia is primarily due to obstruction of the trachea by the endoscope. This can be limited by keeping the procedure short and by administering oxygen through the suction or biopsy channel. Cats can also be pretreated with oxygen prior to endoscopy.

THORACENTESIS AND INSERTION OF CHEST TUBES

Indications

Animals with radiographic or clinical evidence of pneumothorax or pleural effusion are candidates for thoracentesis. The technique allows for the removal of air or fluid from the thoracic cavity and provides relief from respiratory distress. Thoracic masses or cardiac pathology may be more obvious radiographically following thoracentesis. The insertion of chest tubes is indicated in cases of pleural effusion that cannot be adequately drained by needle thoracentesis alone, in cases with recurrent pleural effusion or pneumothorax, or for the administration of intrathoracic medication.

Limitations

Complete drainage of thoracic effusions by simple needle techniques is difficult and time-consuming. Fluid may be difficult or impossible to drain if it is thick with fibrin and purulent debris or if it becomes compartmentalized by pleural adhesions. In these cases an indwelling chest drain is indicated.

Patient Preparation and Technique

Needle Thoracentesis

Manual restraint and local anesthesia are required. The procedure is carried out with the animal standing or in sternal recumbency. It is sometimes helpful to raise the animal's forequarters to encourage gravitation of fluid flow to the caudal ventral aspects of the chest. The area over the seventh to eighth intercostal space near the costochondral junction is shaved and aseptically prepared. Local anesthesia (lidocaine hydrochloride 2%) is infiltrated in the seventh or eighth intercostal space at or just below the costochondral junction. An area one third of the distance from the vertebra may be more appropriate for the aspiration of air. Radiographs will help determine the best location for needle insertion. A 1½-inch, 18- to 20-gauge hypodermic needle, a butterfly needle, or an intravenous catheter (Angiocath [Deseret Medical]) can be used. I prefer an over-the-needle catheter. Once in the chest the needle can be removed and the plastic catheter left in place. Trauma to thoracic structures is less likely with the soft plastic catheter. The needle is inserted at the cranial border of the rib to avoid the intercostal vessels, and advanced into the thoracic space. The needle or catheter is connected to a three-way stopcock and a 30-ml syringe. Fluid is aspirated and categorized as exudate, transudate, modified transudate, chyle, or blood (see Chapter 32). Exudative samples are examined for the presence of bacterial or fungal elements and cultured.

If needle thoracentesis is unsuccessful, the needle is inserted in a different intercostal space and the procedure is repeated. Radiographs following thoracentesis will determine the extent of fluid remaining in the chest and help delineate structures not evident before the procedure was performed. It may be necessary to drain both sides of the chest cavity. If needle thoracentesis is unsuccessful, chest tube drainage is required.

Insertion of Chest Tubes

A soft, flexible feeding tube (20F–22F), Foley catheter (ACMI Foley catheter [American Latex Corp.]), or Argyle trocar catheter (Argyle trocar catheter [Sherwood Medical Industries]) is used. General anesthesia or sedation and local anesthesia is required. The affected sides of the chest are determined radiographically. The animal is placed in lateral recumbency and the area over the eighth to ninth intercostal space is shaved and aseptically prepared. A 2- to 3-cm skin incision is made approximately one third of the distance ventrally from the vertebrae to the sternum. A pursestring suture is placed in the skin incision. The distal end of the catheter is connected to a three-way stopcock and a 30- or 60-ml syringe. The tip of the catheter is grasped with large curved hemostats and tunnelled under the skin two intercostal spaces cranially (Fig. 80–12A). It is pushed and rotated along its axis at a 45-degree angle to the thorax, through the intercostal muscles and parietal pleura. A sudden release of resistance is noted as it enters the chest cavity. The hemostats are opened and the catheter is advanced ventrally to the level of the third sternebra. Alternatively, the skin can be pulled cranially and the hemostats directed perpendicular to the skin incision and advanced through the chest wall into the pleural cavity (Fig. 80-12B). The

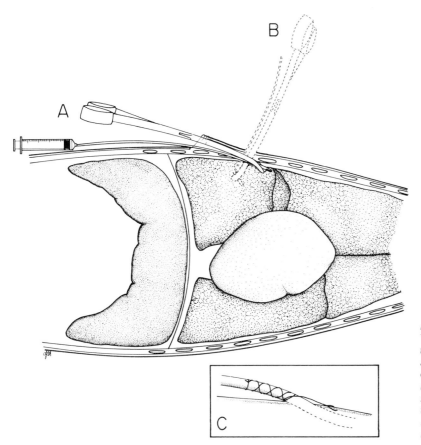

Figure 80–12. *Placement of a chest tube. (A) The catheter tip is grasped with hemostats and tunnelled two or more intercostal spaces cranially under the skin. (B) Alternatively, the skin can be pulled forward and the hemostats directed perpendicular to the chest wall for insertion. (C) Friction suture pattern. Butterfly tape may get wet and allow the tube to slip; this is not a problem with the friction suture technique.*

Argyle catheter comes equipped with a trocar for easy insertion into the chest cavity. The pursestring suture is tied, and the tube secured to the skin with butterfly tapes and sutures or, preferably, a friction suture pattern is tied over and under the catheter to prevent it from slipping out of the chest (Fig. 80-12C). Pleural effusion or air is aspirated.

Continuous chest drainage systems (*e.g.,* Thora-klex chest drainage unit [Davol]) can be also be used to provide continuous suction of air or fluid (Wingfield et al, Additional Reading). These systems are well tolerated in small animals. The Heimlick valve is not routinely recommended for use in cats and dogs under 15 kg. These patients may have difficulty generating sufficient positive intrathoracic pressure necessary to evacuate pleural fluid. Furthermore, proteinaceous material may interfere with the operation of the flutter valve, making close patient monitoring a necessity. Alternatively, continuous

pleural drainage can be accomplished with the three-bottle system (Kagan and Stiff, Additional Reading).

Radiographs are taken to verify the position of the catheter in the chest, and the chest and chest drain are bandaged. Bilateral effusions can usually be drained from one side. In animals with exudative effusions it may be necessary to place drains in both sides of the chest cavity. To remove the tubes, the distal end of the tube is sealed to prevent air from entering the chest cavity, and the tube is gently pulled tube out. The skin wound is then sutured.

Complications and Contraindications

Complications are rare. Blunt trauma or laceration of the lungs, heart, or thoracic vessels is possible. Iatrogenic infection, pneumothorax, and pulmonary edema following rapid drainage of large volumes of chronic effusions have been noted. Pulmonary edema is mild and self-limiting. Subcutaneous hematoma and emphysema also occur on occasion. The only contraindication is the presence of a coagulopathy. Great care must be taken in animals with known cystic lung disease (emphysema, bullae, cysts), as the risk of rupturing associated structures and causing a pneumothorax is greater.

LUNG BIOPSY

Indications

Pulmonary biopsy helps provide a definitive diagnosis in cases of pulmonary parenchymal disease, including neoplasia, allergy, and infection. It is quick and inexpensive. Fine needle biopsy is less traumatic than other pulmonary biopsy techniques (Additional Reading).

Limitations

Fine needle biopsy is not useful in conditions in which tissue architecture is needed to establish a diagnosis (hemangiosarcoma). Solitary lesions may be missed unless guided by the aid of fluoroscopy.

Patient Preparation and Technique

The technique has been well described by Roudebush (Additional Reading). It is summarized here. To guard against undue hemorrhage associated with the procedure, a complete blood count, including platelet numbers and an activated clotting time, should be completed first. Only manual restraint and local anesthesia are required in most cases. In the fractious or uncooperative patient, general anesthesia is recommended.

Solitary lesions are localized radiographically, and the depth of required needle penetration is determined. The site is shaved and made aseptic. The skin, intercostal muscles, and parietal pleura are infiltrated with lidocaine. If the radiographic lesion is diffuse, a point between the seventh to ninth rib at a level two thirds of the distance from the costochondral junction to the vetertebral bodies is chosen. This point should reduce the risk of traumatizing the heart and major blood vessels. In animals under general anesthesia, the lungs are maintained fully expanded to immobilize the lesion for biopsy. A 3-inch spinal needle (Monoject spinal needle [Sherwood Medical Industries]) is directed into the site at the cranial border of the rib space, thus avoiding the intercostal vessels. When the lesion has been entered, the metal stylet is removed and a 12-ml syringe is attached to the needle. Until the syringe is connected, a finger can be placed over the open hub of the needle to prevent air from entering the chest cavity. Continuous suction is applied and the needle is moved back and forth in a stabbing motion over a short distance (0.5–1 cm) to secure a core of tissue. The needle is withdrawn and the tissue sample transferred onto a slide for cytologic interpretation. Samples may also be cultured for bacteria or fungi. If a core sample is obtained, it is fixed in 10% buffered formalin. The procedure is repeated two to five times until adequate samples have been secured. The patient is closely observed for dyspnea for a minimum of 2 hours following the procedure.

Complications and Contraindications

Pulmonary biopsy is an invasive and potentially hazardous procedure. It should not be attempted in animals with bleeding tendencies or pulmonary cavitary lesions (bullae, cysts, emphysema). Pneumothorax, subcutaneous emphysema, hemothorax and intrapulmonary hemorrhage, and iatrogenic infection are possible complications.

SKIN BIOPSY

Indications

Suspect neoplastic, erosive, ulcerated lesions or lesions that are unresponsive to therapy for more than a 3-week period should be biopsied. Impression smears from the biopsy specimen can be stained and examined immediately for cytologic interpretation, and biopsy specimens may be submitted in formalin for histopathologic evaluation. Bacteria, fungi, or parasites may also be identified. Dermatoses in which histopathology is usually diagnostic are listed in Table 80-8. Other dermatoses in which histopathology may be diagnostic are listed in Table 80-9.

Limitations

The punch biopsy (Fig. 80-13) is limited in its usefulness, especially for the biopsy of large pustules, vesicles, bullae, and nodules. These lesions should be removed by excisional biopsy. Erosions and ulcers are best handled with elliptically ori-

ented biopsy (Fig. 80-14). Very early or late lesions may not be diagnostic of the disease process. Skin lesions become less specific and more difficult to interpret with age. The sites chosen for biopsy may not be representative of the principal skin disorder. It is important to have histologic samples evaluated by a veterinary dermatologist or a veterinary pathologist with a specific interest in skin disease.

Patient Preparation and Technique

Manual restraint and local anesthesia will suffice for most patients. General anesthesia may be required for excisional biopsy or biopsy of areas difficult to locally anesthetize (face, nose, footpads). The accuracy of a diagnosis is dependent on the selection of appropriate biopsy sites. At least three different sites should be sampled. Samples taken should include an early lesion (papule or pustule), a fully developed primary lesion (papule, macule), and an older chronic lesion. No normal skin should be included in punch biopsy

Table 80–8 *Dermatoses in Which Histopathology is Usually Diagnostic*

INFECTIOUS

Ringworm
Demodicosis
"Norwegian" type of sarcoptic mange
Pyoderma (superficial and deep)
Mycobacterial granulomas
Blastomycosis and other systemic mycoses with cutaneous lesions
Leishmaniasis

ALLERGIC AND IMMUNE-MEDIATED

Pemphigus
Bullous pemphigoid
Systemic lupus erythematosus
Drug eruption (some)

ENDOCRINOPATHIC

Hyperadrenocorticism (if calcinosis cutis is present)

CONGENITAL AND HEREDITARY

Dermatomyositis
Nodular dermatofibrosis (German shepherd)
Vogt–Koyanagi–Harada syndrome

MISCELLANEOUS

Acral lick dermatitis
Eosinophilic granuloma complex
Plasma cell pododermatitis
Nodular panniculitis
Alopecia areata
Feline follicular mucinosis
Thallium toxicosis

(Yager JA, Wilcock BP. Skin biopsy: Revelations and limitations. Can Vet J 1988; 29:969.)

Table 80–9 *Dermatoses in Which Histopathology may be Diagnostic*

INFECTIOUS

Sarcoptic mange
Atypical mycobacterial granulomas
Sporotrichosis (cats)
Arthropod bites

ALLERGIC AND IMMUNE-MEDIATED

Flea allergy
Bacterial hypersensitivity

ENDOCRINOPATHIC

Hypothyroidism
Growth hormone-responsive dermatosis
Sex-related dermatoses

CONGENITAL AND HEREDITARY

Cutaneous asthenia
Color-mutant alopecia

MISCELLANEOUS

Zinc-responsive dermatoses
Vitamin A-responsive dermatosis
Acne
Sterile pyogranuloma syndrome
Psychogenic alopecia (usually histologically normal)

(Yager JA, Wilcock BP. Skin biopsy: Revelations and limitations. Can Vet J 1988; 29:969.)

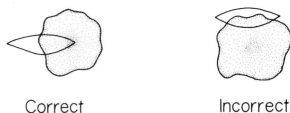

Figure 80–14. *Biopsy of lesions with active or ulcerated borders. The biopsy should be extended to include normal and abnormal tissue so that transitional changes can be observed.*

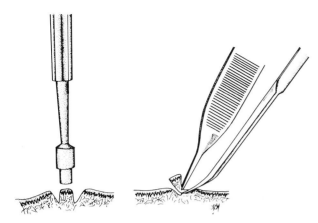

Figure 80–13. *Punch biopsy technique. See text for details. (Withrow SJ, Lowes N. Biopsy techniques for use in small animal oncology. Journal of the American Animal Hospital Association 1981; 17:889.)*

samples. Excoriated, heavily crusted areas or areas recently treated with topical medication should be avoided. If neccessary, the hair over the biopsy site may be clipped, but the clipper blades should never touch the skin. One should not attempt to sterilize the skin prior to biopsy, as this may induce histologic artifact and remove portions of the lesion. If gross contamination is present, the skin can be flushed with warm water and gently blotted dry. Vigorous scrubbing must be avoided, as rough handling of the biopsy area will also induce histologic artifact. Iodine-containing solutions should not be used because they interfere with the staining of histologic sections. Lidocaine hydrochloride 2% with epinephrine (0.5–1 ml) may be injected into the subcutis directly below the biopsy site. Intradermal injection must be avoided to prevent histologic distortion of the sample.

A 6-mm biopsy punch (Acu.Punch [Acuderm], Baker biopsy punch [Key Pharmaceuticals]) is placed over the lesion and rotated in one direction only into the skin until it sinks into the softer fatty tissue below. Single-toothed Adson forceps are used to gently grasp the sample from the underside (dermis or subcutis), raise it, and allow it to be cut free with scissors (see Fig. 80-13). All subcutaneous fat below the incision should be included to allow for histologic examination of deeper structures. The wound may be disinfected at this time if necessary. Simple interrupted sutures are used to close the skin, limit infection, and reduce scarring.

The biopsy sample is gently blotted to remove excess blood, and impression smears may be made. The sample is placed on a wooden tongue depressor or a piece of cardboard (subcutis side down) to prevent curling or distortion, and then placed upside down in the fixative. For routine histology, 10% buffered formalin is used. For direct immunofluorescence testing of suspect immune-mediated skin disease, the sample is cut in half and one half is put into formalin and the other into Michel's fixative. Michel's fixative is preferred for immunofluorescence testing, but cannot be used for routine histologic interpretation. Samples taken for direct immunofluorescence testing may also be satisfactorily preserved in sterile physiologic saline for up to 24 hours.

Excisional biopsy is indicated for vesicles, bullae, or pustules, as the rotation of the punch biopsy tends to shear the epidermal roof from its moorings, causing diagnostic features to be lost. For lesions with active or ulcerative borders, the elliptical biopsy should be extended to include normal tissue so that transitional changes can be observed (see Fig. 80-14). If possible, the ellipse should run parallel to the hair shafts (Fig. 80-15).

Complications and Contraindications

Complications are rare. Local hemorrhage, infection, scarring, and a subsequent change in the hair color over the biopsy site are possible. To prevent trauma to underlying structures, care must be exercised when biopsies are taken of thin-skinned areas overlying vital structures and mucous membranes.

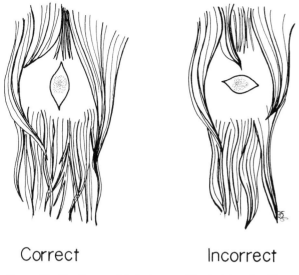

Correct   Incorrect

Figure 80–15. *Biopsy of haired areas. The incision should run parallel to the direction of the hair shafts to help the pathologist evaluate follicular architecture.*

LIVER BIOPSY

Indications

Securing a liver biopsy provides a means for establishing a definitive diagnosis when the clinical, physical, and laboratory data indicate liver pathology. Liver biopsy is indicated in cases of idiopathic hepatomegaly and in clinically normal animals with biochemical abnormalities suggestive of liver disease. It also provides prognostic information and serves as a guide for the response to treatment.

Limitations

Percutaneous liver biopsy is of limited value in focal hepatic disease. Generally, 80% or more of total functional hepatic mass is impaired if clinical signs of liver disease are present, making the chances of securing representative samples excellent. Obese animals and animals with significant ascites are technically more difficult to biopsy. It is advisable to have liver samples interpreted by a veterinary pathologist with an interest in hepatic disease.

Patient Preparation and Technique

A complete blood count, including platelet numbers and a coagulation screen or activated clotting time, should be completed prior to the biopsy. Abdominal radiographs help establish liver size and suitability for percutaneous biopsy. If there is generalized hepatomegaly, a fine needle (20-gauge needle) biopsy may be sufficient to establish a diagnosis in cases of hepatic lipidosis, lymphosarcoma, and histoplasmosis, and should be considered before a core biopsy (Tru-Cut biopsy needle [Travenol Laboratories]) is performed. If a diagnosis cannot be made on the basis of the fine needle aspirate, a core biopsy is recommended.

Animals are starved 12 to 24 hours before the procedure to lessen the chances of traumatizing a full stomach. Some clinicians recommend feeding a fatty meal (10–15 ml of corn oil 30 minutes before biopsy) to contract the gallbladder and make it less susceptible to needle damage. Hardy's studies (Additional Reading) have not documented any beneficial effect of this practice. Local anesthesia with lidocaine and an anesthetic regimen of oxymorphone and acepromazine (0.2 mg/kg and 0.05 mg/kg, respectively, IV), or oxymorphone and diazepam (0.2 mg/kg IV of each drug), or ketamine hydrochloride and acepromazine (5–10 mg/kg and 0.05 mg/kg, respectively, IM) are sufficient to carry out the procedure. Reversal of the oxymorphone component is possible.

The transabdominal percutaneous biopsy as described by Hardy is outlined here. An optional method, the "keyhole" technique, is described by Bunch and associates (Additional Reading). An otoscope permits visual control of the procedure. This approach takes more time, but permits direct visualization of the liver. The approach is otherwise the same as that described here.

Animals are sedated, placed in dorsal recumbency, and rotated about 45 degrees toward their right side. The head is slightly elevated by tilting the table to allow abdominal contents to shift caudally. This positioning should maximize diagnostic yield and minimize trauma to other structures. The area over the xiphoid is shaved and surgically prepared. The puncture site is located midway between tip of the xiphoid and the left costal margin. The site is infiltrated with lidocaine, and a stab incision is made in the skin. Several biopsy needles are available (Menghini needle [Mueller Co.], Jamshidi biopsy needle [Kormed], Tru-Cut biopsy needle [Travenol Laboratories]). Experience dictates the biopsy needle of choice. I prefer a 14-gauge, 11.4-cm-long Tru-Cut biopsy needle. The needle is advanced (30° to 45° to the skin in the dog and about 90° in the cat) through the subcutaneous tissue into the peritoneal cavity and directed slightly craniad and to the animal's left, away from the gallbladder (Fig. 80-16). The liver capsule generally lies next to the parietal peritoneum. To avoid possible trauma to deeper structures, the needle's depth gauge (if

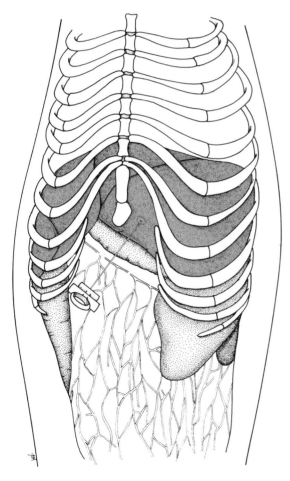

Figure 80–16. *Transabdominal liver biopsy. The needle is inserted midway between the point of the xiphoid and the left costal arch and directed craniad and to the animal's left.*

present) is set at about 1 to 3 cm. The needle is quickly thrust into the liver and then withdrawn from the abdominal cavity. The operator usually does not feel the needle penetrate the liver capsule. Samples are prepared for impression smears, histology sections, and bacterial and fungal culture. The procedure may be repeated two or three times as required to gain the samples needed. Animals are kept quiet and observed for signs of abdominal pain, peritoneal effusion, or vomiting suggestive of abdominal trauma.

An alternative approach is transthoracic hepatic biopsy. It is technically more difficult to perform. Patients are positioned in sternal or left lateral recumbency. Following administration of local anesthesia, the biopsy needle is inserted in the right sixth, seventh, or eighth intercostal space just dorsal to the costochondral junction. It is advanced approximately parallel to the thoracic wall to the diaphragm, where physical resistance is met. At this point the needle may move in phase with respiration. The depth gauge (if present) is set at 1.5 to 2 cm, and the needle is thrust quickly into the liver following a full exhalation (Fig. 80-17).

Complications and Contraindications

Excessively overweight animals and animals with small livers or ascites are technically more difficult to biopsy. Ascitic fluid should be drained before biopsy is carried out. The procedure is contraindicated in animals with bleeding tendencies, vascular hepatic tumors (hemangiosarcoma), hepatic abscesses, dilation of the biliary tree, and diaphragmatic hernia. Complications of the procedure include hemorrhage, laceration of the biliary tree or gallbladder and bile peritonitis, iatrogenic infection, and trauma to the spleen, stomach, pancreas, kidney, diaphragm, or lung.

KIDNEY BIOPSY

Indications

Percutaneous kidney biopsy in the dog and cat helps provide a definitive diagnosis in animals with physical, historical, or laboratory evidence

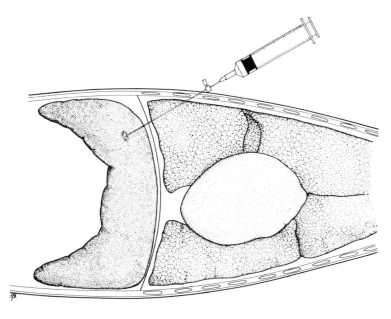

Figure 80–17. *Transthoracic liver biopsy. The needle is inserted in the sixth, seventh, or eighth intercostal space just above the costochondral junction on the right chest wall. It is advanced parallel to the thoracic wall and directed to the diaphragm and into the liver. (Jones BD, Hitt M, Hurst T. Hepatic biopsy. Vet Clin North Am 1985; 39.)*

of renal disease. Evaluation of kidney biopsies can also help establish a prognosis for renal disease, for example, acute renal failure (acute tubular necrosis) vs. chronic renal failure (atrophy, inflammation, mineralization, fibrosis) or severe membranous glomerulonephritis or glomerulosclerosis vs. mild proliferative glomerulonephritis. Kidney biopsies may also provide therapeutic guidance for patients with glomerulonephropathy or proteinuria. Subsequent biopsies may be used to follow the course of therapy. Finally, enlarged, small, or irregularly shaped kidneys may be biopsied to define the cause of structural change.

Limitations

Biopsy specimens may not be representative of focal lesions. Ultrasonography helps determine the suitability of percutaneous renal biopsy in a given patient. Inadequate biopsy specimens (insufficient glomeruli) may preclude a pathologic diagnosis in cases of glomerulonephritis.

Patient Preparation and Technique

Because many animals with renal disease are predisposed to coagulation abnormalities, a coagulation screen should be completed before the procedure is undertaken. Sedation (see Liver Biopsy) and local anesthesia or general anesthesia are required. Ketamine hydrochloride may be used only if renal function is adequate to excrete the drug. An area over the right or left paralumbar fossa just caudal to the last rib and ventral to the lumbar muscles is shaved and aseptically prepared. Blind percutaneous or keyhole kidney biopsy is then performed. Alternatively, a laparotomy and wedge biopsy can be performed. Technically, this is easier to perform and provides pathologists with larger samples of selected tissue.

Blind Percutaneous Kidney Biopsy

The kidney is palpated and grasped by deep palpation. In the dog, usually only the left kidney can be palpated and immobilized by deep digital palpation. Both kidneys can usually be localized and immobilized by digital palpation in the cat. The kidney is secured against the abdominal wall. A biopsy needle (Tru-Cut biopsy needle [Travenol Laboratories], Franklin modified Vim–Silverman biopsy needle [Mueller Co.]) is inserted through a previously made stab incision and directed either into the greater curvature of the kidney or perpendicular to the long axis of the kidney and into either pole (Fig. 80-18). The biopsy needle should be directed away from the

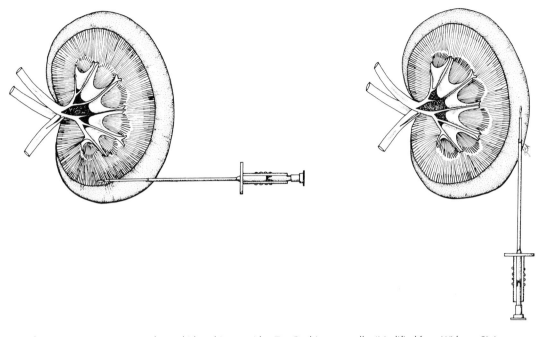

Figure 80–18. *Two approaches to kidney biopsy with a Tru-Cut biopsy needle. (Modified from Withrow SJ, Lowes N. Biopsy techniques for use in small animal oncology. Journal of the American Animal Hospital Association. 1981; 17:889 and Crowe SE, Walshaw SO. Manual of clinical procedures in the dog and cat. Philadelphia: JB Lippincott, 1987: 217.)*

renal pelvis, artery, and vein. Renal blood vessels progressively diminish in size from the medulla to the cortex. To avoid undue hemorrhage, the biopsy should be largely confined to the renal cortex. Biopsy should not be attempted on a kidney that cannot be adequately palpated or immobilized.

Keyhole Kidney Biopsy

In the technique described by Osborne and associates (Additional Reading), an oblique paralumber incision large enough to accommodate the index finger is made caudal to the last rib (Fig. 80-19). In the dog the right kidney is preferred because of the consistency of its location and its firmer attachments to the body wall. Blunt dissection through muscle and fascia to the level of the peritoneal cavity permits digital palpation and examination of the caudal pole of the kidney. The kidney is secured against the body wall with the index finger. As an alternative, a 2.5-cm-wide ribbon malleable retractor can be used to immobilize the kidney and prevent accidental trauma

to the operator's finger by the biopsy needle. The biopsy needle is inserted through a separate stab incision cranial to the paralumbar incision and directed into the caudal pole of the kidney with the index finger. To decrease renal hemorrhage

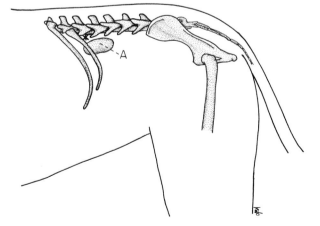

Figure 80–19. *Landmarks for the keyhole kidney biopsy. An oblique paralumbar incision (A) is made at a point equidistant from the ventral border of the lumbar spine and the caudal border of the last rib. The biopsy needle is inserted at a point (*) cranial to the incision.*

after the biopsy, gentle pressure is applied to the biopsy site with the index finger. Biopsy specimens are fixed in 10% buffered formalin or other fixative, as indicated. It is advisable to consult with the pathology laboratory to determine the best manner to fix the tissue samples for light, electron, or immunofluorescence microspcopy prior to fixation.

Complications and Contraindications

A retrospective study documented the potential complications of the technique in dogs and cats over a 10-year period (Jeraj et al, Additional Reading). Renal and perirenal hemorrhage are rare (about 3% of cases) but potentially serious complications even in normal animals. Transient hematuria (2–3 days) is not uncommon.

Animals with bleeding tendencies should not be biopsied by the percutaneous route. Animals with glomerulonephropathies are predisposed to coagulation abnormalities. Hydronephrosis, iatrogenic infection, and retroperitoneal or peritoneal leakage of urine are rare.

ABDOMINAL PARACENTESIS AND LAVAGE

Indications

Trauma, the "acute" painful abdomen, and peritoneal effusion are indications for abdominal paracentesis. If a simple needle tap is unrewarding in securing fluid for analysis, abdominal paracentesis and lavage may be indicated. In addition, continuous and intermittent peritoneal lavage may be used as effective adjunctive therapy in the management of diffuse peritonitis.

Limitations

The accuracy of needle abdominal paracentesis in detecting abnormalities within the peritoneal space is limited by the type and volume of effusion present. Fluid is only likely to be retrieved if the volume present in the abdomen is 5.2 to 6.6 ml/kg or greater. Needle paracentesis may not be helpful in the detection of intra-abdominal injury caused by penetrating wounds. Retroperitoneal injuries, diaphragmatic hernia, and adhesions causing loculation of fluid are causes of false-negative aspirates. Occlusion of the needle by fat, omentum, or viscera may also cause false-negative results. The use of a dialysis catheter increases the chances of fluid retrieval. As little as 1 ml/kg may be detected with the use of a peritoneal catheter.

Patient Preparation and Technique

Needle Paracentesis

Only manual restraint is required in most patients. In the uncooperative animal, local anesthesia or sedation can be achieved as indicated under Liver Biopsy. Prior to abdominocentesis the bladder is emptied. The area over and just caudal to the umbilicus is shaved and surgically prepared. If required, local anesthesia (lidocaine) is infiltrated in an area 2 to 4 cm caudal to the umbilicus along the linea alba. For simple needle paracentesis, a 16- to 18-gauge intravenous catheter (Angiocath [Deseret Medical], or Sovereign intravenous catheter [Sherwood Medical Industries]) is preferred. Extra side holes are cut along the catheter tip to facilitate fluid aspiration. To encourage ventral accummulation of fluid, I prefer to leave animals standing. The catheter is directed through the linea alba and into the abdominal cavity 2 to 4 cm caudal to the umbilicus. Following abdominal puncture the stylet is removed and the catheter is connected to a 3-ml syringe. Aspiration follows. A positive sample is one in which 0.5 ml or more of bloody or opaque fluid is withdrawn. If the tap is unsuccessful, the needle can be withdrawn and redirected for a second attempt.

Alternatively, a four-quadrant abdominal approach is recommended. The abdomen is divided into four areas by bisecting a line drawn through the umbilicus. A small area in each quadrant is shaved and asepticallly prepared for needle insertion and aspiration. If the procedure is unsatisfactory, peritoneal lavage is recommended.

Abdominal Paracentesis and Lavage

For abdominal paracentesis and lavage, sedation and local anesthesia as described under Liver Biopsy is recommended. Animals are placed in dorsal recumbency and the site is aseptically prepared. A small stab incision is made in the skin and an intravenous catheter, 11F peritoneal catheter (Inpersol peritoneal catheter [Abbott Laboratories]), or Parker peritoneal dialysis cannula (DiaLavage [CPA VET]) is inserted into the abdominal cavity. Most peritoneal catheters are supplied with a trocar to facilitate abdominal puncture. Once in the abdominal cavity, the catheter is advanced in a dorsocaudal direction into the paralumbar gutter, where fluid is most apt to collect with patients in this position. Gentle pressure is applied to the abdomen in an attempt to move fluid toward the catheter.

If no fluid is obtained by aspiration, the abdomen is washed. The catheter is connected to an infusion delivery set and approximately 20 ml/kg of warmed physiologic sterile saline is infused into the abdomen. The animal is gently rocked from side to side and the abdomen is gently massaged. Once the calculated volume of fluid has been delivered, the infusion delivery set is placed on the floor and the fluid is allowed to flow by gravity from the abdomen. Usually only 30% to 50% of the infusate is recovered. There is no need to drain all the infusate.

The abdominal fluid is examined on the basis of packed-cell volume, total red and white blood cell counts, amylase, alkaline phosphatase, bilirubin, creatinine, and the presence of bacteria or particulate matter (Table 80-10). A clear sample free of significant numbers of red or white cells and bacteria is considered normal. If clinical signs of abdominal distress continue, the procedure should be repeated. Significant elevations in peritoneal white cell numbers may not occur until 2 to 4 hours following contamination of the abdominal cavity with blood, bile, urine, feces, or gastric or pancreatic secretions. Trauma alone usually does not induce significant elevations in peritoneal white cell numbers. An increase in white cells (greater than 500/μl) in the absence of bacteria, and even in the presence of an elevated peripheral white blood cell count, is not necessarily an indication for exploratory laparotomy. Some clinicians suggest an exploratory laparotomy if any blood is present in the sample. Others recommend surgery in those with a packed-cell volume greater than 2% or a total red cell count in

Table 80–10 Interpretation of Abdominal Fluid

Parameter	Interpretation
Gross appearance	Normal: clear Abnormal: bloody, dark, cloudy, or opaque
Packed-cell volume	<2%: normal 2% to 5%: mild intra-abdominal hemorrhage >10%: significant intra-abdominal hemorrhage
Red blood cell count	Up to 100,000 to 200,000/μl (0.1 to 0.2 × 10^{12}/L): normal >200,000/μl (0.2 × 10^{12}/L): significant intra-abdominal hemorrhage
White blood cell count	Normal: <500/μl (0.5 × 10^9/L) Abnormal: >500/μl or the presence of bacteria and degenerative neutrophils
Amylase	Presence implies possible leakage from pancreas, liver, or small bowel
Alkaline phosphatase	Level greater than serum implies intestinal trauma, ischemia, or leakage
Bilirubin	In nonicteric animals, presence may indicate leakage from biliary tree or proximal bowel
Creatinine	Level greater than serum implies urinary tract leakage

excess of 20,000/μl. Care must be taken not to contaminate the sample with blood from the puncture site.

Complications and Contraindications

The only contraindication to performing abdominal paracentesis and lavage is the presence of a coagulation abnormality. Complications associated with the procedure are rare if it is followed as outlined. Iatrogenic infection or puncture of the bowel, spleen, liver, gallbladder, biliary tree, or urinary bladder are possible. Subcutaneous hematoma and the collection of abdominal fluid in the puncture site may occur, but this will usually resolve spontaneously. With continuous peritoneal lavage, hypokalemia and reductions in packed-cell volume and plasma protein may occur.

PERITONEAL AND PLEURAL DIALYSIS

Peritoneal Dialysis

The large surface area and semipermeable nature of the peritoneum make it an ideal structure for the exchange of solutes between plasma and peritoneal fluid. The movement of solutes from plasma to peritoneal fluid follows concentration gradients, and the movement of fluid follows osmolality gradients. For example, infusion of hypertonic saline into the abdomen would result in plasma water being drawn into the peritoneal space and sodium and chloride diffusing into the plasma. Depending on their size, waste solutes diffuse from plasma to the dialysate.

Indications

The animals that principally benefit from peritoneal dialysis are those in acute oliguric or anuric renal failure that are unresponsive to conventional methods of treatment (see Chapter 43). Renal lesions associated with acute renal failure are often reversible with time. Additionally, viable nephrons can undergo compensatory hypertro-

phy. Peritoneal dialysis can stabilize patients in acute renal failure and buy time for nephron repair and compensation. Animals in compensated chronic renal failure suffering an acute episode of prerenal azotemia from fluid loss (vomiting, diarrhea, hypovolemia) may also benefit from dialysis until renal compensation occurs. Continuous and intermittent peritoneal lavage may also be beneficial as adjunctive therapy in diffuse peritonitis.

Limitations

Peritoneal dialysis is labor-intensive and very costly. Kidney biopsy and confirmation that acute renal failure and a potentially reversible disease is present is recommended before peritoneal dialysis is undertaken. It is not a practical or effective means for treatment of decompensated chronic renal failure. The procedure should not be performed on dehydrated animals.

Patient Preparation and Technique

Sedation and local anesthesia may be required in some animals; however, ketamine hydrochloride should not be used for sedation as it requires adequate renal function for excretion. Animals are placed in lateral recumbency. An area midway between the umbilicus and the pelvic rim is shaved and aseptically prepared. The bladder is emptied. Local anesthetic is infiltrated lateral to the midline and caudal to the umbilicus. The Purdue catheter (Physio Control Corp.) or Lifecath (Quinton Instruments) is implanted alongside the bladder in the lower medial abdominal quadrant (Figs. 80-20 and 80-21). The disk is pulled firmly against the abdominal wall and the peritoneum is closed over the base of the catheter. The abdominal muscles are sutured tightly over the first Dacron velour cuff to prevent fluid leakage and ascending bacterial infection. The free end of the catheter is tunnelled under the skin to exit at a point some distance from the second Dacron velour cuff, which is buried. The catheter is secured to the ventral abdominal body wall and flushed with 20 to 30 ml of heparinized saline (Fig. 80-22). The abdominal wound is closed and the abdomen is bandaged.

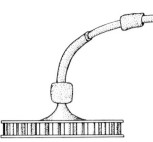

Figure 80–20. *Purdue column disk catheter used in peritoneal dialysis.*

A modified technique has been described by Birchard and associates (Additional Reading). A left paramedian incision is made from a point 4 to 6 cm cranial to the umbilicus to a point 2 to 3 cm cranial to the brim of the pelvis. The rectus muscle layer is bluntly dissected and the remaining muscle layers are incised with Metzembaum scissors. Once in the abdominal cavity, kidney biopsies can be taken. The greater omentum is exteriorized from the abdominal cavity and the caudal two thirds of it is surgically removed. A stab incision is made on the midline of the abdominal wall 2 to 3 cm cranial to the pelvic brim and the catheter tubing is pulled through it. The disk is pulled flush with the peritoneal surface of the ventral abdominal wall. The Dacron cuff closest to the disk should be at the level of the abdominal musculature. A pursestring suture is placed in the rectus fascia around the catheter tubing. A stab incision is created through the skin on the ventral midline 6 to 8 cm cranial to the point where the tubing exits the abdomen, and the disk tubing is tunnelled under the skin to exit at this point. The Dacron cuff farthest from the disk is buried in the subcutaneous tissue. The abdomen is closed and bandaged. This technique eliminates the subcutaneous leakage of dialysate, and removal of two thirds of the omentum helps prevent catheter obstruction. Alternatively, the Parker peritoneal dialysis cannula (DiaLavage [CPA VET]) may be used. Commercial peritoneal dialysis catheter sets are also available (Stylocath and Inpersol peritoneal catheter with stylet [Abbot Laboratories], Diacath [Travenol Laboratories]). Problems of catheter plugging are greater with the use of these systems.

Commercial dialysate solutions (1.5% and 4.5% dextrose) can be used in dogs. The 1.5% solution (Dianeal 137 with 1.5% Dextrose-Viaflex) is preferred. It is moderately hypertonic to plasma (350 mOsm/L). An infusion adaptor is available for the catheter (Dianeal Viaflex Transfer Set Tubing [Travenol Laboratories], Beta-Cap adaptor [Quinton Instruments]). Two milliliters of heparin should be added to every 2 L of solution to prevent fibrin clot formation. The 4.5% solution (490 mOsm/L) is generally reserved for patients with oliguric renal failure and fluid overload. Lactated Ringer's injection with added glucose (1%–2%) is a suitable alternative. The efficiency of peritoneal clearance of solutes can be improved by warming the dialysate to body temperature and decreasing the time the dialysate remains in the peritoneal cavity to as little as 1 hour.

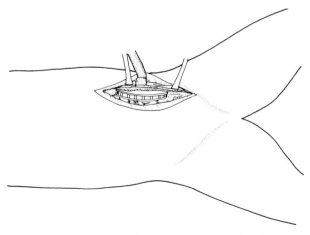

Figure 80–21. *Position of the Purdue catheter in the abdominal cavity of a dog.*

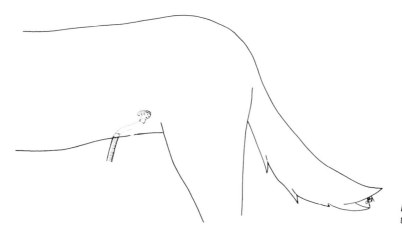

Figure 80–22. *Position of the Purdue catheter in the ventral abdominal wall.*

Warmed dialysate (38°–39°C) should be infused in sufficient volumes to mildly distend the abdomen (30–40 ml/kg). The fluid will empty into the abdomen within a 10-minute period. As the dialysate bag empties, it can be rolled up and taped to the abdomen. The dialysate is left in place for 1 hour and then allowed to drain by gravity into the dialysate bag. The procedure is repeated hourly until acceptable levels of azotemia are reached. This may take 12 to 36 hours. Up to 2 days may be required to stabilize animals in acute uremic crisis. When the animal is stabilized a less intense regimen may be followed. Dialysate may remain in the abdominal cavity for 4 to 6 hours during the day and up to 8 hours at night before an exchange is needed. The volume of fluid instilled and the volume recovered from the abdomen is monitored. Initially, the volume of fluid recovered from the abdomen will be less than that instilled. After a period of time the volumes will equal each other, and, finally, the volume of fluid recovered will exceed that instilled as the dextrose exerts an osmotic effect on plasma.

Dialysate solutions are available in 250-ml, 500-ml, and 1-, 2-, and 3-L plastic bags. Two-liter bags are the bags most readily available; however, in small dogs and cats only a small portion of a 2-L bag is needed, and transferring the remaining solution to other containers increases the risk of peritonitis. To circumvent this problem, a 2-L bag can be placed on a balance scale located above the caged patient and the weight of the bag recorded when full. The weight of the volume of infusion required is calculated (30–40 ml/kg divided by 1000 ml), and this is subtracted from the weight of the bag. The scale is adjusted to the calculated weight and the infusion is started. When the calculated volume has been infused the scale will balance. The infusion is discontinued by closing the roller clamp on the infusion line. After the appropriate dwell time, the peritoneal effluent is drained back into the dialysate bag, where it mixes with fresh dialysate. Repeated dialysis can continue using the mixed solution until the concentration of uremic toxins in the dialysate is equal to that of the blood. Ultrafiltrate or excess body water is measured as the additional volume of fluid osmotically drawn into the dialysate bag.

Complications and Contraindications

Septic or nonseptic peritonitis is the most serious complication. The incidence of peritonitis can be decreased with appropriate aseptic technique and the infusion of dilute iodine solution following each session. Thornhill and associates (Additional Reading) recommends that a volume of physiologic saline equal to that of dialysate be infused following the completion of each dialysis. It is removed immediately and followed by the instillation of saline with iodine (0.2 ml of 2% iodine per liter of saline). This is removed after a 4-minute period. Peritoneal fluid should be evaluated cytologically and, if indicated, by culture and sensitivity for the presence of infection. If peritonitis is diagnosed, 16 mg of tobramycin and 250 mg of cephalothin sodium is added to every 2 L of dialysate, and cephalexin (20 mg/kg three times daily) is given parenterally until results of the bacterial culture are known.

Other complications may include anorexia, reductions in packed-cell volume and plasma protein, electrolyte imbalance, or trauma to abdominal organs.

Pleural Dialysis

An alternative to peritoneal dialysis is pleural dialysis (Shahar and Holmberg, Additional Reading). It is a less expensive technique than peritoneal dialysis because it does not use the costly Purdue catheter. An Argyle catheter (Argyle thoracic catheter [Sherwood Medical Industries]) was implanted as described under Thoracentesis and Insertion of Chest Tubes. The dialysate may be the same as that described for peritoneal dialysis. The recommended volume of dialysate to be infused is 25 to 35 ml/kg. The connection of the catheter to the dialysate bag is as previously described. Complications associated with this approach may include hemothorax, pneumothorax, hypoproteinemia, pleural adhesion, pyothorax, or dyspnea from the use of too large a volume of dialysate.

CYSTOCENTESIS

Indications

Dysuria, hematuria, bacteriuria, pyuria, or decompression of an obstructed bladder are indications for cystocentesis. The technique prevents contamination of the urine by flora from the urethra, genital tract, and skin, and reduces the risk of iatrogenic urinary tract infection associated with urinary catheterization. Consequently, samples for bacterial culture should be taken by this route.

Limitations

The bladder should be palpable through the abdominal wall before an attempt is made to perform the procedure; thus, cystocentesis is difficult in obese or uncooperative animals. Sedation

is required only in the fractious or uncooperative patient.

Patient Preparation and Technique

Cystocentesis can be performed with the animal standing (Fig. 80-23) or in lateral or dorsal recumbency (Fig. 80-24). If the animal remains standing, the area over the lateral abdominal wall just cranial to the pubis is aseptically prepared. Local anesthesia is not required. A 22-gauge, 1½-inch hypodermic needle is directed at a 45-degree angle into the ventral or ventrolateral bladder wall just cranial to the juncture of the bladder and the urethra. The oblique course of the needle aids in closure of the puncture site in the bladder wall when the needle is withdrawn. Samples are collected and submitted for routine urinalysis and bacterial culture (Tables 80-11 and 80-12).

Complications and Contraindications

The only contraindications are an inability to palpate the bladder and the presence of a bleeding disorder. Complications are rare and are generally related to poor technique. Cystocentesis should not be performed on uncooperative animals, as the risk of trauma is too great. Trauma to the bladder and adjacent bowel are possible complications. Leakage of urine into the peritoneal cavity may occur; however, the leakage of small volumes of normal urine into the peritoneal cavity is not a cause for concern.

NASOESOPHAGEAL INTUBATION

Indications

Nasoesophageal intubation may be used for short-term enteral nutrition (less than 1 week), administration of oral liquid medication, aspiration of gastric fluid in the postoperative period, and decompression and prevention of gastric distention. For diagnostic purposes it serves as an access for the administration of contrast material or ammonium chloride. In contrast to pharyngostomy or tube gastrostomy it is less traumatic and

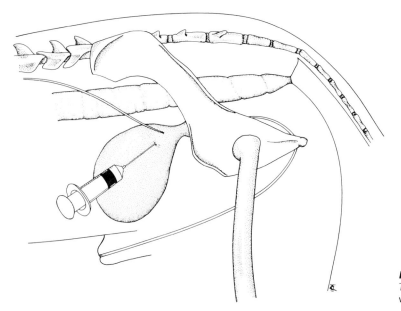

Figure 80–23. *Cystocentesis in the standing dog. The needle is directed at a 45-degree angle into the ventrolateral bladder wall.*

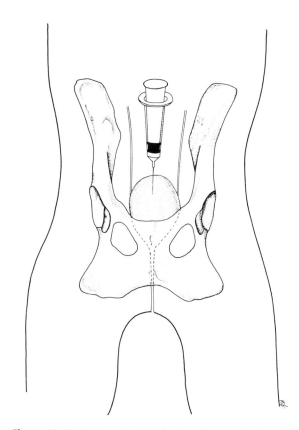

Figure 80–24. *Cystocentesis in the dorsally recumbent animal.*

less expensive, does not require a general anesthetic for placement, requires less time, and presents fewer complications. The same basic technique may be used for the administration of nasal oxygen.

Limitations

The procedure is limited by the size of the animal and the relative diameter of the nares. Consequently, nasoesophageal intubation may not be possible in kittens. The technique cannot be used in animals with nasal obstruction. Nasoesophageal intubation should not be used in animals with esophageal motility disorders, animals that are comatose or lack a gag reflex, or those that are frequently vomiting. The tube itself may become blocked with mucus, food particles, or esophageal or gastric mucosa. To decrease the incidence of this problem, the largest possible tube is chosen and it is periodically flushed with physiologic saline.

Patient Preparation and Technique

The procedure is well described by Crowe (Additional Reading). It is summarized here. Manual restraint and topical nasal anesthesia are re-

Table 80–11 *Physical and Chemical Properties of Normal Urine*

Parameter	Description
Volume	1 to 2 ml/kg/hour or 10 to 20 ml/kg/day
Color	Yellow to amber
Foam	Produces a white foam if shaken
Specific gravity	1.015 to 1.050 (dog)
	1.015 to 1.060 (cat)
Osmolality	750 to 2000 mOsm/kg
Protein	0 to 30 mg/dl, 0 to 1+ on Multistix, or up to 20 mg/kg/day (dog)
	0 to 20 mg/dl or 0 to 1+ on Multistix (cat)
Urine Protein to Creatinine	Normal <0.5 (dog
	Abnormal >1.0 (dog)
	Normal <0.34 (cat)
Glucose	None
Ketones	None
Bilirubin	1+ in 10% to 20% of dogs with high specific gravity
	1+ in 5% of cats with high specific gravity
Urobilinogen	0 to 1 (Ehrlich unit)
	<1:32 (Wallace–Diamond)
pH	5 to 7
Bacteria	Generally no bacteria by cystocentesis; however, up to 1,000 allowed for by contamination
	<10,000/ml by catheterization (dog)
	<1,000/ml by catheterization (cat)
	<100,000/ml free flow (dog)
	<10,000/ml free flow (cat)
Leukocytes	Less than three per high power field by cystocentesis or catheterization
	Less than eight per high power field free flow
Red blood cells	Less than five per high power field
Epithelial cells	Less than two per high power field
Casts	Two to four per low power field
Crystals	Seldom of significance

quired. The head is elevated, and the anesthetic is instilled into the animal's nostril. The dose is five drops of proparacaine hydrochloride (Ophthaine Hydrochloride) in cats and 0.5 to 1 ml of lidocaine hydrochloride in dogs. After a 2- to 3-minute period, the procedure is repeated.

Nasoesophageal tubes are available commercially (Argyle stomach tube [Sherwood Medical Industries], Entron nasogastric feeding tube [Biosearch Medical Products]). Alternatively, an 8F infant feeding tube can be used (American Hospital Supply). The nasogastric tube of choice is based on body size. For animals weighing less than 15 kg, a 5F or 6F polyurethane catheter may be used. In cats, a 19- or 21-gauge butterfly cathe-

ter (with the needle cut off) is an another option. For animals weighing more than 15 kg, a 12F to 18F tube may be used.

The length of tube is estimated by measuring the distance from the external nares to the border of the 11th rib. Unless the purpose of intubation is the removal of gas or gastric fluid, the aboral catheter tip should not extend into the stomach. When the purpose of intubation is enteral nutrition or the administration of medication or contrast material, it is important to retain gastroesophageal sphincter competence and prevent gastroesophageal reflux. If an animal only requires nasal oxygen, the catheter is advanced to the level of the carnassial teeth.

Table 80–12 *Abnormalities in Physical and Chemical Analysis of Urine, and Associated Causes*

Parameter	Interpretation
Volume	<1 ml/kg/hour (oliguria) >50 ml/kg/day (polyuria)
Color	Yellow-brown (urobilin, bilirubin) Red-brown (hemoglobin, myoglobin)
Foam	Excess foam (proteinuria) Green or yellow-brown foam (bilirubinuria) Red-brown foam (hemoglobinuria)
Turbidity	Implies presence of cells or crystals
Odor	Ammonia (bacterial infection) Ketones (diabetes mellitus)
Specific gravity	Dog can normally concentrate to >1.030 Cat can normally concentrate to >1.035 Specific gravity increases only 0.003 unit/g of albumin per 100 ml of urine or every 10 g/L of albumin Specific gravity increases only 0.004 unit/g of glucose per 100 ml of urine or every 550 mmol/L of glucose
Proteinuria	May imply glomerular leakage, reduced tubular absorption, or urinary tract inflammation
Glucosuria	Diabetes mellitus or renal glycosuria
Ketones	Diabetes mellitus
Bilirubinuria	Hepatic or posthepatic biliary tract disease, or, sometimes, severe hemolytic disease
Urobilinogen	Presence implies a patent biliary system Absence may occur with biliary obstruction, polyuria, antibiotic treatment, or diarrhea Increased amounts occur with hemolytic or hepatic disease
pH	Depends on diet, but alkaline urine may be associated with bacterial infection, especially infections caused by proteus or staphylococcus sp.
Occult blood	Positive with hemoglobin or myoglobin, but will not detect hematuria if there is not sufficient red blood cell lysis
Casts	Tubular, epithelial, or glomerular The number of casts does not correlate with the severity of the disease
Crystals	Tyrosine (liver disease) Ammonium urate (portocaval shunt) Calcium oxalate crystals (ethylene glycol toxicity) Cystine (congenital cystinuria)

The tip of the catheter is lubricated with lidocaine jelly (Xylocaine Jelly 2%). The tube is directed ventrally along the ventral nasal meatus, through the pharynx to the distal esophagus (Fig. 80-25). Attempts to pass it through the dorsal or middle meatus will be unsuccessful. The head is slightly elevated. Marked extension of the neck hinders swallowing and may permit the tube to enter the trachea. The position of the tube may be verified by injecting air and listening for gurgling sounds with a stethoscope over the stomach, and by instilling 1 to 2 ml of sterile physiologic saline. If the tube has been inadvertently placed into the trachea the animal should cough, and the procedure will have to be repeated. The tube is secured to the skin near the nares and along the top of the head or along the side of the face with nonabsorbable sutures or Krazy Glue (Krazy Glue Inc.). It is then connected to an intravenous extension set and bandaged to the neck. An Eliz-

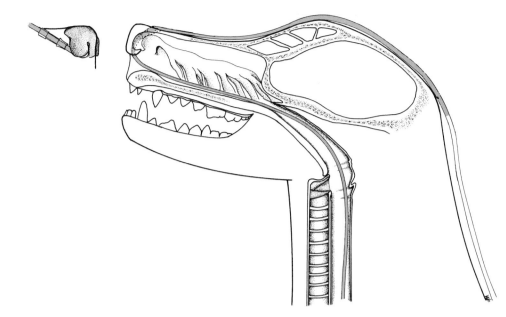

Figure 80–25. Nasoesophageal intubation in a dog. The nasoesophageal tube is passed along the ventral meatus, through the pharynx, and into the distal esophagus.

abethan collar may be required in some animals. To prevent the influx of air into the stomach when the tube is not in use, the end should be capped. To remove the tube, the end is kept sealed to prevent spillage of the tube's contents into the larynx and trachea, the sutures are removed, and the tube is gently pulled out.

Complications and Contraindications

Mild epistaxis on insertion, rhinitis, dacryo-cystitis, and esophageal reflux or vomiting may occur. Trauma to the esophagus and stomach by the tube, reflux esophagitis, and aspiration pneumonia are possible, but rare, sequelae. Animals receiving nasal oxygen are at risk of developing gastric dilatation, and should be monitored for signs of abdominal tympany.

Although the capacity of the stomach in normal dogs and cats is approximately 80 ml/kg, animals anorectic for more than 2 days can only initially tolerate about half this volume at one feeding. The volume of fluid given can be generally increased to normal over a 2 to 3 day period. Excessive intragastric fluid administration may cause vomiting, diarrhea, or abdominal discomfort.

PHARYNGOSTOMY TUBE PLACEMENT

Indications

As with nasogastric intubation, pharyngostomy intubation can be used for the administration of medication or liquid nutrition, the aspiration of gastric fluid in the postoperative period, and the decompression and prevention of gastric distention. It can be used in animals when nasogastric intubation is unsuccessful. The tube can be left in place over a period of weeks without complication.

Limitations

Animals with pharyngeal or esophageal disease or persistent vomiting may be poor candiates for this procedure.

Patient Preparation and Technique

The technique is well described by Crowe (Additional Reading). It is summarized here. General anesthesia is required. Animals are placed in right lateral recumbency and the area over the left lateral cervical area and the angle of the mandible is shaved and aseptically prepared. The index or middle finger of one hand is inserted in the mouth, and the space caudal and dorsal to the hyoid apparatus is palpated (Fig. 80-26). The area is pushed out and a skin incision is made over the area. Previous reports recommended that the tube enter the pharnyx through the piriform recess located between the posterior border of the mandible and the epihyoid cartilage. This site, however, has been associated with laryngeal obstruction, asphyxiation, and aspiration pneumonia (Crowe and Downs, Additional Reading).

Curved Kelly forceps are used to bluntly dissect a tunnel in a slightly caudal direction toward the tip of the finger in the oral cavity. The oral cavity is entered by directing the forceps through the mucous membrane of the pharnyx. The length of tube (14F or larger) (Silastic tubing [Dow Coring Corp.] or Rubber All-Purpose Catheter [Davol], Sovereign Sterile Single-Use Feeding and Urethral Catheter [Sherwood Medical Industries]) is measured from the posterior border of the mandible to the 11th rib. Unless the purpose of intubation is the removal of gas or gastric fluid, the aboral catheter tip should not extend into the stomach. If the purpose of intubation is enteral nutrition or the adminstration of medication or contrast material, it is important to retain gastoesophageal sphincter competence and prevent gastroesophageal reflux.

The tube is placed in the mouth and the esophagus. The end of the tube is beveled, grasped and pulled out through the skin incision with the Kelly forceps. The pharyngostomy tube is secured to the skin with a friction suture technique (see Nasogastric Intubation). When not in use the end is capped to prevent reflux of gastric contents and the aspiration of air. Povidone-iodine ointment is applied to the skin incision and a gauze sponge (cut in half) is used to cover the site. The tube is gently bandaged to the neck, leaving sufficient length uncovered to allow access to the tube. The incision site is cleaned and rebandaged every 24 to 48 hours. To verify correct positioning of the tube in the esophagus, 5 ml of water can be injected into the tube when the animal is conscious. If the animal coughs, the tube should be withdrawn and replaced. Rarely, radiography is necessary to verify correct positioning of the tube. When it is no longer needed, the tube is capped and removed by opening the mouth and withdrawing it into the oral cavity. It is cut at the level of the skin and removed from the mouth. This

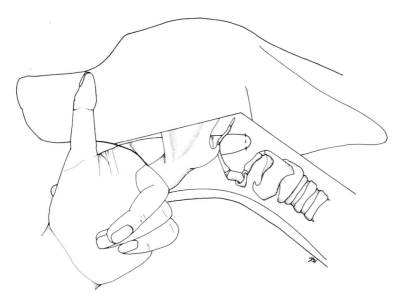

Figure 80–26. Pharyngostomy tube placement. The site for placement of the tube is dorsal and caudal to the hyoid apparatus.

prevents contamination of the pharyngostomy site with gastric contents.

Complications and Contraindications

The tube may become plugged with mucus, food particles, or esophageal or gastric mucosa. To prevent this, the tube should be flushed with water before and after each use. Other complications are rare, but may include reflux esophagitis, esophageal perforation, pharyngitis, laryngitis, laryngeal occlusion, gastritis, vomiting (with tube tips positioned in the stomach), and gastric dilatation with air. Infection of the pharyngostomy site is rare.

SURGICAL TUBE GASTROSTOMY

Indications

Gastrostomy tube placement is indicated in animals with pharyngeal or esophageal disease or facial injury that precludes the use of nasogastric or pharyngeal tube placement. Gastrostomy intubation can be used for the administration of oral liquid medication or liquid nutrition, the aspiration of gastric fluid, and the decompression and prevention of gastric distention. The tube can

be left in place over a period of weeks without major complication.

Limitations

The technique is contraindicated if splenic torsion is present or if the stomach wall is devitalized and prone to rupture. In these cases an exploratory laparotomy is recommended. As with nasogastric intubation and pharyngostomy tube placement, gastrostomy tube placement should be avoided in animals with uncontrolled vomiting, gastric paresis, or gastric outlet obstruction.

Patient Preparation and Technique

The technique has been well described previously (Crowe, Additional Reading). It is summarized here. General anesthesia is required. Animals are placed in right lateral recumbency and the area over the left flank and paracostal region is shaved and aseptically prepared. A 3- to 5-cm vertical skin incision is made 2 cm caudal and parallel to the last rib and 2 to 4 cm below the ventral border of the paravertebral epaxial muscles (Fig. 80-27). The abdominal muscles (external and internal oblique muscle of abdomen and transverse mus-

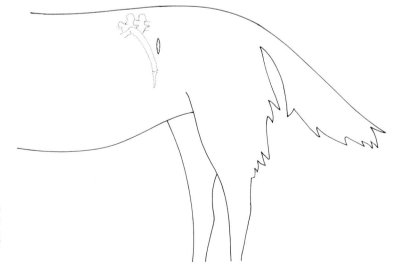

Figure 80–27. *Surgical tube gastrostomy. A 3- to 5-cm vertical incision is made approximately 2 cm caudal and parallel to the last rib and 2 to 4 cm below the ventral border of the paravertebral epaxial muscles.*

cle of abdomen) are separated in the direction of their fibers. The transverse fascia and peritoneum is incised and the stomach is exposed. The stomach is grasped with Allis or Babcock forceps and exteriorized. The left lateral aspect of the body of the stomach or the caudal aspect of the fundus is chosen for the ostomy site. Two full-thickness pursestring sutures of 2-0 or 3-0 nylon, polypropylene, or polydioxanone are placed concentrically through the stomach wall (Fig. 80-28). A stab incision is made in the center of the pursestring suture, and a third pursestring suture is placed in the leading edge of the incision to provide hemostasis. A rubber catheter (18F–22F for cats and 26F–30F for dogs) (Bard Pezzer catheter [C.R. Bard Inc.], Foley urinary catheter [Pharmaseal Laboratories]) is placed into the stomach, and the pursestring sutures are closed and tied. A better seal is provided by placing the catheter through one or more layers of omentum before entering the stomach wall. The stomach is then sutured to the adbominal wall in a simple interrupted or continuous pattern with 2-0 or 3-0

nylon, polypropylene, or polydioxanone suture material. The catheter is brought out through a separate stab incision in the skin and the abdominal wound is closed. The catheter is secured to the skin with a friction suture pattern, and the incision sites are covered with povidone-iodine ointment and a gauze bandage. If a Foley catheter is used, the balloon is filled with saline and pulled against the stomach wall and peritoneum to ensure a tight seal. The tube is then secured to the skin using the friction suture technique (Fig. 80-29). The tube and abdomen are gently bandaged. The site is cleaned and rebandaged every 24 to 48 hours. When not is use, the end of the tube is capped to prevent reflux of gastric contents and the aspiration of air.

When the tube is no longer required, the friction sutures are cut, the fluid in the Foley catheter is removed, and the tube is gently pulled out. Adhesions between the stomach and peritoneum are necessary to prevent leakage of gastric contents into the abdominal cavity, and approximately 8 to 10 days are required for adhesions to form. It is therefore recommended that gastrostomy tubes remain in place for at least this time, or longer if animals are debilitated, hypoalbuminemic, or on corticosteroid therapy.

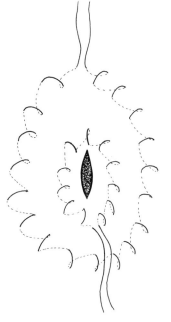

Figure 80–28. *Surgical tube gastrostomy. Two full-thickness pursestring sutures are placed concentrically through the stomach wall. A stab incision is made in the center of the pursestring. (Crowe DT. Enteral nutrition for critically ill or injured patients: Part II. Compendium of Continuing Education 1986; 8:719.)*

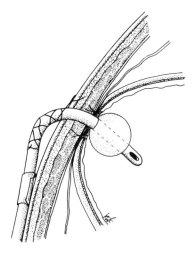

Figure 80–29. *Surgical tube gastrostomy. If a Foley catheter is used, the balloon is filled with saline and pulled against the stomach wall and peritoneum to ensure a tight seal. The tube is then secured to the skin using the friction suture technique. (Crowe DT. Enteral nutrition for critically ill or injured patients: Part II. Compendium of Continuing Education 1986; 8:719.)*

Complications and Contraindications

Peritonitis may result from contamination of the abdominal cavity with gastric contents. Pressure necrosis of the stomach wall and leakage of gastric contents may occur if the gastrostomy tube is pulled too tightly against the gastric mucosa. The tube may become blocked with gastric mucosa or food particles or it may be pulled out by the animal. To prevent plugging of the tube, it can be flushed with water and a small volume of air before and after each use. In some cases, the Foley tip may become digested by gastric contents, causing the tube to fall out prematurely. Vomiting and diarrhea are most often associated with improper feeding practices (too much fluid volume given at any one time), but may be due to gastric irritation from the tube. Infection of the incision sites is also possible.

PERCUTANEOUS TUBE GASTROSTOMY

Indications and Limitations

Same as for Surgical Tube Gastrostomy.

Patient Preparation and Technique

Percutaneous placement of a gastrostomy tube can be done in those practices equipped with a gastroscope (Mathews and Binnington, Additional Reading). The procedure can be carried out in cats with ketamine hydrochloride, in dogs with droperidol-fentanyl (Innovar-Vet), or in both species under general anesthesia. It is a simple, safe, quick, and effective means of delivering food and can be left in place over a period of weeks. Animals have been maintained with percutaneous tube gastrostomy for periods in excess of 320 days. Once in place, owners can be instructed how to feed the animals at home.

The equipment needed includes a soft, 16F de Pezzer (mushroom) catheter, a 200-μl disposable pipette tip (Medical Laboratory Automation), approximately 36 inches of 0 monofilament nylon suture material, and soft rubber tubing. Kits are available for human patients (*e.g.*, Dubhoff PEG, Biosearch). The gastrostomy tube is prepared by cutting off its wide connecting end and the nipple on the mushroom tip (to permit easy passage of food through the catheter). A slit is made in the middle of each of two soft rubber tubes (cut at approximately 3-cm lengths). These tubes will be used as flanges to secure the gastrostomy tube against the abdominal wall in the stomach and to keep the gastrostomy tube in place against the skin. One flange is slipped over the gastrostomy tube and seated next to the mushroom head. The other will be placed over the gastrostomy tube after it has been placed in the stomach.

Animals are starved for at least 12 hours, anesthetized, and placed in right lateral recumbency, and the skin is aseptically prepared. A gastroscope is inserted through the mouth to the level of the stomach. The stomach is gently inflated with air until distention is visible externally. This pushes the abdominal contents away from the gastrostomy site and brings the stomach wall in contact with the abdominal wall. A small (3-mm) incision is made in the skin over the distended stomach immediately caudal to the 13th rib and just ventral to the floating rib. An 18-gauge, 1½-inch needle is then inserted through the skin incision and the abdominal wall, into the distended stomach. The suture material is threaded through the needle into the stomach, visually grasped with biopsy forceps directed through the gastroscope (Fig. 80-30), and brought out through the mouth along with the gastroscope. (Capping the end of the needle with a finger aids endoscopic retrieval of the suture material by keeping the stomach insufflated.) The needle is removed from the abdominal wall and the pipette is passed, tapered end first, over the suture material exiting from the mouth. (Alternatively the tapered Sovereign 16 g Indwelling Catheter may be used instead of the pipette. This product is new and I have not yet had experience with it.) The end of the gastrostomy tube is bevelled at a 60-degree angle, and the suture material secured to the end of the tube farthest away from the mushroom tip. The suture material is grasped and pulled, drawing the gastrostomy tube into the wide end of the pipette (Fig. 80-31). Continuous traction on the suture material exiting from the abdominal wall and maintainance of counterpressure against the skin with the palm of the opposite hand brings

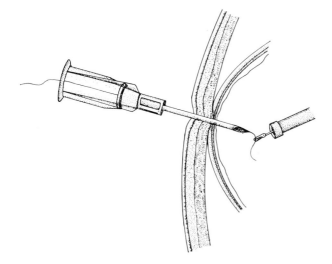

Figure 80–30. *Percutaneous tube gastrostomy. The monofilament suture material is threaded through the needle into the stomach and visually grasped by biopsy forceps directed through the gastroscope.*

the pipette and gastrostomy tube through the mouth, esophagus, stomach, and abdominal incision. The gastroscope is reinserted to ensure proper placement of the gastrostomy tube against the abdominal wall (the mushroom tip and flange should be in loose contact with the stomach wall when gentle traction is applied externally). The gastrostomy tube is fitted externally with a flange of soft rubber tubing to ensure close contact with the skin, and a piece of adhesive tape is wrapped around the tube just behind the flange to prevent it from slipping off the gas-

trostomy tube (Fig. 80-32). The tube is then bandaged to the skin.

The gastrostomy tube should remain in place for no less than 8 to 10 days. To remove it, continuous traction is applied on the tube while counterpressure is maintained with the opposite hand. The inner flange remains in the stomach and is passed in the feces. In larger dogs (more than 10 kg), the catheter may be cut flush with the skin and the mushroom tip allowed to pass in the feces.

Complications and Contraindications

Complications noted with the percutaneous technique are few, but may include pressure necrosis of the stomach wall or skin if the flanges are applied too tightly. Fever may occur in some animals, and is most commonly observed 3 to 4 days after placement of the gastrostomy tube. These animals readily respond to antibiotic therapy. Vomiting has also occurred in some animals.

CEREBROSPINAL FLUID COLLECTION

Indications

Diseases of the central nervous system often result in abnormal cell counts, protein concentrations, and cytology of the cerebrospinal fluid

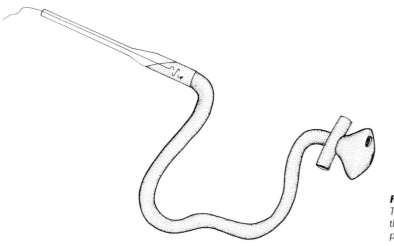

Figure 80–31. *Percutaneous tube gastrostomy. The suture material is grasped and pulled, drawing the gastrostomy tube into the wide end of the pipette.*

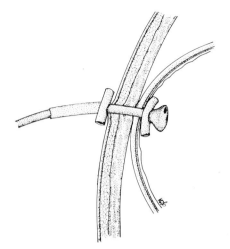

Figure 80–32. *Percutaneous tube gastrostomy. The gastrostomy tube mushroom tip and flange should be in loose contact with the stomach wall. The tube is fitted externally with a flange of soft rubber tubing to ensure close contact with the skin. A piece of adhesive tape is wrapped around the tube just behind the flange to prevent it from slipping off the gastrostomy tube.*

(CSF). Analysis of the CSF can help determine the type and severity of central nervous system disease and monitor its progress.

Limitations

In general, diseases affecting the meninges are more likely to alter the CSF than diseases of the nervous system parenchyma. Some cases exhibiting clinical signs of central nervous system disease may have a normal CSF analysis (metabolic, congenital, nutritional, and toxic encephalopathies and idiopathic epilepsy). Neoplasms of the central nervous system can be difficult to diagnose on CSF analysis. Neoplastic cells are rarely seen in CSF except in dogs with central nervous system lymphosarcoma (Couto et al, Additional Reading). The success of identifying and culturing bacterial organisms in cases of bacterial meningitis is poor (less than half of cases are successfully identified).

Patient Preparation and Technique

General anesthesia is required. The cisterna magna is the preferred site for CSF collection. The caudal lumbar subarachnoid space is not routinely used for the collection of CSF because this space is technically more difficult to puncture, there is less fluid present, and the fluid more often becomes contaminated with peripheral blood. The site is used, however, for myelographic studies of thoracolumbar lesions. The lumbar approach is associated with fewer central nervous system side effects following myelography.

Cisternal Collection

The area from the occipital protuberance to the axis is shaved and aseptically prepared. For right-handed operators, the animal is placed in right lateral recumbency. The head is held parallel to the table and the neck is flexed at a 90-degree angle to the long axis of the spine. A 20- to 22-gauge spinal needle (Monoject spinal needle [Sherwood Medical Industries]) is inserted in the dorsal midline depression, at a point where the midline and a line drawn perpendicular to the cranial edges of the wings of the atlas intersect (Fig. 80-33). The needle is slowly advanced, with frequent stops to check for the presence of CSF before advancing farther. A loss of resistance may be noticed as the needle enters the subarachnoid space. If bone is contacted, the needle is withdrawn and redirected following reassessment of the landmarks for insertion. If frank blood fills the needle, it is withdrawn and the procedure is repeated using a new needle.

If CSF pressure is measured, the spinal needle may be connected to a three-way stopcock and a manometer (Manometer Tray [Pharmaseal Laboratories]) and the maximum elevation of CSF fluid recorded. Care must be taken not to dislodge the spinal needle during the measurement. Compression of the jugular veins causes an elevation in CSF pressure. Changes in CSF pressure also accompany changes in central venous pressure and the anesthetic regimen chosen. Cerebrospinal fluid pressure may also be normal in animals with central nervous system disease. The measurement of CSF pressure is not considered a routine part of the CSF analysis.

One to two milliliters of CSF is allowed to flow by gravity into a serum or EDTA tube (if the sample appears purulent). Aspiration of CSF should not be performed, because even gentle aspiration

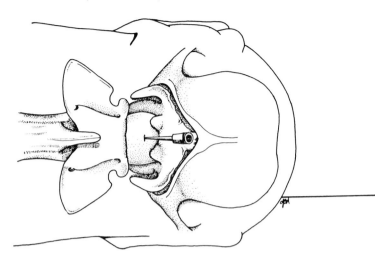

Figure 80–33. *Cisternal cerebrospinal fluid collection. The needle is directed in the dorsal midline, perpendicular to the spine at a point where the midline and a line drawn perpendicular to the cranial wings of the atlas intersect. This drawing denotes the correct position of the needle only. The needle passes into the subarachnoid space; it does not enter spinal cord tissue.*

will induce hemorrhage and alter the interpretation of the sample. Cerebrospinal fluid samples are analyzed on the basis of protein content and cell type and numbers (Tables 80-13 and 80-14). Where appropriate, bacterial or fungal cultures are submitted. Samples for cytologic interpretation must be processed by sedimentation or cytocentrifugation within 30 minutes of collection, and slides for microscopy prepared. The technique for preparation of cytologic samples is described by Mayhew and Beal (Additional Reading).

Lumbar Spinal Collection

Animals are placed in right lateral recumbency, and the caudal lumbar spine is slightly flexed by bringing the forelimbs and hindlimbs together. The area over the lumbosacral spine is shaved and aseptically prepared. The site for lumbar puncture is the space between L-5 and L-6. The needle is inserted at the cranial border of the dorsal spinal process and advanced perpendicular to the spine through the interarcual space and into the subarachnoid space (Fig. 80-34). Penetration of the dura may be signalled by a flinching of the hindlegs. If CSF is not obtained, the needle should be advanced to the ventral spinal floor and slowly retracted into the ventral subarachnoid space. If the tap is unsuccessful, the needle is redirected and a second attempt is made.

Complications and Contraindications

Cisternal puncture, predisposing to tentorial or foramen magnum herniation and subsequent apnea or death, is increased in animals with obvious mentation abnormalities (disorientation,

Table 80–13 *Normal Cerebrospinal Fluid Parameters (Cisterna Magna)*

Parameter	Normal Finding
Appearance	Clear, colorless
Total white cell count	Less than two cells per µl (0.002 × 10⁹/L) Composed primarily of mononuclear cells
Total red cell count	No cells
Protein content	0.1 to 0.3 g/L (10 to 30 mg/dl) (dog) 0.04 to 0.32 g/L (4 to 32 mg/dl) (cat)
Pándy's test	No turbulence
Opening pressure	50 to 180 mm H₂O

Table 80–14 *Common Central Nervous System Disorders and Expected Cerebrospinal Fluid Changes*

Disorder	Appearance	Cell Count	Primary Cell Type	Protein Content
Congenital hydrocephalus	Clear	N	N	N
Bacterial disease	Clear or turbid	I	Neutrophils	I
Viral disease	Clear or turbid	N or I	Small lymphocytes, mononuclears, and few neutrophils	N or I
Fungal disease (cryptococcosis)	Turbid or xanthochromic	I	Neutrophils, mononuclears, and occasional eosinophils	I
Protozoal disease (toxoplasmosis)	N or xanthochromic	I	Neutrophils and macrophages	I
Neoplasia	Clear	N or I	N or occasional mononuclears, and eosinophils	N
Trauma	Clear, xanthochromic, or hemorrhagic	N or I	Neutrophils, lymphocytes variable, red blood cells	I
Fibrocartilaginous myelopathy	Clear	N	N or in acute cases, neutrophils	N or I
Degenerative radiculomyelopathy	Clear	N	N	N or I
Granulomatous meningoencephalitis	Clear or turbid	I	Mononuclears, lymphocytes, and neutrophils	I

(N = normal; I = increased)

stupor, or coma) suggestive of increased intracranial pressure. To avoid accidental trauma to the cervical spinal cord and subsequent respiratory paralysis, the animal must be kept motionless during the procedure. Maintenance of a steady plane of general anesthesia is imperative. Lumbosacral ventral spinal taps are associated with myelomalacia along the tract of needle puncture, but it rarely is associated with detectable neurologic dysfunction.

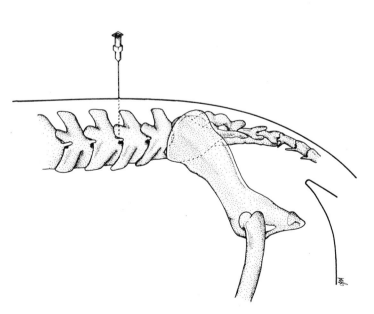

Figure 80–34. *Lumbar spinal tap. The needle is directed perpendicular to the spine at the cranial edge of the dorsal spinal process between L5 and L6.*

ARTHROCENTESIS

Indications

In addition to the physical examination, history, and other ancillary tests, arthrocentesis helps detect the presence and distribution of joint pathology. Analysis of joint fluid differentiates inflammatory (septic and nonseptic) and noninflammatory joint disease. Arthrocentesis is indicated in animals with historical or physical evidence of lameness (even if the joints appear normal on physical examination), joint swelling, stiffness, or fever of unknown origin. Therapeutically, arthrocentesis decompresses distended joints, removes exudate, and allows for the instillation of medication into the joint space. The progress of the disease and the success of therapy can be objectively monitored with repeat joint taps. The technique also provides an access for contrast radiography.

Limitations

The only limitation is technical. Some joints, and especially those with small volumes of fluid are more difficult to aspirate.

Patient Preparation and Technique

In many animals arthrocentesis can be safely accomplished without sedation. For uncooperative patients sedation (see Liver Biopsy) is recommended. It is important that patients remain motionless during the tap. Sudden movement could cause iatrogenic hemorrhage, making interpretation of the sample difficult. Several joints should be aspirated at any one time to help determine the distribution of the problem and increase diagnostic accuracy. The area over the joint (Figs. 80-35 and 80-36) is shaved and surgically prepared. It is gently flexed to open the joint space, and the needle (1- to 1½-inch, 22-gauge hypodermic needle), attached to a 3-ml syringe, is inserted. Joint fluid is gently aspirated. Excessive negative pressure will induce hemorrhage. Normal joints contain 0.01 to 1.0 ml or more of synovial fluid.

Joint fluid is examined on the basis of clarity, color, viscosity, white cell number, and cell type (Table 80-15). Normal joint fluid is clear and colorless to straw-colored. It appears turbid and yellow or bloody in immune-mediated disease and purulent in septic disease. The predominant cell type in the normal joint is the mononuclear cell (predominantly monocytes and macrophages). Neutrophil numbers increase in immune-mediated (nondegenerative) joint disease and septic (degenerative) joint disease. Bacteria may be evident in cases of septic arthritis. Septic cases are cultured for bacteria.

To prepare slides for interpretation, a drop of joint fluid is placed on a glass slide and covered with another glass slide. The joint fluid is allowed to spread, and the slides are drawn apart. The slides are then air dried or cytofixed.

Complications and Contraindications

Animals with coagulation abnormalities are predisposed to hemarthrosis and should generally not undergo arthrocentesis. Possible complications include hemarthrosis, damage to cartilage and bone, iatrogenic infection, and breakage and loss of the needle in the joint space.

BONE BIOPSY

Indications

Closed bone biopsy is indicated in animals with radiographic evidence of bone pathology. It will help differentiate malignancy, infection, trauma,

Figure 80–35. *Arthrocentesis of joints of the forelimb. (A) Left shoulder. The needle enters the scapulohumeral joint proximal to the lateral aspect of the greater tubercle of the humerus, lateral to the supraglenoid tubercle of the scapula, and ventral to the acromion process of the scapula. Alternatively, the needle can enter distal to the acromion process and be directed downward and slightly posterior. (B) Elbow. The elbow is flexed and the needle is directed from the posterolateral aspect, dorsal to the olecranon process and medial to the lateral humeral condyle. (C) Carpus. The carpus is gently flexed and the needle is directed perpendicular to the point of entry. Joint capsules are shaded. (Newton CD, Nunamaker DM. Textbook of small animal orthopaedics. Philadelphia: JB Lippincott, 1985: 1015.)* ▶

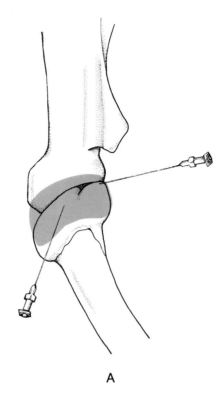

A

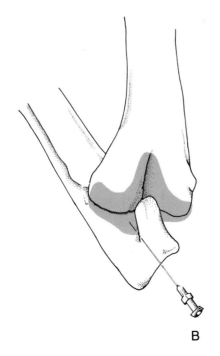

B

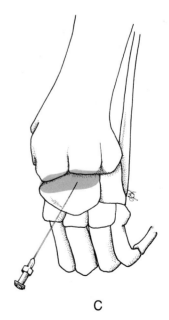

C

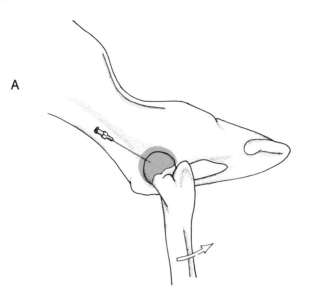

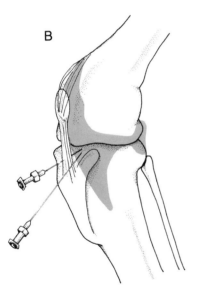

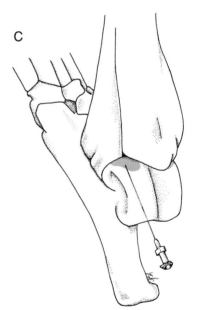

Figure 80–36. *Arthrocentesis of joints of the hindlimb. (A) Hip. To gain access to the hip, the femur is abducted and the leg is extended posteriorly. The needle is advanced in a caudoventral direction, anterior and slightly dorsal to the greater trochanter. (B) Stifle. The stifle and tarsus are gently flexed for arthrocentesis. The stifle joint is entered by inserting the needle medial to, lateral to, or directly through the patellar ligament into the joint space. (C) Left tarsus. To enter the left tarsal joint space, the needle is directed medially from the lateral aspect of the joint parallel to the fibular tarsal bone. Joint capsules are shaded. (Newton CD, Nunamaker DM. Textbook of small animal orthopaedics. Philadelphia: JB Lippincott, 1985: 1015.)*

Table 80–15 *Common Changes in Joint Fluid With Disease*

Condition	Appearance	Viscosity	White Blood Cells per µL†	Cell Type*
Normal	Clear	N	0 to 3,000	Monocytes, lymphocytes 65% to 90%, neutrophils 10%
Degenerative	Clear	N to D	0 to 4,000	Mononuclears 85% to 100%, macrophages increased, neutrophils none to 15%
Traumatic	Clear or turbid	N to D	2,500 to 3,000 +	N, macrophages increased
Septic	Turbid	D	40,000 to 200,000 +	Mononuclears 1% to 10%, degenerate neutrophils, 90% to 99%
Rheumatoid arthritis-like	Turbid	D	3,000 to 40,000 +	Mononuclears 20% to 80%, neutrophils 20% to 80%
Immune-mediated	Turbid	D	100,000 to 300,000	Mononuclears 5% to 85%, neutrophils 15% to 95%

(N = normal, D = decreased)
* *mononuclears include monocytes, lymphocytes, and macrophages*
† *To convert old units (white blood cell count) to SI units, the conversion factor is 10^6. For example, if the total white blood cell count is 3,000 per µl, the same figure in SI units is $3 \times 10^9/L$.*

and degenerative lesions. Histologic diagnosis of tumor type and grade is possible. Samples can also be cultured for bacteria or fungi.

Limitations

Negative biopsy results may be attributed to failure to sample a representative area.

Patient Preparation and Technique

General anesthesia is preferred. Radiographs are used to locate the site of the lesion. Two views are indicated. The radiographic center of the bony lesion provides more accurate samples for a histologic diagnosis than the transition zone or normal bone (Wykes et al, Additional Reading). A 4-inch, 8- to 11-gauge biopsy needle (Jamshidi biopsy needle [Kormed]) is preferred. Use of the Michelle trephine is an alternative (Wykes et al, Additional Reading). However, although it provides samples of larger diameter, it is diagnostically no more accurate than use of the Jamshidi biopsy needle.

The area over the lesion is shaved and aseptically prepared. A stab incision is made in the skin. Soft-tissue structures are retracted to the level of the bone. With the stylet in place the biopsy needle is advanced with a twisting motion through the soft-tissue structures and positioned against the cortex. The stylet is removed and the needle is gently pushed through the cortex into the medullary cavity (Fig. 80-37). The biopsy needle is withdrawn and the tissue sample is pushed out of the cannula with the probe. The needle is redirected and the procedure is repeated. Several tissue samples are obtained. Multiple samples increase diagnostic accuracy. Impression smears can be made, and samples can be submitted for bacterial or fungal culture. Tissue samples are fixed in 10% buffered formalin. The skin is sutured and the area lightly bandaged.

A modified technique described by Tangner (Additional Reading) eliminates sampling errors and improves diagnostic yield. Tangner places a small K-wire through the proposed biopsy site and confirms its position radiographically. The procedure may be repeated with another pin, leaving the first in place to serve as a guide, if the first attempt was not satisfactory. A Michelle trephine is then positioned over the pin and advanced into the bone, and a sample is taken.

Complications and Contraindications

Complications are rare. Subcutaneous hematoma, iatrogenic infection, or pathologic fracture are possible. Biopsy of malignant tissue does not appear to increase the metastatic potential of the tumor. There are no contraindications.

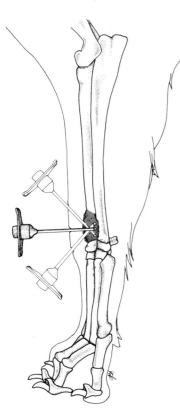

Figure 80–37. *Bone biopsy. The biopsy needle is directed into the radiographic center of the lesion (shaded area). The needle is redirected and the procedure is repeated several times.*

BONE MARROW ASPIRATION AND BIOPSY

Indications

Aspiration or core marrow biopsy is indicated in animals with nonregenerative anemia, thrombocytopenia, leukopenia, atypical peripheral blood cells, or osteomyelitis. It is also used to stage lymphosarcoma and mast cell cancers.

Limitations

The procedure is technically more difficult to complete on obese or very small patients.

Patient Preparation and Technique

The dorsal iliac crest is the preferred site for bone marrow aspiration and biopsy (Fig. 80-38). Other potential sites include the intertrochanteric fossa of the femur, the greater tubercle of the humerus, the sternum, or ribs. Many animals, especially those debilitated by disease, require only local anesthesia. Others require sedation (see Liver Biopsy) or general anesthesia. The area over the

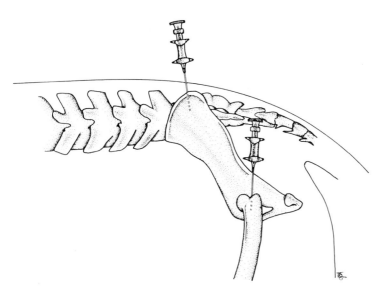

Figure 80–38. *Landmarks for bone marrow biopsy of the iliac crest and intertrochanteric fossa of the femur.*

iliac crest is shaved and aseptically prepared. Local anesthesia (lidocaine hydrochloride 2%) is infiltrated in the skin down to the level of the periosteum.

Bone Marrow Aspiration

A stab incision is made in the skin over the iliac crest approximately 2 to 3 cm from the anterior border of the ilium. A 16- to 18-gauge Rosenthal or Osgood biopsy needle (Becton Dickinson Co.) is used. With the stylet in place, the biopsy needle is directed through soft tissues to the level of the periosteum. The needle is firmly seated at the widest point of the iliac crest and rotated along its axis through the cortex parallel to the wing of the ilium until it is firmly embedded in bone (see Fig. 80-38). Alternatively, the needle can be tapped into the medullary cavity using a hammer. The stylet is removed and a 12-ml syringe attached to the needle, and marrow contents are vigorously aspirated. It is not uncommon to induce pain during this phase of the procedure. When marrow contents appear in the syringe, the needle is removed by twisting and pulling it around its axis. If the tap is unsuccessful, the needle is removed, the stylet replaced, the needle redirected, and aspiration attempted a second time. The contents of the syringe are expelled onto a glass slide held at an angle to allow blood to run off and bony spicules to remain. The slide is covered with another glass slide and the marrow contents allowed to spread. The slides are pulled apart and air dried or cytofixed. The skin wound is sutured as indicated.

Core Bone Marrow Biopsy

When marrow aspiration is unsuccessful (as is frequently the case with myelofibrotic disease), the cell numbers are low, or the diagnosis is in doubt, core marrow biopsy is indicated. Patient preparation and placement of the needle to the level of the periosteum is the same as that described above. With the stylet in place (Jamshidi biopsy needle [Kormed]), the needle is pushed ventrally through the cortex, parallel to the wing of the ilium. When it is firmly embedded in bone

the stylet is removed and the needle is advanced farther to obtain a core of tissue. The needle is rotated in opposite directions around its axis, withdrawn slightly, redirected, and advanced again to break away the tissue sample. The needle is removed by pulling and twisting it in opposite directions around its axis. The sample is expelled with the probe. Impression smears are made and the tissue is fixed in 10% buffered formalin.

Complications and Contraindications

Animals with coagulopathies or thrombocytopenia are predisposed to intramedullary hemorrhage and subcutaneous hematoma. It is my experience that animals with only thrombocytopenia rarely suffer significant bleeding with either procedure. Although rare, iatrogenic infection, soft-tissue trauma, and breakage and lodging of the needle in the bone are potential complications.

CATHETER BIOPSY OF THE URETHRA, BLADDER, AND PROSTATE GLAND

Indications

Catheter biopsy is indicated in animals presented with hematuria, a palpable mass, or radiographic or ultrasonographic evidence of neoplasia of the bladder. The suspect disease is usually transitional cell carcinoma of the urethra or trigonal area of the bladder, but confirmation of the diagnosis has not been possible by urinalysis. The collection of neoplastic cells eliminates the need for laparotomy and biopsy.

Limitations

This technique is generaly only of value in animals with lesions involving the urethra, prostate, or bladder trigone. Failure to collect neoplastic cells does not rule out neoplasia as a cause of disease.

Patient Preparation and Technique

Only manual restraint is required. The largest-diameter urinary catheter (with side holes) that can be advanced into the urethra is chosen. The bladder is catheterized and emptied of urine. The catheter is attached to a 12-ml syringe filled with 3 to 10 ml of normal saline and guided to the level of the lesion, as indicated by radiographs or ultrasonographs or by a finger inserted in the rectum (Fig. 80-39). With a finger in the rectum, the lesion is pushed ventrally against the urinary catheter. Negative pressure is applied by retracting the syringe plunger, and the catheter is rapidly moved back and forth over a short distance to secure a piece of tissue. The negative pressure is gradually released and the catheter is withdrawn. If the lesion involves the prostate gland, it should be massaged rectally prior to and during the aspiration phase. Tissue pieces are fixed in 10% buffered formalin and evaluated histologically. Slides are made of the remaining liquid portion of the sample and examined cytologically.

Samples can also be cultured for microorganisms.

Complications and Contraindications

Although uncommon, it is possible to lacerate the urethra or bladder wall with the catheter.

PROSTATIC MASSAGE, URETHRAL BRUSH TECHNIQUE, AND EJACULATION

Indications

Evaluation of prostatic fluid is indicated in animals presented with prostatic enlargement, pyruria, hematuria, or recurrent urinary tract infection. It may also be indicated in patients with a history of tenesmus or stranguria, and is an important part of a full reproductive examination. The urethral brush technique may be useful for

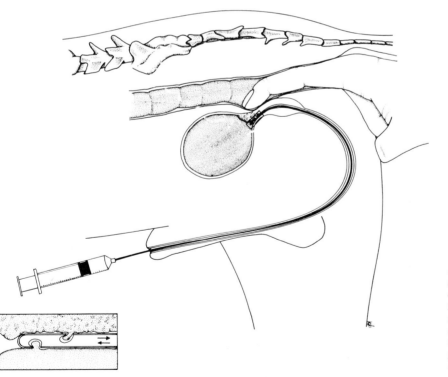

Figure 80–39. *Catheterization and aspiration of a lesion in the neck of the bladder. (Inset) Negative pressure is applied and the catheter is rapidly moved back and forth over a short distance to secure a piece of tissue. The negative pressure is gradually released and the catheter is withdrawn.*

the cytologic diagnosis of prostatic neoplasia, hyperplasia, and bacterial and nonbacterial prostatitis.

Limitations

Ejaculation and prostatic massage may lead to a false-positive diagnosis of prostatic bacterial infection due to contamination with bacteria from the urethra and prepuce. Prostatic massage and wash is not useful in the presence of urinary tract infection. It is also not possible to determine if bacteria and cells originated from the prostate gland, urinary bladder, or urethra with this method. An ejaculate may be difficult to obtain if the animal cannot be aroused. Pain associated with prostatitis may be responsible.

Patient Preparation and Technique

Prostatic Massage

The prepuce and distal part of the penis are retracted and cleansed with a 1 : 1000 dilution of aqueous benzalkonium chloride (Zephiran Chloride). An appropriately sized urinary catheter is passed and the bladder is emptied. This sample should be saved for comparison with the prostatic wash. If bacterial numbers obtained after prostatic massage are a factor of 10^2 per milliliter greater than those obtained prior to massage, the infection is likely to be of prostatic origin (see Chapter 57). The bladder is washed and emptied several times with sterile physiologic saline. The prostate and distal urethra are palpated per rectum. The catheter is then retracted in the urethra just distal to the prostate, where it can be palpated per rectum. Both sides of the prostate gland should be massaged (Fig. 80-40); animals with acute prostatitis may find this painful. A 12-ml syringe of sterile saline is attached, and the urethra is occluded by pressing down on the catheter from the rectum to prevent the retrograde loss of fluid, and then flushed. The catheter is advanced into the bladder and aspiration is performed.

Prostatic massage and wash is indicated in patients without urinary tract infection, in patients in which the urinary tract infection is controlled, or in those in which ejaculation is unsuccesful.

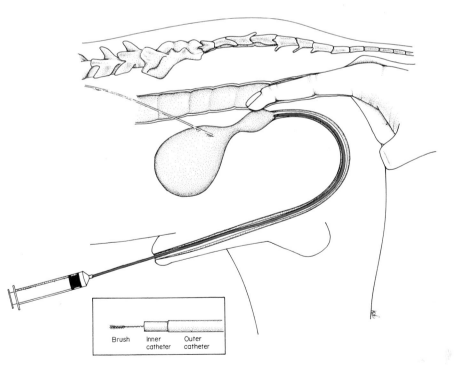

Figure 80–40. *Prostatic massage. A urinary catheter attached to a syringe is advanced just caudal to the prostate gland. The prostate gland is massaged and washed, and the fluid is collected from the bladder. (Inset) Urethral brush. The brush is advanced through the inner catheter.*

Brush   Inner catheter   Outer catheter

Urinary tract infection can be controlled with parenteral ampicillin given 24 hours prior to the collection of the wash. Ampicillin will effectively control the urinary tract infection but will not cross the blood–prostatic barrier. Acute prostatitis may be an exception. In this case the blood–prostatic barrier is more susceptible to penetration by ampicillin.

Urethral Brush Technique

The dog is placed in lateral recumbency and the prepuce and penis are cleansed as described above. A sterile 90-cm microbiologic specimen brush (Microvasive Inc.) is advanced into the urethra to a point just caudal to the prostate gland. The collection brush is protected from distal urethral contamination by a plug within the distal catheter tip of the double-walled catheter. The prostate gland is massaged per rectum, and the inner catheter is then advanced approximately 1 cm forward, dislodging the absorbable catheter plug. The brush is advanced and retracted five or more times to secure representative cytologic material (see Fig. 80-40, inset). The brush and inner catheter are retracted, and the entire device is removed from the urethra. Fluid within the catheter is expelled for cytologic and microbiologic evaluation. The brush is extruded, snipped off with sterile scissors, and mixed into a test tube containing 3 ml of sterile lactated Ringer's injection. Approximately 0.5 ml of this solution is mixed with 0.1 ml of bovine serum albumin in a cyocentrifuge chamber and spun down at 2000 rpm for a 5-minute period, after which samples are prepared for cytologic examination using Wright's stain.

Ejaculation

Culture and sensitivity of prostatic fluid obtained by ejaculation is more accurate for a diagnosis of bacterial prostatitis than samples obtained by prostatic massage and wash, peripheral complete blood counts, or urine cultures. Animals are ejaculated by penile massage. If necessary, a female dog in estrus can be used to arouse the male and facilitate ejaculation. Alternatively, the pheromone p-methyl hydroxybenzoate can be applied to the vulvar area of the anestrus bitch. The efficacy of this chemical agent in arousing the male dog is questionable. Prostatic fluid comprises the third (last) fraction of the ejaculate. It is collected in a sterile glass vial, sterile urinary container, or sterile plastic syringe case and evaluated cytologically and by bacterial culture (see Chapter 57).

Complications and Contraindications

Complications with any of the procedures described are extremely rare. Catheterization predisposes to urinary tract infection. It is possible to initiate a bleeding episode in animals with bleeding abnormalities. If the presenting problem is hematuria with or without other clinical signs of bleeding, an activated clotting time or full coagulation screen should be completed prior to the collection of prostatic fluid. It is possible to rupture an abscess or perforate the rectum if rectal massage is too vigorous. If available, an abdominal ultrasonographic examination will determine the presence of cystic structures before a massage is undertaken.

PROSTATIC BIOPSY

Indications

Biopsy of the prostate gland is indicated in cases of suspect prostatic pathology that cannot be diagnosed by prostatic wash, catheter biopsy, or ejaculation. Suspect neoplastic disease is the most common indication for the procedure.

Limitations

Focal lesions may be missed by the transabdominal, per rectum, or perianal approach. These techniques should not be done on animals if the prostate cannot be palpated per rectum or through the abdominal wall. In these cases a biopsy can be taken by laparotomy.

Patient Preparation and Technique

The prostate gland is evaluated by abdominal radiography and, where available, abdominal ultrasonography prior to the biopsy procedure. It is also recommended that an ejaculate or prostatic wash be collected beforehand in an attempt to identify bacterial prostatitis. The bladder is emptied before biopsy is performed. General anesthesia or local anesthesia and sedation (see Liver Biospy) is recommended. Three approaches are described.

Transabdominal Approach

The animal is placed in lateral recumbency and the prostate gland is immobilized with one hand. The skin over the biopsy site is surgically prepared. A Tru-Cut biopsy needle (Travenol Laboratories) or a 22-gauge 1 1/2-inch spinal needle (Becton Dickinson) attached to a 12-ml syringe is directed into the gland and a sample is collected (Fig. 80-41*A*).

Per Rectum Approach

The rectum is cleansed by an enema, and a Tru-Cut biopsy needle is directed by the palmar aspect of the index finger rectally to the level of the prostate gland. It is advanced into the prostate gland, from which a sample is collected (Fig. 80-41*B*). Alternatively, a 1 1/2- or 3-inch spinal needle can be used, with the sample aspirated with a 12-ml syringe.

Perianal Approach

The skin lateral to either side of the rectum is shaved and surgically prepared. The prostate is palpated per rectum and immobilized laterally against the pelvis. A Tru-Cut biopsy needle or a 22-gauge spinal needle attached to a 12-ml syringe is advanced 2 to 4 cm ventrolateral to the rectum, medial to the tuberischii, and parallel to the rectum to the level of the prostate. A sample is collected (Figs. 80-41*C* and 80-42).

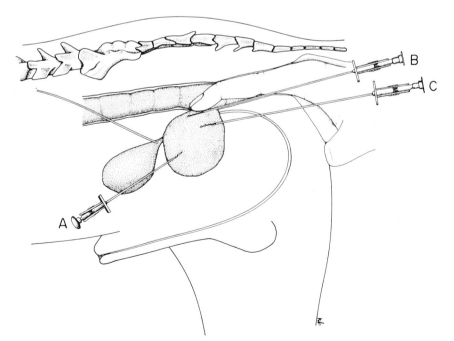

Figure 80–41. *Percutaneous transabdominal (A), per rectum (B), and perineal (C) biopsy approaches to the prostate gland.*

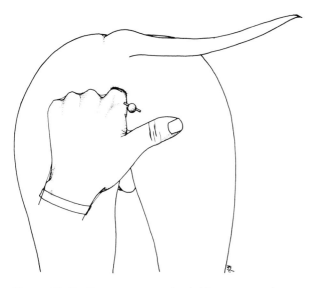

Figure 80–42. *Percutaneous, perineal biopsy approach ventrolateral to the rectum.*

Complications and Contraindications

The presence of a prostatic abscess or cyst is a contraindication to the percutaneous approaches. In these cases laparotomy and biopsy are indicated. Transient, mild hematuria may occur. More serious complications of these procedures are rare, but may include peritonitis, laceration of the urethra, bladder, or intestinal wall, and periprostatic hemorrhage. Animals with bleeding tendencies should not be biopsied.

COLONOSCOPY, MUCOSAL SCRAPING, AND BIOPSY

Indications

Dogs or cats with signs suggestive of chronic or recurrent large bowel disease (tenesmus, mucus-laden stools, increased frequency of defecation, stools with frank blood) are potential candidates for colonoscopy and biopsy. Dietary problems and parasites should be excluded as causes of large bowel disease first. Biopsy should always be a component of the procedure, even if the colon appears to be grossly normal, as changes may be apparent only at a microscopic level.

Limitations

The accurate histologic assessment of colonic tissue depends on the quality of the biopsy material submitted. Small biopsies are difficult to orient for histologic processing and evaluation. Biopsies obtained with forceps may not include the muscularis mucosae, resulting in collapse of epithelial glands. When using biopsy forceps, the clinician should attempt to obtain biopsies that are as large and as deep as is safe. Tissue obtained with a biopsy capsule (described below) is generally easier to evaluate; however, it is very difficult to take directed biopsies with this technique. The optimal situation would be to use forceps for focal lesions and a capsule biopsy instrument for diffuse abnormalities.

Rigid endoscopes usually permit examination of the descending colon only. Examination of the proximal colon and cecum requires a flexible fiberoptic endoscope, the use of which will not be discussed here. Finally, adequate preparation of the colon is essential before colonoscopy and colonic biopsy.

Patient Preparation and Technique

Tests to identify blood clotting abnormalities should be performed before the biopsy procedure.

Food is withheld for a minimum of 24 hours prior to the procedure. A warm-water enema (20 ml/kg) should be administered the evening before and the morning of the procedure. The addition of soap or other additives to the enema water is discouraged, as they may induce artificial changes in the gross and microscopic appearance of the colon. Hypocalcemia may follow the administration of phosphate enemas in cats and small dogs; the use of these enemas is contraindicated in these patients. The animal should be walked immediately before the procedure to encourage it to empty any remaining enema fluid from the colon. Unfortunately, some animals have residual fecal material remaining in the large bowel that hampers the examination.

An oral gastrointestinal lavage solution composed of polyethylene glycol and electrolytes (Golytely, Colyte) safely cleans the large bowel more effectively than repeated enemas. Dogs are given 25 ml/kg of Golytely twice (1 hour apart) through orogastric intubation 12 to 18 hours before proctoscopy. It has been recommended that Colyte be given at a dose of 80 ml/kg, also using orogastric intubation, in two equally divided doses 4 to 6 hours apart in the afternoon of the day preceding the study.

Many animals can be examined and biopsied while they are awake and standing. If the animal is excitable or if the anus is inflamed, sedation (oxymorphone and acepromazine, 0.2 mg/kg and 0.05 mg/kg IV, respectively) may be necessary. General anesthesia is rarely necessary, except with cats and very small dogs, in which the endoscope may be too large to be passed comfortably.

The anus should first be examined for fistulae and fissures, and the anal sacs should be palpated and emptied if necessary. A digital examination of the rectum will help ensure that the animal is properly prepared, and may identify strictures, mass lesions, and rectal diverticula. A rectal mucosal scraping can be performed using a platinum conjunctival spatula (Storz Spatula Platinum Kimura [Ingram and Bell Medical]), and smears can be made for cytologic examination. The procedure is especially rewarding when histoplasmosis is a common complaint.

A rigid fiberoptic endoscope is convenient and easy to use. These are usually sigmoidoscopes designed for use in humans, and a variety of models are available. In cats and dogs weighing less than 10 kg, a pediatric proctoscope 1.5 cm in diameter and 15 cm in length is used. In larger dogs, a sigmoidoscope 2 cm in diameter and 25 cm in length is used. The narrower "stricture" sigmoidoscopes are difficult to see through, are almost impossible to biopsy through, and are not recommended.

The obturator is placed into the endoscope and the instrument is lubricated with water-soluble jelly. The tip of the obturator is held gently against the anus until the anus dilates, then the endoscope is slowly and gently advanced into the rectum. Once in the rectum, the obturator is removed, and any remaining enema fluid is allowed to drain. The door of the endoscope is closed, the colon is gently insufflated, and the endoscope is advanced under visual guidance. The colon is then systematically examined.

Normal mucosa is pink and smooth, although lymphoid aggregates can often be identified as 2- to 3-mm circular to elliptical depressions in the mucosa; these should not be mistaken for ulcers. The operator should attempt to identify erythema, lack of distensibility, ulcers, erosions, masses, parasites, or foreign bodies.

Localized abnormalities should be biopsied with biopsy forceps (ACMI biopsy forceps for colonoscopy [Ingram and Bell Medical]). The door of the endoscope is opened, the biopsy forceps are introduced, and a fold of mucosa is biopsied (Fig. 80-43). The biopsy procedure is usually painless. If no local lesions are seen, at least two to three random biopsies should be obtained. Biopsy tissue should be gently spread out on a small piece of cardboard before immersing in fixative (10% buffered formalin).

Colonic biopsy can also be performed blindly using a suction biopsy capsule (multi-purpose suction biopsy tube [Quinton Instruments]) (Fig. 80-44). This device consists of a cylindrical steel capsule with a side aperture. The capsule is controlled by a long tube. Using a syringe, suction is applied to the capsule, drawing mucosa in through the port. A sliding knife within the capsule is used to cut the tissue. The quality of the biopsy is usually excellent; however, this technique does not allow directed biopsies to be obtained.

The animal should be monitored for several hours after the procedure by following the body temperature and palpating the abdomen. Fever and abdominal pain suggest colonic perforation and peritonitis. In general, animals are discharged the day of the procedure. The owners should be warned that a small amount of blood may be passed when the animal defecates. Feeding can be resumed the same day.

Complications and Contraindications

A bleeding disorder is the major contraindication to biopsy. The major complication is perforation of the colon by the colonoscope or biopsy forceps, leading to peritonitis. This is rare, and is usually associated with severe colonic abnormalities. If signs of peritonitis occur (abdominal splinting,

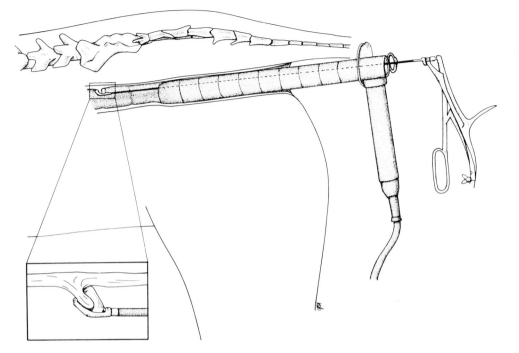

Figure 80–43. *Colonoscopy and biopsy of the colon. The biopsy forceps are advanced through the colonoscope to the level of the lesion, and a fold of mucosa is gently grasped and pulled away from the underlying muscles of the colonic wall (inset). The forceps are closed and the sample is withdrawn from the colon.*

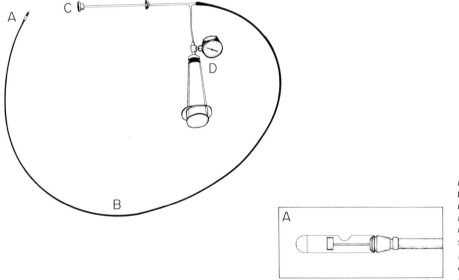

Figure 80–44. *Multi-purpose Suction Biopsy tube (Quinton Instruments). The biopsy capsule (A), flexible tube (B), handle with pull wire used to operate the knife (C), and syringe and vacuum gauge (D) are illustrated. (Inset) Cylindrical biopsy knife and single aperture capsule (same as A, above).*

tenderness and tympany, fever, tachycardia, vomiting), exploratory laparotomy is necessary to repair the rent and to control the infection. Barium studies of the colon should not be performed for 2 weeks following colonic biopsy because the pressure required for the study may cause perforation of the biopsy site.

ADDITIONAL READING

Thoracic Radiography

Burk RL. Radiographic examination of the cardiopulmonary system. Vet Clin North Am 1983; 13:241.

Owens JM. Radiographic interpretation for the small animal clinician. St. Louis, MO: Ralston Purina, 1982: 88.

Root CR, Bahr RJ. The heart and great vessels. In: Thrall DE, ed. Textbook of veterinary diagnostic radiology. Philadelphia: WB Saunders, 1986: 280.

Watters JW. The lungs. In: Thrall DE, ed. Textbook of veterinary diagnostic radiology. Philadelphia: WB Saunders, 1986: 306.

Nonselective Angiocardiography

Fox PR, Bond BR. Nonselective and selective angiocardiography. Vet Clin North Am 1983; 13:259.

Walter PA, Feeney DA, Johnston GR. Diagnosis and treatment of adverse reactions to radiopaque contrast agents. In: Kirk RW, ed. Current veterinary therapy IX. Philadelphia: WB Saunders, 1986: 47.

Echocardiography

Bonagura JD. M-mode echocardiography: Basic principles. Vet Clin North Am 1983; 13:299.

Miles KG. Basic principles and clinical applications of diagnostic ultrasonography. Compendium of Continuing Education 1989; 11:609.

Electrocardiography

Edwards NJ. Bolton's handbook of canine and feline electrocardiography, 2nd ed. Philadelphia: WB Saunders, 1987.

Pericardiocentesis

Sisson DS, Thomas WP, Ruehl WW, Zinkl JG. Diagnostic value of pericardial fluid analysis in the dog. J Am Vet Med Assoc 1984; 184:51.

Nasal Biopsy

Rudd RG, Richardson DC. A diagnostic and therapeutic approach to nasal disease in dogs. Compendium of Continuing Education 1985; 7:103.

Withrow SJ, Susaneck SJ, Macy DW, Sheetz J. Aspiration and punch biopsy techniques for nasal tumors. Journal of the American Animal Hospital Association 1985; 21:551.

Transtracheal Wash

Hoffmann WE, Wellman ML. Tracheobronchial cytology. In: Kirk RW, ed. Current veterinary therapy IX. Philadelphia: WB Saunders, 1986: 243.

Moise NS. Bronchial washings in the cat: Procedure and cytologic evaluation. Compendium of Continuing Education 1983; 5:621.

Tracheobronchoscopy

Amis TC, McKiernan BC. Systematic identification of endobronchial anatomy during bronchoscopy in the dog. Am J Vet Res 1986; 47:2649.

McCarthy GM, Quinn PJ. Bronchoalveolar lavage in the cat: Cytological findings. Canadian Veterinary Journal 1989; 53:259.

Roudebush P. Diagnostics for respiratory diseases. In: Kirk RW, ed. Current veterinary therapy VIII. Philadelphia: WB Saunders, 1983: 222.

Venker-van Haagen AJ. Bronchoscopy of the normal and abnormal canine. Journal of the American Animal Hospital Association 1979; 15:397.

Thoracentesis and Insertion of Chest Tubes

Kagan KG, Stiff ME. Pleural diseases. In: Kirk RW, ed. Current veterinary medicine VIII. Philadelphia: WB Saunders, 1983: 271.

Turner WD, Breznock EM. Continuous suction drainage for management of canine pyothorax: A retrospective study. Journal of the American Animal Hospital Association 1988; 24:485.

Wingfield WE, Bliven MT, Quirk PE. Use of continuous chest drainage in dogs and cats. Journal of the American Animal Hospital Association 1985; 21:29.

Lung Biopsy

Roudebush P. Percutaneous fine needle aspiration of the lung in disseminated pulmonary disease. Journal of the American Animal Hospital Association 1981; 17:109.

Skin Biopsy

Muller GH, Kirk RW, Scott DW. Small animal dermatology, 3rd ed. Philadelphia: WB Saunders, 1983.

Yager JA, Wilcock BP. Skin biopsy: Revelations and limitations. Canadian Veterinary Journal 1988; 29:969.

Liver Biopsy

Bunch SE, Polak DM, Hornbuckle WE. A modified laparoscopic approach for liver biopsy in dogs. J Am Vet Med Assoc 1985; 187:1032.

Hardy RM. Hepatic biopsy. In: Kirk RW, ed. Current veterinary therapy VIII. Philadelphia: WB Saunders, 1983: 813.

Jones BD, Hitt M, Hurst T. Hepatic biopsy. Vet Clin North Am 1985; 15:39.

Kidney Biopsy

Grauer GF, Twedt DC, Mero KN. Evaluation of laparoscopy for obtaining renal biopsy specimens from dogs and cats. J Am Vet Med Assoc 1983; 183:677.

Osborne CA, Low DG, Finco DR. Canine and feline urology. Philadelphia: WB Saunders, 1972: 109.

Jeraj K, Osborne CA, Stevens JB. Evaluation of renal biopsy in 197 dogs and cats. J Am Vet Med Assoc 1982; 181:367.

Withrow SJ, Lowes N. Biopsy techniques for use in small animal oncology. Journal of the American Animal Hospital Association 1981; 17:889.

Abdominal Paracentesis and Lavage

Crowe DT. Diagnostic abdominal paracentesis techniques: Clinical evaluation in 129 dogs and cats. Journal of the American Animal Hospital Association 1984; 20:223.

Hunt CA. Diagnostic peritoneal paracentesis and lavage. Compendium of Continuing Education 1980; 2:449.

Willauer CC, Gregory CR, Parker HR. Treatment of peritonitis with the Parker peritoneal dialysis cannula. Journal of the American Animal Hospital Association 1988; 24:546.

Peritoneal and Pleural Dialysis

Birchard SJ, Chew DJ, Crisp MS, Fossum TW. Modified technique for placement of a column disc peritoneal dialysis catheter. Journal of the American Animal Hospital Association 1988; 24:663.

Shahar R, Holmberg DL. Pleural dialysis in the management of acute renal failure in two dogs. J Am Vet Med Assoc 1985; 187:952.

Thornhill JA. Peritoneal dialysis in the dog and cat. Compendium of Continuing Education 1981; 3:20.

Thornhill JA, Jartmen J, Boon GD et al. Support of an anephric dog for 54 days with ambulatory peritoneal dialysis and a newly designed peritoneal catheter. Am J Vet Res 1984; 45:1156.

Willauer CC, Gregory CR, Parker HR. Treatment of peritonitis with the Parker peritoneal dialysis cannula. Journal of the American Animal Hospital Association 1988;24:546.

Nasogastric Intubation

Crowe DT. Use of nasogastric tube for gastric and esophageal decompression in the dog and cat. J Am Vet Med Assoc 1986; 188:1178.

Pharyngostomy Tube Placement

Crowe DT. Enteral nutrition for critically ill or injured patients: Part II. Compendium of Continuing Education 1986; 8:719.

Crowe DT, Downs MO. Pharyngostomy complications in dogs and cats and recommended technical modifications: Experimental and clinical investigations. Journal of the American Animal Hospital Association 1986; 22:493.

Lantz GC, Cantwell HD, VanVleet JF et al. Pharyngostomy tube induced esophagitis in the dog: An experimental study. Journal of the American Animal Hospital Association 1983; 19:207.

Surgical Tube Gastrostomy

Crowe DT. Enteral nutrition for critically ill or injured patients: Part II. Compendium of Continuing Education 1986; 8:719.

Percutaneous Tube Gastrostomy

Mathews KA, Binnington AG. Percutaneous incisionless placement of a gastrostomy tube utilizing a gastroscope: Preliminary observations. Journal of the American Animal Hospital Association 1986; 22:601.

Cerebrospinal Fluid Collection

Chrisman CL. Problems in small animal neurology. Phildelphia: Lea & Febiger, 1982: 68.

Couto CG, Cullen J, Pedroia V, Turrel JM. Central nervous system lymphosarcoma in the dog. J Am Vet Med Assoc 1984; 184:809.

Kornegay JN. Cerebrospinal fluid collection, examination and interpretation in dogs and cats. Compendium of Continuing Education 1981; 3:85.

Mayhew IG, Beal CR. Techniques of analysis of cerebrospinal fluid. Vet Clin North Am 1980; 10:155.

Arthrocentesis

Fernandez FR, Grindem CB, Lipowitz AJ, Perman V. Synovial fluid analysis: Preparation of smears for cytologic examination of canine synovial fluid. Journal of the American Animal Hospital Association 1983; 19:727.

Werner LL. Arthrocentesis and joint fluid analysis: Diagnostic applications in joint diseases of small animals. Compendium of Continuing Education 1979; 1:855.

Bone Biopsy

Powers BE, LaRue SM, Withrow SJ et al. Jamshidi needle biopsy for diagnosis of bone lesions in small animals. J Am Vet Med Assoc 1988; 193:205.

Tangner CH. A modified technique for closed trephine bone biopsy. Journal of the American Animal Hospital Association 1989; 25:55.

Wykes PM, Withrow SJ, Powers BE, Park RD. Closed biopsy for diagnosis of long bone tumors: Accuracy and results. Journal of the American Animal Hospital Association 1985; 21:489.

Bone Marrow Aspiration and Biopsy

Harvey JW. Canine bone marrow. Normal hematopoiesis, biopsy techniques and cell identification and evaluation. Compendium of Continuing Education 1984; 6:909.

Jain NC. Schalm's veterinary hematology, 4th ed. Philadelphia: Lea & Febiger. 1986: 11.

Catheter Biopsy of the Urethra, Bladder, and Prostate Gland

Barsanti JA. Diagnostic prodedures in urology. Vet Clin North Am 1984; 14:3.

Melhoff T, Osborne CA. Catheter biopsy of the urethra, urinary bladder and prostate gland. In: Kirk RW, ed. Current veterinary therapy VI. Philadelphia: WB Saunders, 1977: 1173.

Prostatic Massage, Urethral Brush Technique, and Ejaculation

Barsanti JA, Finco DR. Evaluation of techniques for diagnosis of canine prostatic diseases. J Am Vet Med Assoc 1984; 185:198.

Kay ND, Ling GV, Nyland TG et al. Cytologic diagnosis of canine prostatic disease using a urethral brush technique. Journal of the American Animal Hospital Association 1989; 25:517.

Ling GV, Branam JE, Ruby AL, Johnson DL. Canine prostatic fluid: Techniques of collection, quantitative bacterial culture, and interpretation of results. J Am Vet Med Assoc 1983; 183:201.

Rogers KS. Diagnostic evaluation of the canine prostate. Compendium of Continuing Education 1986; 8:799.

Thrall MA, Olson PN, Freemyer FG. Cytologic diagnosis of canine prostatic disease. Journal of the American Animal Hospital Association 1985; 21:9

Prostatic Biopsy

Barsanti JA. Diagnostic procedures in urology. Vet Clin North Am 1984; 14:3.

Withrow SJ, Lowes N. Biopsy techniques for use in small animal oncology. Journal of the American Animal Hospital Association 1981; 17:889.

Colonoscopy, Mucosal Scraping, and Biopsy

Burrows CF. Evaluation of a colonic lavage solution to prepare the colon of the dog for colonoscopy. J Am Vet Med Assoc 1989; 195:1719.

Richter KP, Cleveland M. Comparison of an orally administered gastrointestinal lavage solution with traditional enema administration as preparation for colonoscopy in dogs. J Am Vet Med Assoc 1989; 195:1727.

APPENDICES

Conversion Table of Weight to Body Surface Area (in square meters) for Dogs*

Kg	M²	Kg	M²
0.5	0.06	26.0	0.88
1.0	0.10	27.0	0.90
2.0	0.15	28.0	0.92
3.0	0.20	29.0	0.94
4.0	0.25	30.0	0.96
5.0	0.29	31.0	0.99
6.0	0.33	32.0	1.01
7.0	0.36	33.0	1.03
8.0	0.40	34.0	1.05
9.0	0.43	35.0	1.07
10.0	0.46	36.0	1.09
11.0	0.49	37.0	1.11
12.0	0.52	38.0	1.13
13.0	0.55	39.0	1.15
14.0	0.58	40.0	1.17
15.0	0.60	41.0	1.19
16.0	0.63	42.0	1.21
17.0	0.66	43.0	1.23
18.0	0.69	44.0	1.25
19.0	0.71	45.0	1.26
20.0	0.74	46.0	1.28
21.0	0.76	47.0	1.30
22.0	0.78	48.0	1.32
23.0	0.81	49.0	1.34
24.0	0.83	50.0	1.36
25.0	0.85		

* Although the above chart was compiled for dogs, it can also be used for cats. A formula for more precise values follows:

$$BSA \text{ in } M^2 = \frac{K \times W^{2/3}}{10^4}$$

Given that

BSA = body surface area
M² = sq meters
W = weight in gm
K = 10.1 (dogs), 10.0 (cats)

From Ettinger SJ. Textbook of veterinary internal medicine. Vol. I. Philadelphia: WB Saunders, 1975:146.

Note: Many of the drug doses listed are empirical. In some cases, the literature cites two or more dose schedules. The dose, efficacy, and side effects have not been determined for all drugs listed. Many of the drugs have not been approved for use in small animals. Read the product information before using the drug.

APPENDIX I
DRUGS: APPROXIMATE DOSE AND ROUTES OF ADMINISTRATION

Dana G. Allen

DRUG	DOG	CAT
Acetaminophen	10 mg/kg b.i.d. PO	None
Acetazolamide	10 mg/kg q.i.d. PO	Same
Acetohydroxamic acid	10 to 15 mg/kg b.i.d. PO	Unknown
Acetylcholine	6 mg/kg IV	Unknown
Acetylcysteine	50 ml/hour for 30 to 60 minutes b.i.d. by nebulization (respiratory disease)	140 mg/kg (5% solution) PO, IV followed by 70 mg/kg every 4 hours for 3 to 5 treatments (acetaminophen toxicosis)
Acetylpromazine	0.055 to 0.11 mg/kg PO, IV, IM, SC	Same dose PO, IM, SC
Acetylsalicylic acid	10 mg/kg b.i.d.–t.i.d. PO (analgesia) 25 mg/kg t.i.d. PO (antirheumatic) 10 to 25 mg/kg b.i.d. PO or 0.5 mg/kg b.i.d. to 0.5 mg/kg s.i.d. PO (thromboembolic therapy) 7 mg/kg s.i.d. PO (heartworm therapy)	10 mg/kg every other day PO (analgesia) 40 mg/kg every 72 hours (antirheumatic) 25 mg/kg twice weekly PO (thromboembolic therapy)
Albendazole	25 mg/kg b.i.d. PO for 10 days	Same
Albuterol	2 mg t.i.d.–q.i.d. PO	Unknown
Aldactazide	2 mg/kg b.i.d. PO	2.2 to 4.4 mg/kg b.i.d. to every other day PO
Allopurinol	10 mg/kg t.i.d. PO for 1 month, then reduce to 10 mg/kg daily	None
Alpha-Keri	1 capful to 1 to 2 quarts of water for final rinse, or spray aerosol onto wet coat and rub well	Same
Aluminum hydroxide	30 to 90 mg/kg s.i.d.–t.i.d. PO or 300 to 600 mg t.i.d. PO (hyperphosphatemia)	Same 30 to 90 mg/kg in divided doses PO (hyperphosphatemia)

DRUG	DOG	CAT
Aluminum and magnesium hydroxide (Maalox)	5 to 10 ml s.i.d.–q.i.d. PO	Same
Amikacin	5 mg/kg t.i.d. IM, IV, SC	Same
Aminopentamide	0.1 to 0.4 mg b.i.d.–t.i.d. SC, IM or 0.1 mg up to 5 kg 0.2 mg up to 10 kg 0.3 mg up to 20 kg 0.4 mg up to 45 kg	None
Aminophylline	10 mg/kg t.i.d. PO, IM, IV	6.6 mg/kg b.i.d. PO
Aminoproprazine	2 mg/kg b.i.d. IM, SC	Same
Aminosalicylic acid	10 mg/kg bi.d. PO	None
Amitraz	10.6 ml in 2 gallons of water; dip every 2 weeks for 3 treatments, let dry on coat	None
Amitriptyline	2.2 to 4.4 mg/kg s.i.d. PO	5 to 10 mg s.i.d. PO
Ammonium chloride	100 mg/kg b.i.d. PO	20 mg/kg b.i.d. PO or 1 g s.i.d. PO
Amoxicillin	15 to 20 mg/kg b.i.d.–t.i.d. PO 11 mg/kg b.i.d. PO 20 to 50 mg/kg t.i.d. PO, IV, SC, IM	Same 11 to 22 mg/kg s.i.d. PO Same
Amphotericin B	0.15 to 1 mg/kg in 5 to 20 ml of 5% dextrose in water given rapidly IV 3 times weekly for 2 to 4 months; do not exceed 2 mg/kg	Same
Ampicillin	10 to 20 mg/kg q.i.d. PO 5 to 10 mg/kg q.i.d. IV, IM, SC	Same
Amprolium	100 to 200 mg/kg s.i.d. PO for 7 to 10 days	60 to 80 mg/kg s.i.d. PO for 5 days
Amrinone	1 to 3 mg/kg IV followed by 10 to 100 mg/kg/min	Same
Apomorphine	0.04 mg/kg IV 0.08 mg/kg SC, IM	Same
Aprindine	1 to 2 mg/kg t.i.d. PO 100 μg/kg/minute constant infusion	None
Arecoline–acetarsol	5 mg/kg PO once after light meal	Same
Ascorbic acid	100 to 500 mg/day PO (maintenance) 100 to 500 mg t.i.d. PO (urine acidifier)	100 mg/day PO (maintenance) 100 mg t.i.d. PO (urine acidifier) 30 mg/kg q.i.d. PO (acetaminophen toxicosis; support)
Asparaginase	10,000 to 30,000 U/m² IM weekly or 400 U/kg IM once	10,000 U/m² every 1 to 3 weeks IM, SC

DRUG	DOG	CAT
Atenolol	0.5 to 1.0 mg/kg s.i.d.–b.i.d. PO	6.25 to 12.5 mg s.i.d. PO
Atropine	0.02 to 0.04 mg/kg q.i.d. PO, IV, SC, IM	Same
Auranofin	0.05 to 0.2 mg/kg b.i.d. PO	Unknown
Aurothioglucose	1st week: 5 mg IM 2nd week: 10 mg IM Then 1 mg/kg once a week IM decreasing to once a month	1st week: 1 mg IM 2nd week: 2 mg IM Then 1 mg/kg once a week IM decreasing to once a month
Aurothiomalate	Same as for Aurothioglucose	Same
Azathioprine	2 mg/kg s.i.d. PO	1.1 mg/kg every other day PO
Benzoyl peroxide	Bathe every 3 to 14 days p.r.n.; leave on skin for 10 minutes and rinse	Same
Betamethasone	0.15 mg/kg once IM	Topically t.i.d. initially (cream)
Bethanechol	5 to 25 mg t.i.d. PO 2.5 to 10 mg t.i.d. SC	2.5 to 5 mg t.i.d. PO
Bisacodyl	5 to 10 mg s.i.d. PO	5 mg s.i.d. PO
Bismuth subsalicylate	10 to 30 ml every 4 to 6 hours PO or 1 ml/kg s.i.d.–t.i.d. PO	Same with caution
Bunamidine hydrochloride	25 to 50 mg/kg PO once; fast 3 hours before and after administration	Same
Butamisole hydrochloride	2.2 mg/kg SC once	None
Butorphanol tartrate	0.1 to 0.2 mg/kg every 2 to 4 hours IV (analgesia) or 0.2 to 0.4 mg/kg every 2 to 4 hours IM, SC (analgesia) 0.55 mg/kg b.i.d.–q.i.d. PO 0.5 to 1.0 mg/kg b.i.d.–q.i.d. PO (antitussive)	Same None
Butyl chloride	Less than 2.3 kg; 1 ml PO 2.3 to 4.5 kg; 2 ml PO 4.5 to 9 kg; 3 ml PO 9 to 18.2 kg; 4 ml PO More than 18.2 kg; 5 ml PO	None
Calcitonin-salmon	4 to 7 U/kg t.i.d.–q.i.d. SC, IM	Unknown
Calcium carbonate	1 to 4 g/day PO	Same
Calcium chloride (10% solution)	1 ml per 10 kg IV (ventricular asystole)	Same 2 ml/kg/day IV (hypocalcemia)
Calcium gluconate (10% solution)	0.5 to 1.5 ml/kg over 20 to 30 minutes IV	Same or 6 to 8 ml/kg/day IV or up to 750 mg/kg/day PO
Calcium lactate	0.5 to 2 g PO	0.2 to 0.5 g PO or up to 600 mg/kg/day PO
Canex	Apply topically b.i.d. on a 10 day on, 10 day off schedule	Same if diluted 3 : 1 with mineral oil

DRUG	DOG	CAT
Captan powder (50%)	Mix 2 tbsp per gallon of water, apply topically every 3 to 7 days	Same
Captopril	0.5 to 2 mg/kg t.i.d. PO	6.25 mg b.i.d.–t.i.d. PO
Carbamate	Use as a dip every 7 to 14 days; do not rinse off	Same
Carbamazepine	4 to 8 mg/kg b.i.d. PO or 80 to 90 mg/kg divided b.i.d.–t.i.d. PO	Unknown
Carbenicillin	15 mg/kg t.i.d. IV, PO	Same
Carnitine	2 g b.i.d. PO	50 to 100 mg/kg/day PO
Cefoxitin	6 to 40 mg/kg t.i.d. IV, IM, SC	Same
Cephadroxil	10 to 22 mg/kg b.i.d. PO	Same
Cephalexin	10 to 30 mg/kg t.i.d. PO, SC, IM, IV	Same
Cephalothin	20 mg/kg b.i.d.–t.i.d IM, IV	Same
Cephamandole	6 to 40 mg/kg t.i.d.–q.i.d. IM, IV	Same
Cephapirin	10 to 20 mg/kg q.i.d. IM, IV	Same
Cephazolin	20 to 25 mg/kg t.i.d.–q.i.d. IM, IV	Same
Cephradine	20 mg/kg q.i.d. PO 10 mg/kg q.i.d. IM, IV	Same
Charcoal, activated	0.3 to 5 g b.i.d.–t.i.d. PO	Same
Chlorambucil	2 to 8 mg/m² s.i.d. PO for 3 weeks beyond remission, then 1.5 mg/m² s.i.d. PO for 15 days, then every 3rd day	1.5 mg/m², then as for dog
Chloramphenicol	50 mg/kg t.i.d. PO, IV, IM, SC	50 mg/kg b.i.d. PO, IV, IM, SC
Chlordane	Apply 0.5% solution topically	None
Chlorhexidine	Shampoo every 3 to 7 days or apply to lesions s.i.d.–b.i.d.	Same
Chlorothiazide	20 to 40 mg/kg b.i.d. PO	Same
Chlorpheniramine maleate	0.5 to 4 mg/kg b.i.d.–t.i.d. PO	1 to 2 mg/kg b.i.d.–t.i.d. PO
Chlorpromazine hydrochloride	0.5 to 3.3 mg/kg s.i.d.–q.i.d. PO 1.1 to 6.6 mg/kg s.i.d.–q.i.d. IM	Same
Chlorpropamide	10 to 40 mg/kg s.i.d. PO	Unknown
Chlortetracycline	20 mg/kg t.i.d. PO	Same
Cholestyramine	¼ to ½ g b.i.d. PO	Unknown
Chorionic gonadotropin	1000 IU once; half IV, half IM	500 IU once; half IV, half IM
Cimetidine	5 to 10 mg/kg b.i.d.–q.i.d. PO 5 mg/kg b.i.d. IV 3 to 4 mg/kg b.i.d. PO (immunostimulation)	2.5 to 5 mg/kg b.i.d.–t.i.d. PO None Unknown
Ciprofloxacin	10 to 15 mg/kg b.i.d. PO	10 mg/kg b.i.d. PO

DRUG	*DOG*	*CAT*
Cisplatin	30 to 50 mg/m² IV every 3 weeks; pretreat with IV fluids 12 hours before (60 ml/kg); follow with 12 hours of saline diuresis (mannitol not likely required)	None
Clavamox	13.75 mg/kg b.i.d. PO	Same
Clindamycin hydrochloride	5.5 to 11 mg/kg b.i.d. PO	Same
Clindamycin palmitate	3 mg/kg q.i.d. PO	Same
Clindamycin phosphate	5 mg/kg t.i.d. IV, IM	Same
Clonazepam	0.1 to 0.5 mg/kg t.i.d. PO	Unknown
Clorazepate dipotassium	11.25 to 22.25 mg s.i.d.–b.i.d. PO or 2 to 6 mg/kg divided b.i.d.–t.i.d. PO	Unknown
Clotrimazole	Apply to local lesions	Same
Cloxacillin sodium	10 mg/kg q.i.d. PO, IV, IM	Same
Coal tar (0.5% to 8%)	Bathe every 3 to 14 days; leave in contact with skin for 10 minutes and rinse	None
Codeine	1 to 2 mg/kg every 4 to 8 hours PO (cough) 2 mg/kg q.i.d. PO, SC (pain) 0.25 to 0.5 mg/kg t.i.d. PO (diarrhea)	1 to 2 mg/kg b.i.d. PO (cough)
Colchicine	0.03 mg/kg t.i.d. to every other day PO, SC	None
Cortisone acetate	0.2 to 1 mg/kg s.i.d. PO	Same
Cuprimyxin	Apply to lesions b.i.d.	Same
Cyclophosphamide	6.6 mg/kg for 3 days PO then 2.2 mg/kg s.i.d. 10 mg/kg every 7 to 10 days IV or 50 mg/m² s.i.d. PO, IV for 3 to 4 days a week; repeat p.r.n.	Same
Cyclosporine	20 mg/kg s.i.d. PO	Unknown
Cyproheptadine	0.3 to 2 mg/kg b.i.d. PO	4 mg/kg s.i.d. PO
Cytarabine hydrochloride	5 to 10 mg s.i.d. for 2 weeks IV or 30 to 50 mg/kg once a week IV, IM, SC or 100 mg/m² s.i.d. IV, IM for 4 days, then 150 mg/m²	Same
Cythioate	3.3 mg/kg PO every 3rd day or twice weekly (tablets)	0.22 ml/kg PO every 3rd day or twice weekly
Dacarbazine	200 to 250 mg/m² s.i.d. IV for 5 days; repeat every 3 weeks or 300 mg/m² every 3 weeks IV	Same
Danazol	5 mg/kg b.i.d. PO	Unknown

DRUG	DOG	CAT
Dantrolene sodium	1 to 5 mg/kg t.i.d. PO	0.5 to 2 mg/kg b.i.d. PO
Dapsone	1.1 mg/kg t.i.d. PO	50 mg b.i.d. PO
Dehydrocholic acid	10 to 15 mg/kg t.i.d. PO for 7 to 10 days	Same
Derm Caps	1 capsule per 8 kg s.i.d. PO	Unknown
Desmopressin acetate	1 to 2 drops intranasally or in subconjunctival sac s.i.d.–b.i.d. (diabetes insipidus) 1 μg/kg SC, IV (von Willebrand's disease)	Same
Desoxycorticosterone acetate	0.2 to 0.4 mg/kg s.i.d. IM or 1 to 5 mg s.i.d. IM	0.2 mg/kg s.i.d. IM or 0.5 to 1 mg s.i.d. IM
Desoxycorticosterone pivalate	5 to 10 mg once monthly IM	Same
Dexamethasone	0.25 to 1 mg s.i.d. PO, IV, IM 5 mg/kg IV (shock)	0.125 to 0.5 mg s.i.d. PO, IV, IM Same
Dexamethasone sodium phosphate	3 mg/kg IV (shock) 0.5 to 2 mg/kg IV (hypoadrenocorticism)	Same Same
Dextromethorphan	1 to 2 mg/kg q.i.d. PO	Same
Dextrose (5% in water, saline, or Ringer's injection)	40 to 50 mg/kg s.i.d. IV, SC, intraperitoneally	Same
Diazepam	5 to 20 mg IV (repeated up to 3 times) then 5 to 20 mg/hour constant infusion (status epilepticus) 2 to 10 mg t.i.d. PO (relax urinary sphincter)	2.5 to 5 mg PO, IV (seizures) 0.5 to 1 mg/kg PO, IV (stimulate appetite)
Diazoxide	10 to 40 mg/kg/day PO	None
Dichlorophen	300 mg/kg once PO	150 mg/kg once PO
Dichlorvos	27 to 33 mg/kg PO once 11 mg/kg PO once (puppies) Change collars every 4 months	11 mg/kg PO once Same
Diethylcarbamazine	6.6 mg/kg s.i.d. PO (heartworm prevention) 55 to 110 mg/kg PO (treatment of ascarid infection) 3.3 mg/kg s.i.d. PO (ascarid prevention)	None Same
Diethylstilbestrol	0.1 to 1 mg/day PO	0.05 to 0.1 mg/day PO
Digitoxin	0.033 to 0.11 mg/kg PO divided b.i.d.	None
Digoxin	0.01 to 0.02 mg/kg divided b.i.d. PO or 0.22 mg/m² b.i.d. PO (maintenance)	0.007 mg/kg every other day PO

DRUG	DOG	CAT
	0.02 to 0.06 mg/kg divided b.i.d. for 1st day; then go to maintenance or 0.01 to 0.02 mg/kg t.i.d. for 1 day only (rapid oral digitalization) 0.01 to 0.02 mg/kg; give ½ total dose IV, wait 30 to 60 minutes, then give ¼ dose, wait another 30 to 60 minutes, give last ¼ dose if necessary (rapid IV digitalization)	
Dihydrostreptomycin	10 mg/kg t.i.d. IM, SC	Same
Dihydrotachysterol	0.02 to 0.03 mg/kg s.i.d. PO initially, then 0.01 to 0.02 mg/kg every 24 to 48 hours PO	1 to 2 drops s.i.d.–b.i.d. PO or 0.03 mg/kg/day for 3 to 4 days, then 0.01 to 0.02 mg/kg/day PO
Dihydroxyvitamin D_3	0.03 to 0.06 µg/kg s.i.d. PO	Unknown
Diltiazem hydrochloride	1.5 mg/kg t.i.d. PO	0.5 to 2 mg/kg s.i.d.–b.i.d. PO or 3 mg t.i.d. PO
Dimethyl sulfoxide		
Domoso-90	Apply 70% solution topically b.i.d.–t.i.d.	None
Rimso-50	0.5 to 1 g/kg t.i.d. IV of a 10% to 20% solution	
Diphenhydramine	2 to 4 mg/kg t.i.d. PO	Unknown
Diphenoxylate hydrochloride	0.05 to 0.1 mg/kg t.i.d. PO	0.063 mg/kg b.i.d. PO
Dipyrone	25 mg/kg t.i.d. IM, IV, SC	Same
Disophenol	10 mg/kg SC; may be repeated in 2 to 3 weeks	None
Disopyramide	100 mg t.i.d.–q.i.d. PO	None
Dithiazanine	6.6 to 11 mg/kg s.i.d. PO for 7 to 10 days	None
Dobutamine hydrochloride	250 mg in 1 L of 5% dextrose IV to effect or 5 to 20 µg/kg/minute constant infusion	1 to 5 µg/kg/minute constant infusion
Docusate calcium	100 to 150 mg s.i.d. PO	50 to 100 mg s.i.d. PO
Docusate sodium	50 to 200 mg b.i.d. PO	50 mg s.i.d. PO
Domeboro's Solution	1 to 2 tablets/pint of water; apply topically and let soak for 15 to 30 minutes, repeat t.i.d.	Same
Dopamine hydrochloride	40 mg in 500 ml of lactated Ringer's injection IV to effect or 10 µg/kg/minute constant infusion	1 to 5 µg/kg/minute constant infusion
Doxapram	5 to 10 mg/kg once IV	Same

DRUG	DOG	CAT
Doxorubicin hydrochloride	30 mg/m² IV once every 3 weeks, not to exceed total dose of 250 mg/m²	20 mg/m² once every 3 weeks IV
Doxycycline	5 mg/kg b.i.d. PO	Same
Econazole	Apply topically twice daily for 2 to 4 weeks	Unknown
Edrophonium chloride	0.11 to 0.22 mg/kg IV	0.5 to 1 mg/kg IV
EfaVet	1 capsule per 10 kg s.i.d. PO	1 capule per 5 kg s.i.d. PO
Efa-Z Plus	Less than 6.7 kg: 3.7 ml PO 6.7 to 22.5 kg: 7 ml PO More than 22.5 kg: 14 ml	Same
Enalapril	0.25 to 0.5 mg/kg s.i.d.–b.i.d. PO	0.25 to 0.5 mg/kg every other day PO
Enilconazole	Apply 20 mg/kg divided topically b.i.d.	Same
Enrofloxacin	2.5 mg/kg b.i.d. PO, SC or 5 mg/kg s.i.d. PO, SC	Same
Ephedrine hydrochloride	25 to 50 mg b.i.d.–t.i.d. PO	2 to 4 mg/kg b.i.d.–t.i.d. PO
Epinephrine (1 : 1000 solution)	0.1 to 0.5 ml IV, IM, SC, intracardiac	0.1 to 0.2 ml IV, IM, SC, IC
Erythromycin	10 mg/kg t.i.d. PO	Same
Ethacrynic acid	0.2 to 0.4 mg/kg every 4 to 12 hours IV, IM	Unknown
Ethyl alcohol (20%) (ethylene glycol toxicity)	5.5 ml/kg in 5% dextrose in water until comatose, repeat every 4 hours p.r.n.	5 ml/kg with 5 ml/kg sodium bicarbonate in 5% dextrose in water, repeat q.i.d. p.r.n.
Etidronate disodium	5 mg/kg/day PO	Unknown
Etomidate	1 to 3 mg/kg IV	Same
Etretinate	1 mg/kg s.i.d. PO	Unknown
Famotidine	Less than 4.5 kg 5 mg s.i.d.–b.i.d. PO 4.5 to 14 kg 10 mg s.i.d.–b.i.d. PO 14 to 22 kg 20 mg s.i.d.–b.i.d. PO 22 to 36 kg 30 mg s.i.d.–b.i.d. PO	Unknown
Fenbendazole	50 mg/kg s.i.d. PO for 3 days (repeat in 3 weeks)	30 mg/kg s.i.d. PO (for 3 to 6 days)
Fenthion	15 mg/kg SC every 2 weeks for 2 treatments or apply 13.8% solution topically every 2 weeks for 3 treatments (heartworm microfilaricide)	None
Ferrous sulfate	100 to 300 mg/kg s.i.d. PO	50 to 100 mg s.i.d. PO
Flecainide	1 to 5 mg/kg b.i.d.–t.i.d. PO 1 to 2 mg/kg IV slowly	Unknown
Flucytosine	100 mg/kg b.i.d. PO	Same

DRUG	DOG	CAT
Fludrocortisone acetate	0.1 to 0.8 mg divided b.i.d. PO or 0.01 mg/kg divided b.i.d. PO	0.1 to 0.2 mg divided b.i.d. PO
Flumethasone	0.06 to 0.25 mg s.i.d. PO, IV, IM, SC	0.03 to 0.125 mg s.i.d. PO, IV, IM, SC
Flunixin meglumine	1 to 2 mg/kg IV twice at 3- or 12-hour intervals (shock) 1 mg/kg/day IV (analgesia) or 2.2 mg/kg s.i.d. IM (for 3 to 4 days)	None
Fluorouracil	5 mg/kg every 5 to 7 days IV or 200 mg/m² s.i.d. for 3 days IV, then 10 mg/m² IV every other day until signs of toxicity appear, then 200 to 400 mg/m² weekly IV	None
Fluoxymesterone	0.25 to 1 mg/kg/day PO	Same
Flurazepam hydrochloride	0.2 to 0.4 mg/kg every 4 to 7 days	Same
Furosemide	2 to 4 mg/kg b.i.d.–t.i.d. PO	1 to 2 mg/kg b.i.d.–t.i.d. PO (maintenance) 0.5 to 2 mg/kg divided b.i.d.
Gemfibrozil	150 mg b.i.d.–t.i.d. PO for a 10-kg dog	None
Gentamicin	2 mg/kg t.i.d. IM, SC	Same
Glycerin suppositories	1 suppository per rectum	Same
Glycobiarsol	220 mg/kg s.i.d. PO for 5 days	None
Glycopyrrolate	0.005 to 0.01 mg/kg IV, IM 0.01 to 0.02 mg/kg b.i.d.–t.i.d. SC	0.005 to 0.01 mg/kg IM, IV
Gonadotropin releasing hormone	50 μg once IM	25 μg once IM
Griseofulvin	25 to 50 mg/kg s.i.d. PO	Same
Growth hormone Bovine	10 IU every other day SC for 30 days (pituitary dwarf) 2.5 IU every other day for 10 treatments SC (dogs less than 14 kg) and 5 IU every other day for 10 treatments SC (dogs more than 14 kg) (growth hormone-responsive dermatosis)	None
Human	0.15 IU/kg twice weekly SC for 6 weeks (growth hormone-responsive dermatosis)	
Guaifenesin With theophylline	1 capsule per 20 to 30 kg b.i.d.–q.i.d. PO 0.2 to 0.6 ml/kg b.i.d.–q.i.d. PO	None
With oxtriphylline	1 capsule per 20 to 30 kg b.i.d.–q.i.d. PO 0.2 to 0.6 ml/kg b.i.d.–q.i.d. PO	

DRUG	*DOG*	*CAT*
Halothane	Induction: 3% Maintenance: 0.5% to 1.5%	Same
Heparin	Minidose: 10 IU/kg t.i.d.–q.i.d. SC 200 IU/kg IV, then 50 to 100 IU/kg t.i.d.–q.i.d. SC	Same
Hetacillin	10 to 20 mg/kg t.i.d. PO	Same
Hydralazine hydrochloride	1 to 3 mg/kg b.i.d. PO	2.5 mg b.i.d. PO
Hydrochlorthiazide	2 to 4 mg/kg b.i.d. PO	Same
Hydrocodone bitartrate	0.22 mg/kg s.i.d.–q.i.d. PO	2.5 to 5 mg b.i.d.–t.i.d. PO
Hydrocortisone sodium succinate	8 to 20 mg/kg IV 4.4 mg/kg b.i.d. PO (shock) 5 to 20 mg/kg every 2 to 6 hours IV (hypoadrenocortical crisis)	Same Same
Hydrogen peroxide	5 to 10 ml (3% solution) every 15 minutes PO until emesis occurs	Same
Hydroxyurea	80 mg/kg every 3rd day or 40 mg/ kg/day PO	Same
Hydroxyzine	2.2 mg/kg t.i.d. PO	10 mg b.i.d. PO
HY-LYT efa	Apply topically after or between baths p.r.n.	Same
Ibuprofen	10 mg/kg every 24 to 48 hours PO	None
Imipramine hydrochloride	0.5 to 1 mg/kg t.i.d. PO	None
Indomethacin	1 mg/kg divided t.i.d. PO	None
Innovar (fentanyl-droperidol)	0.05 to 0.1 ml/kg IM	None
Insulin		

Regular	0.2 U/kg IM initially, then 0.1 U/kg
	    hourly until glucose is less than
	    250 mg/dl (ketoacidosis)
		Same

Intermediate-acting	0.5 to 1 U/kg s.i.d. SC	0.5 U/kg s.i.d. SC
Protamine zinc	0.5 to 1 U/kg s.i.d. SC	0.5 U/kg s.i.d. SC
Ipecac (syrup)	1 to 2 ml/kg PO	Same
Iron-dextran injection	10 mg/kg in divided doses IM	Same
Isoflurane	Induction: 5% Maintenance: 1.5% to 2.5%	Same
Isopropamide	0.2 to 0.4 mg/kg b.i.d.–t.i.d. PO	None
Isoproterenol hydrochloride	15 to 30 mg every 4 to 6 hours PO 0.1 to 0.2 mg q.i.d. IM, SC 1 mg in 250 ml 5% dextrose IV at a rate of 0.01 µg/kg/minute	Same
Isosorbide dinitrate	0.5 to 2 mg/kg b.i.d.–t.i.d. PO	Unknown
Isotretinoin	1 mg/kg s.i.d.–b.i.d. PO	3 mg/kg s.i.d. PO
Itraconazole	5 mg/kg b.i.d. PO	None

DRUG	DOG	CAT
Ivermectin	0.25 mg/kg PO 2 weeks after adulticide therapy (microfilaricide) 6 μg/kg once a month PO (heartworm prevention)	0.025% once topically
Kanamycin	10 mg/kg q.i.d. PO 7 mg/kg q.i.d. IM, SC	Same
Kaolin–pectin	1 to 2 ml/kg every 2 to 6 hours PO	Same
Ketamine hydrochloride	see under Indications in Appendix II	Restraint: 11 mg/kg IM Anesthesia: 22 to 33 mg/kg IM or 2.2 to 4.4 mg/kg IV
Ketoconazole	10 to 30 mg/kg/day PO up to 40 mg/kg/day PO (nasal and central nervous system infections) 15 mg/kg b.i.d. PO (hyperadrenocorticism)	10 mg/kg s.i.d.–b.i.d. PO
Lactulose	15 to 30 ml t.i.d.–q.i.d. PO or 1 ml/4.5 kg t.i.d. PO, then adjust based on fecal consistency	Same
Levamisole	11 mg/kg s.i.d. PO for 7 to 12 days (microfilaria) 0.5 to 2 mg/kg 3 times weekly PO (immunostimulant)	20 to 40 mg/kg PO every other day for 5 or 6 treatments (lungworms)
Levothyroxine sodium	0.02 mg/kg s.i.d.–b.i.d. PO	0.1 to 0.2 mg s.i.d. or divided b.i.d. PO
Lidocaine hydrochloride (2%)	2 to 4 mg/kg IV over 1 to 2 minutes, then 0.5 to 2 mg/kg every 20 to 60 minutes, then 25 to 80 μg/kg/minute constant infusion	0.25 to 1.0 mg/kg slowly IV with caution
Lime sulfur solution (3%)	Dip once weekly, let dry; use for 4 to 6 weeks	Same
Lincomycin	15 mg/kg t.i.d. PO 10 mg/kg b.i.d. IV, IM	Same
Lindane	Apply 0.025% to 0.1% aqueous solution topically	None
Liothyronine sodium	4 to 6 μg/kg t.i.d. PO	4.4 μg/kg b.i.d.–t.i.d. PO
Lithium carbonate	21 to 26 mg/kg/day PO	Unknown
Loperamide	0.1 to 0.2 mg/kg t.i.d.–q.i.d. PO	None
Magnesium hydroxide	Antacid: 5 to 30 ml s.i.d.–b.i.d. PO Cathartic: 3 to 5 times antacid dose	5 to 15 ml s.i.d.–b.i.d. PO Same
Malathion	Dip in 0.5% weekly for 3 to 4 weeks	Same

DRUG	*DOG*	*CAT*
Mannitol (20% solution)	1 to 2 g/kg every 6 hours IV	Same
Mebendazole	22 mg/kg with food s.i.d. for 3 days	None
Meclofenamate	0.5 to 2 mg/kg t.i.d.–q.i.d. PO	Unknown
Medium-chain triglyceride oil	1 to 2 ml/kg/day PO in food	Same
Medroxyprogesterone acetate	20 mg/kg once IM, SC; repeat at 4 to 6 months if needed (skin) 11 mg/kg p.r.n. IM, SC (behavior)	50 mg SC once; repeat at 3 to 6 months if needed (skin) 10 to 20 mg/kg p.r.n. IM, SC (behavior)
Megestrol acetate	1 mg/kg/day PO (skin) 2.2 to 4.4 mg/kg s.i.d. PO for 2 weeks, reduce to half dose every 2 weeks (behavior)	2.5 to 5 mg/day PO every other day, then once every 1 to 2 weeks (skin) 2.5 mg s.i.d. PO for 7 days, then 2.5 mg weekly (behavior)
Melphalan	0.1 mg/kg s.i.d. PO for 10 days, then 0.05 mg/kg s.i.d. PO	Same
Meperidine hydrochloride	5 to 10 mg/kg p.r.n. IM	1 to 4 mg/kg p.r.n. IM
Mercaptopropionyl glycine (MPG)	15 to 20 mg/kg b.i.d. PO	Unknown
Mercaptopurine	50 mg/m^2 s.i.d. PO or 2 mg/kg s.i.d. PO	None
Metamucil	2 to 10 g s.i.d.–b.i.d. in moistened food	2 to 4 g s.i.d.–b.i.d. in moistened food
Metaproterenol sulfate	0.5 mg/kg q.i.d. PO	Same
Methadone hydrochloride	0.11 to 0.55 mg/kg every 4 hours IM	None
Methandrostenolone	0.25 to 3 mg/kg/day PO	Same
Methenamine mandelate	10 mg/kg q.i.d. PO	None
Methenolone	0.25 to 3 mg/kg/day PO	Same
Methimazole	None	5 mg b.i.d.–t.i.d. PO
Methionine	0.2 to 1 g/kg t.i.d. PO	0.2 to 1 g s.i.d. PO
Methocarbamol	44.4 to 222.2 mg/kg IV (not to exceed a rate of 2 ml/minute) 44.4 mg/kg t.i.d. PO first day, then 22.2 mg/kg to 44.4 mg/kg t.i.d.	Same
Methotrexate	0.06 mg/kg s.i.d. PO 0.3 to 0.8 mg/kg weekly IV 2.5 mg/m^2 once daily PO, IV, IM	Same
Methscopolamine	0.3 to 1.5 mg/kg t.i.d. PO	None
Methylene blue	1 to 2 mg/kg IV; repeat p.r.n. 100 to 300 mg daily PO	None
Methylphenidate hydrochloride	2 to 4 mg/kg s.i.d. PO	None
Methylprednisolone sodium succinate	30 mg/kg IV (shock)	Same

DRUG	DOG	CAT
Metoclopramide hydrochloride	0.2 to 0.4 mg/kg every 6 to 8 hours PO, SC 1 to 2 mg/kg for 24 hours in constant IV infusion	Same
Metoprolol	5 to 60 mg t.i.d. PO	2 to 15 mg t.i.d. PO
Metronidazole	60 mg/kg s.i.d. PO for 5 days (giardiasis) 10 to 15 mg/kg t.i.d.–q.i.d. PO (anti-inflammatory, anaerobic infection)	Same Same
Mexiletine	2 to 5 mg/kg b.i.d.–t.i.d. PO	Unknown
Miconazole	10 mg/kg t.i.d. IV Apply topically b.i.d.	Unknown Same
Midazolam	0.1 to 0.2 mg/kg IM, IV	Same
Milrinone	0.5 to 1 mg/kg b.i.d. PO	Same
Mineral oil	5 to 25 ml b.i.d. PO	2 to 10 ml s.i.d.–b.i.d. PO
Minocycline hydrochloride	25 mg/kg b.i.d. PO	Same
Misoprostol	1 to 3 μg/kg t.i.d.–q.i.d. PO	Unknown
Mithramycin	2 μg/kg s.i.d. for 2 days IV 25 μg/kg in dextrose in water by slow IV infusion once or twice weekly for 3 to 4 weeks	Same
Mitotane	50 mg/kg once daily to effect (approx. 5 to 10 days), then 25 to 50 mg/kg once weekly	None
Mitoxantrone	5 mg/m² once every 3 weeks IV	6.25 mg/m² once every 3 weeks IV
Morphine sulfate	0.25 to 1.0 mg/kg every 4 to 6 hours IM, SC	0.1 mg/kg every 6 to 7 hours IM, SC
Nadolol	0.1 to 1 mg/kg s.i.d.–t.i.d. PO	0.1 to 0.5 mg/kg b.i.d.–t.i.d. PO
Nafcillin sodium	10 mg/kg q.i.d. PO, IM	Same
Nalidixic acid	3 mg/kg q.i.d. PO	Same
Nalorphine	1 mg/kg IV, IM, SC	None
Naloxone	0.04 mg/kg IV, IM, SC 2 mg/kg/hour IV (shock)	0.05 to 0.1 mg/kg IV
Nandrolone decanoate	1 to 1.5 mg/kg/week IM	0.5 to 1.0 mg/kg/week IM
Nandrolone phenylpropionate	1 mg/kg biweekly IM	Same
Neomycin	20 mg/kg q.i.d. PO 3.5 mg/kg t.i.d. IV, IM, SC	Same
Neostigmine	0.5 mg/kg t.i.d. PO 1 to 2 mg p.r.n. IM	0.2 mg p.r.n. IV
Niclosamide	154 mg/kg PO; fast 24 hours before; repeat in 2 to 3 weeks	Same

DRUG	DOG	CAT
Nifedipine	1 mg/kg IV (vasodilator) 0.25 to 0.5 mg/kg sublingually 30 minutes before meals (megaesophagus)	None
Nitroglycerin Ointment	Apply ¼ to 2 inches t.i.d.–q.i.d. topically	Apply ⅛ to ¼ inch t.i.d. topically
Nizatidine	5 mg/kg s.i.d. PO	Unknown
Norethandrolone	0.25 to 3 mg/kg/day PO	0.2 mg p.r.n. IV
Norfloxacin	22 mg/kg b.i.d. PO (systemic infection) 0.5 mg/kg b.i.d. PO (UTI)	Unknown
Noscapine	0.5 to 1 mg/kg t.i.d.–q.i.d. PO	None
Novobiocin	10 mg/kg t.i.d. PO	Same
Nutri-sol efa	1 to 2 ml per 9 kg for 30 to 60 days 1 ml per 3.5 kg for 30 days (puppies)	0.5 ml per 3.5 kg for 30 days
Nystatin	100,000 U q.i.d. PO	Same
Omeprazole	0.5 to 1.5 mg/kg s.i.d. PO	Unknown
Orgotein	5 mg once weekly SC	None
Oxacillin sodium	11 to 22 mg/kg t.i.d. PO	Same
Oxazepam	0.2 to 1 mg/kg s.i.d.–b.i.d. PO (stimulate appetite)	Same
Oxtriphylline	10 to 15 mg/kg t.i.d.–q.i.d. PO	Same
Oxybutynin	5 mg b.i.d.–t.i.d. PO	0.5 mg b.i.d. PO
Oxymetholone	0.25 to 4 mg/kg/day PO or 1 mg/kg s.i.d.–t.i.d. PO	Same
Oxymorphone hydrochloride	0.05 to 0.2 mg/kg every 6 hours IM, IV	0.01 mg/kg every 6 hours IM, IV
Oxytetracycline	20 mg/kg t.i.d. PO 7 mg b.i.d. IV, IM	Same
Paregoric	0.05 to 0.06 mg/kg b.i.d.–t.i.d. PO	None
Pellitol	Apply thin film s.i.d.–b.i.d.	Same
Penicillamine	10 to 15 mg/kg b.i.d. PO	None
Penicillin G benzathine	40,000 U/kg every 5 days IM	Same
Penicillin G sodium or potassium	40,000 U/kg q.i.d. PO 20,000 U/kg every 4 hours IV, IM, SC	Same
Penicillin G procaine	20,000 U/kg s.i.d.–b.i.d. IM, SC	Same
Penicillin V	10 mg/kg t.i.d. PO	Same
Pentazocine	0.5 to 1.0 mg/kg every 2 to 3 hours IM	0.75 to 1.5 mg/kg every 2 to 4 hours IV

DRUG	DOG	CAT
Pentobarbital	2 to 4 mg/kg PO (sedation)	Same
	10 to 30 mg/kg IV (anesthesia)	25 mg/kg IV (anesthesia)
Petrolatum, white	1 to 5 ml s.i.d. PO	Same
Phenobarbital	10 mg/kg t.i.d. IV, IM (status epilepticus)	Same
	1 to 2.5 mg/kg b.i.d. PO (seizures)	4 mg/kg s.i.d. or divided b.i.d. PO
	2 mg/kg b.i.d. PO (sedation)	1 mg/kg b.i.d. PO (sedation)
Phenoxybenzamine	0.25 to 0.5 mg/kg t.i.d.–q.i.d. PO	Same
Phenylbutazone	10 mg/kg b.i.d.–t.i.d. PO	None
Phenylpropanolamine	12.5 to 50 mg t.i.d. PO	12.5 mg t.i.d. PO
Phenytoin	15 to 40 mg/kg t.i.d. PO (seizures)	None
	4 mg/kg IV slowly once (arrhythmias)	
Phosphate enemas (Fleet)	One pediatric enema (medium to large dogs)	None
Phthalofyne	180 mg/kg PO after a 24-hour fast; repeat in 3 months	None
Phthalylsulfathiazole	100 mg/kg b.i.d. PO	Same
Piperazine	110 mg/kg PO; repeat in 3 weeks	Same
Piroxicam	20 mg/kg t.i.d. PO	None
Pitressin Tannate	2.5 to 5 U every 24 to 72 hours SC, IM or	Unknown
	0.5 to 1 ml every other day IM (oil)	Same
Plasminogen activator	Unknown	0.25 to 1 mg/kg/hour IV (total dose 1 to 10 mg/kg)
Polymyxin B	2 mg (20,000 U)/kg b.i.d. IM	Same
Potassium bromide	10 to 20 mg/kg b.i.d. PO	Unknown
Potassium chloride	0.1 to 0.2 mEq/kg/hour IV; not to exceed 0.5 mEq/kg/hour	Same
	1 to 3 g/day PO, IV; not to exceed 10 mEq/hour or 40 mEq/day	0.2 g/day PO
Potassium citrate	60 mEq/day divided b.i.d.–t.i.d. PO	Unknown
Potassium gluconate	5 ml of a 20 mEq/ml solution b.i.d.–t.i.d. PO or	5 to 10 mEq/day PO
	0.65 g (¼ tsp) per 4.5 kg b.i.d. PO (with food)	Same
Potassium iodide	2 to 5 ml every 4 to 6 hours PO	50 to 100 mg/day PO for 7 to 14 days (hyperthyroidism)
Potassium phosphate	0.1 to 0.2 mEq/kg/hour IV; not to exceed 0.5 mEq/kg/hour	Same

DRUG	DOG	CAT
Povidone-iodine	Shampoo every 3 to 7 days p.r.n. (1:4 or 1:6 drug:water solution) or apply to lesions s.i.d.–b.i.d. (cream)	None
	Oral rinse: use 10% solution p.r.n. (oral disease)	None
Praziquantel	5 mg/kg PO, SC, IM once or ½ tablet: less than 2.3 kg 1 tablet: 2.7 to 4.5 kg 1½ tablets: 5 to 6.8 kg 2 tablets: 7.3 to 13.6 kg 3 tablets: 14 to 20.5 kg 4 tablets: 20.9 to 27.3 kg 5 tablets: more than 27.3 kg	½ tablet: less than 1.8 kg 1 tablet: 2.3 to 5 kg 1½ tablets: more than 5 kg
Prazosin hydrochloride	1 mg t.i.d. PO (less than 15 kg) 2 mg t.i.d. PO (more than 15 kg)	None
Prednisolone	10 to 30 mg/kg IV (shock)	Same
	5 to 20 mg/kg IV (hypoadrenocorticism; acute crisis)	Same
	0.2 mg/kg s.i.d. PO (hypoadrenocorticism, maintenance)	Same
	0.5 mg/kg b.i.d. PO, IM (allergy)	1 mg/kg b.i.d. PO, IM (allergy)
	2 to 4 mg/kg/day PO, IM (immune suppression)	Same
	0.5 mg/kg every other day (maintenance)	Same
Prednisone	0.5 mg/kg s.i.d. PO	1 to 4 mg/kg b.i.d. PO (induction dose)
	2 to 4 mg/kg/day PO (immune suppression)	1 to 4 mg/kg every other day PO (maintenance dose)
	0.2 mg/kg s.i.d. PO (hypoadrenocorticism)	Same
Primidone	11 to 22 mg/kg t.i.d. PO	Same
Procainamide hydrochloride	10 to 20 mg/kg t.i.d. PO (Procan SR)	8 to 20 mg/kg t.i.d. PO
	10 to 20 mg/kg q.i.d. PO	3 to 6 mg/kg IV
	11 to 22 mg/kg every 3 to 6 hours IM or 100-mg bolus followed by IV drip at 10 to 40 μg/kg/minute	6 to 10 mg/kg IM
Prochlorperazine	0.13 mg/kg every 6 hours IM	0.13 mg/kg every 12 hours IM
Progesterone	1 to 2 mg/kg once weekly IM (not to exceed 25 mg) 1 week before expected date of fetal loss and continued until 1 week before expected due date or 55 days from 1st breeding	Same

DRUG	DOG	CAT
Propantheline bromide	Small dogs: 7.5 mg t.i.d. PO Medium dogs: 15 mg t.i.d. PO Large dogs: 30 mg t.i.d. PO	7.5 mg s.i.d.–t.i.d. PO
Propionibacterium acnes	Less than 7 kg: 0.25 ml IV twice weekly for 2 weeks, then once weekly 7 to 20 kg: 0.5 ml IV 21 to 34 kg: 1 ml IV More than 34 kg: 2 ml IV	15 µg/kg twice weekly IV for 2 to 3 weeks
Propranolol hydrochloride	0.2 to 1 mg/kg t.i.d. PO 0.04 to 0.06 mg/kg slowly IV	Same 0.25 mg diluted in 1 ml of saline; 0.2-ml boluses IV to effect
Propylthiouracil	None	50 mg b.i.d.–t.i.d. PO
Prostaglandin $F_{2\alpha}$	0.25 mg/kg (diluted in an equal volume of saline) s.i.d. SC for 2 to 7 days	Same
Protamine sulfate	1 mg for each 100 IU of heparin used given over 60 minutes as a 1% solution	Unknown
Pyrantel pamoate	5 mg/kg PO after a meal; repeat in 3 weeks	10 mg/kg PO; repeat in 3 weeks
Pyrethrin	Bathe as needed	Same
Pyridostigmine bromide	0.2 to 2 mg/kg b.i.d.–t.i.d. PO	Unknown
Pyrimethamine	1 mg/kg s.i.d. PO for 3 days, then 0.5 mg/kg s.i.d.	Same
Quinacrine hydrochloride	50 to 100 mg b.i.d. PO	10 mg/kg s.i.d. PO
Quinidine	8 to 20 mg/kg t.i.d.–q.i.d. PO, IM	4 to 8 mg/kg t.i.d. IM
Ranitidine hydrochloride	2.2 to 4.4 mg/kg b.i.d. PO, IM, SC	Same
Rifampin	10 to 20 mg/kg b.i.d. PO or 10 mg/kg s.i.d. PO	Same
Ronnel	Apply to ⅓ of body daily for 8 weeks or longer (generalized demodex)	None
Rotenone	Apply locally s.i.d. (localized demodex)	Same
Salt (table)	1 to 3 teaspoons in warm water PO to induce emesis	Same
Selenium sulfide	Bathe every 3 to 14 days p.r.n.; leave in contact with skin for 10 minutes and rinse	Unknown
Sodium bicarbonate	50 mg/kg b.i.d.–t.i.d. PO (1 teaspoon of powder = 2 g)	Same
Sodium chloride (0.9% solution)	40 to 60 ml/kg/day IV, SC, intraperitoneally	Same

DRUG	DOG	CAT
Sodium chloride (7% solution)	5 ml/kg over 20 to 30 minutes IV (shock)	None
Sodium EDTA	25 to 75 mg/kg/hour IV	Unknown
Sodium iodine (20%)	1 ml per 5 kg b.i.d.–t.i.d. PO, IV or 40 mg/kg t.i.d. PO	0.5 ml per 5 kg s.i.d. PO or 20 mg/kg b.i.d. PO
Sodium nitroprusside	1 to 5 μg/kg/minute constant infusion	None
Sodium polystyrene sulfonate	2 g/kg divided into 3 daily doses (each g suspended in 4 ml of water) or 8 to 15 g t.i.d. PO	Unknown
Sodium sulfate	10 to 25 g PO (purgative)	2 to 4 g PO (purgative) 50 mg/kg every 4 hours of a 1.6% solution (acetominophen toxicity)
Spectinomycin	5.5 to 11 mg/kg b.i.d. IM 22 mg/kg b.i.d. PO	None
Spironolactone	2 to 4 mg/kg s.i.d. PO	Same
Stanozolol	2 to 10 mg b.i.d. PO, IM	1 to 2 mg b.i.d. PO
Streptokinase	Unknown	90,000 IU IV over 20 to 30 minutes, followed by 45,000 IU/hour for 3 hours
Streptomycin	10 mg/kg q.i.d. IM, SC	Same
Styrylpyridium–diethylcarbamazine	N0:20 1 tab/10 kg s.i.d. PO N0:50 1 tab/25 kg s.i.d. PO	Unknown
Sucralfate	½ to 1 tablet t.i.d.–q.i.d. PO	100 to 200 mg/kg t.i.d.–q.i.d. PO
Sulfadiazine	220 mg/kg initial dose PO; then 110 mg/kg b.i.d.	Same
Sulfadimethoxine	25 mg/kg s.i.d.–b.i.d. IV, IM, SC, PO	Same
Sulfadimethoxine-ormetoprim	55 mg/kg s.i.d. PO on day 1, then 27.5 mg/kg s.i.d. thereafter for a maximum of 21 days	None
Sulfamethazine, sulfamerazine, sulfadiazine (triple sulfa)	50 mg/kg b.i.d. PO, IV	Same
Sulfasalazine	10 to 15 mg/kg q.i.d. PO	15 mg/kg divided PO
Sulfisoxazole–sulfamethizole	50 mg/kg t.i.d. PO	Same
Sulfur 2% to 5%	Bathe every 3 to 14 days; leave in contact with skin for 10 minutes and rinse	Same
Tars (shampoo)	Bathe twice weekly until skin is normal, then use only as indicated	None
Taurine	None	500 mg b.i.d. PO
Terbutaline	1.25 to 5 mg b.i.d.–t.i.d. PO	1.25 mg b.i.d.–t.i.d. PO

DRUG	DOG	CAT
Terfenadine	5 to 10 mg/kg b.i.d. PO	Unknown
Testosterone	2 mg/kg s.i.d. PO every 2 to 3 days up to 30 mg total 2 mg/kg every 10 days IM	Same
Tetrachlorethylene	0.22 mg/kg after a 12-hour fast	Same
Tetracycline	20 mg/kg t.i.d. PO 7 mg/kg b.i.d. IV, IM	Same
Tetramine	150 to 300 mg b.i.d. PO	Unknown
Thenium closylate	1 tablet (500 mg) for dogs more than 5 kg ¼ tablet (125 mg) b.i.d. for dogs 2.5 to 5 kg Repeat in 2 to 3 weeks	None
Theophylline	9 mg/kg t.i.d.–q.i.d. PO, IV, IM 20 mg/kg b.i.d. PO (sustained release)	4 mg/kg b.i.d.–t.i.d. PO
Thiabendazole	50 mg/kg s.i.d. PO for 3 days, repeat in 1 month or 20 mg/kg s.i.d. PO for 6 weeks	5 to 10 mg/kg s.i.d. PO 3 times weekly
Thiacetarsamide	2.2 mg/kg b.i.d. IV for 2 days	Same
Thiamylal sodium (4%)	8 to 20 mg/kg IV to effect	5 to 10 mg/kg IV to effect
Thiopental sodium	10 to 25 mg/kg IV to effect	5 to 10 mg/kg IV to effect
Ticarcillin	15 to 25 mg/kg t.i.d. IM, IV	Same
Tiletamine-zolazepam	3 to 5 mg/kg IM	Same
Timolol	0.5 to 5 mg t.i.d. PO	Unknown
Tobramycin sulfate	1 mg/kg t.i.d. IV, IM, SC	Same
Tocainide	5 to 20 mg/kg t.i.d. to q.i.d. PO	None
Toluene	200 mg/kg once PO	Same
Triamcinolone	0.25 to 2.0 mg/kg s.i.d. PO or 0.11 to 0.22 mg/kg IM, SC	Same 0.5 to 1.0 mg/kg s.i.d. PO
Triamterene	2 to 4 mg/kg/day PO	Unknown
Trientine	15 mg/kg b.i.d. PO	None
Triiodothyronine	4 to 6 µg/kg t.i.d. PO	4.4 µg/kg b.i.d.–t.i.d. PO
Trimeprazine	1 to 2 mg/kg t.i.d. PO	Unknown
Trimethobenzamide	3 mg/kg t.i.d. IM	None
Trimethoprim–sulfadiazine	15 mg/kg b.i.d. PO, SC or 30 mg/kg s.i.d. PO, SC	Same
Tylosin	10 mg/kg t.i.d. PO 40 to 80 mg/kg divided t.i.d. PO in food (bacterial overgrowth) 5 mg/kg b.i.d. IV, IM	Same
Valproic acid	60 to 220 mg/kg t.i.d. PO	Unknown

DRUG	DOG	CAT
Vancomycin	5 to 10 mg/kg q.i.d. PO or 20 mg/kg b.i.d. IV	Same Same
Verapamil	1 to 3 mg/kg t.i.d.–q.i.d. PO 0.05 to 0.15 mg/kg IV slowly	None
Vinblastine	2 mg/m² IV weekly, or 0.05 to 0.1 mg/kg IV weekly	Same
Vincristine	0.025 mg/kg IV every 7 to 10 days 0.7 mg/m² IV weekly or twice weekly	Same
Viokase Pancreatic enzymes	1 to 3 tablespoons per pound (454 g) of food or ¾ to 1 teaspoons per meal (i.e., t.i.d.)	Same or ¼ to ¾ teaspoons per meal (i.e., t.i.d.)
Vitamin A	400 U/kg/day PO for 10 days or 10,000 U/day PO	Same
Vitamin E	500 IU s.i.d. PO	10 to 20 IU/kg b.i.d. PO
Vitamin K₁	5 to 20 mg b.i.d. IV, IM, SC or 5 mg/kg initially SC then 2.5 mg/kg divided t.i.d. PO, SC	1 to 5 mg b.i.d. IV, IM, SC Same
Warfarin	0.1 mg/kg s.i.d. PO	0.06 to 0.1 mg/kg s.i.d. PO
Wheat bran	1 to 2 tablespoons per pound (454 g) of food	Same
Xylazine	1 mg/kg IV 1 to 2 mg/kg IM, SC	Same
Zinc acetate	100 to 200 mg b.i.d. PO	None
Zinc methionine	200 to 400 mg s.i.d. PO	None
Zinc oxide	Apply a thin film b.i.d.	Same
Zinc sulfate	100 to 200 mg/kg b.i.d. PO or 10 mg/kg s.i.d. PO in food	None

(IV = intravenously; IM = intramuscularly; SC = subcutaneously; PO = per OS; s.i.d. = once daily; b.i.d. = twice daily; t.i.d. = three times daily; q.i.d. = four times daily; p.r.n. = as indicated)

APPENDIX II
DRUGS: THEIR INDICATIONS AND COMMON SIDE EFFECTS

Dana G. Allen

ACETAMINOPHEN

Indications. Acetaminophen (Tylenol) is an antipyretic, analgesic agent useful in the treatment of mild to moderate pain in dogs. The drug is reported to be as effective as aspirin in the reduction of pain and fever. Acetaminophen is not an anti-inflammatory agent and is not useful in the treatment of rheumatoid arthritis.

Side Effects. The incidence of gastric irritation and hemorrhage is much less than that reported with aspirin. The drug is extremely toxic to cats. Methemoglobinemia, Heinz-body anemia, hepatic necrosis, and cyanosis have been reported in this species (see Chapter 2).

ACETAZOLAMIDE

Indications. Acetazolamide (Diamox) is a carbonic anhydrase inhibitor. It is used in the treatment of metabolic alkalosis and glaucoma. It causes the urinary loss of bicarbonate by inhibiting renal bicarbonate absorption.

Side Effects. Its diuretic action is associated with extracellular volume contraction. Its use may augment potassium loss and potentiate hypokalemia.

ACETOHYDROXAMIC ACID

Indications. Acetohydroxamic acid is a microbial urease inhibitor that should be considered in dogs with persistent urinary tract infection caused by urease-producing bacteria, especially staphylococci. The drug inhibits struvite urolith growth and promotes urolith dissolution. It also has a dose-related bacteriostatic effect against gram-positive and gram-negative bacteria. Acetohydroxamic acid potentiates the effect of trimethoprim, sulfamethoxazole, and methenamine.

Side Effects. Dose-related hemolytic anemia and abnormalties in bilirubin metabolism have been documented. The drug is teratogenic and should not be given to pregnant animals.

ACETYLCHOLINE CHLORIDE

Indications. Acetylcholine choloride (Miochol) is used to obtain miosis. It is also used in the management of ventricular fibrillation.

Side Effects. In humans, slight hyperemia may occur.

ACETYLCYSTEINE

Indications. Acetylcysteine (Mucomyst) is used to help liquify abnormal viscous or inspissated mucous secretions of the respiratory tract. It is also used as antidotal therapy in cases of acetaminophen toxicosis (see Chapter 2).

Side Effects. Bronchospasm may occur with nebulization of the drug, especially in patients with asthma. In these animals an alternative drug is Mucomyst-ISO, a combination of a mucolytic agent (acetylcysteine) and a bronchodilating agent (isoproterenol).

ACETYLPROMAZINE

Indications. Acetylpromazine (Acepromazine) may have a protective effect on epinephrine-induced arrhythmias. It also has sedative and anti-emetic properties.

Side Effects. Constipation, paradoxic aggression, sinus bradycardia, depression of myocardial contractility, hypotension, collapse, and prolongation of pseudocyesis have been reported. Acepromazine lowers the seizure threshold and may precipitate seizure activity in animals with epilepsy. The drug should not be used in animals with tetanus or with strychnine or organophosphate toxicity.

ACETYLSALICYLIC ACID

Indications. Aspirin (acetylsalicylic acid) is an effective analgesic for the management of mild to moderate pain. It is an antipyretic and anti-inflammatory agent. It is not effective in the treatment of visceral pain. It is the drug most often used in the management of degenerative joint disease. The drug is a prostaglandin inhibitor. Aspirin has antiplatelet activity that makes it useful in the prevention of arterial thromboembolization. This property makes it useful as adjunct therapy in the management of feline cardiomyopathy, heartworm disease, and membranoproliferative glomerulonephritis.

Salicylic acid (2%), however, is keratolytic, keratoplastic, mildly antipruritic, and bacteriostatic. It is often used in conjunction with captan and sulfur as a shampoo for seborrhea, pyoderma, and dermatophytosis. When salicylic acid is combined with sulfur, a synergistic effect occurs and the keratolytic effect is enhanced.

Side Effects. Side effects of acetylsalicylic acid are dose-related. Anorexia, vomiting, gastrointestinal ulceration, seizure, and coma have been reported. The presence of food in the stomach may decrease gastric irritation. Chronic high doses of the drug have been associated with the formation of gastric carcinoma in dogs. Buffered aspirin is also associated with gastric irritation, and while enteric-coated aspirin produces fewer gastric side effects, absorption of the drug is less consistent. Concurrent use of glucocorticoids increase the risk of gastrointestinal ulceration. The toxic dose is greater than 25 mg/kg/day in cats and greater than 50 mg/kg every 8 hours in dogs. Severe toxicity is characterized by vomiting, fever, metabolic acidosis, increased respiratory rate, gastrointestinal ulceration and bleeding, depression, seizure, and coma. Serum concentrations are increased in hypoalbuminemia, and drug dosages should be decreased. In cases of toxicity, emesis should be induced and activated charcoal given. Sodium bicarbonate increases the ionization of aspirin in urine and promotes its excretion; it is potentially useful in cases of aspirin toxicity. The drug is contraindicated in animals with gastric ulceration, re-

nal insufficiency, von Willebrand's disease, or asthma, and in those animals undergoing surgery. Aspirin may decrease the vasodilating capabilities of captopril and enalapril and decrease the efficacy of spironolactone. Concurrent administration with digoxin may increase serum digoxin levels. Aspirin may exacerbate clinical signs associated with Scotty cramp. Its antiplatelet activity may be impaired when used concurrently with propranolol. The drug should not be used in pregnant animals. Reproductive anomalies, fetal resorption, and stillbirths have been reported. Salicyclic acid shampoos may be irritating.

ALBENDAZOLE

Indications. Albendazole (Valbazen) is an anthelmintic used in the treatment of ascarid, hookworm, whipworm, and tapeworm (*Taenia* sp.) infections. It has also been effective against filaroidiasis, aelurostrongylosis, and paragonimiasis infections. Efficacy against capillariasis and crenosomiasis is also likely.

Side Effects. Lethargy, depression, and anorexia may occur.

ALBUTEROL

Indications. Albuterol (Ventolin, Salbutamol) is a β_2-adrenergic agonist used for its bronchodilatory effects.

Side Effects. In humans, tremor, nervousness, tachycardia, and arryhthmias are noted. Side effects in small animals are unknown.

ALDACTAZIDE

Indications. Hydrochlorthiazide-spironolactone (Aldactazide) acts at Henle's loop and the proximal and distal convoluted tubules, exerting a synergistic diuretic effect. The main advantage of this combination diuretic is its potassium-sparing action. It is less prone to induce polyuria and polydipsia than furosemide because the onset of action is slower and its effect is longer lasting.

Side Effects. Because the thiazide component causes an increase in renal vascular resistance and a decrease in glomerular filtration rate, the drug should not be used in animals with renal dysfunction. In humans, hyperkalemia is a well-recognized complication.

ALLOPURINOL

Indications. Allopurinol (Zyloprim) is indicated in patients with urate urolithiasis. It inhibits the enzyme xanthine oxidase and blocks the formation and urinary excretion of uric acid.

Side Effects. In humans, use of the drug has occasionally been associated with nausea, vomiting, diarrhea, pancreatitis, and a reversible hepatopathy associated with transient increases in serum alkaline phosphatase, alanine aminotransferase, and aspartate aminotransferase. Rare cases of bone marrow suppression with leukopenia and thrombocytopenia have also been documented.

ALPHA-KERI

Indications. Alpha-Keri is a water-dispersible, antipruritic oil. It contains a dewaxed, oil-soluble, keratin-moisturizing fraction of lanolin, mineral oil, and nonionic emulsifiers. It is indicated for dry, pruritic skin conditions, including seborrhea, to relieve itching and to lubricate and soften the skin.

Side Effects. This agent should not be used if the skin is inflamed.

ALUMINUM HYDROXIDE

Indications. Aluminum hydroxide (Amphojel, Dialume) is an antacid, antiflatulant medication useful in the management of hyperphosphatemia.

Side Effects. The drug is contraindicated in patients with alkalosis. It may interfere with the absorption of iron preparations and tetracyclines. It is poorly palatable and may cause constipation.

ALUMINUM AND MAGNESIUM HYDROXIDE

Indications and Side Effects. Maalox. See Antacid Preparations.

AMIKACIN

Indications and Side Effects. Amikacin sulfate injection (Amikin). See Aminoglycosides.

AMINOGLYCOSIDES

Indications. Aminoglycoside antibiotics (streptomycin, dihydrostreptomycin, neomycin [Biosol], kanamycin [Kantrim], gentamicin [Genticin], tobramycin [Nebcin], amikacin [Amikin]) are indicated in the treatment of gram-negative bacterial infection.

Gentamicin is more effective than kanamycin, but less effective than tobramycin against *Pseudomonas aeruginosa*. Amikacin sulfate injection is especially useful against *Pseudomonas* and *Klebsiella* organisms resistant to gentamicin. Steady-state drug levels of gentamicin are established in 6.5 hours in the dog. Serum concentrations are measured 1 to 2 hours after intramuscular dosing (peak levels) or just before the next dose (trough levels). To establish optimum dosing levels it is desirable to take samples at peak and trough times.

Side Effects. Nephrotoxicity, deafness, vestibular toxicity, respiratory paralysis, and cardiovascular depression have been reported. The aminoglycosides can potentiate the action of neuromuscular blocking agents and lead to respiratory depression, apnea, or muscle weakness, especially in animals with renal insufficiency. The neuromuscular blocking activity can be reversed by neostigmine. Furosemide (Lasix) predisposes to gentamicin-induced deafness. Endotoxemia predisposes to cardiovascular-induced depression. Neomycin is the most toxic and streptomycin the least toxic aminoglycoside.

AMINOPENTAMIDE SULFATE

Indications. Aminopentamide (Centrine) is an antiemetic agent.

Side Effects. Experience with the drug is limited in veterinary medicine, but glaucoma and xerostomia are possible.

AMINOPHYLLINE

Indications. Aminophylline is a bronchodilator used principally for the management of cough due to bronchospasm. It also increases the heart rate and the strength of contractility and has mild diuretic activity.

Side Effects. Side effects are anorexia, vomiting, and nervousness. Serum levels are increased by the concurrent use of cimetidine, erythromycin, and propanolol.

AMINOPROPRAZINE

Indications. Aminoproprazine (Jenotone) is a direct smooth muscle relaxant used in the treatment of urinary (urge) incontinence.

Side Effects. The drug may potentiate the effects of central nervous system depressants, organophosphates, and procaine hydrochloride.

AMINOSALICYLIC ACID

Indications. Aminosalicylic acid (Asacol) is indicated for the treatment of canine colitis.

Side Effects. The lack of a sulfur moiety makes the drug less toxic than sulfasalazine, although keratoconjunctivitis sicca has been reported. The drug should not be given to patients sensitive to salicylates or those with renal dysfunction or pyloric stenosis. Aminosalicylic acid should not be administered concurrently with lactulose. Initial clinical impressions indicate that the drug may not be as effective as sulfasalazine in the management of colitis in the dog.

AMITRAZ

Indications. Amitraz (Mitaban) is a monamine oxidase inhibitor used in the treatment of canine demodicosis and scabies and feline notoedric mange.

Side Effects. Transient sedation (hours, rarely up to 2 days) and transient pruritis have been reported.

AMITRIPTYLINE HYDROCHLORIDE

Indications. Amitryptyline hydrochloride (Elavil) is an anxiolytic agent used in the management of anxiety-related behavioral disorders, including separation anxiety in dogs and anxiety, urine spraying, and excessive grooming in cats. The drug may also have antipruritic properties.

Side Effects. The drug should not be given concurrently or within 14 days following cessation of use of a monoamine oxidase inhibitor, such as amitraz (Mitaban). Sedation may be marked initially. Anticholinergic side effects may include constipation, urine retention, dry mouth, tachycardia, and vomiting. The drug should be used with caution in patients with cardiovascular disease or a history of seizure.

AMMONIUM CHLORIDE

Indications. Ammonium chloride (Uroeze) is used in the treatment of metabolic alkalosis and as an expectorant in the management of cough. The drug is also used to acidify urine, an adjunctive therapy in the treatment of urinary tract infection, feline urologic syndrome, and urolithiasis. It may enhance the antibacterial properties of the penicillins and tetracyclines in the management of urinary tract infection.

Side Effects. Diarrhea, vomiting, and anorexia may occur with oral use of the drug. Ammonia intoxication following intravenous use may occur. Clinical signs include depression, stupor, coma, and seizure.

AMOXICILLIN

Indications and Side Effects. See Penicillins.

AMPHOTERICIN B

Indications. Amphotericin B (Fungizone) is an effective antifungal agent. In decreasing order of susceptibility, it has been used for the treatment of blastomycosis, histoplasmosis, cryptococcosis, and coccidioidomycosis. Aspergillosis is usually resistant.

Side Effects. The most important side effect is renal dysfunction. Serum urea and creatinine should be monitored frequently thoroughout the treatment regimen, and urinalysis should be done often. The simultaneous administration of 12.5 mg of mannitol may help prevent nephrotoxicity. Anorexia, nausea, vomiting, fever, phlebitis, hemolytic anemia, and cardiac arrhythmias have also been documented.

AMPICILLIN

Indications and Side Effects. Ampicillin (Polyflex, Princillin). See Penicillins.

AMPROLIUM

Indications. Amprolium (Corid) is used in the treatment of coccidiosis. The drug is a thiamine inhibitor.

Side Effects. With prolonged use, vomiting, anorexia, diarrhea, and nervous symptoms may occur. In this case the drug should be discontinued and the animal treated with thiamine, calcium gluconate, and fluid therapy.

AMRINONE

Indications. Amrinone (Inocor) is a positive inotropic agent with mild arteriolar-dilating properties. It is of potential use in increasing cardiac output in animals with congestive heart failure or cardiomyopathy.

Side Effects. Although side effects are rare, the drug may cause anorexia, vomiting, tachycardia, and hypotension.

ANABOLIC STEROIDS

Indications. The anabolic androgenic steroids have been used in the treatment of aplastic anemia, myeloproliferative disease, and lymphoma accompanied by a nonregenerative anemia. They are classified into two groups: alkylated agents (methyltestosterone, fluoxymesterone, oxymetholone, methandrostenolone, stanozolol, norethandrolone) and nonalkylated agents (testosterone, methenolone, nandrolone). These drugs stimulate the production of erythropoietin and potentiate its effect, and stimulate an increased production of red cell numbers. Because of the lack of an extrarenal source of erythropoietin, dogs with anemia secondary to renal disease are less likely to respond. It appears that a beneficial effect may be noted in one third of canine and feline patients. In humans a significant increase in red cell mass may take 3 to 6 months.

Side Effects. Virulization of females and skeletal abnormalities in puppies and kittens may occur with prolonged treatment regimens. Cholestatic liver disease accompanied by an increase in bromsulphalein (BSP) retention, an increase in alanine aminotransferase and aspartate aminotransferase enzymes, and jaundice have also been reported. The nonalkylated group is less hepatotoxic, but appears to be less effective in stimulating red cell production. The drugs have also been implicated as a contributing factor in the etiology of hepatic carcinoma.

ANTACID PREPARATIONS

Indications. Orally administered antacids contain aluminum hydroxide (Amphojel, Camalox, Gelusil, Maalox, Mylanta), calcium carbonate (Camalox), or magnesium compounds (Camalox, Gelusil, Maalox, Myalanta, Riopan). These drugs are useful in the management of gastric and duodenal bleeding or ulceration and reflux esophagitis. Aluminum-containing products bind intestinal phosphorus and have been used in the management of hyperphosphatemia associated with renal disease. Antacids reduce the amount of gastric acid and decrease the proteolytic effects of pepsin by inactivating the enzyme when gastric pH is 6 or higher. They have a cytoprotective function through their ability to stimulate the release of prostaglandins and bind bile salts. Astringent properties enhance gastric mucus production. The drugs should be given every 3 to 4 hours for optimal effect. Liquid antacids may be more effective than the tablet form.

Side Effects. Calcium- and aluminum-containing products may be associated with constipation, and magnesium-containing products may be associated with diarrhea. Calcium-containing products may be associated with hypercalcemia and impairment of renal function. Antacids decrease the absorption of orally administered sulfonamides, tetracyclines, phenothiazines, glucocorticoids, cimetidine, phenylbu- tazone, nitrofurantoin, digoxin, aspirin, and phenobarbital.

ANTIHISTAMINES

Indications. Antihistamines (chlorpheniramine, cyproheptadine, diphenhydramine, hydroxyzine, trimeprazine, terfenadine) have been used to help alleviate pruritus in dogs. Chlorpheniramine maleate has also been successfully used for this purpose in the cat. All the drugs listed here are histamine$_1$ antagonists with antihistaminic, anticholinergic, and sedative properties. At low doses they block the release of histamine from mast cells and basophils. At higher doses they may stimulate histamine release. An animal may respond to one drug and not to others, although there is no apparent increased efficacy of one drug over another. These drugs have been used as antiemetics (by depressing the chemoreceptor trigger zone), although they are less effective than the phenothiazines. They may also relieve neuromuscular blockade associated with organophosphate toxicity.

Side Effects. Sedation is a side effect with chlorphenhydramine, cyproheptadine, diphenhydramine, and trimeprazine; sedative effects are mild with hydroxyzine hydrochloride and minimal or nonexistent with terfenadine. Nausea, vomiting, diarrhea, and an increase in pruritus may also occur. With drug overdose, hyperexcitabiltiy, seizure, and death may occur. Some antihistamines are teratogenic and should be avoided during pregnancy.

APOMORPHINE HYDROCHLORIDE

Indications. Apomorphine hydrochloride is a useful and effective emetic agent for dogs and cats. Gastric emptying may be readily induced in cases of recent (less than 4 hours) oral intoxication.

Side Effects. Respiratory depression, sedation, and protracted vomiting have been reported. These signs may be controlled with a narcotic antagonist (naloxone 0.04 mg/kg, levallorphan 0.02 mg/kg, or nalorphine 0.1 mg/kg). Emesis is contraindicated in unconscious animals and in those that have ingested strong acids, bases, petroleum products, tranquilizers, or other antiemetics.

Apomorphine hydrochloride is not available in Canada.

APRINDINE

Indications. Aprindine is useful in the management of supraventricular and premature ventricular contractions. It may be effective in treating ventricular arrhythmias that are unresponsive to quinidine, lidocaine, procainamide, propranolol, or a combination of these drugs. It is less effective in the suppression of supraventricular tachyarrhythmias (atrial fibrillation and flutter).

Side Effects. Tremors, ataxia, blood dyscrasias, and cholestatic jaundice have been reported in humans. It may also decrease cardiac contractility.

ARECOLINE–ACETARSOL

Indications. Arecoline–acetarsol (Nemural) is an anthelmintic used for the elimination of tapeworms (*Taenia, Dipylidium caninum, Echinococcus* sp.).

Side Effects. Severe vomiting, diarrhea, salivation, restlessness, ataxia, and labored breathing may occur. The drug should not be administered to puppies younger than 3 months or to cats younger than 1 year of age or to animals with severe cardiac disease. It should not be administered concurrently with organophosphate compounds. Atropine is an effective antidote for the cholinergic side effects.

ASCORBIC ACID

Indications. Vitamin C is essential for the formation of collagen and intercellular material, and, therefore, the development of bone, cartilage, and teeth as well as wound healing. It may also influence the immune response. Ascorbic acid is used for the treatment of idiopathic methemaglobinemia (acetaminophen toxicosis) and as a urine acidifier. Acetlycysteine, however, is the drug of choice in the management of acetaminophen toxicosis.

Side Effects. In humans large doses may cause diarrhea. Acidification of the urine with ascorbic acid may lead to the precipitation of urate, oxlate, or cysteine stones in the urinary tract.

ASPARAGINASE

Indications. Asparaginase (Elspar) is indicated for the treatment of lymphoma, lymphoblastic leukemia, and idiopathic thrombocytopenia purpura. The drug inhibits the enzyme asparaginase synthetase and depletes asparagine in tumor cells.

Side Effects. Vomiting, diarrhea, hypotension, urticaria, and loss of consciousness have been reported. Anaphylaxis has also been documented. Administration of the drug by the intramuscular route decreases the risk of anaphylaxis. Asparaginase inhibits the activity of methotrexate. These drugs should not be given concurrently.

ATENOLOL

Indications. Atenolol (Tenormin) is a selective β₁-blocking agent equal in potency to propranolol. It is preferred in patients with pulmonary disease (asthma). The drug is useful in the management of supraventricular tachyarrhythmias, ventricular premature contractions, systemic hypertension, and hypertrophic cardiomyopathy in cats.

Side Effects. The drug is excreted through the renal system, and therefore should be used with caution in animals with compromised renal function. Depression, lethargy, bradycardia, impaired atrioventricular conduction, and congestive heart failure have been documented with the use of β-blockers. Glycopyrrolate and dopamine hydrochloride can be used to counter bradycardia.

ATROPINE

Indications. Atropine is indicated in the treatment of sinus bradycardia, sinus block or arrest, and incomplete atrioventricular block. It is also used in the treatment of organophosphate and carbamate poisoning and hyperptyalism, and as a diagnostic test for cataplexy (0.1 mg/kg IV).

Side Effects. Sinus tachycardia and second-degree heart block occur. Atropine also decreases the threshold at which premature ventricular contractions are likely to occur. With drug overdose, respiratory depression and hypotension may occur. The drug should not be given to animals with glaucoma.

AURANOFIN

Indications. Auranofin (Ridaura Capsules) is an oral gold salt (triethylphosphine) that has been used in dogs for the treatment of idiopathic polyarthritis and pemphigus foliaceus. Gold compounds are immunoregulatory rather than immunosuppressive. Auranofin inhibits helper T cell responses without affecting the suppressor T cell population.

Side Effects. An immune-mediated thrombocytopenia may develop. High doses (2.4–3.6 mg/kg/day) result in thrombocytopenia and moderate to severe hemolytic anemia. Rapid reversal of these side effects occurs after cessation of therapy and the administration of glucocorticoids. Dose-dependent diarrhea has been reported in some dogs. It resolves with cessation of therapy or lowering of the dose. Proteinuria has been documented in humans using this drug. The incidence is low. A complete blood count, serum biochemistry profile, and urinalysis should be completed every 2 weeks during the first 2 months of therapy, and then monthly to quarterly as the dose is reduced.

AUROTHIOGLUCOSE

Indications. Sterile aurothioglucose suspension (Solganal) is used in the treatment of pemphigus complex, bullous pemphigoid, rheumatoid arthritis, and, possibly, plasma cell pododermatitis. The drug depresses macrophage phagocytosis, inhibits lysosomal breakdown, stabilizes collagen and lysosomes, interferes with prostaglandin synthesis, supresses cellular immunity, and decreases blood levels of the immunoglobulins. Clinical response should not be expected for 6 to 12 weeks.

Side Effects. Although rare, leukopenia, thrombocytopenia, anemia, renal tubular damage, hepatitis, miliary dermatitis, stomatitis, and anaphylaxis have been reported. A complete blood count, serum biochemistry profile, and urinalysis should be obtained every 2 weeks for the first 2 months of therapy, and then monthly to quarterly as the dose is reduced.

AUROTHIOMALATE

Indications and Side Effects. Gold sodium thiomalate (Myochrysine). Same as for Aurothioglucose.

AZATHIOPRINE

Indications. Azathioprine (Imuran) is a thiopurine antimetabolite immunosuppressive agent used primarily in the treatment of autoimmune disease. It may be used in combination with glucocorticoids or cyclophosphamide. The onset of action is slow, taking 4 to 6 weeks to produce beneficial clinical effects. It is less immunosuppressive than cyclophosphamide, but has fewer side effects. In cats azathioprine has been shown to reverse the neuromuscular blockade induced by tubocurarine chloride and potentiate the neuromuscular blockade induced by succinylcholine chloride.

Side Effects. Leukopenia, anemia, and thrombocytopenia may occur. Cats are especially sensitive to the bone marrow toxicity. White cell counts should be monitored biweekly for the first 8 weeks of therapy, then monthly. If white blood cell counts fall below 4000 per microliter, the drug should be discontinued until the leukopenia is resolved. Other abnormalities associated with the drug have included jaundice, anemia, and poor hair growth.

BARBITURATES

Indications. The barbiturates are used for sedation and general anesthesia. The long-acting drug phenobarbital produces sedation in 70 to 90 minutes, and the effect lasts 6 to 8 hours. Pentobarbital is short-acting, with an onset of action of 30 to 45 minutes and a duration of effect of 4 to 5 hours. Barbiturates provide little analgesia.

Side Effects. At sedative doses, barbiturates have a wide margin of safety with few side effects. Postinduction apnea is common with these drugs. Metabolic acidosis, hypoalbuminemia, uremia, and the administration of nonsteroidal anti-inflammatory agents, certain sulfonamides, or glucose augment the anesthetic effects of barbiturates and potentiate toxicity.

BENZOYL PEROXIDE

Indications. Benzoyl peroxide (Oxydex, Pyoben, Allerderm) is a degreasing, keratolytic, keratoplastic, antipruritic agent useful in the treatment of schnauzer comedone syndrome, canine and feline acne, seborrhea, pyoderma, pruritis, crusts, and scales.

Side Effects. The 5% solutions can be irritating to animals. The gel is often too irritating for use in cats.

BETAMETHASONE

Indications and Side Effects. Betamethasone sodium phosphate (Betasone) and betamethasone valerate (Valisone cream) are long-acting glucocorticoids given intramuscularly in the dog and used topically in the cat. See Glucocorticoids.

BETHANECHOL CHLORIDE

Indications. Bethanechol chloride (Urecholine) is a cholinergic agent used to help stimulate muscular contraction of the bladder.

Side Effects. Vomiting, diarrhea, anorexia, abdominal cramping, increased salivation, and lacrimation may occur.

BISACODYL

Indications. Bisacodyl (Dulcolax) is a laxative used to alleviate constipation and to help cleanse the colon for endoscopy. Following rehydration to soften feces, it is a useful drug for the treatment of severe impaction. The drug generally requires 6 to 12 hours to work effectively.

Side Effects.   Mild cramping has been reported in some patients.

BISMUTH SUBSALICYLATE

Indications.   Bismuth subsalicylate (Pepto-Bismol) is used in the treatment of diarrhea. It has a protective effect, anti-inflammatory, antitoxic, and antiprostaglandin activity on the bowel.

Side Effects.   Stool color may darken with its use. The drug contains salicylate, and may be toxic to cats, especially in the presence of an inflamed bowel (see Acetylsalicylic Acid).

BUNAMIDINE HYDROCHLORIDE

Indications.   Bunamidine hydrochloride (Scolaban) is an anthelmintic used for the eliminaiton of tapeworms (*Taenia* sp., *Dipylidium caninum*, *Echinococcus* sp.).

Side Effects.   Vomiting and mild diarrhea may occur. Collapse and death have been reported. Fatal arrhythmias have been reported in rare cases, and have been associated with exercise within a few hours of treatment. Exercise should therefore be avoided for 24 hours following drug use. Male dogs should not be used for breeding within 28 days of use of the drug. The drug should not be used with butamisole or administered to animals with cardiac or hepatic disease.

BUTAMISOLE HYDROCHLORIDE

Indications.   Butamisole hydrochloride (Styquin) is an anthelmintic used in the treatment of hookworms and whipworms.

Side Effects.   Subcutaneous injection may induce local pain. The drug should not be used in dogs with *Dirofilaria immitis* infection and should not be used concurrently with bunamidine hydrochloride. The drug should not be given to pregnant females prior to the third week of pregnancy.

BUTORPHANOL

Indications.   Butorphanol (Stadol, Torbutrol) is a narcotic antagonist analgesic with potent antitussive activity. Analgesia occurs 30 minutes following intramuscular injection and reaches peak activity in 1 hour. With intravenous injection, the analgesic effect is immediate, with peak activity in 30 minutes. Pain relief lasts 2 to 3 hours. The drug is five times more potent in pain relief than morphine sulfate. Butorphanol tartrate is 15 to 20 times more effective in the management of cough than codeine or dextromethorphan.

Side Effects.   Although rare, side effects may include slight sedation, anorexia, nausea, and diarrhea. Because the drug suppresses the cough reflex, it should not be used in dogs with a productive cough. Moderate to marked cardiopulmonary depression has been reported with intravenous infusions given at a rapid rate (0.2 mg/kg/min). Panting may occur with doses of 0.4 mg/kg IV. In cats mydriasis lasting as long as 3 hours following an intravenous dose of 0.2 mg/kg may occur. It should not be used in pregnant animals or those with liver disease.

BUTYL CHLORIDE

Indications.   Butyl chloride (Nemantic, BuChlorin) is a common anthelmintic used for the elimination of ascarid infection.

Side Effects.   The drug is very safe. A 12-hour fast and the concurrent use of a cathartic increases the efficacy of the drug.

CALCITONIN–SALMON

Indications.   Salmon calcitonin (Calcimar) may be an effective adjunct (in addition to fluid therapy, diuretics, and corticosteroids) to the management of hypercalcemia. The drug inhibits bone resorption and intestinal resorption of calcium and enhances calciuresis.

Side Effects.   Few data are available concerning its use in small animals. In humans, transient nausea, anorexia, and vomiting are most frequently encountered. Resistance to the effects of the drug develop in a small percentage of people.

CALCIUM CARBONATE

Indications and Side Effects.   Large doses may cause alkalosis. It is the preferred calcium preparation for treating hypoparathyroidism. See also Antacid Preparations.

CALCIUM CHLORIDE

Indications.   Calcium chloride is used in cardiac arrest (ventricular asystole and electromechanical dissociation) to stimulate cardiac excitation. It is also used in the treatment of hypocalcemia associated with hypoparathyroidism.

Side Effects.   Hypercalcemia, depression, coma,

and nephrocalcinosis may occur. Extravascular injection causes extensive inflammation and tissue sloughing. All orally administered calcium preparations can cause gastrointestinal upset. Calcium compounds reduce blood levels of orally administered tetracyclines. Concomitant use of these drugs should be spaced 1 hour apart. Calcium chloride should be used with caution in patients receiving digitalis compounds.

CALCIUM GLUCONATE

Indications.   Calcium gluconate (Calcet) is indicated for the treatment of hypocalcemia associated with hypoparathyroidism, with or without hypoglycemia, hyperkalemia, and hyperkalemic myocardial toxicity.

Side Effects.   Intravenous injections must be given slowly to avoid hypercalcemia and potential cardiotoxicity. If the heart rate increases significantly, infusion of the drug should be discontinued until the rate returns to normal, at which time reinfusion can begin. Calcium compounds reduce blood levels of orally administered tetracyclines. Concomitant use of these drugs should be spaced 1 hour apart. Calcium gluconate should be used with caution in patients receiving digitalis compounds. All orally administered calcium preparations can cause gastrointestinal upset.

CALCIUM LACTATE

Indications.   Calcium lactate is indicated in the management of hypocalcemia associated with hypoparathyroidism.

Side Effects.   All orally administered calcium preparations can cause gastrointestinal upset. Calcium compounds reduce blood levels of orally administered tetracyclines. Concomitant use of these drugs should be spaced 1 hour apart. Calcium lactate should be used with caution in patients receiving digitalis compounds.

CANEX

Indications.   Canex contains rotenone and chloroform. It is used for the treatment of demodicosis, canine scabies, and otodectic mange. It may also be used in the ears of cats if diluted 3:1 with mineral oil.

Side Effects.   There are no side effects.

CAPTAN

Indications.   Captan (Orthocide) is an antifungal, bacteriostatic, and relatively nontoxic agent used for the treatment of the dermatophytes.

Side Effects.   It is safe and nontoxic, but may induce contact sensitization in humans.

CAPTOPRIL

Indications.   Captopril (Capoten) is an arterial and venous vasodilator that reduces afterload and preload, leading to increased cardiac output and decreased pulmonary edema in conditions of congestive heart failure and cardiomyopathy. The drug may also have beneficial effects in animals with systemic hypertension. It may be useful in hemorrhagic or endotoxic shock by maintaining peripheral tissue perfusion.

Side Effects.   Because the drug is eliminated by the kidneys, the dose must be reduced in animals with renal failure. Hypotension has been reported. Because captopril may initiate vasodilation simultaneous with decreased circulating blood volume, it should not be used with other vasodilators (hydralazine hydrochloride). In humans, anorexia, cough, bronchospasm, jaundice, pruritis, proteinuria, gastrointestinal upset, deterioration of renal function, and bone marrow-induced neutropenia have also been reported.

CARBAMATE

Indications.   Carbamate shampoo (VIP Flea and Tick Dip) is a cholinesterase inhibitor used in the treatment of fleas, ticks, and cheyletiellic mange. Carbamate is also present in selected flea and tick collars (Mycodex flea collar) and powders. Carbamate derivatives include Sevin and Sendran.

Side Effects.   Resistance develops quickly when the dip is used frequently. Collars lack efficacy on long-haired animals. Carbamate products should not be used on puppies or kittens younger than 4 weeks of age or on pregnant animals. Toxicity results in miosis, salivation, bronchoconstriction, ataxia, incoordination, muscle tremors, convulsions, respiratory depression, paralysis, and possibly death. The phenothiazine tranquilizers may potentiate the adverse effects of carbamate products. In cases of apparent intoxication the skin should be cleansed. If the drug has been ingested, gastric lavage is indicated. Following gastric lavage, activated charcoal should be given by way of stomach intubation. In all cases atropine is given intravenously (0.2 mg/kg) to effect. One fourth of the total dose is given intravenously, and the balance intramuscularly. The use of pralidoxine chloride (2-PAM) is discouraged since it may result in increased toxicity.

CARBAMAZEPINE

Indications. Carbamazepine (Tegretol) has been found in humans to be as effective as phenytoin in the control of seizures.

Side Effects. The drug stimulates its own degradation. Drug doses must, therefore, continue to be increased to maintain efficacy (therapeutic serum concentrations reported in humans are 5–10 μg/ml). The half-life in dogs is short (1–2 hours), and serum levels are difficult to maintain. Other side effects reported in humans include bone marrow suppression and, occasionally, hepatotoxicity. The drug is not recommended for long-term anticonvulsant therapy in the dog. Its usefulness in the cat has not been clarified.

CARBENICILLIN DISODIUM

Indications and Side Effects. Carbenicillin disodium (Geopen). See Penicillins.

CARNITINE

Indications. Carnitine supplementation may be a useful adjunct to, and may eventually replace, some conventional therapies in the treatment of some dogs with dilated cardiomyopathy. The drug may also have a protective effect in myocardial infarction and doxorubicin hydrochloride (Adriamycin)-induced cardiomyopathy. Dietary carnitine supplementation may facilitate hepatic lipid metabolism in cats with idiopathic hepatic lipidosis.

Side Effects. Nausea, vomiting, and diarrhea may occur. D- and L-carnitine have been associated with a myasthenialike syndrome. It is therefore preferable to use the L-isomer (L-carnitine).

CEFOXITIN SODIUM, STERILE

Indications and Side Effects. Cefoxitin sodium, sterile (Mefoxin). See Cephalosporins.

CEPHADROXIL

Indications and Side Effects. Cephadroxil (Cefa Tabs). See CEPHALOSPORINS.

CEPHALEXIN

Indications and Side Effects. Cephalexin (Keflex). See Cephalosporins.

CEPHALOSPORINS

Indications. Cephalosporins are bactericidal to gram-positive bacteria and several gram-negative bacteria. They are used in the treatment of genitourinary, skin, and soft-tissue infections. All are effective against anaerobic infections except *Bacteroides fragilis*. The cephalosporins may be more effective than the penicillins in the treatment of β-lactamase-producing staphylococci. Cephalosporins are usually not effective against resistant strains of *Pseudomonas aeruginosa*. They do not readily diffuse into the cerebrospinal fluid.

First-generation cephalosporins (cephalexin, cephadroxil, cephaloridine, cephradine, cefaclor, cephalothin, cephazolin, cephapirin) are active against gram-positive cocci, including staphylococci, *Escherichia coli*, salmonellae, shigellae, *Proteus*, and *Klebsiella* organisms. They are less expensive than the second- and third-generation products.

Second-generation cephalosporins (cephamandole, cefotiam, cefuroxime, ceforanide, cefoxitin) are useful against gram-negative bacteria that are resistant to first-generation cephalosporins, but their activity against gram-positive organisms is less than that of the first-generation cephalosporins.

Third-generation cephalosporins (cefotaxime, cefoperazone, cefmenoxime, cefsulodin, moxalactam) have increased antibacterial activity to gram-negative organisms, but activity to gram-positive organisms is even less than that of the first- and second-generation drugs. The third-generation drugs do have increased resistance to β-lactamase-producing bacteria and increased activity against *pseudomonas*.

Side Effects. As a group, the cephalosporins are quite safe. Vomiting and diarrhea may occur following oral administration. Administration of the drug with food decreases nausea. Intramuscular injection may be associated with pain. Cephalosporins are potentially nephrotoxic, and although clinical and laboratory evidence is lacking, it is recommended that these drugs be used with caution when administered with other nephrotoxic agents (*e.g.*, aminoglycosides). Cephaloridine has been associated with toxic epidermal necrolysis in a cat.

CEPHALOTHIN

Indications and Side Effects. Cephalothin (Keflin). See Cephalosporins.

CEPHAMANDOLE

Indications and Side Effects. Cephamandole (Mandol). See Cephalosporins.

CEPHAPIRIN SODIUM, STERILE

Indications and Side Effects. Sterile cephapirin sodium (Cefadyl). See Cephalosporins.

CEPHAZOLIN

Indications and Side Effects. See Cephalosporins.

CEPHRADINE

Indications and Side Effects. Cephradine (Velosef). See Cephalosporins.

CHARCOAL, ACTIVATED

Indications. Activated charcoal (Norit, Nuchar, Darco G-60, or compressed tablets) is an excellent absorbant used in the treatment of accidental poisoning. It is often used in conjuction with emetics and gastric lavage. Activated charcoal must be of vegetable origin, not mineral or animal. A slurry is made and administered by a stomach tube. A cathartic (sodium sulfate) is given 30 minutes following the administration of charcoal. Activated charcoal is most useful for mercuric chloride, strychnine, morphine sulfate, atropine, barbiturates, and ethylene glycol poisoning.

Side Effects. The agent is very safe.

CHLORAMBUCIL

Indications. Chlorambucil (Leukeran) is indicated for the treatment of lymphoreticular neoplasia, especially lymphocytic leukemia and macroglobulinemia. The drug has also been used in the treatment of immune-mediated glomerulonephritis that is unresponsive to other immunosuppressive drugs and polycythemia vera.

Side Effects. Bone marrow suppression is possible, but occurs less often than with cyclophosphamide. The complete blood count should be monitored on a regular basis.

CHLORAMPHENICOL

Indications. Chloramphenicol (Chloromycetin) is a bacteriostatic antibiotic with activity against gram-negative and gram-positive bacteria, most anaerobes, mycoplasmas, chlamydiae, rickettsiae, and some protozoa. It is well absorbed following oral administration, widely distributed throughout the body, and excreted in the bile and urine. It is commonly used in the treatment of eye, skin, urinary, and mucous membrane infection. Serum concentrations are monitored just be-

fore the next dose or 6 to 12 hours after last dose, depending on the regimen, and after steady state levels have been attained (21 hours in the dog, 26 hours in the cat).

Side Effects. Chloramphenicol is a hepatic microsomal enzyme inhibitor. It potentiates the activity of barbiturates, codeine, phenytoin, digitalis, and aspirin. Adverse reactions include anemia, thrombocytopenia, dose-related bone marrow suppression and leukopenia, and decreased antibody production. Some dogs may exhibit transient vomiting or diarrhea following oral admistration. Its bacteriostatic action inhibits the bactericidal effects of the penicillins and the cephalosporins.

CHLORDANE

Indications and Side Effects. See Chlorinated Hydrocarbons.

CHLORHEXIDINE

Indications. Chlorhexidine (Nolvasan 2%) is a shampoo with activity against gram-positive and gram-negative bacteria. It is used in the treatment of pyoderma and dermatophyte infection and has been used as an oral rinse in the management of oral disease.

Side Effects. It is nontoxic and nonirritating.

CHLORINATED HYDROCARBONS

Indications. The chlorinated hydrocarbons, including chlordane, lindane, toxaphene, and methoxychlor, are largely banned in many areas because of their persistence in the environment. They have been used in the treatment of mites, fleas, lice, mosquitos, and some ticks in dogs.

Side Effects. All chlorinated hydrocarbons, with the exception of methoxychlor, are toxic to cats. Apprehension, hyperptyalism, hypersensitivity, muscle twitching, and tonic–clonic seizures are possible side effects. Death may result. External stimuli precipitate convulsive activity. Cyanosis is not unusual. Treatment is nonspecific, and includes removal of unabsorbed drug, sedation to control seizures, maintenance of fluid balance, and keeping the animal in a quiet place.

CHLOROTHIAZIDE

Indications. Chlorothiazide (Diuril) is a thiazide diuretic used in the management of congestive heart failure, pulmonary edema, and congenital nephrogenic diabetes insipidus. Thiazide diuretics inhibit sodium and chloride absorption in the disatal tubules. Potassium secretion is promoted, and loss is comparable to that seen with furosemide. The onset of action occurs within 1 hour and peaks in 4 hours. Since thiazide diuretics work in a different part of the kidney than other diuretics, the thiazides and other diuretics are often used in combination.

Side Effects. Diuretic agents should not be used in dehydrated animals. Thiazide diuretics reduce renal blood flow, so should not be used in animals with renal failure.

CHLORPHENIRAMINE MALEATE

Indications and Side Effects. Chlorpheniramine maleate (Chlor-Trimeton, Teldrin) is useful in the management of pruritus in dogs and cats and for treating excessive grooming in cats. The bitter taste makes oral administration difficult in some animals. See also Antihistamines.

CHLORPROMAZINE HYDROCHLORIDE

Indications. Chlorpromazine hydrochloride (Thorazine) is a phenothiazine derivative. It is primarily used as a sedative and as an antiemetic agent. Chlorpromazine hydrochloride raises the threshold for ventricular ectopia and may be used to protect the heart from arrhythmias. Chlorpromazine hydrochloride has been used as adjunct therapy in the management of pulmonary edema by decreasing venous return. It has also been used in the treatment of feline infectious anemia (*Haemobartonella felis*), where it is believed that the drug affects red cell permeability and facilitates detachment of *H. felis* from the red cell membrane.

Side Effects. Constipation, paradoxical aggression, hypotension and collapse, and the initiation of seizure activity in animals with epilepsy has been reported. The drug should not be given to animals with tetanus or with organophosphate or strychnine toxicity.

CHLORPROPAMIDE

Indications. Chlorpropamide (Diabinese) is an oral hypoglycemic agent used in humans in the treatment of diabetes mellitus. In small animals it has been used in the treatment of partial diabetes insipidus, where it potentiates the effect of antidiuretic hormone at the renal tubules and reduces polyuria.

Side Effects. Hypoglycemia is the most common expected side effect. Other side effects are not well documented in small animals. In humans, anorexia, vomiting, weakness, and jaundice have been reported.

CHLORTETRACYCLINE

Indications and Side Effects. See Tetracyclines.

CHOLESTYRAMINE RESIN

Indications. Cholestyramine resin (Questran) is used to lower serum cholesterol levels. The drug binds to bile acids and gastrointestinal toxins and may also be used in the treatment of diarrhea in dogs.

Side Effects. Experience with the drug is limited in veterinary medicine. Nausea, vomiting, diarrhea, constipation, abdominal pain, and distention have been reported in humans.

CHORIONIC GONADOTROPIN

Indications. Chorionic gonadotropin (Follutein) is used to induce ovulation of normal follicles.

Side Effects. No side effects are noted.

CIMETIDINE

Indications. Cimetidine (Tagamet), a histamine (H2) blocking agent, reduces gastric acid secretion and is useful in the management of gastric and duodenal ulceration associated with renal failure, liver disease, mast cell tumor, and gastrinoma. It is less effective than antacids in the treatment of acute gastrointestinal bleeding because it impairs the secretory capacity of the gastric mucosa and decreases bicarbonate concentrations. Histamine (H2) antagonists are not effective in preventing nonsteroidal anti-inflammatory drug-induced gastric ulceration. Cimetidine may also be an effective adjunct to enzyme replacement therapy in pancreatic exocrine insufficiency, by decreasing gastric acid-induced enzyme inactivation. In uremic dogs it decreases the secretion of parathyroid hormone, decreases bone resorption and serum phosphate levels, and increases serum calcium levels. It also has been shown to have some immunomodulating properties. It suppresses T suppressor cell function and has been used in conjunction with antibiotics in dogs with chronic pyoderma and other recurrent infectious dermatoses.

Side Effects. By interfering with hepatic microenzyme systems, cimetidine decreases the metabolism of warfarin-type anticoagulants, phenytoin, theophylline, propranolol, and diazepam, resulting in delayed excretion. Histamine enhances cardiac automaticity; cimetidine blocks histamine and may cause bradycardia, hypotension, and cardiac arrest. Cardiac toxicity is increased with the infusion of lidocaine.

CIPROFLOXACIN

Indications.   Ciprofloxacin (Cipro) is a fluoroquinolone antibiotic with activity against *Escherichia coli*, klebsiellae, *Proteus*, *Pseudomonas*, staphylococci, salmonellae, shigellae, and *Yersinia*, *Camphylobacter*, and *Vibrio* organisms. It has little activity against anaerobic cocci or *Clostridia* or *Bacteroides* organisms. The fluoroquinolones are the preferred drugs in the treatment of complicated urinary tract infections. In humans ciprofloxacin is the preferred drug in the treatment of bacterial prostatitis. See also Quinolone Antibiotics.

Side Effects.   In humans side effects are rare. Primary side effects have been nausea, vomiting, and anorexia. Absorption is hindered by antacid preparations. These drugs are very expensive, but may be considered in cases of resistant bacterial infection.

CISAPRIDE

Indications.   Cisapride (Prepulsid) is chemically related to metoclopramide hydrochloride, and may be used in small animals to improve gastrointestinal motility in cases of primary motility disorders. It improves esophageal transit, increases lower esophageal pressure, and increases gastric emptying rates by increasing acetylcholine chloride release. Although no dose has been established in small animals, a dose of 5 mg three times daily is suggested for adult humans, and a dose of 0.2 mg/kg every 6 to 8 hours has been recommended for children. The drug is given 15 minutes before a meal.

Side Effects.   Diarrhea and loose stools have been reported in some humans.

CISPLATIN

Indications.   Cisplatin (Platinol) is a chemotherapeutic agent that has been used in the treatment of transitional cell carcinoma, squamous carcinoma, adenocarcinoma, and metastatic osteosarcoma, as well as other tumor types.

Side Effects.   Transient vomiting is the most common side effect reported in dogs. Anorexia and diarrhea may also occur; seizure activity has been reported. Granulocytopenia and thrombocytopenia, as well as

renal tubular dysfunction, have been documented. Saline diuresis prior to and following use of the drug is recommended to decrease the incidence of renal pathology. The concurrent use of mannitol does not ameliorate the situation and is not required. Cisplantin also causes local irritation. The drug appears to be quite toxic to cats. Its use has lead to dyspnea and death in this species.

CLAVAMOX

Indications and Side Effects.   Clavamox is an amoxicillin and clavulinic acid preparation. See Penicillins.

CLINDAMYCIN

Indications.   Clindamycin (Antirobe, Cleocin) is a lincosamide antibiotic with activity against gram-positive cocci (staphylococci and streptococci). It is often effective against gram-positive cocci that are resistant to penicillin and the cephalosporins. The drug is also effective against *Actinomyces*, *Nocardia*, *Mycoplasma*, and *Toxoplasma* organisms and anaerobic bacteria (*Bacteroides fragilis*, fusobacteria, peptostreptococci, *Clostridium perfringens*). It has greater antibiotic activity than lincomycin, but is more expensive. Significant concentrations are achieved in most body tissues other than cerebrospinal fluid.

Side Effects.   Adverse effects may include vomiting and hemorrhagic diarrhea in dogs. The drug may potentiate the effects of neuromuscular blocking agents during anesthesia. The safety of its use in pregnant and breeding animals has not been established.

CLONAZEPAM

Indications.   Clonazepam (Clonopin) is a benzodiazepine used in the management of seizure. The drug is potentially useful in the management of status epilepticus. It should not be considered a major anticonvulsant in the dog. It can be used in conjunction with phenobarbital in the treatment of intractable epilepsy.

Side Effects.   Tolerance to the drug develops after a 3- to 9-month period in many dogs. Experience with the drug is limited, but it is anticipated that ataxia and sedation occurs at higher drug dosages.

CLORAZEPATE DIPOTASSIUM

Indications.   Clorazepate dipotassium (Tranxene) is used in the management of behavior problems in dogs (noise phobias).

Side Effects. Excitability, ataxia, lethargy, and tolerance to the drug may occur.

CLOTRIMAZOLE

Indications. Clotrimazole (Lotrimin) in a 1% solution is effective against dermatophytes and *Candida* sp.

Side Effects. It is safe and nontoxic and is associated with little irritation.

CLOXACILLIN SODIUM

Indications and Side Effects. Cloxacillin sodium (Tegopen) is used primarily against gram-positive, β-lactamase-producing bacteria. See also Penicillins.

COAL TAR

Indications. Coal tar shampoos are keratolytic and keratoplastic. They are used in the treatment of seborrhea, pruritis, crusts, and scales.

Side Effects. Coal tar shampoos may be irritating or toxic to cats and are not approved for this species. These products may stain light-coated dogs.

CODEINE

Indications. Codeine is often used with aspirin in the management of moderate pain. It is 10% as potent an analgesic as morphine sulfate. It may be used alone as an antitussive.

Side Effects. Drowsiness, nausea, vomiting, and constipation have been reported.

COLCHICINE

Indications. Colchicine has been used in the dog for the treatment of chronic hepatic fibrosis. The drug works by decreasing collagen formation and promoting its breakdown. It has also been used in the treatment of amyloidosis. It impairs the release of serum amyloid A (SAA) from hepatocytes, prevents the production of amyloid-enhancing factor, and delays tissue deposition of amyloid.

Side Effects. In humans, nausea, vomiting, and diarrhea are most common. Muscular weakness, hematuria, oliguria, agranulocytosis, and anemia have also been reported.

CORTISONE ACETATE

Indications and Side Effects. Cortisone acetate (Cortone, Cortogen). See Glucocorticoids.

CUPRIMYXIN

Indications. Cuprimyxin (Unitop) is a bactericidal, fungicidal, and keratolytic cream useful in the treatment of bacterial skin diseases, dermatophytes, and infection with *Candida albicans*.

Side Effects. It is safe, nontoxic, and nonirritating.

CYCLOPHOSPHAMIDE

Indications. Cyclophosphamide (Cytoxan) is a potent immunosuppressive drug that has been used in the treatment of canine lymphosarcoma, mastocytoma, transmissible venereal tumor, bladder carcinoma, macroglobulinemia, multiple myeloma, and autoimmune diseases that are not responsive to other immunosuppressive agents.

Side Effects. Bone marrow depression, cystitis, and an association with the induction of transitional cell carcinoma have been documented. The complete blood count should be monitored weekly for the first 2 months, and monthly thereafter. Water should be available at all times, and the drug should not be used for more than 4 to 5 months.

CYCLOSPORINE

Indications. Cyclosporine (Sandimmune) is an effective immunosuppressent agent. It inhibits B and T lymphocyte activation. Its exerts its major effect on helper T cells by blocking the release of interleukin-2. It may be useful for the treatment of autoimmune disease and for organ transplants. Susceptibility to infection appears to be less common than that observed for other common immunosuppressive agents. A sterile solution of 2% cyclosporine (optimmune) has been successfully employed to treat idiopathic keratoconjunctivitis sicca (KCS). It does not cure KCS. The drug appears to inhibit T cells within the lacrimal gland from secreting inflammatory mediators that damage lacrimal acini. Lacrimation increases, while superficial pigmentation, vascularization, and granulation decrease.

Side Effects. In dogs, vomiting, diarrhea, anorexia, gingival hyperplasia, pyoderma, bacteriuria, hirsuitism, and papillomatosis have been reported. The incidence of nephrotoxicity and hepatotoxicity appears to be less common in dogs than that reported in humans. Intravenous administration causes acute anaphylactoid reactions in a high percentage of dogs. The ophthalmic preparation has been associated with local irritation in a few cases.

CYPROHEPTADINE

Indications.   Cyproheptadine (Periactin, Vimicon) is an antihistaminic and antiserotonic agent. It is used primarily in the cat to stimulate appetite. It may have antipruritic properties in small animals and may be useful in the treatment of aortic thromboembolism in cats. In humans it has also been used in the management of asthma.

Side Effects.   Sedation, excitation, tremor, hypotension, nausea, vomiting, diarrhea, constipation, and urinary retention have been reported with the use of the drug in humans. About 20% of cats treated with the drug have exhibited extreme excitability and aggression.

CYTARABINE HYDROCHLORIDE

Indications.   Cytarabine and cytarabine hydrochloride (Cytosar-U) have been used for the treatment of lymphoreticular neoplasms, mastocytoma, and myeloproliferative disease, and have been administered intrathecally for the treatment of central nervous system lymphoma.

Side Effects.   Nausea, vomiting, diarrhea, and anaphylaxis have been reported. Bone marrow depression, oral ulceration, hepatotoxicity, and fever have also been documented.

CYTHIOATE

Indications.   Cythioate (Proban) is an oral insecticide used in the management of flea infestation, ticks, and demodicosis. Fleas must ingest the product, and since it is the flea saliva that is allergenic, sensitive animals remain pruritic.

Side Effects.   The margin of safety is good. With drug overdose, muscular tremor, hyperexcitability, vomiting, anorexia, and salivation occur.

DACARBAZINE

Indications.   Dacarbazine (Dtic-Dome) is a chemotherapeutic agent with alkylating and antimetabolite properties. It is primarily used in the treatment of lymphoreticular neoplasia. The drug has minimal activity in malignant melanoma and osteosarcoma.

Side Effects.   Anorexia, vomiting, diarrhea, and cytopenia have been reported. Extravascular injection may cause tissue damage and severe pain.

DANAZOL

Indications.   Danazol (Danocrine) is a modified androgen. It has been shown to be effective in the treatment of canine immune-mediated thrombocytopenia. When combined with corticosteroids, the immunomodulating effects are synergistic. In humans it is also used in the treatment of autoimmune hemolytic anemia, and may be better suited than glucocorticoids in the long-term management of this disease.

Side Effects.   Side effects, although rare in humans, may include virilization and hepatic dysfunction. Side effects in small animals are poorly documented at the present time.

DANTROLENE SODIUM

Indications.   Dantrolene sodium (Dantrium) is a skeletal muscle relaxant useful in reducing external urethral sphincter tone. It is used in the treatment of incontinence due to urethral sphincter hypertonus. The drug is also used in the prevention and treatment of malignant hyperthermia.

Side Effects.   Drug overdose may cause generalized muscle weakness. Hepatotoxicity has been documented in humans following long-term use of the drug.

DAPSONE

Indications.   Dapsone (Avlosulfon) is an anti-inflammatory, antibacterial agent that has been used in the dog for the treatment of dermatitis herpetiformis, subcorneal pustular dermatitis, leprosy, and leukocytoclastic vasculitis.

Side Effects.   Hepatotoxicity, anemia, granulocytopenia, and thrombocytopenia may occur early in the course of therapy. These effects are reversible.

DEHYDROCHOLIC ACID

Indications.   Dehydrocholic acid (Decholin) is used to stimulate the flow of watery bile and help alleviate cholestasis. It is used until bilirubin is no longer present in the urine. Efficacy in small animals is not established.

Side Effects.   It should not be used if there is evidence of complete biliary obstruction.

DEMECLOCYCLINE

Indications and Side Effects.   See Tetracylines. No dose is as yet established for small animals.

DERM CAPS

Indications. Derm Caps is a fatty acid nutritional supplement containing eicosapentaenoic, τ-linolenic, linoleic, and linolenic acids. It has been shown to be of benefit in lessening or eliminating pruritus associated with atopic disease in dogs. The anti-inflammatory action is likely due to the decreased production of inflammatory eicosanoids. The drug has also been successfully used to treat idiopathic seborrhea in dogs, and may be effective in controlling seborrhea and pruritus in cats.

Side Effects. Loose stools and diarrhea may occur in some animals.

DESMOPRESSIN ACETATE

Indications. Desmopressin acetate (DDAVP) is a vasopressin analog used in the management of diabetes insipidus and von Willebrand's disease. It causes an increase in plasma factor VIII activity by stimulating the release of preformed factor VIII from storage sites. The effects of DDAVP in von Willebrand's disease last only 2 to 3 hours. Refractoriness to the drug can develop rapidly, and not all dogs with this disease respond to the drug.

Side Effects. Hypersensitivity reactions and fluid retention leading to hyponatremia may occur.

DESOXYCORTICOSTERONE

Indications. Desoxycorticosterone acetate (Doca Acetate, Percorten, Cortate, Syncort) and desoxycorticosterone pivalate (Percorten Pivalate) are mineralocorticoid preparations used in the management of hypoadrenocorticism. Desoxycorticosterone acetate is used in the acute crisis of the disease, and desoxycorticosterone pivalate is used for maintenace therapy.

Side Effects. Hypokalemia, hypernatremia, muscle weakness, and hypertension are reported in some patients.

DEXAMETHASONE

Indications and Side Effects. Dexamethasone (Azium, Decadron) and dexamethasone sodium phosphate (Decadron Phosphate). See Glucocorticoids.

DEXTROMETHORPHAN

Indications. Dextromethorphan is used in the management of cough.

Side Effects. In humans nausea and drowsiness are infrequent complaints.

DEXTROSE

Indications. Dextrose is indicated in the treatment of hypoglycemia and hypernatremia, and as part of the management of hyperkalemic myocardial toxicity. It also serves as a source of carbohydrates. Following intravenous injection, only one third of the solution remains in the extracellular space (three fourths of this is in the interstitial space, and one fourth in the intravascular space). Two thirds is directed into the intracellular space. This agent should therefore not be used for volume expansion in patients in shock (see Chapter 4).

Side Effects. Dextrose in water should not be used alone for maintenance fluid therapy because continued use may lead to hypokalemia, hyponatremia, hypochloremia, and hypomagnesemia. Intravenous injection of dextrose may cause local thrombophlebitis and thrombosis because of the acidic nature (*p*H 4–5) of the solution. The use of 5% dextrose in water in conjunction with whole blood transfusions should be discouraged because this may cause sludging of the red blood cells and contribute to tissue hypoxia. Dextrose in water should not be given by subcutaneous injection because the hypotonic nature of the solution draws ions from the extracellular space, possibly contributing to a decreased circulating blood volume and shock.

DIAZEPAM

Indications. Diazepam (Valium) is an effective anticonvulsant in the dog and cat. It is also useful in the management of convulsions associated with metaldehyde or methylxanthine (chocolate and caffeine) or salicylate toxicity, in functional urethral obstruction due to a failure of relaxation of the external sphincter muscle, and in canine and feline behavior problems (noise phobias, urine marking, anxiety). The drug is also used to stimulate appetite. It is more effective in cats than in dogs for this purpose. Another benzodiazepine derivative, oxazepam (Serax), is more effective in stimulating appetite. Flurazepam hydrochloride (Dalmane) is also effective and has a longer duration of action. Diazepam is also used in the management of Scotty cramp. Its use in this case decreases the clinical signs associated with the disease and its recurrence.

Side Effects. Dose-related sedation, ataxia, excitement, and sometimes paradoxical aggression are side effects. The benzodiazepines should not be used for more than 2 days to stimulate appetite. Tolerance to the drug may develop, thus limiting its efficacy in the management of epilepsy.

DIAZOXIDE

Indications.   Diazoxide (Proglycem) is an antihypertensive agent. In dogs the drug is used for the management of hypoglycemia associated with islet cell tumor (insulinoma). It inhibits pancreatic insulin secretion, enhances epinephrine-induced glycogenesis, and inhibits glucose uptake by cells. Diazoxide in conjunction with frequent feedings and prednisone (1 mg/kg/day, divided) transiently controls hypoglycemia in most dogs with islet cell neoplasia. Hydrochlorthiazide (2–4 mg/kg/day) may potentiate the hyperglycemic effects of diazoxide if diazoxide alone is not effective.

Side Effects.   Anorexia and vomiting may occur.

DICHLOROPHEN

Indications.   Dichlorophen (Dicestal) is an anthelmintic used in the treatment of infection with *Taenia* sp. and *Dipylidium caninum.*

Side Effects.   Vomiting, diarrhea, and abdominal pain may be associated with the use of this drug.

DICHLORVOS

Indications.   Dichlorvos (Task, Vapona, DDVP) is an anthelmintic cholinesterase inhibitor used for the elimination of hookworms, ascarids, and whipworms. It is also impregnated in collars or tags as a flea repellant.

Side Effects.   See also Organophosphates. Toxicity results in diarrhea, colic, salivation, dyspnea, miosis, muscular fasciculations, weakness, and respiratory paralysis. Atropine (0.2 mg/kg parenterally) alone or in combination with pralidoxime chloride (2 PAM) (20 mg/kg twice daily IM, IV) is generally an effective antidote in cases of toxicity. The drug should not be used in conjunction with other anthelmintics other than diethylcarbamazine, muscle relaxants, or tranquilizers. Dichlorvos should not be given to animals with constipation, intestinal obstruction, or hepatic or cardiac disease. It is also contraindicated in those with *Dirofilaria immitis* infection. In this case, adverse reactions appear similar to those noted above, but atropine is of little benefit as an antidote. In addition to atropine, fluid therapy is given as supportive treatment.

DIETHYLCARBAMAZINE

Indications.   Diethylcarbamazine (Filaribits, Caricide) is recommended for the prevention of heartworm disease. Filaribits Plus is a combination of diethylcar-bamazine and oxibendazole. It is used for the elimination of infection with heartworms, roundworms, hookworms, and whipworms in the dog.

Side Effects.   Vomiting is noted occasionally, and can be avoided by changing to a different formulation. Low sperm counts have been documented in dogs receiving the drug. Fertility returned to normal following cessation of therapy. If given to microfilaremic dogs, it can lead to a hypersensitivity reaction or anaphylaxis and death. Filaribits Plus has occasionally been associated with a hepatopathy that is potentially fatal. The drug should not be given to dogs with a history of liver disease.

DIETHYLSTILBESTROL

Indications.   Diethylstilbestrol is used in the management of estrogen-responsive urinary incontinence in the spayed female, vaginitis, benign prostatic hyperplasia, and perianal adenoma. It is not useful for the termination of pregnancy.

Side Effects.   Thrombocytopenia is observed approximately 2 weeks following the initiation of its use. Leukocytosis with a left shift develops at about 16 to 20 days, and anemia becomes gradually apparent. Leukopenia follows at 22 to 25 days. There is considerable variation in sensitivity to the effects of estrogens. Feminization or the induction of signs of estrus is also possible. Estrogens also cause squamous metaplasia and fibromuscular proliferation of the prostate gland, which predisposes to fluid stasis and infection.

DIGITOXIN

Indications.   Digitoxin (Foxalin) is a cardiac glycoside used in the treatment of supraventricular arrhythmias (atrial flutter or fibrillation), premature atrial contractions and tachycardia. Because it has less parasympathetic activity than digoxin, it is less effective in the management of supraventricular arrhythmias. It is preferred to digoxin in patients with renal dysfunction. Measurement of serum concentrations are taken after steady state levels have been attained (after approximately 5 days of therapy). Normal serum values are between 15 and 35 ng/ml 6 to 8 hours after treatment.

Side Effects.   Anorexia, vomiting, diarrhea, depression, atrioventricular block, ectopia, and junctional tachycardia have been documented.

Patients with hypokalemia, hypernatremia, and hypercalcemia are predisposed to toxic side effects. Because of the exceedingly long half-life in the cat (longer than 100 hours), it is not recommended for use in this species.

DIGOXIN

Indications. Digoxin (Lanoxin) is a positive ino-tropic and negative chronotropic agent. Its chrono-tropic properties make it the drug of choice in the management of supraventricular tachyarrhythmias (atrial fibrillation and flutter) and sinus tachycardia due to congestive heart failure. Its inotropic value is questionable. It is used, however, in an effort to im-prove cardiac output in conditions of congestive heart failure and cardiomyopathy. Samples for the determi-nation of serum drug levels should be taken after a steady state level has been achieved (6–7 days in the dog, 10 days in the cat). Blood samples are taken just prior to the next dose or at least 8 hours after the previous dose. Normal serum concentrations are be-tween 1 and 2 ng/ml, or 1.28 to 2.56 nmol/L. Concurrent measurement of serum electrolytes helps interpret the drug level and its effect on the patient.

Side Effects. Vomiting, diarrhea, anorexia, leth-argy, ataxia, various arrhythmias, and conduction ab-normalities are possible side effects. Toxicity is en-hanced with hypokalemia, decreased glomerular filtration, and hypothyroid and hyperthyroid disease. Furosemide, quinidine, and verapamil may potentiate digoxin toxicity. Serum levels may also increase with the concurrent use of spironolactone, diltiazem, triam-terene, erythromycin, and prazosin. Concurrent ad-ministration of aspirin, furosemide, or digoxin, or a low salt diet predisposes to digitalis intoxication in cats. Drugs that inhibit hepatic microenzymal activity de-crease digoxin excretion and should not be given con-currently (*e.g.,* chloramphenicol, quinidine, tetra-cycline).

DIHYDROSTREPTOMYCIN SULFATE

Indications and Side Effects. See Aminogly-cosides.

DIHYDROTACHYSTEROL

Indications. Dihydrotachysterol (Hytakerol) is used in the management of hypocalcemia due to hypo-parathyroidism. The time required for the drug to exert its maximal therapeutic effects is 1 to 7 days.

Side Effects. Hypercalcemia leading to polyuria, polydipsia, listlessness, depression, anorexia, vomit-ing, nephrocalcinosis, muscle weakness, and trembling or muscle twitching may occur. The time required for

normocalcemia following iatrogenic overdose is 1 to 3 weeks. Serum calcium levels should be monitored ev-ery 2 weeks.

DIHYDROXYVITAMIN D₃

Indications and Side Effects. Dihydroxyvitamin D₃ (Rocaltrol). See Dihydrotachysterol. The time re-quired for the drug to exert its maximal therapeutic effect is 1 to 4 days. The time required for nor-mocalcemia following iatrogenic overdose is 1 day to 2 weeks.

DILTIAZEM HYDROCHLORIDE

Indications. Diltiazem hydrochloride (Cardizem) is a calcium channel blocking agent. It decreases after-load, prolongs atrioventricular conduction (although not as much as verapamil), and is a less potent negative inotrope than verapamil or nifedipine. The drug ap-pears to be useful in the treatment of supraventricular tachycardia and hypertrophic cardiomyopathy. It causes less peripheral arterial vasodilation and reflex tachycardia than verapamil and nifedipine. The drug may also be useful in the treatment of congestive car-diomyopathy, as it decreases ventricular rate response to atrial fibrillation, decreases peripheral resistance and afterload, and has minimal cardiodepressant ef-fects.

Side Effects. Bradycardia appears to be the most common side effect in dogs. Serum levels are increased with the concurrent use of cimetidine. The effects of β-blockers and digoxin on impeding cardiac conduc-tion is also increased.

DIMETHYL SULFOXIDE

Indications. Dimethyl sulfoxide (Domoso) is re-ported to have a number of beneficial properties. It is often used to transport drugs across the skin into the general circulation. It has anti-inflammatory proper-ties. It is a potent diuretic, analgesic, and inotropic agent. Dimethyl sulfoxide inhibits platelet aggregation and the growth of certain bacteria, viruses, and fungi, and decreases fibroplasia. The drug is recommended for topical treatment in dogs with acute and chronic musculoskeletal disease, otitis externa, and ophthal-mic disease. It has also been recommended for the treatment of trauma to the head and spine. Dimethyl sulfoxide has been used in the treatment of renal am-yloidosis in the dog. Improvement in renal function is attributed to the anti-inflammatory properties of the drug, not to any direct effect on amyloid.

Side Effects. Topical application can lead to erythema, edema, and pruritis. Ocular changes, including nuclear cataract, have been reported. Intravascular injection of concentrations greater than 20% leads to severe hemolysis. The drug is potentially teratogenic during the first trimester of pregnancy. Doses for specific indications are not available for small animals.

DIPHENHYDRAMINE

Indications and Side Effects. Diphenhydramine (Benadryl). See Antihistamines.

DIPHENOXYLATE HYDROCHLORIDE

Indications. Diphenoxylate (Lomotil) is indicated for the management of diarrhea and colitis. The drug causes increased segmentation, decreased frequency of bowel movements, decreased abdominal pain, tenesmus, and possibly inhibition of fluid secretion.

Side Effects. Constipation, bloating, and sedation may occur. It should therefore only be used for a 36- to 48-hour period. The drug should not be used in cases of infectious enteritis.

DIPYRONE

Indications. Dipyrone is an anti-inflammatory, antipyretic agent.

Side Effects. Bone marrow suppression, gastrointestinal upset, hepatitis, and nephropathy may occur. It should not be given concurrently with phenothiazine agents, as hypothermia may result.

DISOPHENOL

Indications. Disophenol is an anthelmintic used in the treatment of hookworm and *Spirocerca lupi* infections.

Side Effects. Vomiting and a transient lens opacity have been noted. At higher doses, hyperthermia, labored breathing, polyuria, polydipsia, tachycardia, and tetany may occur. Hyperthermia should be treated with ice baths. Atropine and phenothiazine tranquilizers should be avoided.

DISOPYRAMIDE PHOSPHATE

Indications. Disopyramide phosphate (Norpace) is used for the management of ventricular arrhythmias.

Side Effects. Hypotension, depression of myocardial contractility, and a vagolytic effect that may predispose to accelerated ventricular rhythms in the presence of supraventricular tachycardia are side effects. The drug is contraindicated in the presence of congestive heart failure.

DITHIAZANINE

Indications. Dithiazanine iodide (Dizan) is used for the elimination of ascarids, hookworms, and *Strongyloides stercoralis* and *Dirofilaria immitis* micorfilaria.

Side Effects. Vomiting, diarrhea, anorexia, and weakness may occur. Vomitus or feces may be stained green or purple with the drug. Nephrotoxicity and hepatotoxicity have also been reported.

DOBUTAMINE HYDROCHLORIDE

Indications. Dobutamine hydrochloride (Dobutrex) increases cardiac contractility and cardiac output in patients with congestive heart failure or cardiomyopathy.

Side Effects. Sinus tachycardia and ventricular arrhythmias may occur. Vomiting and seizure activity have been reported in some cats.

DOCUSATE CALCIUM

Indications. Docusate sodium or dioctyl sodium sulfosuccinate (Surfak) is used for the prevention and treatment of constipation. The drug acts at the small and large bowel and generally takes 12 to 72 hours to work effectively.

Side Effects. Mild, transient cramping may rarely occur. It should not be administered with mineral oil, as increased absorption of the oil may occur.

DOCUSATE CALCIUM

Indications. Docusate sodium or dioctyl sodium sulfosuccinate (Surfak) is used for the prevention and treatment of constipation. The drug acts at the small and large bowel and generally takes 12 to 72 hours to work effectively.

Side Effects. Docusate sodium should not be administered with mineral oil, as increased absorption of the oil may result.

DOMEBORO

Indications. Domeboro contains aluminum sulfate and calcium acetate, which when added to water produces aluminum acetate. The product is astringent, drying, soothing, antipruritic, antiseptic, and acidifying. It is useful as a wet dressing for relief of inflammatory conditions of the skin.

DOPAMINE HYDROCHLORIDE

Indications. Same as for dobutamine hydrochloride. Dopamine hydrochloride (Inotropin) also dilates renal and mesenteric vessels and is of use in patients with oliguric renal failure.

Side Effects. Same as for dobutamine hydrochloride. It is more likely than dobutamine hydrochloride to cause tachycardia and peripheral vasoconstriction. Perivascular injection may lead to gangrene secondary to local vasoconstriction.

DOXAPRAM HYDROCHLORIDE

Indications. Doxapram hydrochloride (Dopram) is used to stimulate respiration in patients with postanesthetic respiratory depression or apnea and to encourage the return of laryngopharyngeal reflexes in patients with mild to moderate respiratory and central nervous system depression due to anesthetic overdose.

Side Effects. Cough, dyspnea, and laryngospasm may occur. Nausea and vomiting have also been reported. Excessive doses may initiate hyperventilation and respiratory alkalosis. Arrhythmias and urinary retention occur in some animals, and seizure activity may be provoked in epileptic patients.

DOXORUBICIN HYDROCHLORIDE

Indications. Doxorubicin hydrochloride (Adriamycin) is used in the treatment of lymphomas, thyroid carcinomas, and other solid tumors.

Side Effects. Bone marrow suppression peaks 10 to 14 days after the initiation of treatment, followed by recovery in 21 days. Dose-dependent congestive cardiomyopathy is reported, and nondose-dependent cardiac arrhythmias are observed. It is important not to exceed a cummulative dose of 250 mg/m². Vomiting and diarrhea as well as allergic reactions, including cutaneous hyperemia, pruritis, head shaking, and vomiting, have also been documented. Diphenhydramine (Benadryl) given at a dose of 2.2 mg/kg IM 20 minutes before doxorubicin hydrochloride use has been recommended to prevent anaphylactic reactions. Severe local tissue damage occurs if the drug is injected extravascularly. Because of the nephrotoxicity, the drug is not recommended for routine use in cats.

DOXYCYCLINE

Indications and Side Effects. Doxycycline (Vibramycin). See Tetracyclines.

ECONAZOLE

Indications. Econazole (Spectrazole) is a topical imidazole used in the treatment of localized demodicosis. It is also used in humans in the treatment of dermatophycosis and *Candida* infections.

Side Effects. Occasional local skin irritation occurs.

EDROPHONIUM CHLORIDE

Indications. Edrophonium chloride (Tensilon Chloride) is a cholinesterase inhibitor. It is used in the diagnosis of myasthenia gravis and in the treatment of curare poisoning and unresponsive atrial tachycardia.

Side Effects. Cholinergic reactions, including bradycardia, pupillary constriction, laryngospasm, bronchiolar constriction, nausea, vomiting, diarrhea, and muscle weakness, may occur. In the case of accidental overdose, atropine should be administered.

EFA-VET

Indications. This drug is a combination of vegatable and marine lipids (fatty acid supplement) formulated to have anti-inflammatory properties. The drug may lessen or eliminate seborrhea in dogs and pruritus in atopic dogs, and may be effective in controlling seborrhea and pruritus in cats.

Side Effects. Although rare, fatty acid supplementation may be associated with vomiting, diarrhea, lethargy, urticaria, and increased pruritis.

EFA-Z PLUS

Indications and Side Effects. See EfaVet.

ENALAPRIL MALEATE

Indications. Enalapril maleate (Vasotec) is an angiotensin-converting enzyme inhibitor. Peak concentrations occur 4 to 6 hours after oral administration. It has a longer duration of action than captopril (Capoten). Angiotensin-converting enzyme inhibitors are used for their vasodilatory properties in the treatment of congestive heart failure, systemic hypertension, renal disease, and shock.

Side Effects. In humans, pruritus, proteinuria, gastrointestinal disturbances, hypotension, bone marrow-induced neutropenia, hyperkalemia, and deterioration of renal function have been reported with the use of angiotensin-converting enzyme inhibitors. Because the drug is eliminated by the kidneys, the dose must be decreased in patients with renal dysfunction. There is little information concerning adverse effects with the use of enalapril maleate in veterinary medicine as yet.

ENILCONAZOLE

Indications. Enilconazole (Imaverol) is a topical medication that has been used in the dog for the treatment of nasal aspergillosis (by way of intranasal intubation).

Side Effects. Side effects are rare. Sneezing and salivation occur with topical intranasal appilcation. Inappetence may occur at high doses.

ENROFLOXACIN

Indications and Side Effects. Enrofloxacin (Baytril). See Quinolone Antibiotics.

EPHEDRINE HYDROCHLORIDE

Indications. Ephedrine hydrochloride (Quadrinal, Mudrane GG) stimulates alpha receptors. It is useful for the management of urinary incontinence.

Side Effects. Tachycardia, hypertension, tremors, restlessness, anxiety, hyperexcitability, and urine retention are reported.

EPINEPHRINE

Indications. This drug (Adrenalin) is indicated in cardiac arrest associated with ventricular standstill. It accelerates atrial and ventricular rates.

Side Effects. Hypotension, atrial and ventricular premature contractions, tachycardia, or fibrillation are reported. Epinephrine potentiates halothane-induced arrhythmias, especially with the concurrent use of barbiturate or xylazine anesthesia. Acepromazine given 20 minutes prior to anesthesia may decrease the incidence of epinephrine-induced arrhythmias.

ERYTHROMYCIN

Indications. Erythromycin (Ilotycin) is a macrolide antibiotic used against gram-positive bacteria, some anaerobes, and *Mycoplasma*, *Rickettsia*, and *Chlamydia* organisms. It is effective against penicillinase-producing staphylococci.

Side Effects. Adverse effects are seldom reported in small animals. Nausea, vomiting, and diarrhea may occur following oral administration. Kaolin, pectin, and bismuth decrease gastrointestinal absorption.

ETHACRYNIC ACID

Indications and Side Effects. See Furosemide. Ethacrynic acid (Edecrin) is a loop diruretic similar in action to furosemide. In humans, nausea, vomiting, diarrhea, and abdominal pain occur in a small number of patients with chronic use of the drug. Experience in small animals is limited.

ETHYL ALCOHOL

Indications. This drug is indicated in the management of ethylene glycol (antifreeze) toxicity.

Side Effects. Clincal signs of an overdose of ethyl alcohol include initial excitement, ataxia, weakness, depression, dilated pupils, and a slow heart rate. Vomiting, diarrhea, uremia, anuria, and death due to respiratory failure may follow.

ETIDRONATE DISODIUM

Indications. Etidronate disodium (Didronel) is potentially useful in the management of refractory hypercalcemia.

Side Effects. In humans, diarrhea and loose stools may occur. With drug overdose, hypocalcemia is possible.

ETOMIDATE

Indications. Etomidate (Amidate, Hypnomidate) is used as an anesthetic induction agent.

Side Effects. The drug is considered safe. It has a rapid onset of action, is less of a cardiopulmonary depressive than thiopental sodium or methohexital, and is characterized by a rapid recovery period relative to the prolonged sedation associated with the barbiturates. Side effects of etomidate are dose-dependent, and in dogs include excitement, pain upon injection, myoclonus vomiting, and apnea. The frequency of side effects is decreased with preanesthetic medication (tranquilizers, sedatives, opiods). Transient adrenocortical suppression has also been reported in dogs.

ETRETINATE

Indications. Etretinate (Tegison) is the tri-methylmethoxyphenyl analog of tretinoin ethyl ester. It is useful for disorders of keratinization, abnormalities in follicular keratinization, and quantitative or qualitative disorders of sebaceous gland secretion.

Side Effects. Side effects have included vomiting, conjunctivitis, and cracking of foot pads.

FAMOTIDINE

Indications. Famotidine (Pepcid) is a histamine (H2) receptor anatagonist. Although it is 32 times more potent than cimetidine, no studies to date indicate it is more efficacious than cimetidine or ranitidine in the management of gastric hyperacidity and gastrointestinal ulcers.

Side Effects. Unknown to date in small animals.

FENBENDAZOLE

Indications. Fenbendazole (Panacur) is an anthelmintic used in the treatment of ascarid, *Filaroides* sp., *Aelurostrongylus abstrusus*, *Capillaria plica*, taeniae, *Trichuris vulpis*, and *Paragonimus kellicotti* infections. It has also been shown to reduce burdens of *Ancylostoma caninum* and *Toxocara canis* in newborn pups when the bitch is treated during the last trimester of pregnancy. The drug may also have some efficacy against capillariasis and crensomiasis.

Side Effects. Vomiting is infrequently reported. Pneumothorax from the migration of flukes and anaphylactic reactions rarely occur.

FENTANYL CITRATE–DROPERIDOL

Indications and Side Effects. See Innovar.

FENTHION

Indications. Fenthion (Pro-spot, Spot-on) has been used in dogs for the control of flea infestation. Fleas must ingest the product for it to be efficacious, and since it is the flea saliva that is allergenic, dogs remain pruritic. The drug has also been used in the treatment of demodicosis and heartworm infection (as a microfilaricide). The efficacy of this product for these latter two purposes is unknown.

Side Effects. The drug is an organophosphate, and side effects due to intoxication are the same as those described under Organophosphates. With chronic use (more than 4 weeks, starting at a topical dose of 44 mg/ kg/day for 10 treatments, then 22 mg/kg/day for an additional 13 treatments), clinical signs of toxicity range from ataxia, pelvic limb paralysis, and incontinence to muscle fasciculations, proprioceptive deficits, and pelvic limb "bunny hopping." Most signs appear to be reversible upon cessation of use of the product. This product should not be used at the same time or within 14 days of treatment with other cholinesterase-inhibiting agents. It should not be used concurrently with flea or tick collars. Succinylcholine chloride, procaine hydrochloride, and the aminoglycosides may enhance the toxicity of fenthion. The drug should not be used in puppies younger than 10 days of age or in sick, debilitated animals.

FERROUS SULFATE

Indications. Ferrous sulfate (Fer-in-Sol, Fesofor, Fero-Gard, Slow-Fe) is used for the prevention and treatment of iron deficiency anemia.

Side Effects. Mild gastrointestinal upset may occur in some patients. Oral iron preparations may interfere with the absorption of tetracycline antibiotics. Antacids given concurrently with iron compounds decrease iron absorption.

FLECAINIDE ACETATE

Indications. In humans, flecainide acetate (Tambocor) is effective in controlling ventricular tachycardias and atrial or ventricular premature beats. It is less effective in controlling atrial fibrillation and flutter.

Side Effects. Little information is available concerning its use in small animals. In humans, depression, gastrointestinal upset, hypotension, ataxia, weakness, depression, and seizure have been reported.

FLUCYTOSINE

Indications. Flucytosine or 5-fluorocytosine (Ancabon, Ancotil) is used for the treatment of cryptococcosis and aspergillosis. It has also been used in combination with amphotericin B or ketoconazole for the treatment of cryptococcosis.

Side Effects. Leukopenia, thrombocytopenia, hepatotoxicity, cutaneous eruption, rash, and gastrointestinal upset have been reported. The drug is teratogenic and should not be given to pregnant animals.

FLUDROCORTISONE ACETATE

Indications. Fludrocortisone acetate (Florinef Acetate) is used in the management of hypoadrenocorticism. It promotes sodium retention and urinary potassium excretion. In larger doses it inhibits endogenous cortisol secretion.

Side Effects.   Adverse effects are rare, but may include sodium retention, potassium loss, hypokalemic alkalosis, and muscle weakness.

FLUMETHASONE

Indications and Side Effects.   Flumethasone (Flucort). See Glucocorticoids.

FLUNIXIN

Indications.   Flunixin meglumine (Banamine) is a potent antiprostaglandin agent useful in the treatment of inflammation and pain associated with musculoskeletal disease. Its analgesic properties are considered superior to those of meperidine hydrochloride. It has also been recommended as adjunct therapy in the treatment of shock in the dog. It is not approved for use in small animals.

Side Effects.   Side effects are rare. Gastric ulceration appears common even at recommended therapeutic doses and is exacerbated by the concurrent use of prednisone. At higher doses, salivation, panting, emesis, and tremors have been noted. Kidney necrosis may occur in patients with preexisting renal disease. Intramuscular injection is very irritating.

FLUOROURACIL

Indications.   Fluorouracil (Adrucil) has been used for the treatment of various carcinomas and sarcomas in dogs.

Side Effects.   Nausea, vomiting, and diarrhea may occur. Oral and gastrointestinal ulceration, leukopenia, thrombocytopenia, anemia, neurologic deficits, and alopecia have also been documented. The drug is extremely neurotoxic to cats and should never be used in cats.

FLUOXYMESTERONE

Indications and Side Effects.   Fluoxymesterone (Halotestin, Ultandren). See Anabolic Steroids.

FLURAZEPAM HYDROCHLORIDE

Indications and Side Effects.   Flurazepam hydrochloride (Dalmane) has been used to stimulate appetite. See Diazepam.

FUROSEMIDE

Indications.   Furosemide (Lasix) is a potent loop diuretic that is effective in reducing preload and pulmonary edema in patients with congestive heart failure and cardiomyopathy. It promotes significant sodium and water excretion by inhibiting chloride resorption in the ascending loop of Henle. It also redistributes blood flow from the juxtamedullary region of the kidney to the cortex, and may act as a venous vasodilator by increasing systemic and venous capacitance. The drug is beneficial in the management of systemic hypertension. Activity is noted 5 minutes after intravenous injection and 1 hour after oral use. Peak activity occurs 30 minutes following intravenous injection and 1 to 2 hours after oral use. Duration of action is 2 hours after intravenous injection and 6 hours following oral use.

Side Effects.   Dehydration, hypokalemia, hyponatremia, and hypochloremic alkalosis may occur. Furosemide may enhance the toxic potential of digoxin. With continuous therapy, the loss of water-soluble vitamins is a possibility, and it is therefore recommended that these patients receive concurrent B-complex supplementation.

GEMFIBROZIL

Indications.   Gemfibrozil (Lopid) is used to lower serum triglyceride levels in humans.

Side Effects.   In humans, the incidence of side effects is low. Nausea, vomiting, diarrhea, and abdominal pain may occur. Experience with the drug in veterinary medicine is limited.

GENTAMICIN

Indications and Side Effects.   Gentamicin (Genticin). See Aminoglycosides. Serum concentrations are measured 1 to 2 hours after dosing for peak concentrations, just before the next dose for trough concentrations, and after steady state levels have been attained (6.5 hours in the dog).

GLUCOCORTICOIDS

Indications.   Glucocorticoid agents are recommended for the treatment of allergic and immune-mediated disease and cardiogenic and septic shock. The beneficial effects of these agents include stabilization of lysozymal and capillary membranes, decrease in activation of the complement and clotting cascades, binding of endotoxin, positive inotropic effect, dilation of precapillary sphincters, prevention of gastrointestinal mucosal ischemia in shock, increase in gluconeogenesis, inhibition of the formation of vasoactive substances (kinins, prostaglandins), decrease in collagen and scar formation, and decrease in the accumulation of phagocytes at areas of inflammation. Analgesic activity is related to the inhibition of prostaglandin production.

The glucocorticoids are classified according to their duration of action. Short-acting drugs (less than 12 hours) include hydrocortisone and cortisone acetate. Intermediate-acting drugs (12–36 hours) include prednisone, prednisolone, methylprednisolone, and triamcinolone. Long-acting drugs (more than 48 hours) include paramethasone, flumethasone, betamethasone, and dexamethasone. Topical corticosteroids (Aristocort) are used for their anti-inflammatory, antipruritic, and vasoconstrictive effects.

Side Effects. Polyuria, polydipsia, polyphagia, panting, lethargy, weakness, and bilateral symmetrical alopecia are the most common clinical signs associated with their use. Glucocorticoids may mask the clinical signs of bacterial, viral, fungal, or parasitic disease and potentiate the spread of these diseases. The drugs may decrease the clinical response to bacteriostatic antibiotics by decreasing the inflammatory response and diminishing the phagocytic activity of leukocytes. Hemorrhagic gastroenteritis, pancreatitis, hepatopathy, and iatrogenic hyperadrenocorticism have been reported.

GLYCERIN SUPPOSITORIES

Indications. Glycerin suppositories are used for the treatment of constipation, but bisacodyl (Dulcolax) or suppositories containing docusate sodium are more effective.

Side Effects. No side effects have been noted.

GLYCOBIARSOL

Indications. Glycobiarsol (Milibis-V) is an anthelmintic used in the treatment of whipworms and, occasionally, giardiasis.

Side Effects. The dose should be halved for use in debilitated dogs.

GLYCOPYRROLATE

Indications. Glycopyrrolate (Robinul) is indicated in the treatment of sinus bradycardia, sick sinus syndrome, atrioventricular block, and sinoatrial arrest. It is also used in preanesthetic regimens to reduce salivary, tracheobronchial, and pharyngeal secretions, to reduce the volume and acidity of gastric secretion, and to inhibit cardiac vagal inhibitory reflexes during anesthetic induction and intubation.

Side Effects. Mydriasis, xerostomia, constipation, and, occasionally, tachycardia may be seen with its use. Excretion of the drug may be prolonged in animals with impaired renal or gastrointestinal function. Glycopyrrolate should not be administered to pregnant animals.

GONADOTROPIN RELEASING HORMONE

Indications. Gonadotropin releasing hormone (Cystorelin) is used to induce ovluation of normal follicles.

Side Effects. No side effects are noted.

GRISEOFULVIN

Indications. Griseofulvin (Fulvicin) is used in the treatment of dermatophyte infection. The drug is detectable in the skin within 4 to 8 hours of oral administration. High dietary fat facilitates absorption.

Side Effects. Adverse effects are rare, but may include vomiting, diarrhea, depression, ataxia, pruritis, photosensitization, and depressed spermatogenesis. Leukopenia has also been reported in cats. It is teratogenic to cats and should not be given to pregnant queens. Phenobarbital depresses absorption of the drug.

GROWTH HORMONE

Indications. Growth hormone preparations (other than ovine preparations, which are not effective in dogs) have been used in the treatment of pituitary dwarfism and growth hormone-responsive dermatosis.

Side Effects. Diabetes mellitus due to the gluconeogenic properties of growth hormone is a possible side effect. Hypersensitivity reactions (anaphylaxis) is also possible with the use of this drug.

GUAIFENESIN

Indications. Guaifenesin, or glyceryl guaiacolate, is an expectorant used in the management of dry, unproductive cough. It stimulates gastric receptors that initiate a reflex secretion of bronchial glands, thereby increasing the volume and decreasing the viscosity of bronchial secretions. Its efficacy in improving mucociliary clearance, however, is questionable. The combination of this drug with antitussives, antihistamines, or decongestants appears unjustified.

Side Effects. Nausea, gastric upset, and drowsiness are reported in humans. Guaifenesin may prolong the activated clotting time and impair platelet function. It should be avoided in animals with bleeding tendencies.

HALOTHANE

Indications.   Halothane (Fluothane) is an inhalent drug used for the induction of general anesthesia.

Side Effects.   Dose-dependent hypotension has been documented; it is potentially arrhythmogenic, especially in the presence of epinephrine and the thiobarbiturates.

HEPARIN

Indications.   Heparin may be indicated in cases of aortic and venous thrombosis, pulmonary thromboembolic disease, and disseminated intravascular coagulation. The drug has also been used in the treatment of pemphigus vulgaris at a subcutaneous dosage of 100 U/kg twice daily.

Side Effects.   Prolonged activated partial thrombin time and bleeding may occur with an overdose of the drug.

HETACILLIN

Indications and Side Effects.   Hetacillin (Hetacin). See Penicillins.

HYDRALAZINE HYDROCHLORIDE

Indications.   Hydralazine hydrochloride (Apresoline) is an arterial vasodilator. It increases cardiac output, decreases mitral regurgitation and left atrial size, and alleviates the cough due to left atrial compression of the left principle bronchus. The drug is also used in patients with systemic hypertension, usually in conjunction with a diuretic and a β-blocker.

Side Effects.   Hypotension, increases in heart rate, sodium and water retention, mild gastrointestinal upset, and tolerance to the drug have been described in humans.

HYDROCHLORTHIAZIDE

Indications.   Although hydrochlorthiazide (Hydro-Diuril, Aldoril) is not as potent as furosemide, it is used to decrease pulmonary edema in patients with congestive heart failure and cardiomyopathy.

Side Effects.   Hypokalemia and a loss of water-soluble vitamins may occur.

HYDROCODONE

Indications.   Hydrocodone (Hycodan) is a narcotic antitussive that is especially useful in the control of cough that is not responsive to other agents.

Side Effects.   In humans, adverse reactions may include drowsiness, nausea, vomiting, constipation, and hypotension. The drug is a narcotic, and the potential for abuse by clients must be considered.

HYDROCORTISONE SODIUM SUCCINATE

Indications and Side Effects.   Hydrocortisone sodium succinate (Solu-Cortef). See Glucocorticoids.

HYDROGEN PEROXIDE

Indications.   Hydrogen peroxide (3%) is a useful local antiseptic agent. Although used for the induction of emesis, it is not very effective in this regard.

Side Effects.   No side effects are noted.

HYDROXYUREA

Indications.   Hydroxyurea (Hydrea) is a chemotherapeutic agent used in the treatment of leukemia, mastocytoma, and primary polycythemia (polycythemia vera).

Side Effects.   In the dog, anorexia, vomiting, arrest of spermatogenesis, bone marrow hypoplasia, and sloughing of the nails have been reported. A complete blood count and platelet count should be done every 7 to 14 days until the hematocrit has normalized, and every 3 to 4 months thereafter. If leukopenia, thrombocytopenia, or anemia develops, the drug should be discontinued until blood counts return to normal, and should then be resumed at a lower dosage.

HYDROXYZINE

Indications and Side Effects.   Hydroxyzine (Atarax). See Antihistamines.

HY-LYT EFA

Indications.   HY-LYT efa is a bath oil conditioner containing fatty acids in diluent. It is useful in the treatment of dry skin or following routine or therapeutic shampooing.

IBUPROFEN

Indications.   Ibuprofen (Advil, Motrin, Rufen) is a nonsteroidal anti-inflammatory agent used in the management of joint pain secondary to degenerative joint disease that is unreponsive to aspirin.

Side Effects. Vomiting, gastritis, and renal insufficiency have been associated with the use of this drug.

IMIPRAMINE HYDROCHLORIDE

Indications. Imipramine hydrochloride (Tofranil) is used in the treatment of cataplexy. It may also be of benefit in the management of urinary incontinence, where it acts to increase urethral pressure.

Side Effects. In humans, the use of this drug is sometimes associated with impotency. Hypotension, tachycardia, arrhythmias, anxiety, ataxia, seizure, constipation, mydriasis, urinary retention, pruritis, bone marrow depression leading to granulocytopenia and thrombocytopenia, anorexia, vomiting, diarrhea, and jaundice have also been reported in humans.

INDOMETHACIN

Indications and Side Effects. Indomethacin (Indocin) is a nonsteroidal anti-inflammatory agent recommended by some clinicians in the management of joint pain secondary to degenerative joint disease that is unresponsive to aspirin. It has been associated with hepatotoxicity in dogs and cats and fatal gastrointestinal hemorrhage in dogs, and is not routinely recommended for use in small animals.

INNOVAR

Indications. Innovar-Vet is a combination of droperidol and fentanyl citrate. It is used for its tranquilizing and analgesic properties in dogs as a premed sedative or as an anesthetic induction agent.

Side Effects. Respiratory depression and centrally mediated vagal bradycardia occur. It may cause panting. Patients still respond to loud noises or mechanical stimulation. Behavioural changes including aggression have been noted in some dogs following its use. The drug causes CNS excitation in cats and is not recommended in this species.

INSULIN

Indications. Insulin preparations are used in the management of diabetes mellitus. Regular insulin has the fastest onset of action and the shortest duration. The onset of action is within 15 minutes if the drug is given intramuscularly, within 30 minutes if given subcutaneously, and immediately if given intravenously. Peak effect occurs in ½ hour if given intravenously and in 1 to 6 hours if given intramuscularly or subcutaneously. The duration of effect is 1 to 4 hours (intravenously) or 4 to 10 hours (intramuscularly or subcutaneously).

Intermediate-acting insulins include isophane insulin suspension (NPH) and insulin zinc suspension (Lente Insulin). The onset of action is 1 to 3 hours. Peak activity occurs at 2 to 10 hours with NPH and 4 to 12 hours with Lente. The duration of effect is 8 to 24 hours for both preparations.

The long-acting form of insulin is protamine zinc insulin suspension. Its onset of action is 1 to 4 hours, its peak of activity is 5 to 14 hours, and its duration of effect is 8 to 30 hours.

Side Effects. Overdose may cause hypoglycemia, leading to disorientation, weakness, hunger, seizure, coma, and death. If overdose occurs, the animal should be fed sugar with water or food. If seizures occur, dextrose solutions should be given intravenously until the seizures have stopped.

IPECAC

Indications. Syrup of ipecac is a useful emetic agent. Its mode of action is through gastric irritation and central nervous system stimulation. Only half of the patients will actually vomit with its use. The total dose should not exceed 15 ml (1 tablespoon).

Side Effects. Syrup of ipecac is potentially cardiotoxic. It should not be used concurrently with activated charcoal, since it decreases the activity of this agent.

IRON-DEXTRAN INJECTION

Indications. Iron dextran injection (Imferon) is indicated for the treatment of iron deficiency anemia in cases in which oral therapy is not possible.

Side Effects. Intramuscular injection can be irritating. In humans, allergic reactions and anaphlyaxis have occasionally been reported.

ISOFLURANE

Indications. Isoflurane (Forane) is an inhalant anesthetic agent useful for short surgical procedures. It is especially useful in debilitated patients and those with hepatic or renal impairment. Induction and recovery times are more rapid with isoflurane than with halothane. Isoflurane does not sensitize the heart to epinephrine-induced arrhythmias as does halothane.

Side Effects. Dose-dependent cardiac and respiratory depression occurs.

ISOPROPAMIDE IODIDE

Indications. Isopropamide iodide (Darbid) is an anticholinergic agent that is considered to be effective in the treatment of various forms of heart block.

Side Effects. Atropinelike effects, such as an increase in heart rate, dryness of the mucous membranes, pupillary dilation, and constipation, may occur.

ISOPROTERENOL HYDROCHLORIDE

Indications. Isoproterenol hydrochloride (Isuprel Hydrochloride) is a catecholamine agent useful for the short-term management of heart block, sinus bradycardia, and sick sinus syndrome. It increases atrioventricular conduction and ventricular excitability. It also causes peripheral vascular dilation and bronchial smooth muscle relaxation. Definitive treatment of complete heart block requires pacemaker implantation. Medical managemnent is not successful in these cases.

Side Effects. Vomiting, nervous excitation, sinus tachycardia, and ectopic beat formation are reported.

ISOSORBIDE DINITRATE

Indications. Isosorbide dinitrate (Isordil) is a venous vasodilator useful in the treatment of pulmonary edema associated with congestive heart failure and mitral regurgitation.

Side Effects. Although little information is available concerning its use in small animals, hypotension is a concern.

ISOTRETINOIN

Indications. Isotretinoin (Accutane) appears to be useful for disorders of keratinization, abnormalities in follicular keratinization, and quantitative or qualitative disorders of sebaceous gland secretion.

Side Effects. The incidence of adverse effects appears to be low. Lethargy, anorexia, vomiting, conjunctivitis, pruritus, erythema of the mucocutaneous junctions and feet, hyperactivity, abdominal distention, collapse, and a swollen tongue have been documented in the veterinary literature. All of these were reversible upon discontinuation of the drug. Occasional laboratory abnormalities included increases in serum triglyceride and cholesterol levels, increases in alanine aminotransferase levels, and thrombocytosis. The incidence of adverse effects appears to be higher in cats. Erythema, periocular crusting, epiphora,

blepharospasm, and diarrhea have been recorded. The drug is also reported to be teratogenic in humans.

ITRACONAZOLE

Indications. Itraconazole is more potent than ketoconazole against histoplasmosis, blastomycosis, aspergillosis, and cryptococcosis. Unlike ketoconazole, itraconazole reaches adequate levels in the central nervous system at therapeutic doses. Plamsa testosterone and cortisol levels are not affected by the drug.

Side Effects. Experience with the drug in veterinary medicine is limited, but anorexia, cutaneous vasculitis, gastrointestinal upset, and hepatotoxicity may occur.

IVERMECTIN

Indications. Ivermectin is used for the eradication of demodectic, sarcoptic, otodectic, and *Cheyletiella* mites in dogs. It has also been used for the treatment of *Capillaria aerophilia* and is marketed for the prevention of canine heartworm infection (Heartgard). In cats the drug has been used topically for the treatment of ear mites, *Cheyletiella blakei*, and fleas.

Side Effects. Adverse reactions are uncommon, but mydriasis, tremors, ataxia, vomiting, diarrhea, and death have been reported. Collies and related breeds appear to be predisposed. Microfilaremic dogs may exhibit transient diarrhea with the use of Heartgard.

KANAMYCIN

Indications and Side Effects. Kanamycin (Kantrim). See Aminoglycosides.

KAOLIN—PECTIN

Indications. Kaolin—pectin (Kaopectate) is a gastrointestinal protectant used in the management of diarrhea. It coats the surface of the gut and exerts a mild demulcent and absorbant effect; it may help absorb some bacterial toxins. Efficacy is questionable. It appears to act by adding particulate matter to the feces, which improves consistency until the disease spontaneouly resolves.

Side Effects. It depresses the absorption of lincomycin if given concurrently. The drug may cause constipation in patients with dehydration.

KETAMINE HYDROCHLORIDE

Indications.   Ketamine hydrochloride (Ketaset, Vetalar) is a nonbarbiturate anesthetic used in cats. It may be used for chemical restraint or anesthesia of short duration. It is characterized by a rapid onset of action, profound analgesia, maintenance of normal muscle tone and laryngeal reflex, mild cardiac stimulation, and respiratory depression. Combined with diazepam it is safely used in dogs for sedation.

Side Effects.   Its use is associated with increased muscle tone, and seizures may occur. Dose-dependent respiratory depression and hypotension may occur with larger doses. The drug is eliminated renally and should be used with caution in patients with renal impairment.

KETOCONAZOLE

Indications.   Ketoconazole (Nizoral) has been used in the treatment of *Trichophyton mentagrophytes* infection, coccidioidomycosis, cryptococcosis, blastomycosis, histoplasmosis, and canine nasal aspergillosis. The drug is also used in the treatment of canine hyperadrenocorticism. It lowers serum cortisol and serum testosterone levels and is used in humans in the management of prostatic carcinoma. Therapeutic concentrations are achieved in all body tissues except the brain, testes, and eye. Some authors, however, report that dosages of 30 to 40 mg/kg/day are likely to achieve therapeutic concentrations in the brain and cerebrospinal fluid.

Side Effects.   Nausea, anorexia, vomiting, diarrhea, lightening of the hair coat, transient elevations in liver enzymes, and jaundice are reported. Gastrointestinal side effects may be prevented by administering the drug with food (which may also serve to increase its absorption) and by dividing the daily dose and administering twice to four times daily. Ketoconazole should not be given concurrently with antacids or cimetidine. The drug should not be given to pregnant animals, as its use has been associated with stillbirths and mummified fetuses.

LACTULOSE

Indications.   Lactulose (Cephulac) is a synthetic nonabsorbable disaccharide used in the management of hepatic encephalopathy. Enteric bacteria ferment lactulose to acidic by-products, decrease intraluminal *p*H, and favor the formation of ammonium ions, which are poorly absorbed. It also acts as a mild osmotic laxative, increases the rate of passage of ingesta, and leads to the reduction of bacterial production of ammonia.

Side Effects.   Transient flatulence and abdominal cramping may occur. Excessive dosing often leads to diarrhea.

LEVAMISOLE

Indications.   Levamisole (Ripercol, Tramisol) is used for the elimination of *Dirofilaria immitis* microfilaria. It has also been used for the treatment of filaroidiasis, capillariasis, and aelurostrongylosis, and likely has some efficacy against crenosomiasis. It may help restore immune function by increasing the number and function of T lymphocytes. The drug has also been reported to stimulate antibody production, increase macrophage phagocytosis, inhibit tumor growth, and stimulate suppressor cell activity.

Side Effects.   Vomiting, anorexia, salivation, depression, panting, head shaking, muscular tremors, and agitation are reported. Atropine is only partially effective as an antidote. If toxicity progresses to flaccid paralysis, respiratory assistance should be given and mecamylamine hydrochloride (Inversine), a ganglionic blocking agent, administered at a dose of 1 to 2 mg subcutaneously to effect.

LEVOTHYROXINE SODIUM

Indications.   Levothyroxine sodium (Synthroid) is used for the treatment of hypothyroid disease. Peak serum concentratins are reached in 4 to 10 hours. Some animals require the drug twice daily. Serum levels can be measured after steady state levels have been attained (1 month). For those animals on a once-daily regimen, serum samples should be taken 24 hours after the previous dose. The timing is not as important for those animals receiving the drug twice daily. Levothyroxine sodium (at standard doses) has also been used in the management of dogs with hypothyroidism, von Willebrand's disease, and problems of platelet dysfunction. It causes an increase in vWF : Ag and platelet adhesiveness, corresponding to a correction in bleeding times.

Side Effects.   Thyroid replacement should be undertaken with caution in animals with hypoadrenocorticism, diabetes mellitus, or congestive heart failure. The increase in metabolism may place undue stress on the heart. Increased metabolism of adrenal hormones may precipitate a hypoadrenocortical crisis, and increased metabolism may enhance ketone production and potentiate ketoacidosis in animals with diabetes mellitus. In the case of drug overdose, signs consistent with thyrotoxicosis include polyuria, polydipsia, polyphagia, weight loss, panting, nervousness, and tachycardia. Appropriate adjustment in dosage will alleviate these signs.

LIDOCAINE HYDROCHLORIDE

Indications. Lidocaine hydrochloride (Xylocaine Hydrochloride) is the drug of choice for the management of ventricular premature contractions or tachycardia. Serum concentrations are measured after steady state levels have been attained (5 hours in the dog).

Side Effects. Vomiting, tremors, seizure, excitation, hypotension, and increased atrioventricular conduction with atrial flutter or fibrillation have been reported. The neurologic signs may be controlled with diazepam. Contrary to accepted theory, lidocaine with epinephrine does not appear to provoke ventricular arrhythmias even when hearts are apparently sensitized by halothane. Serum levels are increased with the concurrent use of cimetidine.

LIME SULFUR

Indications. Lime sulfur solution (Lym Dyp) is useful in the treatment of scabies, cheyletiellosis, and dermatophycosis. It is also antiseptic and mildly keratolytic.

Side Effects. The solution can be drying and irritating.

LINCOMYCIN HYDROCHLORIDE

Indications. Lincomycin hydrochloride (Lincocin) is a lincosamide antibiotic with activity directed against gram-positive cocci except enterococci, anaerobes, and mycoplasmas. These drugs are also useful against penicillinase-producing staphylococci. Significant concentrations of the drug are achieved in most tissues of the body other than cerebrospinal fluid. Excretion occurs in the bile and urine.

Side Effects. Vomiting and hemorrhagic diarrhea may occur in dogs. Kaolin, pectin, and bismuth subsalicylate decrease gastrointestinal absorption.

LINDANE

Indications and Side Effects. See Chlorinated Hydrocarbons.

LIOTHYRONINE SODIUM

Indications and Side Effects. See Triiodothyronine.

LITHIUM CARBONATE

Indications. Lithium carbonate (Lithane, Lithotabs) is used in small animals in the treatment of idiopathic aplastic anemia, neutropenia, or thrombocytopenia. It causes an increase in production of all cell lines.

Side Effects. In humans, nausea, diarrhea, vertigo, muscle weakness, fatigue, polyuria, and polydipsia are side effects. Neutrophilia, increases in red cell and platelet numbers, and a decrease in lymphocyte numbers may occur. The drug also may block the release of triiodothyronine and thyroxine, leading to low serum concentrations of each.

LOPERAMIDE

Indications. Loperamide (Imodium) is useful for the management of large and small bowel diarrhea in dogs.

Side Effects. The drug is relatively safe. Dose-dependent vomiting (dose greater than 0.63 mg/kg) may occur. With chronic use, soft stools, vomiting, and weight loss have been reported. The drug should not be used to treat diarrhea in cases with invasive bacterial enteritis, such as with *Salmonella* infection, as decreased intestinal transit time can delay clearance of the pathogen. Loperamide should be discontinued if it has not controlled the diarrhea within 48 hours.

MAGNESIUM HYDROXIDE

Indications and Side Effects. Magnesium hydroxide (Milk of Magnesia). See Antacid Preparationss. The drug also acts as a mild laxative.

MALATHION

Indications and Side Effects. Malathion is an effective and relatively nontoxic organophosphate. An uncommon side effect to overexposure is delayed paralysis of the hindlimbs. See also Organophosphates.

MANNITOL

Indications. Mannitol is an effective diuretic agent. It is used in the prevention and management of oliguria. It is also used in the treatment of cerebral edema.

Side Effects. Volume overload and pulmonary edema are a concern in patients with renal or cardiac insufficiency. Seizures and hyponatremia may also occur in patients receiving large doses.

MEBENDAZOLE

Indications. Mebendazole (Telmintic) is an anthelmintic used for the elimination of ascarids, hookworms, whipworms, and tapeworms (*Taenia* sp.).

Side Effects. Vomiting and diarrhea are the most common side effects reported. Hepatotoxicity is rarely reported.

MECLOFENAMATE SODIUM

Indications. Meclofenamate sodium (Arquel, Meclomen) is a nonsteroidal anti-inflammatory drug with analgesic and antipyretic properties. It is principally used in large animals to treat inflammatory conditions of the musculoskeletal system.

Side Effects. Anorexia, diarrhea with or without occult blood, anemia, depression, and weakness may occur. The drug should not be used in animals with gastrointestinal, hepatic, or renal disease.

MEDIUM-CHAIN TRIGLYCERIDE OIL

Indications. Medium-chain triglyceride oil is used in the management of patients with lymphangiectasia.

Side Effects. The oil is distasteful. It should initially be mixed in small amounts of food. It may lead to signs of hepatic encephalopathy in patients with advanced cirrhosis or portocaval shunts, and should not be used in the presence of these diseases.

MEDROXYPROGESTERONE ACETATE

Indications. Medroxyprogesterone acetate (Depo-Provera) is a progestational compound used in the treatment of feline endocrine alopecia, eosinophilic granuloma complex, psychogenic alopecia and dermatitis, miliary dermatitis, stud tail, intermale aggression, and spraying by male cats. This product is not licensed for use in cats. It is also used in dogs as a contraceptive in countries where it is marketed for this purpose (Depopromone, Perlutex, Anovulin).

Side Effects. Overdosage or prolonged treatment may cause cystic endometritis. Transient or permanent diabetes mellitus, acromegaly, mammary hyperplasia or adenocarcinoma, adrenocortical suppression, immunosuppression (T lymphocytes), suppression of fi-

broblast function (which may delay healing), and pyometra in intact females are other possible side effects. Injections may cause temporary local alopecia, cutaneous atrophy, and pigmentary changes.

MEGESTROL ACETATE

Indications. Megestrol acetate (Ovaban, Megace) is used to postpone estrus in bitches and treat dominance–aggression in dogs. In cats the drug has been used to treat neurodermatitis (psychogenic alopecia), eosinophilic complex, miliary dermatitis, pemphigus foliaceus, endocrine alopecia, hyperesthesia, spraying, intermale aggression, and aggression toward humans. It has also been used in cats to prevent or postpone estrus.

Side Effects. The drug should not be used in bitches with reproductive problems, pregnant bitches, or bitches with mammary tumors. Polyphagia, polydipsia, weight gain, and a change in behavior are common side effects. Overdosage or prolonged treatment may cause cystic endometritis. Transient or permanent diabetes mellitus, mammary hyperplasia or adenocarcinoma, adrenocortical suppression, immunosuppression (T lymphocytes), suppression of fibroblast function (which may delay healing), and pyometra in intact females are other possible side effects.

MELPHALAN

Indications. Melphalan (Alkeran) is indicated in the treatment of lymphoreticular neoplasms, osteosarcoma, mammary and lung tumors, and multiple myeloma.

Side Effects. Nausea, anorexia, and vomiting have been documented. Leukopenia, thrombocytopenia, and anemia may occur. The complete blood count should be monitored on a regular basis.

MEPERIDINE HYDROCHLORIDE

Indications. Meperidine hydrochloride (Demerol Hydrochloride) is used in the treatment of pain. It is only about one eighth as potent as morphine sulfate in pain relief. Given orally, its onset of action is 15 minutes, with a peak effect in 1 hour. The analgesic effect is only one half as effective when given orally rather than parenterally. Given parenterally, the onset of analgesia is 10 minutes and the duration of effect is 2 to 4 hours. As a preanesthetic it reduces the amount of barbiturate required.

Side Effects. Respiratory depression, loss of corneal reflex, and seizure are possible if given to excess. It is quite irritating if injected subcutaneously. It should not be used in animals with head trauma because it increases intracranial pressure. It also causes spasm of the pancreatic and biliary ducts, so should not be used in animals with pancreatic, hepatic, or biliary dysfunction.

MERCAPTOPROPIONYL GLYCINE

Indications. Mercaptopropionyl glycine (Thiola, Tiopronin) increases the solubility of cystine in the urine and has been used for the treatment of cystine urolithiasis in the dog.

Side Effects. Side effects are few. Nonpruritic, vesicular skin lesions that disappeared with the reduction of drug dose have been reported.

MERCAPTOPURINE

Indications. Mercaptopurine (Purinethol) is a chemotherapeutic agent used in the treatment of lymphosarcoma, acute lymphocytic and granulocytic leukemia, and immune-mediated disease.

Side Effects. Nausea, vomiting, and hepatopathy have been reported. Leukopenia is rare.

METAMUCIL

Indications. Metamucil is a hydrophilic colloid (psyllium) used in the treatment of constipation and colitis. It works at the level of the large and small bowel and generally requires 12 to 24 hours to work effectively.

Side Effects. There are no side effects. It should not be used, however, in patients with abdominal pain, vomiting, nausea, or fecal impaction.

METAPROTERENOL SULFATE

Indications. Metaproterenol sulfate (Alupent, Metaprel) is a β_2-adrenergic stimulating agent used as a bronchodilator.

Side Effects. Dose-related skeletal muscle tremors, nervousness, fatigue, and tachycardia may be seen.

METHACYCLINE

Indications and Side Effects. See Tetracyclines. No dose is available for use in small animals.

METHADONE HYDROCHLORIDE

Indications. Methadone hydrochloride (Dolophine Hydrochloride) is a semisynthetic narcotic used in the treatment of pain. Its analgesic potency is two to three times greater than that of morphine sulfate. It is well absorbed following oral administration and has a longer duration of action than morphine sulfate.

Side Effects. The sedative effect is minimal. It causes excitement in cats and is not recommended in this species. It should not be used in animals with head trauma because it increases intracranial pressure. It also causes spasm of the pancreatic and biliary ducts, so should not be used in animals with pancreatic, hepatic, or biliary dysfunction.

METHANDROSTENOLONE

Indications and Side Effects. Methandrostenolone (Dianabol). See Anabolic Steroids.

METHENAMINE MANDELATE

Indications. Methenamine mandelate (Mandelamine) is a urinary antiseptic agent used in the management of urinary tract infection. In the presence of acid urine (*p*H less than 6) the drug is hydrolyzed to formaldehyde.

Side Effects. The drug may cause gastrointestinal upset. It should not be given to patients with renal insufficiency.

METHENOLONE

Indications and Side Effects. Methenolone (Primobolan Acetate). See Anabolic Steroids.

METHIMAZOLE

Indications. Methimazole (Tapazole) is the drug of choice for the medical management of feline hyperthyroid disease. It is safer and more potent than propylthiouracil in blocking thyroid hormone synthesis.

Side Effects. Adverse effects have been observed in a few cats and are generally transient. Anorexia, vomiting, and transient lethargy have been documented in some cats. Serum antinuclear antibodies develop in many cats with long-term use of the drug. A glucocorticoid-responsive pruritus involving the face, ears, and neck may occur. More significantly, hepatopathy, thrombocytopenia, and agranulocytosis have been reported in some cats treated with the drug.

METHIONINE

Indications. Methionine is used to acidify urine. There is no evidence to support its use in the treatment of hepatic lipidosis that is not caused by a choline deficiency (as with pancreatic exocrine insufficiency).

Side Effects. Vomiting may occur. Oral methionine may also potentiate hepatoencephalopathy.

METHOCARBAMOL

Indications. Methocarbamol (Robaxin) is a central-acting muscle relaxant useful as adjunct therapy to rest and physical therapy in the treatment of musculoskelatal injury. The drug has been used to help reduce muscular spasm associated with tetanus or strychnine poisoning.

Side Effects. Excessive salivation, vomiting, muscular weakness, and ataxia have been reported. Extravascular injection may cause tissue necrosis. The drug should not be given to animals with renal dysfunction or to pregnant animals.

METHOTREXATE

Indications. Methotrexate inhibits the conversion of folic acid to folinic acid. The drug is indicated in the treatment of lymphoreticular neoplasms, myeloproliferative disease, and various carcinomas and sarcomas. It has also been used in combination with vincristine sulfate and cyclophosphamide for the treatment of transmissible venereal tumor.

Side Effects. Leukopenia, thrombocytopenia, anemia, stomatitis, destruction of intestinal epithelium causing diarrhea, renal tubular necrosis, and hepatic necrosis have been reported. Leucovorin calcium, a reduced folate, given at 3 mg/m² IM within 3 hours of methotrexate administration helps ameliorate these effects.

METHOXYCHLOR

Indications and Side Effects. See Chlorinated Hydrocarbons.

METHSCOPOLAMINE BROMIDE

Indications. Methscopolamine bromide (Pamine) is an anticholinergic agent used in the treatment of diarrhea and gastrointestinal ulcer.

Side Effects. Dryness of the mouth, urinary retention, constipation, nausea, and tachycardia may occur. The drug is contraindicated in cases of urinary outflow obstruction.

METHYLENE BLUE

Indications. Methylene blue is used in the treatment of methemoglobinemia. It has also been used as a urinary antiseptic and may be useful in the intraoperative identification of parathyroid and pancreatic islet cell tumors in dogs.

Side Effects. Methylene blue may cause Heinz body hemolytic anemia and possibly acute renal failure. Cats are especially sensitive to Heinz-body formation.

METHYLPHENIDATE HYDROCHLORIDE

Indications. Methylphenidate hydrochloride (Ritalin Hydrochloride) is used in the treatment of narcolepsy.

Side Effects. The drug tends to lose its effect over time. In humans, nervousness, anorexia, and tachycardia have been observed. Overdosage may cause vomiting, tremors, muscle twitching, convulsions, tachycardia, arrhythmias, mydriasis, and dryness of the mucous membranes.

METHYLPREDNISONE SODIUM SUCCINATE

Indications and Side Effects. Methylprednisone sodium succinate (Solu-Medrol). See Glucocorticoids.

METOCLOPRAMIDE HYDROCHLORIDE

Indications. Metoclopramide hydrochloride (Maxeran, Reglan) is an antiemetic agent with both central (chemoreceptor trigger zone) and peripheral (gastrointestinal) activity. It contributes to lower esophageal sphincter competence and promotes gastric emptying. It is useful in the management of vomiting, gastroesophageal reflux, and gastric motility disorders.

Side Effects. The drug should not be used in patients with gastric outlet obstruction or a history of epilepsy. Central nervous system reactions include increased frequency of seizure activity, hyperactivity, depression, or disorientation. It should not be used in conjunction with phenothiazines or narcotic analgesics. Atropine will block the effects of the drug on gastrointestinal motility.

METOPROLOL TARTRATE

Indications. Metoprolol tartrate (Lopressor) is a selective β_1-blocking agent equal in potency to propranolol. It is preferred in patients with pulmonary disease, such as asthma. The drug is useful in the management of supraventricular tachyarrhythmias, ventricular premature contractions, and hypertrophic cardiomyopathy in cats.

Side Effects.   The drug is excreted through the renal system, and therefore should be used with caution in animals with compromised renal function. Depression, lethargy, bradycardia, impaired atrioventricular conduction, and congestive heart failure have been documented with the use of β-blockers. Glycopyrrolate and dopamine hydrochloride can be used to counter bradycardia.

METRONIDAZOLE

Indications.   Metronidazole (Flagyl) is used for the treatment of giardiasis, trichomoniasis, amebiasis, balantidiasis, and trypanosomiasis. It is as effective and is better tolerated than quinacrine hydrochloride for the treatment of giardiasis. It is bactericidal to many anaerobic bacteria, as well as *Escherichia coli*, klebsiellae, and *Proteus*, and has been used in the treatment of septicemia, meningitis, peritonitis, biliary infections, colitis, and gingivostomatitis in which anaerobic bacteria are involved. The drug may also have immunosuppressive or immunostimulatory properties.

Side Effects.   Nausea, anorexia, vomiting, and dose-dependent neurologic signs (ataxia, nystagmus, seizure, head tilt) have been documented. It is metabolized in the liver and excreted by the kidneys. Dosage should be adjusted in animals with liver or renal impairment.

MEXILETINE

Indications.   Mexiletine has antiarrhythmic properties similar to those of lidocaine hydrochloride. It is used in the treatment of ventricular arrhythmias.

Side Effects.   Side effects are similar to those reported with lidocaine hydrochloride. However, little information concerning the use of mexiletine in dogs is available. The combination of mexiletine and aminophylline or theophylline may result in ventricular tachycardia or premature ventricular complexes.

MICONAZOLE

Indications.   Miconazole is an antifungal drug used in the treatment of candidiasis, dermatophytosis (Conafite cream), and aspergillosis. It is more valuable than clotrimazole in the treatment of systemic fungal infections.

Side Effects.   Thrombophlebitis, pruritis, nausea, leukopenia, thrombocytopenia, and elevations in hepatic enzymes have been documented in humans, but the drug appears to be safe, nontoxic, and nonirritating in animals.

MIDAZOLAM HYDROCHLORIDE

Indications.   Midazolam hydrochloride (Versed) is a water-soluble benzodiazepine that can be given intramuscularly and is useful as an anesthetic premedicant.

Side Effects.   No significant cardiovascular effects are noted. Dose-dependent sedation occurs. Midazolam hydrochloride is two to three times as potent as diazepam and has a shorter half-life. See also Diazepam.

MILRINONE

Indications.   Indications are the same as for amrinone. Milrinone is a derivative of amrinone, with almost 20 times the inotropic potency of the parent compound and with mild arterial vasodilator activity. It is considered a safer drug than digoxin. It may be used in animals to increase cardiac output. It is therefore of potential use in cardiomyopathy and congestive heart failure.

Side Effects.   Side effects are rare and consist only of clinically manageable ventricular arrhythmias.

MINERAL OIL

Indications.   Mineral oil is used in the treatment of constipation. It softens stools by coating the feces and preventing the colonic absorption of water. The agent acts at the colon and generally takes 6 to 12 hours to work effectively.

Side Effects.   A small amount of oil is absorbed, but this is generally of no concern. Increased absorption of mineral oil may occur if it is given concurrently with docusate sodium or docusate calcium. The principal concern with the use of this product, because of its lack of taste, is the accidental aspiration of the product and subsequent aspiration pneumonia. Mineral oil may interfere with the absorption of fat-soluble vitamins and should only be given between meals.

MINOCYCLINE HYDROCHLORIDE

Indications and Side Effects.   Minocycline hydrochloride (Minocin). See Tetracyclines.

MISOPROSTOL

Indications. Misoprostol (Cytotec) is a synthetic prostaglandin E_1 analog used to prevent gastric ulceration. It is the only medication indicated for the prevention of nonsteroidal anti-inflammatory drug-induced gastric ulceration. It works by decreasing gastric acid secretion and increasing bicarbonate secretion, mucus secretion, epithelial cell turnover, and mucosal blood flow.

Side Effects. The most common side effects reported are dose dependent and include diarrhea, vomiting, and abdominal pain. Abortion may occur in pregnant animals.

MITHRAMYCIN

Indications. Mithramycin (Mithracin) is used to lower serum calcium levels in cases of severe hypercalcemia that is unresponsive to other treatment modalities. The drug is a potent inhibitor of osteoclastic activity.

Side Effects. Nephrotoxicity, hepatotoxicity, myelosuppression, hypocalcemia, and rebound hypercalcemia have been reported in humans. There is little information concerning its use in small animals.

MITOTANE

Indications. Mitotane (Lysodren) has been used for the treatment of hyperadrenocorticism. It causes selective necrosis of cells of the zona fasciculata and reticularis of the adrenal gland. Damage to the zona glomerulosa is slight.

Side Effects. Lethargy, vomiting, weakness, anorexia, and diarrhea are side effects. About 5% of dogs develop hypoadrenocorticism. Although cats appear to be more sensitive to the chlorinated hydrocarbons, the drug has been used in this species. It is well tolerated by 75% of cats and results in adrenocortical suppression in half.

MITOXANTRONE

Indications. Mitoxantrone (Novantrone) is a chemotherapeutic agent related to doxorubicin. It has been used in dogs to treat various malignancies including lymphoma, fibrosarcoma, thyroid carcinoma, squamous cell carcinoma, chondrosarcoma, transitional cell carcinoma, hemangiopericytoma, and renal adenocarcinoma.

Side Effects. The drug is considered safe and effective. It has not been associated with the cardiotoxicity seen with doxorubicin. Adverse effects are dose-related and include depression and gastrointestinal signs. Neutropenia may occur (nadir on day 10).

MORPHINE SULFATE

Indications. Morphine sulfate is a very effective analgesic narcotic. Analgesic effects last 4 to 6 hours following intramuscular injection. In addition to analgesia, it produces central nervous system depression with sedation or sleep. It increases cardiac output, and decreases pulmonary edema associated with congestive heart failure and cardiomyopathy.

Side Effects. In dogs it may produce intial excitement, restlessness, panting, salivation, nausea, vomiting, urination, defecation, and hypotension. Subsequently, central nervous system depression, constipation, urinary retention, bradycardia, respiratory depression, hypothermia, and miosis occur. In cats analgesia and central nervous system depression occur at lower doses (0.1 mg/kg four times daily). At doses of 1 mg/kg, hyperexcitability, aggression, and vomiting may occur. The depressive effects of the drug are antagonized by nalorphine (Nalline) or naloxone (Narcan). The drug should not be used in animals with renal failure or a history of seizures or hypovolemic shock.

NADOLOL

Indications and Side Effects. Nadolol (Corgard) is a nonselective β-blocking drug with a relative potency similar to that of propranolol.

Side Effects. Depression, lethargy, bradycardia, impaired atrioventricular conduction, hypotension, and congestive heart failure have been documented with the use of β-blockers. Glycopyrrolate and dopamine hydrochloride can be used to counter bradycardia. The drug is excreted renally, and should be used with caution in patients with renal impairment.

NAFCILLIN SODIUM

Indications and Side Effects. Nafcillin sodium (Unipen, Nafcil) is used primarily against gram-positive, β-lactamase-producing bacteria. See also Penicillins.

NALIDIXIC ACID

Indications and Side Effects. See Quinolone Antibiotics.

NALORPHINE

Indications.   Nalorphine (Nalline) is a narcotic agonist–antagonist. It reverses the action of opiate and opioid drugs. It is also recommended as adjunct therapy in the treatment of shock (see Chapter 4).

Side Effects.   It produces narcosis in animals that have not received other narcotics.

NALOXONE

Indications.   Naloxone (Narcan) is an narcotic antagonist. It is the preferred agent for reversal of narcotic depression. It is also recommended as adjunct therapy in the treatment of shock (see Chapter 4).

Side Effects.   Its duration of action may be shorter than that of the opioid it is antagonizing, and the animal should be watched for signs of returning narcosis.

NANDROLONE

Indications and Side Effects.   Nandrolone decanoate (Deca-Durabolin) and nandrolone phenpropionate (Durabolin). See Anabolic Steroids.

NEOMYCIN

Indications and Side Effects.   Neomycin (Biosol). See Aminoglycosides.

NEOSTIGMINE

Indications.   Neostigmine (Stiglin, Prostigmin) is an anticholinesterase inhibitor used for the treatment of myasthenia gravis. There is marked variability in response to dose.

Side Effects.   Salivation, urination, diarrhea, or drooling may indicate that the drug dose should be lowered. If a severe overdose occurs, generalized weakness similar in appearance to myasthenia gravis may occur. A test dose of edrophonium chloride will differentiate the two. A cholinergic crisis should be treated with atropine.

NICLOSAMIDE

Indications.   Niclosamide, or Yomesan, is an anthelmintic used for the treatment of tapeworm (*Taenia* sp., *Dipylidium caninum*) infections.

Side Effects.   The drug is well tolerated at therapeutic doses. Some softening of stools is a common side effect.

NIFEDIPINE

Indications.   Nifedipine (Procardia, Adalat) is a calcium channel blocking agent. It is a potent peripheral arterial vasodilator and causes relaxation of smooth muscle. It has no effect in reducing the ventricular response to supraventricular tachyarrhythmias (atrial fibrillation). It has been used in a dog for the management of megaesophagus.

Side Effects.   Dose-dependent hypotension and reflex tachycardia appear to be the most common concerns. The short half-life of the drug (1 hour when administered intravenously) limits its value as a vasodilator. Its effect on decreasing lower esophageal pressure, however, may last 3 to 6 hours.

NITROGLYCERIN

Indications.   Nitroglycerin (Nitrobid, Nitrol) is a venous vasodilator used to treat pulmonary edema.

Side Effects.   In humans, large doses can cause tachycardia and dizziness.

NIZATIDINE

Indications.   Nizatidine (Axid) is a new histamine (H2) receptor antagonist. It inhibits gastric acid secretion and is useful in the treatment of gastrointestinal ulceration.

Side Effects.   There is little experience with the use of the drug as yet in veterinary medicine. In people side effects are rare.

NORETHANDROLONE

Indications and Side Effects.   Norethandrolone (Nilevar). See Anabolic Steroids.

NORFLOXACIN

Indications and Side Effects.   Norfloxacin (Noroxin). See Quinolone Antibiotics.

NOSCAPINE

Indications.   Noscapine (Vetinol, Coscopin) is an antitussive giving temporary relief from dry, irritating, nonproductive coughing.

Side Effects.   In humans, nausea and drowsiness are noted.

NOVOBIOCIN

Indications. Novobiocin (Albamycin) is useful against gram-positive bacteria, including streptococci and staphylococci.

Side Effects. Side effects are unknown to date in small animals.

NUTRI-SOL EFA

Indications and Side Effects. See EfaVet and Derm Caps.

NYSTATIN

Indications. Nystatin (Mycostatin, Nadostine, Nilstat) is indicated for *Candida* infections of the skin, mucous membranes, and intestinal tract. It is only partially effective in the treatment of dermatophytes and aspergillosis.

Side Effects. Rarely, topical application has caused a contact dermatitis. In humans, large oral doses have occasionally been associated with diarrhea, nausea, and vomiting. The drug is too toxic for parenteral use in small animals.

OMEPRAZOLE

Indications. Omeprazole (Losec) is part of a new class of drugs called proton pump inhibitors. It is 10 times more potent than cimetidine and has a long duration of action (24 hours or more). It has cytoprotective (by enhancing mucosal cell prostaglandin production) and acid reducing properties, and may be useful in decreasing gastric hyperacidity and the treatment of gastrointestinal ulcers.

Side Effects. Although the drug is not commercially available, chronic suppression of acid secretion has caused hypergastrinemia in animals leading to mucosal cell hyperplasia, rugal hypertrophy, and the development of carcinoids.

ORGANOPHOSPATES

Indications. The organophosphates (dichlorvos, fenthion, malathion, ronnel, crufomate, parathion, dimpylate) are used for the treatment of cheyletiellic and sarcoptic mange, fleas, ticks, and lice.

Side Effects. These agents, other than malathion, are not approved for use in cats. In dogs, the greyhound appears to be more sensitive to the adverse effects of these drugs. Signs of intoxication include bradycardia, salivation, vomiting, diarrhea, muscle tremors, con-

vulsions, pupillary constriction, bronchoconstriction, respiratory depression, and paralysis. Death may occur. Some organophosphates are associated with a delayed neurotoxicity characterized by muscular weakness and ataxia that progresses to a flaccid paralysis of the hindlimbs and, occasionally, all four limbs 8 to 21 days after administration. Phenothiazine tranquilizers and diazepam potentiate the adverse effects of these drugs. Cats are more sensitive to these agents than dogs.

If topical application has resulted in toxicity, the skin should be cleansed. If the drug was ingested, gastric lavage is indicated, followed by the oral administration of activated charcoal. In all cases, atropine should be given (0.2 mg/kg). One fourth of the total dose is given intravenously and the balance, intramuscularly. In addition, pralidoxime chloride may be useful in the dog and cat (20 mg/kg IM or IV, repeat [2 PAM] every 12 hours as indicated).

ORGOTEIN

Indications. Orgotein (Palosein) is a free radical scavenger. It has been used to treat orthopedic pain, a variety of ophthalmic disorders, and acral lick dermatitis.

Side Effects. Rarely, exacerbation of clinical signs occurs before improvement is noted. Anaphylaxis, although rare, is also possible.

OXACILLIN SODIUM

Indications and Side Effects. Oxacillin sodium (Prostaphilin). The drug has been used in the treatment of staphylococcal infections and infections caused by β-lactamase-producing bacteria. It has been used in the treatment of pyoderma, bacterial endocarditis, and blepharitis. See also Penicillins.

OXAZEPAM

Indications and Side Effects. Oxazepam (Serax) is used to stimulate appetite. See also Diazepam.

OXTRIPHYLLINE

Indications. Oxtriphylline (Choledyl) is a theophylline derivative. It is a bronchodilator used in the management of chronic cough. It is also available in combination with the expectorant guaifenesin.

Side Effects. Anorexia, vomiting, restlessness, tachypnea, arrhythmias, and, rarely, seizures may occur. Serum levels are increased by cimetidine, erythromycin, and propranolol.

OXYBUTYNIN CHLORIDE

Indications.   Oxybutynin chloride (Ditropan) is a direct-acting muscle relaxant that is useful in the management of detrusor hyperreflexia. The drug may take several weeks to be effective.

Side Effects.   In humans, urinary hesitancy and retention, pupillary dilation, tachycardia, syncope, weakness, nausea, vomiting, anorexia, and constipation may occur.

OXYMETHOLONE

Indications and Side Effects.   Oxymetholone (Anadrol-50, Adroyd), or anapolon. See Anabolic Steroids.

OXYMORPHONE HYDROCHLORIDE

Indications.   Oxymorphone hydrochloride (Numorphan) is a narcotic drug useful for sedation and the management of pain in the dog. Pain relief lasts 2 to 4 hours following intramuscular or intraveous injection. It is about 10 times more potent an analgesic than morphine sulfate, causes less sedation, and does not suppress the cough reflex.

Side Effects.   As with morphine sulfate, cats appear to be more sensitive and may exhibit dose-dependent excitement. Respiratory depression is possible. The effects of the drug can be reversed with nalorphine (Nalline) or naloxone (Narcan). It should not be used in animals with head trauma because it increases intracranial pressure. It also causes spasm of the pancreatic and biliary ducts, so should not be used in animals with pancreatic, hepatic, or biliary dysfunction.

OXYTETRACYCLINE

Indications and Side Effects.   See Tetracyclines.

PAREGORIC

Indications.   Paregoric (as in Parepectolin) is a narcotic analgesic used in the control of diarrhea of dogs.

Side Effects.   Excessive doses cause signs similar to those of morphine sulfate intoxication (see Morphine Sulfate).

PELLITOL

Indications.   Pellitol is an antiseptic, analgesic drying ointment. It is used for ear and skin conditions requiring astringent, soothing, antiseptic therapy.

Side Effects.   No side effects are noted.

PENICILLAMINE

Indications.   Penicillamine (Cuprimine) is used in the management of cystine urolithiasis, lead poisoning, and hepatitis associated with progressive copper accumulation. It chelates cystine, lead, and copper and promotes their excretion in urine. In the case of hepatic disease associated with copper toxicosis, clinical improvement may take years of treatment. Tetramine may be an alternative drug to consider.

Side Effects.   Lethargy, vomiting, oral lesions, anorexia, proteinuria, and thrombocytopenia have been reported. The drug decreases the strength of skin wound closure by its effect on collagen, and should only be given after wound healing is complete.

PENICILLINS

Indications.   The penicillins (penicillins G and V, ampicillin, amoxicillin, cloxacillin, carbenicillin, ticarcillin, hetacillin, nafcillin) are effective bactericidal antibiotics for the treatment of gram-positive and gram-negative infections. Penicillin G is effective against most gram-negative organisms and many gram-positive organisms. Penicillin V has the same spectrum but is more reliably absorbed from the gastrointestinal tract. Ampicillin has an extended activity against *Escherichia coli*, shigellae, and *Proteus*. Hetacillin is hydrolyzed to ampicillin in body fluids. Amoxicillin is similar to ampicillin, but is more readily absorbed and persists for a longer time in the body. It is also available in combination with clavulanate potassium (Clavamox), which effectively protects the drug from β-lactamase-producing staphylococci. Cloxacillin sodium is penicillinase-resistant, and is useful in the treatment of staphylococcal infections. Carbenicillin is also active against *Pseudomonas* and *Proteus*. Ticarcillin is more effective than carbenicillin against pseudomonas and can be given at half the dose.

Side Effects.   Toxicity is rare except in guinea pigs and hamsters. Hypersensitivity reactions, including urticaria and anaphylaxis, have been documented in dogs. Sensitivity to one penicillin confers sensitivity to all penicillins. Penicillin and its derivatives may exacerbate clinical signs associated with Scotty cramp. Food and antacids decrease the absorption of orally administered penicillins. The drug should therefore be given 1 hour before or 2 hours after feeding. Neomycin blocks the absorption of oral penicillins.

PENTAZOCINE

Indications.   Pentazocine (Talwin) is a narcotic antagonist used in the management of pain. Its analgesic properties are less than morphine sulfate (one fourth as potent) and equivalent to those of meperidine hydrochloride. It does not depress respiration and produces little or no sedation at therapeutic dosages.

Side Effects. The sedative effect is minimal. Although rare, pentazocine is sometimes associated with salivation in dogs. In cats it appears to cause dysphoria, thus it is not recommended in this species. Its side effects can only be reversed by naloxone. In humans, nausea, vomiting, and sedation are observed; however, these occur less frequently than with meperidine hydrochloride.

PENTOBARBITAL

Indications and Side Effects. Pentobarbital (Nembutal). See Barbiturates.

PETROLATUM, WHITE

Indications. White petrolatum (Laxatone) is a bowel lubricant used to help relieve constipation and to facilitate the removal of hair balls. It exerts its activity in the colon and generally takes 12 to 24 hours to work effectively.

Side Effects. No side effects are noted.

PHENOBARBITAL

Indications. Phenobarbital is an excellent anticonvulsant and sedative agent in dogs and cats. It is reported to be effective in controlling seizures in 60% of dogs when adequate serum concentrations are maintained. See also Barbiturates.

Side Effects. Initially, sedation and ataxia may be noted, especially at higher doses. These effects tend to resolve with continued treatment. Polyuria, polydipsia, and polyphagia have also been documented. Phenobarbital is a hepatic enzyme inducer. It may increase the biotransformation of drugs metabolized by the liver. The drug has also been implicated in hepatotoxicity, especially after chronic use. It is therefore important to monitor serum drug levels after the drug has reached a steady state level (14 days in the dog, 9 days in the cat). Serum samples are collected just prior to the next dose. Effective serum concentrations are in the range of 70 to 170 μmol/L (15–40 mg/dl). Sodium bicarbonate increases the renal excretion of the drug and is potentially useful in cases of overdose.

PHENOXYBENZAMINE HYDROCHLORIDE

Indications. Phenoxybenzamine hydrochloride (Dibenzyline) is an α-adrenergic antagonist. It may of

value in reducing urethral internal sphincter tone, facilitating urine flow. Several days of treatment may be required for a noticeable effect.

Side Effects. Hypotension, reflex tachycardia, weakness, miosis, glaucoma, and vomiting have been reported.

PHENYLBUTAZONE

Indications. Phenylbutazone (Butazolidin) has analgesic, antipyretic, and anti-inflammatory properties useful in the treatment of osteoarthritis, rheumatism, and inflammation of the skin and other soft tissues.

Side Effects. Gastric irritation with vomiting and gastrointestinal ulceration may occur. Thrombocytopenia, leukopenia, and nonregenerative anemia may occur. Effects are unpredictable and unrelated to dosage. Use of phenylbutazone may exacerbate clinical signs associated with Scotty cramp. The drug is toxic to cats and is not recommended in this species.

PHENYLPROPANOLAMINE HYDROCHLORIDE

Indications. Phenylpropanolamine hydrochloride (Ornade, Dexatrim, Triaminic, Propagest) is an α-adrenergic stimulating agent. It is useful in the treatment of urinary incontinence in the dog.

Side Effects. Anorexia, restlessness, irritability, tremors, cardiac arrhythmias, hypertension, and urine retention may occur.

PHENYTOIN

Indications. Phenytoin (Dilantin), or diphenylhydantoin, is an anticonvulsant that is also used in the management of digitalis-induced tachyarrhythmias and atrioventricular block. It may be used in conjunction with other antiarrhythmic agents to control difficult ventricular arrhythmias or in place of lidocaine hydrochloride or procainamide for refractory ventricular arrhythmias. In the control of seizure it stops the propagation and spread of neural excitation. Controversy exists as to its efficacy as a sole agent in the management of epilepsy. Serum concentrations are monitored just before the next dose and after a steady state level has been achieved (22 hours in the dog, 5–6 days in the cat). Effective serum concentrations are in the range of 39.6 to 79.2 μmol/L (10–20 μg/ml).

Side Effects. Vomiting, ataxia, tremors, depression, hypotension, and atrioventricular block are reported. Gingival hyperplasia is an uncommon side effect. The drug is toxic to cats and should not be used in this species. Serum levels are increased by chloramphenicol, cimetidine, and phenylbutazone.

PHOSPHATE ENEMAS

Indications.   Phosphate containing enemas (*e.g.*, Fleet) are used for the treatment of constipation.

Side Effects.   These agents should not be used in the presence of dehydration, abdominal pain, nausea, vomiting, cardiac disease, or severe debility, nor should they be used in small dogs, animals with renal insufficiency, or cats. Clinical signs of toxicity occur within 30 minutes to 1 hour, and may include depression, ataxia, tetany, seizure, vomiting, hemorrhagic diarrhea, tachycardia, pallor of the mucous membranes, or stupor. Associated chemical abnormalities include hyperphosphatemia, hypernatremia, hypocalcemia, hyperglycemia, hyperosmolality, and metabolic acidosis with a high anion gap (increased lactic acid). Death has been reported with the use of these agents in cats.

PHTHALOFYNE

Indications.   Phthalofyne (Whipicide) is an anthelmintic used in the treatment of whipworm infections.

Side Effects.   Vomiting, depression, and ataxia may occur.

PHTHALYLSULFATHIAZOLE

Indications and Side Effects.   Phthalylsulfathiazole (Sulfathalidine, Thalazole) is used for the treatment of enteric infections. The drug is not absorbed from the intestinal tract. See Sulfonamides.

PIPERAZINE

Indications.   Piperazine (Vermizine, Piperate, Pipertab, Piperson, Pipzine, Pipcide) is indicated in the treatment of ascarid infections.

Side Effects.   The drug should not be used in animals with chronic liver or renal disease. At higher doses, vomiting, diarrhea, and ataxia may occur.

PIROXICAM

Indications.   Piroxicam (Feldene) is an nonsteroidal anti-inflammatory agent used in the treatment of joint pain secondary to degenerative joint disease that is unresponsive to aspirin.

Side Effects.   Hemorrhagic gastroenteritis may occur with the use of the drug in humans. The incidence of side effects in small animals is unknown.

PITRESSIN TANNATE IN OIL

Indications.   Pitressin Tannate in Oil is a synthetic form of antidiuretic hormone used in the management of diabetes insipidus.

Side Effects.   Abdominal pain, fluid retention, hyponatremia, pain at injection sites, and the formation of sterile abscesses have been reported.

PLASMINOGEN ACTIVATOR

Indications.   Plasminogen activator (Activase) is a therapeutic thrombolytic agent of potential use in the treatment of feline aortic thromboembolism.

Side Effects.   Death due to reperfusion syndrome (hyperkalemia and metabolic acidosis) occurs in a significant number of treated cats. Congestive heart failure and sudden fatal arrhythmias attributable to embolization of coronary arteries also occur in a number of patients.

POLYMYXIN B

Indications.   Polymyxin B and polymyxin C (Colistin) are used in the treatment of gram-negative bacterial infections, especially those caused by *Pseudomonas*, *Pasteurella* organisms, salmonellae, and shigellae. *Proteus* and *Brucella* organisms are frequently resistant.

Side Effects.   Pain at the injection site, nephrotoxicity, central nervous system signs, and neuromuscular blockade have been documented.

POTASSIUM BROMIDE

Indications.   Potassium bromide (analytical grade) has been used in the management of refractory epilepsy (often in combination with phenobarbital). The drug depresses the central nervous system and has a long half-life (days). Serum levels should be maintained between 1 and 3 mg/ml (9–15 mmol/L).

Side Effects.   Other than sedation, chronic use does not appear to cause serious side effects in the dog. Clinical signs of toxicity may include vomiting, anorexia, constipation, sedation, and incoordination.

POTASSIUM CHLORIDE

Indications.   Potassium chloride is indicated in the treatment of hypokalemia and in the management of supraventricular and ventricular premature contractions. It is used an an antidote in the treatment of digitalis and thallium intoxication.

Side Effects. Cardiac arrest is possible. Because of its potentially serious side effects, potassium chloride is administered only when hypokalemia is considered likely. Other antiarrhythmic agents are preferred.

POTASSIUM CITRATE

Indications. Potassium citrate (Urocit-K) is used for the prevention of calcium oxalate urolithiasis. The citrate complexes with calcium and decreases the urinary concentration of calcium oxalate. Potassium citrate also alkalinizes the urine and increases the solubility of calcium oxalate.

Side Effects. Experience with the drug in veterinary medicine is limited to date; however, hyperkalemia is known to be a potential side effect, especially in animals with renal dysfunction. Nausea, vomiting, and abdominal discomfort have been reported in humans. Other signs of potassium citrate intoxication may include muscular weakness and cardiac arrhythmias, including bradycardia.

POTASSIUM GLUCONATE

Indications. Potassium gluconate (Kaon, Tumil-K) is used in the treatment of hypokalemia in dogs and cats.

Side Effects. Nausea, vomiting, and abdominal discomfort have been reported. Other signs of potassium gluconate intoxication may include muscular weakness and cardiac arrhythmias, including bradycardia. Do not administer to animals with severe renal insufficiency or hypoadrenocorticism. Use the drug with caution in animals receiving concurrent digitalis medication.

POTASSIUM IODIDE

Indications. Potassium iodide (Pima Syrup, SSKI) is used in the treatment of lymphocutaneous sporotrichosis and, occasionally, other subcutaneous opportunistic fungal infections. The drug is also used as an expectorant, in the short-term management of severe feline hyperthyroidism, and for the preoperative induction of euthyroidism.

Side Effects. Anorexia, nausea, salivation, lacrimation, and sneezing are observed. Seborrhea sicca can develop. Cats are very sensitive to iodine compounds. Toxic signs include depression, anorexia, vomiting, muscle spasms, hypothermia, cardiovascular collapse, and death.

POTASSIUM PHOSPHATE

Indications and Side Effects. See Potassium Chloride.

POVIDONE-IODINE

Indications. Povidone-iodine (Betadine) is an antifungal, antibacterial agent that is also useful against the dermatophytes. It is used in the treatment of pyoderma and dermatophyte infection and has been used as an oral rinse in the management of oral disease.

Side Effects. Even the "tamed" iodines can be irritating, especially in cats and in inflammatory conditions of the scrotum and external ear in dogs.

PRAZIQUANTEL

Indications. Praziquantel (Droncit) is the drug of choice for the elimination of tapeworms (*Taenia* sp., *Dipylidium caninum*, *Echinococcus* organisms). The drug has also been used against paragonimiasis.

Side Effects. The drug is very safe, but should not be used in puppies younger than 4 weeks of age or kittens younger than 6 weeks. Marked overdose of the drug may lead to anorexia, vomiting, salivation, diarrhea, and depression.

PRAZOSIN HYDROCHLORIDE

Indications. Prazosin hydrochloride (Minipress) is an arterial and venous vasodilator used to increase cardiac output and decrease pulmonary edema in cases of congestive heart failure and cardiomyopathy. It is also of benefit in patients with systemic hypertension.

Side Effects. Hypotension may occur. Tolerance to the drug has been documented.

PREDNISOLONE

Indications and Side Effects. Prednisolone (Delta-Cortef, Nova-Pred). See Glucocorticoids.

PREDNISONE

Indications and Side Effects. Prednisone (Deltasone). See Glucocorticoids.

PRIMIDONE

Indications. Primidone (Mysoline) is used in the control of seizure activity in the dog. The drug is metabolized to phenobarbital, the most active agent, and phenylethylmalonamide, which contributes about 15% of the anticonvulsant activity of the drug. Primidone works by raising the seizure threshold. Contrary to previous reports, the drug is not exceptionally toxic to cats. Serum concentrations are measured just before the next dose and after steady state levels have been reached (16 days in the dog). Effective serum concentrations (phenobarbital metabolite) are in the range of 68.7 to 206 μmol/L (15–45 μg/ml). Its use for the treatment of epilepsy, however, has been discouraged because it must be administered three times daily to be effective, absorption is poor, clinically it is no more effective than phenobarbital (its active metabolite), and it is associated with a greater incidence of hepatotoxicity than other anticonvulsants.

Side Effects.   Polyuria, polydipsia, and polyphagia are noted during the first few weeks or when the dose is increased. Sedation and ataxia may occur, but tend to resolve with continued treatment. Hepatotoxicity has been recorded, especially with chronic use.

PROCAINAMIDE HYDROCHLORIDE

Indications.   Procainamide hydrochloride (Pronestyl, Procan SR) is second only to lidocaine hydrochloride as the drug of choice in the treatment of ventricular premature contractions and tachycardia. Samples for the measurement of serum drug levels should be taken after a steady state level has been achieved (12 hours in the dog) and before the next dose is administered.

Side Effects.   Hypotension and, rarely, an increase in heart rate, anorexia, vomiting, and diarrhea may occur. Serum levels are increased with cimetidine.

PROCHLORPERAZINE

Indications.   Prochlorperazine (Compazine, Stemetil) is a phenothiazine derivative. It depresses the chemoreceptor trigger zone and is useful in the treatment of vomiting. It is sometimes combined with the anticholinergic agent isopropamide iodide (Darbazine) and used in the management of tenesmus accompanying inflammatory diseases of the rectum and colon.

Side Effects.   Prochlorperazine may prolong the effects of general anesthetics. It should be used with caution in patients with a history of seizure.

PROGESTERONE

Indications.   Progesterone (Repogest) is used in the management of recurrent abortion. Progestogens have also been used in behavorial modification and the treatment of feline endocrine alopecia, eosinophilic granuloma complex, psychogenic alopecia, miliary dermatitis, and "stud tail."

Side Effects.   Polyphagia, polydipsia, weight gain, and a pleasant change in behavior may occur. Progesterone may cause the masculinization of female fetuses and predispose the bitch to pyometra. It may also delay or prevent the onset of parturition if the drug is not discontinued at the due date. Chronic administration of progestogens can cause diabetes mellitus, and has been associated with an increased incidence of mammary hyperplasia and adenocarcinoma in either sex. Local injections may cause temporary alopecia, cutaneous atrophy, and pigmentary changes (dark skin and hair turn white). These drugs also depress testosterone production and spermatogenesis, and should not be used in breeding males. See also Megestrol Acetate and Medroxyprogesterone Acetate.

PROPANTHELINE BROMIDE

Indications.   Propantheline bromide (Pro-Banthine), an anticholinergic agent, is used in the management of detrusor hyperreflexia, sinus bradycardia, atrioventricular block, and sick sinus syndrome.

Side Effects.   Tachycardia, weakness, nausea, vomiting, constipation, and dyness of the mucous membranes may occur. Signs of drug overdose may include urinary retention, excitement, hypotension, respiratory failure, paralysis, and coma.

PROPIONIBACTERIUM ACNES

Indications.   *Propionibacterium acnes* (Immunoregulin) has nonspecific immunostimulatory properties (it induces macrophage activation and lymphokine production, enhances cell-mediated immunity, and increases natural killer cell activity) that may enhance antineoplastic, antiviral, and antibacterial activity and stimulate hemopoiesis. Clinically, this agent has been used in small animals as adjunct therapy to antibiotic treatment for dogs with chronic pyoderma and to increase survival times in dogs with oral melanoma and mastocytoma. It has reportedly been used to help treat immunosuppressed cats with rhinotracheitis and to convert some feline leukemia virus-positive cats to a leukemia virus-negative status.

Side Effects.   The beneficial effects may be negated by the concurrent use of glucocorticoids or other immunosuppressants. Steroids should be discontinued 1 week prior to the use of this drug. Occasionally, fever, anorexia, vomiting, and lethargy may be noted a few hours following its use. Extravascular injection may cause tissue inflammation. The drug has not been evaluated in pregnant animals and should not be given to them. Anaphylaxis is possible. If it occurs the dog should be treated with epinephrine.

PROPRANOLOL HYDROCHLORIDE

Indications. Propanolol hydrochloride (Inderal) is a nonselective β_1- and β_2-blocking agent. It is indicated alone or in conjunction with digoxin in the management of atrial fibrillation. It may be of benefit in the treatment of ventricular premature contractions and systemic hypertension, and is useful in the treatment of arrhythmias caused by digoxin. The antiarrhythmic effects of quinidine, procainamide hydrochloride, and lidocaine hydrochloride are enhanced by simultaneous propranolol hydrochloride therapy. In cats it is also used to manage cases of hypertrophic cardiomyopathy. In humans it has been shown to be of benefit to patients with tetralogy of Fallot. Its value for this purpose in dogs has not been determined.

Side Effects. Bronchoconstriction, hypoglycemia, decreased cardiac contractility, hypotension, bradycardia, peripheral vasoconstriction, and diarrhea may occur. Propranolol hydrochloride should not be used in animals with asthma or clinical evidence of thromboembolic disease. Bronchoconstriction can be treated with terbutaline (2–5 mg orally twice daily) or oxtriphylline (4–8 mg orally three times daily). Lethargy, depression, anorexia, and, occasionally, vomiting and diarrhea have been noted. Congestive heart failure can be treated with dobutamine, furosemide, and oxygen therapy. Glycopyrrolate and dopamine can be used to counter bradycardia. Dextrose can be used to manage hypoglycemia. β-Blocking agents should be gradually withdrawn in patients on long-term regimens because of the possibility of sensitizing the animal to the endogenous release of norepinephrine and epinephrine, resulting in tachycardia, cardiac arrhythmias, and hypertension. Serum levels are increased by cimetidine. Propanolol increases serum lidocaine levels.

PROPYLTHIOURACIL

Indications. Propylthiouracil has been used for the medical management of feline hyperthyroid disease. It has now been essentially replaced by the use of methimazole.

Side Effects. Immune-mediated thrombocytopenia and hemolytic anemia have been documented in cats. Anorexia, vomiting, and lethargy are additional side effects. Serum antinuclear antibodies develop in many cats with long-term use of the drug.

PROSTAGLANDIN F$_{2\alpha}$

Indications. Prostaglandin F$_{2\alpha}$ (Lutalyse) is used in the treatment of pyometra in the dog and cat by causing contraction of the myometrium and relaxation of the cervix. It is also used to hinder conception in animals mistakenly bred.

Side Effects. Restlessness, vomiting, salivation, diarrhea, tachycardia, and panting may occur. These signs occur within the first minute of injection and last approximately 20 to 30 minutes, although they tend to lessen in severity over the course of therapy. Prostaglandin F$_2$ should be used with caution in animals with a closed-cervix pyometra because of the relatively poor therapeutic response and the risk of peritonitis (through retrograde flow of uterine contents through the fallopian tubes) or uterine rupture (from contraction against a closed cervix). The use of estrogens to relax the cervix before the use of prostaglandin F$_2$ is not recommended because estrogens actually enhance the effects of the drug on the uterus.

PROTAMINE SULFATE

Indications. Protamine sulfate is used as an antidote for heparin intoxication.

Side Effects. Anaphylaxis and prolonged bleeding may occur with the use of excessive doses.

PSYLLIUM HYDROPHILIC MUCILLOID FOR ORAL SUSPENSION

Indications and Side Effects. See Metamucil.

PYRANTEL PAMOATE

Indications. Pyrantel pamoate (Nemex) is an anthelmintic used in the treatment of hookworms and ascarids.

Side Effects. Although the drug is very safe, sweating, polypnea, and incoordination may occur at higher doses. Severe toxicity may result in muscular tremors and fasciculation. In cases of severe toxicity, mecamylamine hydrochloride (Inversine), a ganglionic blocking agent, should be administered at a dose of 1 to 2 mg subcutaneously to effect.

PYRETHRINS

Indications. The pyrethrins (Fleavol, KFJ Insecticide Shampoo, Mycodex Pet Shampoo) are volatile oils derived from chrysanthemum flowers. They are used for the treatment of fleas, lice, and cheyletiellic mange.

Side Effects.   These agents are more toxic to cats than dogs. Clinical signs may include salivation, tremors, ataxia, lethargy, dyspnea, coma, and, rarely, death.

PYRIDOSTIGMINE

Indications and Side Effects.   Pyridostigmine (Mestinon). Same as for neostigmine.

PYRIMETHAMINE

Indications.   Pyrimethamine (Daraprim) has been used in combination with the sulfonamides (sulfadiazine) in the treatment of *Toxoplasma* infections. Pyrimethamine appears to increase the activity of the sulfonamide against *Toxoplamosis*.

Side Effects.   Depression, anorexia, and reversible bone marrow suppression (anemia, leukopenia, thrombocytopenia) may occur within 4 to 6 days of initiation of therapy with the pyrimethamine–sulfonamide combination. Bone marrow suppression may be addressed by the addition of folic acid (5 mg/day) or baker's yeast (100 mg/kg/day) to the diet. Leucovorin calcium supplementation (1 mg/kg/day), however, is preferred.

QUINACRINE

Indications.   Quinacrine (Atabrine) is used for the eradication of *Giardia*.

Side Effects.   Yellowing of the skin, anorexia, vomiting, nausea, diarrhea, pruritis, and behavioral changes have been noted. The drug should not be used in pregnant animals. In humans, hepatotoxicity, agranulocytosis, anemia, and hypersensitivity have also been reported.

QUINIDINE

Indications.   Quinidine (Quinaglute, Cardioquin) is indicated for the treatment of ventricular premature contractions, tachycardia, and atrial fibrillation. Serum concentrations are measured just before the next dose and after steady state levels have been reached (28 hours in the dog, 10 hours in the cat).

Side Effects.   Anorexia, vomiting, diarrhea, weakness, hypotension, and decreased cardiac contractility have been reported. A paradoxic acceleration in ventricular rate may occur, especially when the drug is used to treat patients with atrial flutter or fibrillation. In these cases it is often given after patients have first been given a digitalis glycoside. Use of the drug increases serum digoxin levels. Concurrent administration of cimetidine increases serum quinidine levels. Quinidine intoxication can be antagonized by rapid alkalinization of the blood with sodium bicarbonate. Because of these side effects and the availabilty of other effective antiarrhythmic agents, many clinicians do not routinely use the drug.

QUINOLONE ANTIBIOTICS

Indications.   Norfloxacin (Noroxin), enrofloxacin (Baytril), and ciprofloxacin (Cipro) are fluoroquinolone antibiotics with activity against *Escherichia coli*, klebsiellae, *Proteus, Pseudomonas*, staphylococci, salmonellae, shigellae, *Vibrio*, and *Yersinia and Campylobacter* organisms. They have little activity against anaerobic cocci, *Clostridia*, or *Bacteroides* organisms. They have a wider spectrum of activity, greater potency, and less toxicity than nalidixic acid. Nalidixic acid has been used in the treatment of urinary tract infections caused by gram-negative organisms, especially those caused by *Pseudomonas*. The fluoroquinolones are effective in the treatment of respiratory tract infections, bronchopneumonia, enteric infections, bacterial prostatitis, bacterial meningoencephalitis, osteomylelitis, and skin and soft-tissue infections.

Side Effects.   Side effects are rare, but may include vomiting, diarrhea, and hemolytic anemia. The drugs may be teratogenic, and should not be given to pregnant animals. They may also cause erosion of cartilage and a permanent lameness in young dogs, so should not be used in growing animals. Seizure activity may occur at higher dosages. Absorption is hindered by antacid preparations, and nitrofurantoin may impair its efficacy if used concurrently. These drugs are very expensive, but may be considered in cases of resistant bacterial infection.

RANITIDINE HYDROCHLORIDE

Indications.   Ranitidine hydrochloride (Zantac) is a histamine (H2) antagonist used for the treatment of gastrointestinal ulceration. It is more potent (5 to 12 times in inhibiting gastric acid secretion) and has a longer duration of action than cimetidine, but is no more effective. Histamine (H2) antagonists do not prevent nonsteroidal anti-inflammatory drug (NSAID)-induced gastric ulcers, although ranitidine may prevent

NSAID-induced duodenal ulceration. It does not inhibit hepatic microsomal enzymes.

Side Effects. In humans it is reported to have fewer side effects than cimetidine. Nausea and bradycardia may occur with rapid intravenous injection.

RIFAMPIN

Indications. Rifampin (Rifidin, Rimactane) is an antibiotic used alone or in combination with other agents in the treatment of staphylococcal skin diseases, actinomycosis, Coxiella burnetii (Q fever), feline leprosy, listeriosis, Rocky Mountain spotted fever, and tuberculosis.

Side Effects. Hepatopathy and discoloration of tears and urine are reported. Although rare, anorexia, vomiting, diarrhea, thrombocytopenia, hemolytic anemia, and death have been associated with the use of this drug.

RONNEL

Indications. Ronnel (Ectoral) is an organophosphate used for the treatment of *Cheyletiella* and sarcoptic mange, fleas, ticks, and lice.

Side Effects. Ronnel is occasionally associated with weight loss, excessive scaling, vomiting, and hepatotoxicity.

ROTENONE

Indications. Rotenone (2%–10%) (Goodwinol) may be effective against demodectic mites.

Side Effects. Cats are more sensitive than dogs to this product. Clinical signs of toxicity include vomiting, lethargy, tremors, and dyspnea.

SALT

Indications. Table salt has been used as an emetic agent in animals that have ingested toxic compounds. It is not, however, very effective in this regard.

Side Effects. Large amounts of sodium chloride by any route may cause hypokalemia and acidosis. Large oral doses may cause nausea, vomiting, and diarrhea.

SELENIUM SULFIDE

Indications. Selenium sulfide (Selsun Blue, Selsun, Exsel) is a keratolytic, keratoplastic, and degreasing agent useful in the treatment of seborrhea.

Side Effects. It can be drying and irritating and can stain.

SODIUM BICARBONATE

Indications. This drug is indicated for the treatment of metabolic acidosis and in cases of cardiac arrest in which the acidosis lowers the threshold for ventricular fibrillation. It is also used to manage hyperkalemia in cases associated with bradycardia or atrial standstill.

Side Effects. Myocardial depression and peripheral vasodilation leading to hypotension, hyperosmolality, cerebrospinal fluid acidosis, and intracranial hemorrhage have been reported. If sodium bicarbonate is mixed with calcium-containing fluids, insoluble complexes may form. The action of epinephrine is impaired if mixed with sodium bicarbonate.

SODIUM CHLORIDE

Indications. Sodium chloride is recommended for the treatment of hyponatremia and metabolic alkalosis, the restoration of normovolemia, and the promotion of urinary calcium excretion. Hypertonic sodium chloride (3%–5%) is used in cases of sodium depletion associated with a relative increase in body water (syndrome of inappropriate antidiuretic hormone secretion). Isotonic sodium chloride (0.9%) remains in the extracellular space (two thirds in the interstitial space, one third in the intravascular space) following intravenous administration. Half-strength saline (0.45%) is directed into the intracellular space (one third) and extracellular space (two thirds) after intravenous injection. Hypertonic saline (7%) has been successfully used to reverse the pathologic effects of hemorrhagic shock in the dog.

Side Effects. Excessive volumes of 0.9% saline may cause hyperchloremic metabolic acidosis and hypokalemia in those patients with diarrhea in which sodium loss is greater than chloride loss or in those animals in which the kidney cannot excrete the excess chloride load. Volume overload and acute pulmonary edema is a potential problem in patients with cardiac or renal insufficiency. Hypernatremia may also occur and cause irritability, lethargy, weakness, ataxia, stupor, coma, and seizure.

SODIUM EDTA

Indications. Sodium EDTA has been recommended for the treatment of severe hypercalcemia that is unresponsive to other treatment modalities. It reduces the ionized fraction of total serum calcium.

Side Effects. The drug is potentially nephrotoxic.

SODIUM IODIDE

Indications.   Sodium iodide is an antifungal agent used for the treatment of sporotrichosis.

Side Effects.   Depression, lacrimation, and vomiting have been reported in dogs made toxic with the drug. Nausea may be avoided by administering the compound with milk. Cats are especially sensitive to iodide compounds. Toxicity in this species may be manifested by hypothermia, muscle spasms, depression, vomiting, and diarrhea.

SODIUM NITROPRUSSIDE

Indications.   Sodium nitroprusside (Nitropress, Nipride) is an arterial and venous vasodilator that increases cardiac output and decreases pulmonary edema in patients with congestive heart failure and cardiomyopathy. It is also used in the treatment of hypertensive emergencies (retinal detachment).

Side Effects.   Hypotension is a side effect exacerbated with the concurrent use of inhalant anesthetics. Signs of overdosage are similar to those of cyanide poisoning (dyspnea, vomiting, loss of consciousness).

SODIUM POLYSTYRENE SULFONATE

Indications.   Sodium polystyrene sulfonate (Kayexalate) is a sulfonic acid exchange resin. Serum sodium is exchanged with potassium to effectively lower serum potassium levels in hyperkalemic patients.

Side Effects.   Hypokalemia, hypocalcemia, anorexia, nausea, vomiting, and constipation have been noted in humans. Digitalis toxicity may be potentiated with use of this drug. It should not be given concurrently with nonabsorbable cation-donating antacids or laxatives.

SODIUM SULFATE

Indications.   Sodium sulfate, or Glauber's salt, is used as a purgative in the management of oral intoxication in the dog and cat, as a laxative in the dog (one fifth of the purgative dose), and as an antidote to acetaminophen toxicosis in both species.

Side Effects.   Diarrhea may occur.

SPECTINOMYCIN

Indications.   Spectinomycin (Trobicin) is a broad-spectrum antibiotic effective against gram-negative bacteria, including *Escherichia coli*, klebsiellae, salmonellae, proteus, and *Enterobacter* organisms, and gram-positive organisms, including streptococci and staphylococci. It is also effective against mycoplasmas.

Side Effects.   Drug antagonism exists between it and chloramphenicol or tetracycline. Neuromuscular blockade is rare.

SPIRONOLACTONE

Indications.   Spironolactone (Aldactone) is a potassium-sparing diuretic used alone or in conjunction with other diuretics in the management of edema in animals that are unresponsive to other diuretics. It inhibits the action of aldosterone in the distal tubules of the kidney. It is indicated when hypokalemia is a concern. Clinical response of an obvious diuresis generally takes 2 to 3 days to obtain. Clinical effects persist for an additional 2 to 3 days after treatment is ended.

Side Effects.   Hyperkalemia and dehydration may occur. The drug increases serum digoxin levels.

STANOZOLOL

Indications.   Stanozolol (Winstrol) is an anabolic steroid that is potentially useful as an adjunct to the management of catabolic disease processes. It may be used to stimulate erythropoiesis, arouse appetite, promote weight gain, and increase strength and vitality. Prolonged treatment (3–6 months) may be required before a response in the erythron is observed. See also Anabolic Steroids.

Side Effects.   The drug should be used with caution in animals with cardiac or renal insufficiency. It may promote sodium and water retention and exacerbate uremia. The drug is potentially hepatotoxic. It should not be used in animals with neoplastic disease.

STREPTOKINASE

Indications.   Streptokinase (Streptase) is a plasminogen activator that has been used for thrombolysis in cats.

Side Effects.   Minor bleeding often occurs; severe internal bleeding and death are possible.

STREPTOMYCIN

Indications and Side Effects.   See Aminoglycosides.

STYRYLPYRIDINIUM CHLORIDE–DIETHYLCARBAMAZINE

Indications.   Styrylpyridinium chloride with diethylcarbamazine (Styrid-Caricide) is an anthelmintic used in the treatment of ascarid and hookworm infection and in the prevention of heartworm disease.

Side Effects.   It should not be administered to animals with *Dirofilaria immitis* micorfilaria. See also Diethylcarbamazine.

SUCRALFATE

Indications.   Sucralfate (Carafate) accelerates the healing of gastric and duodenal ulcers. The drug forms a complex with proteinaceous exudates that adheres to the ulcer, providing a barrier to the penetration of gastric acid. It stimulates prostaglandin production, increases mucus production and mucosal cell turnover, inactivates pepsin, and absorbs bile acids. Sucralfate does not prevent nonsteroidal anti-inflammatory drug-induced ulceration. The drug is not an antacid. The drug normalizes serum phosphorus levels, which makes it potentially useful in the management of secondary hyperparathyroidism associated with renal failure.

Side Effects.   Sucralfate reduces the bioavailability of digoxin, cimetidine, phenytoin, and tetracycline antibiotics. This can be avoided by administering other drugs 2 hours apart from sucralfate administration. Side effects are rare. Constipation is the only significant problem reported in small animals.

SULFADIAZINE

Indications and Side Effects.   Sulfadiazine (Suladyne). See Sulfonamides.

SULFADIMETHOXINE

Indications and Side Effects.   Sulfadimethoxine (Bactrovet, Albon) and Sulfadimethoxine–Ormetoprim (Primor). See Sulfonamides.

SULFAMETHIZOLE

Indications and Side Effects.   Sulfamethizole (Ultrasul, Urolucosil). See Sulfonamides.

SULFASALAZINE

Indications.   Sulfasalazine (Azulfidine) is used in the management of canine colitis. In the colon, bacteria degrade the drug to release aminosalicyclic acid and sulfapyridine. The aminosalicyclic acid exerts an anti-inflammatory effect by inhibiting prostaglandin synthesis. It may also inhibit the lipoxygenase pathway and hydroxyeicosatetraenoic and leukotriene synthesis. Sulfasalazine may have immunosuppressive properties, especially on B lymphocytes. Other actions include antibacterial effects, scavenging of reactive oxygen, and inhibition of fibrinolysis.

Side Effects.   Vomiting, cholestasis, exacerbation of colitis, fever, oligospermia, anemia, leukopenia, allergic dermatitis, and keratoconjunctivitis sicca have been documented in the dog. An alternative drug, Asacol, contains only the aminosalicyclic acid component, and has been associated with fewer side effects in humans, although keratoconjunctivitis sicca has been reported in the dog. It may not, however, be as effective in the management of colitis in the dog.

SULFISOXAZOLE

Indications and Side Effects.   Sulfisoxazole (Gantrisin). See Sulfonamides.

SULFONAMIDES

Indications.   The sulfonamides are bacteriostatic drugs that are effective against gram-negative and gram-positive bacteria, some chlamydiae, and protozoa (coccidia). They are most often used in the treatment of urinary tract infections due to *Escherichia coli* and infections due to *Proteus mirabilis* and *Klebsiella* organisms. Unfortunately, many organisms are now resistant. The combination of a sulfonamide with trimethoprim or pyrimethamine "potentiated sulfonamides" such as Tribrissen (trimethoprim and sulfadiazine) greatly enhances antimicrobial activity. The enhanced spectrum of activity includes *E. coli, Proteus,* salmonellae, staphylococci, klebsiellae, and streptococci. A recently introduced potentiated sulfonamide (Primor) is a combination of sulfadimethoxine and ormetoprim.

Sulfonamides for systemic use are classified according to the duration of effect. Short-acting sulfonamides (less than 12 hours) include sulfisoxazole, sulfathiazole, and sulfamethizole; intermediate-acting (12–24 hours) include sulfadiazine and sulfamerazine; and long-acting (about 24 hours) include sulfadimethoxine.

Side Effects.   Precipitation and crystalluria are not generally a problem in dogs and cats, but the sulfonamides should be used with caution in patients with pre-existing renal disease, especially if complicated by dehydration or metabolic acidosis. Pruritis and photosensitization have been reported, and alopecia may occur with long-term use. Other reported conditions following the use of sulfonamides and potentiated sulfonamides include polyarthritis, urticaria, facial swelling, fever, hemolytic anemia, polydipsia, polyuria, hepatitis, vomiting, diarrhea, anorexia, seizures, and keratoconjuncititivis sicca. Hypersensitivity, including anaphylactoid reactions, although rare, may also occur.

SULFUR

Indications.   Sulfur as a topical dermatologic agent is keratolytic, keratoplastic, antibacterial, antifungal, antiparasitic, and a mild follicular flushing agent. It may be combined with salicylic acid and coal tar (Mycodex Tar and Sulfur, Thiomar, Lytar) or with sodium salicylate and hexachlorophene (Sebbafon). The shampoo is indicated for the treatment of mites, lice, chiggers, some fleas, dermatophytosis, seborrhea, pyoderma, pruritis, crusts, and scales. When salicylic acid is combined with sulfur, a synergistic effect occurs and the keratolytic effect is enhanced.

Side Effects.   Sulfur may cause scalding if the product is applied to the skin at concentrations greater than 2%. Coal tar may be irritating or toxic to cats. Sebbafon is safe and is approved for cats.

TAURINE

Indications.   Taurine is used in conjunction with other appropriate supportive therapy in the treatment of congestive cardiomyopathy in cats in which dietary taurine deficiency is believed to be responsible for the disease. Taurine may contribute to the inotropic, metabolic, and osmotic function of the myocardium. The drug has also been used alone (at the same dose used to treat cardiomyopathy—500 mg orally twice daily) to successfully treat idiopathic epilepsy in cats.

Side Effects.   No long-term side effects have been noted.

TARS

Indications.   Crude coal tars are used in the management of seborrhea, especially the greasy form of the disease. Tars are keratolytic, keratoplastic, antipruritic, and vasoconstrictive. Most tar shampoos are combined with sulfur and salicylic acid (Lytar, Allerseb T, Mycodex Tar and Sulfur), but some preparations are pure tar shampoos (Pragmatar, Clear Tar).

Side Effects.   Tars are often drying and irritating, and leave an unpleasant odor on the animal. Light-colored hair may be stained. Tar compounds are photosensitizing. Coal tar may be especially irritating or even toxic to cats.

TERBUTALINE SULFATE

Indications.   Terbutaline sulfate (Brethine, Bricanyl Tablets) is indicated for the symptomatic relief of bronchial asthma and reversible bronchospasm in association with bronchitis. It is also used in the treatment of atrioventricular heart block.

Side Effects.   In humans, tremors, nervousness, increased heart rates, and ectopic beats are described.

TERFENADINE

Indications and Side Effects.   Terfenadine (Seldane). See Antihistamines.

TESTOSTERONE

Indications.   Testosterone is indicated for the management of testosterone-responsive urinary incontinence in the neutered male. See also Anabolic Steroids.

Side Effects.   Prostatic enlargement, recurrence or exacerbation of perianal adenoma, or perianal hernia are reported.

TETRACHLORETHYLENE

Indications.   Tetrachlorethylene (Nema) is an anthelmintic used for the elimination of hookworm infections.

Side Effects.   Animals should be put on a fat-free diet 48 hours before treatment and should be starved 12 hours before treatment. The drug is potentially hepatotoxic. It should not be given to nursing animals or ill animals or those with tapeworm infestations.

TETRACYCLINES

Indications.   The tetracycline antibiotics (chlortetracycline, oxytetracycline, tetracycline, demeclocycline, methacycline, doxycycline, minocycline) exert a bacteriostatic activity against gram-positive and gram-negative bacteria. They are especially useful against *Leptospira, Chlamydia, Brucella, Mycoplasma, Pseudomonas, Rickettsia, Actinomyces,* and *Protozoa* organisms. Minocycline and doxycycline are more effective against anaerobes. Diffusion to the eye, brain, cerebrospinal fluid, and prostate gland makes these drugs superior to the other tetracyclines. Minocycline is the most effective of the group against *Nocardia* organisms and *Staphylococcus aureus*.

Side Effects. Tetracyclines, especially chlortetracycline, inhibit protein synthesis. These drugs potentiate the catabolic effects of glucocorticoids and may contribute to cachexia. Nausea, vomiting, diarrhea, dose-related renal tubular damage, and metabolic acidosis have been reported in some dogs. Cats are especially sensitive to these drugs. Fever, vomiting, diarrhea, colic, depression, and anorexia may occur in this species. Discoloration of teeth may occur if these drugs (especially dimethylchlortetracycline and tetracycline) are given to pregnant bitches in the last 2 to 3 weeks of pregnancy or puppies in the first 4 weeks of life. Gastrointestinal absorption is decreased by antacid preparations and dairy or calcium-containing products.

TETRAMINE

Indications. Tetramine tetrahydrochloride is a safe and relatively rapid serum copper chelating agent of potential benefit in the management of dogs with hepatic copper diseases.

Side Effects. There has not been any clinical or laboratory evidence of toxicity associated with the use of the drug.

THENIUM CLOSYLATE

Indications. Thenium closylate (Canopar, Thenatol) is an anthelmintic used for the elmination of hookworm infections.

Side Effects. Vomiting may occur. The drug should not be used in nursing pups or administered with milk or fatty foods or given to dogs weighing less than 2.5 kg. Occasional deaths have been reported in collies and Airdales. In cases of severe toxicity, mecamylamine hydrochloride (Inversine), a ganglionic blocking agent, should be administered at a dose of 1 to 2 mg subcutaneously to effect.

THEOPHYLLINE

Indications. Theophylline (Quibron, Theo-Dur, Quadrinal) is a bronchodilator used in the management of cough. Serum concentrations are monitored just before the next dose and after steady state levels have been attained (30 hours in the dog and 40 hours in the cat).

Side Effects. Restlessness, nausea, vomiting, diarrhea, and tachycardia have been reported. Cardiac arrhythmias, tremors, tachypnea, and seizure activity may be seen at higher doses. Serum levels are increased with cimetidine, erythromycin, and propanolol.

THIABENDAZOLE

Indications. Thiabendazole (Mintezol) is used in the treatment of aspergillosis, penicilliosis, and *Filaroides* (lungworm) infections. The drug is reported to have some immunostimulatory properties. The drug has also been used in cats in the management of the eosinophilic granuloma complex, in which it has been associated with a 75% reduction in the size of the lesion. It is not licensed for use in cats.

Side Effects. Initially, anorexia, vomiting, and diarrhea may be noted. In these patients it is best to stop the drug, wait for several days, and reinstitute the drug at half the dose for a week, then gradually increase the dose.

THIACETARSAMIDE

Indications. Thiacetarsamide (Caparsolate) is currently the adulticide of choice in the treatment of *Dirfilaria immitis* infection. It has also been used to treat symptomatic cases of feline heartworm disease.

Side Effects. Anorexia, vomiting, depression, icterus with elevation of liver enzymes, azotemia, proteinuria, hematuria, and increased numbers of urinary casts may occur. Thromboembolic disease may follow its use, and generally occurs 1 to 2 weeks following adulticidal therapy. An idiosyncratic reaction manifested by acute pulmonary edema and death has been reported in some cats following its use. It is therefore not recommended for use in asymptomatic cats with heartworm disease.

THIAMYLAL SODIUM

Indications. Thiamylal sodium (Surital Sodium, Bio-Tal) is an anesthetic agent. Cardiac arrhythmias occur more frequently with thiamylal sodium than with thiopental sodium. It is more potent, has a shorter duration of action, and is less cummulative than thiopental sodium.

Side Effects. Premature ventricular contractions may occur. Postinduction apnea is common. Metabolic acidosis, uremia, and the administration of glucose augment the anesthetic effects of the drug, potentially leading to toxicity.

THIOPENTAL SODIUM

Indications.   Thiopental sodium (Pentothal Sodium) is an anesthetic of extremely short duration that is suitable for surgical procedures of 10 to 20 minutes' duration. Its short action, smooth recovery, rapid elimination, and minimal side effects are characteristic.

Side Effects.   Postinduction apnea is common. Metabolic acidosis, uremia, and the administration of glucose augment the anesthetic effects of the drug, potentially leading to toxicity.

TICARCILLIN DISODIUM

Indications and Side Effects.   Ticarcillin disodium (Ticar). See Penicillins.

TILETAMINE ZOLAZEPAM

Indications.   Tiletamine zolazepam (Telazol) is an injectable dissociative anesthetic and tranquilizer drug combination useful for sedation and restraint, anesthetic induction, or anesthesia for procedures of short duration (30 minutes) requiring mild to moderate analgesia.

Side Effects.   Rapid intramuscular injection is painful, and salivation may occur. The drug is contraindicated in animals with pancreatic disease. The drug causes an increase in heart rate, arterial blood pressure, cardiac output, and myocardial oxygen consumption, and should not be used in animals with severe cardiac or pulmonary disease. Excretion is renal, so the drug should not be used in animals with compromised renal function. It should not be given to pregnant animals.

TIMOLOL MALEATE

Indications.   Timolol maleate (Blocadren) is a nonselective β-blocking drug with actions and side effects similar to those of propranolol. Timolol maleate, however, is about eight times more potent than propranolol.

Side Effects.   In humans, decreased myocardial contractility may lead to congestive heart failure and pulmonary edema. Syncope, sinus arrest and atrioventricular heart block, hypotension, vomiting, diarrhea, constipation, and weakness have been reported.

TOBRAMYCIN SULFATE

Indications and Side Effects.   Tobramycin sulfate (Nebcin). See Aminoglycosides.

TOCAINIDE

Indications and Side Effects.   Tocainide (Tonocard). Same as for lidocaine hydrochloride and mexiletine.

TOLUENE

Indications.   Toluene (Methacide, Wurm Caps, Vermiplex, Difolin, Anaplex, Paracide) is an anthelmintic used in the treatment of ascarid infection.

Side Effects.   Toxicity results in transient vomiting, incoordination, and depression. It should not be administered concurrently with epinephrine, fats, oils, or alcohol, or administered to severely ill animals.

TRIAMCINOLONE

Indications and Side Effects.   Triamcinolone (Vetalog). See Glucocorticoids.

TRIAMTERENE

Indications.   Triamterene (Dyrenium) is a potassium-sparing diuretic. It may be used in conjunction with other diuretics to promote diuresis in patients that are refractory to one diuretic. The onset of activity occurs within 2 hours, peak activity occurs in 6 to 8 hours, and the duration of activity is 12 to 16 hours.

Side Effects.   Although little information is available on its use in small animals, hypovolemia, hyperkalemia, nausea, anorexia, and vomiting may occur. The drug increases serum digitalis levels.

TRIENTINE HYDROCHLORIDE

Indications.   Trientine hydrochloride (Cuprid) is a serum copper chelating agent of potential use in the treatment of hepatic copper diseases.

Side Effects.   In humans, toxic side effects may include anorexia, gastritits, abdominal pain, melena, and weakness. There is little information concerning its use in small animals to date.

TRIIODOTHYRONINE

Indications.   Triiodothyronine (Cytomel, Cytobin) is a synthetic T_3 replacement agent used in the treatment of hypothyroid disease. It is indicated in animals with impaired ability to convert thyroxine to triiodothyronine or with impaired absorption of thyroxine from the gastrointestinal tract. Peak serum concentrations occur 2 to 5 hours after oral administration. The drug is given 2 to 3 times daily.

Side Effects.   Thyroid replacement should be undertaken with caution in animals with hypoadrenocorticism, diabetes mellitus, or congestive heart failure. The increase in metabolism may place undue stress on the heart. Increased metabolism of adrenal hormones may precipitate a hypoadrenocortical crisis, and increased metabolism may enhance ketone production and potentiate ketoacidosis in animals with diabetes mellitus. In the case of drug overdose, signs consistent with thyrotoxicosis include polyuria, polydipsia, polyphagia, weight loss, panting, nervousness, and tachycardia. Appropriate adjustment in dosage will alleviate these signs.

TRIMEPRAZINE TARTRATE

Indications and Side Effects.   Trimeprazine tartrate (Temaril). See Antihistamines.

TRIMETHOBENZAMIDE HYDROCHLORIDE

Indications.   Trimethobenzamide hydrochloride (Tigan) is an antiemetic with activity directed at the chemoreceptor trigger zone.

Side Effects.   Side effects are rare, but may include depression, hypotension, dizziness, and convulsions.

TRIMETHOPRIM–SULFADIAZINE

Indications.   Trimethoprim–sulfadiazine (Tribrissen) is a bactericidal combination recommended for the treatment of respiratory and urinary tract infections caused by *Escherichia coli*, streptococci, *Proteus*, salmonellae, shigellae, and *Pasteurella* organisms. The drug is less effective against staphlyococci and *Clostridium, Klebsiella, Corynebacterium*, and *Bordetella* organisms. It is especially useful for the long-term, low dose treatment of chronic bacterial urinary tract infections.

Side Effects.   Anemia, leukopenia, thrombocytopenia, anorexia, and ataxia may be noted at higher doses. Dietary supplementation of folinic acid (leucovorin calcium) (0.5–1 mg/day) may protect the patient from the anemia and leukopenia that accompany the interference of folic acid metabolism. This drug combination has also been associated with idiosyncratic reactions that include polyarthritis and fever (especially in Doberman pinchers), cutaneous eruptions, hepatitis, keratoconjunctivitis sicca, glomerulonephropathy, and polymyositis. Signs of polyarthritis and fever typically occur 8 to 20 days after the initiation of therapy. Complete recovery of clinical signs of polyarthritis and fever is generally apparent within 1 week after

withdrawal of the drug. Skin changes resolve within 3 weeks. The drug should not be used for more than 14 days in the cat. Tibrissen may interfere with thyroid function. Excessive salivation may occur in cats given uncoated tablets.

TRIPLE SULFA

Indications and Side Effects.   See Sulfonamides.

TYLOSIN

Indications.   Tylosin (Tylan) is a macrolide antibiotic. It has activity against gram-negative and gram-positive bacteria, spirochetes, chlamydiae, and mycoplasmas. It has been used successfully in the management of canine and feline colitis. The mode of action in this instance is likely related to its antibacterial properties. It is most effective in colitis if used in the powder form (Tylan-Plus Vitamins). It may not be effective in the tablet form for the treatment of colitis.

Side Effects.   Adverse effects are rare.

VALPROIC ACID

Indications.   Valproic acid (Depakene) is an anticonvulsant medication that has been used in dogs. Two metabolites of the drug also appear to have anticonvulsant properties. Efficacy appears to be improved when the drug is used in combination with phenobarbital.

Side Effects.   The drug has a short half-life in the dog (2.8 hours), and must be given at high or frequent doses to achieve adequate steady serum concentrations (220 mg/kg orally three times daily to maintain therapeutic serum concentrations of 50 to 100 μg/ml). In humans, transient nausea, vomiting, and diarrhea are the most common side effects. Thrombocytopenia and minor elevations in hepatic enzymes are rarely reported. It usefulness in the cat is unclear.

VANCOMYCIN HYDROCHLORIDE

Indications.   Vancomycin hydrochloride (Vancocin) is used principally for staphylococcal infections that are unresponsive to other drugs.

Side Effects.   Fever, chills, and phlebitis at the injection site may occur. Leukopenia and eosinopenia have been reported. Nephrotoxicity is an infrequent side effect.

VERAPAMIL

Indications.   Verapamil (Isoptin) is a calcium channel blocking agent useful in the management of atrial fibrillation, flutter, and tachycardia, and, possibly, hypertrophic cardiomyopathy. It is a more potent negative inotropic agent than nifedipine or diltiazem hydrochloride.

Side Effects.   The drug is contraindicated in sick sinus syndrome, pre-exisiting β-blockade, atrioventricular block, and myocardial failure (unless tachycardia is contributing to the failure). Verapamil may increase serum digoxin and theopylline levels.

VINBLASTINE SULFATE

Indications and Side Effects.   Vinblastine sulfate (Velban). See Vinca Alkaloids.

VINCA ALKALOIDS

Indications.   Vincristine sulfate (Oncovin) is used in the management of lymphoid and hematopoietic neoplasms, mammary neoplasms in cats, some sarcomas, transmissible venereal neoplasms in dogs, and immune-mediated disease (thrombocytopenia). Vinblastine sulfate (Velban) is used less frequently in small animals. It is used in combination with other chemotherapeutic agents in the treatment of lymphoreticular neoplasms and disseminated mast cell tumor.

Side Effects.   Perivascular injection will result in severe local irritation and necrosis. If this occurs, aspiration of the drug should be attempted and the area should be infiltrated with sodium bicarbonate (8.4%), dexamethasone, or hyaluronidase (150 μg/ml). In addition, warm compresses should be applied to the area for 1 hour. Dose-related side effects include mucosal necrosis, lymphoid hypoplasia, anemia, leukopenia, and increases in serum aspartate transaminase, alkaline phosphatase, and lactic dehydrogenase levels. Granulocytic depression occurs within 4 to 9 days of administration, with recovery occurring 7 to 14 days later. Peripheral neurotoxicosis is rarely recognized in small animals. Nausea, vomiting, stomatitis, and constipation are more common with vinblastine sulfate.

VINCRISTINE SULFATE

Indications and Side Effects.   Vincristine sulfate (Oncovin). See Vinca Alkaloids.

VIOKASE

Indications.   Viokase is a mixture containing standardized amylase, protease, and lipase activity, as well as esterases, peptidases, nucleases, and elastase of porcine origin. It is used in the management of pancreatic exocrine insufficiency. Powdered forms are usually effective (when mixed in food before eating) even when the same product in tablet form is not. Concurrent use of cimetidine may improve efficacy.

Side Effects.   Overdose can cause diarrhea. Sensitivity to pork protein may develop in some patients.

VITAMIN A

Indications.   The vitamin A compounds or retinoids are used in the management of seborrheic dermatoses to slow down epidermal cell turnover time. Included in this group are retinol, isotretinoin (Accutane), and etretinate (Tegison).

Side Effects.   In humans, numerous adverse effects have been documented with the use of retinoids. Lethargy, depression, anorexia, vomiting, cheilitis, erythema, pruritis, epiphora, conjunctivitis, and hyperactivity have been reported. Abdominal distention, swollen tongues, and collapse have also been noted on occasion. Thrombocytosis and increases in blood cholesterol, serum calcium, alanine aminotransferase, and aspartate aminotransferase have also been documented. Chronic hypervitaminosis A may cause demineralization, cortical hyperostosis, periostitis, and premature closure of the epiphyses.

Dogs treated with retinol over long periods have apparently suffered no ill effects. See also Isotretinoin and Etretinate.

VITAMIN E

Indications.   Vitamin E has been used in dogs in the treatment of Scotty cramp, discoid lupus, pemphigus erythematosus, vitamin E deficiency myositis, and acanthosis nigricans, and in cats in the treatment of steatitis.

Side Effects.   Changes in hair coat color have been documented in a tricolored collie. The drug should be given 2 hours before or after feeding, as the inorganic iron present in most commercial diets interferes with its absorption.

VITAMIN K

Indications.   Vitamin K_1, or phytonadione (Mephyton tablets, Aquamephyton, Konakion, Vet-A-K_1 injectable), is used to treat coagulopathies due to fat-soluble vitamin malabsorption and intoxication of vitamin K antagonists (salicylates, coumarins, indanediones). Vitamin K_3, or menadione, is less expensive, but is also less effective.

Side Effects.   Transient hypotension, dyspnea, and cyanosis rarely have occurred. Anaphylaxis has been reported following intravenous injection of the drug.

WARFARIN

Indications.   Warfarin is used to prevent thromboembolic disease. It augments thrombin inactivation and prevents the conversion of fibrinogen to fibrin.

Side Effects.   Weakness, dyspnea, prostration, and occasionally hematemesis, hematuria, hematachezia, and pale mucous membranes occur. Uncontrolled hemorrhage may lead to death.

WHEAT BRAN

Indications.   Wheat bran is used in the prevention and treatment of constipation. It is cheaper and equally as effective as Metamucil.

Side Effects.   No side effects are noted.

XYLAZINE

Indications.   Xylazine (Rompun) is an anesthetic agent characterized by a rapid onset, good to excellent sedation, excellent analgesia of 15 to 30 minutes' duration, and a smooth recovery.

Side Effects.   Vomiting 1 to 5 minutes after administration (especially in cats), hypotension, bradycardia, second-degree heart block, polyuria, mild respiratory depression, hyperglycemia, and glycosuria may occur. Bradycardia may be prevented by the administration of atropine or glycopyrrolate. Xylazine sensitizes the heart to epinephrine-induced arrhythmias, especially in the face of halothane anesthesia. Yohimbine (Yobine) (dogs: 0.1 mg/kg IV, and cats: 0.5 mg/kg IV) or tolazoline hydrochloride (Priscoline) (dogs: 2–5 mg/kg IV, and cats: 2 mg/kg IV) can be used to antagonize the effects of xylazine and shorten recovery periods and reduce anesthetic-related complications.

ZINC ACETATE

Indications.   Zinc acetate is a hepatic copper chelating agent.

Side Effects.   Clinical signs of zinc toxicity include nausea, vomiting, colic, bloody diarrhea, hypotension, hemolytic anemia, seizure, coma, and, rarely, death.

ZINC METHIONINE

Indications.   Zinc methionine (ZinPro) is used in the management of zinc-responsive dermatoses.

Side Effects.   The most common side effects associated with zinc therapy are nausea, anorexia, and vomiting, which can be controlled by dividing the daily dose into two portions and administering the drug with food. See also Zinc Acetate.

ZINC OXIDE

Indications.   Zinc oxide (Zincofax) is a healing ointment used to sooth, protect, and promote healing of irritated or abraded skin.

Side Effects.   It is safe and nonirritating. If the product is ingested, depression, lethargy, vomiting and, diarrhea may occur. Ingestion of large amounts of the product may cause hemolytic anemia.

ZINC SULFATE

Indications.   Zinc sulfate is used in the management of the zinc-responsive dermatoses in dogs.

Side Effects.   The most common side effects associated with zinc therapy are nausea, anorexia, and vomiting, which can be controlled by dividing the daily dose into two portions and administering the drug with food. See also Zinc Acetate.

ADDITIONAL READING

Booth NH, McDonald LE. Veterinary pharmacology and therapeutics. Iowa City: Iowa University Press, 1988.

Davis LE. Handbook of small animal therapeutics. New York: Churchill Livingstone, 1985.

Kirk RW. Current veterinary therapy X. Philadelphia: WB Saunders, 1989.

Panisset JC. Veterinary pharmaco-therapeutic compendium. St.-Hyacinthe: CDMV Inc., 1987.

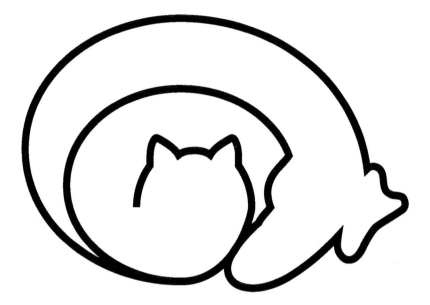

INDEX

Numbers followed by an f *indicate a figure;*
t *following a page number indicates tabular material.*